Lecture Notes in Comput 4

AF760536

Commenced Publication in 1973
Founding and Former Series Editors:
Gerhard Goos, Juris Hartmanis, and Jan

Editorial Board

David Hutchison
Lancaster University, UK
Takeo Kanade
Carnegie Mellon University, Pittsburgh, PA, USA
Josef Kittler
University of Surrey, Guildford, UK
Jon M. Kleinberg
Cornell University, Ithaca, NY, USA
Friedemann Mattern
ETH Zurich, Switzerland
John C. Mitchell
Stanford University, CA, USA
Moni Naor
Weizmann Institute of Science, Rehovot, Israel
Oscar Nierstrasz
University of Bern, Switzerland
C. Pandu Rangan
Indian Institute of Technology, Madras, India
Bernhard Steffen
University of Dortmund, Germany
Madhu Sudan
Massachusetts Institute of Technology, MA, USA
Demetri Terzopoulos
University of California, Los Angeles, CA, USA
Doug Tygar
University of California, Berkeley, CA, USA
Moshe Y. Vardi
Rice University, Houston, TX, USA
Gerhard Weikum
Max-Planck Institute of Computer Science, Saarbruecken, Germany

Nico Karssemeijer Boudewijn Lelieveldt (Eds.)

Information Processing in Medical Imaging

20th International Conference, IPMI 2007
Kerkrade, The Netherlands, July 2-6, 2007
Proceedings

Springer

Volume Editors

Nico Karssemeijer
Radboud University Nijmegen Medical Centre
Dept. of Radiology
P.O. Box 9101, 6500 HB Nijmegen, The Netherlands
E-mail: n.karssemeijer@rad.umcn.nl

Boudewijn Lelieveldt
Leiden University Medical Center
Division of Image Processing (LKEB)
P.O. Box 9600, 2300 RC Leiden, The Netherlands
E-mail: b.p.f.lelieveldt@lumc.nl

Library of Congress Control Number: 2007929386

CR Subject Classification (1998): I.4, I.5, I.2.5-6, J.1, I.3

LNCS Sublibrary: SL 6 – Image Processing, Computer Vision, Pattern Recognition, and Graphics

ISSN 0302-9743
ISBN-10 3-540-73272-1 Springer Berlin Heidelberg New York
ISBN-13 978-3-540-73272-3 Springer Berlin Heidelberg New York

This work is subject to copyright. All rights are reserved, whether the whole or part of the material is concerned, specifically the rights of translation, reprinting, re-use of illustrations, recitation, broadcasting, reproduction on microfilms or in any other way, and storage in data banks. Duplication of this publication or parts thereof is permitted only under the provisions of the German Copyright Law of September 9, 1965, in its current version, and permission for use must always be obtained from Springer. Violations are liable to prosecution under the German Copyright Law.

Springer is a part of Springer Science+Business Media

springer.com

© Springer-Verlag Berlin Heidelberg 2007
Printed in Germany

Typesetting: Camera-ready by author, data conversion by Scientific Publishing Services, Chennai, India
Printed on acid-free paper SPIN: 12082315 06/3180 5 4 3 2 1 0

Preface

The 20th International Conference on Information Processing in Medical Imaging (IPMI) was held during July 2–6, 2007, at Rolduc Abbey, located in Kerkrade in the south of the Netherlands. Following the highly successful IPMI in Glenwood Springs in the Rocky Mountains, Colorado, USA (2005), the conference was the latest in a series of biennial scientific meetings where new developments in acquisition, analysis, and use of medical images are presented. IPMI is one of the longest running conferences in medical imaging. It was started in 1969 by a group of young scientists working in nuclear medicine. With a few iterations the conference expanded to other areas and became established as an important meeting for in-depth discussion of new methodological developments in medical imaging. Nowadays it is widely recognized as one of the most exciting and influential conferences in its field.

At IPMI meetings a wide variety of topics are covered by a relatively small selection of papers presented in single-track sessions. This year, there were 210 manuscripts submitted to the conference. Of these papers, 26 were accepted for oral presentation, and 37 papers were accepted as posters. Papers were carefully judged by three reviewers and two paper selection committee members, with emphasis on originality, methodological development, scientific rigor, and relevance. Selection of papers was difficult, but using the rankings and detailed comments of the reviewers we were able to make a great selection in an objective way. Unfortunately, due to the large number of submissions, it was inevitable that many high-quality papers did not make it into the final program.

One of the key goals of IPMI is to encourage participation of the most promising and talented young researchers in the field, allowing them to explore new ideas with some of the leading researchers in this area. Also this year, active involvement was stimulated by preparation of the sessions in small study groups, in which each conference attendee participated. After reading the papers of their session, the study group members met to discuss the papers before they were presented, and to formulate questions and comments to kick off the discussions. The prestigious Erbsmann award for first time IPMI presenters added an extra stimulus for young researchers to be actively involved in the meeting. Of the accepted papers, 37 were from first time presenters, and 18 of the 26 oral presentations were given by candidates for the prize.

This year we also had a keynote lecture. We were very honored that Freek Beekman from the University Medical Center Utrecht accepted our invitation to present an overview of exciting ongoing research in "high resolution radionuclide imaging". Image acquisition and reconstruction have traditionally been topics that were well represented at earlier IPMIs, before image analysis became the dominant topic. In fact, the speaker who is now a world-leading authority in this field, was attending and contributing to IPMI in his younger years. Therefore we were very pleased that Freek's stimulating lecture brought the innovative recent advances in this area to the attention of the IPMI audience.

IPMI has many traditions and we made every effort we could to maintain its character. The most important tradition is allocation of sufficient time for presentations to allow speakers to give a detailed explanation of their work and to have time for in-depth and lively discussions without time constraints. It has happened that debates have gone on for hours. With the risk of ruining a carefully scheduled program we instructed the session chairs never to cut off a discussion. We strongly believe that it is this unique format that makes IPMI such a remarkable forum for the interchange of ideas in medical imaging..

IPMI is typically situated in a relatively small and sometimes remote location. This year, IPMI was set in a historical location: the abbey Rolduc is a most impressive historical abbey complex that has served as a monastery, where culture, religion and science have gone hand in hand since the 12th century. Since 1970, the major part of the abbey complex has been converted into a unique historical conference venue with modern meeting, lodging and catering facilities. This made Rolduc the perfect setting for the highly informal atmosphere that makes IPMI such a special event. All attendees were housed inside the abbey complex, and the availability of a bar with late opening hours in the abbey basement guaranteed continued scientific, and under the influence of the original Rolduc beer, increasingly non-scientific discussions. On Wednesday afternoon, attendees could explore the beautiful surroundings of Valkenburg on foot, enjoying some of the steepest (and rarest) hills that the Netherlands has to offer. Also, a visit to the beautiful town of Maastricht was organized. Later that evening, everyone joined together for the conference dinner in the magnificent Kasteel Oost, on the river banks of the Geul in Valkenburg. On Thursday, the traditional football (soccer) match, US against "the rest of the world", was played on the Rolduc soccer field. At the time of writing the outcome is still uncertain, but it is expected that the Europeans will continue to dominate this remarkable series of games, with or without impartial refereeing.

In these proceedings all IPMI 2007 papers are published in the order in which they were presented at the meeting. We hope that these papers will form an invaluable source of information for participants, and a reminder of the great conference we had. For those who did not attend the meeting these proceedings provide an excellent overview of some of the best research in medical imaging today. We are already looking forward to IPMI 2009. Use www.ipmi-conference.com to stay informed.

May 2007

Nico Karssemeijer
Boudewijn Lelieveldt

Acknowledgements

The organization of the 20th IPMI conference was only possible due to the efforts and contributions of several organizations and individuals. First of all, the organizers would like to thank the reviewers for providing so many high-quality reviews within a limited time frame. Thanks to these reviews, we were able to make a fair selection of the best papers for the final program. We express our gratitude to the Paper Selection Committee members, who each took on the duty of reading close to 60 papers and the corresponding reviews, and traveling to the Netherlands for the paper selection meeting. Wiro, Christian, Daniel, and Milan, many thanks! We would also like to thank previous IPMI organizers Chris Taylor and Gary Christensen for sharing their experiences with us, and Hans Reiber for his support of the IPMI 2007 organizers.

We are very grateful to Simone Meeuwsen for handling the registrations and other administrative tasks and express our gratitude to Simon Jackson for his assistance with the web-based CAWS conference management system. We also gratefully acknowledge Ilse Brouns from Rolduc for her enthusiasm and constructive brainstorming on the optimal way to set up Rolduc for a meeting like IPMI. Last but not least, we extend our gratitude to the students and post-docs from Nijmegen and Leiden, who were our hands and feet during the conference: they covered quite some distance running around with microphones during the discussions. Finally, we are grateful to the following organizations for their generous financial support:

Stichting Beeldverwerking Leiden
Royal Dutch Academy of Sciences

François Erbsmann Prizewinners

1987 (Utrecht, The Netherlands): **John M. Gauch**, University of North Carolina, Chapel Hill, NC, USA *J.M. Gauch, W.R. Oliver, S.M. Pizer: Multiresolution shape descriptions and their applications in medical imaging.*

1989 (Berkeley, CA, USA): **Arthur F. Gmitro**, University of Arizona, Tucson, AZ, USA *A.F. Gmitro, V. Tresp, V. Chen, Y. Snell, G.R. Gindi: Video-rate reconstruction of CT and MR images.*

1991 (Wye, Kent, UK): **H. Isil Bozma**, Yale University, New Haven, CT, USA *H.I. Bozma, J.S. Duncan: Model-based recognition of multiple deformable objects using a game-theoretic framework.*

1993 (Flagstaff, AZ, USA): **Jeffrey A. Fessler**, University of Michigan, Ann Arbor, MI, USA *J.A. Fessler: Tomographic reconstruction using information-weighted spline smoothing.*

1995 (Brest, France): **Maurits K. Konings**, University Hospital, Utrecht, The Netherlands *M.K. Konings, W.P.T.M. Mali, M.A. Viergever: Design of a robust strategy to measure intravascular electrical impedance.*

1997 (Poultney, VT, USA): **David Atkinson**, GuyâĂŹs Hospital, London, UK *D. Atkinson, D.L.G. Hill, P.N.R. Stoyle, P.E. Summers, S.F. Keevil: An auto-focus algorithm for the automatic correction of motion artifacts in MR images.*

1999 (Visegrad, Hungary): **Liana M. Lorigo**, Massachusetts Institute of Technology, Cambridge, MA, USA *L.M. Lorigo, O. Faugeras, W.E.L. Grimson, R. Keriven, R. Kikinis, C.-F. Westin: Co-dimension 2 geodesic active contours for MRA segmentation.*

2001 (Davis, CA, USA): **Viktor K. Jirsa**, Florida Atlantic University, FL, USA *V.K. Jirsa, K.J. Jantzen, A. Fuchs, J.A. Scott Kelso: Neural field dynamics on the folded three-dimensional cortical sheet and its forward EEG and MEG.*

2003 (Ambleside, UK): **Guillaume Marrelec**, INSERM, France. *G. Marrelec, P. Ciuciu, M. PÂt'elÂt'egrini-Issac, H. Benali: Estimation of the hemodyamic response function in event-related functional MRI: directed acyclic graphs for a general Bayesian inference framework.*

2005 (Colorado, USA) **Duygu Tosun**, Electrical and Computer Engineering, Johns Hopkins University, USA. *T. Duygu, J.L. Prince: Cortical surface alignment using geometry driven multispectral optical flow.*

Conference Committees

Chairs

Nico Karssemeijer	Radboud University Nijmegen Medical Center, The Netherlands
Boudewijn Lelieveldt	Leiden University Medical Center, The Netherlands

Paper Selection Committee

Christian Barillot	IRISA/INRIA, France
Wiro Niessen	Erasmus University Rotterdam, The Netherlands
Daniel Rueckert	Imperial College London, UK
Milan Sonka	University of Iowa, USA

Scientific Committee

Craig K. Abbey	University of California, Davis, USA
Faiza Admiraal-Behloul	Leiden University Medical Center, The Netherlands
Amir A. Amini	University of Louisville, USA
Stephen R. Aylward	KITWARE Inc., USA
Reinhard R. Beichel	University of Iowa, USA
Yves J.C. Bizais	Medical School, UBO, France
Djamal Boukerroui	Université de Technologie de Compiègne, France
Mike Brady	University of Oxford, UK
Aaron Bertrand Brill	Vanderbilt University, USA
Elizabeth Bullitt	University of North Carolina, USA
Gary E. Christensen	University of Iowa, USA
Ela Claridge	University of Birmingham, UK
Timothy F Cootes	University of Manchester, UK
Christos Davatzikos	University of Pennsylvania, USA
Marleen de Bruijne	University of Copenhagen, Denmark
Herve Delingette	INRIA, France
James S. Duncan	Yale University, USA
Alejandro F. Frangi	Universitat Pompeu Fabra, Spain
James C. Gee	University of Pennsylvania, USA
Guido Gerig	University of North Carolina at Chapel Hill, USA
Bram van Ginneken	University Medical Center Utrecht, The Netherlands
Polina Golland	Massachusetts Institute of Technology, USA
Michael L. Goris	Stanford University School of Medicine, USA
Ghassan Hamarneh	Simon Fraser University, Canada

David J. Hawkes	University College London, UK
Pierre Hellier	IRISA/INRIA, France
Kenneth R. Hoffmann	State University of New York at Buffalo, USA
Henkjan Huisman	Radboud University Nijmegen Medical Centre, The Netherlands
Sarang C. Joshi	University of Utah, USA
Jan Kybic	Czech Technical University, Czech Republic
Rasmus Larsen	Technical University of Denmark, DTU, Denmark
Richard M. Leahy	University of Southern California, USA
Gabriele Lohmann	Max-Planck Institute of Cognitive Neuroscience, Germany
Frederik Maes	Katholieke Universiteit Leuven, Belgium
Jean-Francois Mangin	CEA, France
Rashindra Manniesing	Erasmus Medical Center Rotterdam, The Netherlands
Calvin R. Maurer, Jr.	Accuray, Inc., USA
Charles Meyer	University of Michigan, USA
Kyle J. Myers	U.S. Food and Drug Administration, USA
J. Alison Noble	University of Oxford, UK
Xenophon Papademetris	Yale University, USA
Xavier Pennec	INRIA, France
Dzung L. Pham	Johns Hopkins University, USA
Stephen M. Pizer	University of North Carolina at Chapel Hill, USA
Jerry L. Prince	Johns Hopkins University, USA
Anand Rangarajan	University of Florida, USA
Joseph M. Reinhardt	University of Iowa, USA
Torsten Rohlfing	SRI International, USA
Karl Rohr	University of Heidelberg, Germany
Punam Kumar Saha	University of Iowa, USA
Julia A. Schnabel	University College London, UK
Pengcheng Shi	Hong Kong University of Science Technology Hong Kong
Oskar Skrinjar	Georgia Institute of Technology, USA
Colin Studholme	University of California, San Francisco, USA
Martin A. Styner	University of North Carolina at Chapel Hill, USA
Gabor Szekely	Swiss Federal Institute of Technology Zurich, Switzerland
Chris Taylor	University of Manchester, UK
Bart M. ter Haar Romeny	Eindhoven University of Technology, The Netherlands
Andrew Todd-Pokropek	University College London, UK
Carole J. Twining	University of Manchester, UK
Dirk Vandermeulen	Katholieke Universiteit Leuven, Belgium
Baba C. Vemuri	University of Florida, USA

IPMI 2007 Board

Stephen L. Bacharach
Harrison H. Barrett
Yves J.C. Bizais
Aaron B. Brill
Gary E. Christensen
Alan C.F. Colchester
Robert DiPaola
James S. Duncan
Michael L. Goris
Nico Karssemeijer
Richard M. Leahy
Douglas A. Ortendahl
Stephen M. Pizer
Chris Taylor
Andrew Todd-Pokropek
Max A. Viergever

Table of Contents

Segmentation

Cardiovascular Imaging

Detection and Labeling

Poster Session I

Diffusion Tensor Imaging

Registration

Image Reconstruction

Functional Brain Imaging

Poster Session II

Shape Models and Registration

A Shape-Guided Deformable Model with Evolutionary Algorithm Initialization for 3D Soft Tissue Segmentation

Tobias Heimann, Sascha Münzing, Hans-Peter Meinzer, and Ivo Wolf

Div. Medical and Biological Informatics, German Cancer Research Center,
69120 Heidelberg, Germany
t.heimann@dkfz.de

Abstract. We present a novel method for the segmentation of volumetric images, which is especially suitable for highly variable soft tissue structures. Core of the algorithm is a statistical shape model (SSM) of the structure of interest. A global search with an evolutionary algorithm is employed to detect suitable initial parameters for the model, which are subsequently optimized by a local search similar to the Active Shape mechanism. After that, a deformable mesh with the same topology as the SSM is used for the final segmentation: While external forces strive to maximize the posterior probability of the mesh given the local appearance around the boundary, internal forces governed by tension and rigidity terms keep the shape similar to the underlying SSM. To prevent outliers and increase robustness, we determine the applied external forces by an algorithm for optimal surface detection with smoothness constraints. The approach is evaluated on 54 CT images of the liver and reaches an average surface distance of 1.6 ± 0.5 mm in comparison to manual reference segmentations.

1 Introduction

Statistical shape models (SSMs), as introduced by Cootes et al. [1], have become a popular choice for analyzing medical images. Due to their strict constraints on the allowable shapes, they offer robust performance even in case of image artifacts and low signal-to-noise ratio. The price for this robustness, however, is that the limited deformations often impede the exact adaptation to the structure of interest. This holds especially true if the target structure consists of soft tissue with a large amount of natural variability: Besides the systematic variation, there is always a part of essentially random perturbation that cannot be captured adequately by a global deformation model as used in SSMs. A solution to this problem is to combine the SSM with a freely deformable, energy-based model as the original Snake by Kass et al. [2]. In this hybrid approach, the external energy describes the difference to the data and the internal energy is based on the difference between the current shape and the closest SSM [3,4]. The challenge is to balance both forces properly and to ensure that the additional freedom does not affect the robust convergence properties of the SSM.

N. Karssemeijer and B. Lelieveldt (Eds.): IPMI 2007, LNCS 4584, pp. 1–12, 2007.
© Springer-Verlag Berlin Heidelberg 2007

Another critical element when using deformable models is the question of initialization: Although multi-resolution techniques provide a fairly large capture range, the model still has to be roughly aligned and oriented to the structure of interest so that the iterative search procedure can lock onto the target. Apart from the obvious manual initialization, there have been several suggestions how to estimate the target location automatically, e.g. by gray-value thresholding and subsequent morphological operations [5]. While these estimates can work for specialized cases, a more general solution is to conduct an initial global search: In the early 90s, Hill et al. already used a genetic algorithm for this purpose [6], but the method was later given up in favor of the iterative search of the Active Shape Model (ASM). Recently, de Bruijne and Nielsen successfully employed particle filtering for detecting 2D SSMs in radiographs [7]. We are not aware of any former attempts to localize a 3D SSM by global search methods.

In this paper, we present a segmentation method that offers a solution for both of the above presented shortcomings: A reliable initialization of the model using a global search in a down-sampled version of the image, and a robust deformable surface model with enough variability for an accurate segmentation. As an example application, we will employ the case of liver segmentation in abdominal CT datasets.

2 Statistical Model

The foundation of the proposed segmentation approach is a statistical model of the structure of interest, as introduced by Cootes et al. in [1]. It is built from a set of segmented training images and consists of two parts: A geometrical model describing the shape and a local appearance model describing the boundary.

2.1 Geometrical Model

The geometrical model is represented by a point distribution model (PDM), i.e. a dense collection of landmark points on the surface of the object. Each training shape t is described by a single vector $\mathbf{x_t}$ of concatenated landmark coordinates. Averaging all vectors produces the mean shape $\bar{\mathbf{x}}$, and a principal component analysis (PCA) on the covariance matrix yields the principal modes of variation p_m and the respective variances λ_m. Using a limited number of c parameters y_m, all valid shapes $\mathbf{x}$ can then be approximated by

$$\mathbf{x} \cong \bar{\mathbf{x}} + \sum_{m=1}^{c} y_m \mathbf{p}_m \tag{1}$$

A prerequisite for building a shape model is that all landmarks are situated at corresponding locations on all training samples. A number of different methods of how to automatically establish the required correspondences in 3D have been proposed in recent years, including registering mesh to mesh [8], volume to volume [9] or mesh to volume [10]. In this work, we employ a population-based approach for finding correspondences which minimizes a cost function based on the description length of the resulting shape model [11]. As proposed in [12], we utilize continuous landmark resampling during optimization to achieve a homogeneous point distribution over the entire surface.

2.2 Local Appearance Model

To detect the modeled shape in new image data, an additional model of the local gray-value appearance around the boundary is employed. A common method is to sample profiles g_{it} perpendicular to the surface at each landmark i in all training images t. Mean profiles $\bar{g}_i$ and the modes of variation for each landmark can then be determined using PCA. However, due to the essentially non-linear profile distributions in many medical imaging tasks, this method may not be optimal. In [13], an alternative approach to model local appearance based on kNN-classifiers is proposed: In addition to the true profiles g_{it}, a number of shifted profiles (i.e. translated towards the inside and outside of the object) is sampled. During model search, the probability $p(b|g)$ of a profile lying on the boundary can then be estimated by querying the k nearest neighbors to g and calculating the ratio of true profiles $b_k(g)$ among them. To prevent zero probabilities, we use a moderated kNN-classifier [14] and define:

$$p(b|g) = \frac{b_k(g) + 1}{k + 2} \tag{2}$$

Obviously, the accuracy of the classifier improves with the quantity of data available. With a limited number of training images on-hand, clustering landmarks to groups of similar appearance can help to raise the performance.

3 Model Initialization

In this work, we use an algorithm based on the concepts of evolutionary programming [15] and evolution strategies [16] to initialize the shape model. Though these two methods were developed independent from each other, they only differ in details and share most of the important properties. Both are global search algorithms maintaining a population of different solutions which evolve by following the "survival of the fittest" rule: A higher fitness value, as determined by an evaluation function, increases the probability that individual solutions are mutated and reproduced. After several generations (i.e. iterations of the process), the population converges to one or several local maxima (see also Fig. 1). The basic procedure is:

Initialize population
Repeat
  Evaluation of fitness
  Selection by random sampling
  Gaussian mutation
End

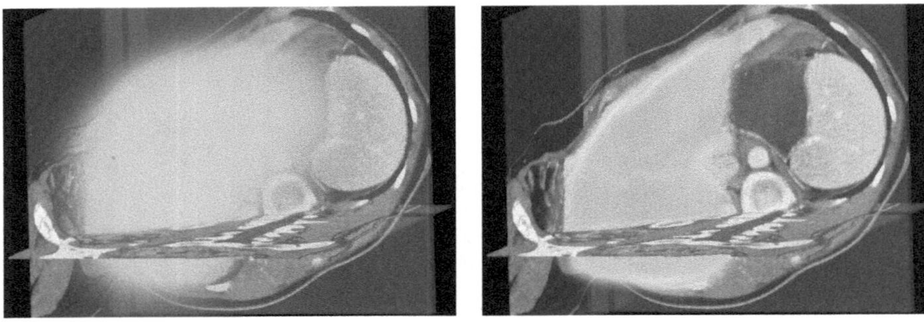

Fig. 1. Shape population in an image after initialization (left) and after convergence (right). All shapes are rendered as transparent solids, overlap increases the density color-coded from light to dark. While the left population is spread widely and only appears as a diffuse cloud, the right population is centered closely around the final solution. Both images display 5000 individual shapes.

The main differences to genetic algorithms [17] that were employed for model matching by Hill et al. [6] are the following: First, solutions do not have to be encoded as bit-strings in artificial chromosomes but are stored as real-valued vectors. Second, there is no cross-over operator for mutation (recombination) and no bit-inversion: Instead, solutions are modified by adding a random vector from a multivariate zero-mean Gaussian distribution.

3.1 Step by Step

One individual in our population represents one possible shape configuration, consisting of a similarity transform and c shape parameters. For initialization, all shape parameters y_m are randomized according to their variance λ_m. The pose parameters (translation, rotation, scale) are estimated from the respective mean values of the training samples (using relative coordinates for location) and are also randomized using a Gaussian distribution.

To evaluate the fitness w_s of an individual shape s, the probabilities $p(b|g)$ from Eq. 2 are estimated for all landmarks i and multiplied:

$$w_s = \exp\left(\frac{v}{n}\sum_i \log p_i(b|g_i)\right) \tag{3}$$

Here, n represents the number of landmarks and v is a constant determining the speed of convergence. We use $v = 5$ for all experiments. The subtle difference to the weighting function used by de Bruijne and Nielsen [7] for particle filtering is that we use the posterior probabilities $p_i(b|g_i)$ instead of the likelihoods $p_i(g_i|b)$. Thus, our fitness function directly expresses the statistical evidence for the individual shape in the image.

The selection process is implemented using a random sampling in which each individual s gets a chance of reproduction proportional to its fitness w_s. Subsequently, all drawn individuals are mutated with the current standard deviation

σ_t. For the next iteration $t+1$, the standard deviation is reduced using $\sigma_{t+1} = 0.95\,\sigma_t$. This corresponds to a reduction in step size of the optimizer and enables us to use a relatively large σ_0 to conduct an exhaustive search in the beginning and still obtain a stable convergence towards the end. After a fixed number of x iterations, we consider the optimization as converged. The individual reaching the maximum fitness during the evolution is the final solution.

3.2 Landmark Reduction

In our segmentation scheme, the evolutionary algorithm is run to find a rough initialization in a strongly down-sampled version of the image. For this purpose, a simplified version of the SSM (i.e. with fewer landmarks) is equally suitable, but considerably faster during the search. The process of choosing the best landmarks for the reduced model is essentially a mesh simplification problem: While we prefer to eliminate landmarks with poorly performing appearance models (details follow in the next section), we have to assure that the reduced landmark set still covers all parts of the surface. Consequently, we do not delete a landmark if the resulting gap would be larger than a certain geodesic radius r, which is estimated by the number of traversed edges in the SSM. For $r = 1$, this means there must exist at least one "surviving" landmark in the direct neighborhood of each deleted one.

3.3 Benchmarking Local Appearance Models

To compare the performance of different appearance models on a per-landmark basis, we propose the following method: In all training images, the probability $p(b|g)$ is estimated at the true boundary position and at $2K$ positions shifted along the respective normal vector. To simulate realistic search conditions and to avoid testing on the actual training data, the true boundary position g_0 is randomized around each landmark i with a uniform distribution in the polygon determined by the direct neighbors of i. In addition, the employed normal vectors are randomized with a standard deviation of $\sigma = 10$ degrees. This way, a number of $R = 30$ tests is run for each landmark in every image. The performance of one test r is evaluated by a weighted sum of differences between the boundary probability at the true position g_{r0} and the ones at shifted positions g_{rk}:

$$f_{ir} = \left(\sum_{k=-K}^{K} |k|^d \left(p_i(b|g_{r0}) - p_i(b|g_{rk})\right) \right) / \left(\sum_{k=-K}^{K} |k|^d \right) \quad (4)$$

where d determines the influence of the shifting distance ($d = 1$ in our case). By averaging the results over all tests, a performance index $f_i \in [-1..1]$ is estimated for each landmark. The obtained benchmark values are used for the mesh simplification from Sect. 3.2.

4 Deformable Model

The deformable model used for the final segmentation is defined as a triangulated mesh $M = (V, E)$ with vertices $p, q \in V$ and edges $[p, q] \in E$. M has the same topology as the statistical shape model, i.e. for each vertex p in the mesh, there is a corresponding vertex $\tilde{p}$ in the SSM. The evolution of the deformable model is controlled by the Lagrangian equation of motion: At every vertex p_i, a regularizing internal force $F_{int}(p_i)$ and a data-driven external force $F_{ext}(p_i)$ are applied. In the following, we will present the derivations for both internal and external forces in detail.

4.1 Internal Forces

The internal forces should keep the shape of the deformable model similar to the one of the underlying SSM. We define this similarity by evaluating differences in edge lengths (also used by Weese et al. in [4]) and differences in angles between neighboring faces. This approach is based on the concepts of tension and rigidity which are also used to define the internal energy of a snake [2].

To implement the tension forces, every edge $[p, q]$ is modeled as a linear spring with the neutral length $|\tilde{p} - \tilde{q}|$, which is the length of $[p, q]$ in the template. Consequently, the tension force on a vertex p in the direction towards q is:

$$F_T(p, q) = \alpha \left(1 - \frac{|\tilde{p} - \tilde{q}|}{|p - q|}\right)(p - q) \quad (5)$$

where α defines the strength of the tension force and is constant for all $[p, q] \in E$. Thus, the total tension force for a vertex is the sum over the forces along all of its edges:

$$F_T(p) = \sum_{[p,q] \in E} F_T(p, q) \quad (6)$$

For the description of rigidity forces, we use the following definitions: For every edge $[p_1, p_2] \in E$, the adjacent triangles $[p_1, p_2, q_1]$ and $[p_2, p_1, q_2]$ form an angle θ that strives towards the corresponding angle $\tilde{\theta}$ in the SSM (see Fig. 2). We call q_1, q_2 the outer vertices of $[p_1, p_2]$; both together form the set $V_O([p_1, p_2])$. The rigidity force for an outer vertex $q \in V_O([p_1, p_2])$ is defined as

$$F_R(q, [p_1, p_2]) = T(q, [p_1, p_2], \beta\delta)) - q \quad (7)$$

where $T(q, [p_1, p_2], \varphi)$ is a rotation of point q around the edge $[p_1, p_2]$ by φ degrees, and β is the strength of the rigidity force. To define δ for both outer vertices, we have to consider the case of a constellation where the distance d_1 between $[p_1, p_2]$ and q_1 is different from d_2. To balance forces on both outer vertices, the triangle with the shorter distance d has to rotate more than the other one:

$$\delta = \frac{d_{op}}{d_1 + d_2} (\theta - \tilde{\theta}) \quad (8)$$

where d_{op} is the distance from $[p_1, p_2]$ to the opposing outer vertex (i.e. d_2 when calculating δ for q_1 and vice versa). An important point to take care of is that the internal forces may not alter the overall position of the deformable surface, i.e. all internal forces must sum up to zero. Therefore, the forces on q_1 and q_2

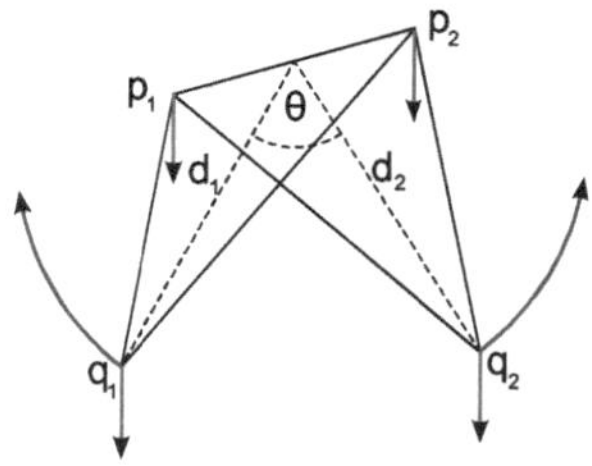

Fig. 2. Two adjacent triangles form the angle θ. Internal rigidity forces striving for a larger angle directly affect the outer vertices q_1 and q_2 (large, curved arrows), but also the edge vertices p_1 and p_2 to maintain the equilibrium of the constellation.

have to be neutralized. The neutralizing force acts equally on all four vertices of a constellation and is defined as

$$F_N([p_1, p_2]) = -\frac{1}{4}(F_R(q_1, [p_1, p_2]) + F_R(q_2, [p_1, p_2])) \tag{9}$$

Overall, this results in a total rigidity force of

$$F_R(p) = \sum_{[p_1,p_2]\in E} \begin{cases} F_R(p, [p_1, p_2]) + F_N([p_1, p_2]) & \text{if } p \in V_O([p_1, p_2]) \\ F_N([p_1, p_2]) & \text{if } p = p_1 \vee p = p_2 \\ \mathbf{0} & \text{else} \end{cases} \tag{10}$$

Finally, the internal force for a given vertex is the sum of tension and rigidity force:

$$F_{int}(p) = F_T(p) + F_R(p) \tag{11}$$

4.2 External Forces

The external forces drive the deformable surface towards the best fit to the data. As in the Active Shape Model search [1], the goodness of fit is evaluated using the local appearance models for all $p \in V$; once at p itself and additional at K positions on each side of the surface. This procedure leads to $2K+1$ probes for each vertex, enumerated as $k \in [-K..K]$. Defining the optimum probe position as $s(p)$, a linear spring force drives the vertex in the corresponding direction:

$$F_{ext}(p) = \gamma(s(p) - p) \tag{12}$$

where γ is the strength of the external forces. Usually, $s(p)$ is determined independently for each vertex p by picking the maximum fitness value, a procedure generating a considerable amount of outliers. Behiels et al. have shown that a smoothness constraint on the allowable changes significantly increases the robustness of deformation in SSMs [18], albeit only for the 2D case. For 3D, no efficient algorithm to adhere to such constraints was known until recently, when Li et al. presented a graph-based approach to detect optimal surfaces [19]. In the following section, we will briefly summarize this algorithm and show how it integrates with our local appearance models.

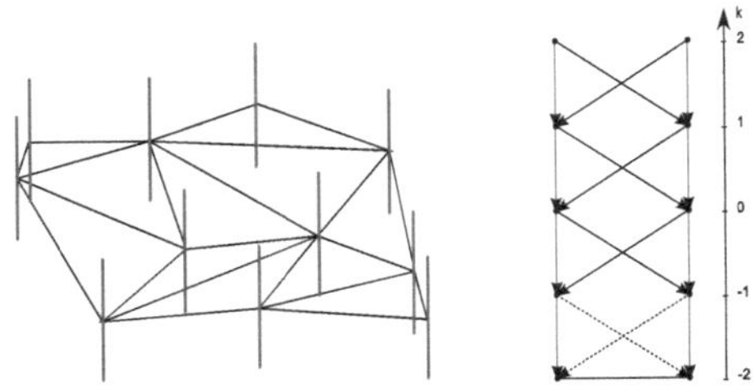

Fig. 3. Optimal surface detection for closed triangle meshes: On the left, a section of the mesh is displayed; the different probe positions for each vertex are displayed by a vertical line. The right side illustrates how two adjacent probe lines are represented in the graph (here for $K = 2$ and $\Delta = 1$). All edges have infinite weight, the dotted connections are optional.

4.3 Optimal Surface Detection

To employ the optimal surface detection algorithm from [19], the first step is to build a directed graph $G = (N, D)$ from the mesh M and its surroundings: For each vertex $p \in V$, $2K + 1$ nodes (corresponding to the probe positions) are inserted into the graph as $n(p, k)$. These nodes are connected by directed edges of infinite weight from $n(p, k)$ to $n(p, k - 1)$ for $k > -K$ and form a so-called column. Next, directed edges between neighboring columns $col(p_1)$ and $col(p_2)$ are added from $n(p_1, k)$ to $n(p_2, \max(-K, k - \Delta)$, where Δ is the smoothness constraint and specifies how many steps adjacent probes may shift against each other during deformation. $col(p_1)$ and $col(p_2)$ count as adjacent if $[p_1, p_2] \in E$. A simplified visualization of this graph structure is given in Fig. 3.

The next step is to assign a weight $w(p, k)$ to each $n(p, k) \in N$. Assuming that the costs for each probe are stored in $c(p, k)$, weights are computed as

$$w(p,k) = \begin{cases} c(p,k) & \text{for } k = -K \\ c(p,k) - c(p,k-1) & \text{for } k > -K \end{cases} \tag{13}$$

Since the algorithm finds the solution that minimizes the sum of costs, we have to transform the probabilities $p(b|g)$ from Eq. 2 accordingly. As in the weight calculation for the evolutionary algorithm (3), we want to maximize the posterior probability of the shape, i.e. the product of all boundary probabilities. Thus, we define the costs as

$$c(p,k) = -\log p_p(b|g_{pk}) \tag{14}$$

Subsequently, an additional source node n_s and a sink node n_t are added to the graph. All previously inserted nodes are connected to these two in the following way: Every node with $w(p, k) \geq 0$ is connected to n_t by a directed edge of weight $w(p, k)$, and n_s is connected to every node with $w(p, k) < 0$ by a directed edge of weight $-w(p, k)$. Employing an s-t cut algorithm like the one presented in [20], the graph can now be divided into a source set S with $n_s \in S$ and sink set T with $n_t \in T$. The optimal displacements $s(p)$ are given by the largest k with $n(p, k) \in S$.

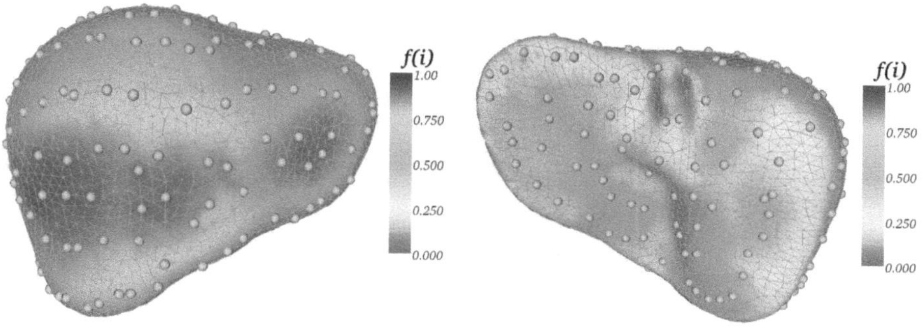

Fig. 4. Reduced set of landmarks on the shape model of the liver (front and back view): The performance f_i of the local appearance models is color-coded over the entire surface. The full set of landmarks is displayed using a triangular grid, the reduced set is shown as small spheres. The maximum gap-radius r is 2. It is clearly visible how landmarks evade the low-performance sections of the surface by grouping around them.

5 Experiments and Results

We chose the task of liver segmentation as an example to validate our approach: An automatic segmentation of this organ without prior shape information is prone to fail due to the low contrast to neighboring structures. However, the large amount of anatomical variation makes it particularly challenging to model and detect using classical SSMs.

5.1 Image Data and Model Generation

All used images are contrast-enhanced CT volumes of the abdomen with an in-plane resolution of 512x512 pixels and 60 to 130 slices (spacing ~0.7x0.7x3mm). In most cases the anatomy is pathologic, i.e. interspersed with tumors. Additionally, the data was acquired using different protocols, which should allow a reliable prediction of the clinical performance of the presented segmentation scheme.

Out of 86 volumes, 32 were selected as training data for the statistical model, which was built using 2562 equally distributed landmarks. The remaining 54 volumes were used for evaluation. Appearance models as described in Sect. 2.2 were generated for five different resolutions R_0 (original resolution) to R_4 (four times down-sampled), featuring a profile-length of 7 pixels and a pixel-spacing of 1mm in R_0. The k-Means algorithm [21] was employed to group all landmarks into 22–42 clusters (depending on the resolution) and to improve the accuracy of the kNN-classifiers. After that, the performance of the appearance models for the lowest resolution R_4 was benchmarked with the method from Sect. 3.3. The obtained results were used to create a reduced set of 204 landmarks for the evolutionary algorithm (see Fig. 4).

5.2 Segmentation Workflow and Parameter Values

The segmentation of one image consisted of three major steps: To find the initial position and shape parameters of the SSM, the evolutionary algorithm was

Table 1. Parameter values used in the different phases of the deformable model segmentation: Convergence criteria are either the maximum vertex movement per iteration d_{max} or the number of iterations I

Resolution	Convergence criterion	α	β	γ	Δ
3	$d_{max} < 0.3$mm	0.125	0.25	0.01	1
2	$d_{max} < 0.4$mm	0.125	0.25	0.02	2
2	$d_{max} < 1.0$mm	0.125	0.25	0.05	2
2	$I = 50$	0.125	0.25	0.10	2
1	$I = 50$	0.125	0.25	0.10	2
0	$I = 20$	0.125	0.25	0.10	2

run with a population of 1000 individuals over 40 iterations. Fitness was evaluated on the 204 reduced landmarks in R_4. The initial standard deviation for mutation σ_0 was set to 0.4, resulting in a final σ_{40} around 0.05. After that, a normal ASM search (i.e. without allowing extra deformation) was conducted to improve the solution if possible. It was first run in R_4 until the maximum vertex movement D_{max} was less than 4mm, then in R_3 until $D_{max} < 2mm$. Finally, the deformable model search was started in R_3 down to R_0. As in the previous steps, the underlying SSM used 10 modes of variation. To improve the runtime of the algorithm, the external forces were updated every 10 iterations. For an overview over the used parameter values, see Table 1.

5.3 Results

All 54 generated segmentations were compared to manual delineations by radiological experts using three different error metrics: Symmetric average surface distance D_{avg}, symmetric RMS surface distance D_{RMS} and volumetric error V_D. V_D is based on the Dice coefficient and is calculated as $V_D = 1-(2\cdot|A\cap B|)/(|A|+|B|)$ for two sets of voxels A and B. The results achieved by the presented deformable model, a standard ASM search with 30 modes of variation after manual initialization and two other approaches from literature are summarized in Table 2. The three worst segmentations (V_D>10% for the deformable model) were treated as outliers and omitted from the statistics. For a visual performance assessment, the image featuring the median average surface distance is displayed in Fig. 5. The computation time on a 3GHz desktop PC is approximately 10 minutes per image, of which the automatic initialization requires the major part of 6 minutes.

6 Conclusion

We have presented an automated segmentation procedure combining techniques from statistical shape models and deformable surfaces. Main contributions are the initialization of a 3D SSM using an evolutionary algorithm on a simplified model and a robust deformation scheme by means of a constrained optimal surface detection. Fitting costs for both searches are estimated by the posterior

Table 2. Segmentation error in comparison with a standard ASM and numbers from previous work (customized ASM [22] and deformable simplex mesh [5]), given as $\mu \pm \sigma$

Segmentation method	$D_{avg}[mm]$	$D_{RMS}[mm]$	$V_D[\%]$
Deformable model	1.6 ± 0.5	3.3 ± 1.2	5.1 ± 1.4
Active Shape Model	2.9 ± 1.1	5.2 ± 2.3	8.9 ± 2.4
Lamecker et al. [22]	2.3 ± 0.3	3.1 ± 0.5	7.0 ± 1.8
Soler et al. [5]	2±?	*n.a.*	*n.a.*

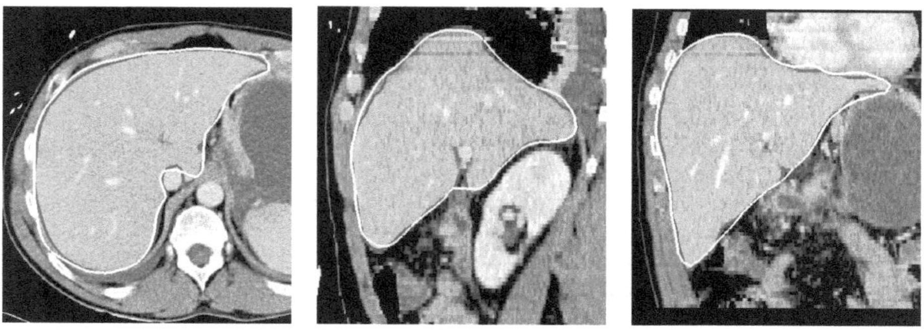

Fig. 5. Transversal, sagittal and coronal slices for the image with median average surface error. The result of the deformable model is displayed in white, the manually traced reference contour in dark gray.

probability for the model given the data. The obtained results on liver CT images are excellent and encourage us to employ the approach for other soft tissue objects in the near future.

Acknowledgements

This work was supported by the German Research Foundation DFG under grant WO 1218/2-1.

References

1. Cootes, T.F., Taylor, C.J., Cooper, D.H., Graham, J.: Active shape models – their train- ing and application. Computer Vision and Image Understanding 61(1), 38–59 (1995)
2. Kass, M., Witkin, A., Terzopoulos, D.: Snakes: Active contour models. International Journal of Computer Vision 1(4), 321–331 (1988)
3. Shen, D., Davatzikos, C.: An adaptive-focus deformable model using statistical and geometric information. IEEE Trans. Pattern Analysis and Machine Intelligence 22(8), 906–913 (2000)
4. Weese, J., Kaus, M., Lorenz, C., Lobregt, S., Truyen, R., Pekar, V.: Shape constrained deformable models for 3D medical image segmentation. In: Insana, M.F., Leahy, R.M. (eds.) IPMI 2001. LNCS, vol. 2082, pp. 380–387. Springer, Heidelberg (2001)

5. Soler, L., Delingette, H., Malandain, G., Montagnat, J., Ayache, N., et al.: Fully automatic anatomical, pathological, and functional segmentation from ct scans for hepatic surgery. In: Proc. SPIE Medical Imaging, pp. 246–255 (2000)
6. Hill, A., Taylor, C.J., Cootes, T.F.: Object recognition by flexible template matching using genetic algorithms. In: Sandini, G. (ed.) ECCV 1992. LNCS, vol. 588, pp. 852–856. Springer, Heidelberg (1992)
7. de Bruijne, M., Nielsen, M.: Shape particle filtering for image segmentation. In: Barillot, C., Haynor, D.R., Hellier, P. (eds.) MICCAI 2004. LNCS, vol. 3216, pp. 168–175. Springer, Heidelberg (2004)
8. Subsol, G., Thirion, J.P., Ayache, N.: A scheme for automatically building three-dimensional morphometric anatomical atlases: application to a skull atlas. Medical Image Analysis 2(1), 37–60 (1998)
9. Frangi, A.F., Rueckert, D., Schnabel, J.A., Niessen, W.J.: Automatic construction of multiple-object three-dimensional statistical shape models: application to cardiac modeling. IEEE Trans. Medical Imaging 21(9), 1151–1166 (2002)
10. Kaus, M.R., Pekar, V., Lorenz, C., Truyen, R., Lobregt, S., Weese, J.: Automated 3-D PDM construction from segmented images using deformable models. IEEE Trans. Medical Imaging 22(8), 1005–1013 (2003)
11. Davies, R.H., Twining, C.J., Cootes, T.F., Waterton, J.C., Taylor, C.J.: 3D statistical shape models using direct optimisation of description length. In: Heyden, A., Sparr, G., Nielsen, M., Johansen, P. (eds.) ECCV 2002. LNCS, vol. 2352, pp. 3–20. Springer, Heidelberg (2002)
12. Heimann, T., Wolf, I., Meinzer, H.P.: Optimal landmark distributions for statistical shape model construction. In: Proc. SPIE Medical Imaging: Image Processing. vol. 6144, pp. 518–528 (2006)
13. de Bruijne, M., van Ginneken, B., Viergever, M.A., Niessen, W.J.: Adapting active shape models for 3D segmentation of tubular structures in medical images. In: Taylor, C.J., Noble, J.A. (eds.) IPMI 2003. LNCS, vol. 2732, pp. 136–147. Springer, Heidelberg (2003)
14. Kittler, J., Alkoot, F.M.: Moderating k-NN classifiers. Pattern Analysis & Applications 5(3), 326–332 (2002)
15. Fogel, L.J., Owens, A.J., Walsh, M.J.: Artificial Intelligence through Simulated Evolution. John Wiley, New York (1966)
16. Schwefel, H.P.: Evolution and Optimum Seeking. John Wiley & Sons, Inc, New York (1995)
17. Holland, J.H.: Adaptation in natural and artificial systems. University of Michigan Press, Ann Arbor (1975)
18. Behiels, G., Maes, F., Vandermeulen, D., Suetens, P.: Evaluation of image features and search strategies for segmentation of bone structures in radiographs using active shape models. Medical Image Analysis 6(1), 47–62 (2002)
19. Li, K., Millington, S., Wu, X., Chen, D.Z., Sonka, M.: Simultaneous segmentation of multiple closed surfaces using optimal graph searching. In: Christensen, G.E., Sonka, M. (eds.) IPMI 2005. LNCS, vol. 3565, pp. 406–417. Springer, Heidelberg (2005)
20. Boykov, Y., Kolmogorov, V.: An experimental comparison of min-cut/max-flow algorithms for energy minimization in vision. IEEE Trans. Pattern Analysis and Machine Intelligence 26(9), 1124–1137 (2004)
21. Hartigan, J.A., Wong, M.A.: A K-means clustering algorithm. Applied Statistics 28, 100–108 (1979)
22. Lamecker, H., Lange, T., Seebass, M.: Segmentation of the liver using a 3D statistical shape model. Technical report, Zuse Institute, Berlin, Germany (2004)

Shape Regression Machine

Shaohua Kevin Zhou and Dorin Comaniciu

Integrated Data Systems Department,Siemens Corporate Research
755 College Road East, Princeton NJ 08540

Abstract. We present a machine learning approach called *shape regression machine* (SRM) to segmenting in real time an anatomic structure that manifests a deformable shape in a medical image. Traditional shape segmentation methods rely on various assumptions. For instance, the deformable model assumes that edge defines the shape; the Mumford-Shah variational method assumes that the regions inside/outside the (closed) contour are homogenous in intensity; and the active appearance model assumes that shape/appearance variations are linear. In addition, they all need a good initialization. In contrast, SRM poses no such restrictions. It is a two-stage approach that leverages (a) the underlying medical context that defines the anatomic structure and (b) an annotated database that exemplifies the shape and appearance variations of the anatomy. In the first stage, it solves the initialization problem as object detection and derives a regression solution that needs just one scan in principle. In the second stage, it learns a nonlinear regressor that predicts the nonrigid shape from image appearance. We also propose a boosting regression approach that supports real time segmentation. We demonstrate the effectiveness of SRM using experiments on segmenting the left ventricle endocardium from an echocardiogram of an apical four chamber view.

1 Introduction

Deformable shape segmentation is a long-standing challenge in medical imaging. Numerous algorithms have been proposed in the literature to tackle the problem, among which there are three important approaches: the deformable model or snake [1], the Mumford-Shah variational method [2], and the active appearance model (AAM) [3].

The deformable model or snake [1] seeks a parameterized curve $\mathtt{C}(s)$ that minimizes the cost function $\mathcal{E}_{snake}(\mathtt{C})$:

$$\mathcal{E}_{snake}(\mathtt{C}) = \int_0^1 \{-\mu|\nabla \mathtt{I}(\mathtt{C}(s))|^2 + w_1(s)|\mathtt{C}'(s)|^2 + w_2(s)|\mathtt{C}''(s)|^2\}ds, \quad (1)$$

where μ controls the magnitude of the potential, ∇ is the gradient operator, $\mathtt{I}$ is the image, $w_1(s)$ controls the tension of the curve, and $w_2(s)$ controls the rigidity of the curve. The implicit assumption of the snake model is that edge defines the curve due to the use of the gradient operator.

N. Karssemeijer and B. Lelieveldt (Eds.): IPMI 2007, LNCS 4584, pp. 13–25, 2007.
© Springer-Verlag Berlin Heidelberg 2007

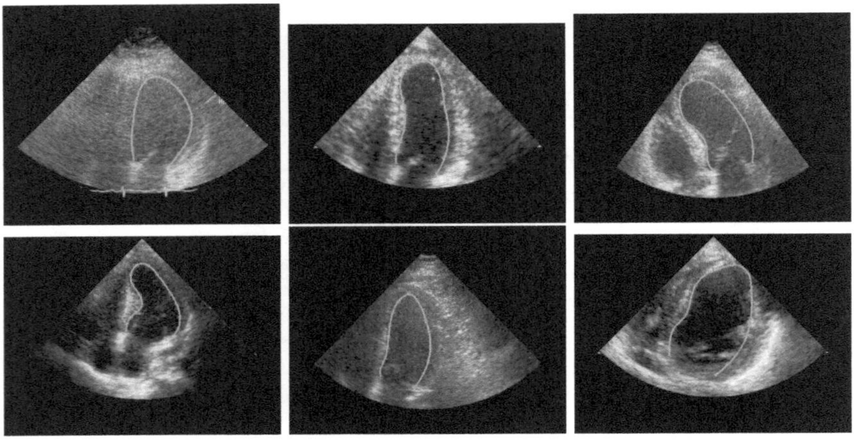

Fig. 1. Examples of A4C echocardiogram. The expert annotation of the LV endocardium is marked by the green line. The shape is represented by 17 landmarks and the cubic spline is used for intepolation.

In the Mumford-Shah variational method [2], the minimal partition problem is mostly studied, where a curve $\mathtt{C}$ is sought to minimize the cost function $\mathcal{E}_{ms}(\mathtt{C})$:

$$\mathcal{E}_{ms}(\mathtt{C}) = \int_{\Omega_i} |\mathtt{I}(x,y) - u_i|^2 dxdy + \int_{\Omega_o} |\mathtt{I}(x,y) - u_o|^2 dxdy + \mu\mathcal{L}(\mathtt{C}), \qquad (2)$$

where Ω_i and Ω_o denote the inside and outside regions, respectively, with respect to the curve $\mathtt{C}$, u_i and u_o are piecewise constants for the two regions, and $\mathcal{L}(\mathtt{C})$ is the length of the curve. The region homogeneity is assumed here.

The AAM [3] jointly characterizes the appearance $\mathtt{I}$ and shape $\mathtt{C}$ using a linear generative model:

$$\mathtt{C} = \bar{\mathtt{C}} + \mathtt{Q}_c\mathtt{a}; \quad \mathtt{I} = \bar{\mathtt{I}} + \mathtt{Q}_i\mathtt{a}, \qquad (3)$$

where $\bar{\mathtt{C}}$ is the mean shape, $\bar{\mathtt{I}}$ the mean appearance in a normalized patch, and $\mathtt{a}$ is the blending coefficient vector shared by both the shape and appearance. The model parameter $\mathtt{a}$, along with a similarity transformation parameter, is found by fitting the AAM to the observed image using the mean square error criterion.

However, the above assumptions are easily violated in practice. Consider the problem of segmenting the left ventricle (LV) endocardium from an echocardiogram of an apical four chamber (A4C) view. The echocardiogram is an ultrasound image of human heart and the A4C view is a canonical view in which all four heart chambers are visible. Fig. 1 presents several A4C examples that manifest the following facts: (i) The LV endocardium is not defined by the edge. For example, it cuts the papillary muscle attached to the LV; (ii) The region homogeneity is severely violated due to ultrasound imaging artifacts and signal dropouts; and (iii) The shape and appearance variations are hardly linear due to differences in instrument, patient, and sonograher, respiratory interferences, unnecessary probe movements, etc. Furthermore, the above three methods need a good initialization and different initializations might yield very different results due to the attraction of local minima.

In this paper, we present a machine learning approach called shape regression machine (SRM), which poses none of the above restrictions. It deals with deformable contour not necessarily supported by the edge, allows region inhomogeneity, and utilizes nonlinear models to characterize shape and appearance in a discriminative manner. In addition, it is fully automatic with no manual initialization and runs in real time. SRM is mostly appropriate for segmenting an anatomical structure. The core of SRM is to effectively leverage the underlying *structural context* present in medical images and, using regression, to extract knowledge from an *annotated database* that exemplifies the shape and appearance variations. Section 2 depicts the principle of the SRM approach and section 3 elaborates an image-based boosting regression method that underpins SRM. Section 4 presents the experimental results of segmenting the LV endocardium from the A4C echocardiogram.

2 Shape Regression Machine

The shape $\mathtt{C}$ is represented by two parts: rigid and nonrigid. The rigid transformation is parameterized by θ and the nonrigid part by $\mathtt{S}$. If the rigid similarity transformation is used, then the above shape representation reduces to Kendall's interpretation. To rigidly align the LV shape in the A4C echocardiogram more accurately, we use a 5D-parameterization $\theta = (t_x, t_y, \log(s_x), \log(s_y), \alpha)$, with (t_x, t_y) for translation, α for orientation, and (s_x, s_y) for scale (or size) in both x- and y-directions. Due to the multiplicative nature of the scale parameter, we take the logarithm operator to convert it to additive. Fig. 2(a) illustrates the meaning of the five parameters.

SRM is a two-stage approach. It first solves the rigid transformation θ as object detection and then infers the nonrigid part $\mathtt{S}$, both using the machine learning technique of regression.

2.1 Regression-Based Object Detection

A promising approach to medical anatomy detection is to use the classifier-based object detection approach like [4]: It first trains a binary classifier, discriminating the anatomic structure of interest from the background, and then exhaustively scans the query image for anatomy targets. In [4], the so-called integral image is proposed to enable real time evaluation of the classifier when applied for searching the translation parameter exhaustively and the scale parameter sparsely. No orientation is scanned. However, the medical anatomy such as LV often manifests arbitrary orientation and scale. To give an accurate account of orientation and scale, which is required for subsequent tasks like LV endocardial wall segmentation, the detection speed is sacrificed if a dense set of orientations and scales is tested. In general, the computational complexity of the classifier-based approach linearly depends on the image size (for the translation parameter), and the number of tested orientations and scales. Also, multiple integral images according to different rotations need to be computed. Therefore, the bottleneck of the classifier-based detection approach lies in its exhaustive scanning native. To avoid exhaustive scanning, we propose a regression-based detection approach. By leveraging the anatomical structure that manifests regularization and context in geometry and appearance, we formulate a novel regression task that, in theory, necessitates *only one scan.* Also, we compute *only one integral image.*

Basic idea. Fig. 2(b) demonstrates the basic idea of the regression-based medical anatomy detection. For illustrative purpose only, we address only the translation parameter θ as in Fig. 2(b). In other words, we are only interested in finding the center position $\theta_0 = (t_{x,0}, t_{y,0})$ of the LV in an A4C echocardiogram, assuming that the orientation of the LV is upright and the scale/size of the LV is fixed. It is straightforward to extend the 2D case to the 5D-parameterization.

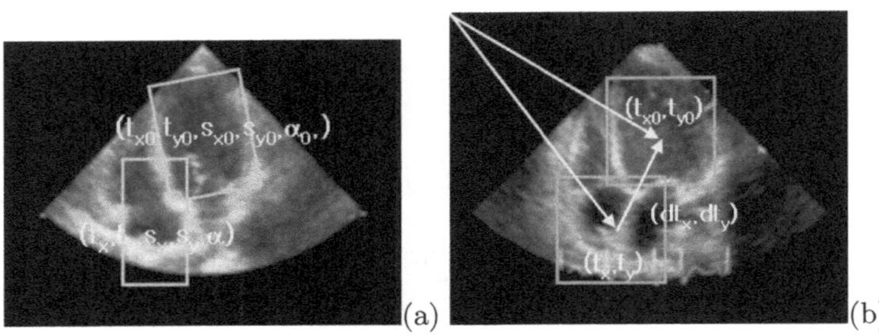

Fig. 2. (a) The regression setting of a 5D parameter space: (t_x, t_y) is the LV center, (s_x, s_y) the LV size, and α the LV angle. (b) A graphical illustration of regression-based medical anatomy detection based on a 2D translation parameterization.

Suppose that, during running time, we confront an image patch $\mathtt{I}(\theta)$ centered at position $\theta = (t_x, t_y)$. If there exists an oracle $\mathcal{F}_1$ that does the following: given an image patch $\mathtt{I}(\theta)$, it tells the difference vector $d\theta$ between the current position θ and the target position $\theta_0 = (t_{x,0}, t_{y,0})$, i.e., $d\theta = \theta_0 - \theta$, then we achieve the detection using *just one* scan. In other words, through the oracle that defines a mapping $\mathcal{F}_1 : \mathtt{I} \rightarrow d\theta$, the ground truth position $\hat{\theta}_0$ is estimated as follows.

$$d\theta = \mathcal{F}_1(\mathtt{I}(\theta)), \quad \hat{\theta}_0 = \theta + d\theta = \theta + \mathcal{F}_1(\mathtt{I}(\theta)). \tag{4}$$

Learning the function $\mathcal{F}_1(\mathtt{I}(\theta))$ is referred to as *regression* in machine learning.

Does such an oracle $\mathcal{F}_1$ exist? Since the anatomic structure of interest is tied with human body atlas, there is a known number of objects appearing within geometric and appearance contexts. Often only one object is available. For example, in the A4C echocardiogram, there is only one target LV available and its relation with respect to other structures such as left atrium, right ventricle and right atrium is geometrically fixed (that is why they are called left/right ventricle/atrium). Also there exists a strong correlation among their appearances. By knowing where the LA, RV, or RA is, we can predict the LV position quite accurately. In principle, by knowing where we are (i.e., knowing θ) and then looking up the map/atlas that tells the difference to the target (i.e., telling $d\theta$ through the oracle), we can reach the target instantaneously in a virtual world.

Medical atlas is widely used in the literature [5,6]. However, the methods in [5,6] use the atlas as an *explicit* source of prior knowledge about the location, size, and shape of the anatomic structures and deform it to match the image content for registration, segmentation, tracking, etc. In this paper, we take an *implicit* approach, that is, embedding the atlas in a learning framework. After learning, the atlas knowledge is fully absorbed and the atlas is no longed kept.

How to learn the oracle $\mathcal{F}_1$? We leverage machine learning techniques, based on an annotated database. As in Fig. 3, we first collect from the database input-output pairs (as many as possible) as training data. By varying the location, we crop out different local image patches while recording their corresponding difference vectors. Similarly, for the 5D parameterization, we can extract the training data. We now confront a multiple regression setting with a multidimensional output, which is not well addressed in the machine learning literature. In this paper, we propose the image-based boosting regression (IBR) algorithm to fulfill the learning task.

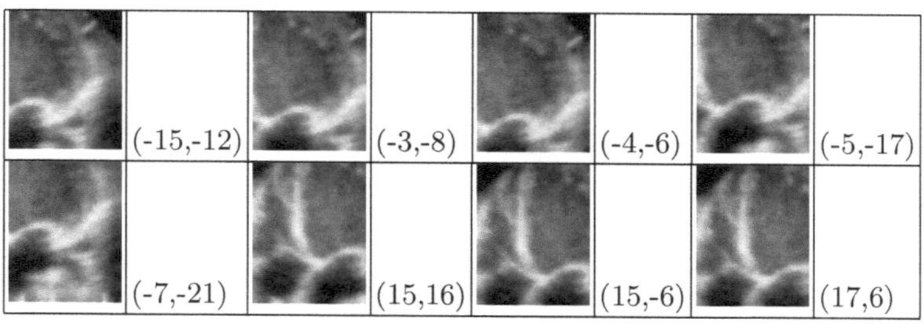

Fig. 3. Training image examples (generated based on the image in Fig. 2(b)): image $\mathtt{I}$ and its associated rigid transformation parameter $d\theta = (dx, dy)$

Detection algorithm. In theory, only one scan is needed to find the target; in practice, we conduct a sparse set of random scans and then estimate the parameter using fusion. Suppose that in total M random samples are scanned at positions $\{\theta^{<1>}, \theta^{<2>}, \ldots, \theta^{<M>}\}$. For each $\theta^{<m>}$, we invoke the regressor to predict the difference parameter $d\theta^{<m>}$ and, subsequently, the target parameter $\theta_0^{<m>}$ as follows:

$$d\theta^{<m>} = \mathcal{F}_1(\mathtt{I}(\theta^{<m>})), \;\; \theta_0^{<m>} = \theta^{<m>} + d\theta^{<m>}, \;\; m = 1, 2, \ldots, M. \quad (5)$$

We also learn a binary classifier (or detector) $\mathcal{D}$ that separates the object from the background and use its posterior probability $p_d(\mathtt{I})$ of being positive as a confidence scorer. After finding the mth prediction $\theta_0^{<m>}$, we apply the detector $\mathcal{D}$ to the image patch $\mathtt{I}(\theta_0^{<m>})$. If the detector $\mathcal{D}$ fails, we discard the mth sample; otherwise, we keep the confidence score $p_d^{<m>}$. This way, we have a weighted set

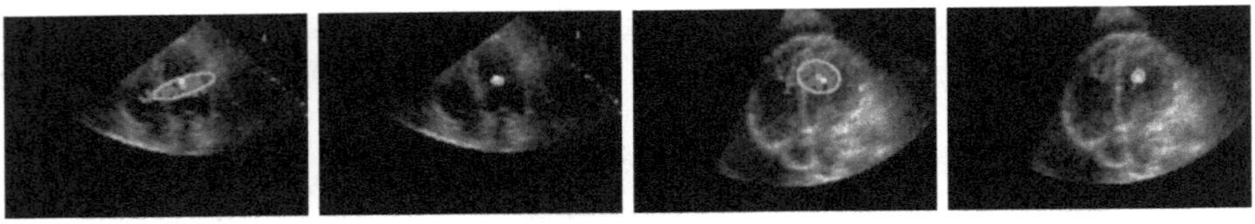

Fig. 4. The odd-indexed images show the 100 predicted target outputs (red) and the even-indexed images show only the predicted target outputs (red) passing the detector. The green point is the final estimate of the target position, the green curve is the 95% confidence curve, and the yellow point indicates the ground truth position. Note that the region bounded the 95% confidence curve on the even-indexed images is significantly smaller than that on the odd-indexed images.

$\{(\theta_0^{<j>}, p_d^{<j>}); j = 1, 2, \ldots, J\}$ (note that $J \leq M$ as samples might be dropped), based on which we calculate the weighted mean as the final estimate $\hat{\theta}_0$

$$\hat{\theta}_0 = \{ \sum_{j=1:J} p_d^{<j>} \theta_0^{<j>} \} / \{ \sum_{j=1:J} p_d^{<j>} \}. \tag{6}$$

In practice, we stop scanning when $J \geq J_{valid}$ in order to further save computation. If there is no sample $\theta_0^{<m>}$ passing $\mathcal{D}$, then we use the unweighted mean of $\theta_0^{<m>}$ as the final estimate.

Combining the regressor and binary detector yields an effective tool for medical anatomy detection; empirical evidence tells that, when compared with the method using only the regressor, it needs only a smaller number of scans to reach a better performance. Fig. 4 demonstrates the intuition behind this improvement using the 2-D translational case. Two example images are shown along with their $M = 100$ predicted target positions (the red points). The majority of the prediction is close to the ground truth position (the yellow point) although there are outliers. Fig. 4 also shows the predicted points passing the detector: All the outliers are eliminated, thereby significantly improving the precision of the estimate as evidenced by the smaller region bounded by the 95% confidence curve.

2.2 Regression-Based Nonrigid Shape Inference

After the first stage that finds the bounding box (parameterized by θ) to contain the object, we have the object rigidly aligned. In the second stage, we are interested in inferring the nonrigid part $\mathtt{S}$. In this paper, we assume that $\mathtt{S}$ consists of N landmark points, i.e., $\mathtt{S} = [x_1, y_1, \ldots, x_N, y_N]^{\mathsf{T}}$. Other shape representations can be used with no difficulty.

Basic idea. We formulate the nonrigid shape inference again as a regression problem. In other words, we seek an oracle $\mathcal{F}_2$ that tells the shape $\mathtt{S}$ based on the image patch $\mathtt{I}$ that is known to contain the object.

$$\mathtt{S} = \mathcal{F}_2(\mathtt{I}). \tag{7}$$

Does such an oracle $\mathcal{F}_2$ exist? Because we deal with one particular anatomic structure (say LV), it is obvious that a regularity exists in terms of its appearance

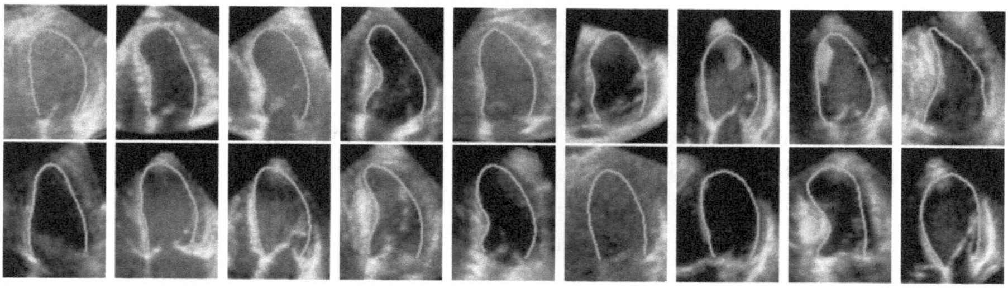

Fig. 5. Training image examples: image I and its associated nonrigid shape S. The first six images correspond to those in Fig. 1. The image size is 104 by 80.

and shape although the variations in them can be quite significant. Fig. 5 displays several images with corresponding shapes that are rigidly aligned to the mean shape. As mentioned earlier, a linear modeling of the appearance and shape is insufficient. One goal of the paper is to provide a nonlinear modeling of the shape and appearance.

How to learn the oracle $\mathcal{F}_2$? Given an annotated database, we extract corresponding pairs of (already rigidly aligned) shape and appearance as in Fig. 5. We also slightly perturb the rigid parameter to accommodate imperfect localization derived from the first stage. We now again confront a multiple regression setting with a multidimensional output, except that this time the output cardinality is even higher.

Inference algorithm. To improve robustness, we slightly perturb the bounding box[1] to generate K random samples $\{\mathtt{I}^{<1>}, \mathtt{I}^{<2>}, \ldots, \mathtt{I}^{<K>}\}$ and apply the regressor to obtain shape estimates $\{\mathtt{S}^{<1>}, \mathtt{S}^{<2>}, \ldots, \mathtt{S}^{<K>}\}$, where $\mathtt{S}^{<k>} = \mathcal{F}_2(\mathtt{I}^{<k>})$. We also build a nonparametric density $p_s(\mathtt{S})$ based on the prior shape examples and use it as a confidence scorer. Finally, we output the weighted mean as the final estimate $\hat{\mathtt{S}}$ for the shape parameter (we empirically choose $K = 10$):

$$\hat{\mathtt{S}} = \{ \sum_{k=1:K} p_s^{<k>} \mathtt{S}^{<k>} \} / \{ \sum_{k=1:K} p_s^{<k>} \}. \quad (8)$$

3 Image-Based Boosting Regression

The underpinning of the above two stages of SRM is a regression procedure that takes an image as input and outputs a multidimensional variable. In this section, we invoke the influential boosting framework [7,8] to derive a novel regression algorithm called image-based boosting regression (IBR).

We denote a scalar by a, a column vector by $\mathbf{a}$, and a matrix by $\mathtt{A}$. We also denote the input by $\mathtt{x} \in \mathcal{R}^d$, the output by $\mathtt{y}(\mathtt{x}) \in \mathcal{R}^q$, the regression function by $\mathtt{g}(\mathtt{x}) : \mathcal{R}^d \rightarrow \mathcal{R}^q$ and the training data points by $\{(\mathtt{x}_n, \mathtt{y}_n); n = 1, 2, ..., N\}$.

[1] The perturbation is limited to translation and scaling as they share one integral image. There is no perturbation in rotation.

Further, we denote $\mathtt{x}^{\top}\mathtt{x} = \|\mathtt{x}\|^2$ and $tr(\mathtt{X}^{\top}\mathtt{X}) = \|\mathtt{X}\|^2$. In SRM, $\mathtt{x}$ is the image $\mathtt{I}$, $\mathtt{y}$ is the difference vector $d\theta$ in the first stage and the nonrigid shape parameter $\mathtt{S}$ in the second stage, and the regression function $\mathtt{g}(\mathtt{x}) = \mathcal{F}(\mathtt{I})$ is the oracle.

IBR minimizes the following cost function, which combines a regression output fidelity term and a regularization term:

$$J(\mathtt{g}) = \sum_{n=1:N} \{\|\mathtt{y}(\mathtt{x}_n) - \mathtt{g}(\mathtt{x}_n)\|^2\} + \lambda R(\mathtt{g}), \tag{9}$$

where λ is a *regularization coefficient* and $R(g)$ is the regularization term that will be subsequently defined. As in any boosting procedure [7,8], IBR assumes that the regression output function $\mathtt{g}(\mathtt{x})$ takes an additive form:

$$\mathtt{g}_t(\mathtt{x}) = \mathtt{g}_{t-1}(\mathtt{x}) + \mathtt{h}_t(\mathtt{x}) = \sum_{i=1:t} \mathtt{h}_i(\mathtt{x}), \tag{10}$$

where each $\mathtt{h}_i(\mathtt{x}) : \mathcal{R}^d \rightarrow \mathcal{R}^q$ is a weak learner (or weak function) residing in a *dictionary* set $\mathcal{H}$, and $\mathtt{g}(\mathtt{x})$ is a strong learner (or strong function).

Boosting [7,8] is an iterative algorithm that leverages the additive nature of $\mathtt{g}(\mathtt{x})$: At iteration t, one more weak function $\mathtt{h}_t(\mathtt{x})$ is added to the target function $\mathtt{g}(\mathtt{x})$ to maximally reduce the cost function. Because we associate each weak function with visual features (as shown next), boosting operates as a *feature selector* that singles out relevant features to the regression task.

Weak function. We use a bank of over-complete features to represent the image $\mathtt{x}$. In particular, we use the Haar-like local rectangle features [4], whose rapid evaluation is enabled by the use of integral image. As shown in [4], (i) it is easy to construct numerous local rectangle features and (ii) the local rectangle feature, whose response is normalized by the standard deviation of the image patch, is relatively robust to appearance variation. Each local rectangle feature $f(\mathtt{x}; \mu)$ has its own attribute μ, namely feature type and window position/size.

Based on the local rectangle features, we construct one-dimensional (1D) regression stumps as primitives of the dictionary set $\mathcal{H}$. A regression stump $h(\mathtt{x}; \mu)$, illustrated in Fig. 6(a), is defined as

$$h(\mathtt{x}; \mu) = \sum_{k=1:K} w_k \, [f(\mathtt{x}; \mu) \in R_k] = \mathtt{e}(\mathtt{x}; \mu)^{\top}\mathtt{w}, \tag{11}$$

where $[.]$ is an indicator function and $\{R_k;\ k = 1, 2 \ldots, K\}$ are K evenly spaced intervals (except that R_1 and R_K go to ∞). The interval boundary points are empirically determined. We first find the minimum and maximum responses for the feature and then uniformly divide them. In (11), all the weights w_k are compactly encoded by a vector $\mathtt{w}_{K\times 1} = [w_1, w_2, \ldots, w_K]^{\top}$ and the vector $\mathtt{e}(\mathtt{x}; \mu)$ is some column of the identity matrix: only one element is 1 and others are 0.

A weak function is constructed as a q-dimensional (q-D) regression stump $\mathtt{h}(\mathtt{x})_{q\times 1}$ that stacks q different 1D regression stumps, i.e.,

$$\mathtt{h}(\mathtt{x}; \mu_1, \ldots, \mu_q) = [h_1(\mathtt{x}; \mu_1), ..., h_q(\mathtt{x}; \mu_q)]^{\top} = [\mathtt{e}_1(\mathtt{x}; \mu_1)^{\top}\mathtt{w}_1, ..., \mathtt{e}_q(\mathtt{x}; \mu_q)^{\top}\mathtt{w}_q]^{\top}, \tag{12}$$

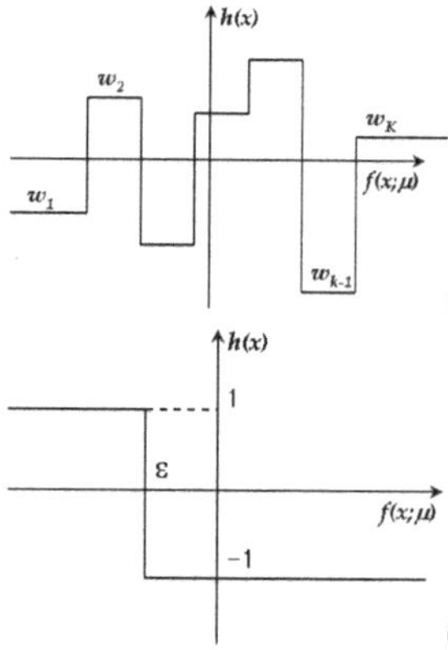

(a)

(b)

1. Initialization $t = 0$.
   (a) Set λ (the regularization coefficient) and η (the shrinkage factor).
   (b) Set the values related to the stopping criteria: T_{max} (the maximum number of iterations) and J_{min} (the minimum cost function).
   (c) Set initial values for $t = 0$: $\mathtt{g}_0(\mathtt{x}) = 0$ and $\mathtt{r}_0(x) = \mathtt{y}(\mathtt{x})$.
2. Iteration $t = 1, \ldots, T_{max}$
   (a) Find the optimal $\hat{\mathtt{h}}_t$ that solves (13).
   (b) Form the new function $\mathtt{g}_t(\mathtt{x}) = \mathtt{g}_{t-1}(\mathtt{x}) + \eta\hat{\mathtt{h}}_t(\mathtt{x})$.
   (c) Evaluate the approximation error $\mathtt{r}_t(\mathtt{x}) = \mathtt{y}(\mathtt{x}) - \mathtt{g}_t(\mathtt{x})$ and the cost function $J(\mathtt{g}_t)$.
   (d) Check convergence, e.g., see if $J(\mathtt{g}_t) < J_{min}$.

(c)

Fig. 6. (a) Regression stump. (b) Binary decision stump. The regression stump carries more representational power than the decision stump. (c) The proposed image-based boosting regression (IBR) algorithm.

where $\mathtt{w}_j$ is the weight vector for the jth regression stump $h_j(\mathtt{x}; \mu_j)$. We further encode the weights belonging to all regression stumps into a *weight matrix* $\mathtt{W}_{K\times q} = [\mathtt{w}_1, \mathtt{w}_2, \ldots, \mathtt{w}_q]$. A binary decision stump is used in [4]. Fig. 6(a,b) compares the regression and binary decision stumps.

Boosting ridge regression. The model complexity of the regression output function $\mathtt{g}_t(\mathtt{x}) = \sum_{i=1:t} \mathtt{h}_i(\mathtt{x})$ now depends on its weight matrices $\{\mathtt{W}_i, i = 1, \ldots, t\}$. We incorporate the ridge regression principle [9] (also known as Tikhonov regularization) into a boosting framework to penalize overly complex models. Because boosting regression proceeds iteratively, at the tth boosting iteration, we set up the following ridge regression task that only involves the weight matrix $\mathtt{W}_t$:

$$\arg\min_{\mathtt{W}_t}\{J_t(\mathtt{g}) = \sum_{n=1:N} \{\|\mathtt{r}_t(\mathtt{x}_n) - \mathtt{h}_t(\mathtt{x}_n)\|^2\} + \lambda\|\mathtt{W}_t\|^2\}, \tag{13}$$

where $\mathtt{r}_t(\mathtt{x}_n) = \mathtt{y}(\mathtt{x}_n) - \mathtt{g}_{t-1}(\mathtt{x}_n)$ is the residual.

As the weight vectors $\{\mathtt{w}_1, \mathtt{w}_2, \ldots, \mathtt{w}_q\}$ in the matrix $\mathtt{W}_t$ are associated with q different local rectangle features, the optimization in (13) implies two subtasks:

1. Given a set of q features with attributes $\mu_1, \ldots, \mu_q$, respectively, find the optimal matrix $\hat{\mathtt{W}}_t(\mu_1, \ldots, \mu_q)$ and its minimum cost $\hat{J}_t(\mu_1, \ldots, \mu_q)$;
2. Find the optimal set of q features with respective attributes $\hat{\mu}_1, \ldots, \hat{\mu}_q$ that minimizes the cost $\hat{J}_t(\mu_1, \ldots, \mu_q)$. This corresponds to feature selection.

However, to transform the above optimization into an efficient implementation, there is a computational bottleneck: The second subtask necessitates a greedy feature selection scheme, which is too expensive to evaluate given a large local rectangle feature pool. In practice, approximate non-greedy solutions [10] can be derived to speedup the feature selection process; however, this is beyond the scope of the paper. Finally, IBR invokes shrinkage [9] to derive a smooth output: $\mathbf{g}_t(\mathbf{x}) = \mathbf{g}_{t-1}(\mathbf{x}) + \eta \mathbf{h}_t(\mathbf{x})$. Fig. 6(c) summarizes the IBR algorithm.

4 Experimental Results and Discussions

We applied the SRM approach to segmenting the LV endocardium from 2D echocardiograms. We had in total 527 A4C sequences. Though we had video sequences, we focused on detecting the LV at the end of diastole (ED) frame, when the LV dilates to its maximum. We randomly selected 450 ED frames for training and used the remaining 77 for testing.

4.1 Rigid Object Detection

In this experiment, we tested the first stage of SRM to detect the LV using the 5-D parameterization. Figure 1 shows six ED images with the unaligned LV present. The range of the five parameters is empirically found as: $t_x \sim [43, 118]$, $t_y \sim [24, 70]$, $s_x \sim [26, 86]$, $s_y \sim [37, 92]$ and $\alpha \sim [-25, 35]$. We scanned the image following the above range. The average image size is 111×151.

There are several tuning parameters in the IBR algorithm. For the number of threshold levels K of a weak function, the regularization coefficient λ and the shrinkage coefficient η, we empirically tested different combinations and decided to use the following: $K = 64$, $\lambda = 0.1/K$, and $\eta = 0.1$. We trained the regressor based on 450 randomly selected ED frames, each yielding 30 image patches; in total we had 13,500 training data. It takes more than two days to train the regressor (on a high-end workstation with four Xeon 3GHz CPUs and 3GB RAM), which consists of 10,000 local rectangle features or 200 weak functions. Training the detector $\mathcal{D}$ is not straightforward because here the image rotation is involved. To avoid computing integral images for all rotations, we followed [11] to train the detector, which is able to simultaneously classify the object as well as infer its rotation yet using only one integral image.

We implemented three scanning methods: "IBR", "IBR+Det", and "Det". The "IBR" means that we randomly scanned the image within the prior range using the learned IBR function and used the unweighted average as the final estimate of the target position. The "IBR+Det" means that we further equipped the "IBR" method with the trained detector and used (6) as the final estimate. We also set $J_{valid} = 10$ to enable early exit when scanning. The "Det" means that we exhaustively scanned the image within the same range using the detector and used the parameter that maximizes the detector response as the final estimate. For the "Det" method, we exhaustively scanned the image every 4 pixels in both translations and every 4 pixels in both scales.

Table 1(a) compares the three scanning methods[2]. The error in scale is measured as $s_{detected}/s_{groundtruth} - 1$. Because we did not observe significant performance difference between training and testing, we pooled them together and

[2] To count the number of effective scans in Table 1, we excluded those scans if their associated image patches have less than 40% of their pixels inside the known fan.

Table 1. (a) Detection performance comparison of the three methods for the 5-parameter case. (b) Segmentation performance comparison of four regression methods.

(a)

Method	IBR	IBR+Det	Det
# of features	10000	10000+1201	1201
median err. in t_x (pixels)	0.32 ± 3.13	0.65 ± 2.07	1.69 ± 3.40
median err. in t_y (pixels)	0.67 ± 2.40	1.25 ± 1.95	0.84 ± 3.73
median err. in s_x	0.02 ± 0.12	0.04 ± 0.12	0.05 ± 0.17
median err. in s_y	0.01 ± 0.08	0.02 ± 0.08	0.04 ± 0.15
median err. in α (degree)	-1.76 ± 7.17	-0.98 ± 6.39	0.22 ± 6.74
# of eff. scans	200	38	29383
avg. speed (ms)	704	118	6300

(b)

Method	SRM	KRR	NPR	AAM
25% seg. err. (pixels)	1.778	1.695	2.013	2.323
median seg. err. (pixels)	2.207	2.372	2.482	2.734
75% seg. err. (pixels)	2.753	3.347	3.101	4.002
avg. speed (ms)	≤ 1	692	865	30

jointly reported the results. The speed was recorded on a laptop with a Pentium 2.1GHz CPU and 2GB RAM. The "IBR+Det" achieves appealing detection performance while running the fastest. It runs about 7 times faster than the "IBR" method and more than 50 times faster than the "Det" method, while yielding comparable performance to the "IBR" in terms of bias and improving the localization precision. The slowest "Det" method does not always yield the best performance in terms of either bias or variance because it does not exhaust all possible configurations. Fig. 7(a) shows example images with estimated and ground truth boxes overlaid.

4.2 Nonrigid Shape Inference

In this experiment, we invoked the complete SRM approach to automatically delineate the LV endocardium. The above "IBR+Det" algorithm was first used to locate the LV and then the second stage of SRM was applied. The shape $\mathtt{S}$ is parameterized by 17 landmark points and PCA was used to reduced the shape dimensionality from 34 to 20. Through random perturbations, we generated 6,750 training data points (one data point is a pair of image and shape) based on 450 ED frames and trained an IBR model consisting of 20,000 local rectangle features or 1,000 weak functions.

For comparison, we implemented three other regression methods: "KRR", "NPR", and "AAM" where kernel rigid regression (KRR) and nonparametric kernel regression (NPR) are two off-the-shelf nonlinear regression methods [9], and AAM is from [3]. In AAM, the appearance and shape are assumed to be jointly Gaussian, which amounts to multiple linear regression [9]. The number of principal components was chosen to keep 95% of the energy in AAM. When comparing different nonrigid shape regressors, we fixed the detection part.

To quantify the shape segmentation performance, we measured the average pixel error for the landmark points: $\sqrt{||\mathtt{C}_1 - \mathtt{C}_2||^2/34}$. We did this measurement on the aligned domain of size 104 by 80 to overcome the difference in physical

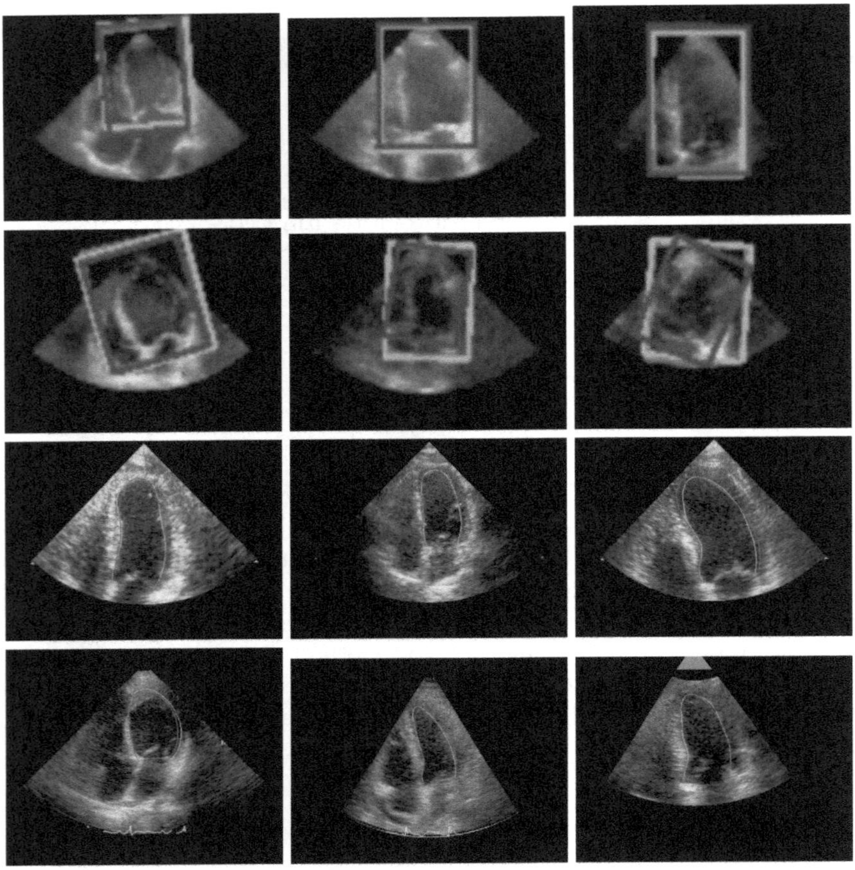
(a)

(b)

Fig. 7. (a) The estimated LV box versus the ground truth. The red box is from the "IBR" method, the green is from the "IBR+Det" method, and the blue is the ground truth. (b) The inferred LV endocardium versus the ground truth. The red contour is from the SRM approach and the green is the ground truth.

units of difference images. Table 1(b) shows the error statistics and computational time (only for the regression part though). We collected the error statistics for all testing images and reported their 25% percentile, median, and 75% percentile. From Table 1(b), we observe that the proposed SRM approach achieves favorable contour localization performance over other methods while running significantly faster. The AAM method that uses linear models performs the worst, implying the need for nonlinear modeling of the appearance and shape. The KRR and NPR methods are slow because they require comparing the query image with the whole database, while the IBR absorbs the database knowledge into the weak functions whose rapid evaluation is guaranteed by using the integral image. In sum, *it takes less than 120ms on the average to automatically localize the LV endocardium in an A4C echocardiogram with a better accuracy.* Fig. 7(b) visualizes the ground truth and predicted contours.

5 Conclusion

We have presented a machine learning approach called shape regression machine for fast medical anatomy detection and segmentation. SRM effectively utilizes the structural context in medical images with annotations to eliminate unfavorable restrictions posed by conventional deformable shape segmentation methods. In particular, the detection solution in SRM replaces the exhaustive scanning of the query image required by the classifier-based detector by a sparse scanning and reaches improved detection accuracy with significantly less computation and no need for image rotation. In terms of shape inference, the IBR solution in SRM outperforms other regression methods such as kernel ridge regression, nonparametric kernel regression, and active appearance model. In the future, we will apply the SRM approach to other medical applications such as organ segmentation from a full body 3D CT scan. We will also address the scalability and trainability issues related to learning the regression function.

References

1. Kass, M., Witkin, A., Terzopoulos, D.: Snakes: Active contour models. Int. J. Computer Vision 1, 321–331 (1988)
2. Mumford, D., Shah, J.: Optimal approximations by piecewise smooth functions and associated variational problems. Comm. Pure Appl. Math. 42, 577–685 (1989)
3. Cootes, T.F., Edwards, G.J., Taylor, C.J.: Active appearance models. IEEE Trans. Pattern Anal. Machine Intell. 23, 681–685 (2001)
4. Viola, P., Jones, M.: Rapid object detection using a boosted cascade of simple features. In: Proc. CVPR (2001)
5. Cootes, T., Beeston, C., Edwards, G., Taylor, C.: A unified framework for atlas matching using active appearance models. In: IPMI (1999)
6. Mazziotta, J., Toga, A., Evans, A., Lancaster, J., Fox, P.: A probabilistic atlas of the human brain: Theory and rational for its development. Neuroimage 2, 89–101 (1995)
7. Freund, Y., Schapire, R.: A decision-theoretic generalization of online learning and an application to boosting. J. Computer and System Sciences 55, 119–139
8. Friedman, J., Hastie, T., Tibshirani, R.: Additive logistic regression: a statistical view of boosting. Ann. Statist. 28, 337–407 (2000)
9. Hastie, T., Tibshirani, R., Friedman, J.: The Elements of Statistical Learning. Springer, Heidelberg (2001)
10. Zhou, S., Georgescu, B., Zhou, X., Comaniciu, D.: Image-based regression using boosting method. In: Proc. ICCV (2005)
11. Zhang, J., Zhou, S., Comaniciu, D.: Joint real-time object detection and pose estimation using probabilistic boosting network. In: Proc. CVPR (2007)

Active Mean Fields: Solving the Mean Field Approximation in the Level Set Framework

Kilian M. Pohl[1,2], Ron Kikinis[1], and William M. Wells[1,2]

[1] Surgical Planning Laboratory, Harvard Medical School and Brigham and Women's Hospital, Boston, MA, USA
{pohl,kikinis,sw}@bwh.harvard.edu
http://www.spl.harvard.edu

[2] Computer Science and Artificial Intelligence Lab, Massachusetts Institute of Technology, Cambridge, MA, USA

Abstract. We describe a new approach for estimating the posterior probability of tissue labels. Conventional likelihood models are combined with a curve length prior on boundaries, and an approximate posterior distribution on labels is sought via the Mean Field approach. Optimizing the resulting estimator by gradient descent leads to a level set style algorithm where the level set functions are the logarithm-of-odds encoding of the posterior label probabilities in an unconstrained linear vector space. Applications with more than two labels are easily accommodated. The label assignment is accomplished by the Maximum *A Posteriori* rule, so there are no problems of "overlap" or "vacuum". We test the method on synthetic images with additive noise. In addition, we segment a magnetic resonance scan into the major brain compartments and subcortical structures.

1 Introduction

Many clinical researchers rely on automatic segmentation techniques to analyze medical images [1]. Popular approaches for this task are curve evolution methods, which evolve the boundary of an object coupling image data with smoothness constraints of a zero-level set [2,3,4,5,6,7,8,9]. Some of these methods evolve multiple zero-level sets but they usually do not provide a simple interpretation for overlapping curves. We address this issue by using an alternative representation called LogOdds that views the entire level set function as a representation of posterior probabilities of label maps.

We derive the corresponding curve evolution framework, called Active Mean Fields (AMF), by revisiting the Mean Field approximation; a method frequently used in medical imaging for estimating the posterior probabilities of label maps [10,11]. When estimating the solution to the Markov Random field model [12], simplifications result from approximating some random field variables by their mean value. Similar to other approximations of Markov Random field models [13,14,15] the methods by [10,11] lack the notion of objects' boundaries – this often leads to fragmented label maps. We address this issue by incorporating a curve length prior into the Mean Field model. This results in the AMF algorithm, which approximates the solution via a level set framework in the LogOdds space.

N. Karssemeijer and B. Lelieveldt (Eds.): IPMI 2007, LNCS 4584, pp. 26–37, 2007.
© Springer-Verlag Berlin Heidelberg 2007

The contributions of this paper are three-fold. First, we derive a new level set representation based on multinomial Logarithm-of-Odds (LogOdds). For the probability p of a binary variable, the LogOdds (also called logit) is the logarithm of the ratio between the probability p and its complement $1-p$. As a generalization of [16], here LogOdds defines a vector space structure that relates the evolution of multiple curves in the level set formulation to space conditioned probabilities. An advantage of this new representation is that it replaces the potentially ambiguous interpretation of overlapping zero-level sets with a simpler Maximum *A Posteriori* (MAP) Probability criteria.

Second, we compute the Mean Field solution of the posterior probabilities of label maps via a level set formulation. We do so by projecting the probabilities into the vector space of LogOdds maps and determining the solution via gradient descent. This, combined with our choice of prior model, results in a curve evolution algorithm coupling the curve shortening prior from the level set model with the posterior probabilities traditionally associated with the Mean Field approximation. The resulting curve evolution, called AMF, not only updates the zero-level set but also evolves the entire family of curves, as it is common in the level set community, which now correspond to levels of the posterior probabilities of labels.

Third, to the best of our knowledge, this is the first time for a level set framework to simultaneously segment 3D MR images into the three major brain compartments and subcortical structures. As we show in our example, if AMF is initialized by a noisy automatic segmentation [17] it can improve the 3D segmentations by removing outliers and islands that violate the smoothness constrains of the prior model.

This paper is organized as follows. In Section 2, we provide the mathematical definition of LogOdds, as well as their relationship with discrete probabilities. In Section 3, we derive the AMF which approximates the Mean Field solution via a level set framework. In Section 4, we apply AMF to synthetic and medical images.

2 Multinomial LogOdds

In this section, we generalize the binomial LogOdds representation discussed in [16] to discrete distributions, which we call multinomial LogOdds. We show that the LogOdds space has a one-to-one mapping to the space of discrete probabilities and defines a vector space. These two properties are very important for the derivations in Section 3 where we determine an approximation for the Mean Field solution via gradient descent.

LogOdds are an example of a class of functions that map the space of discrete distributions [18] to the Euclidean space. Let $\mathbb{P}_M$ be the open probability simplex for M labels $\mathbb{P}_M = \left\{p \,|p = (p_1,\ldots,p_{M-1}, 1-\sum_{i=1,\ldots,M-1} p_i) \in (0,1)^M\right\}$. Note that $\mathbb{P}_M$ is an M-1 dimensional space as the Mth entry is defined by the first M-1 entries. Furthermore, the space is open avoiding distributions that are certain about the assignment. For the specific case of M = 2, $\mathbb{P}_2 = \{(p, 1-p)|p \in (0,1)\}$ is the Bernoulli distribution [19]. Many binary classification problems use the Bernoulli distribution where p represents the probability that a voxel belongs to a particular anatomical structure and its complement $\bar{p} = 1-p$ represents the probability of the voxel being in the background.

The multinomial LogOdds function $\text{logit}(\cdot) : \mathbb{P}_M \longrightarrow \mathbb{R}^{M-1}$ of a discrete distribution $p \in \mathbb{P}_M$ is defined as the logarithm of the ratio between the ith and last entry of p:

$$[\text{logit}(p)]_i \triangleq \log\left(\frac{p_i}{p_M}\right),$$

with $i \in \{1,\ldots,M-1\}$. The inverse of the log odds function $\text{logit}(\cdot)$ is the generalized logistic function

$$[\sigma(t)]_i \triangleq \begin{cases} \frac{e^{t_i}}{Z} & \text{, for } i \in \{1,\ldots,M-1\} \\ \frac{1}{Z} & \text{, if } i = M \end{cases}, \tag{1}$$

where $Z \triangleq 1 + \sum_{j=1,\ldots,M-1} e^{t_j}$ is the normalization factor. Having defined $\text{logit}(\cdot)$ and $\sigma(\cdot)$, we now induced from $\mathbb{P}_M$ the M-1 dimensional space of LogOdds $\mathbb{L}_{M-1} \triangleq \{\text{logit}(p)|p \in \mathbb{P}_M\}$. Note that $\mathbb{L}_{M-1}$ is equivalent to (M-1) dimensional real vector space. In Appendix A, we make use of this vector space structure to induce a vector space on $\mathbb{P}_M$.

3 Approximating the Mean Field Solution Via Curve Evolution

We now combine the Mean Field approximation with the level set framework by using the LogOdds parametrization. We do so by embedding the Mean Field parameters into the LogOdds space. We then determine the optimal parameters via gradient descent which we is realized in the level set formulation. This results in the AMF algorithm which computes space conditioned probabilities while incorporating regional as well as boundary properties of objects.

3.1 Using Gradient Descent

We now derive a model for segmenting medical images via the Mean Field approximation. The segmentation problem can be described as assigning each voxel of the image I to an anatomical compartment, which results in the label map $\mathcal{T}$. Without priors, the relationship between the label map $\mathcal{T}$ and the image I is generally unclear as the image might not visualize some anatomical boundaries or is corrupted by noise and other image artifacts. Some of these difficulties can be addressed by the use of prior models. This results in estimating posterior probabilities which can, in some cases, be accomplished via the Mean Field approximation [11,15].

The Mean Field approach makes the problem of estimating the posterior probabilities $P(\mathcal{T}|I)$ feasible by approximating $P(\mathcal{T}|I)$ as a factorized distribution $Q(\mathcal{T};\theta) = \prod_x Q_x(\mathcal{T}_x;\theta)$, where θ are the parameters defining $Q(\mathcal{T};\theta)$. The approach now computes the parameter setting $\widehat{\theta}$ that minimize Kullback-Leibler (KL) divergence between the true posterior probability $P(\mathcal{T}|I)$ and the approximation $Q(\mathcal{T};\theta)$

$$D(Q(\mathcal{T};\theta)||P(\mathcal{T}|I)) = E_Q\left(\log\frac{Q(\mathcal{T};\theta)}{P(\mathcal{T}|I)}\right) = \sum_{\mathcal{T}\in\mathbb{T}} Q(\mathcal{T};\theta)\log\frac{Q(\mathcal{T};\theta)}{P(\mathcal{T}|I)},$$

where $\mathbb{T}$ is the space of all label maps $\mathcal{T}$ and $E_Q(\cdot)$ is the expected value. In a nutshell, the Mean Field approximation determines the solution to

$$\widehat{\theta} \triangleq \min_\theta D(Q(\mathcal{T};\theta)||P(\mathcal{T}|I)). \tag{2}$$

Frequently, the multinomial distribution $Q(\mathcal{T};\theta)$ is parametrized by the component probabilities, in which case Equation (2) is a constrained minimization problem. We obtain an unconstrained problem by using the LogOdds parametrization. $\theta \triangleq (\theta_1,\ldots,\theta_n) \in \mathbb{L}_M^n$ parametrizes the multinomial distribution Q_x as $Q_x(\mathcal{T}_x = j;\theta_x) = [\sigma(\theta_x)]_j$. Equation (2) is now an unconstrained problem whose solution can be approximated via the following gradient descent:

$$\theta^{(k+1)} = \theta^{(k)} - \lambda \cdot \frac{\partial}{\partial\theta} D(Q(\mathcal{T};\theta)||P(\mathcal{T}|I))_{|\theta=\theta^{(k)}},$$

where λ is the step size parameter.

In the remainder of this section we derive the update term, which can be rewritten using the expected value $E_Q[\log(P(\mathcal{T}))]$ of the log prior of the label map $\log(P(\mathcal{T}))$, and the KL divergence $D(Q(\mathcal{T};\theta)||P(I|\mathcal{T}))$ of the estimated probability distribution $Q(\mathcal{T};\theta)$ and label likelihood $P(I|\mathcal{T})$. For notational convenience, we will continue to use the KL divergence even when its second argument is a not a probability distribution over $\mathcal{T}$. (We also note that the likelihood could be re-normalized without affecting the solution).

$$\begin{aligned}\frac{\partial}{\partial\theta} D(Q(\mathcal{T};\theta)||P(\mathcal{T}|I)) &= \frac{\partial}{\partial\theta} E_Q[\log(Q(\mathcal{T};\theta)) - \log(P(\mathcal{T}|I))] \\ &= \frac{\partial}{\partial\theta} E_Q[\log(Q(\mathcal{T};\theta)) - \log(P(I|\mathcal{T}))] - \frac{\partial}{\partial\theta} E_Q[\log(P(\mathcal{T}))] \quad (3) \\ &= \frac{\partial}{\partial\theta} D(Q(\mathcal{T};\theta)||P(I|\mathcal{T})) - \frac{\partial}{\partial\theta} E_Q[\log(P(\mathcal{T}))].\end{aligned}$$

The first term drives the estimate $Q(\mathcal{T};\theta)$ towards the normalized label likelihood $P(I|\mathcal{T})$. The prior $P(\mathcal{T})$ is defined in Section 3.3 in such a way that the second term $\frac{\partial}{\partial\theta} E_Q[\log(P(\mathcal{T}))]$ encourages smoothness along the boundary of the object.

3.2 The Derivative of the KL Divergence of $Q(\mathcal{T};\theta)$ and $P(I|\mathcal{T})$

To simplify the computation of the derivative of the KL divergence $D(Q(\mathcal{T};\theta)||P(I|\mathcal{T}))$ we assume that the likelihood of the label map $P(I|\mathcal{T}) = \prod_{x\in\mathbb{I}} P(I_x|\mathcal{T}_x)$ is factorized over the image domain $\mathbb{I}$, which is typically a valid assumption. In this case, $D(Q(\mathcal{T};\theta)||P(I|\mathcal{T}))$ is the sum of KL divergences over $\mathbb{I}$:

$$D(Q(\mathcal{T};\theta)||P(I|\mathcal{T})) = \sum_{x\in\mathbb{I}} D(Q_x(\mathcal{T}_x;\theta_x)||P(I_x|\mathcal{T}_x))$$

For temporary convenience, we omit the voxel index x. If we now denote the probability of label i according to the parameter $\theta \triangleq (\theta_1,\ldots,\theta_M)$ with $q_i \triangleq Q(\mathcal{T}=i;\theta) = [\sigma(\theta)]_i$ and the normalized likelihood of label i as $p_i \triangleq P(I|\mathcal{T}=i)$ then the derivative of the KL divergence with respect to θ_i is

$$\frac{d}{d\theta_i} D(Q(\mathcal{T};\theta)||P(I|\mathcal{T})) = \frac{d}{d\theta_i} q_i \log\frac{q_i}{p_i} + \frac{d}{d\theta_i} q_m \log\frac{q_m}{p_m} + \sum_{j\neq\{i,m\}} \frac{d}{d\theta_i} q_j \log\frac{q_j}{p_j}. \quad (4)$$

The derivative of q_j is $\frac{d}{d\theta_i} q_j = \frac{d}{d\theta_i} \frac{e^{\theta_j}}{1+e^{\theta_i}+\sum_{j\neq i} e^{\theta_j}} = \begin{cases} -q_j q_i & ,j \neq i \\ q_i(1-q_i) & ,i=j \end{cases}$

and $\frac{d}{d\theta_i} q_j \log \frac{q_j}{p_j} = \begin{cases} -q_j q_i(1+log\frac{q_j}{p_j}) & ,j \neq i \\ q_i(1-q_i)(1+log\frac{q_i}{p_i}), & i=j \end{cases}$ so that Equation (4) can be rewritten as

$$\begin{aligned} & q_i(1-q_i)(1+\log\frac{q_i}{p_i}) - q_i(1-q_i-\sum_{j\neq\{i,m\}} q_j)(1+\log\frac{q_m}{p_m}) - q_i \sum_{j\neq\{i,m\}} q_j(1+\log\frac{q_j}{p_j}) \\ =& q_i \cdot (1-q_i) \cdot (\log\frac{q_i}{p_i} - \log\frac{q_m}{p_m}) - q_i \sum_{j\neq\{i,m\}} q_j \cdot (\log\frac{q_j}{p_j} - \log\frac{q_m}{p_m}) \\ =& [\sigma(\theta)]_i (1-[\sigma(\theta)]_i)(\theta_i - [\text{logit}(p)]_i) \quad - \sum_{j\neq\{i,m\}} [\sigma(\theta)]_i [\sigma(\theta)]_j (\theta_j - [\text{logit}(p)]_j) \end{aligned} \tag{5}$$

When used within gradient descent, the derivative of KL divergence combines a driving force towards the LogOdds of the label likelihood $[\text{logit}(p_x)]_i$ with a second term, which we call the *coupling* term. In areas with high uncertainty ($q_{x_i} \approx 0.5$) the equation weighs heavily to move towards the LogOdds function $[\text{logit}(p_x)]_i$. However, if θ_{x_i} has high certainty about the label ($q_{x_i} \approx 0$ or $q_{x_i} \approx 1$) then the likelihood term is less important.

Unlike with binary representations of curves, our method allows zero-contours to overlap as the curves now represent level set of the posterior probabilities $Q(\mathcal{T};\theta)$, where $Q(\mathcal{T};\theta)$ is a multinomial distribution in $\mathbb{P}^n_m$. In $\mathbb{P}^n_m$, the probability maps indicate a label map via the MAP criteria.

3.3 Determining the Smoothing Term

We now compute $\frac{\partial}{\partial\theta} E_Q[\log(P(\mathcal{T}))]$, the second term of Equation (3). First, we define the probabilistic model for the label map prior $P(\mathcal{T})$ as a distribution preferring smooth boundaries in $\mathcal{T}$. We do so by making the prior $P(\mathcal{T})$ a function of the arc length of the binary maps that is defined by $\mathcal{T}$ [20]. For this purpose, we define $\mathcal{T}$ as a vector of indicator random variables $\mathcal{T}_x \in \{e_1,\ldots,e_m\}$ with the indicator $[e_j]_j = 1$ and zero otherwise. We can then extract from $\mathcal{T}$ a binary map $[\mathcal{T}]_i \triangleq (\mathcal{T}_{1_i},\ldots,\mathcal{T}_{n_i})$ for each label i. The arc length $L([\mathcal{T}]_i)$ of the binary map $[\mathcal{T}]_i$ is defined as the length of the boundaries in $[\mathcal{T}]_i$. Based on the arc length for each label we can then specify the prior as $P(\mathcal{T}) \triangleq \frac{1}{Z} e^{-\sum_i L([\mathcal{T}]_i)} = \frac{1}{Z}\prod_i e^{-L([\mathcal{T}]_i)} \sim \prod_i P([\mathcal{T}]_i)$ and rewrite the derivative of the expected value as

$$\begin{aligned} \frac{\partial}{\partial\theta} E_{Q(\mathcal{T};\theta)}[\log(P(\mathcal{T}))] &= -\sum_{i=1,\ldots,m} \frac{\partial}{\partial\theta} E_{Q(\mathcal{T};\theta)}[L([\mathcal{T}]_i)] \\ &= -\sum_{i=1,\ldots,m} \frac{\partial}{\partial\theta} E_{Q([\mathcal{T}]_i;\theta)}[L([\mathcal{T}]_i)]. \end{aligned}$$

It is intractable to compute $E_{Q([\mathcal{T}]_i;\theta)}$ as we have to sum over all possible label maps $[\mathcal{T}]_i$ with $i = 1,\ldots,m$. According to Lemma 2 of Appendix B, however, an approximation for the expected value is

$$\begin{aligned} E_{Q([\mathcal{T}]_i;\theta)}[L([\mathcal{T}]_i)] &\approx -\int_{-\infty}^{\infty} \sigma(\alpha)(1-\sigma(\alpha)) L(\mathcal{H}([\theta]_i - \alpha)) d\alpha \\ &= -\int_{-\infty}^{\infty} \sigma(\alpha)(1-\sigma(\alpha)) \iint_{\mathbb{I}} \delta(\theta_{x_i} - \alpha) dx\, d\alpha, \end{aligned}$$

where $\mathcal{H}(y) \triangleq \{1 \text{ for } y > 0, 0 \text{ otherwise}\}$ is the Heaviside Function, $\delta(\cdot)$ the Dirac Delta function, and $[\theta]_i \triangleq (\theta_{1_i}, \ldots, \theta_{n_i})$ are the parameters of label i. The above approximation would be accurate if $L([\mathcal{T}]_i)$ were a sum of functions (or $P(\mathcal{T})$ were independent in space) as outlined in Lemma 2.

We compute the derivative of the above approximation by applying the Euclidean curve shortening flow [21], which states that $\frac{d}{d\theta}\iint_{\mathbb{I}} \delta(\theta-\alpha)dx = \kappa_\alpha(\theta)|\nabla_\alpha(\theta)|\delta(\theta-\alpha)$, where $\nabla_\alpha(\theta)$ is the derivative of the LogOdds map θ with respect to the α-contour in θ and $\kappa_\alpha(\theta) = div(\frac{\nabla_\alpha(\theta)}{|\nabla_\alpha(\theta)|})$ is the corresponding curvature. Thus, we approximate the derivative of the expected value as the weighted integral over the curve shortening flow of all contours in the LogOdds map θ,

$$\frac{\partial}{\partial\theta}E_Q[\log(P(\mathcal{T}))] \approx -\int_{-\infty}^{\infty} \sigma(\alpha)(1-\sigma(\alpha))\kappa_\alpha(\theta)|\nabla_\alpha(\theta)|\delta(\theta-\alpha)d\alpha.$$

The derivative for each voxel location x and label i is defined as

$$\frac{\partial}{\partial\theta_{x_i}}E_Q[\log(P(\mathcal{T}))] \approx -\sigma(\theta_{x_i})\cdot(1-\sigma(\theta_{x_i}))\kappa_{\theta_{x_i}}(\theta_{x_i})|\nabla_{\theta_{x_i}}(\theta_{x_i})|. \tag{6}$$

Combining the results of this section, we compute the solution to the Mean Field approximation as defined in Equation (2) through the following curve evolution

$$\begin{aligned}\theta_{x_i}^{(k+1)} = \theta_{x_i}^{(k)} - \lambda\cdot\Big(&[\sigma(\theta_x^{(k)})]_i\cdot(1-[\sigma(\theta_x^{(k)})]_i)\cdot(\theta_{x_i}^{(k)} - [\text{logit}(p_x)]_i)\\ &-\textstyle\sum_{j\neq\{i,m\}}[\sigma(\theta_x^{(k)})]_i\cdot[\sigma(\theta_x^{(k)})]_j\cdot(\theta_{x_j} - [\text{logit}(p_x)]_j)\\ &+\sigma(\theta_{x_i}^{(k)})\cdot(1-\sigma(\theta_{x_i}^{(k)}))\cdot\kappa_{\theta_{x_i}^{(k)}}(\theta_{x_i}^{(k)})|\nabla_{\theta_{x_i}^{(k)}}(\theta_{x_i}^{(k)})|\Big).\end{aligned} \tag{7}$$

This update function defines the AMF algorithm. In a level set framework, the first term of the update formulation corresponds to the image coupling term. This coupling term is defined by the LogOdds of the corresponding normalized likelihoods, which are normally determined beforehand (e.g. with Gaussian classification techniques as in Section 4.3). The second part of our method defines the curve shortening flow, which controls the smoothness of the boundary. Both terms are weighted by the product $[\sigma(\theta_x^{(k)})]_i\cdot(1-[\sigma(\theta_x^{(k)})]_i)$ or $[\sigma(\theta_x^{(k)})]_i\cdot[\sigma(\theta_x^{(k)})]_j$ so that it may be possible to use the "narrow-band" style frequently discussed in the level set community.

The above derivations are greatly simplified by embedding θ in the vector space of LogOdds. The more usual parametrization requires each entry of θ to be confined to the interval $[0,1]$ and each vector θ_x needs to sum up to one. The corresponding gradient descent would therefore need to map each update to the manifold of discrete probabilities. Another advantage of the LogOdds representation is that our algorithm can simultaneously evolve multiple curves. The curves are level sets of LogOdds maps, which define posterior probabilities in our case. Applying MAP rule, each voxel is clearly assigned to a label. AMF is therefore free of complications with overlap or vacuum, which is a common problem in other multi-label level set formulations.

This completes our derivation of the AMF method. The resulting algorithm combines local constraints at each voxel location with global smoothness constraints of the boundaries.

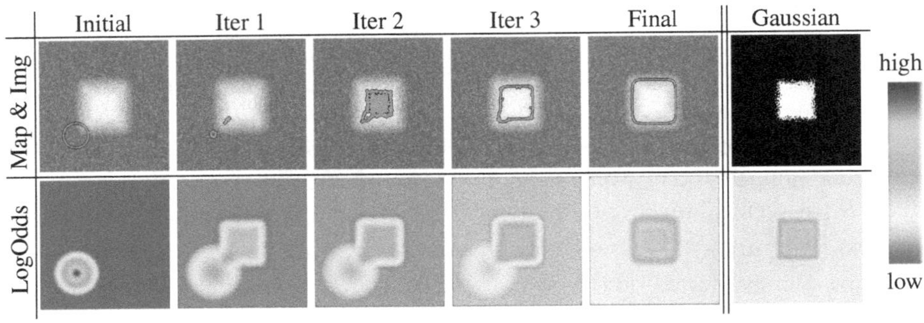

Fig. 1. Our level set evolution (green line) over a noisy image with corresponding LogOdds maps. The fragmented maps (last column) are obtained from a Gaussian likelihood model. In comparison, our results are smooth and connected even though the initial curve did not overlap with the square.

4 Experiments

We now apply the AMF to two examples. We first discuss the curve evolution of our algorithm on a noisy image that was segmented by a Gaussian classifier into a fragmented label map. The corresponding probability maps are the inputs to our algorithm, which robustly identifies the boundary of the structure. The second experiment includes real MRI images, in which AMF automatically segments the major brain compartments as well as subcortical structures. Due to the LogOdds parametrization, our method naturally evolves families of curves.

4.1 Segmenting Noisy Images

We now apply the AMF algorithm of Section 3 to a noisy image of a square (see top row of Figure 1). Before doing so, we compute the likelihood through a Gaussian intensity model, which results in a noisy LogOdds map (bottom, right) and, when thresholded, in a fragmented segmentation (top, right). The robustness of the classifier is greatly impacted by the noise as the approach ignores dependencies between neighboring voxels.

We initialize our curve evolution with the distance map of a small circle (see black circle in top, left image and distance map below) and the input is the noisy LogOdds map of the normalized likelihood (bottom, right). The initial curve is disconnected from the square forcing our method to split the zero-level set into two separate curves by Iteration 1. The circle connected to the square is expanding while the other curve is shrinking. Our curve evolution further evolves both curves until the connected curve converges to the shape of the square and the disconnected curve vanishes.

The evolution produces the LogOdds maps shown in the bottom row of Figure 1. Initially, the dark blue region shrinks, i.e. the number of voxels with high certainty about the presence of the square is decreasing. The shrinking is due to the discrepancy between the initial LogOdds map and the input label likelihoods. As the method progresses, the blue region assimilates towards the predefined LogOdds map. Unlike the segmentation produced through thresholding the initial likelihoods, our level set method

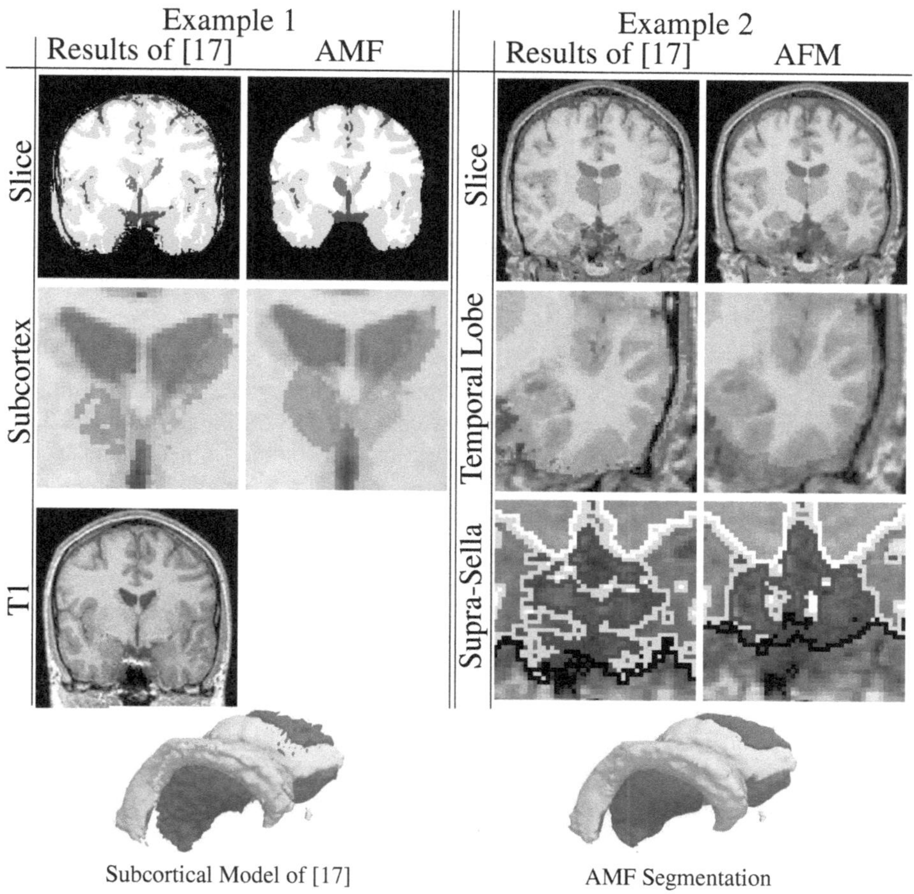

Fig. 2. The subcortical 3D models and two samples slices of the 3D data set segmented by [17] and AMF. The maps of [17] are fragmented and show many falsely identified regions. AMF produces smoother segmentations where most of the outliers are removed.

filters out the noise. The final LogOdds map is smooth and the binary map shows the square as one connected region.

4.2 Segmenting Magnetic Resonance Images

In this experiment, we apply the AMF algorithm to a real 3D Magnetic Resonance (MR) scan (T1-weighted, matrix=256×256×124, dimension=0.9375×0.9375×1.5mm) to automatically segment the scan into the major brain compartments (gray matter = dark gray, white matter = white, cerebrospinal fluid = dark) as well as the ventricles (light gray), the thalamus (darker gray), and the caudate (gray). Figure 2 shows example slices of the segmentations, which were produced in 1.8 hours on a PC (dual processor Xoen, 3.0 GHz, 2 gig ram). We also segmented the scan using the approach of [17]. We

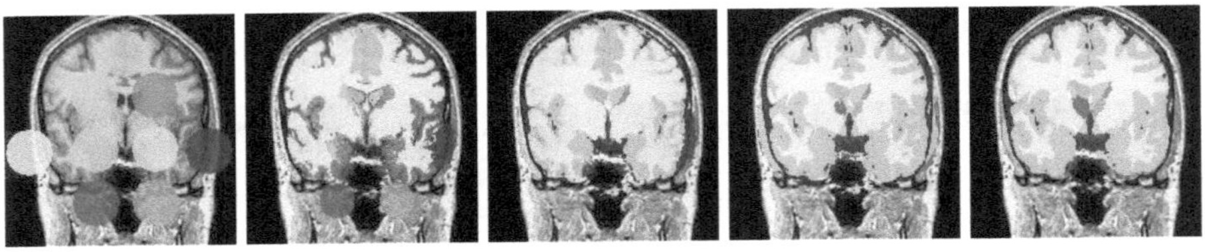

Initial → Final

Fig. 3. Revisiting Example 1 of Figure 2, where the level set framework is initialized by nine circles. The resulting level set evolution is very similar to the segmentation of Figure 2.

determined the accuracy of each subcortical segmentation by computing its Dice score with respect to the manually generated label maps, which we view as ground truth.

The segmentation of [17] received a Dice Score of 0.778 for the left caudate, 0.770 for the right caudate, 0.895 for the left thalamus, and for the right thalamus 0.896. The label map is fragmented and has many misclassified regions. For example, in the temporal region a part of the skull is identified as gray matter. The segmentation AMF improves this segmentation using the corresponding space conditioned probabilities of [17] for the definition of the label likelihoods p_x in Equation (7). This improvement is also reflected in the Dice score, which is higher for each structure (left caudate: 0.789, right caudate: 0.774, left left thalamus: 0.897, right thalamus: 0.906).

The second and forth column of Figure 2 show example slices of the label map generated by our method. Our curve evolution model is not only robust enough to simultaneously segment the 3D Volume into 10 compartments, but also produces a much smoother label map with fewer islands than [17]. Unlike in the results of [17], the 3D model and slice of Example 1 show a subcortical region composed of oval-shaped structures, which closely match the expected anatomy in that region. In addition, the skull is properly separated from the brain (see temporal region in Example 2). Furthermore, the label map in the supra-sella region does not seem to be influenced by the noise in the image.

In the final experiment, we test the robustness of AMF by again segmenting the 3D MR image scan of Figure 2. This time the approach is initialized with a set of LogOdds maps representing nine circles as shown in Figure 3. Figure 3 shows the segmentation corresponding to the MR image of Example 1 of Figure 2. The method converges again to a solution that is very similar to the previously discussed results. Based on the these results, joining the Mean Field approach with the smoothness constraints of the level set formulation seems to be a robust framework for removing outliers and islands.

5 Conclusion

We described a new approach for estimating the posterior probabilities of tissue labels. We combined conventional likelihood models with a curve length prior on boundaries, and obtained posterior distributions by way of the Mean Field method. We used the LogOdds parametrization to facilitate optimization of the estimator by gradient descent, and with our choice of prior model, the influence of the prior is defined by the curve shortening flow. As demonstrated by our experiments, the approach can robustly segment multiple 3D objects in MR scans.

We tested the accuracy of our model by automatically identifying a single square in a noise synthetic image. In the final experiment, our approach segmented a 3D MR scan into the major brain compartments and subcortical structures; to our knowledge, this is the first time for a level set approach achieved this. The AMF algorithm accurately identified the structures and generated a smooth segmentation.

Acknowledgments. We thank Karl Krissen [22] for his level set implementation in the 3D Slicer (www.slicer.org), which we used as a starting point for our AMF implementation. We also appreciate the valuable comments by Sylvain Bouix, Torsten Rohlfing, Mert Sabuncu, and Kinh Tieu. This research was supported by the NIH (NIBIB NAMIC U54-EB005149, NCRR NAC P41-RR13218, NINDS R01-NS051826, NCRR mBIRN U24-RR021382, U41-RR019703), the NSF (JHU ERC CISST), US Army (SBIR W81XWH-04-C0031), and the Brain Science Foundation.

References

1. Fischl, B., van der Kouwe, A., Destrieux, C., Halgren, E., Segonne, F., Salat, D., Busa, E., Seidman, L., Goldstein, J., Kennedy, D., Caviness, V., Makris, N., Rosen, B., Dale, A.: Automatically parcellating the human cerebral cortex. Cerebral Cortex 14, 11–22 (2004)
2. Yezzi, A., Kichenassamy, S., Kumar, A., Olver, P., Tannenbaum, A.: A geometric snake model for segmentation of medical imagery. IEEE Transactions on Medical Imaging 16(2), 199–209 (1997)
3. Krissian, K., Malandain, G., Ayache, N., Vaillant, R., Trousset, Y.: Model based detection of tubular structures in 3d images. Computer Vision and Image Understanding 80(2), 130–171 (2000)
4. Leventon, M., Grimson, W., Faugeras, O.: Statistical shape influence in geodesic active contours. In: IEEE Conference on Computer Vision and Pattern Recognition, 1316–1323 (2000)
5. Tsai, A., Yezzi, A., Wells, W., Tempany, C., Tucker, D., Fan, A., Grimson, W., Willsky, A.: A shape-based approach to the segmentation of medical imagery using level sets. IEEE Transactions on Medical Imaging 22(2), 137–154 (2003)
6. Rousson, M., Paragios, N., Deriche, R.: Active shape models from a level set perspective. Technical Report 4984, Institut National de Recherche en Informatique et en Automatique (2003)
7. Yang, J., Staib, L.H., Duncan, J.S.: Neighbor-constrained segmentation with level set based 3D deformable models. IEEE Transactions on Medical Imaging 23(8), 940–948 (2004)
8. Xu, M., Thompson, P., Toga, A.: An adaptive level set segmentation on a triangulated mesh. IEEE Transactions on Medical Imaging 23(2), 191–201 (2004)
9. Yushkevich, P., Piven, J., Hazlett, H., Smith, R., Ho, S., Gee, J., Gerig, G.: User-guided 3D active contour segmentation of anatomical structures: significantly improved efficiency and reliability. NeuroImage 31(1), 1116–1128 (2006)
10. Kapur, T.: Model based three dimensional Medical Imaging Segmentation. PhD thesis, Massachusetts Institute of Technology (1999)
11. Van Leemput, K., Maes, F., Vandermeulen, D., Suetens, P.: Automated model-based tissue classification of MR images of the brain. IEEE Transactions on Medical Imaging 18(10), 897–908 (1999)
12. Besag, J.: On the statistical analysis of dirty pictures. Journal of the Royal Society. Series B. 48(3), 259–302 (1986)

13. Fischl, B., Salat, D., Busa, E., Albert, M., Dieterich, M., Haselgrove, C., van der Kouwe, A., Killiany, R., Kennedy, D., Klaveness, S., Montillo, A., Makris, N., Rosen, B., Dale, A.: Whole brain segmentation: Automated labeling of neuroanatomical structures in the human brain. Neuron 33 (2002)
14. Zhang, Y., Brady, M., Smith, S.: Segmentation of brain MR images through a hidden Markov random field model and the expectation-maximization algorithm. IEEE Transactions on Medical Imaging 20(1), 45–57 (2001)
15. Marroquin, J., Santana, E., Botello, S.: Hidden Markov measure field models for image segmentation. IEEE Transactions on Pattern Analysis and Machine Intelligence 25, 1380–1387 (2003)
16. Pohl, K., Fisher, J., Shenton, M., McCarley, R.W., Grimson, W., Kikinis, R., Wells, W.: Logarithm odds maps for shape representation. In: Larsen, R., Nielsen, M., Sporring, J. (eds.) MICCAI 2006. LNCS, vol. 4191, pp. 955–963. Springer, Heidelberg (2006)
17. Pohl, K.M., Fisher, J., Grimson, W., Kikinis, R., Wells, W.: A Bayesian model for joint segmentation and registration. NeuroImage 31(1), 228–239 (2006)
18. Kendall, M.G., Buckland, W.R.: A Dictionary of Statistical Terms. Longman Group (1976)
19. Evans, M., Hastings, N., Peacock, B.: 4: Bernoulli Distribution. In: Statistical Distributions, 3rd edn., pp. 31–33. Wiley, Chichester (2000)
20. Taron, M., Paragios, N., Jolly, M.P.: Modelling shapes with uncertainties: Higher order polynomials, variable bandwidth kernels and non-parametric density estimation. In: IEEE International Conference on Computer Vision (2005)
21. Grayson, M.: The heat equation shrinks embedded plane curves to round points. Journal of Differential Geometry 26(2), 285–314 (1987)
22. Krissian, K., Westin, C.: Fast sub-voxel re-initialization of the distance map for level set methods. Pattern Recognition Letters 26(10), 1532–1542 (2005)

Appendix A Define a Vector Space for Discrete Probabilities

The function $\text{logit}(\cdot)$ and its inverse comprise a homeomorphism between $\mathbb{P}_M$ and $\mathbb{L}_{M-1}$ so that we can borrow the vector space structure on $\mathbb{L}_{M-1}$ to induce one on $\mathbb{P}_M$.

A.1 Addition in $\mathbb{P}_M$

The *probabilistic addition* $p_a \oplus p_b$ in $\mathbb{P}_M$ is constructed by mapping p_a and p_b into LogOdds space, performing the addition between $\text{logit}(p_a)$ and $\text{logit}(p_b)$, and then mapping the result back into $\mathbb{P}_M$ via the logistic function. This operation is equivalent to a normalized multiplication of two discrete probabilities within $\mathbb{P}_M$:

$$p_a \oplus p_b \triangleq \sigma(\text{logit}(p_a) + \text{logit}(p_b)) = \frac{1}{\sum_{i=1,\ldots,M} p_{a_i} \cdot p_{b_i}} (p_{a_1} \cdot p_{b_1}, \ldots, p_{a_M} \cdot p_{b_M}). \quad (8)$$

$(\mathbb{P}_M, \oplus)$ with the zero element being the uniform distribution $(\frac{1}{M}, \ldots, \frac{1}{M})$ forms an Abelian group as the *probabilistic addition* $\oplus$ is closed in $\mathbb{P}_M$. The additive inverse of a discrete probability $p \in \mathbb{P}_M$ is its complement $\bar{p}$, defined as $\bar{p}_i \triangleq \frac{1}{1+\sum_{j\neq i} \frac{p_i}{p_j}}$, for all $i \in \{1, .., M\}$. Similar to [16], it can be shown that for certain probabilistic models of p_a and p_b the *probabilistic addition* carries out the arithmetic of Bayes' rule.

A.2 Scalar Multiplication in $\mathbb{P}_M$

For $\mathbb{P}_M$ to be a vector space we also need to define a scalar multiplication operator. As with the probabilistic addition, the *probabilistic scalar multiplication* $\alpha \circledast p$ in $\mathbb{P}_M$ is defined as the logistic function of the product between α and the LogOdds $\text{logit}(p)$:

$$\alpha \circledast p \triangleq \sigma(\alpha * \text{logit}(p)) = \frac{1}{\sum_{i=1,\ldots,M} p_i^\alpha}(p_1^\alpha, \ldots, p_M^\alpha).$$

This operation is equivalent to exponentiating the discrete distribution with α and normalizing it. The technique of exponentiating and normalizing probabilities is frequently used in areas such as Markov Random fields [12] for controlling the "sharpness" of discrete distributions. As shown for the Binomial case in [16], α can also represent the certainty in the boundary location within an image space.

This completes our discussion of vector space $(\mathbb{P}_M, \oplus, \circledast)$ with 1 as the identity element of the scalar multiplication and $\bar{p} = -1 \circledast p$ the complement of p. By construction, this vector space is equivalent to $(\mathbb{L}_{M-1}, +, *)$ and its addition and scalar multiplication can be used to perform statistical computations in $\mathbb{P}_M^n$.

Appendix B Define the Expected Value Via the Heaviside Function

Lemma 1: If Y is a random variable with Bernoulli distribution $P(Y=1) = p \in [0,1]$ then the expected value of $F(\cdot) : \{0,1\} \to \mathbb{R}$ with respect to Y can be defined by the integral over the LogOdds space and the Heaviside function $\mathcal{H}(y) \triangleq \{1 \text{ for } y > 0, 0 \text{ otherwise}\}$: $E_{P(Y)}(F(Y)) = \int_{-\infty}^{\infty} \sigma(\alpha) \cdot (1-\sigma(\alpha)) \cdot F(\mathcal{H}(\text{logit}(p) - \alpha)\, d\alpha.$

Proof: $E_{P(Y)}(F(Y)) \triangleq pF(1) + (1-p))F(0) = \int_0^p F(1) d\beta + \int_p^1 F(0) d\beta$

$$= \int_0^1 F(\mathcal{H}(p-\beta)) d\beta = \int_{-\infty}^{\infty} F(\mathcal{H}(\text{logit}(p) - \alpha)) \left(\frac{d}{d\alpha}\sigma(\alpha)\right) d\alpha$$

$$= \int_{-\infty}^{\infty} \sigma(\alpha) \cdot (1-\sigma(\alpha)) \cdot F(\mathcal{H}(\text{logit}(p) - \alpha))\, d\alpha \qquad \blacksquare$$

Lemma 2: If $Y = (y_1, \ldots, y_n)$ is a vector of independent random variable with Bernoulli distribution $P = (p_1, \ldots, p_n)$ where $P(y_x = 1) = p_x \in [0,1]$ for $x \in \mathbb{I} = \{1, \ldots, n\}$ and the function $F(\cdot)$ is defined as $F(Y) = \sum_{x \in \mathbb{I}} f_x(y_x)$ then the expected value of F with respect to Y is defined within the LogOdds space as

$$E_{P(Y)}(F(Y)) \triangleq \int_{-\infty}^{\infty} \sigma(\alpha)(1-\sigma(\alpha)) F(\mathcal{H}(\text{logit}(P) - \alpha))\, d\alpha$$

Proof: $E_{P(Y)}(F(Y)) = \sum_{x \in \mathbb{I}} E_{P(Y_x)}(F(Y_x))$. Then according to Lemma 1

$$E_{P(Y)}(F(Y)) = \sum_{x \in \mathbb{I}} \int_{-\infty}^{\infty} \sigma(\alpha) \cdot (1-\sigma(\alpha)) \cdot f_x(\mathcal{H}(\text{logit}(p_x) - \alpha))\, d\alpha$$

$$= \int_{-\infty}^{\infty} \sigma(\alpha) \cdot (1-\sigma(\alpha)) \sum_{x \in \mathbb{I}} f_x(\mathcal{H}(\text{logit}(p_x) - \alpha))\, d\alpha$$

$$= \int_{-\infty}^{\infty} \sigma(\alpha) \cdot (1-\sigma(\alpha)) F(\mathcal{H}(\text{logit}(P) - \alpha)\, d\alpha \qquad \blacksquare$$

Liver Segmentation Using Sparse 3D Prior Models with Optimal Data Support

Charles Florin[1], Nikos Paragios[2], Gareth Funka-Lea[1], and James Williams[3]

[1] Imaging & Visualization Department,
Siemens Corporate Research, Princeton, NJ, USA
[2] MAS - Ecole Centrale de Paris,
Chatenay-Malabry, France
[3] Siemens Medical Systems
Forchheim, Germany

Abstract. Volume segmentation is a relatively slow process and, in certain circumstances, the enormous amount of prior knowledge available is underused. Model-based liver segmentation suffers from the large shape variability of this organ, and from structures of similar appearance that juxtapose the liver. The technique presented in this paper is devoted to combine a statistical analysis of the data with a reconstruction model from sparse information: only the most reliable information in the image is used, and the rest of the liver's shape is inferred from the model and the sparse observation. The resulting process is more efficient than standard segmentation since most of the workload is concentrated on the critical points, but also more robust, since the interpolated volume is consistent with the prior knowledge statistics. The experimental results on liver datasets prove the sparse information model has the same potential as PCA, if not better, to represent the shape of the liver. Furthermore, the performance assessment from measurement statistics on the liver's volume, distance between reconstructed surfaces and ground truth, and inter-observer variability demonstrates the liver is efficiently segmented using sparse information.

1 Introduction

Computerized medical imaging analysis aims at detecting and delineating anatomical structures for surgery planning and diagnosis. It has gained significant importance in hepatic procedures, specially in oncology to detect tumors and lesions, quantify the ratio of tumors' volume and liver's volume (future liver remnant volume and total liver volume), their localization with respect to the liver's vasculature and the different lobes of the liver [12][15]. Also, in the context of liver transplantation, graft from living donors is increasingly performed due to the shortage of cadaveric donors. This particular procedure requires a pre-operative quantification of the donor's liver volume [6]. However, the segmentation of the liver is an arduous task for two main reasons. First, the liver's appearance and shape has a large inter-patient variability; it is one of the largest organ of the human body, after the skin, and imaged patients may suffer from heavy diseases such as cancer. Second, the neighboring structures have similar appearance in CT and MR, and may juxtapose the liver in a way that corresponds to a statistical shape

N. Karssemeijer and B. Lelieveldt (Eds.): IPMI 2007, LNCS 4584, pp. 38–49, 2007.
© Springer-Verlag Berlin Heidelberg 2007

variation, or without clear edge between the two. In this paper, we propose a novel method for liver segmentation that combines a statistical analysis of the data with a reconstruction model from sparse information: only the most reliable information in the image is used, and the rest of the liver's shape is inferred from the model and the sparse observation.

Given the difficulty of segmenting the liver, a model is commonly used, either as a localization, a shape or an appearance constrain. In [20], a cascading segmentation scheme sequentially detects the different abdominal structures for hepatic surgery planning. In [13][19], the liver is detected by a classification procedure based on the pixels intensity. A semiautomatic procedure is presented in [18] where a live-wire based on dynamic programming assists the user in drawing the liver's contour slice by slice. In the context of deformable models, the reason for using prior knowledge is that this segmentation method is a local optimization, and therefore is sensitive to local minima. Therefore, the prior work on liver segmentation includes models based on shape variations, and constrains on pixel intensities learned from classification. Intensity based methods are used in [10] with snakes segmenting the liver's contour in a slice-by-slice fashion. However, the vicinity of the liver to neighboring structures of similar appearance makes models attractive for this task [5]. The models used in [5] are based on Cootes et al.'s Active Shape Models [1]. The results obtained in [5] demonstrate Active Shape Models may represent to a certain extent the liver's shape. However, they fall short of accurately segmenting the liver because of the large shape variability of this organ. Furthermore, Active Shape Models are highly dependent on initialization, a problem the authors deal with using multi-resolution. Nonlinear models, such as shape-based Kernel PCA [2] or Fourier coefficients [3], are also a solution that have been investigated more recently for segmentation. The main limitation of these methods (linear or non-linear) is the explicit assumption of the data distribution that, for example, forms a linear subspace in the case of PCA. These methods process the total amount of data and find the optimum trade-off between an image term and a prior term. Furthermore, the quality of image support is at no point taken into account; it is assumed that should an image region quality be low, another region would compensate. Most of these methods treat segmentation as a statistical estimation problem, where the quality and the support of the training set's exemplars is often ignored. Instead, the approach presented in this paper relies on observation at key locations, and on a reconstruction model ; both the key locations and the reconstruction models are learned from prior knowledge. This technique gives better results because the segmentation is only supported by the data with the strongest image support, and is also of low complexity because it uses the data in an optimal fashion.

Interpolation models have been studied before. The simplest and most common method is to use a spline or piecewise polynomial function [14,21] that interpolates the contour between explicit points. Other methods use an implicit representation of the contour (a continuous function that takes a zero value on the contour) and interpolating functions such as thin-plate splines [22]. An example of surface reconstruction is the work of Hoppe *et al.* [7] who computed a signed distance function in 3D which is the distance in $\mathbb{R}^3$ to any input point. Then, from the zero levelset of this function is extracted the surface using the Marching Cubes [11]. At last, deformable models [9] are used to minimize an energy function of the mesh by deforming the mesh so that the mesh is simultaneously attracted to the data by an image term, kept smooth by a tension term and by an optional prior term.

The approach we propose here is different: we propose a liver model that encodes the shape variations using a small number of carefully chosen key-slices where the organ's contours can be optimally recovered. First, the image or shape to reconstruct is discretized along the longitudinal axis, and all the liver exemplars are registered so that they fit into the same reference region. Then, a set of slice indices are determined so that it minimizes three different criteria: image support, quality of the reconstruction and sensibility to variations in the projection's subspace. Finally, the reconstruction operator itself is learned over the given liver exemplars. To present this approach, section (2) contains a rather generic formulation of Sparse Information Models. Then, section (3) is devoted to explicit this model to the particular problem of 3D liver segmentation. To validate the methodology, section (4) aims at proving the liver's shape is indeed well recovered from few contours at key-slices, and quantifying the quality of the segmentation obtained in this way.

2 Choice of Sparse Information

Let us consider a shape $\mathbf{x}$ and its partition into m elements $\mathbf{x} = (\mathbf{x}_1, ..., \mathbf{x}_m)$ (see figure (1)) associated to m measures $\mathbf{w} = (\mathbf{w}_1, ..., \mathbf{w}_m)$ which reflect the data support for the observations. Without loss of generality, we assume the m sub-elements are obtained by a discretization process along one or several axis $\mathbf{v}_0$ using an operator $\rho : [\Omega_r \times \mathbb{R}] \rightarrow \Omega_r/\mathbf{v}_0$:

$$\forall\, k \in [1, m], \;\; \mathbf{x}_k = \rho(\mathbf{x}, k) \tag{1}$$

In the remaining of the paper, this continuous parameterization is assumed when not specified. The aim of our approach is to recover a minimal description length set of $|\mathcal{B}|$ sub-elements $\mathcal{B} = \{\mathbf{x}_{t_k}\}_{k \in [|1,K|]}$ with K small compared to m, and a continuous operator ϕ, from which the whole data $\mathbf{x}$ is deducted:

$$\forall\, k \in [1, m], \;\; \phi(\mathbf{x}_{t_1}, ..., \mathbf{x}_{t_K}, k) = \mathbf{x}(k). \tag{2}$$

2.1 Optimal Reconstruction of the Data

Let us consider a training set of P exemplars $\mathcal{X} = \{\mathbf{x}^1, \mathbf{x}^2, ..., \mathbf{x}^P\}$ registered in a reference space Ω_r. Toward optimal reconstruction of the training set from the basis $\mathcal{B}$, the distance between the reconstruction and the existing samples is minimized. To this end, let a metric $\psi : [\Omega_r \times \Omega_r] \rightarrow \mathbb{R}^+$ measures the distance between two sub-elements. Then, assuming the number of components of the training set is fixed, such reconstruction minimizes

$$E_{int}(\mathcal{B}, \phi) = \sum_{p=1}^{P} \sum_{i=1}^{m} \psi\left(\mathbf{x}_i^p, \phi_i(\mathbf{x}_{t_1}^p, ..., \mathbf{x}_{t_K}^p)\right). \tag{3}$$

Such an approach is purely geometric and does not account for the image support of each sub-element.

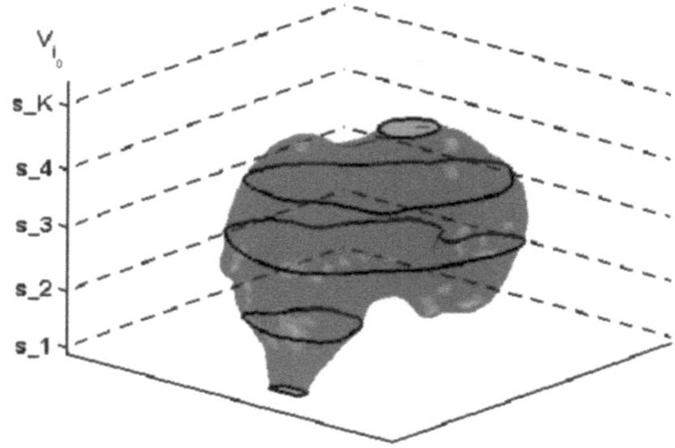

Fig. 1. Example of a 3D liver surface $\mathbf{x}$ whose subcomponents $(\mathbf{x}_1, ..., \mathbf{x}_m)$ are obtained by intersecting the 3D shape with the axial plane (dark contours) at specific slice indices $s_1, s_2, ...s_K$.

2.2 Optimal Image Support

We recall that the sub-elements of a given exemplar $\mathbf{x}^p$ have some underlying image support noted $\mathbf{w}^p = (\mathbf{w}_1^p, ..., \mathbf{w}_m^p)$. The optimum basis $\mathcal{B}$ consists of elements that are confidently extracted from the data; therefore, the basis minimizes

$$E_{sup}(\mathcal{B}) = \sum_{p=1}^{P} \sum_{k=1}^{K} g\left(\mathbf{w}_k^p\left(\mathcal{T}_\theta^{-1}(\mathbf{x}_{t_k}^p)\right)\right) \tag{4}$$

where g is a monotonically decreasing function, and $\mathcal{T}_\theta^{-1}(\mathbf{x}_{t_k}^p)$ is the inverse mapping between the basis $\mathcal{B}$ and the observation space. The use of such inverse mapping is also to be considered during the application of the model to new data. Therefore, it is critical to have a selection of $\mathcal{B}$ that is relative robust to errors when locating the basis elements in a new exemplar.

2.3 Robustness to Parameters Variability

Let us consider a slight variation on the selection of the basis, noted $\delta\mathbf{x}_t$. For the interpolation precision of the model not to be significantly affected,

$$\lim_{|\delta\mathbf{x}_t| \to 0} \frac{E_{int}(\mathcal{B}, \phi) - E_{int}(\mathcal{B} + \delta\mathbf{x}_t, \phi)}{\delta\mathbf{x}_t} = 0 \tag{5}$$

that is reformulated in terms of a cost by defining a smoothness function $\eta()$, like the error-two norm,

$$E_{var}(\mathcal{B}, \phi) = \eta\left(\nabla_{\mathcal{B}} E_{int}(\mathcal{B}, \phi)\right). \tag{6}$$

Such a penalty term introduces robustness in the basis selection step, as well to the reconstruction process. Now, one integrates these three constraints into a single cost function: $E(\mathcal{B}, \phi) = E_{int}(\mathcal{B}, \phi) + \alpha E_{sup}(\mathcal{B}) + \beta E_{var}(\mathcal{B}, \phi)$ where α and β are problem-specific normalizing constants (results have shown little sensibility to small variations of α and β). The cost function E is minimized with respect to the interpolation function ϕ and the basis $\mathcal{B}$. Such a process cannot be described in a general fashion, but a gradient descent is an excellent choice when considering linear interpolation models, while more advanced non-linear optimization methods like neural networks can be considered for non-linear cases. Last, but not least the residual cost that characterizes the *Sparse Information Model* is used to determine the best number K of key components that optimizes the Minimum Description Length. In order to demonstrate the efficiency of such a model for volumetric organ segmentation, we consider the particular case of liver segmentation in CT images. The same approach is easily adapted to any other organ, in any dimension.

3 Sparse Knowledge-Based Segmentation

Knowledge-based segmentation is one of the dominant approaches to organ extraction from 3D images. First, the Sparse Model is built by selecting a minimal set $\mathcal{B}$ of 2D contours (represented in an explicit or an implicit fashion) along with an interpolation function ϕ to reconstruct the whole 3D surface in the reference space Ω_r. During the segmentation, the global transformation $\mathcal{T}_\theta$ that relates the reconstructed model to the observation volume is to be determined, along with the set $\mathcal{B}$ of 2D contours that fits the observation.

3.1 Model Construction

The experiment is conducted on segmentation for medical imaging for the case of liver in Computed Tomography (CT). We represent the training set exemplars $\mathbf{x}$ by 3D distance maps to the closed surface Γ defined by the liver's edge $\mathcal{C}$ in the volumetric data:

$$\forall p \in \Omega, \ \mathbf{x}(p) = \begin{cases} 0, & p \in \mathcal{C} \\ +D(p) \geq 0, & p \in \Gamma \\ -D(p) < 0, & p \in \bar{\Gamma} \end{cases} \tag{7}$$

Such a selection is motivated from its implicit nature, as well as the ability to introduce surface-based as well as area based criteria in the segmentation process. Classic explicit parameterizations like triangulated surfaces, or other form of parametric snakes can also be considered.

The acquisition process guides our choice for the definition of the sub-elements: since the image volume is reconstructed slice by slice, with maximum resolution in the slice plane, the axis of projection $\mathbf{v}_{i_0}$ (see section (2)) is the longitudinal axis. Therefore, a sub-element $\mathbf{x}_i$ corresponds to a particular slice (see figure (1)). The geometric transformation T_θ is a translation-scaling that sets $\mathbf{x}$ in a reference space Ω_r with m slices $(\mathbf{x}_1, \ldots \mathbf{x}_m)$.

In order to determine the best possible interpolation class, different models for ϕ have been tested. We have concluded that generalized linear interpolation for each slice

i is a good compromise between complexity and interpolation quality. In other words, the solution (2D contour) at each slice $\mathbf{x}_i$ is reconstructed using a particular linear combination $\mathbf{H}_i$ of the key contours $\mathbf{x}_{t_1}, ...\mathbf{x}_{t_K}$. This notation is kept in the remaining of the paper: $\phi = \mathbf{H}$. The interpolation quality is defined according to sum of square difference between the reconstructed distance map and the observed shape's distance map in the reference space Ω_r:

$$E_{int}(\mathcal{B}, \mathbf{H}) = \sum_{i=1}^{m} \int_{\Omega_r} \left| \mathbf{H}_i \left[\mathbf{x}_{t_1}, ...\mathbf{x}_{t_K} \right]^T - \mathbf{x}_i \right|^2 \tag{8}$$

E_{int} is a quadratic function with global minimum, and since the reference space Ω_r is a continuous space, the minimization of E_{int} benefits from the large literature on quadratic functions minimization.

The image support $\mathbf{w}_i$ at slice i is defined by the Kullback-Leibler distance between the pixels intensity distributions inside and outside the 2D contour and the a priori learned histograms. Knowing a priori the normalized histogram h_{in} (resp. h_{out}) of the pixels intensity inside (resp. outside) the liver, and computing the pixels intensity distribution p_{in} and p_{out} inside and outside of the reconstructed shape on the key slices,

$$E_{sup}(\mathcal{B}) = \sum_{k=1}^{K} \int h_{\text{in}}(k,s) \log\left(\frac{h_{\text{in}}(k,s)}{p_{\text{in}}(k,s)}\right) ds + \sum_{k=1}^{K} \int h_{\text{out}}(k,s) \log\left(\frac{h_{\text{out}}(k,s)}{p_{\text{out}}(k,s)}\right) ds. \tag{9}$$

Finally, the key contours are chosen so as to minimize the impact of little variations in their position, and of little errors in the contours extraction in the key slices. Since a continuous interpolation of the 2D contours is introduced in equation (1), the impact of an infinitesimal change ∂k in the slice index may be written as the squared magnitude of the gradient of $\mathbf{x}_{t_k}$ with respect to t_k: $\|\nabla_{t_k} \mathbf{x}_{t_k}\|^2$. In practice, since the contours are represented using distance functions (see equation (7)), the derivative of the distance function at index t_k, with respect to the index, is a field of 2d vectors whose squared magnitude is $\|\nabla_{t_k} \mathbf{x}_{t_k}\|^2$. Therefore, the key contours are chosen so as to minimize the integral over the image space of the distance map's gradient at the key locations:

$$E_{\text{var}}(\mathcal{B}) = \sum_{k=1}^{K} \int_{\Omega_r} \|\nabla_{t_k} \mathbf{x}_{t_k}\|^2 . \tag{10}$$

In order to determine the number K, the indices of the key contours $t_1, ...t_K$ as well as the interpolation operator $\mathbf{H}$, a gradient descent optimization method is used and combined with the Schwarz Bayesian criterion [4] to determine the optimum cardinality of the basis. After registering the volumes with $m = 100$ slices, the optimum number of key slices is 5.

3.2 Model-Based Segmentation

With sparse model in hand, the volumetric segmentation is boiled down to the segmentation of the shape at key slices; in other words, the whole 3D segmentation problem is reduced to a small set of parallel 2D contours to be segmented at specific locations. Therefore, one needs to optimize an image-based cost function with respect to both the set of key contours $\mathcal{B} = \mathbf{x}_{t_1}, ...\mathbf{x}_{t_K}$ in the reference space and the transformation $\mathcal{T}_\theta$ simultaneously. In an iterative optimization scheme, the transformation $\mathcal{T}_\theta$ at a given iteration is used to relate the current set of 2D contours $\mathbf{x}_{t_1}, ...\mathbf{x}_{t_K}$ to the image so that both the transformation and the sparse set of contours are optimized concomitantly.

To this end, the cost function consists of the intensity-based likelihood of each pixel, assuming that normalized histograms inside (h_{in}) and outside (h_{out}) the liver are available (if not, one recovers them on-the-fly). Then, the posterior likelihood of the partition with respect to the two classes is maximized to obtain the key contours $\mathcal{B}$ and the transformation $\mathcal{T}_\theta$:

$$\begin{aligned} E_{seg}\left(\mathcal{B}, \mathcal{T}_\theta\right) = \sum_{k=1}^{K} \int_\Omega -\log\left(h_{\text{in}}(I(s))\right) \mathcal{H}(\mathbf{x}_{t_k}(\mathcal{T}_\theta(s)))\, ds \\ + \sum_{k=1}^{K} \int_\Omega -\log\left(h_{\text{out}}(I(s))\right)\left(1 - \mathcal{H}(\mathbf{x}_{t_k}(\mathcal{T}_\theta(s)))\right)\, ds, \end{aligned} \tag{11}$$

where $\mathcal{H}(\mathbf{x}_{t_k}(s))$ denotes the Heaviside function that is equal to 1 inside the contour $\mathbf{x}_{t_k}$, and 0 outside. During the sparse model's construction the image support has been taken into account in the selection of the key slices. This information has been inherited to the segmentation and, in principle, the slices where one best separates liver from the rest of the background are used (see equation (9)). When $(\mathcal{B}, \mathcal{T}_\theta)$ have reached the energy minimum, the whole volumetric shape **x** is reconstructed in Ω_r by applying the linear combination $\mathbf{H}_i$ for each slice i. Finally, the inverse of T_θ is used to transform the reconstructed volume from Ω_r to the image space Ω. In a subsequent step, one may consider refining the results by locally optimizing the solution **x** on each slice i, using the sparse model's result as a prior such as [**?**].

4 Experimental Validation

4.1 Dimensionality Reduction Using Sparse Information Model

Before proving Sparse Information Models are efficiently used to segment an organ in volumetric data, one needs to quantify the error introduced by the Sparse Models dimension reduction and compare it with common techniques such as PCA. The volumetric data is acquired on Sensation 16 CT scanners, with an average resolution of 1 mm in axial plane and 3 mm along the longitudinal axis. 31 volumes (different oncology patients, with or without pathologies such as tumors) are used in our experiments on a leave-one-out basis: 30 volumes are used to build the models (sparse and PCA) and the last one is used for testing.

Table (1) summarizes the error introduced by dimensionality reduction for PCA (30 modes), linear interpolation and Sparse Information Model with 5 slices. This error measure is defined as the symmetric difference [18] between the two volumes V_1 and V_2:

$$\epsilon = 1 - \frac{|V_1 \cap V_2|}{0.5 * (|V_1| + |V_2|)} \tag{12}$$

Table 1. Results table showing the median, maximum and minimum symmetric difference between ground truth volumes and reconstructed volumes using PCA (30 modes), linear interpolation from 5 key slices and Sparse Information Model (SIM) with 5 key slices

method	PCA	Linear interp.	SIM
median symmetric diff.	11.70%	10.72%	8.35%
maximum symmetric diff.	23.32%	16.13%	13.14%
minimum symmetric diff.	6.56%	7.69%	6.28%

The results demonstrate that the Sparse Information Model with 5 key elements provides the same reconstruction quality than linear PCA with 30 modes of variation. However, the PCA results have a large variance because diseased organs are poorly represented by a Gaussian model in the linear PCA space. Nevertheless, a larger study with different pathologies could demonstrate kernel PCA [8] best represents the shapes.

Figure (2) illustrates different error measures for liver segmentation with linear PCA, liner interpolation and Sparse Information Model. The quality assessment is performed with four error measures: the volumetric error in %, the average surface distance, the RMS distance, and the percentage of surface father than 5mm from the ground truth.

4.2 Sparse Information Model for Segmentation

The second step consists in demonstrating Sparse Information Models can efficiently be used for segmentation. For that purpose, it is assumed an expert (i.e. either a human expert, or an expert system such as the ones described in the literature) roughly initializes the rigid transformation and the key contours. When no user interaction is available, a preprocessing step, such as exhaustive search or coarse-to-fine search, is to be developed. In the case of PCA [16], the segmentation problem is solved by minimizing the cost function resulting from the intensity-based likelihood of each pixel in the volumetric image:

$$
\begin{aligned}
E_{seg} &= \sum_{k=1}^{m} \int_{\Omega} -\log\left(h_{\text{in}}(I(s))\right) \mathcal{H}(\mathbf{x}_k(T_\theta(s)))\, d\Omega \\
&+ \sum_{k=1}^{m} \int_{\Omega} -\log\left(h_{\text{out}}(I(s))\right) \left(1 - \mathcal{H}(\mathbf{x}_k(T_\theta(s)))\right)\, d\Omega,
\end{aligned}
\tag{13}
$$

As in [16], equation (13) is minimized in the PCA's parametric space, where the shapes' distribution is modeled using kernels. The kernels are justified by the poor modeling of the samples distribution by a Gaussian. For the PCA segmentation, all the m slices of the volume are used, whereas the Sparse Information Model only segments the K slices determined during the model construction (see equation (11)).

Table (2) summarizes the symmetric difference (see equation (12)) between ground truth and the segmented liver obtained using the Sparse Information Model and PCA [16] (see figure (3)). Neighboring structures of similar intensities juxtapose the liver in a way that PCA estimates as a shape variation. On the contrary, the Sparse Model ignores the regions with low support, and reconstructs the information in these regions based on

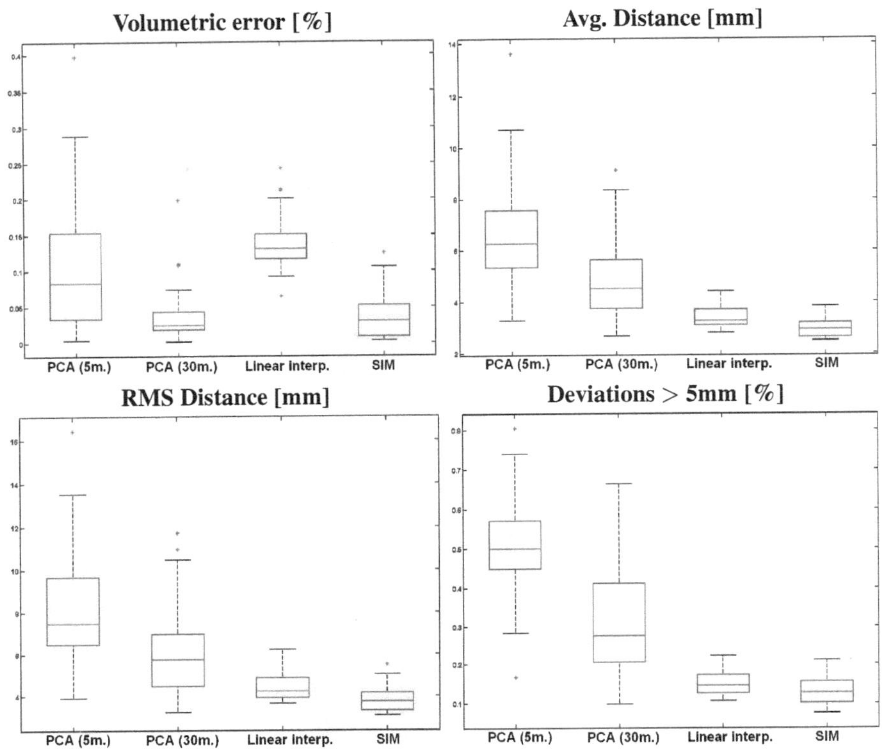

Fig. 2. Segmentation result boxplots comparing PCA (5 and 30 modes), linear interpolation and Sparse Information Model. The box has lines at the lower quartile, median, and upper quartile values. The whiskers are lines extending from each end of the box to show the extent of the rest of the data. Outliers are data with values beyond the ends of the whiskers.

other visual clues elsewhere in the image. For information, the inter-observer symmetric difference in table (2) indicates the symmetric difference between livers segmented by different experts using the same semi-automatic tool. Overall, when compared with [5], the results seem to demonstrate Sparse Information Models outperform Active Shape Models. Nevertheless, it must be underlined that the training and evaluation datasets are different. Furthermore, in [5], the shape model is built from smoothed surface meshes, while the training shapes used in this paper are represented by distance functions (see

Table 2. Results table showing the average symmetric difference and maximum symmetric between hand-segmented livers and automatic segmentation with PCA and Sparse Information Model (SIM). Also, is also given the Inter-Observer Variability (IOV) statistics.

method	PCA	SIM	IOV
median symmetric diff.	26.41%	11.49%	5.56%
maximum symmetric diff.	36.84%	17.13%	7.83%
minimum symmetric diff.	16.68%	9.49%	2.96%

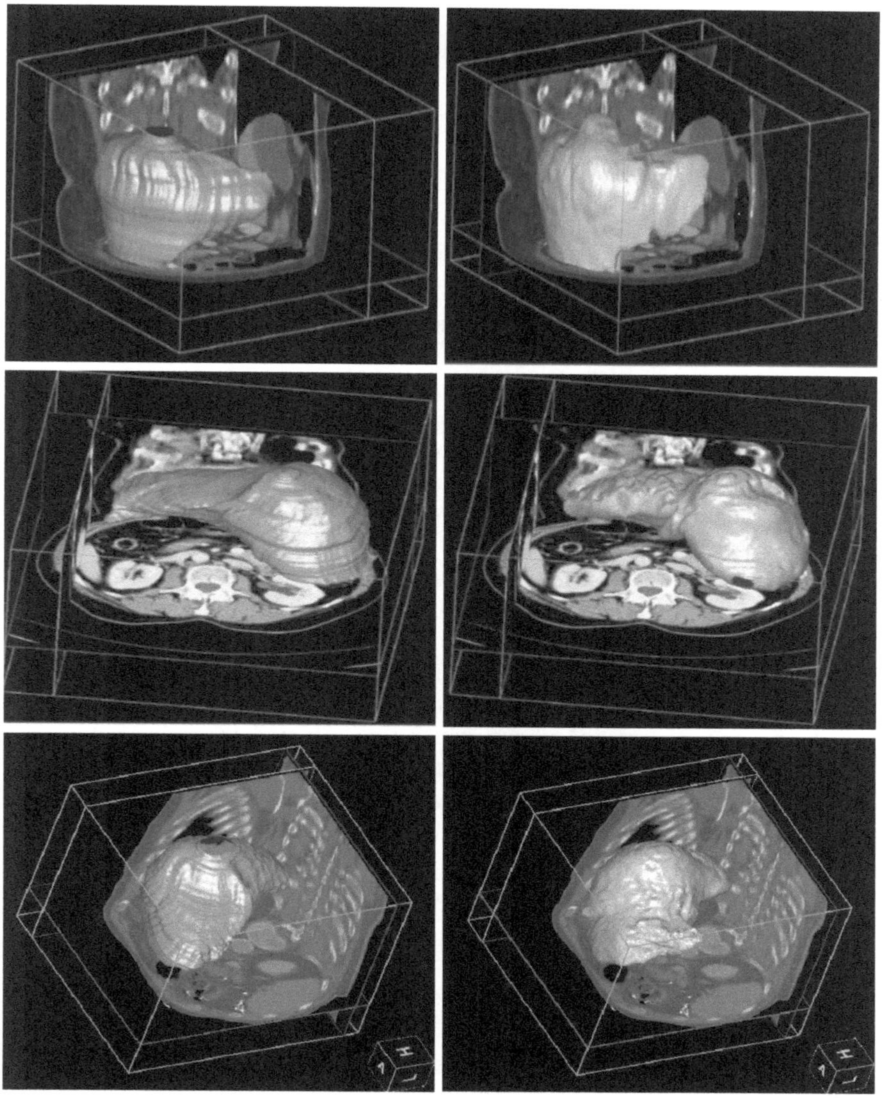

Fig. 3. Comparison of liver segmentation obtained by SIM (left column) and expert segmentation (right column)

equation (7)) and are not smoothed. However, as one suspects, Sparse Information Models are sensitive to initialization. To quantify this, two different Sparse Segmentations were performed by segmenting by hand the key slices in the datasets, and comparing the reconstruction results with the ground truth. The difference in quality (symmetric difference with ground truth) between the different reconstructions ranges from 0.02% to 6.73%. Moreover, this variance is not correlated to the IOV (correlation coefficient of 0.47); otherwise stated, a volume with high inter-observer variability may be segmented by the SIM in a way that is robust to initialization, and reciprocal may be true. Indeed, the IOV depends on the whole organ's structure while the SIM's quality only depends on the key slices. Furthermore, the maximum quality difference of 6.73% is below the maximum IOV symmetric difference (7.83% in table (2)).

5 Conclusion

In this paper, we have introduced a novel family of dimension reduction techniques based on intelligent selection of key sub-elements with respect to reconstruction quality, image support and variability of these key sub-elements. It is demonstrated that Sparse Information Models can be used for dimensionality purposes, and can efficiently be integrated into a segmentation framework in the context of volumetric organ segmentation. We have applied this technique to the problem of liver segmentation in volumetric images with successful results compared to common dimensionality reduction techniques based on linear projections and kernel distributions. On top of interpolation and segmentation quality, this method is also very fast since only the most important and most reliable information is processed for the reconstruction of the whole information. However, as noted in [5], a statistical shape model may not be sufficient to represent the exact shape of the liver ; in a post-processing step, a local optimization - using active contours for instance - may be necessary for better results. This local optimization would not be computed from Sparse Information. Further work will investigate the use of non-linear models for the interpolation function, as well as a subsequent refinement step that will locally adjust the reconstruction from the model to the actual image information by taking into account the confidence in the reconstruction. More advanced prior models using axial coronal and sagittal sparse information would be an interesting extension of our approach, as it would diminish the quality difference between two differently initialized segmentations. Last, but not least, the use of such methods for feature extraction, classification and content-based image indexing and retrieval is a natural extension on the application side.

References

1. Cootes, T., Taylor, C., Cooper, D., Graham, J.: Active shape models - their training and application. Computer Vision and Image Understanding 61, 38–59 (1995)
2. Dambreville, S., Rathi, Y., Tannenbaum, A.: Shape-based approach to robust image segmentation using kernel pca. In: CVPR, pp. 977–984, Washington, DC, USA (2006)
3. Derrode, S., Chermi, M., Ghorbel, F.: Fourier-based invariant shape prior for snakes. In: ICASSP 2006 (2006)
4. Hansen, M.H., Yu, B.: Model selection and the principle of minimum description length. Journal of the American Statistical Association 96(454), 746–774 (2001)
5. Heimann, T., Wolf, I., Meinzer, H.P.: Active shape models for a fully automated 3d segmentation of the liver - an evaluation on clinical data. In: Larsen, R., Nielsen, M., Sporring, J. (eds.) MICCAI 2006. LNCS, vol. 4191, pp. 41–48. Springer, Heidelberg (2006)
6. Hermoye, L., Laamari-Azjal, I., Cao, Z., Annet, L., Lerut, J., Dawant, B., Van Beers, B.: Liver segmentation in living liver transplant donors: comparison of semiautomatic and manual methods. Radiology 234(1), 171–178 (2005)

7. Hoppe, H., DeRose, T., Duchamp, T., McDonald, J., Stuetzle, W.: Surface reconstruction from unorganized points. In: SIGGRAPH '92: Proceedings of the 19th annual conference on Computer graphics and interactive techniques, pp. 71–78 (1992)
8. Leventon, M., Grimson, E., Faugeras, O.: Statistical Shape Influence in Geodesic Active Controus. In: IEEE Conference on Computer Vision and Pattern Recognition, pp. I:316–322 (2000)
9. Liao, C.W., Medioni, G.: Surface approximation of a cloud of 3d points. Graph. Models Image Process 57(1), 67–74 (1995)
10. Liu, F., Zhao, B., Kijewski, P., Wang, L., Schwartz, L.: Liver segmentation for ct images using gvf snake. Medical Physics 32(12), 3699–3706 (2005)
11. Lorensen, W., Cline, H.: Marching cubes: A high resolution 3d surface construction algorithm. In: SIGGRAPH '87: Proceedings of the 14th annual conference on Computer graphics and interactive techniques,NewYork,NY,USA, pp. 163–169. ACM Press, New York (1987)
12. Meinzer, H.P., Thorn, M., Cardenas, C.: Computerized planning of liver surgery-an overview. Computer and Graphics 26(4), 569–576 (2002)
13. Park, H., Bland, P., Meyer, C.: Construction of an abdominal probabilistic atlas and its application in segmentation. IEEE Trans. Med. Imaging 22(4), 483–492 (2003)
14. Pham, B.: Quadratic b-splines for automatic curve and surface fitting. C&G 13, 471–475 (1989)
15. Reitinger, B., Bornik, A., Beichel, R., Schmalstieg, D.: Liver surgery planning using virtual reality. IEEE Comput. Graph. Appl. 26(6), 36–47 (2006)
16. Rousson, M., Cremers, D.: Efficient kernel density estimation of shape and intensity priors for level set segmentation. In: Duncan, J.S., Gerig, G. (eds.) MICCAI 2005. LNCS, vol. 3750, pp. 757–764. Springer, Heidelberg (2005)
17. Rousson, M., Paragios, N.: Shape Priors for Level Set representations. In: European Conference on computer Vision, pages II: 78–93, Copenhangen, Denmark, 2002(2002)
18. Schenk, A., Prause, G., Peitgen, H.: Efficient semiautomatic segmentation of 3d objects in medical images. In: Delp, S.L., DiGoia, A.M., Jaramaz, B. (eds.) MICCAI 2000. LNCS, vol. 1935, pp. 186–195. Springer, Heidelberg (2000)
19. Seo, K.S., Kim, H.B., Park, T., Kim, P.K., Park, J.A.: Automatic liver segmentation of contrast enhanced ct images based on histogram processing. In: ICNC (1), pp. 1027–1030 (2005)
20. Soler, L., Delingette, H., Malandain, G., Montagnat, J., Ayache, N., Koehl, C., Dourthe, O., Malassagne, B., Smith, M., Mutter, D., Marescaux, J.: Fully automatic anatomical, pathological, and functional segmentation from CT scans for hepatic surgery. Computer Aided Surgery (CAS), vol. 6(3), August 2001 (2001)
21. Tehrani, S., Weymouth, T.E., Schunck, B.: Interpolating cubic spline contours by minimizing second derivative discontinuity. In: ICCV, pp. 713–716, 90
22. Turk, G., O'brien, J.: Modelling with implicit surfaces that interpolate. ACM Trans. Graph. 21(4), 855–873 (2002)

Adaptive Non-rigid Registration of Real Time 3D Ultrasound to Cardiovascular MR Images

Weiwei Zhang, J. Alison Noble, and J. Mike Brady

Wolfson Medical Vision Lab, Department of Engineering Science, University of Oxford, Parks Road, Oxford OX1 3PJ, United Kingdom
{weiwei,noble,jmb}@robots.ox.ac.uk

Abstract. We present a new method to non-rigidly co-register a real-time 3D ultrasound volume slice to a cardiovascular MR image. The motivation for our research is to assist a clinician to automatically fuse the information from multiple imaging modalities for the early diagnosis and therapy of cardiac disease. The local phase presentation of both images is utilized as an image descriptor of the "featureness". The local deformation of ventricles is modeled by a polyaffine transformation. The anchor points (or control points) used in the polyaffine transformation are automatically detected and refined by calculating a local mis-match measure based on phase mutual information. The registration process is built in an adaptive multi-scale framework to maximize the phase-based similarity measure by optimizing the parameters of the polyaffine transformation. Registration results have demonstrated that this novel method is superior to our prior work [1], yielding an accurate registration to local cardiac regions.

1 Introduction

Cardiovascular disease is one of the world's leading causes of death. With the aid of advanced imaging techniques, the cardiovascular examination has helped to improve early diagnosis and therapy. Among the existing imaging techniques, cardiovascular magnetic imaging (CMR) and real-time three-dimensional echocardiography (RT3DUS) are receiving a lot of attention at the current time [2].

Due to the 3D nature of the heart and its complex motion in 3D space, the RT3DUS is well-suited for 3D analysis of the cardiac disease. However, RT3DUS has lower specificity and sensitivity than the high spatial resolution CMR, which makes it difficult to interpret. Therefore the comparison and fusion of information from multiple cardiac image modalities is of increasing interest in the medical community for physiological understanding and diagnostic purposes. In this paper, our objective is to non-rigidly register the RT3D echocardiography to CMR images from the same patient. Current cardiac image registration methods can be divided into two main categories: 1) those based on geometric image features and 2) those based on voxel similarity measures [3]. When considering the feature-based method, there exist only few salient anatomical landmarks due to the complex shape of the heart. Moreover, in certain pathological conditions, the

N. Karssemeijer and B. Lelieveldt (Eds.): IPMI 2007, LNCS 4584, pp. 50–61, 2007.
© Springer-Verlag Berlin Heidelberg 2007

functional alterations may also hide a sparse set of anatomical landmarks, which makes it difficult to accurately identify the same landmarks in both modality images [3]. Voxel similarity measures have an important advantage that no a priori segmentation of the registered features is required. These methods are based on the assumption that the registered images are strongly correlated by the pixel (voxel) values. Mutual information based registration methods have proved particularly promising for inter-modality voxel based image registration such as MR-CT, CT-PET and MR-PET in the area of neurology, since no assumptions are made regarding the nature of the relation between the image intensities in the registered images [4]. However, its application to cardiovascular non-rigid image registration, especially to the RT3D-CMR image registration, has not been reported before.

Even though US-MR image registration is a challenging task, some authors have proposed to pre-processed both US and MR images with a 'feature transform', so that the appearance of features is approximately compatible. For instance, Roche et al [5] present a novel correlation ratio to incorporate the US intensity with both MR intensity and MR gradient magnitude. For this rigid registration case applied to intra-operative US and pre-operative MR images, he maximized the bi-variate extension of the correlation ratio. In other work, Penney and Black et al [6] report a method to register a pre-operative MR volume to a sparse set of intra-operative US slices of abdominal images. Liver vessels were detected as the main feature to be registered. The grayscale intensity images of both modalities were transformed into a probability image where intensity values represented the probability of a voxel containing a vessel. This rigid registration was then carried out by maximizing the normalized cross-correlation between the vessel probability images of both modalities. Extending these methods to non-rigid registration has not been done to our knowledge.

In our prior work [1], we proposed a registration method to align a RT3DUS volume slice with a CMR image using a differential transformation technique, but the deformation was limited to the global affine transformation. In this paper, we extend our previous work to non-rigid registration that combines the best aspects of both feature-based and intensity-based image registration methods. In our new method, the mutual information of local phase is derived as the similarity measure to capture the feature relationship between both modality images. The polyaffine transformation, a diffieomorphic transformation, which mixes several local displacements via an ordinary differential equation (ODE), is adopted to model the local deformation of ventricles. By calculating the mismatch measure based on phase mutual information, the anchor points (or control points) of polyaffine transformation is automatically identified where the most misaligned region is located. The registration proceeds in an adaptive and multiscale manner to reduce computation. In the following sections, we will first detail our method in section 2, followed by the adaptive non-rigid registration algorithm presented in section 3. In section 4, the result and validation of one volunteer dataset is demonstrated. Finally, section 5 summarizes the proposed work and describes possible future work.

2 Method

Our method consists of three main steps. First of all, both modality images are transformed into their corresponding phase maps. A local mis-match measure using phase mutual information then automatically identifies the centers of several misaligned regions that act as the anchor points (the regional parameter) for a polyaffine transformation. Finally, the parameters of the polyaffine transformation are adaptively tuned in a multi-scale framework in order to reduce the expensive computation of non-rigid registration. In this section, we present the different stages of our method.

2.1 Monogenic Signal and Phase Mutual Information

Most image registration methods use the intensity as the natural image descriptor, while local phase is an alternative image descriptor that better describes image structure (rather than signal magnitude). It has previously been argued as a good representation for ultrasound image analysis [7,8]. Local image phase can be efficiently estimated using the monogenic signal [9], which is derived by a pair of vector valued filters H_1 and H_2 that are odd and distributed with isotropic energy in the frequency domain:

$$. H_1(u,v) = \frac{u}{\sqrt{u^2+v^2}}i, H_2(u,v) = \frac{v}{\sqrt{u^2+v^2}}i \tag{1}$$

where u, v are the Fourier domain coordinates. Let I be the image, then in the space domain, local phase ϕ can be caculated using the filer in equation (1) and the bandpass filtered image $g = f * I$ (where f is the bandpass filter) as:

$$\phi(x,y) = \tan^{-1}\left(\frac{g}{\sqrt{(h_1 \bigotimes g)^2 + (h_2 \bigotimes g)^2}}\right) \tag{2}$$

The local phase can thus be interpreted as a qualitative description of a detected feature, such as the edge or ridge in a signal.

It should be noted that it is necessary to carefully choose a zero mean bandpass filter for affine (or non-rigid) registration as some bandpasss filters are not affine invariant, which make it difficult to accurately predict the effect of an increment to the affine transformation so as to bring about a desired change in phase. We propose to use the scale invariant filter to estimate the local phase, which reduce this problem significantly [8]. Figure 1 shows the phases estimated from a 2D CMR image and a RT3DUS volume slice.

It is now straightforward to extend the intensity based mutual information to one based on phase:

$$MI(\phi_I, \phi_J) = \sum \mathcal{P}(\phi_I, \phi_J) \ln\left(\frac{\mathcal{P}(\phi_I, \phi_J)}{\mathcal{P}(\phi_I)\mathcal{P}(\phi_J)}\right) \tag{3}$$

where $\mathcal{P}(\phi_I, \phi_J)$ is the phase joint probability and $\mathcal{P}(\phi_I), \mathcal{P}(\phi_J)$ is the individual phase probability. Replacing the intensity-based mutual information with the

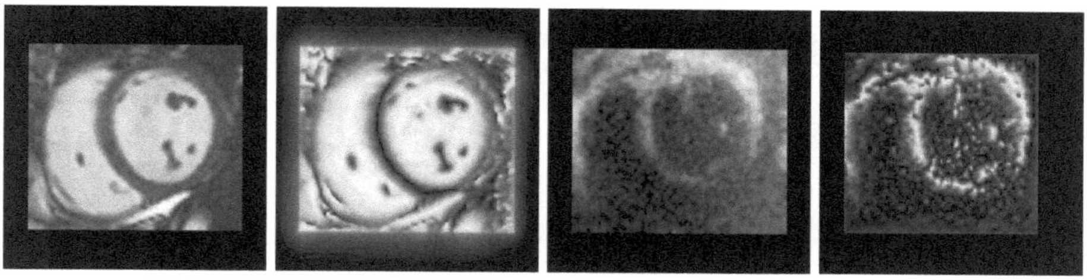

Fig. 1. An example of the phase representation with scale invariant filter. From left to right: CMR image and its phase representation; RT3DUS slice and its phase representation.

local phase one can detect a meaningful structural relationship between the local shapes of an image pair. Furthermore, the mutual information of local phase avoids the intensity changes cross multi-modalities and makes no assumption of a like-with-like correspondence, which make it well-suited for cardiovascular image registration.

2.2 Polyaffine Transformation

The heart is undergoing a spatially varying motion during the cardiac cycle. Even at the same phase of the cardiac cycle, multi-modal cardiac images exhibit local differences due to the motion between the examinations and the different ways to acquire and slice the datasets, which are not easily modeled by only a rigid transformation. In this paper, we assume that the deformation of the ventricles in multi-modal cardiac images is composed of locally affine transformations.

In order to model the deformation that presents several local behaviours, we propose to employ the polyaffine frame work to obtain a globally non-rigid transformation [10]. The idea behind the polyaffine transformation is to weight the sum of local displacements according to a weight function for each arbitrary image region:

$$T_{global}(x) = \frac{\sum_i w_i(x) T_i(x)}{\sum_i w_i(x)} \tag{4}$$

where $T_{global}(x)$ denotes the globally weighted transformation for a point x in the image domain; w_i and T_i denote the weight function and the local displacement for an image region i respectively.

In equation 4, the local displacement is obtained via an ODE to guarantee the invertibility property as all transformations induced by an ODE are reversible [11]. Therefore it can avoid the "folding" effect that a traditional spline-based transformation tends to produce at the high image resolution [12,13]. More precisely, if the locally affine transformation is associated with the speed vector field of a first order ODE, a point x under its motion can be considered as a trajectory governed by the following ODE:

$$\frac{\partial(x)}{\partial(s)} = V_i(x,s) = T_i(x,s) = (A_i + \exp(sA_i) S_i \exp(-sAi)).(x - st_i) + t_i \tag{5}$$

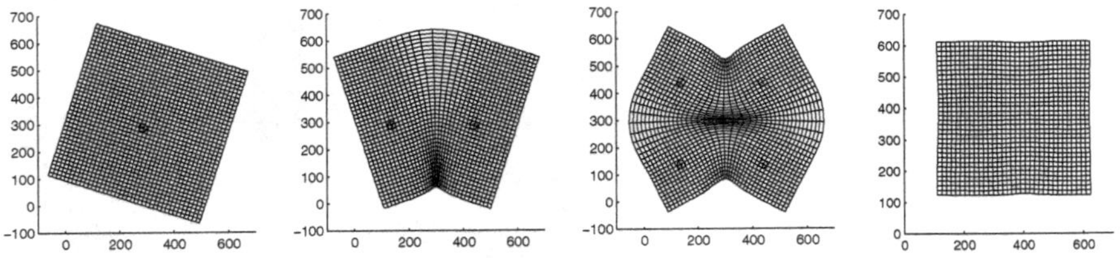

Fig. 2. An example of polyaffine transformation. From left to right: regular grids (in green) deformed by the polyaffine transformation with one, two and four anchor points respectively and the inversed grid (in blue).

where $V_i(x, s)$ is the speed vector field characterized by a time parameter s varying between 0 and 1 and defined to be smooth with respect to x. The last term in equation 5 is obtained by differentiating the trajectory equation $x(s) = \exp(sA_i).\exp(sS_i) + st_i$ with respect to the time parameter s, where M_i and t_i are the deformation (rotation, scaling and shearing) and translation parts in the locally affine transformation respectively; A_i and S_i are the real skew square matrix and symmetric matrix respectively.[1] The local displacement T_i is then obtained by continuously integrating the flow in speed vector between time 0 and time 1.

The local displacement in an arbitrary image region affects the global transformation unequally and its influence needs to be weighted. A weight function can act as a pre-defined shape for each region and play an important role in modeling its influence in the image space. The globally weighted transformation can encompass all the weighted influences of each region. In this paper, we propose to adopt the Gaussian model to define the weight function:

$$w_i(x) = p_i \sum_{i=1}^{n_i} G_{(a_i^j, \sigma_i^j)}(x) \tag{6}$$

where p denotes the relative weight that ranks the global influence of each region, σ denotes the standard deviation that controls the smoothness of the weighted transformation and a indicates the anchor point that describes how each region of core influence is geometrically anchored. In each region i, it can have its own number of j anchor points which are obtained either by automatic identification or by manual selection. In summary, there are two categories of parameters of

[1] To define the local polyaffine transformation, it is required that there exists a real logarithm of M_i and a real skew square matrix A_i, which satisfy the relationship $M_i = \exp(A_i)$. Unfortunately, for a locally affine transformation, this can not be satisfied since not all real invertible matrices M_i admit a real logarithm. However, Wustner point out that any element of a real connected Lie Group is equal to the product of two exponentials [14]. Thus the deformation part can be represented as $M_i = \exp(A_i)\exp(S_i)$ by the singular value decomposition (SVD).

the polyaffine transformation for any registration task: the local deformation parameters defined in the speed vector field and the regional parameters defined in the weight function.

2.3 Local Mis-match Measure

In the polyaffine frame work, it would be desirable for the anchor point to carry some information about where the misaligned regions are located so that the polyaffine transformation can effectively adjust these control points to make them aligned and correct the spatial difference. Further more, the automatic identification of these anchor points can be adapted from the grid refinement methods that use the gradient of the mutual information or the local entropy of the image to put an irregular grid of control points on the image pair [15,16,17].

In this paper, we extended the local mis-match measure proposed by Park et al [15] to automatically identify the anchor point (the centre of local misaligned region) of a polyaffine transformation by using the local phase mutual information. If a region between an image pair is observed to have a low phase MI, it is said that the region is less correlated by local features. On the other hand, a low phase MI may imply that either a corresponding region has low entropy or is devoid of features. A region with low entropy is less "interesting" as it contains fewer features such as the image background and noise. Therefore those regions with high local entropy and a low phase MI are found to be the most misaligned. These notions are formalized in a normalized measure:

$$M_\phi = 1 - \frac{MI(\phi_I, \phi_J)}{\min(H(\phi_I), H(\phi_J))} \tag{7}$$

where $MI(\phi_I, \phi_J)$ is the phase mutual information between two images and $H(\phi_I), H(\phi_J)$ are the local phase entropy of the images. If the phase MI goes down to zero or the phase MI is relatively smaller than $\min(H(\phi_I), H(\phi_J))$, the mis-match measure gets the largest value (close to one), which implies a less aligned or a featureless region needs to be corrected by the proposed transformation.

All the values of the mis-match measure are locally computed on a finite sub-block across the whole image. The measure yields the best performance on detecting the misaligned region whose scale is similar to the sub-block size. Therefore the size of the sub-block can be viewed as the scale parameter that determines the range of locally misaligned region. If the sub-block size is defined to be larger, the detected centre of the misaligned region might be less reliable since the mis-match measure has to calculate over a larger sub-block than the real deformation and the most misaligned location may be blurred by a larger sub-block. On the contrary, multiple detected locations will occur within the same deformation if we employ the local mis-match measure on a smaller sub-block size. Thus in practice some prior knowledge about the expected deformation is needed. In this paper, we use a sub-block size of 31×31 pixels.

3 The Algorithm

The proposed adaptive non-rigid registration operates on multi-scales from coarse to fine. There are two loops in the algorithm. The outer loop is controlled by the standard deviation σ of the weight function, whose value determines the density of the global transformation. For the coarse scale, we set a large value σ to ensure the smoothness of the global transformation. However, for the finer scale, we set a small value σ to model a dense local deformation. The inner loop adaptively tunes the deformation parameter of the polyaffine transformation and places extra anchor points, followed by the maximization of the global phase mutual information.

For the first iteration, affine registration is performed to ensure that the global registration has taken effect before attempting the further local deformation. For the subsequent non-rigid registration, only the angle of local rotation and the anchor points of each region are respectively increased until the algorithm reaches a pre-defined threshold of optimal phase mutual information.

For both registrations, the local phase maps of both modality images are firstly estimated using the monogenic signal. In the initialization step when the initial affine registration is done, $N \geq 4$ initial anchor points are placed where the maximum misalignment occurs between the divided N regions of the image pair, based on an estimate of the local misaligned measure using phase mutual information. The polyaffine transformation is then estimated by iteratively adding an increment to the angle of the local rotation vector ranged from 0.1π to 0.2π(we have limited the full range of the local deformation to reduce computational cost). At each iteration, the optimization of the transformation is performed by maximizing the global phase mutual information. If the optimized global phase mutual information tends to increase but does not arrive at the user defined threshold, which implies that tuning the angle of rotation vector can no longer recover more localized deformation, an extra anchor point is placed in each pre-divided region for the next iterations at the higher resolution level.

When there is a need to place an extra anchor point in the misaligned region, we seek a minimum distance constraint to avoid placing two anchor points at the same location and to determine the distance between the extra anchor point and the existing anchor point. The minimum distance constraint is similar to the deformation scale, whose value determines the scale of local deformation that can be corrected. Therefore the sub-block size used to calculate the mis-match measure is the best choice to define the distance between any two anchor points. We suggest that the minimum distance constraint should be smaller than the sub-block size so that the extra anchor points can correct the local deformation only within the sub-block.

4 Results

One volunteer dataset was used in the experiments. The CMR images were acquired using a 1.5 Tesla Siemens Sonata. A 20 slice acquisition was used with a

Algorithm 1. Adaptive Non-Rigid Multi-Modal Registration

```
Ensure: affine registration
Require: transform both modality images into their corresponding local
  phase maps
Require: place N ≥ 4 anchor points where the maximum misalignment occurs
  in the pre-divided regions, based on an initial estimate of the local
  mis-match measure
  for S = large σ to small σ do
    for R = 0.1π to 0.2π do
      Tune the rotation vector of the polyaffine transformation
      Calculate the global phase mutual information
    end for
    if  the global phase mutual information increases but is smaller than
    the user defined threshold then
      Add one more anchor point to the maximum misaligned region
      according to the minimum distance constraint
    end if
  end for
```

280×340 mm field of view, a 1.8×1.8 mm in-plane resolution and a 7.5 mm slice thickness with a 7.5mm gap between slices. ECG gating was used and breath-hold commands issued via the intercom system. The short axis (SA) slices were automatically aligned with the heart axis with one localizer sequence, using the method presented by Jackson et al [18]. One of the cropped SA slice was arbitrarily selected as the reference image. The RT3D echocardiography was acquired using a Philips Sonos 7500. The SA slice was taken from a RT3D apical acquisition. The volunteer dataset had 17 frames in one cardiac cycle. One slice from one of the frames was visually identified to match the ECG gated end-diastole MR reference image and the two matched to estimate the transformation parameters (i.e. every 104th slice from frame 1 of volunteer's scan). The estimated transformation was then applied to each slice of the ultrasound frames.

4.1 Global Affine Registration

The global affine registration is the special case of the polyaffine transformation, in which the image is not split into several regions; therefore the mismatch measure is calculated across the whole image domain. In addition to the global rotation, the affine transformation considers the translation between the RT3DUS slice and CMR image, which is achieved by using two common landmarks between the image pair. The landmark in the RT3DUS slice is the centre of the maximum misaligned region. In figure 3, the identified location is marked as the red star in the RT3DUS slice, whose Euclidean coordinate is (176, 156). The other landmark in CMR image is the equivalent point to the one found in the RT3DUS (this is generally easy to do in the example we have considered). The translation vector is simply calculated as the Euclidean distance between the two landmarks, while the rotation vector is adaptively tuned by adding a small increment, following an optimization of the global phase mutual information at each iteration.

Figure 3 illustrates the registered RT3DUS slice superimposed with the CMR image and the CMR contour for visual comparison. Although the result gets close to the optimal transformation, there are still misalignments around the left ventricle and the papillary muscle, which implies a need for further local deformation to correct for the spatial difference. The value of the global phase mutual information increases from 0.93 to 1.18 after the affine registration. By comparison of our previous work [1], the new global affine transformation has less parameters to optimize (the differential transformation was working on a regular size grid of 64x64 pixels). Therefore it is very efficient to compute.

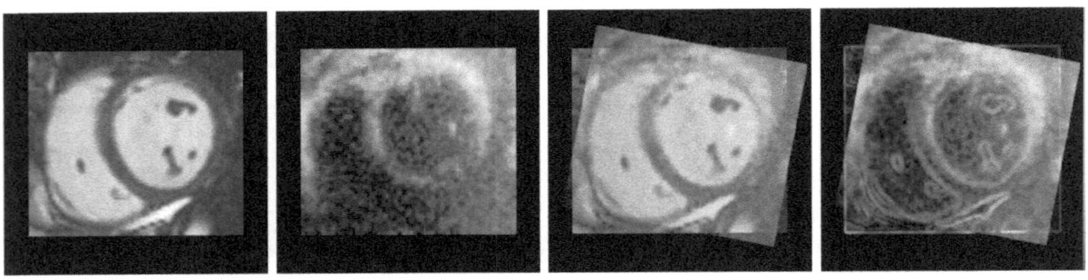

Fig. 3. Illustrating the result of the global affine registration. From left to right: the reference image (cardiovascular MR image) on, the floating image (RT3DUS volume slice) with one anchor point (in red star) and the registered ultrasound images superimposed by the reference image and the contour estimated by Canny edge detector.

4.2 Adaptive Non-rigid Registration

Following the affine registration and the initialization step, the adaptive non-rigid registration starts from the coarse scale and continues to the finest scale. In figure 4, four anchor points marked as red stars in the RT3DUS slice are identified in the initialization step at the coarse scale ($\sigma = 100$). Three additional anchor points marked as to blue stars are placed in the divided regions at the next finer scale ($\sigma = 60$), according to the minimum distance constraint. At the third and finest scale ($\sigma = 40$), only one more anchor point marked as the yellow star has been placed in the maximum misaligned region. Although more localized deformations can be modeled by adding more anchor points, we propose to reduce the number of additional anchor points at each scale. This is because some local misalignment can be well corrected by using only one anchor point. Moreover, a large number of anchor points at the finest scale iteration would demand expensive computation and cause "shearing" which produces an unrealistic warped image. Therefore, after each inner loop, we recalculate the mis-match measure and accordingly place the extra anchor points only where the misaligned regions is not well recovered from lower scale iterations.

Figure 4 shows the registered RT3DUS slice superimposed with the CMR image and the CMR contour at the coarse scale and the finest scale respectively.

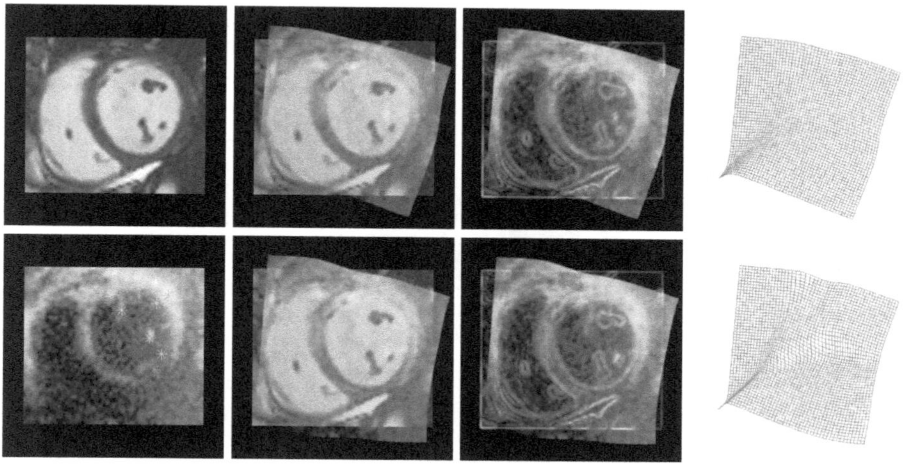

Fig. 4. Illustrating the result of the adaptive non-rigid registration. Left column: the reference image and the floating image with anchor points calculated by the local mismatch measure at scale 2 and 3. Middle columns: the registered images superimposed by the reference image and the edge contours.

Only four anchor points have already recovered most spatial difference of the myocardium around the left ventricle between the image pair. However, the papillary muscle still appears off aligned. By adding extra anchor points at the finest scale, the spatial difference of the papillary muscle is corrected to some extent.

5 Validation

Validation of registration accuracy is a difficult task, because the ground truth is not generally available. In cardiovascular image registration, a global measure of registration accuracy is not really what is required; the main interest is the target registration error in the cardiac area. Registration methods are also often validated by using external marks, anatomical landmarks, or external fiducial frames as gold standards and we use this method here. In our work, the anatomical landmarks in cardiovascular images, such as, the conjoint of the anterior and anterior septum, the conjoint of the septum and inferior PPM, and the APM, were carefully identified by an experienced clinical expert in the RT3DUS slice. The identified anatomical landmarks were registered to the CMR image as the reference standard. The measure of the registration accuracy is defined as the root mean square error (RMS) distance of the identified anatomical landmarks between the registered RT3D slice and the reference standard. The results of the registration accuracy were 2.32mm and 3.47mm for the adaptive non-rigid registration and the global affine registration respectively. Alternatively, we provide the visual (qualitative) assessment of alignment by superimposing the registered RT3D slice with the reference standard.

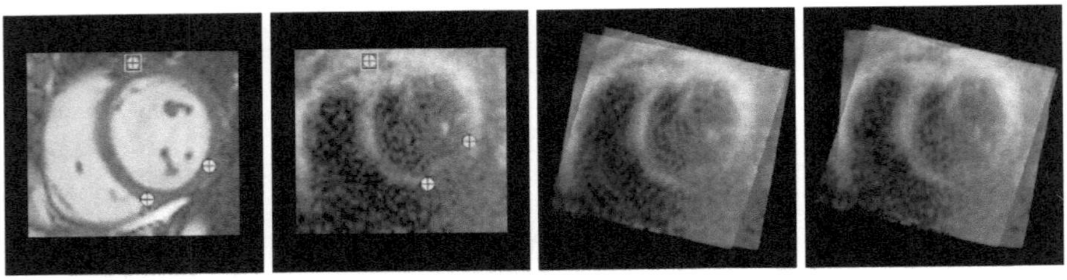

Fig. 5. Illustrating the result of the registration accuracy. Left to right: the reference image and the floating image with expert-identified landmarks; the globally affine registered and adaptively non-rigid registered RT3DUS slices superposed by the reference standard.

6 Discussion

In this paper, a novel algorithm has been presented to solve the problem of non-rigidly registering a pair of US and MR images. The deformation is modeled by a polyaffine transformation. Small local deformation particular cardiac regions, e.g. the papillary muscle between the image pair, can be recovered by adding extra anchor points to the maximal misaligned regions. The anchor point is automatically identified by the local mis-match measure using the phase mutual information. Adopting the local phase as the image descriptor is shown to increase the accuracy of non-rigid registration in terms of the information theory based similarity measure. In particular, the RMS TRE (non-rigid registration) is better than the one found in related research on MR-US registration (Penney et al. [6]), but in a very different clinical domain.

In this initial work we have assumed temporal alignment of multi-modal frames so registration has been reduced to a static image registration problem. For the complex motion of the heart, we expect an accurate spatial-temporal non-rigid registration result with the polyaffine transformation. We are looking at this in current work together with extending the method to RT3DUS to multi-slice CMR registration which will be computationally more demanding but enable correlation of 3D information between these two modalities. Challenges here relate to the difference in spatial and temporal resolution and producing a final method that is fast enough to be useful in clinical practice. Clinical uses of the alignment will also be explored.

Acknowledgements. We thank the Oxford Centre for Clinical MR Research (Dr Matthew Robson) and the Oxford John Radcliffe Hospital Cardiology Department (Dr Harold Becher) for providing the clinical motivation and data.

References

1. Zhang, W.W., Noble, J.A., Brady, J.M.: Real time 3d ultrasound to mr cardiovascular image registration using phase-based approach. In: Proc. ISBI. (2006)
2. Panza, J.A.: Real-time three-dimemsional echocardiography: An overview. Int. J. Cardiovasc. Imag. 17, 227–235 (2001)

3. Makela, T.J., et al.: A review of caridac image registration methods. IEEE Trans. Med. Imag. 21, 1011–1021 (2002)
4. Pluim, J.P., Maintz, J.B.A., Viergever, M.A.: Mutual information based registration of medical images: A survey. IEEE Trans. Med. Imag. 22, 986–1004 (2003)
5. Roche, A., Pennec, X., Malandin, G., Ayache, N.: Rigid registration of 3d ultrasound with mr images: A new approach combining intensity and gradient information. IEEE Trans. Med. Imag. 20, 1038–1049 (2001)
6. Penny, G.P., Blackhall, J.M., et al.: Registration of freehand 3d ultrasound and magnetic resonance liver images. Med. Imag. Anal. 8, 81–91 (2004)
7. Mulet-Parada, M., Noble, J.A.: 2d+t acoustic boundary detection in echocardiography. Med. Imag. Anal. 4, 21–30 (2000)
8. Mellor, M., Brady, J.M.: Phase mutual information as a similarity measure for registration. Med. Imag. Anal. 9, 330–343 (2005)
9. Felsberg, M., Sommer, G.: new extension of linear signal processing for estimating local properties and detecting features. In: Proc. DAGM, pp. 195–202 (2000)
10. Arsigny, V., Pennec, X., Ayache, N.: Polyrigid and polyaffine transformations: A novel geometrical tool to deal with non-rigid deformations - application to the registration of histological slices. Med. Imag. Anal. 9, 507–523 (2005)
11. Tenebaum, M., Pollard, H.: Ordinary differential equations. Dover (1985)
12. Rueckert, D., et al.: Non-rigid registration using free-form deformation: Application to breast mr images. IEEE Trans. Med. Imag. 18, 712–721 (1999)
13. Meyer, C.R.: Demonstration of accuracy and clinical versatility of mutual information for automatic multimodality image fusion using affine and thin plate spline warped geometric deformations. Med. Imag. Anal. 1, 195–206 (1997)
14. Wustner, M.: A connected lie group equals the square of the exponential image. J. Lie Theory. 13, 307–309 (2003)
15. Park, H., Bland, P.H., Brock, K.K., Meyer, C.R.: Adaptive registration using local information measures. Med. Imag. Anal. 8, 465–473 (2004)
16. Schnabel, A., et al.: A generic framework for non-rigid registration based on non-uniform multi-level free form deformations. In: Niessen, W.J., Viergever, M.A. (eds.) MICCAI 2001. LNCS, vol. 2208, pp. 573–581. Springer, Heidelberg (2001)
17. Rohde, G.K., Aldroubi, A., Dawant, B.M.: The adaptive bases algorithm for intensity-based non-rigid registration. IEEE Trans. Med. Imag. 22, 1470–1479 (2003)
18. Jackson, C.E., Robson, M.D., Francis, J.M., Noble, J.A.: Computerised planning of the acquisition of cardiac mr images. Comp. Med. Imag. Grap. 28, 411–418 (2004)

Multi-slice Three-Dimensional Myocardial Strain Tensor Quantification Using *z*HARP

Khaled Z. Abd-Elmoniem[1], Matthias Stuber[1,2], and Jerry L. Prince[1,2]

[1] Electrical and Computer Engineering department, Johns Hopkins University, Baltimore MD 21218, USA
khaled@jhu.edu

[2] Department of Radiology and Radiological Sciences, School of Medicine, Johns Hopkins School of Medicine, Baltimore, MD 21287, USA

Abstract. In this article we propose a novel method for calculating cardiac 3-D strain. The method requires the acquisition of myocardial short-axis (SA) slices only and produces the 3-D strain tensor at every point within every pair of slices. Three-dimensional displacement is calculated from SA slices using *z*HARP which is then used for calculating the local displacement gradient and thus the local strain tensor. There are three main advantages of this method. First, the 3-D strain tensor is calculated for every pixel without interpolation; this is unprecedented in cardiac MR imaging. Second, this method is fast, in part because there is no need to acquire long-axis (LA) slices. Third, the method is accurate because the 3-D displacement components are acquired simultaneously and therefore reduces motion artifacts without the need for registration. This article presents the theory of computing 3-D strain from two slices using *z*HARP, the imaging protocol, and both phantom and in-vivo validation.

1 Introduction

Magnetic resonance imaging (MRI) of cardiac regional function has gained a wide acceptance in the diagnosis of cardiac diseases that are related to abnormal cardiac mechanics. Regional cardiac imaging methods, e.g., MR tagging [1,2] and DENSE [3], encode 1-D or 2-D in-plane displacement components. These displacements are used to calculate in-plane strain. Harmonic phase (HARP) imaging[4,5] is a fast method to acquire and calculate in-plane displacement and strain from tagged data. Strain-encoding (SENC) imaging is used to directly image the through-plane strain of a particular slice. Extending strain quantification from 1-D or 2-D to the quantification of the 3-D strain tensor for each material point has been a challenging task because of the prohibitively long scan times and its susceptibility to mis-registration caused by patient motion, breathing, and heart rate variation.

A quick but incomplete 3-D strain quantification is done by acquiring SENC and tagging for the same imaged slice. The technique is less accurate because

N. Karssemeijer and B. Lelieveldt (Eds.): IPMI 2007, LNCS 4584, pp. 62–73, 2007.
© Springer-Verlag Berlin Heidelberg 2007

both tagging and SENC are insensitive to through-plane tilting and SENC is not a slice-following procedure. Other methods proposed applying tagged MRI to an SA slice and as many LA slices as possible in order to produce 3-D strain at the intersection lines of the SA and LA slices[6,7,8,9,10]. Three-dimensional displacement tracking from a single slice (zHARP) [11,12] has been recently developed for simultaneous tracking of the 3-D displacement of every material point within the acquired slice.

In this article, we propose a method that overcomes the limitations of the previous 3-D strain quantification methods. The method produces the full 3-D strain tensor for every material point in N slices for every $N+1$ zHARP parallel SA slices. A complete 3-D strain tensor covering the whole left ventricle is therefore possible in as few as fourteen breath-hold scans[1]. Results from a compressible phantom and in-vivo experiments show a strong correlation between the proposed method and a conventional 3-D method both visually and from linear regression and Bland-Altman statistics.

2 Background

2.1 Definitions

A region $\mathcal{S}$ of tissue is assumed to be the *reference configuration* of a moving object in Euclidean space $\mathcal{E}$. Points $\mathbf{p} \in \mathcal{S}$ are called *material points.* A *motion* of $\mathcal{S}$ is a class C^3 function

$$\mathbf{X} : \mathcal{S} \times \mathbb{R} \rightarrow \mathcal{E}$$

with $\mathbf{X}(\cdot, t)$. For each fixed time t, $\mathbf{X}$ is a *deformation* of $\mathcal{S}$. The spatial position occupied by the material point $\mathbf{p}$ at time t is given by

$$\mathbf{x}=\mathbf{X}(\mathbf{p}, t), \text{ where } \mathbf{x} \equiv [x, y, z]^T \tag{1}$$

and the region of space occupied by the object at time t is

$$\mathcal{S}_t = \mathbf{X}(\mathcal{S}, t)\,.$$

At each t, $\mathbf{X}(\cdot, t)$ is a one-to-one mapping of $\mathcal{S}$ onto $\mathcal{S}_t$; hence it has an inverse $\mathbf{P}(\cdot, t) : \mathcal{S}_t \rightarrow \mathcal{S}$ such that $\mathbf{P}(\mathbf{X}(\mathbf{p}, t)) = \mathbf{p}$ and $\mathbf{X}(\mathbf{P}(\mathbf{x}, t)) = \mathbf{x}$. The spatial vector $\mathbf{u}(\cdot,\ t) : \mathcal{S}_t \rightarrow \mathcal{E}$

$$\mathbf{u}\left(\mathbf{x}, t\right) \equiv \left[u_x, u_y, u_z\right]^{\mathbf{T}} = \mathbf{x} - \mathbf{P}\left(\mathbf{x}, t\right),$$

is called the spatial (Eulerian) *displacement vector* and $\nabla\mathbf{u}$ is called the *displacement gradient* and is given by

$$\nabla\mathbf{u}\left(\mathbf{x}, t\right) = \begin{pmatrix} \frac{\partial u_x}{\partial x} & \frac{\partial u_x}{\partial y} & \frac{\partial u_x}{\partial z} \\ \frac{\partial u_y}{\partial x} & \frac{\partial u_y}{\partial y} & \frac{\partial u_y}{\partial z} \\ \frac{\partial u_z}{\partial x} & \frac{\partial u_z}{\partial y} & \frac{\partial u_z}{\partial z} \end{pmatrix} \tag{2}$$

The deformation gradient $\mathbf{F}$ is defined by

$$\mathbf{F}^{-1} = \left(\mathbf{I} - \nabla\mathbf{u}\right)\,. \tag{3}$$

[1] Using seven zHARP slices. Each of them is acquired in two breath-hold scans.

2.2 *z*HARP Pulse Sequence

*z*HARP is an MRI tagging pulse sequence that is an extension of slice-following CSPAMM (SF-CSPAMM)[13,14]. Instead of only encoding the in-plane displacement of the imaged slice as it is the case in SF-CSPAMM, *z*HARP also encodes the through-plane displacement, which allows tracking the 3-D path-lines of any point in the image plane. As shown in Fig. 1, *z*HARP is a segmented *k*-space pulse sequence that requires $4R$ heartbeats where R is the number of segments per cine data set. Each cine data set contains Q time-frames. The four cine

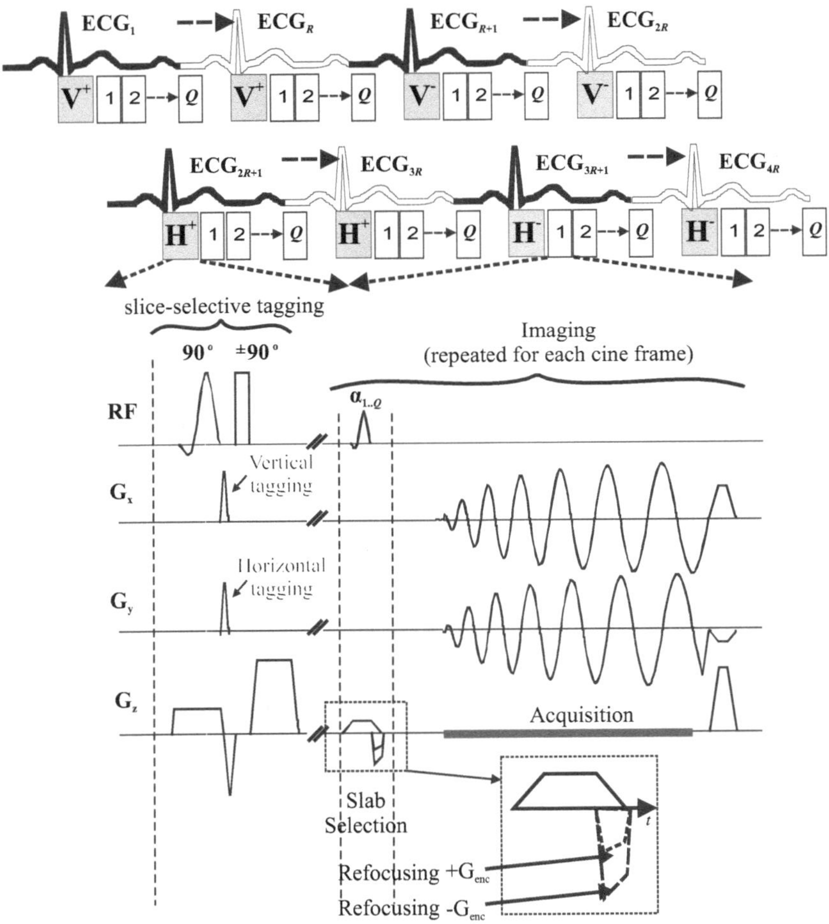

Fig. 1. Single-slice *z*HARP pulse sequence

data sets are tagged with vertical cosine, vertical minus cosine, horizontal cosine, and horizontal minus cosine tagging patterns, respectively. A gradient G_{enc} in the slice-select direction is turned on before the acquisition with positive and negative polarities in the vertical and horizontal tagging, respectively. After the complex addition of the vertical and the horizontal data sets, separately, we end up with the two data sets

$$\begin{aligned} I_v(x,y,t) &\approx \rho(\mathbf{x},t)\, e^{j\varphi_e(\mathbf{x})} e^{\,j\kappa z} \cos\left(\omega\left(x-u_x(\mathbf{x},t)\right)\right), \\ &= \frac{\rho(\mathbf{x},t)}{2}\left[e^{j(\varphi_e+\kappa z+\omega u_x-\omega x)} + e^{j(\varphi_e+\kappa z-\omega u_x+\omega x)}\right] \end{aligned} \quad (4)$$

$$\begin{aligned} I_h(x,y,t) &\approx \rho(\mathbf{x},t)\, e^{j\varphi_e(\mathbf{x})} e^{-j\kappa z} \cos\left(\omega\left(y-u_y(\mathbf{x},t)\right)\right), \\ &= \frac{\rho(\mathbf{x},t)}{2}\left[e^{j(\varphi_e-\kappa z+\omega u_y-\omega y)} + e^{j(\varphi_e-\kappa z-\omega u_y+\omega y)}\right] \end{aligned} \quad (5)$$

where ρ is the spin density, ω is the tag frequency, $\kappa \equiv \gamma G_{enc}$ is the z-encode frequency, γ is the gyromagnetic ratio, and φ_e is the artefactual phase caused by susceptibility and general field inhomogeneity.

2.3 zHARP 3-D Displacement Extraction

The Fourier transform of each of I_v and I_h consists of two distinct harmonic spectral peaks and no peaks at the origin. Therefore, applying HARP filtering to these four peaks produces four distinct HARP phases

$$\phi_A \equiv \varphi_e + \varphi_z - \varphi_x$$

$$\phi_B \equiv \varphi_e + \varphi_z + \varphi_x$$

$$\phi_C \equiv \varphi_e - \varphi_z - \varphi_y$$

$$\phi_D \equiv \varphi_e - \varphi_z + \varphi_y$$

where φ_x, φ_y, and $\varphi_z$are the elements of the the 3-D harmonic phase vector map $\mathbf{\Phi}$, defined as

$$\mathbf{\Phi}(\mathbf{x},t) \equiv \begin{pmatrix} \varphi_x \\ \varphi_y \\ \varphi_z \end{pmatrix} = \mathcal{W}\left(\begin{pmatrix} \omega & 0 & 0 \\ 0 & \omega & 0 \\ 0 & 0 & \kappa \end{pmatrix} \begin{pmatrix} u_x \\ u_y \\ u_z \end{pmatrix} \right). \quad (6)$$

The operator $\mathcal{W}(\cdot)$ is the wrapping function

$$\mathcal{W}(\theta) = \mathrm{mod}(\theta + \pi, 2\pi) - \pi .$$

Upon solving for φ_x, φ_y, and φ_z, we get

$$\begin{aligned} \varphi_x &= (\phi_B - \phi_A)/2 , \\ \varphi_y &= (\phi_D - \phi_C)/2 , \\ \varphi_z &= [(\phi_A + \phi_B) - (\phi_C + \phi_D)]/4 . \end{aligned}$$

3 Theory

3.1 Three-Dimensional Strain

The *Eulerian strain tensor* $E(\mathbf{x}, \mathrm{t})$ is defined by[15]

$$E(\mathbf{x}, t) \equiv \begin{pmatrix} \varepsilon_{xx} & \varepsilon_{xy} & \varepsilon_{xz} \\ \varepsilon_{yx} & \varepsilon_{yy} & \varepsilon_{yz} \\ \varepsilon_{zx} & \varepsilon_{zy} & \varepsilon_{zz} \end{pmatrix} \quad \text{,where } \varepsilon_{ij} = \varepsilon_{ji} \; .$$

It is related to the deformation gradient $\mathbf{F}$ by

$$E = \frac{1}{2}\left[\mathbf{I} - \left(\mathbf{F}^{-1}\right)^T \mathbf{F}^{-1}\right]. \tag{7}$$

3.2 *z*HARP 3-D Displacement Gradient

Restoration of the actual displacement $\mathbf{u}(\mathbf{x}, t)$ requires a sophisticated unwrapping algorithm that is not necessary for strain calculation. Instead $\nabla\mathbf{u}$ is readily computed using

$$\nabla\mathbf{u}(\mathbf{x}, t) = \begin{pmatrix} \omega^{-1} & 0 & 0 \\ 0 & \omega^{-1} & 0 \\ 0 & 0 & \kappa^{-1} \end{pmatrix} \nabla^{\star}\mathbf{\Phi}(\mathbf{x}, t) \tag{8}$$

where

$$\nabla^{\star}\mathbf{\Phi}(\mathbf{x}, t) \equiv \begin{pmatrix} \nabla^{\star}\varphi_x \\ \nabla^{\star}\varphi_y \\ \nabla^{\star}\varphi_z \end{pmatrix}$$

and

$$\nabla^{\star}\varphi_k \equiv \begin{cases} \nabla\varphi_k & \|\nabla\varphi_k\| \le \|\nabla\mathcal{W}(\varphi_k + \pi)\| \\ \nabla\mathcal{W}(\varphi_k + \pi) & \text{otherwise} \end{cases}, \; k = x, y, z. \tag{9}$$

3.3 *z*HARP 3-D Strain Algorithm

Given two parallel *z*HARP slices, the following steps are used to calculate the pixel-wise 3-D strain tensor $E(\mathbf{x}, \mathrm{t})$.

Step1. Extract the the 3-D harmonic phase vector maps $\mathbf{\Phi}(\mathbf{x}^{(1)}, t)$ and $\mathbf{\Phi}(\mathbf{x}^{(2)}, t)$ on an equidistant mesh of points of size N covering the myocardium region-of-interest where

$$\mathbf{x}^{(n)} \equiv \mathbf{x}^{(n)}(i, j) \equiv \begin{pmatrix} x^{(i)} \\ y^{(j)} \\ z^{(n)}\left(x^{(i)}, y^{(j)}\right) \end{pmatrix}, \; 1 \le i, j \le N$$

Step2. Given $\mathbf{\Phi}\left(\mathbf{x}^{(1)},t\right)$ and $\mathbf{\Phi}\left(\mathbf{x}^{(2)},t\right)$, calculate $\nabla^{\star}\mathbf{\Phi}\left(\mathbf{x}^{(1.5)},t\right)$ as in Eq. (9) using finite difference scheme such that

$$\nabla\varphi_k\left(\mathbf{x}^{(1.5)},t\right)=\frac{1}{2}\left[\nabla\varphi_k\left(\mathbf{x}^{(1)},t\right)+\nabla\varphi_k\left(\mathbf{x}^{(2)},t\right)\right]$$

where

$$\nabla\varphi_k\left(\mathbf{x}^{(n)},t\right)\approx\begin{pmatrix}\varphi_k\left(\mathbf{x}^{(n)}\left(i+1,j\right)\right)-\varphi_k\left(\mathbf{x}^{(n)}\left(i,j\right)\right)\\ \varphi_k\left(\mathbf{x}^{(n)}\left(i,j+1\right)\right)-\varphi_k\left(\mathbf{x}^{(n)}\left(i,j\right)\right)\\ \varphi_k\left(\mathbf{x}^{(2)}\left(i,j\right)\right)\quad-\varphi_k\left(\mathbf{x}^{(1)}\left(i,j\right)\right)\end{pmatrix}^T$$

Step3. Compute $E(\mathbf{x},\mathrm{t})$, the Eulerian strain tensor, by substituting the output of Eq. (9) into Eqs. (8) and (7).

3.4 3-D Strain Tensor Tracking

The *strain tensor* $E(\mathbf{x},\mathrm{t})$ is calculated pixel-by-pixel in the spatial coordinate system. To track the 3-D strain tensor of a specific material point $\mathbf{p}$ the following steps are used:

Step1. Compute $E(\mathbf{x},\mathrm{t}_q)$ as described in Sec. 3.3 at all cardiac phases t_q, $1\leq q\leq Q$

Step2. Consider a given material point $\mathbf{p}$ from the myocardium at the cardiac phase t_1[2]. The path-line or the trajectory $\mathcal{T}(\mathbf{p})$, defined as

$$\mathcal{T}(\mathbf{p})\equiv\left\{(\mathbf{x},t_q)\,|\mathbf{P}(\mathbf{x},t_q)=\mathbf{p},1\leq q\leq Q\right\},\tag{10}$$

is calculated by tracking $\mathbf{p}$ throughout the entire cardiac cycle using zHARP tracking algorithm [11].

Step3. Compute the 3-D strain time-profile $E(\mathcal{T}(\mathbf{p}))$

$$E(\mathcal{T}(\mathbf{p}))\equiv\left\{E(\mathbf{x},t_q)\,|\,(\mathbf{x},t_q)\in\mathcal{T}(\mathbf{p})\right\}.\tag{11}$$

This is done using bi-linear interpolation of $E(\cdot,\mathrm{t}_q)$ of the four closest points to $(\mathbf{x},\mathrm{t}_q)$.

4 Methods

The zHARP pulse sequence was implemented on a Philips 3.0T Achieva MRI scanner (Philips Medical Systems, Best, NL). A six-channel phased array cardiac receiver coil is used in the experiments. Channels are distributed between the anterior and the posterior sides surrounding the chest for human subjects and 35 cm apart for phantom experiments.

[2] In general, any time frame t_q can be chosen as the reference time frame. To simplify mathematical manipulation, t_1 is selected here as such.

4.1 Phantom Experiments

The goal of these experiments was to show that it is possible to measure 3-D strain from parallel image slices.

Setup. A gel phantom was built using Sylgard® 527 Silicone Dielectric Gel (Dow Corning, Midland, Michigan) with 33% of material A and 67% of material B which experimentally possesses magnetic properties (T1 and T2) and elasticity similar to in-vivo muscular tissues.

As shown in Fig. 2, the deformable phantom had a rectangular shape (70 × 50 × 60mm) and was tightly contained in a rigid plastic box except on one side where there was an air-bag and from the top where the gel phantom was allowed to bulge in the y-direction when it got compressed. The air-bag was made to periodically inflate and deflate in the x-direction at a fixed rate of 30 cycles/min. A TTL pulse simulating the R-wave of the heart was generated at the beginning of each compression cycle in order to trigger the air-bag inflation and the MRI scanning simultaneously.

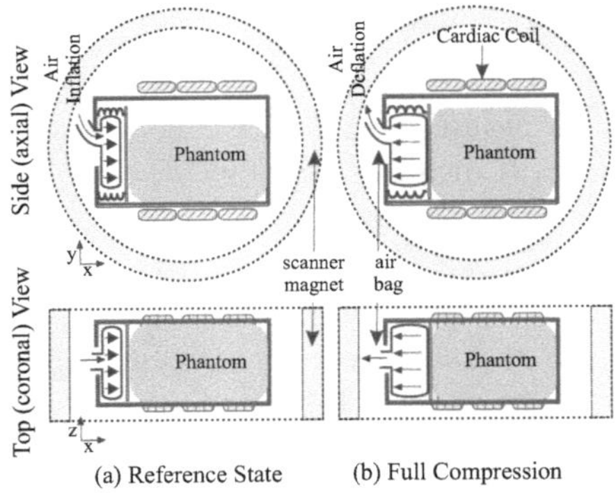

Fig. 2. Phantom Setup in the original and the full-compression states

Data Acquisition. Two phantom experiments were done in which the images were acquired in three orthogonal orientations. The imaging orientations are the sagittal, coronal, and the axial planes. Sagittal planes are orthogonal to the

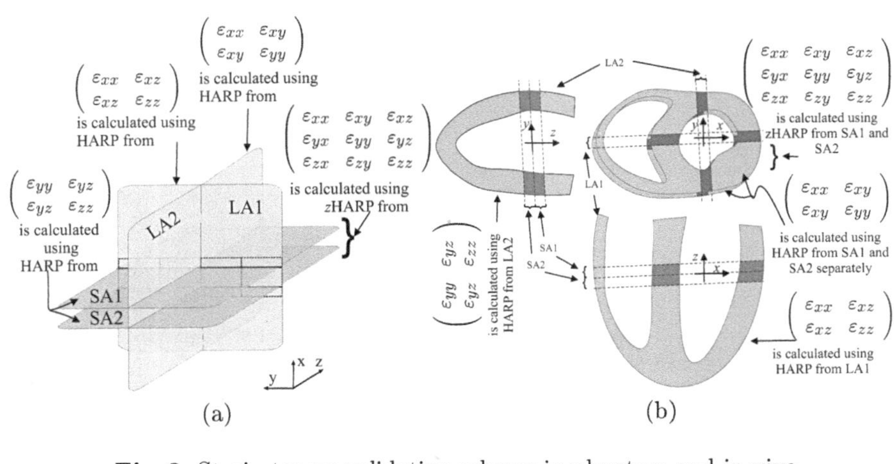

Fig. 3. Strain tensor validation scheme in phantom and in-vivo

x-direction are hence called short-axis (SA) planes. Axial and coronal planes are orthogonal to the SA plane and hence called long-axis (LA) planes. Ten contiguous SA zHARP slices were acquired with $\kappa = \frac{2\pi}{33}$ rad/mm, FOV=160 mm, and slice-thickness=8 mm. For the validation of the through-plane strain components, twenty contiguous LA SF-CSPAMM slices were acquired (10 axial and 10 coronal).

Analysis and Validation. In each SA slice, a fine mesh of points was created covering the whole phantom area in the slice. The 3-D strain tensor $E(\mathbf{x}, \mathrm{t})$ was then calculated and tracked for each point in the mesh in all the SA slices using zHARP as described in Sec. 3.4. For validation, the intersection region between every SA slice and LA slice was divided into three segments. The 3-D strain in each segment is calculated as the average 3-D strain from all the points in the segment. The segmental though-plane strain (calculated from SA slice) was again calculated from the corresponding LA slice using conventional HARP (see Fig. 3). As an example of the method's performance, linear regression and Bland-Altman plots were generated comparing the through-plane strain component ε_{zz} as calculated from SA and LA slices using zHARP and regular HARP, respectively.

4.2 In Vivo Experiments

Three or four SA zHARP slices were acquired from basal to apical position. Slices were 8 mm thick and 8 mm spaced (center-to-center) with a 35 ms temporal resolution, a FOV of 300 mm and 15 cardiac phases. Four radially-spread LA SF-CSPAMM were acquired for validation. From every two contiguous SA slices, a mesh of points were created. The strain tensor $E(\mathbf{x}, \mathrm{t})$ was calculated and tracked throughout the cardiac cycle. The intersection regions between SA and LA slices were used for comparison and validation similar to the phantom procedure.

5 Results

5.1 Phantom Results

Images of the SA and LA slices are shown in Fig. 4(a,b). Notice that the compression is shown in the SA slice as a bulging of tag lines while in the LA slice it is shown as in-plane narrowing of the tag lines. As shown in 4(c,d), ε_{zz} in the SA slice agrees with ε_{xx} from the LA slice at the intersection line (shown dotted). The complete list of the 3-D strain tensor components is shown in Fig. 5. Notice the bulging of the phantom is represented in the SA slice as stretching in the ε_{xx} and ε_{yy} components. The 3-D position and tracking of representative SA and LA slices are also shown in Fig. 6. The agreement is further shown quantitatively using linear regression and Bland-Altman plots (Fig. 7).

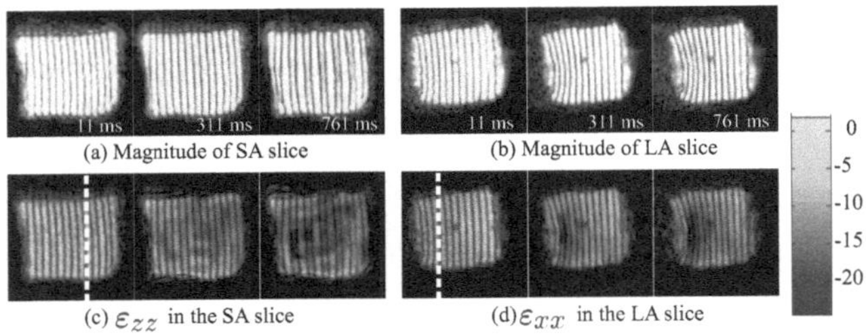

Fig. 4. ε_{zz} in a SA slice and the corresponding ε_{xx} in an orthogonal LA slice. The dotted line represents the location of the other slice.

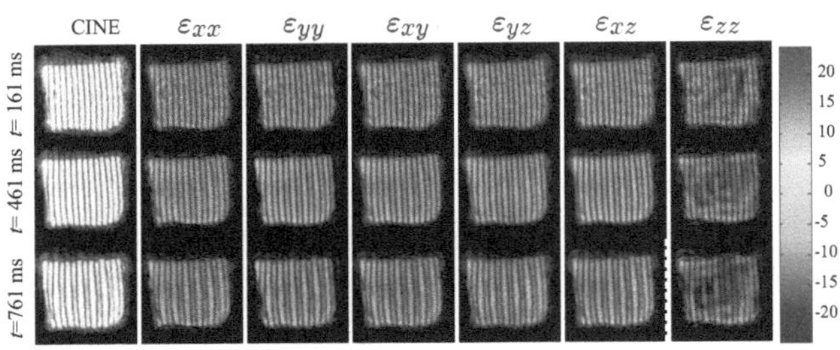

Fig. 5. 3-D strain tensor components in the compressible phantom

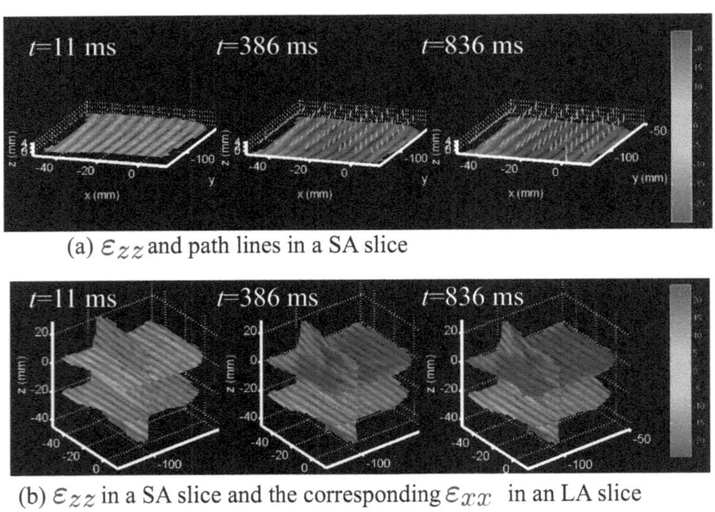

Fig. 6. 3-D representation of ε_{zz} and path line tracking in a compressible phantom SA slice and the corresponding ε_{xx} in a LA slice

5.2 In Vivo Results

The 3-D strain tensor components in a basal SA are shown in Fig. 8. A 3-D representation of ε_{zz} in the SA slice and the corresponding ε_{xx} in the LA slice are

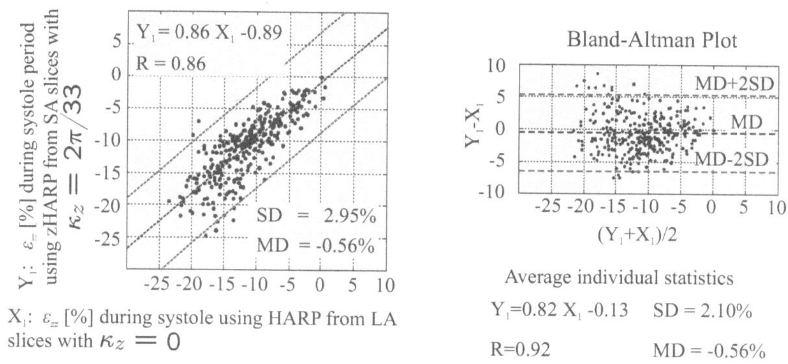

Fig. 7. Linear regression and Bland-Altman plots for the compressible phantom SA ε_{zz} strain and the corresponding LA ε_{xx}

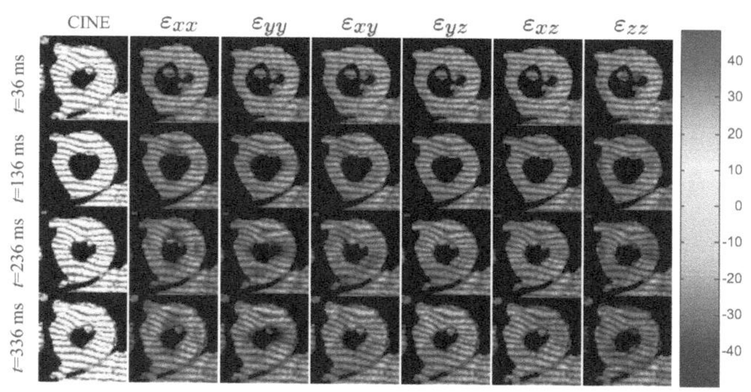

Fig. 8. In-vivo tagged SA slice and its 3-D strain tensor components

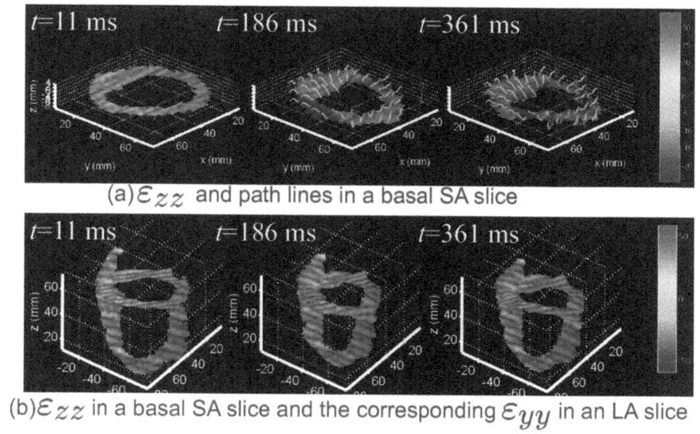

Fig. 9. 3-D representation of ε_{zz} in the SA slice and the corresponding ε_{xx} in a LA slice

shown in Fig. 9. Finally, the quantitative comparison shows a strong correlation (R¿0.85) between ε_{xx}, ε_{yy}, ε_{zz} calculated using zHARP and conventional HARP (Fig. 10).

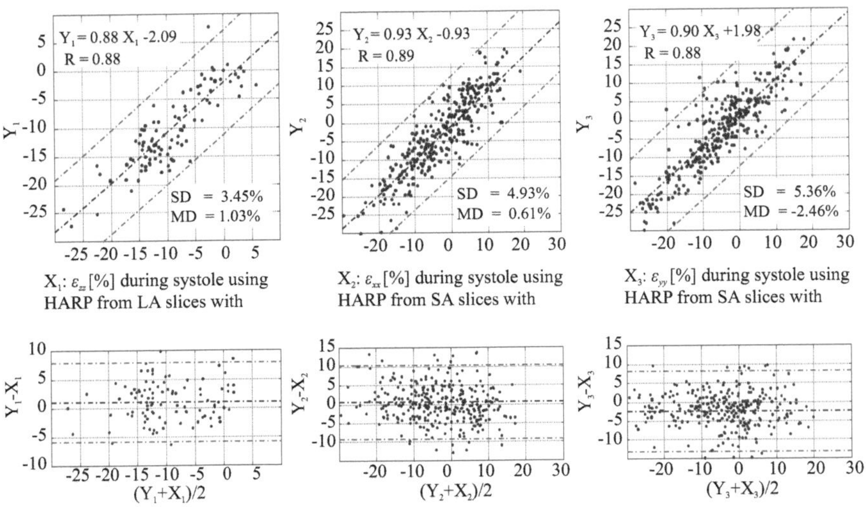

Fig. 10. In-vivo linear regression and Bland-Altman plots for the three diagonal strain tensor components. Y_1, Y_2 and Y_3 are the ε_{zz}, ε_{xx}, and ε_{yy} during systole in zHARP SA slices with $\kappa = \frac{2\pi}{33}$ rad/mm.

6 Discussion and Conclusion

We developed a cine multi-slice zHARP imaging scheme dedicated for fast 3D strain tensor quantification using only SA slices with the result being a point-by-point 3-D displacement and 3-D strain tensor maps. In addition, the sequence follows the exact excited slice and therefore the measured quantities are properties of the original material point not just the apparent point.

The scheme has potential clinical application when there is needs for full heart scan coverage and 3-D functional quantification. With the rich amount of information, another potential scientific application is in 3-D cardiac modeling where accurate modeling requires as much information as possible given that the registration error is minimized compared to conventional imaging methods that acquire multi-orthogonal slices. In addition, combining point tracking with 3-D strain measurement allowed the display of the strain of every point as it moves throughout the cardiac cycle.

The scheme was validated against typical SF-CSPAMM approach. The in-plane and through-plane strain components compare well with that measured from conventional tagging in both compressible phantom and in-vivo. Since no LA slices are required, the scheme has the potential to significantly abbreviate a 3D cardiac strain imaging as compared to more conventional approaches

Acknowledgments

This research was funded by the National Heart, Lung, and Blood Institute under grant R01HL47405 and a Biomedical Engineering Grant from the Whitaker Foundation (RG-02-0745).

Notice — Jerry Prince and Matthias Stuber are founders of and own stock in Diagnosoft, Inc., a company that seeks to license the HARP technology. The terms of this arrangement are being managed by the Johns Hopkins University in accordance with its conflict of interest policies.

M. Stuber is compensated as a consultant by Philips Medical Systems NL, the manufacturer of equipment described in this presentation. The terms of this arrangement have been approved by the Johns Hopkins University in accordance with its conflict of interest policies.

References

1. Zerhouni, E.A., Parish, D.M., Rogers, W.J., Yang, A., Shapiro, E.P.: Human heart: tagging with mr imaging: a method for noninvasive assessment of myocardial motion. Radiology 169, 59–63 (1988)
2. Axel, L., Dougherty, L.: Heart wall motion: improved method of spatial modulation of magnetization for mr imaging. Radiology 172, 349–350 (1989)
3. Aletras, A.H., Ding, S., Balaban, R.S., Wen, H.: Dense: displacement encoding with stimulated echoes in cardiac functional mri. Journal of magnetic resonance (San Diego, Calif.: 1997) 137(1), 247–252 (1999)
4. Osman, N.F., Kerwin, W.S., McVeigh, E.R., Prince, J.L.: Cardiac motion tracking using cine harmonic phase (harp) magnetic resonance imaging. Magnetic Resonance in Medicine 42, 1048–1060 (1999)
5. Osman, N.F., McVeigh, E.R., Prince, J.L.: Imaging heart motion using harmonic phase mri, vol. 19, pp. 186–202 (2000)
6. O'Dell, W.G., Moore, C.C., Hunter, W.C., Zerhouni, E.A., McVeigh, E.R.: Three-dimensional myocardial deformations: calculation with displacement field fitting to tagged mr images. Radiology 195(3), 829–835 (1995)
7. Young, A.A.: Model tags: direct three-dimensional tracking of heart wall motion from tagged magnetic resonance images. Medical image analysis 3(4), 361–372 (1999)
8. Ryf, S., Spiegel, M.A., Gerber, M., Boesiger, P.: Myocardial tagging with 3d-cspamm. Journal of magnetic resonance imaging: JMRI 16(3), 320–325 (2002)
9. Pan, L., Prince, J.L., Lima, J.A., Osman, N.F.: Fast tracking of cardiac motion using 3d-harp. IEEE transactions on bio-medical engineering 52(8), 1425–1435 (2005)
10. Sampath, S., Prince, J.L.: Automatic 3d tracking of cardiac material markers using slice-following and harmonic-phase mri. Magnetic Resonance Imaging 25(2), 197–208 (2007)
11. Abd-Elmoniem, K.Z., Osman, N.F., Stuber, M., Prince, J.L.: Zharp: Three-dimensional motion tracking from a single image plane. In: Christensen, G.E., Sonka, M. (eds.) IPMI 2005. LNCS, vol. 3565, pp. 639–651. Springer, Heidelberg (2005)
12. Abd-Elmoniem, K.Z., Osman, N.F., Prince, J.L., Stuber, M.: Magnetic resonance myocardial motion tracking from a single image plane. Magnetic Resonance in Medicine (accepted)
13. Fischer, S.E., McKinnon, G.C., Maier, S.E., Boesiger, P.: Improved myocardial tagging contrast. Magnetic resonance in medicine 30(2), 191–200 (1993)
14. Fischer, S.E., McKinnon, G.C., Scheidegger, M.B., Prins, W., Meier, D., Boesiger, P.: True myocardial motion tracking. Magnetic resonance in medicine 31(4), 401–413 (1994)
15. Lai, W.M., Rubin, D., Krempl, E.: Introduction to continuum mechanics. Pergamon Press, New York (1993)

Bayesian Tracking of Elongated Structures in 3D Images

Michiel Schaap, Ihor Smal, Coert Metz, Theo van Walsum, and Wiro Niessen

Biomedical Imaging Group Rotterdam,
Departments of Radiology and Medical Informatics
Erasmus MC - University Medical Center Rotterdam
{michiel.schaap,i.smal,c.metz,t.vanwalsum,w.niessen}@erasmusmc.nl

Abstract. Tracking of tubular elongated structures is an important goal in a wide range of biomedical imaging applications. A Bayesian tube tracking algorithm is presented that allows to easily incorporate a priori knowledge. Because probabilistic tube tracking algorithms are computationally complex, steps towards a computational efficient implementation are suggested in this paper.

The algorithm is evaluated on 2D and 3D synthetic data with different noise levels and clinical CTA data. The approach shows good performance on data with high levels of Gaussian noise.

Keywords: Bayesian tracking, efficient, high noise, CTA.

1 Introduction

Tracking of tubular elongated structures is an important goal in a wide range of biomedical imaging applications. For example, vessel tracking in medical images has received considerably attention, as it can be used as a preprocessing step towards stenosis evaluation and grading, by generating multi-planar reformatted images [1]. For a review of several vessel tracking methodologies, we refer to papers of Kirbas and Quek [2], Suri et al. [3], and Florin et al. [4].

State-of-the-art methods to track elongated structures use a priori knowledge of the tubular appearance in the image and the geometry of the tube. Appearance information include zeroth, first and second order image intensity information (e.g. in [5]) and geometric measures include the minimal surface curvature of the tracked tube (see, for example, [6]).

Until recently only deterministic approaches were presented, which take only one assumption of the track configuration into account during tracking. The path is found by updating the track to the most probable configuration at each iteration of the method. This may lead to situations where imaging data that locally does not meet the a priori assumptions, e.g. owing to pathologies, corrupted or missing data, can steer the track to incorrect configurations.

By taking into account multiple hypotheses during tracking this problem can be circumvented. Probabilistic approaches to track elongated structures using Monte Carlo sampling (particle filtering)[4,7] have been presented in order to

N. Karssemeijer and B. Lelieveldt (Eds.): IPMI 2007, LNCS 4584, pp. 74–85, 2007.
© Springer-Verlag Berlin Heidelberg 2007

search globally for the path that reflects the priors as good as possible. It has been reported that these methods can better overcome corrupted and missing data than deterministic approaches. Because the probabilistic methods track multiple hypotheses at once, they are computationally more complex than deterministic approaches.

The novelty of the current paper is twofold. First, it presents a Bayesian tracking approach which allows to easily incorporate a priori knowledge. It is shown that this approach enables tracking of tubular structures, even in the case of very high noise levels. Second, to overcome the computational complexity of probabilistic tracking algorithms, a computationally efficient implementation is proposed.

2 Bayesian Tracking of Elongated Structures

In this section the iterative Bayesian tracking approach is presented. We will first discuss the tubular model that we employ. Subsequently we will describe the observation model, hypotheses prediction and update step.

2.1 Tube Model

Out tracking method will consider a tube as a series of tube segments. A tube segment at iteration t is described by its location $\boldsymbol{p}_t = (x_t, y_t, z_t)^T$, orientation $\boldsymbol{v}_t = (\theta_t, \phi_t)$, radius r_t, and average intensity I_t. Thus each tube segment is characterized by a state vector $\mathbf{x}_t = (\boldsymbol{p}_t, \boldsymbol{v}_t, r_t, I_t)^T$. This results in a tube configuration described by $\mathbf{x}_{0:t} \triangleq \{\mathbf{x}_0, \ldots, \mathbf{x}_t\}$, see Figure 1(a).

With every tube segment we associate a region of interest, defined by the components $\boldsymbol{p}_t$, r_t, and $\boldsymbol{v}_t$ of $\mathbf{x}_t$ (see Fig. 1b). Subsequently, we let $\mathbf{z}_t$ denote the image measurements within this ROI. Hence, all measurements corresponding to tube $\mathbf{x}_{0:t}$ are denoted with $\mathbf{z}_{0:t}$. As an example, the image intensity within the tube and outside the tube (I_{in} and I_{out}) are computed, using nearest neighbor interpolation, from $\mathbf{z}_t$, see Figure 1(b).

2.2 Observation Model

In our observation model, we assume tubes to be bright relative to their background. Given the tube segment $\mathbf{x}_t$ and the measurements $\mathbf{z}_t$, the likelihood of the measurements given the state $\mathbf{x}_t$, $p(\mathbf{z}_t|\mathbf{x}_t)$, is constructed as follows:

$$p(\mathbf{z}_t|\mathbf{x}_t) \propto p(\mathbf{z}_t|\boldsymbol{p}_t, \boldsymbol{v}_t, r_t, I_t) = p(I_{\text{in}}, I_{\text{out}})\mathcal{N}(I_{\text{in}}|I_t, \sigma_\varsigma^2), \tag{1}$$

where

$$p(I_{\text{in}}, I_{\text{out}}) = \begin{cases} (\frac{I_{\text{in}} - I_{\text{out}}}{I_c})^s, & I_{\text{in}} > I_{\text{out}}, \\ 0, & I_{\text{in}} \leq I_{\text{out}}. \end{cases} \tag{2}$$

with I_c and s contrast regulating parameters and $\mathcal{N}(.|\mu, \sigma^2)$ a real normal distribution with mean μ and variance σ^2. The term $\mathcal{N}(I_{\text{in}}|I_t, \sigma_\varsigma^2)$ describes the

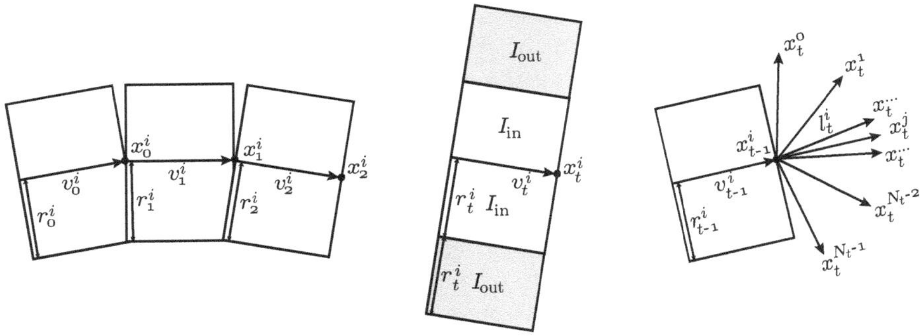

(a) (b) (c)

Fig. 1. Figure (a) shows a part of the tube configuration $\mathbf{x}_{0:t}$. Figure (b) demonstrates how the values I_{in} and I_{out} are obtained from patch $\mathbf{z}_t$. The prediction of new tubular segments, as explained in Section 2.3, is presented in Figure (c).

likelihood that the measured intensity I_{in} resembles the intensity I_t, which is predicted from the previous iterations using the Kalman filter described in Section 2.4.

2.3 Prediction

Using the Bayesian rule, the probability density function (pdf) $p(\mathbf{x}_{0:t}|\mathbf{z}_{0:t})$, that describes the posterior probability of the tube configuration, having all the observations up to iteration t can be estimated with the following recursion [8]

$$p(\mathbf{x}_{0:t}|\mathbf{z}_{0:t}) \propto p(\mathbf{x}_t|\mathbf{x}_{t-1})p(\mathbf{z}_t|\mathbf{x}_t)p(\mathbf{x}_{0:t-1}|\mathbf{z}_{0:t-1}), \tag{3}$$

where the transition prior $p(\mathbf{x}_t|\mathbf{x}_{t-1})$ is assumed to be Markovian ($\mathbf{x}_t$ only depends on $\mathbf{x}_{t-1}$ and not on any other past states) and is factorized as

$$p(\mathbf{x}_t|\mathbf{x}_{t-1}) = p(\boldsymbol{p}_t, \boldsymbol{v}_t|\boldsymbol{p}_{t-1}, \boldsymbol{v}_{t-1})p(r_t|r_{t-1})p(I_t|I_{t-1}), \tag{4}$$

The likelihood $p(\mathbf{z}_t|\mathbf{x}_t)$ relates the conditionally independent measurements at iteration t to the state $\mathbf{x}_t$, as defined in equation (1).

At each iteration step, we represent the probability of the tube configuration with a set of N_t weighted states $\boldsymbol{X}_{0:t} = \{\mathbf{x}_{0:t}^i, w_t^i\}_{i=1}^{N_t}$, thus

$$p(\mathbf{x}_{0:t}|\mathbf{z}_{0:t}) = \sum_{i=1}^{N_t} w_t^i \delta(\mathbf{x}_{0:t} - \mathbf{x}_{0:t}^i), \tag{5}$$

where $\delta(\cdot)$ is the Dirac delta function and the weights are normalized such that $\sum_{i=1}^{N_t} w_t^i = 1$.

In each iteration we use the variance of the weights w_t^i to determine how many and which hypotheses should be kept in the next iteration. The N_e most probable hypotheses are kept according to the weights $w_t^i, i \in \{1, ..., N_t\}$, where

$$N_e = \frac{1}{\sum_i^{N_t} (w_t^i)^2} \tag{6}$$

From each of these states, $N_t^i = \text{nint}(w_t^i N)$ new states are created, where nint(.) denotes a nearest integer round and N is pre-defined and describes the maximum number of hypotheses created. This approach will keep only the relevant hypotheses and effectively distribute them according to the described pdf.

2.4 Update

In the update step, prior knowledge on the curvature of the centerline, the variance of the tube radius along the centerline, the intensity variance in the tube and the contrast-to-noise ratio in the image are incorporated. This is achieved as follows.

The formation of the N_t^i new hypotheses $\mathbf{x}_t^j$, $j = \{0, ..., N_t^i - 1\}$, at iteration t from the previous hypothesis $\mathbf{x}_t^i$ consist of a transition to a new position $\boldsymbol{p}_t$, which is deterministically defined by

$$\boldsymbol{p}_t^j = \boldsymbol{p}_{t-1}^i + R_z(\theta_{t-1}) R_y(\phi_{t-1}) R_z(\vartheta_t^j) R_y(\varphi_t^j)(0, 0, l_t^i)^T \tag{7}$$

where $R_z(.)$ and $R_y(.)$ are rotation matrices around the z- and y-axis [9]. The length of a tube segment l_t^i depends on the radius of the tube r_{t-1}^i and a predefined parameter α.

$$l_t^i = \frac{r_{t-1}^i}{\tan(\alpha)} \tag{8}$$

Figure 1(c) gives a schematic explanation of the transition in eq. (7). The angles $(\vartheta_t^j, \varphi_t^j)$ describe a point in the local spherical coordinate system with the z-axis orientated in the direction of $\boldsymbol{v}_{t-1}^i$ and origin at $\boldsymbol{p}_{t-1}$. Therefore, the angle φ_t^j is equal to the enclosed angle between $\boldsymbol{v}_{t-1}$ and $\boldsymbol{v}_t$. The two angles $(\vartheta_t^j, \varphi_t^j)$ are constructed with an algorithm that uniformly distributes points on a sphere, as described by Saff and Kuijlaars [10]. This algorithm is used to distribute the N_t^i new hypotheses uniformly on the half sphere in front of $\boldsymbol{p}_{t-1}$ oriented in the direction of $\boldsymbol{v}_{t-1}$. In this case, the transition density $p(\boldsymbol{p}_t, \boldsymbol{v}_t | \boldsymbol{p}_{t-1}^i, \boldsymbol{v}_{t-1}^i)$ is given by

$$p(\boldsymbol{p}_t, \boldsymbol{v}_t | \boldsymbol{p}_{t-1}^i, \boldsymbol{v}_{t-1}^i) = \sum_{j=0}^{N_t^i - 1} \tilde{\omega}_j \delta(\boldsymbol{p}_t - \boldsymbol{p}_t^j) \tag{9}$$

where the weight $\tilde{\omega}_j$ of a given enclosed angle is given by

$$\tilde{\omega}_j = \frac{\omega(\phi_j)}{\sum_{k=0}^{N_t^i} \omega(\phi_k)} \tag{10}$$

$$\omega(\varphi) = N(\varphi | 0, \sigma_\varphi^2) \tag{11}$$

with σ_φ being a pre-defined parameter.

The transition of r_t and I_t is assumed to be Markovian and described by

$$r_t = r_{t-1} + \eta_t, \tag{12}$$

$$I_t = I_{t-1} + \xi_t \tag{13}$$

where η_t and ξ_t are uncorrelated Gaussian random variables with variances σ_r^2 and σ_I^2, respectively. In this case

$$p(r_t|r_{t-1}) = \mathcal{N}(r_t|r_{t-1}, \sigma_r^2) \tag{14}$$
$$p(I_t|I_{t-1}) = \mathcal{N}(I_t|I_{t-1}, \sigma_I^2) \tag{15}$$

The observation model for the intensity I_t is a linear (conditional on the rest of the state parameters) Gaussian model given by

$$I_{\text{in}} = I_t + \varsigma_t \tag{16}$$

where $\varsigma_t \sim \mathcal{N}(\varsigma|0, \sigma_\varsigma^2)$. The model (13),(16) is a linear Gaussian model that can be solved analytically using the Kalman filter [8]

$$I_{t|t-1} = I_{t-1}, \qquad I_t = I_{t|t-1} + K_t(I_{\text{in}} - I_{t|t-1}),$$
$$P_{t|t-1} = P_{t-1} + \sigma_I^2 \qquad P_t = (1 - K_t)P_{t|t-1}$$

where P_t denotes the estimated variance of I_t and the Kalman gain $K_t = \frac{P_{t|t-1}}{P_{t|t-1}+\sigma_\varsigma^2}$.

For each prediction $I_{t|t-1}^j$ of the Kalman filter for the intensity I_{t-1}^i we estimate the radius of the tube segment r_t^j as follows

$$\hat{r}_t^j = \underset{r_t}{\text{argmax}}\, p(\mathbf{z}_t|\boldsymbol{p}_t^j, \phi_t^j, r_t, I_{t|t-1})p(r_t|r_{t-1}) \tag{17}$$

Then, the Kalman update is performed for the intensity I_t with the new measurement I_{in}. If no a priori knowledge about the image intensity distribution is available, the Kalman filter is not used in the first iteration, then I_1^i is set to I_{in}.

3 Implementation Details

Each of the possible new states $\mathbf{x}_t^j$ is described by a relative angle $\boldsymbol{v}_t^j$ and a radius r_t, where $r_t \in (0..R)$, with $R = r_{t-1} + \sigma_r$ being the maximum evaluated tube radius.

For each voxel in a patch around $\boldsymbol{p}_{t-1}^i$ we can easily calculate to which angle and radius combination it belongs. Using these measurements it is possible to quickly calculate for all the possible $N_t^i \times R$ combinations the values I_{in} and I_{out}. The advantage of this procedure is that each voxel in the image is accessed only once per state $\mathbf{x}_{t-1}^i$ and several redundant computations are avoided, which has computational benefits.

4 Evaluation

In this section, the developed probabilistic tracking algorithm is evaluated on 2D and 3D synthetic data, simulated computed tomography angiography (CTA) data and real CTA data.

4.1 Parameters

For all the evaluations we used fixed parameter settings that were empirically selected based on experiments on synthetic data not belonging to the test set. In these studies it was observed that the method was not sensitive to parameter changes. The following parameter settings were used, $N = 500$, $I_c = 1.0$, $s = 1.0$, $\sigma_\varphi^2 = 1.5$, $\sigma_r^2 = 2$, $\sigma_I^2 = 1000$, $\sigma_\varsigma^2 = 10$, and $\alpha = 0.25$.

4.2 Initialization

The algorithm is initialized with a seed point and a radius estimation. The set of state vectors $\mathbf{X}_0$ contains two state vectors, with locations $\boldsymbol{p}_0^0$ and $\boldsymbol{p}_0^1$ equal to the seed point and radii r_0^0 and r_0^1 equal to the estimated radius. The orientations are initialized with $\boldsymbol{v}_0^0 = (0, 0)$ and $\boldsymbol{v}_0^1 = (\pi, 0)$.

4.3 2D Synthetic Data

In order to investigate the accuracy of the developed method as a function of image noise, a quantitative study on 2D synthetic data was carried out.

Rose has introduced a distinguishability measure $\text{MD} = \text{CNR}\sqrt{A}$ in [11], where CNR is the ratio of the contrast between an object and its background and the standard deviation of the noise in the image and A denotes the amount of voxels of the object.

For our experiments, four random tubes were created with radii and distinguishability values of respectively $r = \{2.5, 5.0, 7.5, 10\}$ pixels and $\text{MD} = \sqrt{2}\{0.5, 1.0, 1.5, 2.0\}$ pixels, resulting in 64 different test images.

These synthetic tubes were created by fitting 3rd order splines through five randomly selected points in a 2D grid of 512×512 pixels. Tubes were excluded if a part of the tube had a distance to other parts of the tube, not being direct neighbors, of less than 100 pixels or if the maximum curvature of the tube centerline was higher than 0.04 pixels^{-1}. See Figure 3(a) for an example tube.

The tubes were tracked automatically and manually which allows comparison between the obtained accuracy and the human capabilities of tracking tubes in noisy data. Four observers each annotated centerlines in 16 of the 64 images. The different radii and noise levels were equally distributed over the four observers.

In the automatic tracking, the radius was initialized at the average size of the synthetic tubes evaluated, being 6.25 pixels. It is believed that this simulates typical a priori knowledge of an expected tube size.

As an evaluation criterion we determine the root mean squared distance (RMSD) between the automatically or manually tracked tube and the centerline of the golden standard. This number is divided by the radius of the tube in order to present the accuracy of tracking relative to the tube size (RMSD/r).

Only distances for paths where at least 95% of the track is found at a distance within twice the radius of the golden standard are taken into account. In this way the ability of tracking the tube and the accuracy of tracking is presented.

4.4 3D Synthetic Data

A 3D synthetic evaluation was carried out to evaluate the performance of the algorithm for tracking 3D tubes with varying radius and high image noise. A 3D synthetic tube with varying radius from $r = 4$ voxels to $r = 10$ voxels is created and Gaussian noise is added, resulting in a CNR value of 0.25 and thereby distinguishability measures of MD = 1.8 to MD = 4.4 voxels. The algorithm was initialized with a seed point at the beginning of the tube and radius was set to 7 voxels. The performance of the algorithm is evaluated by measuring the RMSD to the centerline of the synthetic tube.

4.5 Simulated CTA Data

To simulate clinical data with high noise, a computed tomography angiography (CTA) artery segmentation was manually extracted from CTA data. The segmentation was given a contrast of 200 intensity units to its background, similar to the contrast of arteries in CTA. This segmentation was smoothed with a Gaussian kernel with standard deviation of 1 voxel, similar to the point spread function of CT. Afterward Gaussian noise was added, with a standard deviations of 240 intensity units, approximately eight times higher than the clinical noise value of 30 intensity units. The algorithm was initialized with a seedpoint at the approximate beginning of the tube and the radius was set to twice the (approximate) average radius of the simulated vessel. The RMSD difference to a manual tracked centerline is used as a performance measure.

4.6 Tracking in Real CTA Data

In order to demonstrate the applicability of the algorithm on real data, we have used the algorithm to track two arteries in a CTA dataset. We used a dataset where the imaged patient had a chronic total occlusion, meaning that an artery was blocked and (almost) no blood was passing the point of occlusion. Such a dataset is problematic for conventional deterministic algorithms, because of the lack of local image contrast. The algorithm was initialized by putting a seedpoint in the vessels and setting the radius to approximately twice the radius of the vessel.

5 Results

5.1 2D Synthetic Data

The results of the evaluation on 2D synthetic data are shown in Figure 2 and Table 1. Figure 2 shows the relation between the accuracy of the manually and

Table 1. Evaluation results for the evaluation with 2D synthetic data. A tube is found if at least 95 percent of the length of the path was tracked at a distance to the golden standard of less than two times the radius of the tube. For tubes that were found both manually and automatically, the root mean squared difference (RMSD) and the root of the average of the squared ratio between distance and radius RMSD/r is shown.

	Manual			Automatic		
$\frac{MD}{\sqrt{2}}$	#found	RMSD	RMSD/r	#found	RMSD	RMSD/r
0.5	14/16	3.12	0.40	5/16	2.85	0.39
1.0	16/16	1.37	0.25	16/16	1.72	0.31
1.5	16/16	1.11	0.21	16/16	1.60	0.30
2.0	16/16	1.05	0.19	16/16	1.52	0.28

automatically tracked paths. Table 1 shows the performance of the manual and automatic trackings, for the four different distinguishability measures.

For the automatically tracked path that had an overlap of less than 95%, the overlap was always less than 45%. Two of these tracks were also not found manually with an overlap of at least 95% (respectively 85% and 88%). An example of the input data and the automatic tracking is presented in Figure 3.

5.2 3D Synthetic Data

The algorithm tracked the full length of the path in the 3D synthetic tube. The RMSD to the golden standard was 2.3 voxels. Figure 4 visualizes this result.

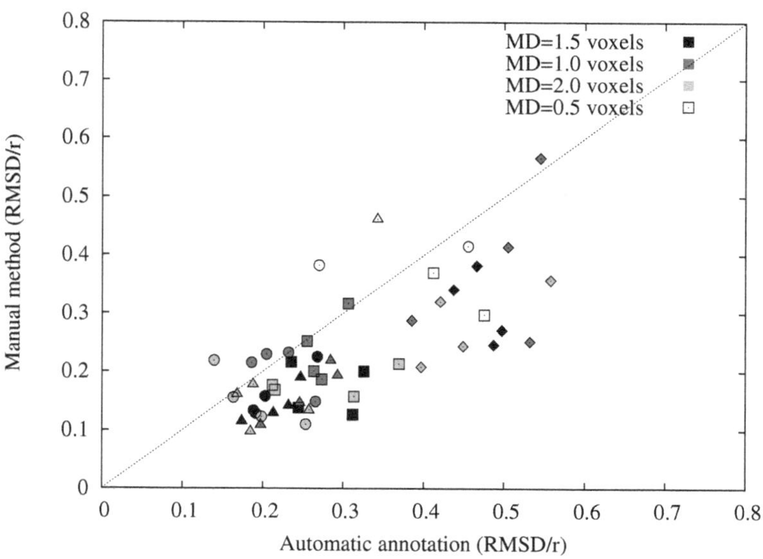

Fig. 2. Scatter plot demonstrating the relation between the accuracy, measured in RMSD/r, of the manually and automatically tracked tube centerlines. The different symbols denote different radii (◊ = 2.5, □ = 5.0, ○ = 7.5, △ = 10.0, all in voxels), and different colors denote different noise levels.

(a) (b) (c)

Fig. 3. An example of the data and results of the 2D synthetic evaluation. Figure (a) is a randomly created tube with radius of 5 voxels and 200 intensity units contrast. Figure (b) is the image after Gaussian noise with a standard deviation of 894 was added, resulting in CNR = 0.224 and $M_d = 0.5\sqrt{2}$. Figure (c) shows the tracking result of the algorithm.

5.3 Simulated CTA Data

The automatically found track in the simulated CTA dataset was found with a RMSD of 1.7 voxels to the manually annotated reference standard. Figure 5 shows the simulated CTA dataset, found path and reference standard.

5.4 Clinical Examples

The two clinical examples are shown in Figure 6. Both trackings were visually evaluated and found to be well within the boundary of the vessel.

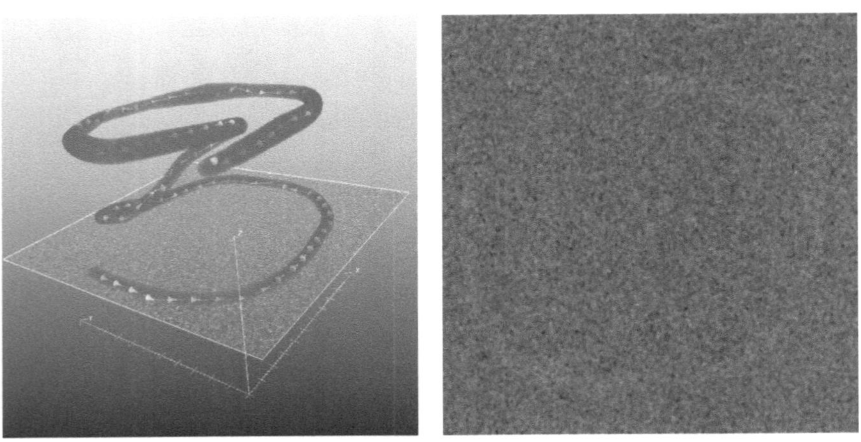

(a) (b)

Fig. 4. A demonstration of tracking with the developed algorithm of a 3D synthetic tube with radius varying between 5 and 10 voxels and CNR of 0.25. In (a) the tracking result in 3D is shown with the tube without noise and a slice of the volume with noise. (b) shows the noisy slice in 2D.

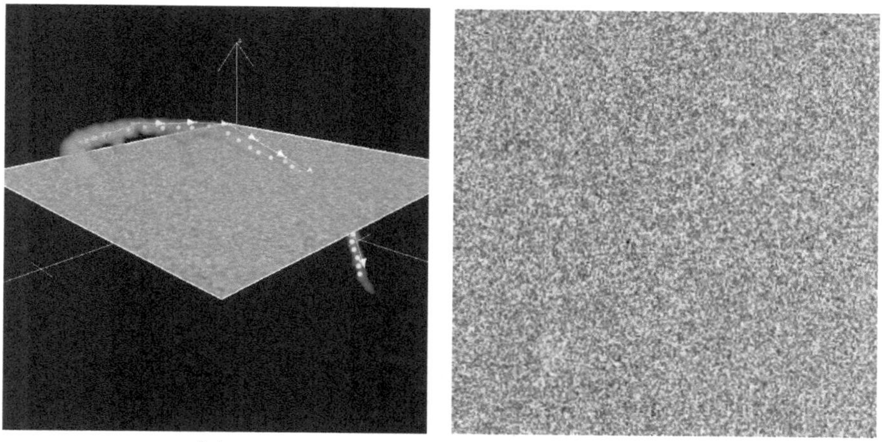

(a) (b)

Fig. 5. (a) An automatically found track (shown with arrows) in a simulated CTA dataset displayed together with the simulated dataset without noise, manual reference standard (white dots), and a slice from the dataset with noise. (b) shows the slice with noise in 2D.

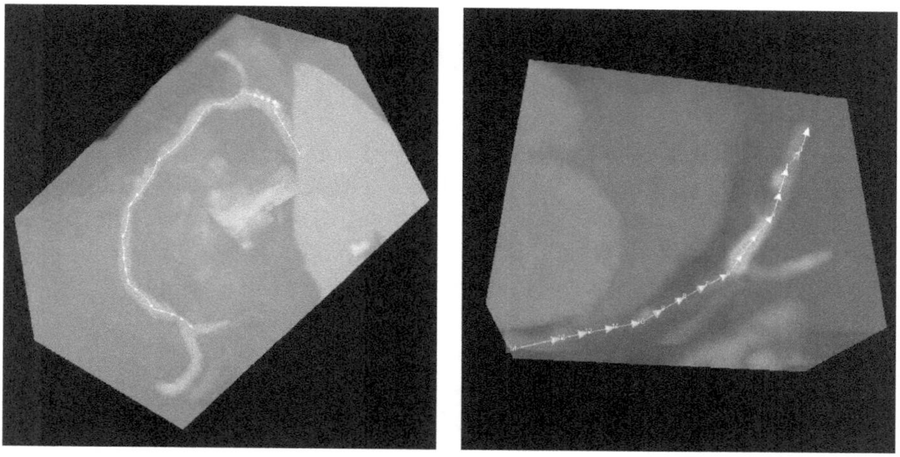

(a) (b)

Fig. 6. Examples of clinical applications of the probabilistic tracking algorithm. (a) shows a tracked right coronary artery in a CTA dataset. In (b) it is shown that an artery with a chronic total occlusion (CTO) in a CTA dataset is successfully tracked.

6 Discussion

The evaluation on 2D synthetic data showed that the algorithm was capable of tracking tubes with a distinguishability measure MD of 1.4 with accuracies that were in the same order of magnitude as the tracking results of the human observers.

As a reference for values of MD we would like to refer to [5] and [12] for respectively tube enhancement and tracking. In [12] it is reported that straight tubes were successfully enhanced at MD > 5.3. The values presented in [5] are more difficult to compare, because varying tube radii were used, but indicative values can be obtained from this article.

The algorithm is also applied to 3D synthetic data (with a CNR of 0.25) and simulated high noise CTA data. Both tracks were found automatically with a RMSD of approximately 2 voxels to the reference standard. Furthermore, tracking results in real CTA data are presented, to demonstrate the clinical applicability of the proposed algorithm. The accuracy of the method is sufficient for using it as a first processing step in automated vessel quantification techniques.

Because probabilistic tube tracking algorithms are computationally complex, several computational improvements are suggested in this paper.

The development of automatic stopping criteria, bifurcation detection, and a comparison with existing deterministic and probabilistic algorithms are subject to future work.

The results are already promising for a wide variety of applications, but it should be noted that when using the presented algorithm for a specific application more a priori knowledge can be incorporated, such as expected intensity distributions and more specific observation models, and thereby probably improving the results.

7 Conclusion

A probabilistic tube tracking algorithm is presented in this article. The algorithm was evaluated on 2D synthetic data and tubes with $\text{CNR}\sqrt{\text{radius}} = 1.0$ were all successfully tracked with accuracies that were in the same order of magnitude as the tracking results of the human observers. Furthermore, the approach was applied, with good performance, to 3D synthetic and clinical data.

Acknowledgment

This work was sponsored by the Dutch Foundation for Scientific Research, NWO, STW.

References

1. Caussin, C., Larchez, C., Ghostine, S., Pesenti-Rossi, D., Daoud, B., Habis, M., Sigal-Cinqualbre, A., Perrier, E., Angel, C.-Y., Lancelin, B., Paul, J.-F.: Comparison of coronary minimal lumen area quantification by sixty-four-slice computed tomography versus intravascular ultrasound for intermediate stenosis. American Journal of Cardiology 98(7), 871–876 (2006)
2. Kirbas, C., Quek, F.: A review of vessel extraction techniques and algorithms. ACM Computing Surveys 36(2), 81–121 (2004)

3. Suri, J.S., Liu, K., Reden, L., Laxminarayan, S.: A review on MR vascular image processing algorithms: acquisition and prefiltering: part I. IEEE Trans Inf. Technol Biomed 6(4), 324–337 (2002)
4. Florin, C., Paragios, N., Williams, J.: Globally optimal active contours, sequential monte carlo and on-line learning for vessel segmentation. In: Leonardis, A., Bischof, H., Pinz, A. (eds.) ECCV 2006. LNCS, vol. 3953, pp. 476–489. Springer, Heidelberg (2006)
5. Aylward, S., Bullit, E.: Initialization, noise, singularities, and scale in height ridge traversal for tubular object centerline extraction. IEEE Transactions on Medical Imaging 21(2), 61–75 (2002)
6. Lorigo, L.M., Faugeras, O.D., Grimson, W.E.L., Keriven, R., Kikinis, R., Nabavi, A., Westin, C.-F.: Curves: Curve evolution for vessel segmentation. Medical Image Analysis 5, 195–206 (2001)
7. Myatt, D., Nasuto, S., Maybank, S.: Towards the automatic reconstruction of dendritic trees using particle filters. In: Linear Statistical Signal Processing Workshop (on CD-ROM) (2006)
8. Doucet, A., Godsill, S., Andrieu, C.: On Sequential Monte Carlo Sampling Methods for Bayesian Filtering. Statistics and Computing 10, 197–208 (2000)
9. Weisstein, E.W.: Rotation Matrix. From MathWorld–A Wolfram Web Resource
10. Saff, E., Kuijlaars, A.: Distributing many points on a sphere. The Mathematical Intelligence 19(1), 5–11 (1997)
11. Rose, A.: Vision: Human and Electronic. Plenum Press, New York (1973)
12. Manniesing, R., Niessen, W.: Multiscale vessel enhancing diffusion in CT angiography noise filtering. In: Christensen, G.E., Sonka, M. (eds.) IPMI 2005. LNCS, vol. 3565, pp. 138–149. Springer, Heidelberg (2005)

Effective Statistical Edge Integration Using a Flux Maximizing Scheme for Volumetric Vascular Segmentation in MRA

Ali Gooya[1], Hongen Liao[2], Kiyoshi Matsumiya[1], Ken Masamune[1], and Takeyoshi Dohi[1]

[1] Graduate School of Information Science and Technology, the University of Tokyo,
[2] Graduate School of Engineering, the University of Tokyo,
7-3-1, Hongo, Bunkyo, Tokyo, 113-8656
{gooya,liao,dohi}@atre.t.u-tokyo.ac.jp

Abstract. Evolutionary schemes based on the level set theory are effective tools for medical image segmentation. In this paper, a new variational technique for edge integration is presented. Region statistical measures and orientation information from ramp-like edges, are fused within an energy minimization scheme that is based on a new interpretation of edge concept. A region driven advection term simulating the edge strength effect is directly obtained from this minimization strategy. We have applied our method to several real Magnetic Resonance Angiography data sets and comparison has been made with a state-of-the-art vessel segmentation method. Presented results indicate that using this method a significant improvement is achievable and the method can be an effective tool to extract vessels in MRA intracranial images.

1 Introduction

Magnetic Resonance Angiography (MRA) is increasingly used to provide volumetric information of vascular system. Accurate assessment of MRA images requires that the vessel structures to be extracted from MRA data sets. Currently, a number of techniques have been developed for vessel segmentation based on the advanced level set evolutionary methods. Lorgio *et al* [1] has proposed CURVES using image gradient strength information, and the surface minimum curvature as the smoothing term. Also capillary active contours is invented by Yan *et al.* [2], a method that is based on the capillary force acting on the free fluid surface through a capillary tube. In [3], based on the natural continuity of vessel a shape prior is introduced that forces the surface to expand anisotropically so that it can pass over small noise speckels. A shape prior has been introduced in [4] for minimizing the leakage from noisy edges. Despite of relative success from some of these methods, segmentation of long thin structures is still considered as a delicate task. Edge intensity based methods fail to capture elongated low contrast structures well. Ramp-like pattern of edge observed in many non-contrast agent vascular imaging techniques, such as phase contrast

N. Karssemeijer and B. Lelieveldt (Eds.): IPMI 2007, LNCS 4584, pp. 86–97, 2007.
© Springer-Verlag Berlin Heidelberg 2007

and time-of-flight MRA data sets, prevents the custom geodesic active contours model to fit the problem effectively. On the other hand, gradient information inside the vessels is rather week and even gets singular. In this paper, based on textured regional measures, such as mean value, a new "statistical" interpretation of edge is presented. To obtain the optimum performance, it is combined with flux maximizing framework [5], to take the advantage of directional information. By this means, statistical information from both regions are fused into orientation information available on the border of object.

1.1 Related Work

In a related work to our algorithm, a level set method is introduced by Vasilevsky [5] that integrates the directions of gradient vectors into the evolution equation so that the gradient flux through the evolving curve is maximized. Since estimation of flux requires that the divergence of image to be calculated, this may be problematic at locations where the image gradient is becoming singular, such as blood vessels. Therefore rather than explicitly calculating the divergence, a multi-scale method is used. This can be slow and needs a prior knowledge of the scale of the vessel. In another closely related paper for segmentation of thin structures, a combinational method is proposed by Gazit *et al.*[6], using Haralik edge detector and Chan-Vese minimal variance functional and geodesic active contours [7]. In their work, minimization of topological variation inside the vessels needs the second order of image intensity derivations to be computed. This can be singular inside the vessels. Also, their proposed functional still relies on Geodesic active contours model to provide advection term. We show that, information provided by Chan-Vese model can be effectively used to regularize "edge areas". Our new energy functional mimics the geodesic active contours model by providing a new advection term driven by the statistical information obtained from both regions. Update algorithm of regional parameters is unique and benefits from the edge information. By this means, we have also eliminated using the geodesic active contours.

2 Formation of Energy Functional

Assume for a given open region D, the evolving surface is represented as the zero level of the level set function $\phi(x)$ where $\phi(x) < 0$ for inside of the object, and $\phi(x) > 0$ for outside. $H(x)$ is representing Heaviside function such that $H(x) = 1$ if $x \geq 0$ otherwise $H(x) = 0$. Also $\delta(x) = \frac{d}{dx}H(x)$ is the Dirac delta function. Further, we assume that $I(x) : \Omega \to [0, 1]$ is a grey level given image that the object of interest appears brighter than background

2.1 Statistical Edge Detector

In this section based on a new definition of edge, we develop optimization functional. The distance of a point from a set is a general concept. It is a useful way of determining similarity of an unknown sample set to a known one and differs from Euclidean distance. For example, Mahalanobis distance of a point from a given set, is defined using the covariance and mean value of the set. In this paper, such general function is considered in our definition.

We consider the edge as the area with maximum statistical distance from both regions. If, for example, $0 \leq d_1(x) \leq 1$ and $0 \leq d_2(x) \leq 1$ represent some statistical distance functions of point x from outside and inside regions respectively,

Definition 1 (Statistical Edge). *we say that x on the surface S (in three dimension) is placed on the (statistical) edge if:*

$$d(x) = d_1(x)d_2(x) \tag{1}$$

attains a maximum along the normal vector to S.

In the frame work of level set theory, this means that norm of the vector $d(x)\nabla\phi$ is maximized. Straight functional development based on this fact can consist of maximization of this functional:

$$E_s(\phi) = \int [-\alpha + d(x)]\delta(\phi(x))|\nabla\phi|dx \tag{2}$$

Where $\alpha > 0$ enforces the smoothness. Using principles outlined in [8], it is easy to see that in this case Euler-Lagrange equation of the above equation is:

$$\frac{\partial\phi}{\partial t} = -\delta(\phi)\{\nabla d \cdot \nabla\phi + (-\alpha + d)\nabla \cdot (\frac{\nabla\phi}{|\nabla\phi|})\} \tag{3}$$

Since the ∇d has the same and opposite directions of $\nabla\phi$ inside and outside the object respectively, ($d(x)$ has a maximum on the border), the first term is an advection term that fixes the contour on the most admissible place. By this means based on the regional properties, we implicitly eliminate necessity of a separate edge detector operator as is the case for [9]. Therefore an enhancement can be obtained for low contrast edges, e.g, thin vessel structures. On the other hand the second term, enforces the smoothness provided that α is chosen to be a large enough positive value.We remind that although in this paper we utilize a simple form of distance function- basically distance to mean value- it can be any other general form.

2.2 Flux Maximizing Flow

Flux maximizing edge integration method finds the image location where $|\nabla I \cdot \nabla\phi|$ is maximized [5]. Therefore, no matter how $|\nabla I|$ is faint, it has ability to obtain the edge using angular information between these two vectors. The functional to be minimized in this case can be witten in a similar variational framework:

$$E_f(\phi) = \int \delta(\phi(x))\nabla\phi(x) \cdot \nabla I dx \tag{4}$$

Here we remind that it is assumed that on the object border $\nabla I \cdot \nabla \phi < 0$, therefore this integration is an estimation of in-ward flux. The Euler-Lagrange equation can be easily shown to be:

$$\frac{\partial \phi}{\partial t} = \delta(\phi)\nabla \cdot (\nabla I) \tag{5}$$

Evolution over time, results in a flux inward maximizing flow, that takes the advantageous of directional information provided by the image gradient. However, leakage happens if the divergence term is not effectively computed using a multi-scale method as explained in [5].

2.3 Enhanced Edge Detection Framework

Statistical edge detectors as defined in section 2.1, can be effectively combined with flux maximizing framework. The idea is to maximize the norm of dot product of $d(x)\nabla\phi$ and ∇I. In this case enhanced edge detection energy functional be written as:

$$E_{nf}(\phi) = \int \delta(\phi) d(x) \nabla\phi \cdot \nabla I dx \tag{6}$$

Therefore, this formulation combines regional properties through $d(x)$ and directional information provided by ∇I on the border. The EL equation for the minimization of eq.(6) can be obtained by applying Frechet derivate in the direction of a test function ψ:

$$< E_{nf}, \psi >= \int \psi\delta'(\phi)d(x)\nabla\phi(x) \cdot \nabla I dx + \int \delta(\phi)d(x)\nabla\psi(x) \cdot \nabla I dx$$

Where using Green's formula:

$$\begin{aligned}\int \delta(\phi)d(x)\nabla\psi(x) \cdot \nabla I dx &= -\int \psi(x)\nabla \cdot (\delta(\phi)d(x)\nabla I)dx \\ &= \int -\psi\{\delta'(\phi)d(x)\nabla\phi(x) \cdot \nabla I + \delta(\phi)\nabla \cdot (d(x)\nabla I)\}dx\end{aligned}$$

From above we have:

$$< E_{nf}, \psi >= -\int \psi(x)\delta(\phi)\nabla \cdot (d(x)\nabla I)\}dx$$

This should vanish for every ψ, therefore by using gradient decent method we obtain:

$$\frac{\partial \phi}{\partial t} = \delta(\phi)\nabla \cdot (d(x)\nabla I) \tag{7}$$

this can be further expanded to:

$$\frac{\partial \phi}{\partial t} = \delta(\phi)\{\nabla d(x) \cdot \nabla I + d(x)\Delta I) \tag{8}$$

Since we are assuming that the object of interest is brighter than the background as it is the case with MRA images), i.e, $\nabla I \cdot \nabla \phi < 0$, it easy to see that the first term has a similar advection property as described in equation (3). The effect of multiplication of $d(x)$ at ΔI is damping of divergence term from the current estimate of the border (where $d(x)$ is maximized) toward both regions. Here, we remind that one may not consider eq.(8) as a subclass of general divergence equation outlined in [5], since $d(x)$ is a regional dependent measure that changes along with the evolution of both regions.

3 Distance from Mean Values

In this section we first briefly review Chan-Vese model, and then represent our complete evolutionary equation for vessel segmentation.

3.1 Chan-Vese Model

Chan and Vese in [10], proposed a measure based on the minimal variance criteria. The image is divided in two regions, the anterior and exterior of the closed surface. This model minimizes the variance in each segment. Given a gray level image, Chan and Vese proposed to use a minimal variance criterion given by the functional:

$$E_{cv}(\phi, c_1, c_2) = \int \delta(\phi)|\nabla\phi|dx +$$
$$\alpha \int H(\phi)(I(x) - c_1)^2 dx + \alpha \int H^*(\phi)(I(x) - c_2)^2 dx \tag{9}$$

Where $H^*(\phi) = 1 - H(\phi)$ indicates inside the contour and α determines the regularization level. While minimizing this functional, c_1 and c_2 obtain the mean intensity values outside and inside the contour. The optimal curve would separate the interior and exterior with respect to their expected values.

3.2 Combinational Model

For the sake of simplicity, we propose to set: $d_1(x) = |I(x) - c_1|$ and $d_2(x) = |I(x) - c_2|$, where c_1 and c_2 are the mean intensity values outside and inside the contour. Therefore according to (1) d can be written as:

$$d(x) = |I(x) - c_1||I(x) - c_2| \tag{10}$$

If we assume a ramp profile for edge, so that the gray levels on the edge are between the mean values of both regions, i.e., $c_1 < I(x) < c_2$, on the border we can set: $d(x) = -(I(x) - c_1)(I(x) - c_2) > 0$, this reduces the non-linearity from gradient operator applied on $d(x)$. In the next step we will need to set mean values constraint in both regions. A Lagrangian application of this constraint can be regarded as the combination of our proposed functional E_{nf} with E_{cv}. In other word, our functional to be minimized is:

$$E_{cvf}(\phi, c_1, c_2) = E_{cv} + \rho E_{nf} \tag{11}$$

Where ρ is a user defined positive constant and E_{nf} is defined according to equation (6) as:

$$E_{nf}(\phi, c_1, c_2) = \int \delta(\phi)(I(x) - c_2)(c_1 - I(x))\nabla\phi(x).\nabla I dx \tag{12}$$

The function $(I(x) - c_2)(c_1 - I(x))$ is maximized by: $I(x) = \frac{c_1+c_2}{2}$ (a nominal value for edge) and reaches at zero in c_1 and c_2 respectively. Regularized version of $\delta(\phi)$ has a vanishing effect far from the current border. Therefore, the proposed functional will be selective on the current edge. Minimization of E_{cvf}, according to equations (9) and (8) can be easily achieved by the following evolutionary equation:

$$\frac{\partial\phi}{\partial t} = \delta(\phi)\{\rho\nabla\cdot(d(x)\nabla I) - \alpha(I(x) - c_1)^2 + \alpha(I(x) - c_2)^2 + \nabla\cdot(\frac{\nabla\phi(x)}{|\nabla\phi(x)|})\} \tag{13}$$

However the term $\nabla \cdot (d(x)\nabla I)$ can be written as:

$$\nabla.(d(x)\nabla I) = 2(c_1 + c_2 - 2I)|\nabla I|^2 + f(I)\Delta I \tag{14}$$

Equation eq.(14) has interesting property: $(c_1 + c_2 - 2I)$ inside the object is negative and causes expansion while outside becomes a contraction term. Therefore similar to advection term property in geodesic active contour model, it can reduce the leakage from spurious noisy edges. The term $\frac{\nabla\phi(x)}{|\nabla\phi(x)|}$ is the mean curvature of the evolving surface, however, since we are segmenting thin structures, this is replaced by the surface minimum curvature $\hat{k_2}$ as explained in [1]. In the next step we need to estimate unknown mean values.

3.3 Estimation of Parameters

Estimation of c_1 and c_2 takes the advantage of directional gradient information on the border and is basically interconnected to later. Since $E_{cvf}(\phi, c_1, c_2)$ is not a convex functional, estimation of unknown parameters is not trivial. One should guarantee energy minimization while update of these values. We propose algorithm 1 that guarantees the minimization of E_{cvf} at every iteration of eq.(13) with a given level set function ϕ^n.

3.4 Implementation

For prevention of convergence into local minimum implementation of the eq. (13) is achieved using $C^\infty(\bar{\Omega})$ regularization of H (and $\delta_\varepsilon = H'_\varepsilon$) introduced in [10]:

$$\begin{aligned} H_{2,z} &= \frac{1}{2}(1 + \frac{2}{\pi}arctan(\frac{z}{\varepsilon})) \\ \delta_{2,z} &= \frac{\varepsilon}{\pi(\varepsilon^2 + z^2)} \end{aligned} \tag{15}$$

Algorithm 1. Estimation of c_1 and c_2

$E^n \leftarrow E_{cvf}(\phi^n, \mathbf{c}^n)$;
$\alpha \leftarrow -1$
$flag \leftarrow 1$
$\mathbf{g}^n \leftarrow [\frac{\partial E_{cvf}(\phi,\mathbf{c})}{\partial c_1}, \frac{\partial E_{cvf}(\phi,\mathbf{c})}{\partial c_2}]^t|_{\mathbf{c}^n}$
while $flag = 1$ **do**
  $\mathbf{c}^{n+1} \leftarrow \mathbf{c}^n + \alpha \frac{\mathbf{g}^n}{|\mathbf{g}^n|}$
  $E \leftarrow E_{cvf}(\phi^n, \mathbf{c}^{n+1})$;
  if $(E^n < E)$ **then**
    $\alpha \leftarrow 0.5\alpha$
  else
    $flag \leftarrow 0$
  end if
end while

Computation of advection terms such as $\nabla\phi \cdot \nabla I$ involved in estimation of c_1 and c_2, is done using up-winding schemes. We need also to compute the surface minimum curvature $\hat{k_2}$. To that end, the Hessian matrix $\nabla^2(\phi)$, is first projected into the tangential direction of the underlining curve [11]:

$$J = \frac{1}{|\nabla(\phi)|} P_{\nabla(\phi)} \nabla^2(\phi) P_{\nabla(\phi)} \tag{16}$$

Where the projection operator is defined as below:

$$P_{\nabla(\phi)} = I - \frac{\nabla(\phi) \otimes \nabla(\phi)}{|\nabla(\phi)|^2} \tag{17}$$

Thus the first nonzero minimum eigenvalue of J, is taken as the surface min-curvature $\hat{k_2}$. For the numerical computation of curvature we use central differencing scheme. The solution of eq.(13) is achieved using forward Euler method and optimized using the narrow band level set method. Every few iterations ϕ is reinitialized to the signed distance function of the zero level set by solving:

$$\phi_t = sign(\phi)(1 - |\nabla\phi|) \tag{18}$$

using the method described in [12].

4 Experimental Results

Figure 1, is an illustration of a sample evolution under equation eq.(13). A finite length 3D cross cylinder is taken as the target shape as shown in part (b). Uniform intensities inside and outside of the model are smoothed by a Gaussian low pass filter and added with a Gaussian noise as indicated in part (a). Evolution starts from an initial volume specified inside the object. As it can be seen by comparing part (c) and (d) while minimization of $E_{cv} + \rho E_f$ model in (c) has produced a "convolved version" of the object, our functional, i.e, $E_{cv} + \rho E_{nf}$ is able to utilize edge information to better specify the object by closer estimates of the object border.

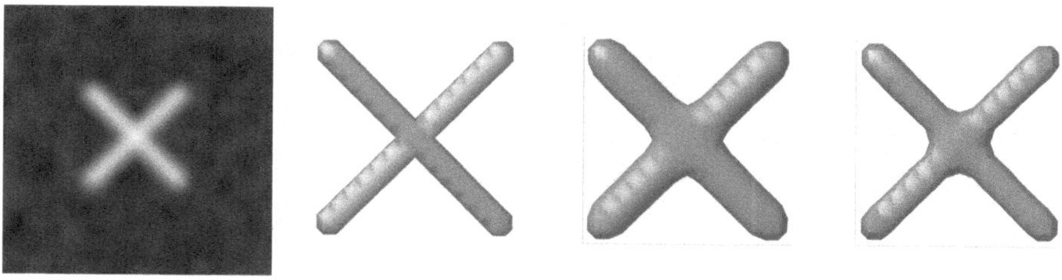

(a) (b) (c) (d)

Fig. 1. (a)Noise added slice from the midst of the model, (b) Final shape to be recovered, (c) Recovered shape from by minimization of $E_{cv} + \rho E_f$, (d) Recovered shape by minimizing E_{cvf}

4.1 Vessel Segmentation in MRA Images

In this section we have used our method to segment the brain vessels in MRA images. We have applied our method to several Time-of-Flight (TOF) and Phase-Contrast (PC) MRA data sets and consistently obtained robust extraction of vascular structures. Some typical examples are presented here. The first experiment is a qualitative evaluation study for different values of α and fixed amount of ρ. Figure 2 is a ROI selected from a PCMRA data set with the size of 256×256×60 voxels and spacing of 0.625×0.625×0.9 mm^3, that is obtained from a 0.4 Tesla MR scanner. Column (a) indicates maximum intensity projections (MIP) of a selected ROI from three different views. Initial segmentation is obtained with a user specified threshold value. Column (b) and (c) are the segmentations after approximately 300 iterations of eq.(13) for $\alpha = .03$ and $\alpha = .035$ As it can be seen, although extracted structures are smoother in part (c), vessels with lower contrast is obtained better in part (b). Typically, depending on the noise level one can select for the best value of α for a given type of data set. During our experiments, we observed that for higher noise levels, α to should be set to slightly higher values. We have compared the output of our model to the well-established CURVES method [1]. CURVES is an evolutionary level set method that its energy functional is based on the geodesic active contours $E_g = \int \delta(\phi(x)).g(x)|\nabla\phi(x)|dx$ where $g(x) = g(|\nabla I(x)|)$ is a uniform decreasing function of the image gradient. The final level set equation of CURVES algorithm is:

$$\frac{\partial \phi}{\partial t} = \delta(\phi)\{\hat{k_2} + \rho(\nabla\phi.\nabla I)\frac{\nabla g}{g}.\frac{\nabla \phi}{|\nabla \phi|}\} \tag{19}$$

where introducing $\rho(\nabla\phi.\nabla I)$ is heuristic and required for successful segmentation of vessels. The data set shown in figure 3 is a PCMRA data set with the same specifications as above. Colmun (a) is showing the MIP from three different views. Segmentation using CURVES algorithm is indicated in column (b) and (c) shows the obtained result using our proposed method by choosing α and ρ to positive user selected values. For this low Tesla data set, while both methods

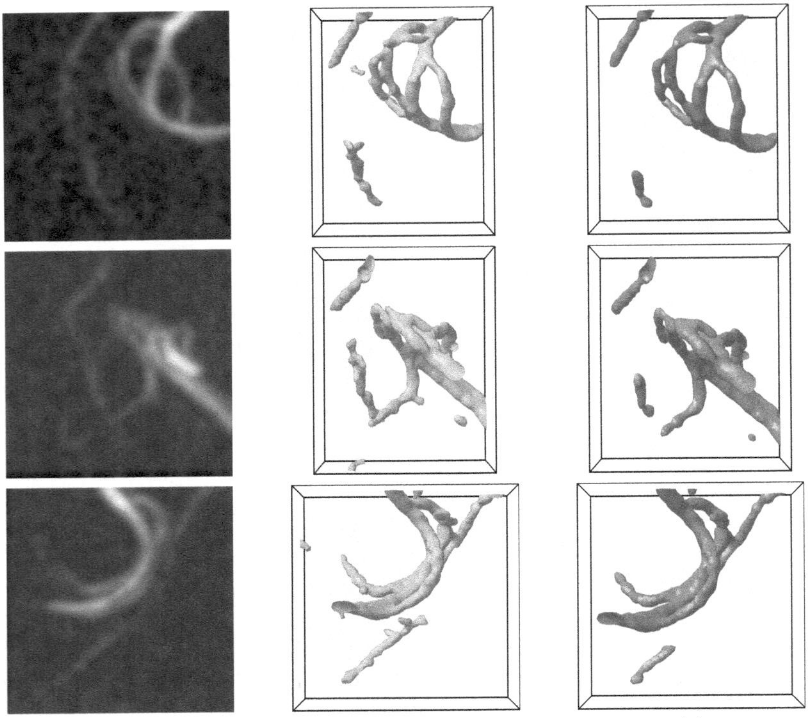

(a) (b) (c)

Fig. 2. Segmentation of ROI from a sample PCMRA data set, (a) MIP images in different directions, (b) Segmented vessels using $\alpha = 0.03$, (c) Segmented structures using $\alpha = 0.035$

have extracted the main vascular structures, by visual comparison to MIP images we observe that in low-contrast areas our method has produced more continuous and longer structures.

The data set shown in figure 4 is a TOF 256×256×120 matrix with spacing of 0.625×0.625×0.7 mm^3, obtained from a 0.3 Tesla MR scanner. MIPs are indicated from three different orientation. Segmentation using CURVES algorithm and our proposed algorithm is indicated in column (b) and (c) respectively. Note that elongation of segmented structures is achieved better in (c) compared to (b). Comparison of these two figures reveals that our proposed can be very useful to improve the continuity of the extracted vessels.

5 Discussion and Future Work

The main contribution of this paper is introduction of a new segmentation functional using both region statistics and gradient information available on the borders. Our method can be regarded as a new extention to flux maximizing

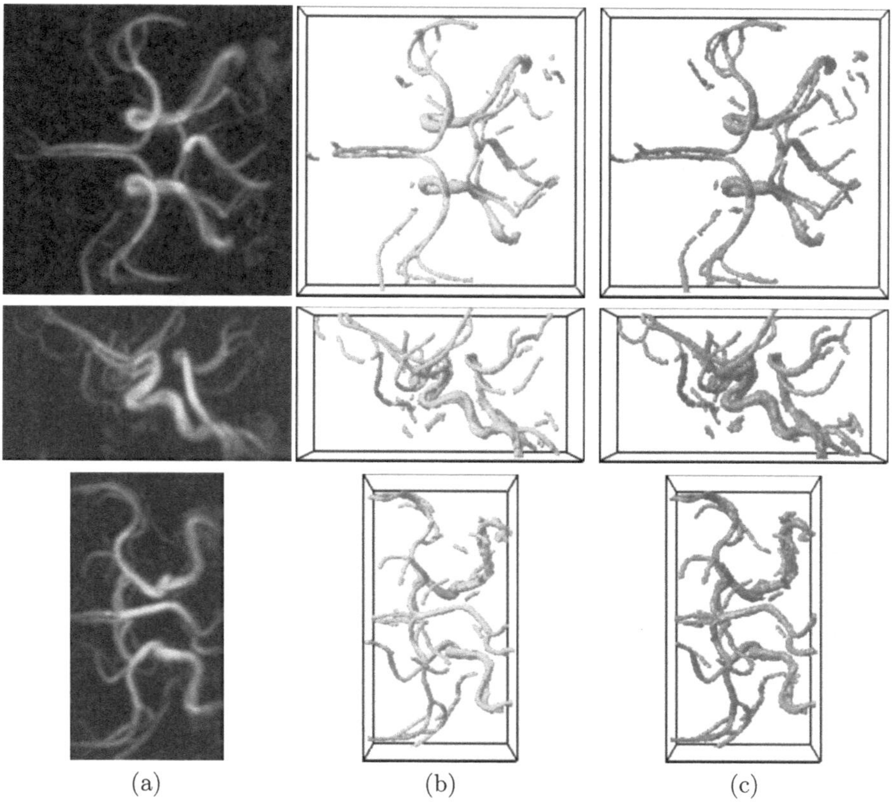

Fig. 3. Segmentation of a PCMRA data set, (a) MIP images in different directions, (b) Segmented vessels using CURVES, (c) Segmented structures using our proposed method

method. While the later requires a multi-scale computation of image divergence, our method eliminates such computation by integrating a statistical distance measure. Several application of our method to real MRA images, reveals its efficiency to robust extraction of vessels even in low Tesla MRA data sets. Also, the method is qualitatively compared to CURVE algorithm. Though both methods use the minimum surface curvature as a regularization term, tangential expantion along thin vessels in our proposed method is more efficient. This results in better elongation of these structures. A usefull direction for future work would include quantitative validation as well as comparison to other methods. We hope to gain access to the data sets used in previous works. Although, we used Chan-Vese model as our statistical model, outlined concept of statistical edge, in the framework of variational level set methods, can be extended to include non-parametrical probability distance functions. This will be a challenging formulation, since in that case the distance functions are explicitly defined using level set heavy side functions. We are currently developing such explained frame work.

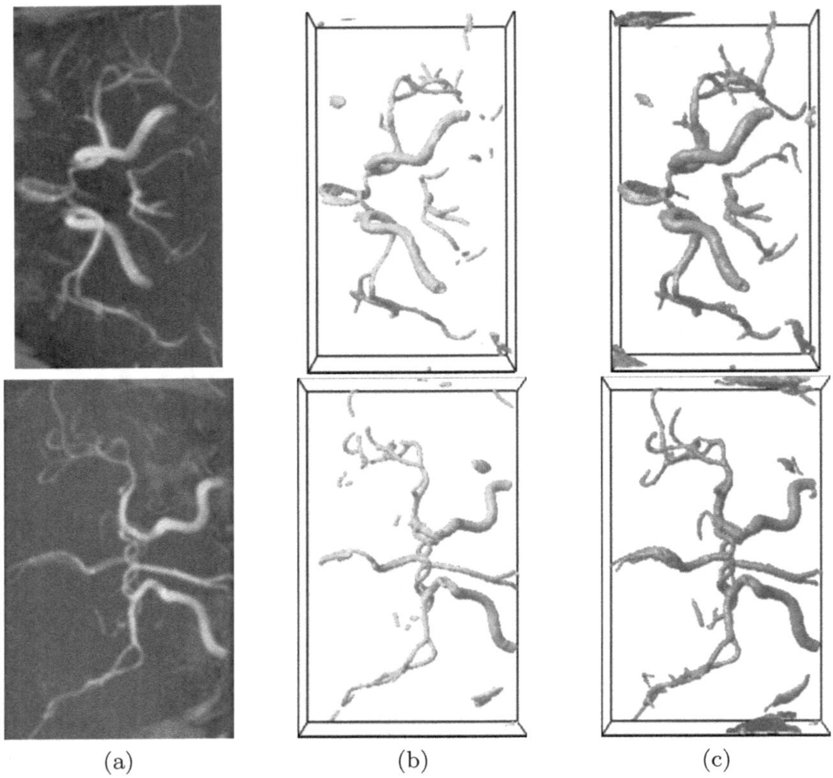

Fig. 4. Segmentation of a TOFMRA data set, (a) MIP images in different directions, (b) Segmented vessels using CURVE , (c) Segmented structures using our proposed method

Acknowledgment

This study was supported in part by the Grant-in-Aid of the Ministry of Education, Culture, Sport, Science and Technology in Japan (to H. Liao), and the Grant-in-Aid of the Japan Society for the Promotion of Science (to T.Dohi).

References

1. Lorgio, L.M., Faugeras, O.D., Grimson, W.E.L., Kerivan, R., Kikinis, R., Nabavai, A., Westin, C.F.: CURVES: Curve evolution for vessel segmentation. Medical Image Analysis 5, 195–206 (2001)
2. Yan, P., Kassim, A.A.: Segmentation of volumetric MRA images by using capillary active contour. Medical Image Analysis 10(3), 317–329 (2006)
3. Gooya, A., Liao, H., Matsumiya, K., Masamune, K., Dohi, T.: A shape induced anisotropic flow for volumetric vascular segmentation in mra, In: The Fourth IEEE International Symposium on Biomedical Imaging ISBI 2007 (to appear)

4. Nain, D., Yezzi, A., Turk, G.: Vessel segmentation using a shape driven flow. In: Barillot, C., Haynor, D.R., Hellier, P. (eds.) MICCAI 2004. LNCS, vol. 3216, pp. 51–59. Springer, Heidelberg (2004)
5. Vasilevsky, A., Siddiqi, K.: Flux maximizing geometric flows. IEEE Trans. Pat. Anal. Mach. Intel. 24(12), 1565–1578 (2002)
6. Gazit, M.H., Kimmel, R., Peled, N., Goldsher, D.: Segmentation of thin structures in volumetric medical images. IEEE Trans. Image Proc. 15(2), 354–363 (2006)
7. Caselles, V., Kimmel, R., Sapiro, G.: Geodesic Active Contours. Int. Journal of Computer Vision 22(1), 61–79 (1997)
8. Zaho, H.K., Chan, T., Merriman, B., Osher, S.: A variational level set approach to multiphase motion. Journal of Computational Physics 127, 179–195 (1996)
9. Paragios, N., Deriche, R.: Geodesic Active Regions: A new paradagim to deal with frame partition problems in computer vision. Int. Journal of Visual Communiation and Image Representation 13, 249–268 (2002)
10. Chan, T.F., Vese, A.: Active contours without edges, IEEE Trans. Imag. Proc., vol. 10, pp. 266–277 (2001)
11. Ambrosio, L., Soner, H.M.: Level set approach to mean curvature flow in arbitrary codimension. J.Differential Geometry 43, 693–737 (1996)
12. Peng, D., Merriman, B., Osher, S., Zhao, H.-K., Kang, M.: A pde based fast local level set method. J.Comput. Phys 155, 410–438 (1995)

Joint Sulci Detection Using Graphical Models and Boosted Priors

Yonggang Shi[1], Zhuowen Tu[1], Allan L. Reiss[2], Rebecca A. Dutton[1], Agatha D. Lee[1], Albert M. Galaburda[3], Ivo Dinov[1], Paul M. Thompson[1], and Arthur W. Toga[1]

[1] Lab of Neuro Imaging, UCLA School of Medicine, Los Angeles, CA, USA
{yshi,ztu,ivo.dinov,thompson,toga}@loni.ucla.edu
[2] School of Medicine, Stanford University, Stanford, CA, USA
[3] Harvard Medical School, Boston, MA, USA

Abstract. In this paper we propose an automated approach for joint sulci detection on cortical surfaces by using graphical models and boosting techniques to incorporate shape priors of major sulci and their Markovian relations. For each sulcus, we represent it as a node in the graphical model and associate it with a sample space of candidate curves, which is generated automatically using the Hamilton-Jacobi skeleton of sulcal regions. To take into account individual as well as joint priors about the shape of major sulci, we learn the potential functions of the graphical model using AdaBoost algorithm to select and fuse information from a large set of features. This discriminative approach is especially powerful in capturing the neighboring relations between sulcal lines, which are otherwise hard to be captured by generative models. Using belief propagation, efficient inferencing is then performed on the graphical model to estimate each sulcus as the maximizer of its final belief. On a data set of 40 cortical surfaces, we demonstrate the advantage of joint detection on four major sulci: central, precentral, postcentral and the sylvian fissure.

1 Introduction

Cortical sulci are important landmarks in human brain mapping because they encode rich information about the convolution patterns of human brains[1] and provide guidance for registration tasks[2], but the variability of the brain morphometry poses serious challenges for their automatic detection, thus manual annotation remains the golden standard in practice. In this paper, we propose a novel approach to incorporate prior knowledge from manual tracing by modeling the relation of major sulci with boosting techniques and detect them *jointly* via the solution of an inference problem on graphical models.

Many algorithms were proposed for sulci detection in previous works. Curvature features were used in [3,4,5] to detect sulci semi-automatically with the need of manually inputing the starting and ending points. Depth features with respect to a shrink wrap surface were also used for sulci detection on surfaces[6,7]. The extraction of sulci from volume images were proposed in [8,9,10], but human interactions are still necessary to pick out specific sulci from the results.

N. Karssemeijer and B. Lelieveldt (Eds.): IPMI 2007, LNCS 4584, pp. 98–109, 2007.
© Springer-Verlag Berlin Heidelberg 2007

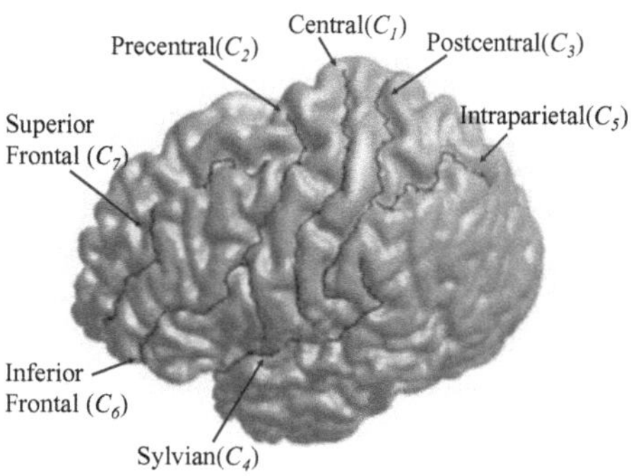

(a)

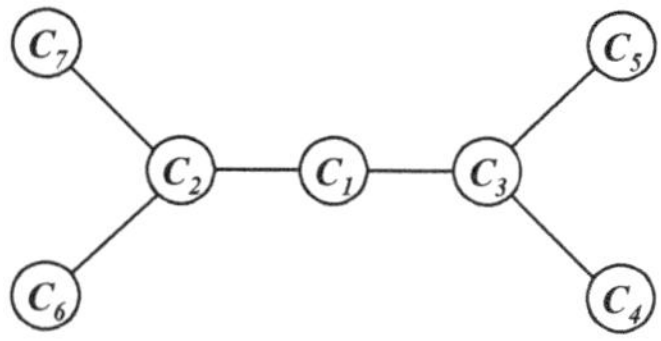

(b)

Fig. 1. An illustration of joint sulci detection. (a) Seven major sulci on a cortical surface. (b) A graphical model representing the local dependency between neighboring sulci.

To address this challenge, learning-based approaches were introduced into the detection process. Because of its simplicity, techniques based on the principal component analysis(PCA) of point sets[11] were used in[12,13]. Graphical models and neural networks were used in [14] for automatic recognition of sulcal ribbons, which only identify subsets of major sulci. A learning-based technique based on probabilistic boosting trees[15] was proposed in [16] for the automatic detection of cortical sulci from volume images, but each sulcus was detected separately.

We propose in this work to detect multiple sulci jointly with graphical models. From the experience of manual tracing, this seems a natural choice as the knowledge about the relative location of sulci is frequently utilized for the correct identification of these curves. Modeling the relation of multiple objects has also been shown useful in medical image segmentation[17]. As an example, seven major sulci are plotted on the lateral surface of a cortex in Fig. 1(a). Even though we can see that most parts of sulci follow furrows of high curvature, choices have to be made at intersections of multiple furrows because of the variability of the cortex. What makes this task more difficult is that the gyral regions have to be crossed sometimes to ensure a continuous curve is generated for each sulcus. To counter this kind of complications, protocols are defined in practice on how to use *local* dependency of sulcal lines for manual annotation. For the example in Fig. 1(a), the precentral sulcus has to cross a gyrus to meet the requirement that it should follow a path as parallel as possible to the central sulcus. In determining the inferior portion of postcentral sulcus that is highly variable, its relation with respect to the tail of the sylvian fissure also helps to provide critical information.

There are two main challenges, however, to formulate a tractable inference problem over graphical models for joint sulci detection. (1) With each node of the graph representing a sulcus, the random variables of interest here live in high dimensional shape spaces and it is generally hard to do inferences directly over such spaces. (2) Every major sulcal curve observes flexible shape and it is hard to capture their individual as well as joint regularity by a good prior.

In our joint detection framework, we tackle these challenges by first constructing a sample space containing a finite number of candidate curves at each node of the graph. These sample spaces greatly reduce the search range of inference algorithms and they are generated automatically based on the Hamilton-Jacobi skeleton of sulcal regions on triangulated cortical surfaces. We then use boosting techniques[18] to learn discriminative shape models of each sulcus and their neighboring relations. The advantages are twofold. (1) The algorithm is able to automatically select and fuse a set of informative shape features, characterizing unary as well as binary relationships of the sulcal curves, from a large set of candidate features. (2) The priors are learned directly from the training data and there is no parameter to tune for different sucal curves. Traditional generative model based algorithms, e.g. PCA, have difficulty in modeling such complicated priors due to its Gaussian assumptions. In making the inference, a belief propagation algorithm[19,20] is used to perform inferences efficiently on these sample spaces for joint sulci detection.

In the rest of the paper, we first propose our joint detection framework with graphical models in section 2. The generation of sample spaces for each node of the graph is then described in section 3. After that, we develop a boosting approach in section 4 to learn potential functions in graphical models for sulci of interest. In section 5, experimental results on the joint detection of four major sulci: central, precentral, postcentral and the sylvian fissure on 40 cortical surfaces are presented. Finally, conclusions are made in section 6.

2 The Joint Detection Framework

For the detection of a set of major sulci $C_1, C_2, \cdots, C_L$ on a cortical surface $\mathcal{M}$, we assume an undirected graphical model $G = (V, E)$ that represents the Markovian relation among sulci, where $V = \{C_1, C_2, \cdots, C_L\}$ are the set of nodes, and E is the set of edges in the graph. As an example, a graphical model for the seven sulci in Fig. 1(a) is shown in Fig. 1(b). Because the number of major sulci is small on the cortical surface, it is straightforward to construct the graph structure of such models and this only needs to be done once for the same detection task.

To perform inferences on sulcal lines with graphical models, it is critical to first specify a proper sample space for each node as the general space of curves is infinite dimensional. One possible solution is to reduce the dimension of shape spaces with PCA, but there is no guarantee that these parameterized curves will live on the cortical surface and follow the bottom of sulcal regions. To overcome this problem, we generate a set of candidate curves S_i automatically for each sulcus C_i using a novel algorithm that will be developed in section 3. These candidate curves are weighted geodesics on the cortical surface and follow the skeleton of sulcal regions closely. By adopting the set of candidate curves S_i as

Table 1. The AdaBoost algorithm[18]

Given training data: $(x_1, y_1, w_1^1), \cdots, (x_n, y_n, w_n^1)$ where x_i are the sample data, $y_i \in \{-1, 1\}$ are the corresponding class labels, and w_i^1 are the initial weights.

For $t = 1, \cdots, T$

- Train a weak classifier h_t given the current weights.
- Compute the weighted error rate ϵ_t of the classifier h_t.
- Update the weights:

$$w_i^{t+1} = \frac{w_i^t e^{-\alpha_t y_i h_t(x_i)}}{Z_t}$$

where $\alpha_t = \log((1 - \epsilon_t)/\epsilon_t)/2$ and Z_t is a normalization constant such that $\sum_{i=1}^n w_i^{t+1} = 1$.

Output the final classifier $H = sign(f)$ with the decision function $f = \sum_{t=1}^T \alpha_t h_t$.

the sample space for each node C_i, we are able to model each sulcus as a discrete random variable with values in a finite set and this makes the inference on the graphical model computationally tractable.

Over the sample spaces of all the nodes in a graphical model, we define two types of potential functions to complete the construction of the graphical model: the local evidence function $\phi_i : S_i \rightarrow \mathbb{R}$ at each node C_i and the compatibility function $\psi_{i,j} : S_i \times S_j \rightarrow \mathbb{R}$ for $(C_i, C_j) \in E$. To incorporate shape priors about individual sulcus and their relations, we propose a discriminative approach using AdaBoost[18] in section 4 to learn both types of potential functions from manually annotated training data. Given input data x, the discriminative method learns the posterior probability $p(y|x)$ of a label y. With the discriminative approach, there is no need of specifying parametric forms for prior models of sulcal lines and their neighboring relations. Instead we use a large set of features derived from training data and selectively combine information from these features with boosting techniques. The central idea of AdaBoost, as listed in Table I, is the formation of a strong classifier through the combination of a series of weak classifiers. Using the decision function f generated from AdaBoost, an approximate posterior can then be defined and used as the potential function.

With the graphical model defined, we can write down the joint distribution of all the sulci as:

$$p(C_1, \cdots, C_L) = \frac{1}{Z} \prod_{(C_i, C_j) \in E} \psi_{i,j}(C_i, C_j) \prod_{C_i \in V} \phi_i(C_i) \quad (1)$$

where Z is the partition function for normalization. For sulci detection, we use belief propagation to compute the marginal distribution of each sulcus from the joint distribution because it is applicable to graphs both with and without cycles. With belief propagation, each node in the graph receives and sends out messages at every iteration of the algorithm. For a node C_i, the message it sends to its

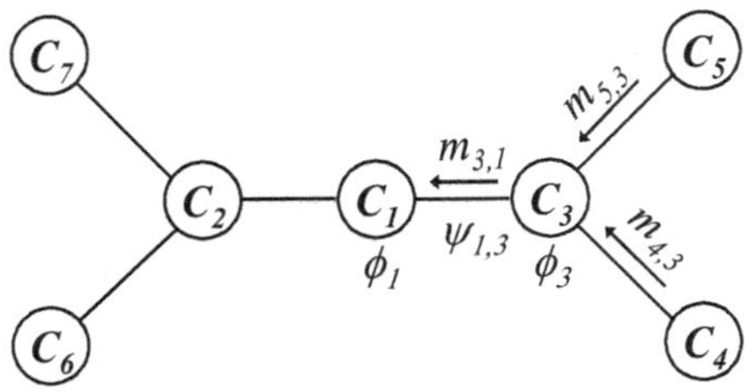

Fig. 2. An example of message passing in the graphical model of Fig. 1(b)

neighbor C_j is defined as:

$$m_{i,j}(C_j) = \sum_{C_i \in S_i} \psi_{i,j}(C_i, C_j)\phi_i(C_i) \prod_{C_k \in \mathcal{N}(C_i) \setminus C_j} m_{k,i}(C_i) \tag{2}$$

where $\mathcal{N}(C_i)$ are neighbors of C_i in the graph. This message takes into account not only the local evidence ϕ_i and the compatibility function $\psi_{i,j}$, but also the messages the node C_i received from its neighbors except C_j. As an illustration, we show in Fig. 2 the flow of messages from the node C_4 and C_5 to C_3, and then to C_1 in the graphical model shown in Fig. 1(b). If we continue this message passing process until it converges, i.e., when the messages stop changing, we obtain the final belief at each node of the graph as:

$$b_i(C_i) = \phi_i(C_i) \prod_{C_j \in \mathcal{N}(C_i)} m_{j,i}(C_i) \quad i = 1, 2, \cdots, L. \tag{3}$$

Using belief propagation, we collect information from all the nodes to form the final belief for every sulcus. For graphs without cycles[19], such as trees, the final belief function corresponds to the marginal distribution of each sulcus derived from the joint distribution in (1), thus we can detect a sulcus by maximizing the final belief:

$$C_i^* = \arg\max_{C_i \in S_i} b_i(C_i) \quad i = 1, 2, \cdots, L. \tag{4}$$

Even for graphs with cycles, belief propagation is known to frequently perform well and generate excellent results[20], most notably for its near Shannon limit performance in turbo decoding[21]. Thus the above equation is also applicable for joint sulci detection in the case that the graphical model has loops.

3 Generation of Sample Spaces

Given a cortical surface, there are three main stages in our algorithm of sample space generation for each node of a graphical model: skeletonization of sulcal regions, a learning-based approach that picks out candidates for the starting and ending point of the sulcus, and the generation of member curves of the sample space as weighted geodesics on the cortical surface.

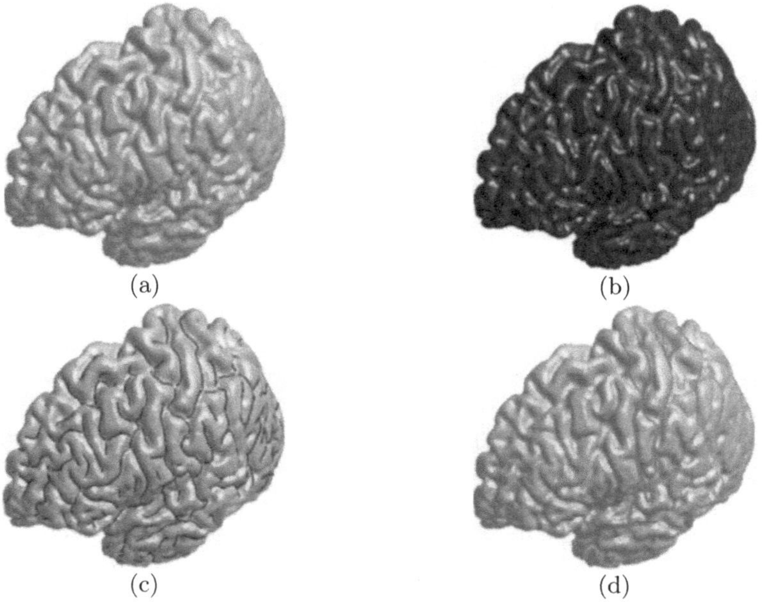

Fig. 3. The process of generating sample spaces for sulci detection. (a) The original cortical surface. (b) Mesh segmentation results. Red: sulcal regions; blue: gyral regions. (c) The skeleton of sulcal regions plotted in black. (d) Curves from the sample space of the central sulcus plotted in red.

In the first stage, we compute the skeleton of sulcal regions with the method we reported in[22]. For completeness we briefly review the main steps of this algorithm. We represent the cortical surface $\mathcal{M}$ as a triangular mesh and first compute the principle curvatures at each vertex. Using the curvature features, the cortical surface is then partitioned into sulcal and gyral regions using graph cuts. As an illustration, we show in Fig. 3(b) the result of the partition algorithm for the cortical surface in Fig. 3(a). Finally an extension of the method of Hamilton-Jacobi skeleton[23] is used to calculate the skeleton of sulcal regions as shown in Fig. 3(c). For all vertices of $\mathcal{M}$ in the skeleton, we classify them into three types using the neighboring system of the triangular mesh:

- End points: vertices with one neighbor in the skeleton.
- Knot points: vertices with three or more neighbors in the skeleton.
- Middle points: vertices with two neighbors in the skeleton.

We learn a two-class classifier with AdaBoost in the second stage to pick a set of candidate points from the union of end and knot points in the skeleton for the starting and ending point of each sulcus. We use a set of K cortical surfaces with manually labeled sulci for the construction of our training data. These cortical surfaces are assumed to be registered to a common coordinate space such as ICBM. To learn the classifier for the starting point of a sulcus C_i, we construct the training data as follows. The starting point of the manually labeled sulcus C_i on the K cortical surfaces are assigned label 1 and weight $1/2K$. The union of all the knot and end points from the skeletons of the K cortical surfaces are assigned label -1 and weight $1/2\tilde{N}$ where $\tilde{N}$ is the total number of points in this set. At each iteration of AdaBoost, we train a perceptron as the weak classifier using the pocket algorithm with ratchet[24]. As shown in Table I, the final decision function generated from AdaBoost is of the following form:

$$f = \sum_{t=1}^{T} \alpha_t h_t \tag{5}$$

where $h_t : \mathbb{R}^3 \to \{-1, 1\}$ is the weak classifier at the t-th iteration of AdaBoost and α_t is the weight for this weak classifier. Applying the decision function f to all the end and knot points in the skeleton of a cortical surface, we pick the candidates for the starting point of C_i as M points with the largest f values. Typically we choose $M = 10$ in our experiments and this generates a sufficiently large candidate set for the final detection of sulcal lines according to our experience. Similarly, a candidate set of M points can also be generated for the ending point of C_i.

Given the candidate set for the starting and ending points of the sulcal line C_i, we connect them with weighted geodesics on $\mathcal{M}$ to generate the sample space S_i. The weights are derived from the geodesic distance transform d of the skeleton on $\mathcal{M}$ generated in the first stage. We compute these geodesics with the fast marching algorithm on triangular meshes[25]. For a candidate of starting point X_s and a candidate for the ending point X_e, we connect them through a weighted geodesic with the weight defined as

$$F = e^{-d^2/2\sigma^2} \tag{6}$$

to encourage the weighted geodesic overlapping as much as possible with the skeleton of sulcal regions. To find this geodesic, we first compute a weighted distance transform d^w on $\mathcal{M}$ by solving the Eikonal equation

$$\nabla d^w F = 1 \tag{7}$$

intrinsically over the cortical surface and trace backward from X_e to X_s in gradient descent directions. This geodesic is then added to the sample space S_i. We choose the parameter $\sigma = 1, 2, 3, 4, 5$ to cover a wide range of possible routes. So overall the sample space S_i of C_i is composed of $5M^2$ curves. As an illustration, all the candidate curves in the sample space of the central sulcus on the cortical surface in Fig. 1(a) are plotted in Fig. 1(d) and we can see that the true central sulcus is included in this sample space.

4 Learning Potential Functions Using AdaBoost

In this section, we describe our learning-based approach for the construction of the potential functions in graphical models to take into account individual and joint shape priors of major sulci. Our approach is discriminative and learns both the local evidence functions ϕ_i and the compatibility functions $\psi_{i,j}$ with AdaBoost. For each potential function, we construct a set of features and learn a strong two-class classifier by combining with AdaBoost a series of weak classifiers on these features. It is shown in [26] that AdaBoost approximates logistic regression and its result can be used to estimate the probability of a class label, which we then use to define the potential function.

For a sulcus C_i we learn its local evidence function ϕ_i from a training data set of K cortical surfaces with the sulcus manually labeled on each surface. We also assume these cortical surfaces are registered to the same common coordinate system as in section 3. For the same sulcus, we generate a sample space on each of the cortical surface in the training data. All curves are parameterized with N (typically 100) uniformly sampled points such that one-to-one correspondences are established between curves. In the training data set, all manually labeled sulcus for C_i on the K cortical surfaces are assigned label 1 and weight $1/2K$ and all the curves in the sample spaces are assigned a label -1 and weight $1/10KM^2$. The same perceptron in section 3 is used as our weak classifier. At each iteration of AdaBoost, we train N perceptrons $P_n(1 \leq n \leq N)$ with the n-th point from all the curves and pick the one with the best performance as the weak classifier h_t. By combining all the weak classifiers, we obtain the final decision function $f(C_i) = \sum_{t=1}^{T} \alpha_t h_t(C_i)$. Following [26], we define the local evidence function for C_i as:

$$\phi_i(C_i) = \frac{e^{2f(C_i)}}{1 + e^{2f(C_i)}} \quad \forall C_i \in S_i. \tag{8}$$

The local evidence function approaches the value 1 at curves in the sample space that are similar to the manually labeled sulcus in the training data, indicating intuitively that they exhibit strong evidence to be the sulcus we want to detect.

To learn the compatibility function between two sulci C_i and C_j, we define the feature used for training as $d_{i,j} = C_i - C_j$, which is the difference between the two curves. For each cortical surface in the training data, the manually labeled sulci for C_i and C_j are used to construct the feature vector $d_{i,j}$ with label 1 and weight $1/2K$. From the sample spaces of C_i and C_j on the K cortical surfaces, we randomly pick $5KM^2$ pairs to construct the negative sample data with label -1 and weight $1/10KM^2$. The same boosting process as above is applied to learn a decision function for the compatibility between the two sulci $f(C_i, C_j) = \sum_{t=1}^{T} \alpha_t h_t(d_{i,j})$ and we can define the compatibility function between C_i and C_j as:

$$\psi_{i,j}(C_i, C_j) = \frac{e^{2f(C_i,C_j)}}{1 + e^{2f(C_i,C_j)}} \quad \forall C_i \in S_i, C_j \in S_j. \tag{9}$$

With AdaBoost, we have developed a common solution for the learning of both local evidence functions and compatibility functions. Even though we used only features derived from coordinate information in our current work, the boosting method for learning priors is general and allows the inclusion of more features in future work. By inserting the potential functions into graphical models, the belief propagation process can then be used for the joint detection of major sulci.

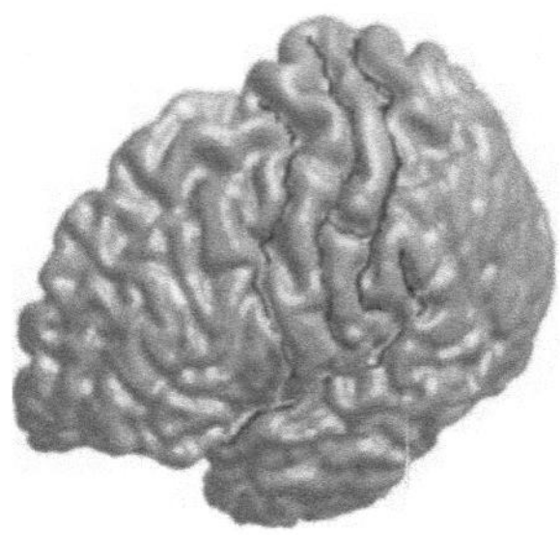

(a) Without graphical models.

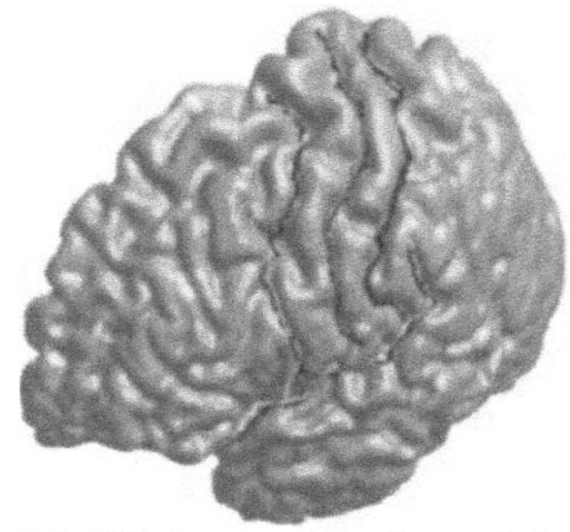

(b) With graphical models.

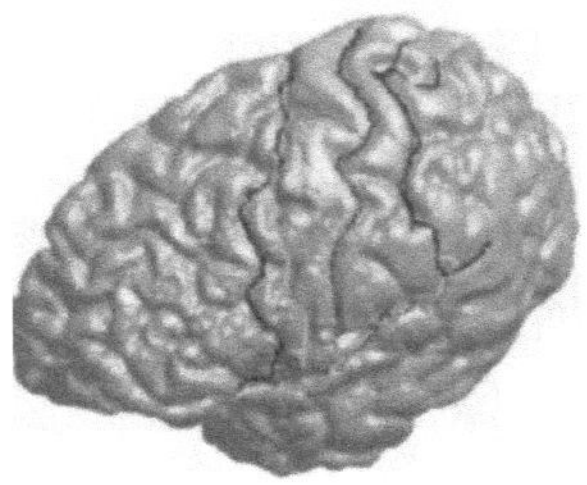

(c) Without graphical models.

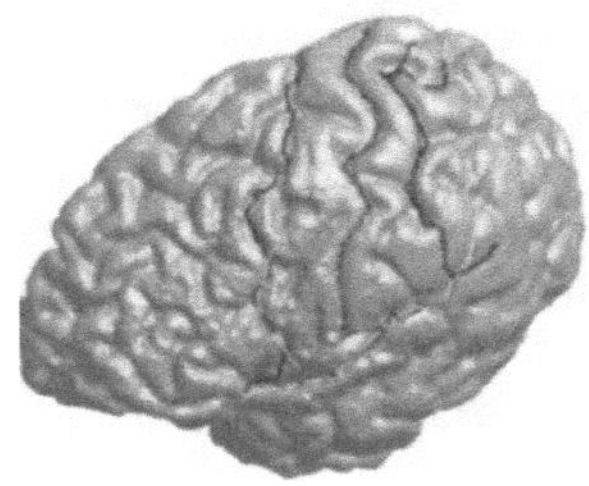

(d) With graphical models.

Fig. 4. Sulci detection results on two cortical surfaces. (a) and (b) show results from a surface in the training data. (c) and (d) show results from one of the surface in the testing data. For all the results, manually labeled results are plotted in black for comparison. The detected curves for the central, precentral, postcentral, and sylvian fissure are plotted in red, green, blue and cyan.

5 Experimental Results

In this section we present preliminary experimental results for the joint detection of four major sulci: the central, precentral, postcentral sulcus and sylvian fissure. The graphical model used for the joint detection of these four sulci is the subgraph in Fig. 1(b) that includes the nodes C_1, C_2, C_3 and C_4.

In our experiments, we have a dataset of 40 cortical surfaces with the four sulci manually labeled. We used 20 of them as the training data and the other 20 for testing. During the training stage, we first computed the skeleton of sulcal regions for the 20 training data. Decision functions were then learned for each sulcus such that a set of candidate points can be generated for both of its starting and ending point. After that, a sample space was generated for each sulcus with weighted geodesics as described in section 3. With these sample spaces, the local evidence functions and the compatibility functions between neighboring vertices in the graphical model were learned using the boosting method developed in section 4. For every cortical surface in the testing data, the sample space of each sulcus was generated with the same classifier learned from the training data.

Once all the potential functions and sample spaces were constructed, we applied the joint detection algorithm with graphical models in section 2 to detect the four sulci on all 40 cortical surfaces. As a comparison, we also detected each sulcus independently without using graphical models. This is realized by simply picking the curve in the sample space that maximizes the local evidence function. To illustrate the advantage of the joint detection algorithm, we show in Fig. 4 the detection results on two cortical surfaces, one from the training data and the other from the testing data, using these two different methods. For the first surface, the results without using graphical models is shown in Fig. 4(a) and we can see the inferior part of the postcentral sulcus overlaps with the central sulcus and this is clearly undesirable. In the joint detection results shown in Fig. 4(b), it is easy to see the postcentral sulcus is correctly detected. Thanks to the compatibility functions learned with boosting, the tail of the sylvian fissure detected in Fig. 4(b) also agrees better with manually labeled results than the sylvian fissure detected in Fig. 4(a). In results of the second surface shown in Fig. 4(c) and (d), improved results were also obtained with graphical models for the central and precentral sulcus as compared to the results detected independently.

We next perform a quantitative analysis of the performance of our sulci detection algorithm by comparing with manually labeled curves. For two curves $\tilde{C}_1$ and $\tilde{C}_2$ that are parameterized with N points, we define two distances:

$$D_a(\tilde{C}_1, \tilde{C}_2) = \frac{1}{N} \sum_{x_n \in \tilde{C}_1} \min_{y_m \in \tilde{C}_2} \| x_n - y_m \| \tag{10}$$

and

$$D_h(\tilde{C}_1, \tilde{C}_2) = \max_{x_n \in \tilde{C}_1} \min_{y_m \in \tilde{C}_2} \| x_n - y_m \| . \tag{11}$$

The distance D_a is an average of the distance from points on $\tilde{C}_1$ to $\tilde{C}_2$, while D_h measures the Hausdorff distance from $\tilde{C}_1$ to $\tilde{C}_2$. For a detected sulcus C_i and its manually labeled result $\overline{C}_i$, we use four distances to measure the difference between them: $D_a^1 = D_a(C_i, \overline{C}_i)$, $D_a^2 = D_a(\overline{C}_i, C_i)$, $D_h^1 = D_h(C_i, \overline{C}_i)$, and $D_h^2 = D_h(\overline{C}_i, C_i)$.

Quantitative comparisons to manually labeled results were performed for both the sulci detected jointly with graphical models and independently without graphical models. For these two different groups of results, the average of the four distances over the training and testing data were computed and listed separately for each sulcus in Table 2. Overall we have 32 average distances for each group of results. The advantage of the jointly detected results are clear as they outperform results without graphical models in 28 of the 32 distances. A more detailed analysis shows that we achieve very good performance with our joint sulci detection algorithm in terms of D_a^1 and D_a^2 for all four sulci, and the results are especially encouraging for the central sulcus where an average distance of around 1mm is obtained to the manually annotated curves. The relatively large distances in terms of D_h^1 and D_h^2 are mostly due to the variability of the starting and ending part of sulci. Considering the lack of consensus among manual tracers on these parts, it might be interesting to use other metrics in our future research to measure how well the main body of each sulcal curve is detected.

Table 2. Differences between sulci detected jointly with graphical models and independently as compared to manually annotated results (in millimeters)

	Without graphical models				With graphical models			
Sulci	D_a^1	D_a^2	D_h^1	D_h^2	D_a^1	D_a^2	D_h^1	D_h^2
Central (training)	1.86	1.91	7.88	8.40	0.99	1.36	5.64	6.98
Precentral (training)	3.01	2.50	11.48	11.87	2.57	2.56	10.03	11.13
Postcentral(training)	5.65	5.00	15.34	14.58	2.90	3.26	11.75	12.19
Sylvian (training)	2.68	2.55	11.14	13.05	2.88	2.32	11.15	10.83
Central (testing)	3.04	2.98	10.52	11.01	1.10	1.59	6.59	8.55
Precentral (testing)	4.37	4.48	13.19	14.75	2.92	3.41	10.55	12.60
Postcentral (testing)	2.80	3.10	11.33	11.80	2.50	3.04	10.16	12.42
Sylvian (testing)	3.07	2.75	13.41	13.59	2.65	2.48	12.09	12.55

6 Conclusions

A general framework for the joint detection of major sulci was proposed in this paper. Using boosting techniques, we integrated discriminative shape priors of each sulcus and their Markovian relations into graphical models and transformed sulci detection into a tractable inference problem over sample spaces of candidate curves. The boosting approach is flexible and allows the inclusion of new features to capture more detailed priors in future work. We are also testing the joint detection of more major sulci with our algorithm.

Acknowledgment

This work was funded by the National Institutes of Health through the NIH Roadmap for Medical Research, Grant U54 RR021813 entitled Center for Computational Biology (CCB).

References

1. Ono, M., Kubik, S., Abarnathey, C.: Atlas of the Cerebral Sulci. Thieme Medical Publishers (1990)
2. Thompson, P.M., Hayashi, K.M., Sowell, E.R., Gogtay, N., Giedd, J.N., Rapoport, J.L., de Zubicaray, G.I., Janke, A.L., Rose, S.E., Semple, J., Doddrell, D.M., Wang, Y., van Erp, T.G.M., Cannon, T.D., Toga, A.W.: Mapping cortical change in alzheimers disease, brain development, and schizophrenia. NeuroImage 23, S2–S18 (2004)
3. Khaneja, N., Miller, M., Grenander, U.: Dynamic programming generation of curves on brain surfaces. IEEE Trans. Pattern Anal. Machine Intell. 20(11), 1260–1265 (1998)
4. Bartesaghi, A., Sapiro, G.: A system for the generation of curves on 3D brain images. Human Brain Mapping 14, 1–15 (2001)
5. Lui, L.M., Wang, Y., Chan, T.F., Thompson, P.M.: Automatic landmark and its application to the optimization of brain conformal mapping. In: Proc. CVPR. vol. 2, pp. 1784–1792 (2006)
6. Rettmann, M.E., Han, X., Xu, C., Prince, J.L.: Automated sulcal segmentation using watersheds on the cortical surface. NeuroImage 15(2), 329–244 (2002)

7. Kao, C., Hofer, M., Sapiro, G., Stern, J., Rotternberg, D.: A geometric method for automatic extraction of sulcal fundi. In: Proc. ISBI 2006, pp. 1168–1171 (2006)
8. Lohmann, G.: Extracting line representations of sulcal and gyral patterns in MR images of the human brain. IEEE Trans. Med. Imag. 17(6), 1040–1048 (1998)
9. Zhou, Y., Thompson, P.M., Toga, A.W.: Extracting and representing the cortical sulci. IEEE Computer Graphics and Applications 19(3), 49–55 (1999)
10. Mangin, J.F., Frouin, V., Bloch, I., Régis, J., López-Krahe, J.: From 3d magnetic resonance images to structural representations of the cortex topography using topology preserving deformations. Journal of Mathematical Imaging and Vision 5(4), 297–318 (1995)
11. Cootes, T., Taylor, C., Cooper, D., Graham, J.: Active shape models-their training and application. Computer Vision and Image Understanding 61(1), 38–59 (1995)
12. Lohmann, G., Cramon, D.: Automatic labelling of the human cortical surface using sulcal basins. Medical Image Analysis 4, 179–188 (2000)
13. Tao, X., Prince, J., Davatzikos, C.: Using a statistical shape model to extract sulcal curves on the outer cortex of the human brain. IEEE Trans. Med. Imag. 21(5), 513–524 (2002)
14. Rivière, D., Mangin, J., Papadopoulos-Orfanos, D., Martinez, J., Frouin, V., Régis, J.: Automatic recognition of cortical sulci of the human brain using a congregation of neural networks. Medical Image Analysis 6, 77–92 (2002)
15. Tu, Z.: Probabilistic boosting-tree: learning discriminative models for classification, recognition, and clustering. In: Proc. ICCV 2005, vol. 2, pp. 1589–1596 (2005)
16. Zheng, S., Tu, Z., Yuille, A., Reiss, A., Dutton, R., Lee, A., Galaburda, A., Thompson, P., Dinov, I., Toga, A.: A learning-based algorithm for automatic extraction of the cortical sulci. In: Larsen, R., Nielsen, M., Sporring, J. (eds.) MICCAI 2006. LNCS, vol. 4190, pp. 695–703. Springer, Heidelberg (2006)
17. Pizer, S., Jeong, J., Lu, C., Joshi, S.: Estimating the statistics of multi-object anatomic geometry using inter-object relationships. In: Proc. DSSCV 2005, pp. 60–71 (2005)
18. Freund, Y., Schapire, R.: A decision-theoretic generalization of on-line learning and an application to boosting. Journal of Computer and System Sciences 55(1), 119–139 (1997)
19. Perl, J.: Probabilistic Reasoning in Intelligent Systems. Morgan Kaufman, San Mateo (1988)
20. Yedidia, J., Freeman, W., Weiss, Y.: Understanding Belief Propagation and Its Generalizations, pp. 239–269. Morgan Kaufmann Publishers Inc, San Francisco (2003)
21. Berrou, C., Glavieus, A., Thitimajshima, P.: Near Shannon limit error-correcting coding and decoding: Turbo-codes. In: Proc. IEEE Int. Conf. on Communications, pp. 1064–1070 (1993)
22. Shi, Y., Reiss, A., Lee, A., Dutton, R., Bellugi, U., Galaburda, A., Korenberg, J., Mills, D., Dinov, I., Thompson, P., Toga, A.: Hamilton-Jacobi skeletons on cortical surfaces with applications in characterizing the gyrification pattern in Williams syndrome. In: Proc. ISBI 2007 (2007)
23. Siddiqi, K., Bouix, S., Tannebaum, A., Zuker, S.: Hamilton-Jacobi skeletons. Int'l Journal of Computer Vision 48(3), 215–231 (2002)
24. Gallant, S.: Perceptron-based learning algorithms. IEEE Trans. Neural Networks 1(2), 179–191 (1990)
25. Kimmel, R., Sethian, J.A.: Computing geodesic paths on manifolds. Proc. Natl. Acad. Sci. USA 95(15), 8431–8435 (1998)
26. Friedman, J., Hastie, T., Tibshirani, R.: Additive logistic regression: a statistical view of boosting. Ann. Statist. 28(2), 337–407 (2000)

Rao-Blackwellized Marginal Particle Filtering for Multiple Object Tracking in Molecular Bioimaging

Ihor Smal[1,*], Katharina Draegestein[2], Niels Galjart[2], Wiro Niessen[1], and Erik Meijering[1]

[1] Departments of Radiology and Medical Informatics
[2] Department of Cell Biology
Erasmus MC – University Medical Center Rotterdam
P. O. Box 2040, 3000 CA Rotterdam, The Netherlands
i.smal@erasmusmc.nl

Abstract. Modern live cell fluorescence microscopy imaging systems, used abundantly for studying intra-cellular processes in vivo, generate vast amounts of noisy image data that cannot be processed efficiently and accurately by means of manual or current computerized techniques. We propose an improved tracking method, built within a Bayesian probabilistic framework, which better exploits temporal information and prior knowledge. Experiments on simulated and real fluorescence microscopy image data acquired for microtubule dynamics studies show that the technique is more robust to noise, photobleaching, and object interaction than common tracking methods and yields results that are in good agreement with expert cell biologists.

Keywords: Bayesian estimation, particle filtering, multiple object tracking, Rao-Blackwellization, microtubule dynamics, fluorescence microscopy.

1 Introduction

Live cell imaging using time-lapse fluorescence microscopy has rapidly advanced in the past decade and has opened new possibilities for studying intra-cellular dynamic processes in vivo. Motion analysis of nanoscale objects, such as proteins, vesicles, or microtubules (Fig. 1), requires tracking of large and time-varying numbers of spots in noisy image sequences [1, 2, 3]. Manual analysis of such image data is laborious and often produces results with poor accuracy and/or reproducibility. Hence, the development of automated tracking methods is of great importance. Commonly used tracking methods fail to yield reliable results in the case of poor imaging conditions (SNR<5) [4], because the detection is usually based on simple intensity thresholding or model fitting, and available temporal information and prior knowledge are largely ignored. Alternative techniques, based on spatiotemporal segmentation [5], are also prone to errors in the case of very noisy images containing many objects at high densities.

* Corresponding author.

N. Karssemeijer and B. Lelieveldt (Eds.): IPMI 2007, LNCS 4584, pp. 110–121, 2007.
© Springer-Verlag Berlin Heidelberg 2007

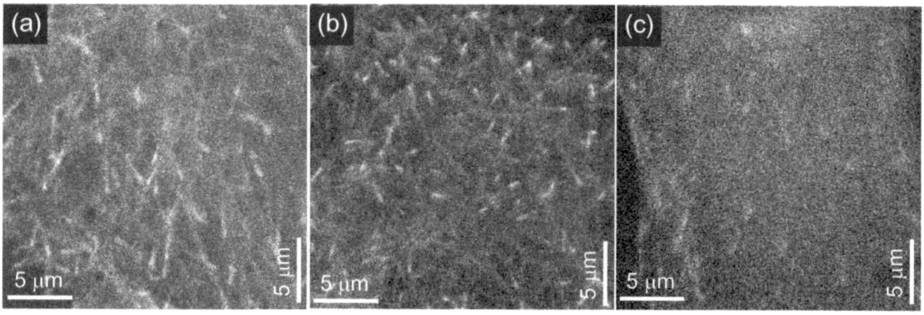

Fig. 1. Microtubules tagged with fluorescently labeled plus end tracking proteins (bright spots) and imaged using fluorescence confocal microscopy. The images are single frames from three 2D time-lapse studies, acquired under different experimental conditions. The quality of the images ranges from SNR≈5–6 (a) to ≈2–3 (c).

Recently, sequential Monte Carlo (SMC) methods [6], also known as particle filters (PF) [7], have become a popular tool to perform tracking in many fields. In this paper we extend our previous PF approach [8] and present a substantially more efficient Rao-Blackwellized marginal particle filter (RBMPF) for robust and accurate tracking of multiple nanoscale targets in two-dimensional (2D) and three-dimensional (3D) fluorescence microscopy image sequences. The RBMPF takes into account the analytical structure of the modeled processes and makes it possible to reduce the variance of the estimates in the case of high-dimensional state spaces, where standard PF fails. We compare the performance of standard PF and RBMPF with manual tracking using simulated as well as real image data acquired for microtubule dynamics studies.

2 Tracking Framework

Bayesian estimation for tracking aims at inferring knowledge about the unobserved state $\mathbf{x}_t$ of an object, which changes over time, using noisy measurements $\mathbf{z}_{1:t} \triangleq \{\mathbf{z}_1, \ldots, \mathbf{z}_t\}$ up to time t. The state evolution is modeled as a Markov process of initial distribution $p(\mathbf{x}_0)$ and transition prior $p(\mathbf{x}_t|\mathbf{x}_{t-1})$. The idea is to sequentially estimate the time evolving joint filtering distribution $p(\mathbf{x}_{0:t}|\mathbf{z}_{1:t})$ or the marginal filtering distribution $p(\mathbf{x}_t|\mathbf{z}_{1:t})$ and associated features, such as expectation. A recursive formula for the former is given by [6]

$$p(\mathbf{x}_{0:t}|\mathbf{z}_{1:t}) \propto p(\mathbf{z}_t|\mathbf{x}_t)p(\mathbf{x}_t|\mathbf{x}_{t-1})p(\mathbf{x}_{0:t-1}|\mathbf{z}_{1:t-1}). \tag{1}$$

It is assumed that the initial pdf, $p(\mathbf{x}_0|\mathbf{z}_0) \equiv p(\mathbf{x}_0)$ is available ($\mathbf{z}_{1:0} = \mathbf{z}_0$ being the set of no measurements). The distribution $p(\mathbf{x}_t|\mathbf{z}_{1:t})$ follows from (1) as

$$p(\mathbf{x}_t|\mathbf{z}_{1:t}) \propto p(\mathbf{z}_t|\mathbf{x}_t)\int p(\mathbf{x}_t|\mathbf{x}_{t-1})p(\mathbf{x}_{t-1}|\mathbf{z}_{1:t-1})d\mathbf{x}_{t-1}. \tag{2}$$

The optimal Bayesian solutions defined by the recurrence relations (1) and (2) are analytically tractable only in a restrictive set of cases [7]. For most practical models of interest, SMC methods [7,9] are used as an efficient numerical approximation. Here, the required posterior, $p(\mathbf{x}_{0:t}|\mathbf{z}_{1:t})$, is represented as a set of N_s random samples (particles), and associated weights $\{\mathbf{x}_{0:t}^{(i)}, w_t^{(i)}\}_{i=1}^{N_s}$:

$$p(\mathbf{x}_{0:t}|\mathbf{z}_{1:t}) \approx \textstyle\sum_{i=1}^{N_s} w_t^{(i)} \delta(\mathbf{x}_{0:t} - \mathbf{x}_{0:t}^{(i)}), \tag{3}$$

where $\delta(\cdot)$ is the Dirac delta function and the weights are normalized such that $\sum_{i=1}^{N_s} w_t^{(i)} = 1$. These samples and weights are propagated through time to give an approximation of the filtering distribution at subsequent time steps. The weights $w_t^{(i)}$ are chosen using sequential importance sampling (SIS) [10], which applies when auxiliary knowledge is available in the form of an importance density $q(\mathbf{x}_t|\mathbf{x}_{0:t-1}, \mathbf{z}_{1:t})$ describing which areas of the state-space contain most information about the posterior. In order to calculate the weights recursively, the importance density is factorized as $q(\mathbf{x}_{0:t}|\mathbf{z}_{1:t}) = q(\mathbf{x}_t|\mathbf{x}_{0:t-1}, \mathbf{z}_{1:t})q(\mathbf{x}_{0:t-1}|\mathbf{z}_{1:t-1})$. The particle representation of the posterior at time t is obtained by augmenting the set of existing particles $\mathbf{x}_{0:t-1}^{(i)}$ with the new state $\mathbf{x}_t^{(i)} \sim q(\mathbf{x}_t|\mathbf{x}_{0:t-1}^{(i)}, \mathbf{z}_{1:t})$. A detailed formulation of $q(\cdot|\cdot)$ is given in Section 3.4. The weights $w_t^{(i)}$ in (3) may be recursively updated as [10]

$$w_t^{(i)} \propto \frac{p(\mathbf{x}_{0:t}|\mathbf{z}_{1:t})}{q(\mathbf{x}_{0:t}|\mathbf{z}_{1:t})} = \frac{p(\mathbf{z}_t|\mathbf{x}_t^{(i)})p(\mathbf{x}_t^{(i)}|\mathbf{x}_{t-1}^{(i)})}{q(\mathbf{x}_t^{(i)}|\mathbf{x}_{0:t-1}^{(i)}, \mathbf{z}_{1:t})} w_{t-1}^{(i)}. \tag{4}$$

In order to obtain the particle representation of $p(\mathbf{x}_t|\mathbf{z}_{1:t})$, only $\mathbf{x}_t^{(i)}$ need to be stored and the *path* $\mathbf{x}_{0:t-1}^{(i)}$ can be discarded. Each particle at time t, used to augment the previous state, is a draw from the joint space $p(\mathbf{x}_{0:t}|\mathbf{z}_{1:t})$, sampled sequentially. At each time step, the dimension of the sampled paths is increased by the dimension of the state space, n_x, quickly resulting in a very high-dimensional space. Because of the sequential nature of the algorithm, the variance of the importance weights can only increase (stochastically) over time [10], leading to most paths having vanishingly small probability. The degeneracy effect can be reduced by a good choice of importance density (Section 3.4) and by resampling [7,10] to eliminate particles with small weights. Additionally, it can be reduced by using the marginal particle filter (MPF) [11], where the filtering is performed directly on the marginal distribution $p(\mathbf{x}_t|\mathbf{z}_{1:t})$ defined by (2) instead of on the joint state. Having a representation of $p(\mathbf{x}_t|\mathbf{z}_{1:t})$ in the form of (3), we can approximate the integral in (2) as the weighted kernel estimate $\sum_{j=1}^{N_s} w_{t-1}^{(j)} p(\mathbf{x}_t|\mathbf{x}_{t-1}^{(j)})$. The importance weights are now on the marginal space:

$$w_t^{(i)} \propto \frac{p(\mathbf{x}_t|\mathbf{z}_{1:t})}{q(\mathbf{x}_t|\mathbf{z}_{1:t})} = \frac{p(\mathbf{z}_t|\mathbf{x}_t^{(i)}) \sum_{j=1}^{N_s} w_{t-1}^{(j)} p(\mathbf{x}_t^{(i)}|\mathbf{x}_{t-1}^{(j)})}{q(\mathbf{x}_t^{(i)}|\mathbf{z}_{1:t})}. \tag{5}$$

The variance of the importance weights is less than or equal to the variance of the standard SIS scheme [11]. By using particle representations, statistical inferences such as expectation, maximum a posteriori, and minimum mean square error (MMSE) estimators, can easily be approximated. For example,

$$\hat{\mathbf{x}}_t^{\mathrm{MMSE}} = \int \mathbf{x}_t p(\mathbf{x}_t|\mathbf{z}_{1:t}) d\mathbf{x}_t \approx \sum_{i=1}^{N_s} \mathbf{x}_t^{(i)} w_t^{(i)}. \tag{6}$$

Straightforward generalization of SMC methods to the problem of multiple object tracking leads to an increase in dimensionality and an exponential explosion of computational demands [6]. We represent the multi-modal posterior distribution, in which multiple modes are caused by ambiguity about the object state due to either insufficient measurements or measurements coming from multiple objects being tracked, by an M-component mixture model [12]:

$$p(\mathbf{x}_t|\mathbf{z}_{1:t}) = \sum_{m=1}^{M} \pi_{m,t} p_m(\mathbf{x}_t|\mathbf{z}_{1:t}), \tag{7}$$

with $\sum_{m=1}^{M} \pi_{m,t} = 1$ and a non-parametric model is assumed for the individual mixture components. In this case, the particle representation of the filtering distribution, $\{\mathbf{x}_t^{(i)}, w_t^{(i)}\}_{i=1}^{N}$ with $N = MN_s$ particles, is augmented with a set of component indicators, $\{c_t^{(i)}\}_{i=1}^{N}$, with $c_t^{(i)} = m$ if particle i belongs to mixture component m. This representation can be updated in the same fashion as the standard Bayesian sequential estimation [12].

3 Tailoring the Framework

3.1 State-Space and Dynamics

In this paper the framework is tailored towards microtubule (MT) tracking. MTs are cylindrical structures (diameter ~25 nm) in the cytoskeleton that play a crucial role in several cellular processes [13]. We approximate the dynamic behavior of the visible ends of MTs by a nearly constant velocity model [14] with the state vector $\mathbf{x}_t = (x_t, \dot{x}_t, y_t, \dot{y}_t, z_t, \dot{z}_t, \sigma_{\max,t}, \sigma_{\min,t}, \sigma_{z,t}, I_t)^T$, where $(\sigma_{\max,t}, \sigma_{\min,t}, \sigma_{z,t})^T \triangleq \mathbf{s}_t$ is the object shape feature vector (Section 3.2), $(x_t, y_t, z_t)^T \triangleq \mathbf{r}_t$ is the radius vector, $\dot{\mathbf{r}}_t \triangleq \mathbf{v}_t$ velocity, and I_t object intensity.

In practice, the analysis of time-lapse fluorescence microscopy image sequences is complicated by photobleaching, a light-induced chemical process by which fluorescent proteins lose their ability to fluoresce. The two commonly used approximations of the process are given by [15]

$$I(t) = Ae^{-at} + B, \qquad \text{and} \qquad I(t) = I_0\left(1 + (t/L)^k\right)^{-1}, \tag{8}$$

where A, B, a, I_0, L, k are experimentally determined constants. Photobleaching is ignored by common tracking techniques but in many practical cases it is necessary to model it so as to increase robustness. To conveniently incorporate the photobleaching effect into our framework, we approximate it as a first-order Gauss-Markov process, $I_t = (1 - \alpha)I_{t-1} + u_t$, where u_t is zero-mean Gaussian noise and $\alpha \leq 1$ an experimentally obtained rate of photobleaching, which can be estimated from image data, using (8), by model fitting.

In summary, in our implementation, the state evolution $p(\mathbf{x}_t|\mathbf{x}_{t-1})$ is a linear Gaussian model [10], which can easily be evaluated pointwise in (4):

$$p(\mathbf{x}_t|\mathbf{x}_{t-1}) \propto \exp\left(-\frac{1}{2}(\mathbf{x}_t - \mathbf{F}\mathbf{x}_{t-1})^T \mathbf{Q}^{-1}(\mathbf{x}_t - \mathbf{F}\mathbf{x}_{t-1})\right), \tag{9}$$

with process transition matrix $\mathbf{F} = \text{diag}[\mathbf{F}_1, \mathbf{F}_1, \mathbf{F}_1, 1, 1, 1, 1-\alpha]$ and covariance matrix $\mathbf{Q} = \text{diag}[\mathbf{Q}_1, \mathbf{Q}_1, \mathbf{Q}_1, q_2T, q_2T, q_2T, q_3T]$. Here,

$$\mathbf{F}_1 = \begin{pmatrix} 1 & T \\ 0 & 1 \end{pmatrix}, \qquad \mathbf{Q}_1 = \begin{pmatrix} \frac{q_1}{3}T^3 & \frac{q_1}{2}T^2 \\ \frac{q_1}{2}T^2 & q_1T \end{pmatrix},$$

where q_1, q_2 and q_3 denote the level of process noise in object motion, appearance and intensity, respectively, and T is the sampling interval. The proposed model correctly approximates small accelerations in object motion and fluctuations in object appearance and intensity. To obtain a more realistic motion model and avoid track coalescence in the case of multiple objects, we explicitly model object interaction using a Markov random field (MRF) [8, 16]. The model (9) can also be successfully used for tracking structures with higher motion nonlinearity, by adapting the process noise level, defined by $\mathbf{Q}$.

3.2 Observation Model

The image formation process can be modeled as a convolution of the true, unobserved 3D image with the point-spread function (PSF) of the microscope. The PF framework can accommodate any PSF that can be calculated pointwise. Despite its minor imperfection, the 3D Gaussian approximation of the PSF [3] is commonly favored over the more accurate Gibson-Lanni model [1], for its computational advantages. To model the shape of the intensity profile of an imaged object, one would have to use the convolution with the PSF for every state $\mathbf{x}_t^{(i)}$. To overcome this computational overload, we model the PSF together with object shape using a 3D Gaussian approximation. The elongation in the intensity profile of MTs can be modeled by utilizing the velocity components from $\mathbf{x}_t$ as parameters in the PSF. In this case, for an object of intensity I_t at position $\mathbf{r}_t$, the intensity contribution to pixel (i, j, k) is approximated as

$$h_t(i, j, k; \mathbf{x}_t) = a_t(i, j, k; \mathbf{r}_t, \mathbf{v}_t, \mathbf{s}_t)I_t + b_t, \tag{10}$$

where b_t is the background intensity and

$$a_t(i, j, k; \mathbf{r}_t, \mathbf{v}_t, \mathbf{s}_t) = \exp\left(-\frac{1}{2}\mathbf{m}_t^T \mathbf{R}^T \mathbf{\Sigma}_t^{-1} \mathbf{R}\mathbf{m}_t - \frac{(k\Delta_z - z_t\|\mathbf{m}_t\| \tan\theta_t)^2}{2\sigma_{z,t}^2}\right) \tag{11}$$

with $\sigma_{z,t}$ ($\approx$ 235nm) modeling the axial blurring, z_t denoting the measured intensity, and $\mathbf{R} = \mathbf{R}(\phi_t)$ denoting a rotation matrix

$$\mathbf{R}(\phi_t) = \begin{pmatrix} \cos\phi_t & \sin\phi_t \\ -\sin\phi_t & \cos\phi_t \end{pmatrix}, \quad \mathbf{\Sigma}_t = \begin{pmatrix} \sigma_{\mathrm{m},t}^2(\theta_t) & 0 \\ 0 & \sigma_{\mathrm{min},t}^2 \end{pmatrix}, \quad \mathbf{m}_t = \begin{pmatrix} i\Delta_x - x_t \\ j\Delta_y - y_t \end{pmatrix},$$

$$\sigma_{\mathrm{m},t}(\theta_t) = \sigma_{\mathrm{min},t} - (\sigma_{\mathrm{min},t} - \sigma_{\mathrm{max},t}) \cos\theta_t,$$

$$\tan\theta_t = \frac{\dot{z}_t}{\sqrt{\dot{x}_t^{\,2} + \dot{y}_t^{\,2}}}, \quad \tan\phi_t = \frac{\dot{y}_t}{\dot{x}_t}, \quad -\pi < \phi_t, \theta_t \leq \pi.$$

In these formulae, each pixel (i, j, k) is assumed to correspond to a rectangular volume of dimensions $\Delta_x \times \Delta_y \times \Delta_z$ nm^3. The parameters $\sigma_{\mathrm{max},t}$ and $\sigma_{\mathrm{min},t}$ represent the amount of blurring and, at the same time, model object elongation along the direction of motion. For subresolution structures such as vesicles, $\sigma_{\mathrm{min}} = \sigma_{\mathrm{max}} \approx 80$nm, and for the elongated MTs, $\sigma_{\mathrm{min}} \approx 100$nm and $\sigma_{\mathrm{max}} \approx 300$nm. For the background level estimate b_t we use the average image intensity at time t, taking into account the contribution of object intensity values to the total image intensity (mainly formed by background structures with lower intensity) is negligible. For a typical 2D image of size $10^3 \times 10^3$ pixels containing a thousand objects, the number of object pixels is only about 1%.

3.3 Rao-Blackwellization and Likelihood

As mentioned in Section 2, in the case of high-dimensional state spaces (in our case n_x=10), the SIS becomes inefficient and leads to variance increase of the estimator. However, when the transition and observation models have an analytically tractable structure, the size of the state space can be drastically reduced by analytical marginalization of some of the state variables, also called Rao-Blackwellization [6]. In our case, for each realization of state variable $\mathbf{y}_t = (\mathbf{r}_t, \mathbf{v}_t, \mathbf{s}_t)^T$, we have a linear Gaussian transition and observation model for the intensity I_t. For such models the optimal solution can be obtained analytically using the Kalman filter. We therefore combine a PF to compute the distribution of the discrete states $\mathbf{y}_t$ with a bank of Kalman filters to compute exactly the distribution of the continuous state. With the factorization

$$p(\mathbf{y}_t, I_t|\mathbf{z}_{1:t}) = p(I_t|\mathbf{y}_t, \mathbf{z}_{1:t})p(\mathbf{y}_t|\mathbf{z}_{1:t}), \tag{12}$$

the density $p(I_t|\mathbf{y}_t, \mathbf{z}_{1:t})$, which is Gaussian, can be computed analytically by applying the Kalman filter:

$$p(I_t|\mathbf{y}_t, \mathbf{z}_{1:t}) = \mathcal{N}(I_t|I_{t|t}, P_{t|t}), \tag{13}$$

with $\mathcal{N}(\cdot|\mu, \sigma^2)$ the normal distribution with mean μ and variance σ^2,

$$\begin{aligned} I_{t|t-1} &= (1-\alpha)I_{t-1|t-1}, & I_{t|t} &= I_{t|t-1} + K_t(Z_t - H_t I_{t|t-1}), \\ P_{t|t-1} &= (1-\alpha)^2 P_{t-1|t-1} + q_3 T, & P_{t|t} &= P_{t|t-1} - K_t H_t P_{t|t-1}, \\ S_t &= H_t P_{t|t-1} H_t^T + R_t, & K_t &= P_{t|t-1} H_t^T S_t^{-1}, \end{aligned}$$

and the vectors H_t and Z_t are formed as

$$H_t = (\ldots, a_t(i,j,k; \mathbf{r}_t, \mathbf{v}_t, \mathbf{s}_t), \ldots)^T, \quad Z_t = (\ldots, z(i,j,k) - b_t, \ldots)^T, \tag{14}$$

for all triplets $(i,j,k) \in C(\mathbf{x}_t)$, where $C(\mathbf{x}_t)$ is the region of pixels that are affected by the object with state $\mathbf{x}_t$ and is defined as $C(\mathbf{x}_t) = \{(i,j,k) \in \mathbb{Z}^3 : a_t(i,j,k;\mathbf{r}_t,\mathbf{v}_t,\mathbf{s}_t) > 0.1\}$. The covariance matrix of the measurement noise R_t models the Poisson noise, the main source of noise in fluorescence microscopy imaging, and is given by $R_t = \text{diag}[\ldots, h_t(i,j,k;\mathbf{x}_t), \ldots]$. The recursive Bayesian solution is applicable as long as the statistics of the measurement noise is known for each pixel. Thus, we need to estimate only $p(\mathbf{y}_t|\mathbf{z}_{1:t})$, using a PF, in a space of reduced dimension, which satisfies the alternative recursion

$$p(\mathbf{y}_t|\mathbf{z}_{1:t}) \propto p(\mathbf{y}_{t-1}|\mathbf{z}_{1:t-1})p(\mathbf{z}_t|\mathbf{y}_t,\mathbf{z}_{1:t-1})p(\mathbf{y}_t|\mathbf{y}_{t-1}). \tag{15}$$

The likelihood $p(\mathbf{z}_t|\mathbf{y}_t,\mathbf{z}_{1:t-1})$ does not simplify to $p(\mathbf{z}_t|\mathbf{y}_t)$ because there is a dependency on past values through $I_{0:t}$. For conditionally linear models, we have $p(\mathbf{z}_t|\mathbf{y}_t,\mathbf{z}_{1:t-1}) = \mathcal{N}(b_t + H_t I_{t|t-1}, S_t)$ [6]. The variance of the importance weights for RB(M)PF is lower than for (M)PF [11]. Also, for the same performance, fewer MC particles are needed. This is because the dimension of $p(\mathbf{y}_t|\mathbf{z}_{1:t})$ is smaller than that of $p(\mathbf{x}_t|\mathbf{z}_{1:t})$. Another reason is that optimal algorithms are used in order to estimate the linear state variables.

3.4 Data-Dependent Sampling

Basic PFs [9,7], which use the proposal distribution $q(\mathbf{x}_t|\mathbf{x}_{t-1},\mathbf{z}_t) = p(\mathbf{x}_t|\mathbf{x}_{t-1})$, usually perform poorly because too few samples are generated in regions where the desired posterior $p(\mathbf{x}_t|\mathbf{z}_{1:t})$ is large. In order to construct a proposal distribution which alleviates this problem and takes into account the most recent measurements $\mathbf{z}_t$, we propose to transform the image sequence into probability distributions. True spots are characterized by relatively high intensities with convex profiles. Noise-induced local maxima typically exhibit a random distribution of intensity changes in all directions, leading to a low local curvature [3]. These two discriminative features (intensity and curvature) are used to construct an approximation of the likelihood $L(\mathbf{z}_t|\mathbf{x}_t)$, using the image data available at time t. For each object we use the transformation

$$\tilde{p}_m(\mathbf{r}_t|\mathbf{z}_t) = \frac{(G_\sigma * \tilde{z}_t(\mathbf{r}_t))^r \kappa_t^s(\mathbf{r}_t)}{\int_{C_{m,t}} (G_\sigma * \tilde{z}_t(\mathbf{r}_t))^r \kappa_t^s(\mathbf{r}_t) dx dy dz}, \qquad \forall \mathbf{r}_t \in C_{m,t}, \tag{16}$$

where G_σ is the Gaussian kernel with scale σ, $\tilde{z}_t$ denotes a first-order interpolation of z_t, $C_{m,t}$ is the circular region (with radius defined by the covariance matrix of $p(\mathbf{x}_t|\mathbf{x}_{t-1})$, e.g. 3-standard-deviation level) centered at the object position predicted from the previous time step, the curvature κ_t is given by the determinant of the Hessian matrix $\mathbf{H}$ of the intensity $\tilde{z}_t$:

$$\kappa_t(\mathbf{r}_t) = \det(\mathbf{H}(\mathbf{r}_t)), \qquad \mathbf{H}(\mathbf{r}_t) = \nabla \cdot \nabla^T \tilde{z}_t(\mathbf{r}_t), \tag{17}$$

and the exponents $r > 1$ and $s > 1$ weigh each of the features and determine the peakedness of the likelihood. Using this transformation, we define the new data dependent proposal distribution for object m as

$$\tilde{q}_m(\mathbf{y}_t|\mathbf{y}_{t-1},\mathbf{z}_t) = \tilde{p}_m(\mathbf{r}_t|\mathbf{z}_t)\mathcal{N}(\mathbf{v}_t|\mathbf{r}_t - \hat{\mathbf{r}}_{m,t-1}^{\text{MMSE}}, \mathbf{\Sigma}_\mathbf{v})\mathcal{N}(\mathbf{s}_t|\mathbf{s}_{m,t-1}^{\text{MMSE}}, q_2 T), \tag{18}$$

where the covariance matrix $\mathbf{\Sigma_v} = \text{diag}[q_1T, q_1T, q_1T]$. Contrary to the original proposal distribution, which fails if the likelihood is too peaked, (18) generates samples that are highly consistent with the most recent measurements in the predicted (using the information from the previous time step) regions $C_{m,t}$. A mixture of both proposal distributions gives excellent results:

$$q_m(\mathbf{y}_t|\mathbf{y}_{t-1}, \mathbf{z}_t) = \gamma p(\mathbf{y}_t|\mathbf{y}_{t-1}) + (1-\gamma)\tilde{q}_m(\mathbf{y}_t|\mathbf{y}_{t-1}, \mathbf{z}_t),$$

where $0 < \gamma < 1$. Compared to the regular one, this proposal distribution scales much better to smaller sample sizes.

3.5 Track Initialization and Management

The initialization of the proposed RBMPF can be done by manually specifying the objects of interest in the first frame, or by using a completely automatic initialization procedure [8]. The latter, also used for detection of newly appearing objects in subsequent frames, divides the image space into rectangular 3D cells and samples N_s particles according to importance function (16). The number of sampled particles in each cell represents the degree of belief in object birth. In cells (not containing any of the M existing objects) with counts larger than some threshold N_{td}, new tracks are initiated with initial mixture weights π_{bd}. The threshold N_{td} can be estimated experimentally and depends on N_s, cell volume and the number of bright spots in the image data.

Whenever objects pass close to one another, the object with the best likelihood score typically "hijacks" particles of nearby mixture components. This problem is partly solved using the MRF model for object interactions [8]. To better resolve the ambiguity in such situations, the Hough transform is used for each spatiotemporal ROI of 3-5 frames, $C_{m,t-T:t+T}$, to correctly model velocity changes. If object m passes close to a new object, the distribution $p_m(\mathbf{x}_t|\mathbf{z}_{1:t})$ becomes too diffuse in a few time steps and the reclustering procedure $(\{c'^{(i)}_t\}, M') = F(\{\mathbf{x}^{(i)}_t\}, \{c^{(i)}_t\}, M)$ [12] is performed to initiate new tracks. Merging of objects does not occur in our application and is therefore forbidden. If the mixture weight $\pi_{m,t}$ is below some predefined threshold level π_{td}, component m is removed from the mixture and the track terminated.

4 Experimental Results

4.1 Evaluation on Synthetic Data

The RBMPF was first evaluated and compared to the standard PF using synthetic but realistic 2D image sequences (20 frames of 512×512 pixels) of moving MT-like objects ($10-20$ objects per frame), generated according to (9) and (10), for different SNRs (Fig. 2) in a range around SNR=4, which has been identified by previous studies [4] as a critical level at which several popular tracking techniques break down. Object velocities ranged from 200 to 700 nm/sec, representative of published data [13]. The PFs used 300 samples per object and

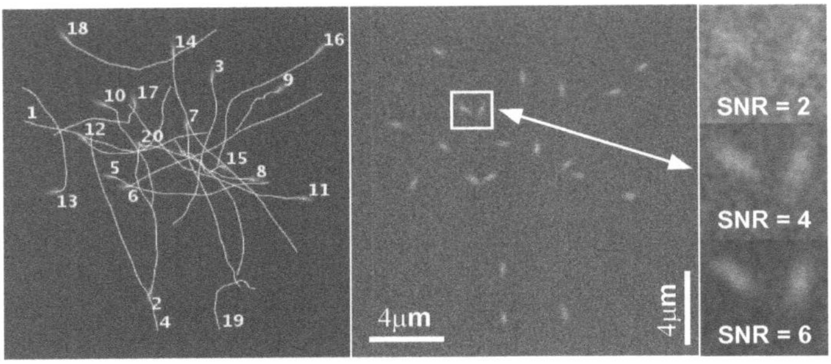

Fig. 2. Examples of synthetic images used in the experiments. The left image is a frame from one of the sequences (SNR=7) with the trajectories of the 20 moving objects superimposed, illustrating the motion patterns allowed by the linear state evolution model (9). The right image is a frame from another sequence (SNR=4), giving an impression of object appearance. The insets show zooms at different SNRs.

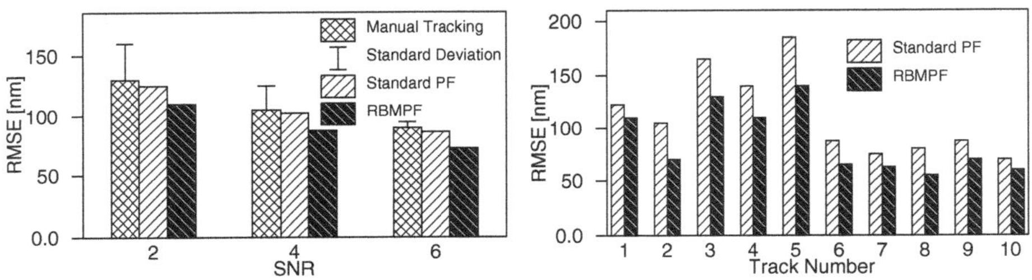

Fig. 3. Average RMSE (left) for different SNRs, and RMSE per track (right, SNR=4), for manual and automatic tracking in the described synthetic data sets.

the algorithm parameters were as follows: $\sigma_{\max} = 250$ nm, $\sigma_{\min} = 100$ nm, $\Delta_x = \Delta_y = 50$ nm, $r = 5$, $s = 1$, $q_1 = 3$, $\alpha = 10^{-3}$ and $q_2 = 0.04$, $q_3 = 1$, $T = 1$ sec. SNR is defined as the difference in intensity between the object I_o and background I_b, divided by the object noise, $\sigma_o = \sqrt{I_o}$ [4]. Tracks were initialized manually in desired regions of interest in the first frame, or automatically using the described procedure, giving similar results.

Having the ground truth for the synthetic data, we evaluated the accuracy of the tracking and compared the PF techniques and manual tracking (done by five independent expert observers). To quantify the localization error, we used the traditional root mean square error measure [3]. Figure 3 shows the RMSE in the object position estimates as a function of SNR for the manual tracking and using the PF techniques. The localization error of our algorithm is in the range of errors made by experts. The error bars represent interobserver variability and indicate that manual tracking performance degrades significantly for low SNRs. The figure also shows the reduction of the variance when the RBMPF is used, compared to the standard PF. The RBMPF was also evaluated on 3D synthetic image sequences, with 20 optical slices, $\sigma_z = 250$ nm, Δ_z =200 nm. The RMSE

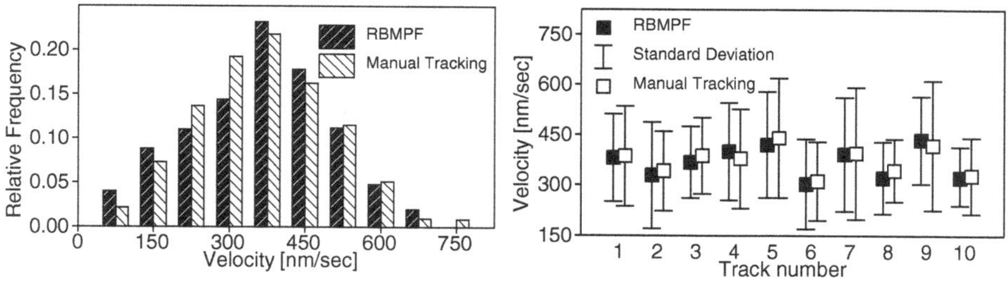

Fig. 4. Examples of velocity distributions (left) and velocity estimation for 10 representative MT objects (right) obtained with our RBMPF-based automatic tracking algorithm versus manual tracking applied to real fluorescence microscopy image sequences of growing MTs (data set in Fig. 1(a), SNR≈5).

in this case was higher (about 300-400 nm), due to the approximately three times lower optical resolution of the modeled imaging system in the axial direction, and the variance reduction by using RBMPF was not significant, due to the increase of the state space dimension for the PF from 6 to 9.

4.2 Evaluation on Real Data

The algorithm was also applied to real 2D fluorescence confocal microscopy image sequences acquired for MT dynamics studies [13]. Three representative

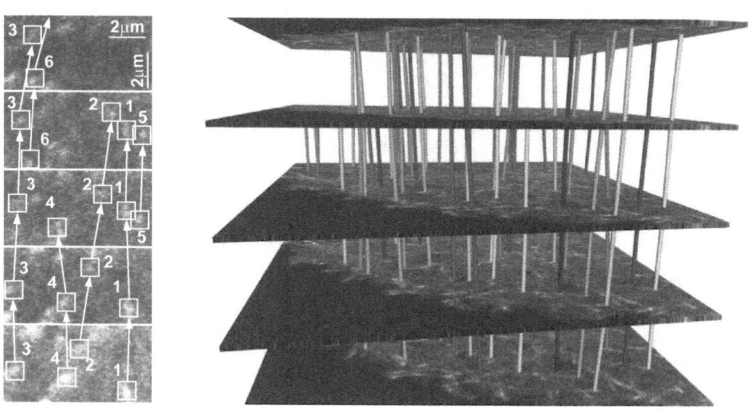

Fig. 5. Left: Results (six tracks) of automatically tracking MTs in the presence of photobleaching, illustrating the capability of our algorithm to capture newly appearing objects (tracks 5 and 6) and to detect object disappearance (track 4). It also shows the robustness of the algorithm in the case of closely passing objects (tracks 1 and 5). Right: Visualization of tracking results produced by our algorithm in the case of the real data of Fig. 1(a). Shown are five frames (time is increasing from bottom to top) with the trajectories rendered as small tubes.

data sets (of size 512×512 pixels, 30 time frames, examples of which are shown in Fig. 1) were preselected from larger volumes by manually choosing the regions of interest. In these experiments, the parameters of the algorithm were fixed to the same values as in the case of the synthetic data. Using the automatic track initiation procedure, the tracker simultaneously followed 10–30 spots during 3–20 consecutive frames until their disappearance.

Lacking ground truth for the real data, we evaluated the performance of our algorithm by comparison with manual tracking results from two expert cell biologists. Distributions of instant velocities estimated using our RBMPF-based algorithm versus manual tracking for SNR$\approx$5 are presented in Fig. 4. Application of a paired Student t-test per track revealed no statistically significant difference between the results of our algorithm and that of manual tracking, for both expert human observers ($p \gg 0.05$ in all cases). The difference in average velocity (over 10 tracks) between automatic and manual tracking was less than 1%, for both observers. Our velocity estimates are also comparable to those reported previously based on manual tracking in the same type of image data [13]. Two different example visualizations of real data together with the results of tracking using our algorithm are given in Fig. 5.

5 Discussion and Conclusions

We have presented a Rao-Blackwellized marginal particle filter for tracking of multiple objects in molecular bioimaging data. The proposed approach contains several improvements over previous PF-techniques. Specifically, the robustness and reproducibility of the algorithm are improved by means of a new importance function for data-dependent sampling and by using marginalization for both the filtering distribution and selected variables from the state vector. These modifications reduce the number of MC samples required for tracking from $10^5 - 10^6$ [8] to $10^2 - 10^3$. Compared to existing deterministic approaches, which perform object detection prior to linking using non-Bayesian maximum likelihood or least squares estimators, the proposed estimator optimally exploits temporal information and prior information about the parameters, resulting in lower variance. As the experiments show, even in data with SNR as low as 2 (which is not uncommon in practice), our algorithm still yields reliable tracking results, whereas common frame-by-frame approaches break down at SNR<4–5 [4].

The results of the experiments on synthetic image data suggest that our algorithm is potentially more accurate than manual tracking by expert human observers. The experiments on real fluorescence microscopy image sequences from MT dynamics studies showed comparable performance. This is explained by the fact that in the latter experiments, we were limited to comparing distributions and averages (Fig. 4), which may conceal small local discrepancies, especially when the objects' velocities vary over time. Instant velocities were also analyzed per track but could not be quantitatively validated due to the lack of ground truth. Nevertheless, the results indicate that our algorithm may replace laborious manual procedures. Currently we are evaluating the method also for other biological applications to further demonstrate its advantages over current means of manual and automated quantification of subcellular dynamics. Our findings encourage use of the method to analyze complex biological image sequences not only for obtaining statistical estimates of average velocity and life span, but also for detailed analyses of complete life histories.

References

1. Meijering, E., Smal, I., Danuser, G.: Tracking in molecular bioimaging. IEEE Signal Process. Mag. 23(3), 46–53 (2006)
2. Gerlich, D., Mattes, J., Eils, R.: Quantitative motion analysis and visualization of cellular structures. Methods 29(1), 3–13 (2003)
3. Thomann, D., Rines, D.R., Sorger, P.K., Danuser, G.: Automatic fluorescent tag detection in 3D with super-resolution: Application to the analysis of chromosome movement. J. Microsc. 208(1), 49–64 (2002)
4. Cheezum, M.K., Walker, W.F., Guilford, W.H.: Quantitative comparison of algorithms for tracking single fluorescent particles. Biophys. J. 81(4), 2378–2388 (2001)
5. Sage, D., Neumann, F.R., Hediger, F., Gasser, S.M., Unser, M.: Automatic tracking of individual fluorescence particles: Application to the study of chromosome dynamics. IEEE Trans. Image Process. 14(9), 1372–1383 (2005)
6. Doucet, A., de Freitas, N., Gordon, N.: Sequential Monte Carlo Methods in Practice. Springer-Verlag, Berlin (2001)
7. Arulampalam, S.M., Maskell, S., Gordon, N., Clapp, T.: A tutorial on particle filters for online nonlinear/non-Gaussian Bayesian tracking. IEEE Trans. Signal Process. 50(2)174–188 (2002)
8. Smal, I., Niessen, W., Meijering, E.: Advanced particle filtering for multiple object tracking in dynamic fluorescence microscopy images. In: Proceedings of the IEEE International Symposium on Biomedical Imaging (April 2007)
9. Isard, M., Blake, A.: CONDENSATION – Conditional density propagation for visual tracking. Int. J. Comput. Vis. 29(1), 5–28 (1998)
10. Doucet, A., Godsill, S., Andrieu, C.: On sequential Monte Carlo sampling methods for Bayesian filtering. Statistics and Computing 10, 197–208 (2000)
11. Klaas, M., de Freitas, N., Doucet, A.: Toward practical N^2 Monte Carlo: The marginal particle filter. In: Proceedings of the 21th Annual Conference on Uncertainty in Artificial Intelligence (UAI-05) 2005, pp. 308–331. AUAI Press (2005)
12. Vermaak, J., Doucet, A., Pérez, P.: Maintaining multi-modality through mixture tracking. In: Proceedings of the 9th IEEE International Conference on Computer Vision 2003, pp. 1110–1116 (2003)
13. Stepanova, T., Slemmer, J., Hoogenraad, C.C., Lansbergen, G., Dortland, B., De Zeeuw, C.I., Grosveld, F., van Cappellen, G., Akhmanova, A., Galjart, N.: Visualization of microtubule growth in cultured neurons via the use of EB3-GFP (end-binding protein 3-green fluorescent protein). J. Neurosci. 23(7), 2655–2664 (2003)
14. Li, X.R., Jilkov, V.P.: Survey of maneuvering target tracking. Part I: Dynamic models. IEEE Trans. Aerosp. Electron. Syst. 39(4), 1333–1364 (2003)
15. Song, L., Hennink, E.J., Young, I.T., Tanke, H.J.: Photobleaching kinetics of fluorescein in quantitative fluorescence microscopy. Biophys. J. 68(6), 2588–2600 (1995)
16. Khan, Z., Balch, T., Dellaert, F.: MCMC-Based particle filtering for tracking a variable number of interacting targets. IEEE Trans. Pattern Anal. Machine Intell. 27(11), 1805–1819 (2005)

Spine Detection and Labeling Using a Parts-Based Graphical Model

Stefan Schmidt[1,2], Jörg Kappes[2], Martin Bergtholdt[2], Vladimir Pekar[1], Sebastian Dries[1], Daniel Bystrov[1], and Christoph Schnörr[2]

[1] Philips Research Europe - Hamburg, Germany
[2] CVGPR Group, University of Mannheim, Germany
Stefan.Schmidt@ti.uni-mannheim.de

Abstract. The detection and extraction of complex anatomical structures usually involves a trade-off between the complexity of local feature extraction and classification, and the complexity and performance of the subsequent structural inference from the viewpoint of combinatorial optimization. Concerning the latter, computationally efficient methods are of particular interest that return the globally-optimal structure.

We present an efficient method for part-based localization of anatomical structures which embeds contextual shape knowledge in a probabilistic graphical model. It allows for robust detection even when some of the part detections are missing. The application scenario for our statistical evaluation is spine detection and labeling in magnetic resonance images.

1 Introduction

Problem Description. We investigate a new method for automatically locating the human vertebral column (spine) and for simultaneously labeling the intervertebral disks in 3D T1-weighted magnetic resonance (MR) survey images of total spine. The method provides robust input for further automatic processing, e.g. initialization of vertebra models to segment individual vertebrae or extraction of regions of interest for subsequent image acquisition or processing.

The human spine typically consists of 24 vertebrae (7 cervical: C1-C7, 12 thoracic: T1-T12, 5 lumbar: L1-L5) with in-between situated intervertebral disks, aligned in a double-S shaped curve. In T1-weighted fast field-echo (FFE) images, the disks typically appear as bright structures, and the vertebrae themselves give virtually no signal and appear dark. We therefore use the disks as high level features (parts) for localizing the spine column and individual vertebrae. Integration of spatial context is essential, however, for coping with erroneous local detections and missing features, in order to label vertebrae anatomically.

There are several pathologies that may significantly affect the appearance of the spine such as fracture, neoplasm, deformity (e.g. scoliosis) and degeneration. Also the number of vertebrae may differ from 24, e.g. by lumbalization of the cranial sacral segment into an L6. Our objective is the design of a probabilistically sound model for reliably detecting and localizing the spine column, that copes with the complexity of the depicted anatomy and the variability in image quality. In this paper, we concentrate on the standard case of 24 vertebrae.

N. Karssemeijer and B. Lelieveldt (Eds.): IPMI 2007, LNCS 4584, pp. 122–133, 2007.
© Springer-Verlag Berlin Heidelberg 2007

Approach. We use a probabilistic graphical model for representing both the appearance of local parts and the shape of the anatomy in terms of geometric relations between parts. Features for detecting parts are learned from a set of training data in manually marked image regions.

In the detection stage, a multi-class classifier is applied to detect potential locations for each part in a new image. In a subsequent step, the graphical model provides a contextual decision by fusing these data with the geometrical prior knowledge and inferring the globally optimal configuration of the parts.

2 State of the Art and Contribution

Related Work. At present, not many fully automated methods for locating the spine in MR images have been reported in the literature.

Peng et al. [1] detect the intervertebral disks in MR images in connection with segmenting the whole spine column. The detector used convolves a gray value template of a disk with the image, followed by searching for the disk centers and further local postprocessing. The method is not 3D but processes (sagittal) 2D slices only which may not intersect the whole spine. Furthermore, the approach does not model and employ contextual (non-local) prior knowledge. The study reports good results for 5 subjects, but the performance of the method for low-quality scout data, or when local disk detection fails, is unclear.

Weiss et al. [2] propose a semi-automatic algorithm for localizing the spine and for labeling the intervertebral disks. Operator assistance is used to provide a single seed point in the C2-3 disk. The procedure relies on intensity thresholds for detecting the remaining disks, rendering the method highly dependent on image quality and intensity correction in a preprocessing step. This also applies to the approach of Vrtovec et al. [3] who locate the spinal canal by searching for circular areas of homogeneous intensity in axial slices.

A well-known class of approaches that exploits geometrical prior knowledge for anatomy segmentation tasks is based on the Active Shape Model (ASM) [4]. ASMs are known for their dependency on a good search initialization, and on the reliability of local feature detection. Despite using a non-local shape model, the optimization strategy is merely local. If the search is misled by ambiguous landmarks, the optimization process cannot recover. In principle, the same criticism applies to the Active Appearance Model (AAM) [5,6], that extends the ASM by additionally representing the texture within the shape.

Recently, a combination of ASM and robust point-matching (RPM) has been proposed [7], that uses soft-assign for matching the model and image features. This work is closer to our approach regarding the ability to revise erroneous local decisions through contextual prior knowledge. The success of the method for finding the globally optimal configuration depends crucially on the annealing schedule that is used in the nonconvex energy minimization whereas the inference algorithm that combines local and global information in our approach guarantees global optimality.

Our model can be regarded as an instance of the object recognition framework suggested in [8] that describes the image as a deformable configuration of local parts. While this work only considers tree-structured constellations for computational efficiency, we use a fully interconnected model which enables the efficient detection of missing parts. Other instances of this class of approaches include [9], [10] and [11] where the geometry is described by a multivariate normal distribution of part positions relative to a non-occluded reference part. Our model does not rely on any particular reference part and is invariant against translation and rotation. The graphical shape templates proposed by Amit [12] for anatomy detection are defined by potential functions on triples of parts, and require a *decomposable* graph structure enabling the application of a dynamic programming algorithm for second order Markov chains. The specific graph structure causes the approach to be sensitive to missing part detections, a limitation which is overcome in our formulation.

Contribution. The basic features of our approach are:

- The design of the part detectors is completely determined by learning from the data. It does *not* involve any model assumptions (e.g., template).
- Local information is fused with non-local geometrical prior information and results in a globally optimal configuration. Favorable consequences of this globally optimal inference are (i) that problems due to a poor initialization are obsolete, and (ii) that evaluations of the result only judge the model and cannot be misinterpreted as poor local minima.
- Missing parts are explicitly taken into account by the probabilistic graphical model. In case of failure of a local detector, we are still able to predict the most probable position of a missing part.
- Any further available information, e.g., identification of the up-most intervertebral space (C1-2) as anchor point, can be easily integrated and fully exploited during inference.

3 Methods

Graphical Model. Our probabilistic model represents the image appearance of single parts as well as the relative geometry of *pairs* of parts, in terms of vertices V and edges E of a graph $G = (V, E)$. Each vertex $s \in V$ indexes a random variable x_s that assigns to the part its unknown image location. Accordingly, $x = \{x_1, x_2, \ldots, x_{|V|}\}$ denotes a *configuration* of parts.

Given an image I, the objective is to localize the object of interest by determining the most probable configuration x that maximizes

$$P(x|I, \theta) = P^A(x|I) P^S(x|\theta) , \tag{1}$$

where P^A represents the appearance of parts and P^S captures shape information using a set of parameters θ. We model $P(x|I, \theta)$ by the Gibbs distribution

$$P(x|I,\theta) = \frac{1}{Z} \exp(-\mathcal{E}(x|I;\theta)) , \quad \mathcal{E}(x|I;\theta) = \sum_{s \in V} \psi_s(I, x_s) + \alpha \sum_{(s,t) \in E} \psi_{st}(x_s, x_t; \theta), \tag{2}$$

whose components will be detailed below.

Part Appearance Potentials. The unary potential functions ψ_s in (2) are directly given by the output probability $P(x_s|I)$ provided by the classifier that is used to detect candidates for part s in an image, as described below. Note that we assumed mutual independence of *local* detections in (2).

Relative Geometry of Part Pairs. The potential functions ψ_{st} in (2) represent the relative geometry of pairs s, t of parts.

We evaluate two alternative models: The first version models the distance of the parts by the 1D Gaussian,

$$\psi_{st}(x_s, x_t) = \frac{(\|x_s - x_t\| - \mu_{st})^2}{2\sigma_{st}^2} . \tag{3}$$

This representation is invariant against joint translations and rotation of both parts. The second version uses instead of (3) a multivariate normal distribution to represent the part locations relative to each other:

$$\psi_{st}(x_s, x_t) = \frac{1}{2}(x_s - x_t - \mu_{st})^\top \Sigma_{st}^{-1}(x_s - x_t - \mu_{st}) . \tag{4}$$

This variant captures the geometry more accurately but is no longer rotational invariant. In applications where the absolute orientation of the structure of interest does not vary too much relative to the image frame (i.e. scanner axis), this second formulation is preferable.

In connection with spine detection, it is undesirable to allow disks to overlap. To account for this, we truncate the Gaussians by multiplying them with the indicator functions $I_{C_{st}}(x_s, x_t)$ that take the value 1 inside the sets $C_{st} := \{(x_s, x_t) \,|\, a_{st} \le \|x_s - x_t\| \le b_{st}\}$, where the parameters a_{st} and b_{st} are determined in relation to the minimum and maximum lengths in the training set. Hence, overlapping parts and pairs too far apart are assigned a pairwise probability of 0 and effectively are no longer considered together.

We point out that, while truncated Gaussian distributions are appropriate for the application studied in this paper, the model adopted from [13] also copes with more general, e.g. multimodal, local distributions.

Part Detection. Randomized classification trees allow for fast evaluation and can be used to detect points of interest [14]. Training such a classifier amounts to creating a set of decision trees and collecting the statistics of the training data under the trees' classifications. The branching tests at tree nodes are chosen at random from a set of very simple tests, each involving only few feature space dimensions.

For our application, we use sub-volumes of 15x15x15 voxels as local feature vectors. The tree tests are plain comparisons of two of their dimensions, translating to simple "brighter than resp. darker than" decisions for pairs of voxels in a neighborhood. The overall performance and robustness against noise results from the aggregation of the statistics over a large number of such tests, that are distributed over the ensemble of decision trees used. As only the ordering of intensity is taken into account, the resulting detector is insensitive to intensity distribution variation as commonly observed in MR images.

Local rotation and scale tolerance is achieved by augmenting the training set by resampled copies of the training images, which have been randomly transformed to vary within the expected range of orientation and scale changes.

Applying the classifier to an image yields a probability volume for each class (Fig. 1). After sorting by descending probability, we pick candidates for each class, starting with the most probable location, and add further candidates as long as a specified number of candidates and a given probability threshold are not exceeded. We impose a minimum spacing constraint between a class's candidate points to suppress non-maxima, and to restrict further the set of candidates.

Modeling Undetected Parts. Missing detections of individual parts are handled by introducing an artificial candidate for each node of the graphical model, the location and appearance of which is declared "hidden". As its position is not known, we would need to marginalize the associated potentials over the image domain, which is computationally infeasible. Instead, we approximate this marginalization by setting the hidden candidate's potentials to their expectation with respect to the training data plus a penalty for the miss:

$$\psi_s(\cdot) = -\log \beta\, \mathbb{E}_{x_s}\big[\exp(-\psi_s(x_s))\big]\,,\ \ \psi_{st}(\cdot,\cdot) = -\log \gamma\, \mathbb{E}_{x_s,x_t}\big[\exp(-\psi_{st}(x_s,x_t))\big] \tag{5}$$

Here, $\mathbb{E}_{x_s}$ resp. $\mathbb{E}_{x_s,x_t}$ denote the expectation with respect to the ground truth training data, and the parameters β, γ are empirically determined from the training set such that these "hidden"-probabilities indeed incur a penalty for omitting parts in the majority of training cases.

Inference Algorithm. We use the graphical model as specified above to infer the most likely configuration x (position and overall pose) of the model in any novel image I. This maximum a posteriori (MAP) estimate

$$\hat{x} = \arg\max_{x \in \Omega} P(x|I,\theta) \tag{6}$$

is obtained by searching over all configurations consistent with detected part candidate points. This is done using the A^* algorithm [15] based on a tight upper-bound estimate for efficiently pruning the search space. This estimate is computed by exact inference on a tree-structured subgraph and guarantees not to miss the global optimum [13]. As described below, it turned out empirically that A^*-search terminates after reasonable computation time. Therefore, we preferred this method over alternative approaches to *approximate* graphical inference based on *non*convex optimization [16].

Missing Part Postprocessing. We can estimate the approximate location of parts detected as missing in a postprocessing step. This is done by greedily searching for these locations while keeping the already inferred parts fixed. For each missing part h, treated individually now, we predict its position by aggregating the evidence from all neighbors N_h of h that have been successfully identified. Specifically, using the learned distributions $x_t - x_s \sim \mathcal{N}(\mu_{st}, \Sigma_{st})$ and the identity $\mathcal{N}(a,A) \cdot \mathcal{N}(b,B) \propto \mathcal{N}(c,C)$ where $C = (A^{-1}+B^{-1})^{-1}$, $c = CA^{-1}a + CB^{-1}b$

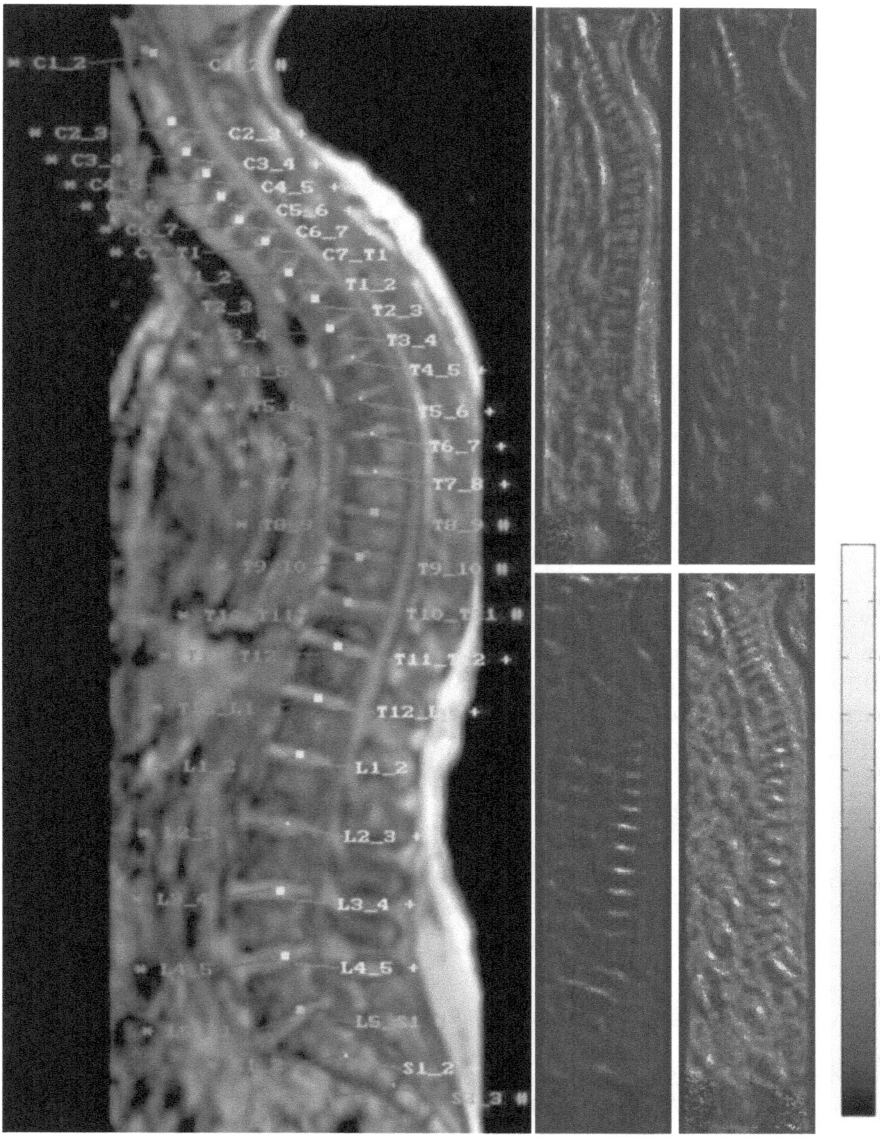

Fig. 1. Left: Labeling result. Yellow labels denote the graphical model's MAP estimate(+), green labels represent parts found by postprocessing(#), and blue labels show the ground truth annotation(*). Larger dots indicate positions located in the viewing plane and smaller dots positions next to it. **Right: Classifier probability maps** for four classes in a new image, produced by the randomized tree classifier that was trained on independent datasets. Clockwise, the corresponding classes are C1-2, C2-3, L1-2, and S1-2. The depicted slices from the probability volumes were normalized for visualization such that the value 1 represents the most likely pixels with respect to these classes. Note that particularly in case of the L1-2 class, the neighboring disks are highly similar in appearance. Thus, local classification cannot discriminate between them, but has to be complemented by "geometrical context" as studied in this paper.

for the multiplication of Gaussians, we compute the maximum at the mean of the product

$$\hat{x}_h = \max_{x_h} \prod_{s \in N_h} \mathcal{N}(x_s + \mu_{sh}, \Sigma_{sh}) = (\sum_{s \in N_h} \Sigma_{sh}^{-1})^{-1} (\sum_{s \in N_h} \Sigma_{sh}^{-1}(x_s + \mu_{sh})) . \quad (7)$$

Optionally, we incorporate the appearance term by multiplying the product of Gaussians by the classifier's probability map of the missing part, and then locate the maximum.

Scale Estimation and Invariance. The learned geometry representation exhibits a high variance if the training examples are not normalized in scale. Hence, tighter geometry constraints are obtained if both training and test data are on a common scale. For training images, this can be achieved by Procrustes analysis, for instance. But for the test images, the scale information is not readily available, because the correspondences have not been established prior to detection.

In order to compensate for global changes in scale in a new image, we extend our algorithm by a second run of the graphical model inference. After the first run, which is performed with the original geometry model without scale normalization, we obtain an estimate for the global scale correction parameter as follows: For each pair of detected parts, the ratio of their distance to the model's mean distance is entered into a weighted histogram $H(\frac{(||x_s - x_t||}{\mu_{st}}; \frac{1}{\sigma_{st}})$ with the weight derived from the model's standard deviation, so that less reliable pairs of parts have lesser influence on the estimate. After smoothing the histogram H using kernel density estimation with a Gaussian kernel, we use its mode as the global scale compensation parameter for this image.

A second inference run is then performed using the scale-compensated inter-part geometry together with a geometry model learned from scale-normalized training examples. The scale estimates for the training data needed to build this latter model are extracted using the same histogram-based procedure, using ground truth pairs of parts instead of part detections.

4 Experimental Results

We evaluate the performance of our graphical model and its components for spine detection and localization, based on annotated ground truth data.

Data Sets. T1-weighted MR images were acquired on a Philips 1.5T Achieva scanner with a multi-station 3D FFE sequence. These 30 datasets each consist of two station scans (224 × 224 × 180 voxels of extent 1.96mm × 1.96mm × 1.5mm), which were combined into a single image and resampled to obtain an isotropic voxel size of 2mm edge length. The image quality of these MR acquisitions varied greatly. Artefacts and intensity distribution fluctuations due to field inhomogeneities as well as pathologies such as vertebra fractures were present in these data.

Training and Parameter Values. The tree classifiers were trained on 5000 positive examples for each of the 26 classes (intervertebral disks C1-2 to S2-3)

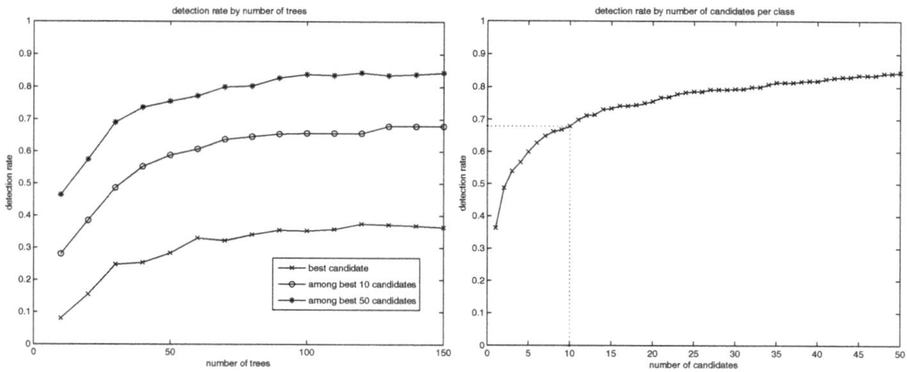

Fig. 2. Local detection performance. A part is detected if any of the best k candidates is within 14mm of the ground truth location. **Left:** Detection performance increases as more classification trees are used. Searching among the best 10 candidates for each class gives about 70% detection rate with 150 trees. **Right:** Producing more candidates increases the probability of detection, shown here for 150 trees. The line indicates our choice of 10 candidates used in subsequent experiments. Note that using a single local decision (the best candidate only) yields a poor detection rate of 36%.

and 50000 background examples (randomly picked patches from other image regions), all generated by resampling from a training set of 16 images. During resampling, the images were anisotropically scaled ($\pm 20\%$) and rotated ($\pm\pi/4$) about a randomly defined axis.

For scale detection, we always used model (4). It identifies sufficiently many parts such that the estimated scale correction factor differs from an estimate using ground truth by at most 4%. Further parameters used were $\beta = 0.01$ and $\gamma = 0.1$ in Eq. 5. In (2), we set $\alpha = \frac{2}{|V|}$. The parameters a_{st}, b_{st} for truncating the Gaussians (3) and (4) were determined by multiplying by 0.8 (1.15) the minimum (maximum) distance between parts observed in the training data.

Part Detector Performance. The part detectors are parametrized by the number of trees and the tree depth. We limited the maximum tree depth to 30 and pruned at branches with less than 10 training samples, so that most branches are actually much shorter. In order to set the number of trees to a reasonable value, we conducted a series of experiments for assessing the detection accuracy relative to annotated ground truth positions.

A detection is considered as "correct" if it occurs within a radius of 14mm from the ground truth annotation, resulting in good overall localization.[1] Fig. 2, left, shows the results.

Another important parameter is the number of candidate points we produce for each part class. This number determines the average running time of the inference algorithm based on the graphical model. Motivated by the experimental findings (cf. Figs. 2 right, and Fig. 3), we set the number of candidates per class

[1] This value equals the minimum intervertebral disk distance in our data.

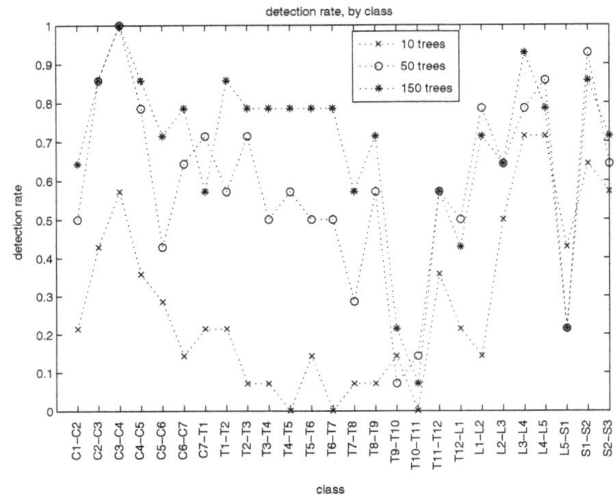

Fig. 3. Local detection performance for each part. While the detection probability increases with the numbers of trees, it varies significantly for different parts. The subsequent non-local inference using the graphical model is therefore essential in order to cope with parts that are more difficult to detect.

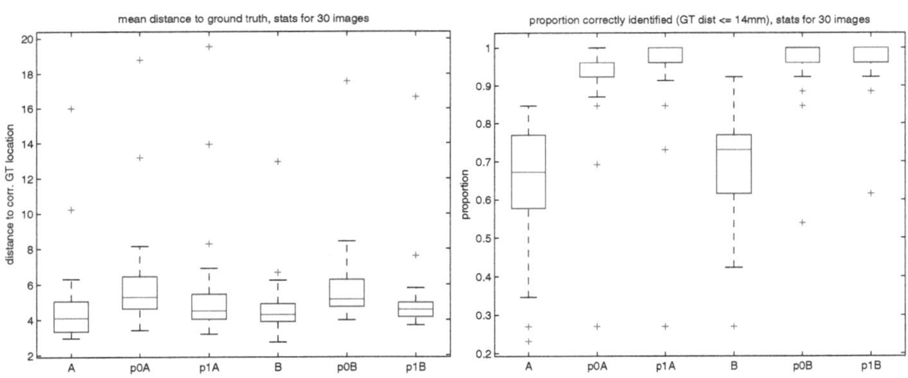

Fig. 4. Localization accuracy of the overall model variants. The box plots show the median (center line), the lower and upper quartiles (box), and the extent of the data (whiskers extending by at most 1.5 times the interquartile distance) excluding outliers, which are separately plotted as crosses. Symbol A indicates the use of orientation information in the geometry model (4); symbol B indicates the rotational invariant geometry model (3). Symbol p1 indicates missing-part postprocessing with appearance information, and p0 without. **Left:** Distances to ground truth locations, averaged over all classes, for each model variant A, p0A, p1A, B, p0B, p1B. **Right:** Proportion of correctly identified parts for each model variant.

to 10 in all subsequent experiments. An obvious modification is to let this number vary for different part classes. We did not investigate this option, however.

Overall Performance and Cross Validation. We determined the localization accuracy and robustness of the complete model by leave-one-out cross validation with 30 annotated images. In each of the 30 runs, 29 datasets were used for training the randomized tree classifier as well as either of the two geometry models (3) and (4), and the remaining dataset was used for testing the resulting model, utilizing the classifier together with graphical model inference, scale estimation, and missing part postprocessing.

Localization accuracy results are summarized in Fig. 4. Due to the restriction to interest points on the voxel grid as candidate locations, our model is not expected to yield sub-voxel accuracy. Nevertheless, Fig. 4, left, shows that most detected part locations are within a few millimeters of the ground truth position.

Using the geometry model with orientation (4) yielded an average ground truth distance of 6.2mm (lower quartile 4.6mm, upper quartile 6.5mm) and a part detection rate of 0.91. The rotational invariant model (3) resulted in an average ground truth distance of 5.8mm (lower quartile 4.8mm, upper quartile 6.3mm) and a part detection rate of 0.95. Including appearance in the search for missing parts improved this to 5.5mm and 5.1mm (part detection rates 0.94 and 0.97), respectively. Fig. 5 shows the localization errors for each class separately.

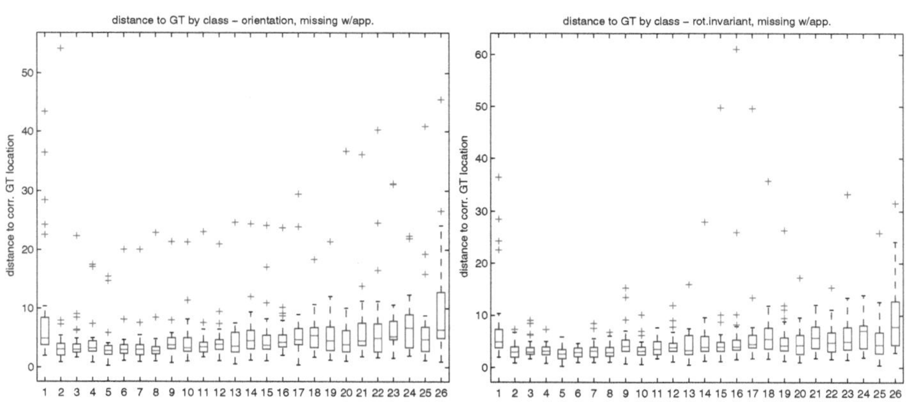

Fig. 5. Localization accuracy for each part class. The class numbers correspond to intervertebral disks C1-2 (class 1) to S2-3 (class 26). **Left:** Model using a geometry model with orientation, and missing part postprocessing with appearance information. **Right:** Rotational invariant geometry model, and missing part postprocessing with appearance information.

Using the rotational invariant geometry model results in more accurate localizations with less outliers. An example result of the overall model fit, i.e. the most probable configuration x, is visualized in Fig. 1.

Generalization to Novel Images. We tested the algorithm also on a set of 37 new images, that were not used for training nor for optimizing the parameters. Using the rotational invariant geometry model and appearance information in the search for missing parts, yielded an average ground truth distance of 7.8mm (lower quartile 5.3mm, upper quartile 9.5mm). This indicates that our models generalizes well to novel data.

Semi-automated Incorporation of Expert Knowledge. We investigate if, and to what extent the incorporation of expert knowledge (as used in semi-automatic algorithms by "clicking" on relevant anatomical structures) improves the localization accuracy. We repeated the same series of experiments as described above, but replaced the candidates for C1-2 with the expert's annotation (ground truth) and assigned to them an appearance probability of 1, while disallowing to declare it as missing. The results improved slightly: The model including orientation yielded an average ground truth distance of 5.8mm (lower quartile 3.9mm, upper quartile 5.5mm) and a part detection rate of 0.94. The rotational invariant model resulted in an average ground truth distance of 5.7mm (lower quartile 4.2mm, upper quartile 5.3mm) and also a part detection rate of 0.94.

5 Conclusion and Further Work

We presented a probabilistic graphical approach to the localization of spinal structures, by fusing local part detection with non-local geometrical context. The latter enables to revise local detections in case of ambiguous image data or missing features. The inference algorithm returns always the globally optimal configuration of parts conditioned on the observed image data, and does therefore not suffer from initialization problems.

While our approach enables robust localization and appears to generalize well to novel image data, it fails in cases of severe fractures that lead to geometrical configurations not covered by the training data. Enlarging the latter will most likely fix this problem.

Surprisingly, regarding computational complexity, the limiting component of our current implementation are the local part detectors. For a full volume, they take several minutes computation time. The subsequent combinatorial search for the optimal configuration, on the other hand, runs below 1 second on the average, despite the size of 10^{26} possible configurations. This proves empirically the tightness of our upper-bound estimate used within the A^*-algorithm.

Our approach can be extended in several ways. For example, subvoxel localization can be achieved by fitting more elaborate part models in a post-processing step. Reduction of the processing time mainly depends on a more sophisticated implementation of the part detectors. We also would like to point out, that our model is sufficiently flexible to be adapted to the localization of other anatomical structures.

An important topic of our future work concerns to handle also cases where the total number of vertebrae differs from the standard of 24. The latter can be achieved by extending the graphical model to include a latent unknown variable that represents the major cases of anatomy deviation and has to be inferred as part of the overall process.

Acknowledgements. The MR images used in this work were kindly provided by Rene Bergmans und Chiel den Harder (Philips Medical Systems, Best, The Netherlands).

References

1. Peng, Z., Zhong, J., Wee, W., Lee, J.h.: Automated vertebra detection and segmentation from the whole spine MR images. In: Proc. Engineering in Medicine and Biology, IEEE-EMBS 2005, pp. 2527–2530 (2005)
2. Weiss, K.L., Storrs, J.M., Banto, R.B.: Automated spine survey iterative scan technique. Radiology 239(1), 255–262 (2006)
3. Vrtovec, T., Ourselin, S., Gomes, L., Likar, B., Pernus, F.: Generation of curved planar reformations from magnetic resonance images of the spine. In: Larsen, R., Nielsen, M., Sporring, J. (eds.) MICCAI 2006. LNCS, vol. 4191, pp. 135–143. Springer, Heidelberg (2006)
4. Cootes, T., Taylor, C., Cooper, D., Graham, J.: Active shape models – their training and application. Comp. Vision Image Underst. 61(1), 38–59 (1995)
5. Cootes, T.F., Edwards, G.J., Taylor, C.J.: Active appearance models. In: Burkhardt, H., Neumann, B. (eds.) ECCV 1998. LNCS, vol. 1407, pp. 484–498. Springer, Heidelberg (1998)
6. Matthews, I., Baker, S.: Active appearance models revisited. International Journal of Computer Vision 60, 135–164 (2004)
7. Abi-Nahed, J., Jolly, M.P., Yang, G.Z.: Robust active shape models: A robust, generic and simple automatic segmentation tool. In: Larsen, R., Nielsen, M., Sporring, J. (eds.) MICCAI 2006. LNCS, vol. 4191, pp. 1–8. Springer, Heidelberg (2006)
8. Felzenszwalb, P.F., Huttenlocher, D.P.: Pictorial structures for object recognition. International Journal of Computer Vision 61, 55–79 (2005)
9. Pham, T.V., Smeulders, A.W.M.: Object recognition with uncertain geometry and uncertain part detection. Computer Vision and Image Understanding 99(2), 241–258 (2005)
10. Weber, M., Welling, M., Perona, P.: Unsupervised learning of models for recognition. In: ECCV (1) 2000, 18–32 (2000)
11. Fergus, R., Perona, P., Zisserman, A.: Object class recognition by unsupervised scale-invariant learning. In: IEEE Computer Society Conference on Computer Vision and Pattern Recognition (CVPR). vol. 2, p. 264 (2003)
12. Amit, Y.: Graphical shape templates for automatic anatomy detection with applications to MRI brain scans. IEEE Trans. Med. Imaging 16(1), 28–40 (1997)
13. Bergtholdt, M., Kappes, J.H., Schnörr, C.: Learning of graphical models and efficient inference for object class recognition. In: Franke, K., Müller, K.-R., Nickolay, B., Schäfer, R. (eds.) Pattern Recognition. LNCS, vol. 4174, pp. 273–283. Springer, Heidelberg (2006)
14. Lepetit, V., Fua, P.: Keypoint recognition using randomized trees. IEEE Trans. Pattern Anal. Mach. Intell. 28(9), 1465–1479 (2006)
15. Minoux, M.: Mathematical programming: theory and algorithms. Wiley, Chichester (1986)
16. Pakzad, P., Anantharam, V.: Estimation and marginalization using Kikuchi approximation methods. Neural Computation 17(8), 1836–1873 (2005)

Lung Nodule Detection Via Bayesian Voxel Labeling

Paulo R.S. Mendonça[1], Rahul Bhotika[1], Fei Zhao[2], and James V. Miller[1]

[1] GE Global Research, One Research Circle, Niskayuna, NY 12309, USA
[2] University of Iowa, Department of Electrical Engineering, Iowa City, IA 52246, USA

Abstract. This paper describes a system for detecting pulmonary nodules in CT images. It aims to label individual image voxels in accordance to one of a number of anatomical (pulmonary vessels or junctions), pathological (nodules), or spurious (noise) events. The approach is orthodoxly Bayesian, with particular care taken in the objective establishment of prior probabilities and the incorporation of relevant medical knowledge. We provide, under explicit modeling assumptions, closed-form expressions for all the probability distributions involved. The technique is applied to real data, and we present a discussion of its performance.

1 Introduction

There are significant clinical motivations for the pursuit of computer-aided detection (CAD) systems for lung cancer, which is the leading cause of cancer deaths worldwide. According to the GLOBOCAN survey [1] the global death toll in 2002 was over 1.1 million people and 1.3 million new cases were diagnosed. The overall survival rate of a lung cancer patient is about 14% [2], a figure that can be improved to 70% for early-stage patients that undergo a lung resection [3]. The medical community sees CAD as a necessary tool for meeting the demands of a CT screening program for lung cancer [4].

The choice of a *Bayesian* voxel labeling technique to address the problem of pulmonary nodule detection is justified for several reasons. The uncertainty inherent to the detection problems commonly faced in medical imaging is best accounted for through statistical techniques. Moreover, there often is useful medical knowledge that can be utilized to regularize or bound the solution of such problems. Bayesian methods are therefore a natural choice, due to their ability to incorporate informative prior probabilities (or simply *priors*) that encode and account for pertinent data and meta-data, such as patient family history or prior medical examinations. Besides, as nicely put in [5], the use of priors forces the explicit acknowledgment of otherwise hidden assumptions.

As for the choice of a voxel labeling scheme for nodule detection, it should be contrasted with the alternative method of generating candidate detections through segmentation followed by classification of the segmented regions ([6] is a good example). This is a perfectly sound approach, with potential advantages over voxel labeling — in particular, it eases the reckoning of spatial information. However, such detection systems are hostages of the segmentation step. First, the detection rate of the segmentation step places an upper bound on the detection rate of the complete system. Even if the segmentation provides a full partition of the image, in our experience undersegmentation (common with small and vascularized nodules) and oversegmentation (common with large and complex nodules) occur frequently. This issue could perhaps be tackled by

N. Karssemeijer and B. Lelieveldt (Eds.): IPMI 2007, LNCS 4584, pp. 134–146, 2007.
© Springer-Verlag Berlin Heidelberg 2007

a joint segmentation and detection algorithm, but the state of the art on such tasks [7] assumes a few discrete data sources, unsuitable to describe a space of segmentations. Voxel labeling bypasses such issues by incorporating information from neighboring pixels in a predefined way and making decisions only at a local level.

There is a wealth of research in the area of CAD systems applied to the detection of lung nodules from CT exams [34]. Local shape analysis of the 3D data was presented in [8]. A 2½D technique was employed in [6], with solid results on noisy low-dose screening data. Nonetheless, the method uses 2D segmentation to generate candidates and the number of false positives grows with the use of thinner CT slices. The distribution of surface normals at the air-tissue interface was used in [9]; the algorithm was tested on only eight images and results were reported for nodules larger than the minimum size of 4 mm for which a follow up is recommended [10]. Recent works [11] report strong results, but the dose violates the requirements of current screening protocols [10].

At a high level, this work applies a Bayesian statistical framework akin to that of [6] to the problem of local shape analysis. It departs from that work by not requiring a training step, avoiding image segmentation, building statistical models from geometric abstractions of label classes rather than data, and making extensive use of available medical data to generate priors for the parameters of the models. It is also distinct from previous works in differential shape analysis [8,12] that follow a purely deterministic approach. Great care was taken in developing rigorous statistical models, in avoiding the often hasty adoption of off-the-shelf Gaussian likelihoods, uniform priors and maximum likelihood estimators; concessions to mathematical simplicity were made in generating a practical solution to the problem, but less so in the problem statement. We make specific choices of features, models and priors, but acknowledge that different choices are possible and that such choices are paramount to algorithm performance.

The next section will introduce the mathematical framework of this paper. Sections 3-5 describe the relevant models and probability distributions. Implementation and results are discussed in section 6.

2 The Voxel Labeling Problem from a Bayesian Perspective

The symbol $P(A)$ denotes the probability of the event A in an adequate probability space. The symbol $p_X(x)$ denotes the value of the probability density of the random variable X at x. We omit the subscript X in $p_X(x)$ when doing so is not ambiguous.

Let $\{\mathscr{M}_i, i = 1, \ldots, N\}$ be a set of parametric models, a model being a mathematical description of an object. Each $\mathscr{M}_i$ has parameters $\mathbf{m}_i$ in the domain $\mathbf{M}_i$. Given a choice of $\mathscr{M}_i$, if $\mathscr{D}$ can be *assumed* to be a set $\mathscr{D} = \{\mathscr{D}_j, j = 1, \ldots, M\}$ of *independent* datum $\mathscr{D}_j$ associated with voxel $\mathbf{x}$, we have, using Bayes' law and marginalizing over the model parameters,

$$
\begin{aligned}
P(\mathscr{M}_i|\mathscr{D},\mathbf{x}) &= p(\mathscr{D}|\mathscr{M}_i,\mathbf{x})\frac{P(\mathscr{M}_i|\mathbf{x})}{p(\mathscr{D}|\mathbf{x})} = M! \times \prod_{j=1}^{M} p(\mathscr{D}_j|\mathscr{M}_i,\mathbf{x})\frac{P(\mathscr{M}_i|\mathbf{x})}{p(\mathscr{D}|\mathbf{x})} \\
&= M! \times \prod_{j=1}^{M} \int_{\mathbf{M}_i} p(\mathscr{D}_j|\mathbf{m}_i,\mathscr{M}_i,\mathbf{x})p(\mathbf{m}_i|\mathscr{M}_i,\mathbf{x})\,d\mathbf{m}_i \frac{P(\mathscr{M}_i|\mathbf{x})}{p(\mathscr{D}|\mathbf{x})}. \qquad (1)
\end{aligned}
$$

The independence assumption embedded in (1) is admittedly strong, but there is little hope that a practical solution can be achieved under weaker hypotheses. The integral in (1) is complicated enough; without this assumption, it would be unmanageable.

In the first line of the derivation of (1) the *posterior*, *likelihood*, and *prior* terms are $P(\mathcal{M}_i|\mathcal{D},\mathbf{x})$, $p(\mathcal{D}|\mathcal{M}_i,\mathbf{x})$, and $P(\mathcal{M}_i|\mathbf{x})$, respectively. The independence assumption allows for the factorization of the likelihood term and $M!$ must be included because $\mathcal{D}$ is a set of M individual datum $\mathcal{D}_j$, not an M-tuple. The marginalization step underscores the distinction between the problems of detection and that of joint detection and *fitting*. While in the latter the parameters of the selected model are also estimated, in the former they are simply nuisance parameters whose values are accounted for, but not explicitly computed. The identity $p(\mathbf{m}_i|\mathcal{D}_j,\mathcal{M}_i,\mathbf{x}) = \frac{p(\mathbf{m}_i|\mathcal{M}_i,\mathbf{x})}{p(\mathcal{D}_j|\mathcal{M}_i,\mathbf{x})} p(\mathcal{D}_j|\mathbf{m}_i,\mathcal{M}_i,\mathbf{x})$ justifies referring also to $p(\mathcal{D}_j|\mathbf{m}_i,\mathcal{M}_i,\mathbf{x})$ and $p(\mathbf{m}_i|\mathcal{M}_i,\mathbf{x})$ as likelihood and prior terms, and it is to indicate these probability densities that these words are henceforth reserved. Whenever a reference to $p(\mathcal{D}|\mathcal{M}_i,\mathbf{x})$ and $P(\mathcal{M}_i|\mathbf{x})$ is made, we will avoid confusion by using the terms *data likelihood* and *model prior* instead.

2.1 Modeling the Likelihood Term

To compute the likelihood term $p(\mathcal{D}_j|\mathbf{m}_i,\mathcal{M}_i,\mathbf{x})$ in (1) we first need to define the parametric model $\mathcal{M}_i$ and the datum $\mathcal{D}_j \in \mathcal{D}$ for the set $\mathcal{D}$ associated to the voxel $\mathbf{x}$. We consider four models: a *nodule model* $\mathcal{M}_1$, a *vessel model* $\mathcal{M}_2$, a *vessel junction model* $\mathcal{M}_3$, and an *outlier model* $\mathcal{M}_4$. The first three are jointly referred to as *anatomical models*, as they are representative of structures found in lungs; the last model is a catchall for everything that does not correspond to any of the anatomical models.

The above choices are reasonable if one considers the anatomy and pathology of the lungs, but what constitutes a good choice of $\mathcal{D}$ is less clear. A number of works in computer-aided detection of lung nodules [8,12] or colonic polyps [13,14] have demonstrated that differential operators such as the Hessian or the structure tensor can be efficiently used to discriminate between round and elongated structures in images. A comparison of differential operators was carried out in [12], suggesting an advantage for the curvature tensor. In view of this we choose to use principal curvatures $\boldsymbol{\kappa} = (\kappa_1, \kappa_2)$, with $\kappa_1 \leq \kappa_2$, as the datum $\mathcal{D}_j \in \mathcal{D}$. This, in turn, makes geometric representations a natural choice for our anatomical models. The likelihood term $p(\mathcal{D}_j|\mathbf{m}_i,\mathcal{M}_i,\mathbf{x}) = p(\boldsymbol{\kappa}|\mathbf{m}_i,\mathcal{M}_i,\mathbf{x})$ is thus defined as the probability density of the random vector $\mathbf{K}^i$ which maps a voxel $\mathbf{x}$ to a pair (κ_1, κ_2), given the geometric model $\mathcal{M}_i$ with parameters $\mathbf{m}_i$.

2.2 Modeling the Prior

At the heart of the still ongoing philosophical debate on the validity of Bayesian methods [15] is the alleged subjectivism with which prior distributions are selected. Since Jeffreys [16], however, there are firm grounds to reject such criticism, and there are now a number of objective methods to elicit prior probabilities [17]. Of these, the *maximum entropy principle* [18] is particularly attractive to our problem, due to its amenability to the incorporation of external information. In a nutshell, the maximum entropy principle prescribes as the prior the distribution p of maximal entropy $S = -\int p(x) \log p(x)\,dx$, subject to the available constraints, expressed in the form $\int p(x) f_k(x)\,dx = c_k$ for given functions f_k and constants c_k. We therefore obtain p through the solution of a standard variational problem.

Bringing medical scholarship into the design of the prior distribution of the model parameters is of fundamental importance in this work. A popular alternative is the learning of parameter distributions from training data [19,20], where prior knowledge is encoded in the form of prelabeled data samples. In this work, the probability distributions of the model parameters are inferred from data in the medical literature. Obviously, both approaces have merits. In many situations, particularly in more exploratory research, the very point of the work is to gain medical knowledge by understanding the parameters of a given model [21], in which case data-driven learning techniques are the best option.

Volume Normalization. The procedure above computes $p(\mathbf{m}_i|\mathscr{M}_i)$, *not* $p(\mathbf{m}_i|\mathscr{M}_i,\mathbf{x})$. But once $p(\mathbf{m}_i|\mathscr{M}_i)$ is obtained, $p(\mathbf{m}_i|\mathscr{M}_i,\mathbf{x})$ can be found with the help of the identity $p(\mathbf{m}_i|\mathscr{M}_i,\mathbf{x}) = p(\mathbf{x}|\mathbf{m}_i,\mathscr{M}_i)p(\mathbf{m}_i|\mathscr{M}_i)/p(\mathbf{x}|\mathscr{M}_i)$. Taking a frequentist detour from our Bayesian orthodoxy we argue that $p(\mathbf{x}|\mathbf{m}_i,\mathscr{M}_i)/p(\mathbf{x}|\mathscr{M}_i)$ is proportional to the volume $\mathrm{V}(\mathbf{m}_i,\mathscr{M}_i)$, since, all else being equal, we are more likely to sample a voxel from the instance of $\mathscr{M}_i$ that has more voxels. Therefore, given $p(\mathbf{m}_i|\mathscr{M}_i)$, $p(\mathbf{m}_i|\mathscr{M}_i,\mathbf{x})$ can be obtained as $p(\mathbf{m}_i|\mathscr{M}_i,\mathbf{x}) = p(\mathbf{m}_i|\mathscr{M}_i)\mathrm{V}(\mathbf{m}_i,\mathscr{M}_i)/\int_{\mathbf{M}_i} p(\mathbf{m}_i|\mathscr{M}_i)\mathrm{V}(\mathbf{m}_i,\mathscr{M}_i)\,d\mathbf{m}_i$. This frequentist argument can also be used to determine $P(\mathscr{M}_i|\mathbf{x})$.

The Bayesian Horizon. The constraints on the priors are, in general, not directly accessible from medical literature, but must themselves be inferred from available information. This estimation problem could, in turn, be tackled with the introduction of *hyperpriors* [35], a process that should not be iterated indefinitely; the *ad hoc* point at which one stops is one's *Bayesian horizon* (a term, to our knowledge, coined by Nils Krahnstoever [22]).

2.3 Overview of the Modeling Procedure

We can now describe the general steps of the modeling procedure. *All* of these steps must be adapted to the particular model under consideration and are prescribed here only as general guidelines. They are: (i) selection of a geometric representation for $\mathscr{M}_i$, (ii) design of the priors $p(\mathbf{m}_i|\mathscr{M}_i,\mathbf{x})$ and $P(\mathscr{M}_i|\mathbf{x})$, (iii) derivation of the likelihood $p(\boldsymbol{\kappa}|\mathbf{m}_i,\mathscr{M}_i,\mathbf{x})$, and (iv) marginalization of $p(\boldsymbol{\kappa}|\mathbf{m}_i,\mathscr{M}_i,\mathbf{x})$ over $p(\mathbf{m}_i|\mathscr{M}_i,\mathbf{x})$.

The marginalization is further broken down into two steps: simplification of the integrand and solution of the simplified integral. The integral in (1) is, in general, intractable, and a conservative variant of Laplace's method [23] is employed to simplify it. The procedure affects only the likelihood term, resulting in

$$p(\boldsymbol{\kappa}|\mathbf{m}_i,\mathscr{M}_i,\mathbf{x}) \approx \sum_{j=1}^{J} w_j \delta(\kappa_1 - g_j(\kappa_2,\mathbf{m}_i,\mathscr{M}_i)) p_j(\kappa_2|\mathbf{m}_i,\mathscr{M}_i,\mathbf{x}), \qquad (2)$$

where the number of terms J, the weights w_j, with $\sum_j^J w_j = 1$, the functions g_j and the densities p_j depend on $p(\kappa_1|\kappa_2,\mathbf{m}_i,\mathscr{M}_i,\mathbf{x})$. The roles of κ_1 and κ_2 may be exchanged as long as the necessary modifications in g_j and p_j are made. While most variants of Laplace's method completely replace the integral in (1) with an integral-free term, our approximation only reduces the number of nested integrals, resulting in an expression that can be solved in closed form.

3 The Nodule Model

The model $\mathscr{M}_1$ chosen to represent a nodule is a solid ellipsoid with similar concentric ellipsoidal isosurfaces such that the outermost isosurface has semi-axes a, b and c with $a = b \leq c$, i.e.,

$$\begin{aligned} \mathscr{M}_1 : \Pi \times \Theta \times \Phi &\to \mathbb{R}^3 \\ (\rho, \theta, \phi) &\mapsto \mathbf{x} = \begin{bmatrix} a\rho \cos\theta \cos\phi \\ a\rho \sin\theta \cos\phi \\ c\rho \sin\phi \end{bmatrix}, \end{aligned} \tag{3}$$

where $\Pi = [0,1]$, $\Theta = [0, 2\pi)$, $\Phi = [-\pi/2, \pi/2]$. The parameters of the model are $\mathbf{m}_1 = (a, c)$, with domain $\mathbf{M}_1 = \{(a,c) \in \mathbb{R}^2 | 0 < a \leq c\}$. Each choice of $\rho \in \Pi$ defines a different isosurface, at any point of which the principal curvatures can be computed. Moreover, using standard results from differential geometry [24], it can be shown that

$$\rho = (c/a^2)\sqrt{\kappa_1/\kappa_2^3} \text{ and } \sin^2\phi = (c^2 - a^2(\kappa_2/\kappa_1))/(c^2 - a^2). \tag{4}$$

3.1 Design of the Priors

Let A and C be random variables that map a nodule to the half-size of its minor and major axes (a, c). Assuming that nodules have non-negative dimensions with an average diameter of $2/\lambda$, as yet to be determined, the choice of an exponential distribution for A is supported by both the principle of maximum entropy and data from the medical literature [25]. The same is true for the random variable C, but now the additional constraint that $0 < A \leq C$ must be satisfied. Observe that the second inequality is arbitrary: A and C are *chosen* from the pair (A', C') with $0 < A' < \infty$ and $0 < C' < \infty$ so that $A \leq C$. Therefore, the maximum entropy principle can be first applied to (A', C'), resulting in a probability density for the pair (A', C') given by $p(a', c') = \lambda^2 e^{-\lambda(a'+c')} \mathbb{I}_{(0,\infty)}(a') \mathbb{I}_{(0,\infty)}(c')$, where $\mathbb{I}_X$ is the indicator function of the set X, i.e., $\mathbb{I}_X(x) = 1$ if $x \in X$ and 0 otherwise. This expression implies that A' and C' are independent, which, in the absence of contrary evidence, is the maximum entropy solution. The joint distribution for (A, C) can then be obtained via the transformation $A = \min(A', C')$, $C = \max(A', C')$, resulting in $p(\mathbf{m}_1 | \mathscr{M}_1) = p(a, c) = 2\lambda^2 e^{-\lambda(a+c)} \mathbb{I}_{\mathbf{M}_1}(\mathbf{m}_1)$. Given the volume $\mathrm{V}(a, c) = 4\pi a^2 c/3$ of an instance of $\mathscr{M}_1$, following the procedure discussed in Section 2.2 we obtain the desired prior $p(\mathbf{m}_1 | \mathscr{M}_1, \mathbf{x})$ for $\mathbf{m}_1 = (a, c)$ as

$$p(\mathbf{m}_1 | \mathscr{M}_1, \mathbf{x}) = (8/5)\lambda^5 a^2 c e^{-\lambda(a+c)} \mathbb{I}_{\mathbf{M}_1}(\mathbf{m}_1). \tag{5}$$

Using data from [25], a maximum likelihood estimation of λ results in $\lambda \approx 0.5\ \mathrm{mm}^{-1}$. To determine $P(\mathscr{M}_1 | \mathbf{x})$ we again used the data in [25], which places the likelihood of finding a nodule in a given exam of a screening cohort as 60%, with average nodule volume of 0.033 ml.

3.2 Derivation of the Likelihood

Let $\mathbf{x}$ be a point in the range $\mathcal{M}_1(\Pi \times \Theta \times \Phi) = \mathcal{R}_1 \subset \mathbb{R}^3$ of $\mathcal{M}_1$, randomly chosen according to a uniform distribution on $\mathcal{R}_1$. Define now the random variables Π_1, Φ_1 and $\mathbf{K}^1 = (K_1^1, K_2^1)$, given by

$$\begin{array}{llll} \Pi_1 : \mathcal{R}_1 \to \mathbb{R} & \Phi_1 : \mathcal{R}_1 \to \mathbb{R} & \text{and} & \mathbf{K}^1 : \mathcal{R}_1 \to \mathbb{R}^2 \\ \quad \mathbf{x} \mapsto \rho(\mathbf{x}) \in \Pi, & \quad \mathbf{x} \mapsto \phi(\mathbf{x}) \in \Phi & & \quad \mathbf{x} \mapsto \boldsymbol{\kappa}(\mathbf{x}) = (\kappa_1, \kappa_2). \end{array} \tag{6}$$

The joint probability density function of Π_1 and Φ_1 can be computed from the fractional volume element $d\mathbf{x}/dV$ in polar coordinates and is given by

$$p(\rho, \phi) = (3/2)\rho^2 \cos\phi \mathbb{I}_\Pi(\rho)\mathbb{I}_\Phi(\phi). \tag{7}$$

Using (7) and the Jacobian of (4), the joint probability density $p(\boldsymbol{\kappa}|\mathbf{m}_1, \mathcal{M}_1, \mathbf{x})$ of $\mathbf{K}^1$ can be computed via a simple transformation of random variables, yielding

$$p(\boldsymbol{\kappa}|\mathbf{m}_1, \mathcal{M}_1, \mathbf{x}) = 3c^3 \left(2a^4 \sqrt{\kappa_2^9 (c^2 - a^2)(c^2\kappa_1 - a^2\kappa_2)} \right)^{-1} \mathbb{I}_{\mathcal{K}_1}(\boldsymbol{\kappa}), \tag{8}$$

where $\mathcal{K}_1 = \left\{ \boldsymbol{\kappa} \in \mathbb{R}^2 \middle| \frac{a}{c^2} \leq \kappa_1 \text{ and } \max\left(\kappa_1, \left(\frac{c^2\kappa_1}{a^4} \right)^{1/3} \right) \leq \kappa_2 < \frac{c^2}{a^2}\kappa_1 \right\}$.

3.3 Marginalization over the Model Parameters

The probability density in (8) is sharply peaked (in fact, infinite) on the set $\mathcal{K}_1^\infty = \{\boldsymbol{\kappa} \in \mathcal{K}_1 | c^2\kappa_1 - a^2\kappa_2 = 0\}$, and quickly falls as the distance $d(\boldsymbol{\kappa}, \mathcal{K}_1^\infty)$ grows. Therefore, at the isosurface of $\mathcal{M}_1$ defined by a given ρ, the expressions

$$\kappa_1(\rho) \triangleq E[K_1^1|\rho] = \int_\Phi \kappa_1(\phi, \rho)p(\phi|\rho)\, d\phi = h_1(\rho) = (c\rho)^{-1}, \tag{9}$$

$$\kappa_2(\rho) \triangleq E[K_2^1|\rho] = \int_\Phi \kappa_2(\phi, \rho)p(\phi|\rho)\, d\phi = h_2(\rho) = \frac{c \arccos(a/c)}{a\rho\sqrt{c^2 - a^2}}, \tag{10}$$

which suppress the dependence of κ_1 and κ_2 on ϕ, are excellent approximations for the actual values of κ_1 and κ_2. From (9) and (10) one can write

$$\kappa_2 \approx g(\kappa_1, \mathbf{m}_1, \mathcal{M}_1) = \kappa_1 \frac{c^2 \arccos(a/c)}{a\sqrt{c^2 - a^2}} \approx \kappa_1(4c - a)/(3a). \quad \textit{(Taylor series)} \tag{11}$$

Furthermore, computing the marginal probability density $p_{\Pi_1}(\rho)$ of Π_1 from (7) and using the Jacobian of (9), we obtain $p(\kappa_1|\mathbf{m}_1, \mathcal{M}_1, \mathbf{x}) = p_{\Pi_1}(h_1^{-1}(\kappa_1))dh_1^{-1}(\kappa_1)/d\kappa_1 = 3/(c^3\kappa_1^4)\mathbb{I}_{\{1/c \leq \kappa_1\}}(\kappa_1)$. Using this result together with the expression for $g(\kappa_1, \mathbf{m}_1, \mathcal{M}_1)$ defined by (11), we obtain the simplified likelihood term

$$p(\boldsymbol{\kappa}|\mathbf{m}_1, \mathcal{M}_1, \mathbf{x}) \approx \frac{3\delta(\kappa_2 - \kappa_1(4c - a)/(3a))}{c^3\kappa_1^4} \mathbb{I}_{[1/c, \infty)}(\kappa_1)\mathbb{I}_{[0, \kappa_2]}(\kappa_1). \tag{12}$$

Using the approximation in (12) and the prior (5), the integral in (1) can be computed, resulting in

$$p(\boldsymbol{\kappa}|\mathcal{M}_1, \mathbf{x}) \approx 4608\lambda^3 e^{-\frac{\lambda(5\kappa_1 + 3\kappa_2)}{\kappa_1(\kappa_1 + 3\kappa_2)}} \frac{\kappa_1(\kappa_1 + 3\kappa_2) + \lambda(5\kappa_1 + 3\kappa_2)}{5\kappa_1^2(\kappa_1 + 3\kappa_2)^3(5\kappa_1 + 3\kappa_2)^2} \mathbb{I}_{[0, \kappa_2]}(\kappa_1). \tag{13}$$

4 The Vessel Model

The vessel model $\mathscr{M}_2$ is represented as a section of a solid torus with similar concentric isosurfaces such that the outermost isosurface has minor and major radii r and R with $r \leq R$, i.e.,

$$\mathscr{M}_1 : \Pi \times \Theta_0 \times \Psi \to \mathbb{R}^3$$
$$(\rho,\theta,\psi) \mapsto \mathbf{x} = \begin{bmatrix} (R+r\rho\cos\psi)\cos\theta \\ (R+r\rho\cos\psi)\sin\theta \\ r\rho\sin\psi \end{bmatrix}, \tag{14}$$

where $\Pi = [0,1]$, $\Theta_0 = [0,\theta_0]$, $\Psi = [-\pi/2, 3\pi/2)$, and each choice of $\rho \in \Pi$ defines a different isosurface. The parameters of the model are $\mathbf{m}_2 = (\theta_0, r, R)$, with domain $\mathbf{M}_2 = \{(\theta_0, r, R) \in \mathbb{R}^3 | 0 < \theta_0 < 2\pi \text{ and } 0 < r \leq R\}$. The principal curvatures (κ_1, κ_2) at any point $\mathbf{x}$ in the torus can be expressed in terms of the model parameters (ρ, θ, ψ) as

$$\rho = 1/(r\kappa_2) \text{ and } \cos\psi = \kappa_1\kappa_2 R/(\kappa_2 - \kappa_1). \tag{15}$$

4.1 Design of the Priors

The first step in determining the priors on the parameters $\mathbf{m}_2$ of the vessel model is examining available clinical data. Murray's work on vessel structures [26] provides the basis for deriving several mathematical relationships between the vessel model parameters. Two particular corollaries of Murray's law are a power-law distribution for vessel radius, $p(r) \propto 1/r^3$ [27], and a linear relationship between vessel length and diameter, $\theta_0 R \propto r$ [28], with the latter implying that the vessel volume is proportional to r^3. The volume normalization step produces a prior $p(r|\mathbf{x}) \propto 1$, which is improper. To address this issue we assume an upper bound for r and take one further step in our Bayesian horizon. Invoking the maximum entropy principle under the appropriate constraints, we obtain as a hyperprior for $r_{\max}$ a gamma distribution with shape parameter 1 and scale parameter t, such that $E[r_{\max}] = t$. We then marginalize the bounded prior over $r_{\max}$, yielding $p(r|\mathbf{x}) = e^{-r/t}/t$, where t is the average maximum radius of a pulmonary vessel ($\approx$ 15 mm using the radius of the aorta).

Now, a probability distribution on R must satisfy the constraint $R \geq r$ and expert advice [29] indicated that pulmonary vessels tend to be straight, i.e., $R \approx \infty$, suggesting a better representation for the model parameters as $(I_R = 1/R, r)$, with $0 \leq I_R \leq 1/r$. The maximum entropy distribution for I_R is simply the *uniform distribution*, i.e., $p(I_R|r) = r\mathbb{I}_{[0,1/r]}(I_R)$, and therefore $p(R|r) = (r/R^2)\mathbb{I}_{[r,\infty)}(R)$, which combined with $p(r|\mathbf{x})$ yields

$$p(\mathbf{m}_2|\mathscr{M}_2,\mathbf{x}) = (r/(R^2 t))e^{-r/t}\mathbb{I}_{\mathbf{M}_2}(\mathbf{m}_2). \tag{16}$$

Finally, $P(\mathscr{M}_2|\mathbf{x})$ is proportional to the volume of the pulmonary tree ($\approx$ 300 ml [30]).

4.2 Derivation of the Likelihood

We omit the derivation of the likelihood term, $p(\boldsymbol{\kappa}|\mathbf{m}_2,\mathscr{M}_2,\mathbf{x})$ for the vessel model, because it follows exactly the same steps as that of the nodule model. The final result is

$$p(\boldsymbol{\kappa}|\mathbf{m}_2,\mathscr{M}_2,\mathbf{x}) = \frac{2R/(\pi r^2)}{(\kappa_2-\kappa_1)^2\sqrt{(\kappa_2-\kappa_1)^2-(\kappa_1\kappa_2 R)^2}}\mathbb{I}_{\mathscr{K}_2}(\boldsymbol{\kappa}), \tag{17}$$

where $\mathscr{K}_2$ is the set $\mathscr{K}_2 = \left\{\boldsymbol{\kappa} \in \mathbb{R}^2 \middle| 1/r \leq \kappa_2 \text{ and } \frac{\kappa_2}{1-R\kappa_2} \leq \kappa_1 \leq \frac{\kappa_2}{1+R\kappa_2}\right\}$.

4.3 Marginalization over the Model Parameters

The probability density in (17) is infinite on the set $\mathscr{K}_2^\infty = \mathscr{K}_2^{\infty,-} \cup \mathscr{K}_2^{\infty,+}$, where $\mathscr{K}_2^{\infty,-} = \{1/r \le \kappa_2 \text{ and } \kappa_1 = \kappa_2/(1-\kappa_2 R)\}$ and $\mathscr{K}_2^{\infty,+} = \{1/r \le \kappa_2 \text{ and } \kappa_1 = \kappa_2/(1+\kappa_2 R)\}$ and falls sharply as the distance $d(\boldsymbol{\kappa}, \mathscr{K}_2^\infty)$ grows. Observe that the sets $\mathscr{K}_2^{\infty,-}$ and $\mathscr{K}_2^{\infty,+}$ are disjoint, and using (15) they can be identified with the sets $\Psi^- = [\pi/2, 3\pi/2)$ and $\Psi^+ = (-\pi/2, \pi/2]$, with $\Psi = \Psi^- \cup \Psi^+$. Analogous to the case of the simplified nodule model, we have, for a given ρ defining a specific isosurface,

$$\kappa_1^-(\rho) \triangleq E[K_1^1|\rho, \psi \in \Psi^-] = \frac{\int_{\Psi^-} \kappa_1(\psi,\rho) p(\psi|\rho)\, d\psi}{\int_{\Psi^-} p(\psi|\rho)\, d\psi} = h_1^-(\rho) = \frac{-2}{R\pi - 2r\rho}, \tag{18}$$

$$\kappa_1^+(\rho) \triangleq E[K_1^1|\rho, \psi \in \Psi^+] = \frac{\int_{\Psi^+} \kappa_1(\psi,\rho) p(\psi|\rho)\, d\psi}{\int_{\Psi^+} p(\psi|\rho)\, d\psi} = h_1^+(\rho) = \frac{2}{R\pi + 2r\rho}, \tag{19}$$

which approximate κ_1 in Ψ^- and Ψ^+, despite suppressing its dependence on ψ. There is no need to approximate κ_2, since we see from (15) that it is already independent of ψ. From (18), (19) and (15) we obtain

$$\kappa_1^- \approx g_1(\kappa_2, \mathbf{m}_2, \mathscr{M}_2) = \frac{2\kappa_2}{2 - R\pi\kappa_2} \text{ and } w_1 = \int_{\Psi^-} p(\psi)\, d\psi = \frac{1}{2} - \frac{2r}{3\pi R} \tag{20}$$

$$\kappa_1^+ \approx g_2(\kappa_2, \mathbf{m}_2, \mathscr{M}_2) = \frac{2\kappa_2}{2 + R\pi\kappa_2} \text{ and } w_2 = \int_{\Psi^+} p(\psi)\, d\psi = \frac{1}{2} + \frac{2r}{3\pi R}. \tag{21}$$

Proceeding as with the nodule model and again using (15), we have $p(\kappa_2|\kappa_1, \mathbf{m}_2, \mathscr{M}_2, \mathbf{x}) = 2/(\kappa_2^3 r^2)\mathbb{I}_{\kappa_2 \ge 1/r}(\kappa_2)$ and finally

$$p(\boldsymbol{\kappa}|\mathbf{m}_2, \mathscr{M}_2, \mathbf{x}) \approx \left(\left(1 - \frac{4r}{3\pi R}\right) \delta\left(\kappa_1 - \frac{2\kappa_2}{2 - R\pi\kappa_2}\right) + \left(1 + \frac{4r}{3\pi R}\right) \delta\left(\kappa_1 - \frac{2\kappa_2}{2 + R\pi\kappa_2}\right) \right) \frac{1}{\kappa_2^3 r^2} \mathbb{I}_{\kappa_2 \ge 1/r}(\kappa_2). \tag{22}$$

The integral in (1) for the vessel model can now be estimated, using the approximation in (22) and the prior in (16), resulting in

$$p(\boldsymbol{\kappa}|\mathscr{M}_2, \mathbf{x}) \approx \pi \left(\frac{\kappa_1 \left(e^{\frac{-1}{t\kappa_2}} - e^{\frac{2(\kappa_1 - \kappa_2)}{t\pi\kappa_2|\kappa_1|}} \right)}{3(\kappa_2 - \kappa_1)^3} - \frac{\mathrm{Ei}\left(\frac{-1}{t\kappa_2}\right) - \mathrm{Ei}\left(\frac{2(\kappa_1 - \kappa_2)}{t\pi\kappa_2|\kappa_1|}\right)}{2t\kappa_2(\kappa_2 - \kappa_1)^2} \right) \mathbb{I}_{\mathscr{K}_2^*}(\boldsymbol{\kappa}), \tag{23}$$

where $\mathscr{K}_2^* = \{\boldsymbol{\kappa} \in \mathbb{R}^2 \,|\, \kappa_2 \ge 0, -2\kappa_2/(\pi - 2) \le \kappa_1 \le 2\kappa_2/(\pi + 2)\}$ and Ei denotes the exponential integral function.

5 The Vessel Junction and Outlier Models

Junction detection is an interesting problem on its own and the derivation of the junction model is quite involved. Here, we limit ourselves to a superficial discussion of its prior and likelihood terms and refer the reader to [36] for details.

By appropriately "slicing" and "stitching" three tori with parameterizations as in (14) but different values for R, we obtain the object $\mathscr{M}_3$ depicted in Figure 1. Vessel junctions are often described as the most common source of false positives in lung CAD systems aimed at detecting nodules [31,32], and to account for that we fill the gap between the three tori with an ellipsoid. For the joint prior of this structure, we have

$$p(\mathbf{m}_3|\mathscr{M}_3,\mathbf{x}) = \delta(a - c_0^{3/2}/c^{1/2}) \times \frac{\mu^2 c e^{-\mu(c-c_0)}}{1+\mu c_0} \times \frac{e^{-r/t}}{t} \mathbb{I}_{\mathbf{M}_3}(\mathbf{m}_3), \tag{24}$$

where $\mathbf{m}_3 = (a,c,r)$, $c_0 = \alpha r$, $\alpha \approx 0.41$ (an exact form is available), $\mathbf{M}_3 = \{\mathbf{m}_3 \in \mathbb{R}^3 | r \geq 0, 0 \leq a \leq c_0 \leq c\}$, and t is the same as in (16). For the likelihood term we have

$$p(\boldsymbol{\kappa}|\mathbf{m}_3,\mathscr{M}_3,\mathbf{x}) = (1 - \omega_2 - \omega_3)p_1(\boldsymbol{\kappa}|a,c) + \omega_2 p_2(\boldsymbol{\kappa}|r) + \omega_3 p_3(\boldsymbol{\kappa}|r), \tag{25}$$

where p_1 is given by (12), p_2 is given by (22) with $R = r$, p_3 is also given by (22), but with $R = r\sin\beta/(1+\sin\beta)$, $\beta = \arccos(2^{-1/3})$, $\omega_2 \approx 0.25$, and $\omega_3 \approx 0.69$, for which exact but lengthy expressions are available. The result of the marginalization is an enormous expression that can be obtained with the aid of a symbolic computation package.

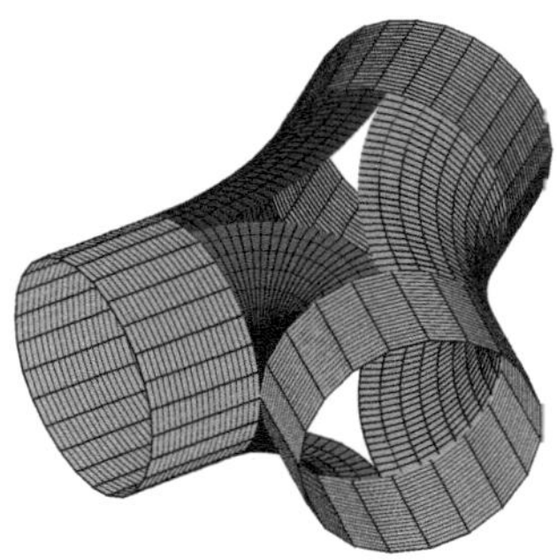

Fig. 1. Three tori with adequate parameters form the junction model. The cylinders are included for clarity.

The outlier model does not comply with the steps provided in Section 2; there is no deterministic shape on which we can base its computation. Instead, we adapt recent results in the theory of Gaussian random fields [33], which directly establish the joint probability distribution of *random isosurfaces* of an initially spatially uncorrelated Gaussian random field after smoothing by an isotropic kernel. For our purpose, we choose this kernel to be Gaussian with zero mean and scale parameter σ_0, and the resulting probability distribution is

$$p(\boldsymbol{\kappa}|\mathscr{M}_4,\mathbf{x}) = \frac{256\sigma_0^3(\kappa_2 - \kappa_1)}{\pi(4 + 3\sigma_0^2\kappa_2^2 - 2\sigma_0^2\kappa_2\kappa_1 + 3\sigma_0^2\kappa_1^2)^3}\mathbb{I}_{[0,\kappa_2]}(\kappa_1). \tag{26}$$

6 Algorithm and Results

An algorithm for lung nodule detection in CT volumes using the models described in sections 3 to 5 was implemented with the Insight Toolkit [37]. The volume image is first smoothed with a Gaussian kernel to reduce the effect of noise in the computation of derivatives. The lung volume is automatically extracted to obtain a region of interest (ROI) for all subsequent operations. Given a voxel $\mathbf{x}$ in the extracted ROI, the principal curvatures $\boldsymbol{\kappa}(\mathbf{x})$ of the implicit isosurface at $\mathbf{x}$ are computed directly from the image intensities [14,12]. Given the curvatures, the probabilities $p(\boldsymbol{\kappa}|\mathbf{m}_i,\mathscr{M}_i,\mathbf{x})$ are computed at each voxel $\mathbf{x}$ for each model $\mathscr{M}_i$. The probability distributions involve parameters such as the expected nodule diameter and the expected maximum vessel radius that

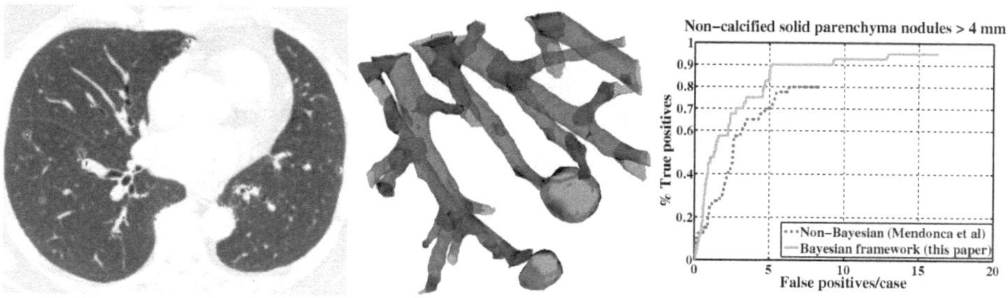

(a) (b) (c)

Fig. 2. (a) A 2D slice of a high-resolution CT scan with nodule labels overlaid in green on the intensity image. (b) A 3D rendering of the voxel labeling for a small region from the same case showing nodules (green), vessels (red), and junctions (blue). (c) FROC curves comparing performance of the Bayesian voxel labeling framework to a curvature-based non-probabilistic approach given in [12].

were set to typical anatomical values. The curvatures at every voxel in a neighborhood $\mathcal{N}$ centered at $\mathbf{x}$ are used to define the set $\mathcal{D}$ and $p(\mathcal{D}|\mathcal{M}_i,\mathbf{x})$ is computed as the product $\prod_{j\in\mathcal{N}} p(\mathcal{D}_j|\mathbf{m}_i,\mathcal{M}_i,\mathbf{x})$. The neighborhood shape is a simple cube with size set to 4 mm, the diameter of the smallest nodule of interest [10]. Finally, multiplying by the model prior probabilities, $P(\mathcal{M}_i|\mathbf{x})$, yields the individual posterior probabilities, $P(\mathcal{M}_i|\mathcal{D},\mathbf{x})$.

The posterior model probabilities can be used to design a utility function over misclassification errors (false negatives and false positives) but this can be quite involved in the case of distinguishing between more than two alternatives or models [38]. Since the target application is nodule detection, we reduce the decision problem to two classes (nodule and non-nodule) by combining all model posteriors other than $P(\mathcal{M}_1|\mathcal{D},\mathbf{x})$ into a single probability and evaluating the Bayes factor [23] for the nodule model as $P(\mathcal{M}_1|\mathcal{D},\mathbf{x})/P(\mathcal{M}_i \neq \mathcal{M}_1|\mathcal{D},\mathbf{x})$. Figure 2(a-b) shows results of the Bayesian voxel labeling using this scheme on a high resolution 0.625 mm slice thickness CT scan of a patient with over 80 nodules due to metastatic lung cancer.

Validation of the algorithm was performed against ground truth provided by three radiologists through FROC analysis. A dataset of 50 low-dose CT scans of asymptomatic high-risk subjects, acquired via a screening protocol (40 mAs, 120 kVp, slice thickness of 1.25 mm), was used to validate the proposed lung nodule detection algorithm. Ground truth was defined as all nodules with diameter greater or equal to 4 mm marked by at least 2 out of 3 radiologists, and included 60 non-calcified solid parenchymal nodules. For performing the FROC analysis, a connected component algorithm was run to group neighboring voxels as a single detection. After applying a diameter threshold of 3 mm to remove small, clinically irrelevant detections, the average Bayes factor over the constituent voxels of each detection was used as the threshold parameter to generate the FROC curve. The algorithm achieved 90% sensitivity at 5.1 false positives per case. In comparison, the algorithm from [12] which uses the ratio κ_1/κ_2 as the decision threshold gave only 70% sensitivity at the same false positive rate. The corresponding FROC curves are shown in Figure 2(c). The Bayesian framework shows better specificity and achieves a much higher overall maximum sensitivity (95%).

7 Conclusions and Future Work

This paper introduces a Bayesian technique for lung nodule detection. The emphasis is on careful development of likelihood and prior probability distribution using geometry, available clinical knowledge, and physical principles. Assumptions made in model construction are directly motivated by the clinical application and always incorporated explicitly into the resulting probability distributions. The prior probabilities are quite general and have applications to any lung CAD algorithm for which the size and shape of nodules and the diameter of vessels are relevant parameters [6,11]. In future work, we plan to extend the Bayesian framework to account for variations in acquisition protocol and include models for other pulmonary lesions such as subsolid nodules, and also to validate the algorithm on larger datasets.

Acknowledgement

This publication was supported by the DOD and the Medical University of South Carolina under DOD Grant no. W81XWH-05-1-0378. Its contents are solely the responsibility of the authors and do not necessarily represent the official views of the DOD or the Medical University of South Carolina.

References

1. Ferlay, J., Bray, F., Pisani, P., Parkin, D.M.: GLOBOCAN 2002: Cancer incidence, mortality and prevalence worldwide. Technical report, IARC CancerBase No. 5. version 2.0, IARC-Press (2004)
2. Fry, W.A., Menck, H.R., Winchester, D.P.: The national database report on lung cancer. Cancer 77, 1947–1955 (1996)
3. Flehinger, B.J., Kimmel, M., Melamed, M.R.: The effect of surgical treatment on survival from early lung cancer: Implications for screening. Chest 101(4), 1013–1018 (1992)
4. Mulshine, J.L.: Clinical issues in the management of early lung cancer. Clin. Cancer Res. 11(13), 4993s–4998s (2005)
5. Torr, P.H.S.: Bayesian model estimation and selection for epipolar geometry and generic manifold fitting. Int. Journal of Computer Vision 50(1), 35–61 (2002)
6. McCulloch, C.C., Kaucic, R.A., Mendonça, P.R.S., Walter, D.J., Avila, R.S.: Model-based detection of lung nodules in computed tomography exams. Academic Radiology 11(3), 258–266 (2004)
7. Dobigeon, N., Tourneret, J.Y., Scargle, J.D.: Joint segmentation of multivariate astronomical time series: Bayesian sampling with a hierarchical model. IEEE Trans Signal Processing 55(2), 414–423 (2007)
8. Sato, Y., Westin, C., Bhalerao, A., Nakajima, S., Shiraga, N., Tamura, S., Kikinis, R.: Tissue classification based on 3D local intensity structures for volume rendering. IEEE Trans. Visualization and Computer Graphics 6(2), 160–180 (2000)
9. Paik, D.S., Beaulieu, C.F., Rubin, G.D., Acar, B., Jeffrey, Jr.,R.B., Yee, J., Dey, J., Napel, S.: Surface normal overlap: A computer-aided detection algorithm with application to colonic polyps and lung nodules in helical CT. IEEE Trans. Med. Imag. 23(6), 661–675 (2004)
10. ELCAP : International early cancer action program — Protocol (2003) `http://icscreen.med.cornell.edu/ielcap.pdf`

11. Farag, A.A., El-Baz, A., Gimel'farb, G.G., El-Ghar, M.A., Eldiasty, T.: Quantitative nodule detection in low dose chest CT scans: New template modeling and evaluation for CAD system design. In: Duncan, J.S., Gerig, G. (eds.) MICCAI 2005. LNCS, vol. 3749, pp. 720–728. Springer, Heidelberg (2005)
12. Mendonça, P.R.S., Bhotika, R., Sirohey, S., Turner, W.D., Miller, J.V., Avila, R.S.: Model-based analysis of local shape for lesion detection in CT scans. In: In: Duncan, J.S., Gerig, G. (eds.) MICCAI 2005. LNCS, vol. 3749, pp. 688–695. Springer, Heidelberg (2005)
13. Yoshida, H., Näppi, J.: Three-dimensional computer-aided diagnosis scheme for detection of colonic polyps. IEEE Trans. Med. Imag. 20(12), 1261–1274 (2001)
14. Vos, F.M., Serlie, I.W.O., van Gelder, R.E., Post, F.H., Truyen, R., Gerritsen, F.A., Stoker, J., Vossepoel, A.M.: A new visualization method for virtual colonoscopy. In: Niessen, W.J., Viergever, M.A. (eds.) MICCAI 2001, LNCS, vol. 2208 pp. 645–654. Springer, Heidelberg (2001)
15. Efron, B.: Bayesians, frequentists, and scientists. J. Amer. Stat. Assoc. 100(469), 1–5 (2005)
16. Jeffreys, H.: An invariant form for the prior probability in estimation problems. In: Proc. Royal Soc. London A 186(1007), pp. 453–461(1946)
17. Kass, R.E., Wasserman, L.: The selection of prior distributions by formal rules. J. Amer. Stat. Assoc. 91(435), 1343–1370 (1996)
18. Jaynes, E.T.: Probability Theory: The Logic of Science. Cambridge University Press, New York (2003)
19. Martin, J., Pentland, A., Sclaroff, S., Kikinis, R.: Characterization of neuropathological shape deformations. PAMI 20(2), 970–1112 (1998)
20. Ow, W., Golland, P.: From spatial regularization to anatomical priors in fMRI analysis. In: Christensen, G.E., Sonka, M. (eds.) IPMI 2005. LNCS, vol. 3565, pp. 88–100. Springer, Heidelberg (2005)
21. Gerig, G., Styner, M., Shenton, M.E., Lieberman, J.A.: Shape versus size: Improved understanding of the morphology of brain structures. In: Niessen, W.J., Viergever, M.A. (eds.) MICCAI 2001. LNCS, vol. 2208, pp. 24–32. Springer, Heidelberg (2001)
22. Krahnstoever, N.: Personal communication. http://vision.cse.psu.edu/krahnsto/index.html
23. Kass, R.T., Raftery, A.E.: Bayes factors. J. Amer. Stat. Assoc. 90(430), 773–795 (1995)
24. do Carmo, M.P.: Differential Geometry of Curves and Surfaces. Prentice-Hall, Englewood Cliffs (1976)
25. Swensen, S.J., Jett, J.R., Hartman, T.E., Midthun, D.E., Sloan, J.A., Sykes, A.M., Aughenbaugh, G.L., Clemens, M.A.: Lung cancer screening with CT: Mayo clinic experience. Radiology 226(3), 756–761 (2003)
26. Murray, C.D.: The physiological principle of minimum work. I. The vascular system and the cost of blood flow. Proc. Natl. Acad. Sci. 12(3), 207–214 (1926)
27. Bennett, S.H., Eldridge, M.W., Puente, C.E., Riedi, R.H., Nelson, T.R., Beotzman, B.W., Milstein, J.M., Singhal, S.S., Horsfield, K., Woldenberg, M.J.: Origin of fractal branching complexity in the lung. Preprint (2000)
28. Karau, K.L., Krenz, G.S., Dawson, C.A.: Branching exponent heterogeneity and wall shear stress distribution in vascular trees. Am. J. Physiol. — Heart Circ. Physiol. 280(3), 1256–1263 (2001)
29. Piacsek, K.L.: Personal communication (XX)
30. Singhal, S., Henderson, R., Horsfield, K., Harding, K., Cumming, G.: Morphometry of the human pulmonary arterial tree. Circ. Res. 33(2), 190–197 (1973)
31. van Ginneken, B., ter Haar Romeny, B.M., Viegever, M.A.: Computer-aided diagnosis in chest radiography: A survey. IEEE Trans. Med. Imag. 20(12), 1228–1241 (2001)

32. Rubin, G.D., Lyo, J.K., Paik, D.S., Sherbondy, A.J., Chow, L.C., Leung, A.N., Mindelzun, R., Schraedley-Desmond, P.K., Zinck, S.E., Naidich, D.P., Napel, S.: Pulmonary nodules on multi-detector row CT scans: Performance comparison of radiologists and computer-aided detection. Radiology 234(1), 274–283 (2005)
33. Mendonca, P.R.S., Bhotika, R., Miller, J.V.: Probability distribution of curvatures of isosurfaces in gaussian random fields. arXiv:math-ph/0702031v2 (February 2007) http:// www.citebase.org/abstract?id=oai:arXiv.org:math-ph/0702031
34. Sluimer, I., Schilham, A., Prokop, M., van Ginneken, B.: Computer analysis of computed tomography scans of the lung: A survey. IEEE Trans. Med. Imag. **25**(4), 385–405 (2006)
35. Bernardo, J.M., Smith, A.F.M.: Bayesian Theory. Wiley (2004)
36. Zhao, F., Mendonça, P.R.S., Bhotika, R., Miller, J.V.: Model-based junction detection with applications to lung nodule detection. In: ISBI. (April 2007)
37. Ibáñez, L., Schroeder, W., Ng, L., Cates, J.: The ITK Software Guide. Second edn. (Nov 2005) http://www.itk.org/ItkSoftwareGuide.pdf
38. He, X., Metz, C.E., Tsui, B.M.W., Links, J.M., Frey, E.C.: Three-class ROC analysis — A decision theoretic approach under the ideal observer framework. IEEE Trans. Med. Imag. 25(5), 571–581 (2006)

Functional Interactivity in fMRI Using Multiple Seeds' Correlation Analyses – Novel Methods and Comparisons

Yongmei Michelle Wang[1,2,3] and Jing Xia[1]

Departments of Statistics[1], Psychology[2], Bioengineering[3]
University of Illinois at Urbana-Champaign, Champaign, IL 61820, USA
ymw@uiuc.edu

Abstract. This paper presents novel statistical methods for estimating brain networks from fMRI data. Functional interactions are detected by simultaneously examining multi-seed correlations via multiple correlation coefficients. Spatially structured noise in fMRI is also taken into account during the identification of functional interconnection networks through non-central F hypothesis tests. Furthermore, partial multiple correlations are introduced and formulated to measure any additional task-induced but not stimulus-locked relation over brain regions so that we can take the analysis of functional connectivity closer to the characterization of direct functional interactions of the brain. Evaluation for accuracy and advantages of the new approaches and comparison with the existing single-seed method were performed extensively using both simulated data and real fMRI data.

Keywords: Functional connectivity, fMRI, partial correlation, multiple correlation, spatial noise modeling, time series analysis, hypothesis testing.

1 Introduction

Recent advances in functional magnetic resonance imaging (fMRI) provide an unparalleled opportunity for measuring and characterizing brain function in humans. A thorough understanding of the neural mechanisms not only requires the accurate delineation of activation regions but demands precise description of function in terms of the information flow across networks of areas. Various approaches have been proposed to extract information of interaction from fMRI datasets, most of which rely on either functional or effective connectivity [7]. In this work, we present novel statistical methods for robust estimation of functional connectivity or interactivity. In addition, we provide comprehensive comparisons of our proposed multi-seed based methods using multiple and partial correlation analyses of fMRI data with the existing single-seed based method using marginal correlation.

For functional connectivity study, a common approach is to calculate the temporal correlation coefficients of a signal from a selected voxel or region (so called "seed", or "seed region") in a region of interest with all other voxels in the brain. Each correlation map is resulting from the cross-correlation of only one seed region. However, when areas with quite different time series patterns are used as seed regions for brain connectivity inference, they should not be grouped as a single region; in

N. Karssemeijer and B. Lelieveldt (Eds.): IPMI 2007, LNCS 4584, pp. 147–159, 2007.
© Springer-Verlag Berlin Heidelberg 2007

some applications, functional co-activation to multiple seeds rather than a single one would be of particular interest. Multiple seeds can be chosen to calculate multiple correlation maps to separately discover the functional connectivity to different seeds. But how to reasonably integrate multiple connectivity maps for brain function inference is still unresolved and ambiguous. Furthermore, it is often forbidding to examine all pair-wise correlations. Thus, it is desirable to have a single correlation map resulting from the cross-correlation of multiple seed regions simultaneously.

Dynamic connections in fMRI are thought to be reflected by high temporal correlations of the time series. The strong correlation between the time series of each region in the network with that of another distant region implied by the functional interactions may be related to the spatially structured noise in fMRI. The spatial correlations of the noise must therefore be taken into account when dealing with the robust inference of the network. Recently, an approach for large-scale network identification in fMRI was proposed in [2] by considering the noise structure in the data. However, this method is again entirely restricted to connectivity detection between pair-wise (one to one) brain areas through regular Pearson's correlation (i.e. marginal correlation) analysis and can not handle multiple regions simultaneously.

Brain functional connectivity based on marginal correlation can be dominated by the stimulus-locked responses. For example, if visual and auditory stimuli are presented concurrently, the stimulus-locked neural responses would cause increases in the BOLD signal in the primary auditory cortex (A1) and the primary visual cortex (V1) simultaneously. Correlation between A1 and V1 would thus be high, though not due to any intrinsic task-induced functional couplings but due to the responses in both regions to externally driven stimuli. Partial correlation is the conditional correlation which estimates any remaining correlation between time series after taking into account the relationship of each to one or more reference time series. This allows us to measure any additional task-induced, but not stimulus-locked relation over brain regions. Recently, methods using partial correlation (or coherence) have been proposed [9, 8], though they are for pair-wise correlation / coherence analysis and not applicable to multiple seeds. In addition, the partial correlation in [8] is for subtracting and removing mutual dependencies on common influences from other brain areas rather than from stimulus-locked responses. How to mathematically compute and estimate the partial correlation to multiple seed regions and how to apply this to brain connectivity are challenging and have not yet been pursued in the literature.

The aim of the present paper is to develop new statistical methods to estimate brain networks based on multiple correlations and partial multiple correlations of fMRI data. To the best of our knowledge, this work shows for the first time an innovative and successful application of multiple and partial multiple correlation analyses to study brain connectivity caused by multiple seed regions.

2 Methods and Formulations

In this section, we present our methods and our mathematical formulations for functional connectivity inference based on multiple seeds using multiple correlations (section 2.2) and partial multiple correlations (section 2.3).

2.1 Determining Multiple Homogeneous Seed Regions

We select multiple seed regions based on their respective homogeneity as well as their known involvement in the functional or behavioral task and our interest in characterizing their interactions with other regions of the brain. The homogeneity is achieved with a region growing algorithm, which can start from a peak activation voxel during categorical comparisons, and grows by merging with other neighboring voxels based on a similarity criterion, such as the Pearson's linear correlation between the time series of the peak voxel and the candidate voxel considered to be merged. In this way, we can find the regions of interest, i.e. seed regions, $S_1, S_2, \cdots S_P$, where P is the total number of regions. For subsequent statistical analysis, the *mean time series* of any seed region is utilized as the time series of that seed, and the centroid of any seed region is considered to be the position of that seed.

2.2 Method 1 – Functional Connectivity Using Multiple Correlations

2.2.1 Estimating Temporal/Sample Multiple Correlations

The temporal or sample multiple correlation coefficient considers the fMRI time series correlation between a given voxel X and a combination of seed regions, $S_1, S_2, \cdots S_P$. Its estimation is based on the variance-covariance matrix:

$$\hat{\boldsymbol{\Sigma}}_{tem} = \begin{bmatrix} \hat{\text{var}}_X & \hat{\text{cov}}_{X,S_1} & \cdots & \hat{\text{cov}}_{X,S_P} \\ \hat{\text{cov}}_{S_1,X} & \hat{\text{var}}_{S_1} & \cdots & \hat{\text{cov}}_{S_1,S_P} \\ \vdots & \vdots & \vdots & \vdots \\ \hat{\text{cov}}_{S_P,X} & \hat{\text{cov}}_{S_P,S_1} & \cdots & \hat{\text{var}}_{S_P} \end{bmatrix} = \begin{bmatrix} \hat{\text{var}}_X & \hat{\textbf{cov}}_{XS}' \\ \hat{\textbf{cov}}_{XS} & \hat{\boldsymbol{\Sigma}}_{SS} \end{bmatrix},$$

where var_X and var_{S_p} are the time series variances for voxel X and seed s_p ($p = 1,2,\cdots P$), respectively; and cov_{X,s_p} is their covariance. Their estimation can be achieved through time series samples of size T. The temporal multiple correlation coefficient $\hat{R}_{tem}$ between voxel X and the multiple seeds $[S_1, S_2, \cdots S_P]'$ can be calculated as [1]:

$$\hat{R}_{tem} = \sqrt{\frac{\hat{\textbf{cov}}_{XS}' \cdot \hat{\boldsymbol{\Sigma}}_{SS}^{-1} \cdot \hat{\textbf{cov}}_{XS}}{\hat{\text{var}}_X}}.$$

2.2.2 Estimating Spatial Multiple Correlations in Noise

Main factors contributing to the spatial correlation of the noise include fMRI data preprocessing, partial volume effect, non-white measurement noise, and motion-related artifacts. Despite the strategies and efforts to reduce such structured noise [10, 11], some residual and further corrections are still essential for robust fMRI data analysis.

2.2.2.1 Voxel-Based Spatial Correlograph of Noise. We assume the spatial noise is stationary and has a multivariate Gaussian distribution with variance-covariance matrix $\Sigma = (\sigma_{i,j})_{i,j=1}^{M}$, where M is the total number of voxels; σ_i and σ_j are positive standard deviations for voxels X_i and X_j. The spatial correlations in noise then depend only on the spatial distance between voxels: $\sigma_{ij} = \sigma_i \sigma_j \rho(\| i - j \|)$, where $\| i - j \|$ denotes the spatial distance or lag between X_i and X_j; and ρ is the spatial correlogram, a real-valued function that satisfies $\rho(0) = 1$ and is bounded by -1 and 1. Such a spatial model is valid if and only if the resulting variance-covariance matrix $\mathbf{\Sigma}$ is positive-definite [5].

Since it is unknown what voxels or regions are predominantly influenced by the noise, the entire set $D_h = \{(X_i, X_j) \mid \|i - j\| = h\}$ of pairs of voxels at lag h over the whole brain area is considered for the non-parametric estimate based on the median: $\hat{\rho}(h) = median\{r_{ij}, (X_i, X_j) \in D_h\}$, where r_{ij} is the Pearson's linear correlation between the time series of the two voxels. As in general the empirical estimator $\hat{\rho}$ of the correlogram does not provide a positive-definite correlation matrix, we focus on a parametric class of valid matrices, based on the empirical values $\hat{\rho}$ estimated from the fMRI data. The rational-quadratic model $\rho_\theta(h)$ in [5, 2] is utilized for such purpose with $\rho_\theta(0) = 1$ (θ is the involved parameter). The derived spatial correlogram of noise, $\rho_\theta(h)$, decreases rapidly from a correlation level between nearby voxels, ρ_{0+}, towards an asymptotic correlation, ρ_∞. A critical distance h_∞ can be determined beyond which the correlogram is almost equal to the asymptote.

2.2.2.2 Spatial Multiple Correlations in Noise. The spatial multiple correlations of the noise consider the correlations between any voxel X and a combination of multiple seeds $S_1, S_2, \cdots S_P$. Suppose the distances between the voxel X and the seeds $S_1, S_2, \cdots S_P$ are respectively $h_1, h_2, \cdots h_P$, and the distances between any pair-wise seeds are h_{ij} (for S_i and S_j, $h_{ij} = h_{ji}$). The noise spatial correlation matrix for $[X, S_1, S_2, \cdots S_P]'$ can then be constructed as:

$$\mathbf{\Lambda}_{spa} = \begin{bmatrix} 1 & \rho_\theta(h_1) & \cdots & \rho_\theta(h_P) \\ \rho_\theta(h_1) & 1 & & \rho_\theta(h_{1P}) \\ \vdots & \vdots & \ddots & \vdots \\ \rho_\theta(h_P) & \rho_\theta(h_{P1}) & \cdots & 1 \end{bmatrix} = \begin{bmatrix} 1 & \boldsymbol{\rho}_S' \\ \boldsymbol{\rho}_S & \mathbf{\Lambda}_{SS} \end{bmatrix}$$

where $\rho_\theta(h)$ is the correlogram estimated above. Let σ_X^2 and $\sigma_{S_p}^2$ respectively denote the noise variance for voxel *X*, and seed S_p $p = 1, 2, \cdots P$ (see Appendix for their estimation). Then the corresponding variance-covariance matrix is:

$$\mathbf{\Sigma}_{spa} = \begin{bmatrix} \sigma_X^2 & \rho_\theta(h_1) \cdot \sigma_X \cdot \sigma_{S_1} & \cdots & \rho_\theta(h_P) \cdot \sigma_X \cdot \sigma_{S_P} \\ \rho_\theta(h_1) \cdot \sigma_{S_1} \cdot \sigma_X & \sigma_{S_1}^2 & \cdots & \rho_\theta(h_{1P}) \cdot \sigma_{S_1} \cdot \sigma_{S_P} \\ \vdots & \vdots & \ddots & \vdots \\ \rho_\theta(h_P) \cdot \sigma_{S_P} \cdot \sigma_X & \rho_\theta(h_{P1}) \cdot \sigma_{S_P} \cdot \sigma_{S_1} & \cdots & \sigma_{S_P}^2 \end{bmatrix} = \begin{bmatrix} \sigma_X^2 & \boldsymbol{\sigma}_{XS}' \\ \boldsymbol{\sigma}_{XS} & \mathbf{\Sigma}_{SS} \end{bmatrix}$$

The spatial multiple correlation coefficient of the noise between any voxel X and the seeds $[S_1, S_2, \cdots S_P]'$ is estimated as: $R_{spa} = \sqrt{\frac{\boldsymbol{\sigma}_{XS}' \cdot \boldsymbol{\Sigma}_{SS}^{-1} \cdot \boldsymbol{\sigma}_{XS}}{\sigma_X^2}}$, and can be simplified to:

$$R_{spa} = \sqrt{\boldsymbol{\rho}_S' \cdot \boldsymbol{\Lambda}_{SS}^{-1} \cdot \boldsymbol{\rho}_S} \tag{1}$$

2.2.3 Identifying Functional Connectivity of the Brain

We would like to test whether the temporal multiple correlation $\hat{R}_{tem}$ is likely to be found only by chance from the noise correlation. Under the null hypothesis that the temporal multiple correlation, $\hat{R}_{tem}$, arises from a population whose multiple correlation equals the spatial multiple correlation of the noise, R_{spa}, the following quantity is a non-central F [1, pp. 153-154]:

$$F = \frac{\hat{R}_{tem}^2}{1 - \hat{R}_{tem}^2} \cdot \frac{T - 1 - P}{P} \tag{2}$$

Here, the degrees of freedom are P and $T - 1 - P$, and the noncentrality parameter is $\frac{(T-1)\boldsymbol{\sigma}_{XS}' \boldsymbol{\Sigma}_{SS}^{-1} \hat{\boldsymbol{\Sigma}}_{SS} \boldsymbol{\Sigma}_{SS}^{-1} \boldsymbol{\sigma}_{XS}}{(1 - R_{spa}^2)\sigma_X^2}$, where we condition on the seeds' time series. In the present work, due to the simplified R_{spa} in Eq. (1), the noncentrality parameter can be shown to be: $\frac{(T-1)\boldsymbol{\rho}_S' \boldsymbol{\Lambda}_{SS}^{-1} \boldsymbol{\Psi} \hat{\boldsymbol{\Sigma}}_{SS} \boldsymbol{\Psi} \boldsymbol{\Lambda}_{SS}^{-1} \boldsymbol{\rho}_S}{1 - \boldsymbol{\rho}_S' \cdot \boldsymbol{\Lambda}_{SS}^{-1} \cdot \boldsymbol{\rho}_S}$, where $\boldsymbol{\Psi}$ is a $P \times P$ diagonal matrix with diagonal element $1/\sigma_{S_p}$, for $p = 1, 2, \ldots, P$. In this way, the p-value for each voxel can be calculated from this noncentral F distribution. A voxel shall be included in the functional connectivity network if the corresponding p-value is smaller than a pre-chosen type I error α (note: $\alpha = 0.05$ is used in this paper).

It can also be shown that under the null hypothesis of the population multiple correlation, R_{spa}, is zero, the F in Eq. (2) [1, pp. 149-150] is a central F, with P and $T - 1 - P$ degrees of freedom. In fact, this is equivalent to multiple correlation analysis of multi-seed functional connectivity but without taking the spatial correlations of the noise into consideration.

A departure from the temporally i.i.d. (independent and identically distributed) assumption due to the temporal autocorrelation will result in an increase in the degrees of freedom in the above hypothesis testing. To correct such possible bias, we estimate the effective degrees of freedom T_{eff}. This can be achieved through the context of the general linear model [12]. We then use the estimated T_{eff} to replace the T-1 in the F statistic's calculation in Eq. (2).

Furthermore, we have to perform numerous tests equal to the total number of voxels over the brain area. In order to correct this multiple testing problem, we apply a Bonferroni correction for simplicity. Other more advanced techniques can also be employed for this purpose.

2.3 Method 2 – Functional Interactivity Using Partial Multiple Correlations

2.3.1 Estimating Temporal Partial Multiple Correlations

The temporal partial multiple correlation coefficient considers the fMRI time series correlation between a given voxel X and a combination of seed regions $S_1, S_2, \cdots S_P$ conditioned on fixed stimuli (experimental paradigms or reference functions) $V_1, V_2, \cdots V_N$. Its estimation is based on the matrix:

$$\begin{bmatrix} \hat{\text{var}}_X & \hat{\text{cov}}_{X,S_1} & \cdots & \hat{\text{cov}}_{X,S_P} & \hat{\text{cov}}_{X,V_1} & \cdots & \hat{\text{cov}}_{X,V_N} \\ \hat{\text{cov}}_{S_1,X} & \hat{\text{var}}_{S_1} & & \hat{\text{cov}}_{S_1,S_P} & \hat{\text{cov}}_{S_1,V_1} & \cdots & \hat{\text{cov}}_{S_1,V_N} \\ \vdots & \vdots & \vdots & \vdots & \vdots & \vdots & \vdots \\ \hat{\text{cov}}_{S_P,X} & \hat{\text{cov}}_{S_P,S_1} & \cdots & \hat{\text{var}}_{S_P} & \hat{\text{cov}}_{S_P,V_1} & \cdots & \hat{\text{cov}}_{S_P,V_N} \\ \hat{\text{cov}}_{V_1,X} & \hat{\text{cov}}_{V_1,S_1} & \cdots & \hat{\text{cov}}_{V_1,S_P} & \text{var}_{V_1} & \cdots & \text{cov}_{V_1,V_N} \\ \vdots & \vdots & \vdots & \vdots & \vdots & \vdots & \vdots \\ \hat{\text{cov}}_{V_N,X} & \hat{\text{cov}}_{V_N,S_1} & \cdots & \hat{\text{cov}}_{V_N,S_P} & \text{cov}_{V_N,V_1} & \cdots & \text{var}_{V_N} \end{bmatrix} = \begin{bmatrix} \hat{\text{var}}_X & \hat{\mathbf{cov}}_{XS}' & \hat{\mathbf{cov}}_{XV}' \\ \hat{\mathbf{cov}}_{XS} & \hat{\boldsymbol{\Sigma}}_{SS} & \hat{\boldsymbol{\Sigma}}_{SV} \\ \hat{\mathbf{cov}}_{XV} & \hat{\boldsymbol{\Sigma}}_{SV}' & \boldsymbol{\Sigma}_{VV} \end{bmatrix}$$

$$= \begin{bmatrix} \hat{\boldsymbol{\Sigma}}_{\{XS\}\{XS\}} & \hat{\boldsymbol{\Sigma}}_{\{XS\}V}' \\ \hat{\boldsymbol{\Sigma}}_{\{XS\}V} & \boldsymbol{\Sigma}_{VV} \end{bmatrix},$$

where var_{V_n} is the time series variances of the stimulus V_n $(n = 1, 2, \cdots N)$; cov_{X,V_n} is the covariance between voxel X and V_n, and cov_{S_p,V_n} is the covariance between the seed S_p and V_n. Their estimation can be achieved through time series and reference function samples of size T, though they are not technically variances and covariances because the V_n are fixed stimuli. With the assumption that the conditional distribution $(X, S_1, \cdots, S_P | V_1 = v_1, V_2 = v_2, \cdots V_N = v_N)'$ is a multi-normal distribution [1], its variance-covariance matrix can be calculated as: $\hat{\boldsymbol{\Sigma}}^*_{tem} = \hat{\boldsymbol{\Sigma}}_{\{XS\}\{XS\}} - \hat{\boldsymbol{\Sigma}}_{\{XS\}V}' \cdot \boldsymbol{\Sigma}_{VV}^{-1} \cdot \hat{\boldsymbol{\Sigma}}_{\{XS\}V}$. Let the components of $\hat{\boldsymbol{\Sigma}}^*_{tem}$ be divided into four groups, $\begin{bmatrix} \hat{\text{var}}^*_X & \hat{\mathbf{cov}}^{*\prime}_{XS} \\ \hat{\mathbf{cov}}^*_{XS} & \hat{\boldsymbol{\Sigma}}^*_{SS} \end{bmatrix}$, where $\hat{\text{var}}^*_X$ and $\hat{\boldsymbol{\Sigma}}^*_{SS}$ are variances of voxel X and the seeds holding the reference functions (stimuli) fixed, $\hat{\mathbf{cov}}^*_{XS}$ is their corresponding covariance under the same condition. Based on section 2.2.1, the temporal partial multiple correlation is thus: $\hat{R}_{tem \cdot \mathbf{V}} = \sqrt{\frac{\hat{\mathbf{cov}}^{*\prime}_{XS} \cdot \hat{\boldsymbol{\Sigma}}^{*-1}_{SS} \cdot \hat{\mathbf{cov}}^*_{XS}}{\hat{\text{var}}^*_X}}$

2.3.2 Estimating Spatial Partial Multiple Correlations in Noise

In section 2.2.2.1, we estimate the voxel-based spatial correlograph of noise using the median of Pearson's linear correlation, i.e. marginal correlation. Here, we take the similar approach but replace the marginal correlation with partial correlation because the stimuli are now considered to be fixed, i.e., $\hat{\rho}^*(h) = median\{r_{ij\cdot V}, (X_i, X_j) \in D_h\}$, where $r_{ij\cdot V}$ is the partial correlation coefficient between voxels X_i and X_j holding $V_1, V_2, \cdots V_N$ fixed, and its calculation is as below. Let the variance-covariance matrix of $(X_i, X_j, V_1, \cdots, V_N)'$ be $\begin{bmatrix} \hat{\Sigma}_{XX} & \hat{\Sigma}_{XV} \\ \hat{\Sigma}_{XV} & \Sigma_{VV} \end{bmatrix}'$. $(X_i, X_j | V_1 = v_1, V_2 = v_2, \cdots V_N = v_N)'$ is assumed to be multi-normal and its variance-covariance matrix is calculated as: $\hat{\Sigma}_{X\cdot V} = \hat{\Sigma}_{XX} - \hat{\Sigma}_{XV}' \cdot \Sigma_{VV}^{-1} \cdot \hat{\Sigma}_{VX} = \begin{bmatrix} \hat{\sigma}_{i\cdot V}^2 & \hat{\sigma}_{ij\cdot V}' \\ \hat{\sigma}_{ij\cdot V} & \hat{\sigma}_{j\cdot V}^2 \end{bmatrix}$. The partial correlation coefficient is thus given by $r_{ij\cdot V} = \frac{\sigma_{ij\cdot V}}{\sigma_{i\cdot V} \cdot \sigma_{j\cdot V}}$ [1]. The corresponding parametric correlogram $\rho_\theta^*(h)$ based on $r_{ij\cdot V}$ can then be estimated as in section 2.2.2.1.

The noise spatial partial correlation matrix for $[X, S_1, S_2, \cdots S_P]'$ holding $V_1, V_2, \cdots V_N$ fixed can be constructed as:

$$\Lambda_{spa}^* = \begin{bmatrix} 1 & \rho_\theta^*(h_1) & \cdots & \rho_\theta^*(h_P) \\ \rho_\theta^*(h_1) & 1 & & \rho_\theta^*(h_{1P}) \\ \vdots & \vdots & \ddots & \vdots \\ \rho_\theta^*(h_P) & \rho_\theta^*(h_{P1}) & \cdots & 1 \end{bmatrix} = \begin{bmatrix} \mathbf{1} & \boldsymbol{\rho}_S^{*\prime} \\ \boldsymbol{\rho}_S^* & \boldsymbol{\Lambda}_{SS}^* \end{bmatrix}$$

where $\rho_\theta^*(h)$ is the correlogram estimated above. Let $\sigma_{S_p}^*$ denote the residual standard deviation of the noise for seed S_p, $p = 1, 2, \cdots P$, holding $V_1, V_2, \cdots V_N$ fixed (see Appendix for its estimation). As in section 2.2.2.2, the spatial partial multiple correlation coefficient of the noise between any voxel X and the seeds $[S_1, S_2, \cdots S_P]'$ holding the stimuli fixed is estimated as: $R_{spa\cdot V} = \sqrt{\boldsymbol{\rho}_S^{*\prime} \cdot \boldsymbol{\Lambda}_{SS}^{*\,-1} \cdot \boldsymbol{\rho}_S^*}$.

2.3.3 Identifying Conditional Functional Connectivity of the Brain

We would like to test whether the temporal partial multiple correlation $\hat{R}_{tem\cdot V}$ is likely to be found only by change from the noise correlation. The hypothesis is $H_0 : R_{tem.V} = R_{spa\cdot V}$ vs $H_1 : R_{tem.V} > R_{spa\cdot V}$. Here, we can show that $\frac{\hat{R}_{tem.V}^2}{1 - \hat{R}_{tem.V}^2} \cdot \frac{(T-1) - N - P}{P}$ is a non-central F, with the degrees of freedom P and $T - 1 - N - P$, and the noncentrality parameter $\frac{(T-1)\boldsymbol{\rho}_S^{*\prime} \boldsymbol{\Lambda}_{SS}^{*-1\prime} \boldsymbol{\Psi}^{*\prime} \hat{\boldsymbol{\Sigma}}_{SS}^{*} \boldsymbol{\Psi}^* \boldsymbol{\Lambda}_{SS}^{*-1} \boldsymbol{\rho}_S^*}{1 - \boldsymbol{\rho}_S^{*\prime} \boldsymbol{\Lambda}_{SS}^{*-1} \boldsymbol{\rho}_S^*}$, where we condition on the seeds' time series; ψ^* is a $P \times P$ diagonal matrix with diagonal element $1/\sigma_{S_p}^*$, for $p = 1, 2, \cdots P$. Note that the effective degrees of freedom and the multiple testing problem mentioned in section 2.2.3 shall also be applied here.

3 Experiments and Results

3.1 Simulated Data

The simulated time series were composed of time- and space-correlated noise on a base 3D brain image with size 64x64x20. The space correlation was based on a rational-quadratic parameter model, with $\rho_{0+}=0.4$, $\rho_{\infty}=0.001$, and $h_{\infty}=20$ mm. The spatial Gaussian noise was generated using a Cholesky decomposition of the space correlation matrix [5, pp. 201-203]. The time series (T=128) have added to them ARMA(1,1) temporal noise, resulting in separable space-time correlation structure. In addition, some randomly selected regions were further summed with different types of signal time series (boxcar functions convolved with the hemodynamic response function as defined by the SPM software package; signal amplitude: 3%~5%) to simulate functional networks with multiple seed regions. We generated the data at four different noise levels.

3.1.1 Validation of Our Multi-seed Method Using Multiple Correlations

In this experiment, two types of networks were simulated, highly correlated with the two types of seed regions respectively. We used receiver operating characteristic (ROC) analysis for evaluation. The essence of ROC analysis is the comparison of true positive rates (TPR, proportion of voxels correctly detected as significant to all voxels with added connectivity) obtained with different analysis techniques for a given false positive rate (FPR, proportion of voxels incorrectly detected as significant to all voxels without added connectivity). The ROC curves in Fig. 1 indicate that our multiple correlation method can robustly detect the true multi-seed connectivity when the signal-to-noise ratio (SNR) is greater than or equal to -1.5dB, though the performance increases for increased SNR.

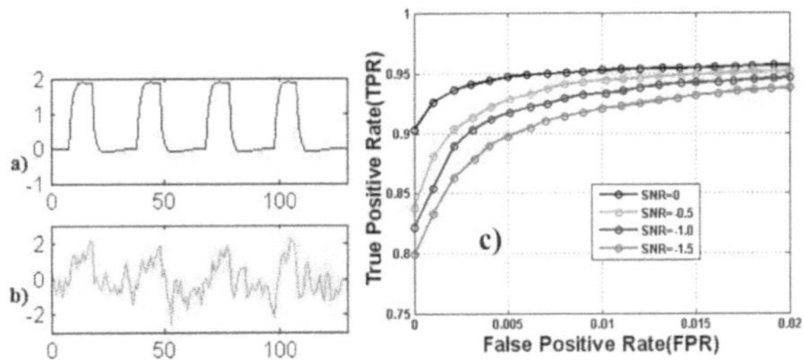

Fig. 1. (a): Ground truth of a simulated seed; **(b):** Normalized time series of an associated connectivity voxel at SNR = -0.5dB. Note SNR is defined as: $SNR(dB) = 10\log_{10}\left(Var_{signal} / Var_{noise} \right)$. **(c):** ROC curves at SNR (in dB) = 0.0, -0.5, -1.0, -1.5 (top to bottom).

3.1.2 Comparison of Our Multi-seed Method and the Single-seed Method

In Fig. 2, three types of networks were simulated, with the green region highly correlated to seed 1, the blue region highly correlated to seed 2, and the brown having medium (relatively low) correlation to both of the two seed regions. Fig. 2 shows that the identified connectivity (at $\alpha = 0.05$, corrected) by our multi-seed method and by the single seed method (spatial correlations in noise also considered using the technique in [2]): i) With our multi-seed method using multiple correlations, all three types of connectivity are detected, both the highly correlated ones to the seeds (green and blue) and the medium correlated one (brown). ii) Using any one seed alone, only the corresponding one type of highly correlated connectivity is detected in each case; in addition, compared to our multi-seed method, the significance level is lower, and there are more false negatives and false positives; the correlation over the brown region is not high enough in either of the cases to be shown as significant when using any single seed alone.

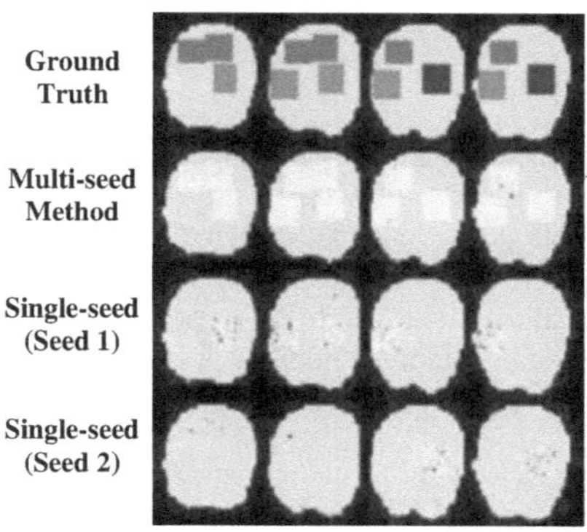

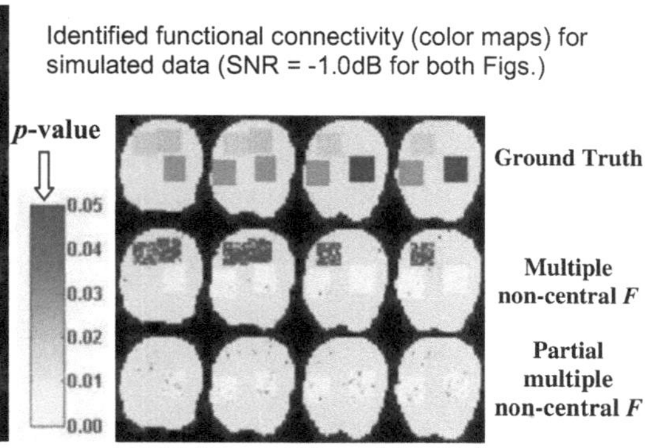

Fig. 2. Comparison of our muti-seed method (multiple correlation) and the sindle-seed method(with spatial noise considered, too).

Fig. 3. comparison of our multi-seed methods using multiple and partial multiple correlations

3.1.3 Comparison of Our Methods: Multiple vs. Partial Multiple Correlations

We also generated simulated data with four different types of connectivity (see Fig. 3): light green and light blue denote the stimulus-locked activation regions to the type 1 and type 2 seeds respectively; dark green and dark blue denote the stimulus-locked activation plus the task-induced functional coupling to the type 1 and type 2 seeds respectively. With the multiple correlations, all four types of regions are shown as significant, though at different significance levels. However, using partial multiple correlations, only the regions imbedding task-induced functional coupling (dark green and dark blue) are identified as significant because the partial correlation analysis is able to adjust for the stimulus-locked effects.

3.2 Real fMRI Data

The real fMRI dataset (53x63x46x360) was obtained from the SPM data site (*http://www.fil.ion.ucl.ac.uk/~wpenny/datasets/attention.html*) with a visual motion task (see [4] for the detailed description). The subject was scanned during four runs, with 90 image volumes in each run. Four conditions – 'fixation', 'attention', 'no attention', and 'stationary' – were used, and there were 10 multi-slice volumes per condition. The structural model for the dorsal visual pathway is shown in Fig. 4. Here we examine the functional interactions by using the different seed regions: V1, or V5 or both V1 and V5, and by using different methods. The seed regions were defined through categorical comparisons using a t-test and their anatomical coordinates listed in [4], followed by a region growing strategy described in Section 2.1.

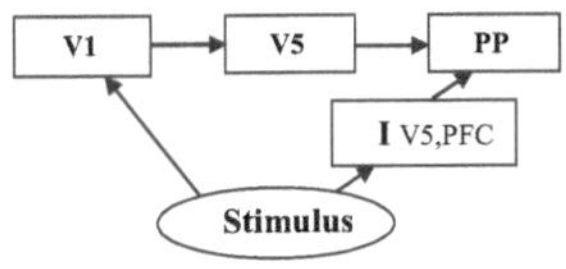

Fig. 4. Structural model for the dorsal visual stream (modified from [4]), including primary visual cortex (V1), V5, posterior parietal cortex (PP), and modulatory interaction term involving dorsolateral prefrontal cortex (PFC)

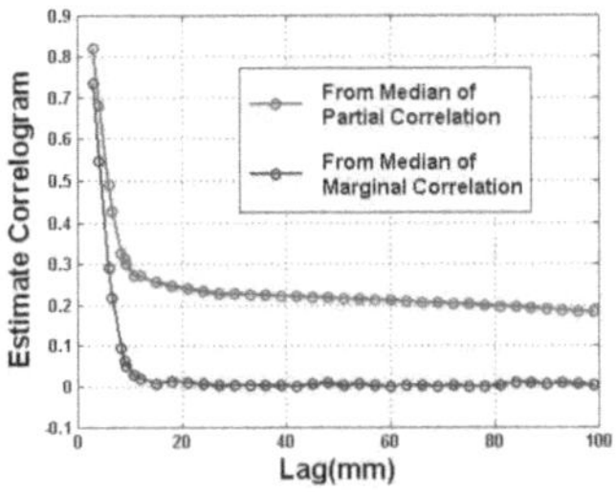

Fig. 5. Estimated correlograms from the real fMRI data, showing the asymptotic correlation, ρ_∞, in $\rho_\theta(h)$ (marginal correlation) is lower than the one in $\rho^*_\theta(h)$ (partial correlation). This might be closely related to the "default mode" network of the human brain investigated in [6].

3.2.1 Partial Correlation Effects – Multiple vs. Partial Multiple Correlations

From Fig. 6 (a) and (b), we can see that using multiple correlation (2nd row), both stimulus-locked and task-induced networks are identified, with all the involved regions in Fig. 4 shown as highly significant (yellow). However, using partial

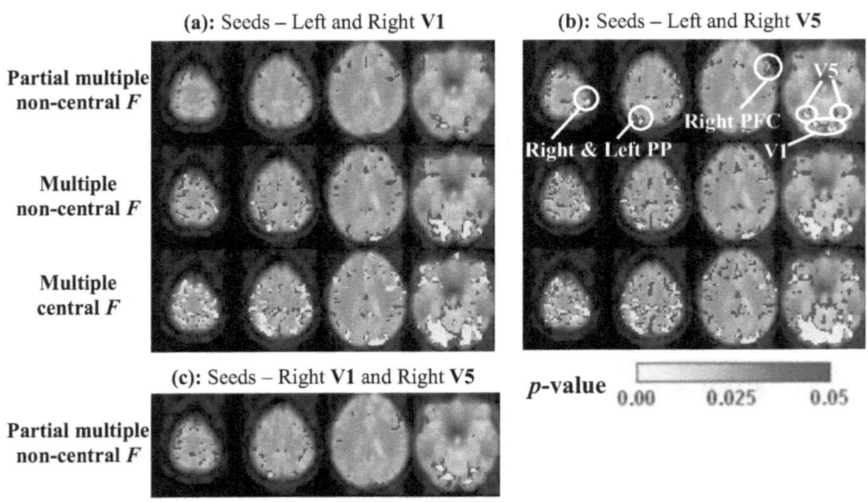

Fig. 6. Comparison of functional interaction maps for the real fMRI data

multiple correlation (1st row), since the stimulus-locked effects are accounted for, the network regions and their sizes are considerably reduced. Specifically: i) with V1 as seed regions (Fig. 6(a), 1st row), mainly the low level visual network is identified as highly significant implying task-induced coupling among the visual areas, such as V1 to V5; ii) withV5 as seed regions (Fig. 6(b), 1st row), the two PP and the right PFC regions are still shown as highly significant, suggesting the involved task-induced coupling of attention to motion modulation described in Fig. 4, after taking account of the stimulus-locked effects.

3.2.2 Effects of Multiple Seeds - Comparison Using Both V1 and V5 as Seeds

The partial multiple correlation results using V1 or V5 (Fig. 6 (a) and (b), 1st row) as seed regions have been illustrated in the above section. With a combination of a V1 and a V5 as seed regions (Fig. 6(c)), using partial multiple correlation, we can not only detect the highly significant low level visual network regions (as in Fig. 6(a) and (b), 1st row, last slice), but also identify the highly significant attention to motion modulation PP areas (as in Fig. 6(b), 1st row; also compare to Fig. 6(a), 1st row), achieving the combined effects of multiple seed regions involving both V1 and V5. Note that since only one V5 is used here, the region sizes and significance levels for the PP and right PFC are not as large as the ones using both V5 regions in Fig. 6(b) (1st row).

3.2.3 Effects of Spatial Noise - Comparison of Non-central and Central *F*-Tests

The results without taking the spatial noise correlations into consideration (central *F*-test) are shown in Fig. 6 (a) and (b), 3rd row, with many unjustified areas identified as functionally correlated with the V1 and/or V5 seed regions due to the spatial structured noise in the fMRI data.

4 Conclusions

This paper presents novel statistical methods for robust inference of brain connectivity from fMRI based on multiple and partial multiple correlation analyses and multiple seed regions. The networks of functional interconnections are found by comparing the temporal multiple (and/or partial multiple) correlations against a model of the spatial multiple (and/or partial multiple) correlations in the noise. Compared with the existing single-seed method, using multiple seeds can not only lead to more robust inference of functional connectivity, but also more sensitive identification of functional co-activation networks or regions to multiple seeds that may not be detected in the single-seed method. The use of the partial multiple correlation has the interesting features of providing a convenient summary of conditional independences and hence of being more closely related to the direct functional interactions (i.e. effective connectivity) of the brain than marginal correlation. Experimental results from both simulated and real fMRI data demonstrate that the proposed approaches allow detecting and differentiating in robust and sensitive way functional networks in the working brain caused by stimulus-locked and/or task-induced responses.

Acknowledgments

We would like to thank Dr. John Marden for the valuable discussion and for proofreading of this paper.

References

1. Anderson, T.W.: An Introduction to Multivariate Statistical Analysis, 3rd edn. John Wiley and Sons Inc., New Jersey (2003)
2. Bellec, P., et al.: Identification of large-scale networks in the brain using fMRI. NeuroImage 29, 1231–1243 (2006)
3. Brockwell, P.J., Davis, R.A.: Introduction to Time Series and Forcesting. Springer, New York (2002)
4. Buchel, C., Friston, K.J.: Modulation of connectivity in visual pathways by attention: Cortical inferences evaluated with structural equation modeling and fMRI. Cerebral Cortex 7, 768–778 (1997)
5. Cressie, N.: Statistics for Spatial Data. John Wiley and Sons, New York (1993)
6. Greicius, M.D., Krasnow, B., Reiss, A.L., Menon, V.: Functional connectivity in the esting brain: A network analysis of the default mode hypothesis. PNAS 100, pp. 253–258 (2003)
7. Horwitz, B.: The elusive concept of brain connectivity. Neuroimage 19, 466–470 (2003)
8. Marrelec, G., et al.: Partial correlation for functional brain interactivity investigation in functional MRI. Neuroimage 32, 228–237 (2006)
9. Sun, F.T., Miller, L.M., D'Esposito, M.: Measuring interregional functional connectivity using coherence and partial coherence analyses of fMRI data. Neuroimage 21, 647–658 (2004)
10. Wang, Y.M., Schultz, R.T., Constable, R.T., Staib, L.H.: Nonlinear estimation and modeling of fMRI data using spatio-temporal support vector regression. In: Taylor, C.J., Noble, J.A. (eds.) IPMI 2003. LNCS, vol. 2732, pp. 647–659. Springer, Heidelberg (2003)
11. Wang, Y.M.: Modeling and nonlinear analysis in fMRI via statistical learning. In: Advanced Image Processing in Magnetic Resonance Imaging, pp. 565–586 (2005)
12. Worsley, K.J., Friston, K.J.: Analysis of fMRI time-series revisited – again. Neuroimage 2, 173–181 (1995)

Appendix – Estimation of Noise Variance

Let σ^2 denote the noise variance for each individual voxel in the fMRI data. It can be estimated with an ARMA(1,1) model. First, we use the general linear model to take away the part related to neural activity. The residual noise error is assumed to be the ARMA(1,1) process, generated from a temporally i.i.d. $N(0,\sigma^2)$. $\hat{\sigma}^2$ can then be estimated as in [3] through a parametric fitting, which is the estimated noise variance at each individual voxel.

Let σ_S^2 denote the noise variance for a seed region S (i.e., the noise variance for the mean time series of this seed region). Suppose there are w voxels in S, and the voxels within this region are correlated rather than independent. In order to estimate σ_S^2 , we first calculate the $w \times w$ variance-covariance matrix, *A*. The diagonal elements in *A* are σ_i^2 $(i = 1,2, \cdots w)$, the variance of the noise at voxel *i* estimated above; and the off diagonal elements in *A* are $\rho_\theta(d_{ij}) \cdot \sigma_i \cdot \sigma_j$ $(i, j = 1,2,\ldots, w)$, where $\rho_\theta(d_{ij})$ is the correlogram estimated in section 2.2.2.1 for lag d_{ij}, the spatial distance between voxel *i* and *j*. Let the entries in matrix *A* be a_{ij}. We then have: $\sigma_S^2 = \frac{\sum_{i=1}^{w}\sum_{j=1}^{w} a_{ij}}{w^2}$, which is used as the noise variance of the seed region *S*, needed in the *F* statistic's calculation in section 2.2.3 (multiple correlation case). If we replace the $\rho_\theta(d_{ij})$ with $\rho_\theta^*(d_{ij})$ (see section 2.3.2) in matrix *A*, using the same procedure, we can estimate σ_S^*, the residual standard deviation of the noise for seed region *S* holding the stimuli fixed, which is needed in the *F* statistic's calculation in section 2.3.3 (partial correlation case).

Learning Best Features and Deformation Statistics for Hierarchical Registration of MR Brain Images

Guorong Wu[1,2], Feihu Qi[1], and Dinggang Shen[2,*]

[1] Department of Computer Science and Engineering
Shanghai Jiao Tong University, Shanghai, China 200240
{grwu, fhqi}@sjtu.edu.cn

[2] Section of Biomedical Image Analysis, Department of Radiology
University of Pennsylvania, Philadelphia, PA 19104
dinggang.shen@uphs.upenn.edu

Abstract. A fully learning-based framework has been presented for deformable registration of MR brain images. In this framework, the entire brain is first adaptively partitioned into a number of brain regions, and then the best features are learned for each of these brain regions. In order to obtain overall better performance for both of these two steps, they are integrated into a single framework and solved together by iteratively performing region partition and learning the best features for each partitioned region. In particular, the learned best features for each brain region are required to be identical, and maximally salient as well as consistent over all individual brains, thus facilitating the correspondence detection between individual brains during the registration procedure. Moreover, the importance of each brain point in registration is evaluated according to the distinctiveness and consistency of its respective best features, therefore the salient points with distinctive and consistent features can be hierarchically selected to steer the registration process and reduce the risk of being trapped in local minima. Finally, the statistics of inter-brain deformations, represented by multi-level B-Splines, is also hierarchically captured for effectively constraining the brain deformations estimated during the registration procedure. By using this proposed learning-based registration framework, more accurate and robust registration results can be achieved according to experiments on both real and simulated data.

1 Introduction

Deformable registration for medical images is very important for many clinical applications. So far, many registration algorithms [1-4], based on image intensities or features, have been developed. Generally, the same type of features is used for all points in the entire images, and each point is equally treated during the whole registration procedure. For regularizing the deformations estimated between two images under registration, simple smoothness constraints such as Laplacian smoothness term are typically employed. As indicated next, many previous methods are limited at several aspects.

* Corresponding author.

N. Karssemeijer and B. Lelieveldt (Eds.): IPMI 2007, LNCS 4584, pp. 160–171, 2007.
© Springer-Verlag Berlin Heidelberg 2007

First, the same type of image features is not always effective in distinguishing different parts of images. For example, in registering MR brain images of different subjects, the cortical regions might need very different types of features to distinguish themselves, compared to the uniform white matter regions. Also, the distinctiveness of features is highly related to the size of neighborhood used for the calculation of features. As clearly demonstrated in [5, 6], the best-scale Geometric Moment Invariants (GMIs) show better performances in brain image registration, compared to GMIs of the identical scale used in the HAMMER algorithm [4]. Therefore, it is important to investigate the best scales as well as the best types of features for different brain regions, in order to best differentiate each brain region during the registration procedure.

Second, equally treating each point during the registration procedure might eventually undermine the registration performance. Actually, some brain regions, such as roots of sulci and crowns of gyri, are more reliable to be distinguished, compared to other regions. Therefore, it is important to develop methods for differentiating those reliable regions and hierarchically using them to steer the brain image registration.

Third, simple constraints on the smoothness of voxel-wise deformation fields might be not effective for registration. Actually, the statistics of deformations among different brain images can be captured from a set of training samples, by performing PCA on each band of wavelet coefficients (wavelet-PCA) of deformations [7] or performing PCA on the parameters of control points of B-Splines [8]. It has been shown that, by using this statistical constraint on deformation fields, the performance of registration algorithm can be greatly improved [7, 9]. It is worth noting that B-splines can efficiently represent the deformation fields, while wavelet-PCA can effectively capture both global and local statistical information of deformations. Therefore, it is important to integrate the advantages of both methods [7, 8], for efficiently and effectively capturing the deformation statistics.

Accordingly, a learning-based registration framework for MR brain images is presented in this paper. To overcome the first limitation, a systematic approach is proposed to adaptively learn the best scale and the best types of image features for each brain region. This is achieved by requiring the learned best features consistent across the correspondences of individual brains, while distinctive from those of neighboring points. The former actually requires the consistency of learned best features, while the latter requires the saliency of learned best features. Both consistency and saliency measures can be integrated and used as an important guide for selecting the reliable points to primarily drive the image registration especially during the initial registration stages, thus overcoming the second limitation of treating different points equally in the registration. Moreover, to integrate the advantages of both methods [7, 8] mentioned above, multi-level B-splines [10] with adaptively placed control points are employed to efficiently represent the deformation fields in multiple levels, and thus different levels of deformation statistics (i.e., both global and local) can be captured by performing separate PCAs on each level of control points.

Compared to the method presented in [11], the steps of learning best features and deformation statistics have been significantly improved. In particular, the partition of brain region and the selection of best features are integrated into a single framework in this paper, since these two steps intimately depend on each other. This formulation potentially overcomes the limitation by *ad hoc* brain region partition method used in [11]. Moreover, multi-level B-Splines, instead of single-level B-Splines, are used to represent the deformation fields, thereby facilitating the adaptive placement of control points and capturing the deformation statistics from coarse to fine levels.

Promising results have been obtained on both real and simulated data. For real data, good registration results have been achieved in warping subject brains to the template space. On the other side, our method out-performs HAMMER in the aspect of registration consistency when independently warping longitudinal data. For simulated data, the average deformation error is decreased from 0.92 mm by HAMMER to 0.72 mm by the proposed method.

2 Method

2.1 Learning the Best Features

In this subsection, we will first demonstrate the importance of using best feature in point matching. Then, we present a systematical approach of adaptively learning the best scales and best types of features for different brain regions, by iteratively repeating the steps of brain region partition and best features determination, according to some heuristic criteria.

Importance of Learning Best Features: For each point v in an image I, different local image descriptors can be used to calculate local features from its local spherical neighborhoods with different scales. Without loss of generality, three typical image descriptors, i.e., RIFT [12], SPIN [12], and local spatial histograms [13], are employed. RIFT, standing for *Rotation Invariant Feature Transform*, is a generalization of famous SIFT descriptor [14], and it can be efficiently calculated without the determination of dominant orientation of the local patch. SPIN is another rotation invariant descriptor, which can capture the distribution of image intensities along the radial direction of the point v. Local spatial histograms capture the overall intensity distributions within neighborhoods of different scales, thus preserving spatial information simultaneously [13].

In order to obtain the compact feature representation on each point, the statistical features, i.e., mean and variance, are collected for each of these three local image descriptors. Therefore, totally six features, i.e., two for each local image descriptor, are obtained. Since scale is highly related to the distinctiveness of features, each local image descriptor is calculated from spherical neighborhoods of four scales, i.e., 4, 8, 12, and 16mm, around the point v. Thus, totally M=6×4=24 features, i.e., $G(v)=\{g_k(v)|k=1...M\}$, are obtained for each point v, and can be used as attributes for this point. Notice that $G(v)$ includes six types of features at four different scales.

It is worth noting that no single type of features can be used as a universal signature to reliably distinguish all brain regions, as demonstrated by Fig. 1. For example, by using RIFT, SPIN, and local-histogram features calculated in a scale of 8mm, the similarities between the red-crossed points in Fig. 1(a) and all points in Fig. 1(b) can be calculated, as color-coded and shown in Figs. 1(c)-(e), respectively. Dark red denotes high similarity, while deep blue denotes low similarity. It can be observed that the corresponding points can not be distinguished. On the contrary, by using the best features that will be selected by the method described next, we can successfully distinguish correspondences, as shown in Fig. 1(f). This example demonstrates the importance of learning the best features for each brain region, in order to maximally distinguish all brain regions simultaneously.

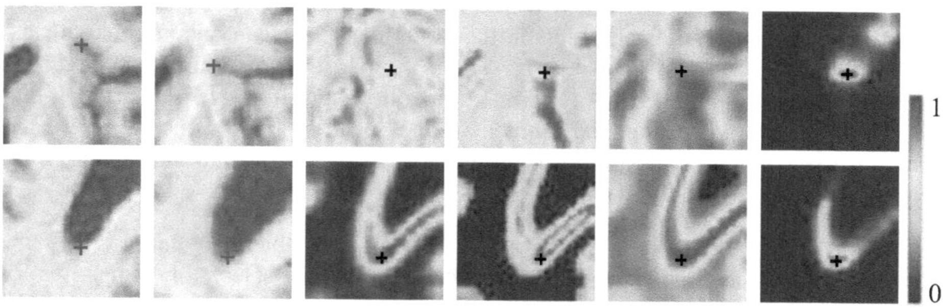

(a) Model (b) Subject (c) By RIFT (d) By SPIN (e) By Histo . (f) By Best Features

Fig. 1. The similarities between each red-crossed point in (a) and all points in (b), measured by RIFT, SPIN, local histograms, and our best features, respectively. The color-coded similarity maps in (c)-(f) indicate the importance of using best features for image registration.

Method: To learn the best features for different brain regions, the step of adaptive brain region partition and the step of best features determination should be completed simultaneously. This is because the partition of brain regions depends on the best features selected for each brain location, while the determination of best features also depends on the partition of brain regions since each brain region is reasonable to have the same set of best features. In particular, we iteratively perform (1) the partition of brain regions based on the tentatively estimated best features, and (2) the selection of best features for each tentatively partitioned brain region, until the algorithm converges.

It is worth noting that, the statistics of the selected best features for each brain point can also be estimated from all training samples. This information can be used to statistically measure the similarity between the best features of two points under comparison during the registration procedure, thus helping look for correct correspondences.

***Partition of Brain Regions*:** Brain partition is achieved by adaptively grouping the neighboring points with the similar image features into various regions. Notice that the similarity between image features of neighboring points highly depends on the particular features used, which will be determined by a learning step detailed in the next. For convenience, a weighting vector $\omega(v)=(\omega_1(v), \ldots,\omega_k(v), \ldots,\omega_M(v))$ is designed for each point v, to represent whether a particular feature $g_k(v)$ is selected (if $\omega_k(v)=1$) or not (if $\omega_k(v)=0$). After brain partition, all points in the same brain region should have the same weighting vector, since they are required to have the same set of best features.

To achieve brain partition, we can first calculate for each point v the difference of tentatively selected best features between this point and the points in its neighborhood $N(v)$. The difference degree $s(v)$ can be defined as follows:

$$s(v) = \sum_{all\ samples} \left(\sum_{u \in N(v)} \sum_{k=1}^{M} \omega_k(v)(g_k(v) - g_k(u))^2 \right) \quad (1)$$

Notice that $s(v)$ will be small if features are similar in the neighborhood, while large if features are very different in the neighborhood. By calculating the feature difference measure $s(v)$ for all points in the brain image, we can obtain a map of feature difference measures, $\{s(v) \mid v \in I\}$. Then, the partition of brain regions can be straightforwardly completed by a region competition algorithm [15], or a graph cutting algorithm [16], or watershed segmentation algorithm [17]. In this paper, we use watershed segmentation algorithm to partition the entire brain into various brain regions, i.e., $\{R_i\}$.

Selection of Best Features: As mentioned, it is required that all points in the same brain region, R_i, have the same set of best features. But the selected best features for each brain region R_i should make all points in this region as distinctive as possible, for facilitating the feature-based image registration. The distinctiveness can be measured by both saliency and consistency of features on each point v in R_i. The saliency evaluates whether the selected best features on this point v are different from those on nearby points. The consistency evaluates whether the selected best features on this point are statistically similar across its corresponding points of individual subjects.

For convenience, the saliency and the consistency can be first measured for each feature $g_k(v)$ on each point v. Jenson-Shannon (*JS*) divergence and entropy (*E*) can be used to formulate the saliency $Sal(g_k(v))$ and the consistency $Con(g_k(v))$ of each feature $g_k(v)$, respectively:

$$Sal(g_k(v)) = JS\left(H(g_k; N_1(v)), H(g_k; N_2(v))\right), \qquad Con(g_k(v)) = -E\left(H(g_k; N_1(v))\right) \quad (2)$$

where N_1 denotes a small neighborhood around the point v and N_2 denotes the ring neighborhood outside of N_1. $H(g_k; N(v))$ denotes for the histogram of feature g_k in the neighborhood $N(v)$, calculated from all samples with different weights that will be iteratively updated in each round of *adaboosting* as described next.

Then, the saliency and the consistency of all features on each point v can be obtained as follows:

$$Sal(G(v)) = \sum_{k=1}^{M} \omega_k(v) \cdot Sal(g_k(v)), \qquad Con(G(v)) = \sum_{k=1}^{M} \omega_k(v) \cdot Con(g_k(v)) \quad (3)$$

where ω_k represents whether feature g_k is currently selected.

Thus, the overall saliency and consistency measurement of a brain region, R_i, can be obtained by integrating all saliency and consistency measures over all points in the region, as given next:

$$E(R_i) = \sum_{v \in R_i} \left(\sum_{k=1}^{M} \omega_k(v) \cdot (Sal(g_k(v)) + \lambda \cdot Con(g_k(v))) \right) \quad (4)$$

where λ is a parameter used to balance between saliency and consistency measurements, and it is set to 1.0 in our study. $E(R_i)$ is a function of weights $\{\omega_k\}$. By finding a suitable set of weights $\{\omega_k\}$ for all points in the region, we can minimizing $E(R_i)$ with the result of obtaining the best features for this region.

To more effectively optimizing $E(R_i)$, we might also need to treat different point samples within neighborhoods $N_1(v)$ and $N_2(v)$ adaptively. *First*, given the current weight for each point sample, we can conveniently calculate the integrated saliency and consistency measurement for each feature according to the definition of $E(R_i)$. This measurement can be used to rank all features, thus allowing us to select the top ranked features as best features. *Second*, by considering the points in $N_1(v)$ as positive samples and points in $N_2(v)$ as negative samples for the point v, we classify both positive and negative samples by using each of the best features currently selected. The *adaboosting* strategy can be used to update the weights for these samples, i.e., weights on correctly classified samples will be decreased while weights on wrongly classified samples will be increased. By repeating the above two steps until convergence, we can finally select a set of best features, i.e., selecting the top ranked features in each round of adaboosting. In our study, four best features are selected for each brain region.

Results: In order to evaluate the selected best features by our method, Fig. 2 shows the detailed distributions of various features selected in a cross-sectional brain image. Fig. 2(b) provides the average scales used by the selected best features for the template in Fig. 2(a). As expected, small scales are used for boundary areas, while large scales are used for uniform regions. The right panel of Fig. 3 shows the selection result for a rectangular region in Fig. 2(a), with red color designating the selection of particular feature at particular position. It can be observed that RIFT features, which are based on edge orientation, are often selected for the points around the boundaries. Local histogram based features, often calculated from large scales, are selected for the points in the uniform regions. Overall, these results indicate that our learning-based method can well utilize the characteristics of each type of features.

2.2 Learning Active Points

Two main measurements are considered, when selecting the reliable and salient points, called as active points, to hierarchically steer the image registration. The first measurement is the saliency of a point v, i.e., $Sal(G(v))$, which is defined in Eq. (3). The large saliency value means that the point v can be easily distinguished from its nearby points, thus reducing the ambiguity in image matching. The second measurement is the consistency of the best features of the point v across different individuals, i.e., $Con(G(v))$, which is also defined in Eq. (3). The large consistency measurement means that it is relatively easy to find the correspondence of point v in the other brain images. By combining these two measurements into a single measurement, i.e., $A(v)=Con(G(v))+\lambda\cdot Sal(G(v))$, we can rank all brain points according to their overall measurements, $\{A(v)\}$.

Fig. 3 demonstrates the hierarchical selection of active points during image registration. In the initial stage of registration, only the most reliable and salient points are selected, as shown in Fig. 3(a). It can be observed that most active points locate at roots of sulci, crowns of gyri, and boundaries of ventricles, all of which can be distinguished reliably from others. With the progress of registration, more and more points are selected as active points and gradually added into the registration process, as shown by green and yellow in Figs. 3(b) and 3(c). By hierarchically focusing these active points during the registration procedure, the registration performance can be greatly improved, as demonstrated latter by our experimental results.

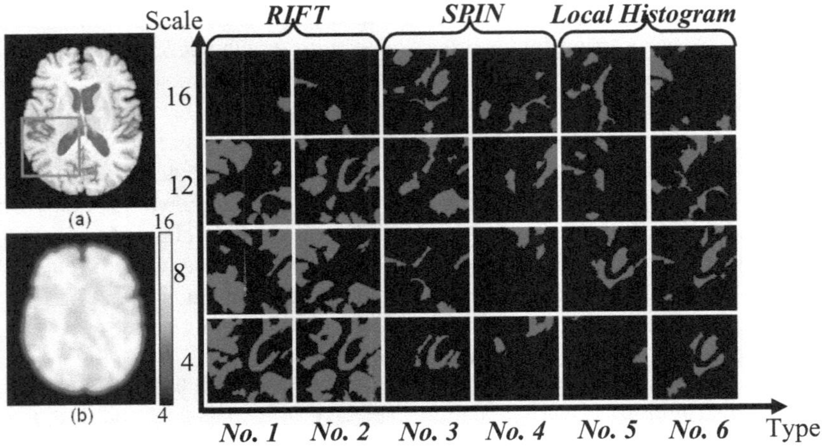

Fig. 2. The selected best features for the template brain in (a). The average scale used to calculate the best features is displayed in (b). To visually appreciate the actual features finally selected for each point in the pink block of (a), the selection results on all 24 features, from 4 scales and 6 features of 3 types, are displayed in the right panel.

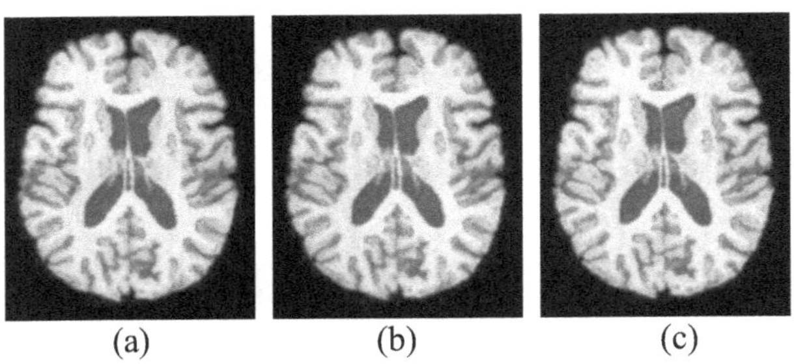

Fig. 3. Hierarchical selection of active points for a template brain. Initial active points are shown in red (a) and gradually added ones are shown in green (b) and yellow (c), respectively.

2.3 Learning Deformation Statistics

We propose to build up the statistical model on deformation parameters to regularize the deformation fields estimated during the registration procedure. There are three major properties with this model. *First*, multi-level B-Splines are used to represent the deformation fields from coarse to fine levels, thus potentially overcoming the limitation of using single-level B-Splines, i.e., high dimensionality. *Second*, at each level, the control points are adaptively placed according to both deformation approximation degree and overall saliency & consistency measurement around the control points. *Third*, the statistical model is built up at each level, for capturing the statistics of deformations at each particular level, thus facilitating both efficient and effective representation of deformation fields. All of these three properties are explained in detail below.

Multi-Level Representation: Let $\Omega=\{(x,y,z)|0\le x<X, 0\le y<Y, 0\le z<Z\}$ be the domain of deformation fields in the *xyz* coordinate system, and $\Phi(\delta)=\{\varphi_{i,j,k}|0\le i<N_x,\ 0\le j<N_y,\ 0\le k<N_z\}$ be the mesh of control points with uniform spacing δ overlaid on Ω. The deformation $d(x,y,z)$ of each point (x,y,z) in Ω can be represented as $d_\delta(x,y,z)$ by a set of cubic B-spline functions B:

$$d_\delta(x,y,z)=\sum_{l=0}^{3}\sum_{m=0}^{3}\sum_{n=0}^{3}B_l(u)B_m(v)B_n(w)\varphi_{i+l,j+m,k+n},\quad \varphi_{i+l,j+m,k+n}\in\Phi(\delta) \tag{5}$$

where $i=[x/\delta]$-1, $j=[y/\delta]$-1, $k=[z/\delta]$-1, $u=x/\delta$-$[x/\delta]$, $v=y/\delta$-$[y/\delta]$, and $w=z/\delta$-$[z/\delta]$. $[x/\delta]$ returns the maximum integer less than x/δ, and B_r, B_s, B_t are uniform cubic B-spline basis functions as defined next:

$$B_0(u)=(1-u)^3/6,\quad B_1(u)=(3u^3-6u^2+4)/6,\quad B_2(u)=(-3u^3+3u^2+3u+1)/6,\quad B_3(u)=u^3/6 \tag{6}$$

The parameters on $\varphi_{i,j,k}$ can be estimated from all known deformations $\{d(x,y,z)\}$ of the points $\{(x,y,z)\}$ within the neighborhood $P_{i,j,k}(\delta)$:

$$P_{i,j,k}(\delta)=\{(x,y,z)|(i\text{-}2)\cdot\delta\le x<(i+2)\cdot\delta,\ (j\text{-}2)\cdot\delta\le y<(j+2)\cdot\delta,\ (k\text{-}2)\cdot\delta\le z<(k+2)\cdot\delta\}$$

In order to represent deformation field $d(x,y,z)$ from coarse to fine levels, multi-level B-Splines are used. Using a mesh of control points with large uniform spacing, i.e., δ_0, the deformation field $d(x,y,z)$ can be represented as $d_{\delta 0}(x,y,z)$, with the residual deformation field as $e(x,y,z)=d(x,y,z)\text{-}d_{\delta 0}(x,y,z)$. The residual deformation field $e(x,y,z)$ can be represented by a mesh of control points with small uniform spacing, i.e., $\delta_0/2$, resulting in a representation of $e(x,y,z)$ as $f_{\delta 0/2}(x,y,z)$ and a new residual as $e(x,y,z)=e(x,y,z)\text{-}f_{\delta 0/2}(x,y,z)$. Notice that $f_{\delta 0/2}(x,y,z)$ can be estimated from $e(x,y,z)$ similarly according Eq. (5). By repeatedly halving the spacing, i.e., δ_0/h (with h=4,8,…), we can obtain various new representation $f_{\delta 0/h}(x,y,z)$ for new residuals. Accordingly, the deformation field $d(x,y,z)$ can be represented as:

$$d(x,y,z)\approx d_{\delta_0}(x,y,z)+\sum_{h=2,4,\ldots}f_{\delta_0/h}(x,y,z) \tag{7}$$

In our case, total four levels of B-Splines with spacing $\{\delta=\delta_0/h \mid h=1,2,4,8\}$ are used. Notice that, in the application stage, the parameters on $\varphi_{i,j,k}$ of each level will be estimated from the given deformations on the active points, which actually provides a new way of statistically interpolating the entire deformation fields by multi-level B-Splines, using the deformations available only on a small number of active points.

Adaptive Placement of Control Points: The control points of B-Splines can be adaptively placed at each level according to two criteria described next, by taking the advantage of multi-level representations. *First*, if the residual error around a particular control point is below a certain threshold, it is not necessary to split the current cube into smaller cubes in the next levels. *Second*, if the overall measurement of image saliency and consistency around a particular control point is higher than a certain value, it is worth splitting the current cube into smaller cubes, considering the saliency and importance of images in the current cube. By applying these two criteria, about 50% of control points can be discarded in the coarsest level, with most of them as background points. Also, nearly 85% of the control points are not necessarily kept in the finest level, since deformations on those locations have been well represented by the previous levels. Accordingly, the dimensionality of our statistical model can be significantly reduced. Fig. 4 shows the adaptive lattices at three levels (a)~(c), using the spacing of control points 16mm, 8mm, and 4mm, respectively. Fig. 4(d) shows the overlay of all control points from three different levels, indicating dense control points in the complex areas and sparse control points in the uniform regions.

Statistical Regularization: Due to significant dimensionality reduction at each level, it is feasible to use a PCA to learn the statistics of $\Phi(\delta)$ at each level, based on a relatively small number of training samples. The learned statistics can be used to reasonably constrain the deformation fields estimated during the image registration procedure. In particular, the regularization of tentatively estimated deformation fields can be achieved as follows:

- The parameter of each $\varphi_{i,j,k}$ on $\Phi(\delta)$ at current level is computed from the residual error within neighborhood $P_{i,j,k}$.
- The statistical model of this level is applied to statistically constraining the parameters on $\Phi(\delta)$.
- Update residual error, and repeat the above two steps until the total number of levels is reached.

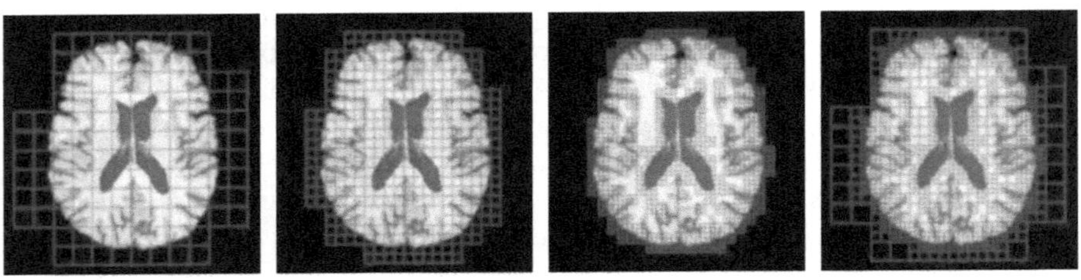

(a) spacing: 16mm (b) spacing: 8mm (c) spacing: 4mm (d) all levels overlaid

Fig. 4. Adaptively placed control points at three different levels, with the spacing of 16mm, 8mm, and 4mm, respectively. The overlay of all control points from all levels, as shown in (d), indicates the control points are dense in the complex areas and sparse in the uniform regions.

2.4 Summary of Our Learning-Based Registration Framework

Our registration framework includes two parts, i.e., training stage and application stage. In the training stage, the best features are learned from a pool of features by *adaboosting*, and active points are hierarchically selected according to the overall saliency and consistency measures. The multi-level statistical models are learned from the deformation fields represented by multi-level B-Splines.

In the application stage, the most salient points are initially selected as active points to drive the registration. The deformations on other brain points are statistically interpolated by the multi-level B-Splines with learned parameters. With the progress of registration, other less salient points are gradually added and used as active points to start driving the registration. In the procedure of point matching, the learned best features are used to achieve better correspondence detection. In the end of each iterative registration, the tentatively estimated deformation fields are represented by multi-level B-splines, and the parameters of control points at each level are statistically constrained by their respective statistical models learned at that level.

3 Experiments

Our learning-based registration method has been extensively evaluated on both real and simulated data, and its performances are also compared with those of the HAMMER algorithm. It's worth noting that our learning-based registration method is developed for achieving similar performance as HAMMER's, but avoiding tissue segmentation as required before the HAMMER registration algorithm. For real data, our learning-based registration method obtained the similar accuracy of registration as HAMMER's, but it is more robust in registering the longitudinal data as demonstrated next. For simulated data, our learning-based registration method produced 0.72 mm registration error, which is less than 0.92 mm produced by HAMMER.

For all experiments described next, total 18 MR brain images are used to learn both the best features and the active points, while 100 deformation fields from [18] are used to learn the deformation statistics. It's worth noting that all results reported in the next are obtained from the testing samples, which are not included in the training set.

3.1 Experiments on Real Data

In the first experiment, both our learning-based registration method and HAMMER are tested on a number of real brain images obtained from our datasets. According to visual inspection, most registration results by these two methods are very similar. However, in some special cases, as shown in Fig. 5, our learning-based registration method produces better results than HAMMER, i.e., circled regions in Fig. 5.

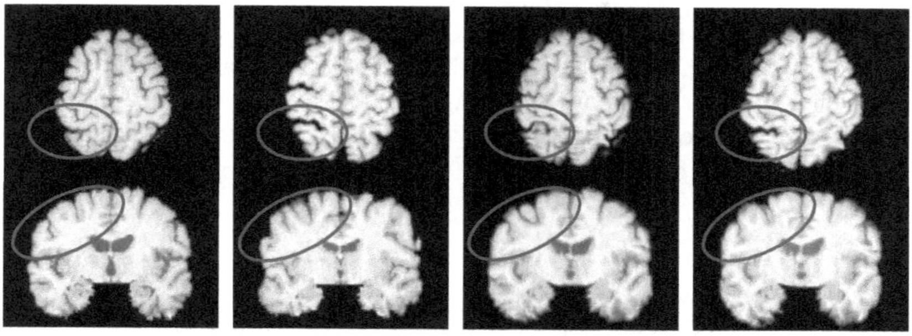

(a) Template (b) Linear registration (c) HAMMER (d) Our method

Fig. 5. Results produced by linear method, HAMMER, and our method, respectively

In the second experiment, the consistency of both methods in registering different time-point images of the same subject is evaluated. Since the warping consistency is very important to measure longitudinal brain changes, it is expected that the corresponding points in different time-point images of the same subject are consistently warped to the same location in the template space. Fig. 6 shows the warping results of five different year images of the same subject, produced by HAMMER 6(a) and our method 6(b), respectively. For better comparison of warping results on the cortex, 3D renderings of all warped different-year images are provided, with the dotted curves in the same spatial locations placed as landmarks to facilitate the visual comparison. For the region indicated by a green arrow in the year 4 image of Fig 6(a), its warping result is inconsistent with those in other years. On the contrary, the warping results on this region are relatively consistent by our method.

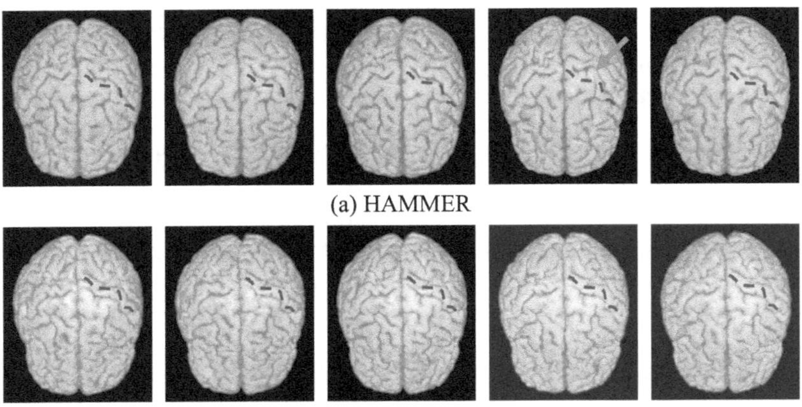

(a) HAMMER

(b) Our Method

Fig. 6. The warped results by HAMMER and our method are shown in (a) and (b) respectively, where the warping in the year 4 seems inconsistent by HAMMER in the region indicated by a green arrow.

3.2 Experiments on Simulated Data

The accuracy of our learning-based registration method is quantitatively evaluated by simulated data. For our method, the average registration error is 0.72mm, while, for HAMMER, its average registration error is 0.92mm. This indicates nearly 25% of error reduction by our method.

4 Conclusion

A fully learning-based framework has been developed for deformable registration of MR brain images. Learning methods have been designed to learn (1) the best features to enhance the accuracy of correspondence detection, (2) the active points to hierarchically steer the image registration, and (3) the multi-level deformation statistics to constrain the deformations. By using this learning-based registration framework, both registration accuracy and robustness have been achieved by our method. Our future work will include the investigation of more image features into our framework and the extension of our framework to other registration problems.

Reference

[1] Wang, Y., Staib, L.H.: Elastic model-based non-rigid registration incorporating statistical shape information. In: Wells, W.M., Colchester, A.C.F., Delp, S.L. (eds.) MICCAI 1998. LNCS, vol. 1496, pp. 1162–1173. Springer, Heidelberg (1999)
[2] Gee, J.C., Reivich, M., Bajcsy, R.: Elastically deforming 3D atlas to match anatomical brain images. Journal of Computer Assisted Tomography 17, 225–236 (1993)
[3] Christensen, G.E., Johnson, H.J.: Consistent Image Registration. IEEE Transactions on Medical Imaging 20, 568–582 (2001)
[4] Shen, D., Davatzikos, C.: HAMMER: Hierarchical attribute matching mechanism for elastic registration. IEEE Transactions on Medical Imaging 21, 1421–1439 (2002)
[5] Wu, G., Qi, F., Shen, D.: Learning Best Features for Deformable Registration of MR Brains. In: Duncan, J.S., Gerig, G. (eds.) MICCAI 2005. LNCS, vol. 3750, pp. 179–187. Springer, Heidelberg (2005)
[6] Wu, G., Qi, F., Shen, D.: Learning-Based Deformable Registration of MR Brain Images. IEEE Trans. on Medical Imaging 25, 1145–1157 (2006)
[7] Xue, Z., Shen, D., Davatzikos, C.: Statistical Representation of High-Dimensional Deformation Fields with Application to Statistically-Constrained 3D Warping Medical Image Analysis. Medical Image Analysis 10, 740–751 (2006)
[8] Rueckert, D., Frangi, A.F., Schnabel, J.A.: Automatic construction of 3D statistical deformation models of the brain using non-rigid registration. IEEE Trans. on Medical Imaging 22, 1014–1024 (2003)
[9] Xue, Z., Shen, D.: Statistically-Constrained Deformable Registration of MR Brain Images. In: Fourth IEEE International Symposium on Biomedical Imaging (ISBI 2007), Metro Washington, D.C., USA (2007)
[10] Lee, S., Wolberg, G., Shin, S.Y.: Scattered Data Interpolation with Multilevel B-Splines. IEEE Transactions on Visualization and Computer Graphics 3, 228–224 (1997)
[11] Wu, G., Qi, F., Shen, D.: A General Learning Framework for Non-rigid Image Registration, In: International Workshop on Medical Imaging and Augmented Reality (MIAR'06), Shanghai, China 2006, pp. 219–227 (2006)
[12] Lazebnik, S., Schmid, C., Ponce, J.: A Sparse Texture Representation Using Local Affine Regions. IEEE Trans. on Pattern Analysis and Machine Intelligence 27, 1265–1278 (2005)
[13] Shen, D.: Image Registration by Local Histogram Matching. Pattern Recognition 40, 1161–1172 (2007)
[14] Lowe, D.: Distinctive Image Features form Scale-Invariant Key-points. International Journal of Computer Vision 2, 91–110 (2004)
[15] Zhu, S., Yuille, A.: Region Competition: Unifying Snake/balloon, Region Growing and Bayes/MDL/Energy for multi-band Image Segmentation. IEEE Trans. on Pattern Analysis and Machine Intelligence 18, 884–900 (1996)
[16] Shi, J., Malik, J.: Normalized Cuts and Image Segmentation. IEEE Trans. on Pattern Analysis and Machine Intelligence 22, 888–905 (2000)
[17] Vincent, L., Soille, P.: Watersheds in digital spaces: An efficient algorithm based on immersion simulations. IEEE Transactions in Pattern Analysis and Machine Intelligence 13, 583–598 (1991)
[18] Xue, Z., Shen, D., Karacali, B., Stern, J., Rottenberg, D., Davatzikos, C.: Simulating Deformations of MR Brain Images for Evaluation of Registration Algorithms. Neuroimage 33, 855–866 (2006)

Information-Theoretic Analysis of Brain White Matter Fiber Orientation Distribution Functions

Ming-Chang Chiang[1], Andrea D. Klunder[1], Katie McMahon[2], Greig I. de Zubicaray[2], Margaret J. Wright[3], Arthur W. Toga[1], and Paul M. Thompson[1]

[1] Laboratory of Neuro Imaging, Department of Neurology, UCLA School of Medicine, Los Angeles, CA 90095, USA
[2] Centre for Magnetic Resonance, University of Queensland, Brisbane, Queensland 4072, Australia
[3] Genetic Epidemiology Lab, Queensland Institute of Medical Research, PO Royal Brisbane Hospital, Queensland 4029, Australia

Abstract. We propose a new information-theoretic metric, the symmetric Kullback-Leibler divergence (sKL-divergence), to measure the difference between two water diffusivity profiles in high angular resolution diffusion imaging (HARDI). Water diffusivity profiles are modeled as probability density functions on the unit sphere, and the sKL-divergence is computed from a spherical harmonic series, which greatly reduces computational complexity. Adjustment of the orientation of diffusivity functions is essential when the image is being warped, so we propose a fast algorithm to determine the principal direction of diffusivity functions using principal component analysis (PCA). We compare sKL-divergence with other inner-product based cost functions using synthetic samples and real HARDI data, and show that the sKL-divergence is highly sensitive in detecting small differences between two diffusivity profiles and therefore shows promise for applications in the nonlinear registration and multi-subject statistical analysis of HARDI data.

1 Introduction

High angular resolution diffusion imaging (HARDI) is a variant of conventional MRI that uses multiple radially-distributed gradients to encode directional profiles and orientations of water diffusion [1]. In conventional diffusion tensor imaging (DTI), the 3D diffusion profile of water molecules at each point in the brain is considered to have an ellipsoidal profile, which can be modeled using a second-rank tensor. Theoretically, 7 diffusion-encoding gradients are sufficient for fitting a tensor. By contrast, HARDI applies many more diffusion-encoding gradients to measure diffusivity at high angular resolution, revealing the detailed orientation profile for water diffusion within each voxel. Diffusivity profiles can be resolved more clearly in brain regions where fiber tracts cross, providing more accurate information for fiber-tracking (tractography), disease detection, and analysis of anatomical connectivity.

Several successful algorithms exist for linear and nonlinear registration of DTI [2-4]. Registration of HARDI data has not been widely studied, perhaps because HARDI yields high-dimensional datasets, often with 30-100 observations per voxel

N. Karssemeijer and B. Lelieveldt (Eds.): IPMI 2007, LNCS 4584, pp. 172–182, 2007.
© Springer-Verlag Berlin Heidelberg 2007

(corresponding to the number of gradient directions), compared with 6 independent parameters per voxel in DTI. Modeling and comparing diffusivity profiles is therefore computationally expensive, but vital for guiding alignment (registration) of HARDI data across subjects or time, prior to multisubject statistical analysis.

Several cost functions have been proposed for DTI registration, such as Euclidean or log-Euclidean distance between two diffusion profiles, or the multichannel sum of squared differences (SSD) [5]. Here we evaluate a new information-theoretic metric, the symmetric Kullback-Leibler divergence (sKL-divergence), for measuring differences between diffusivity profiles in HARDI. Information theory is relevant for estimating diffusivity profiles and also for measuring anisotropy (e.g., the cumulative residual entropy method [6, 7]). Vemuri [8] successfully used the sKL-divergence to measure the distance between two Gaussian tensors, for DTI segmentation. Here we compute sKL-divergence from spherical harmonic expansions of the orientation-dependent diffusion functions (ODFs). Spherical harmonic series are widely used in HARDI visualization and regularization [9, 10]; they can help in efficiently computing the diffusion displacement probabilities [11], and visualizing the ODF at each voxel [12]. We show that sKL-divergence is more robust than standard inner product measures for detecting small rotational deviations between HARDI data, at various diffusion weights and noise levels, making it an attractive measure for HARDI registration.

2 Methods

2.1 Kullback-Leibler Divergence of Two Diffusivity Functions

In HARDI, the signal attenuation in a specific direction, g, is given by the Stejskal-Tanner equation [13]:

$$S(g) = S_0 \exp(-bD(g)). \tag{1}$$

where b is the diffusion weighting factor, D is the scalar diffusivity (apparent diffusion coefficient) and g is the diffusion-encoded gradient direction, with $g = g(\theta,\phi) = \begin{bmatrix}\sin\theta\cos\phi & \sin\theta\sin\phi & \cos\theta\end{bmatrix}^T$; θ and ϕ are the polar and azimuthal angles. Inspired by [14], we model the diffusivity function as a probability density function (pdf), by normalizing its integral over the spherical angle Ω to 1:

$$\begin{aligned} p(\theta,\phi) &= D(\theta,\phi)/gtr(D), \\ gtr(D) &= \int_\Omega D(\theta,\phi)d\Omega, \end{aligned} \tag{2}$$

where gtr is the generalized trace of D [14]. For two diffusivity functions D_p and D_q, we define the symmetric KL-divergence based on the corresponding pdfs $p(\theta, \phi)$ and $q(\theta, \phi)$:

$$sKL(p,q) = \frac{1}{2}\left\{ \int_\Omega p\log(\frac{p}{q})d\Omega + \int_\Omega q\log(\frac{q}{p})d\Omega \right\}$$

$$= \frac{1}{2}\left\{ \begin{matrix} \int_\Omega p\log(p)d\Omega - \int_\Omega p\log(q)d\Omega + \int_\Omega q\log(q)d\Omega \\ - \int_\Omega q\log(p)d\Omega \end{matrix} \right\} \quad (3)$$

Applying Eq (2) to the integrals in Eq (3), for example,

$$\begin{aligned} \int_\Omega p\log(q)d\Omega &= \int_\Omega \frac{D_p}{gtr(D_p)}\left[\log(D_q) - \log(gtr(D_q))\right]d\Omega \\ &= \left[\frac{1}{gtr(D_p)}\int_\Omega D_p \log(D_q)d\Omega\right] - \log(gtr(D_q)), \end{aligned} \quad (4)$$

we then have

$$sKL(p,q) = \frac{1}{2}\left\{ \begin{matrix} \frac{1}{gtr(D_p)}\left[\int_\Omega D_p\log(D_p)d\Omega - \int_\Omega D_p\log(D_q)d\Omega\right] \\ + \frac{1}{gtr(D_q)}\left[\int_\Omega D_q\log(D_q)d\Omega - \int_\Omega D_q\log(D_p)d\Omega\right] \end{matrix} \right\}. \quad (5)$$

Direct estimation of sKL in Eq (5) is computationally expensive, but is faster if we expand the diffusivity functions $D(\theta, \phi)$ as a spherical harmonic (SH) series [9, 10]:

$$\begin{aligned} D(\theta,\phi) &= \sum_{l=0}^{\infty}\sum_{m=-l}^{l} c_l^m Y_l^m(\theta,\phi), \\ Y_l^m(\theta,\phi) &= \sqrt{\frac{(2l+1)}{4\pi}\frac{(l-m)!}{(l+m)!}}P_l^m(\cos\theta)e^{im\phi}; \end{aligned} \quad (6)$$

here $P_l^m(\cos\theta)$ are the associated Legendre polynomials. $D(\theta, \phi)$ is real and radially symmetric, so it is sufficient to adopt a real basis function set Y_{lm} while retaining the orthonormality of Y_l^m [10]:

$$\begin{aligned} D(\theta,\phi) &= \sum_{l=0,even}^{\infty}\sum_{m=-l}^{l} c_{lm}Y_{lm}(\theta,\phi), \\ Y_{lm} &= \begin{cases} \frac{\sqrt{2}}{2}\left((-1)^m Y_l^m + Y_l^{-m}\right), \text{ if } -l \le m < 0 \\ Y_l^0, \text{ if } m = 0 \\ \frac{\sqrt{2}i}{2}\left((-1)^{m+1} Y_l^m + Y_l^{-m}\right), \text{ if } 0 < m \le l \end{cases} \quad l = 0, 2, 4, \ldots \end{aligned} \quad (7)$$

As the Y_{lm} are orthonormal, the inner product of the real functions D_1 and D_2 can be expressed in terms of their SH coefficients ($c_{lm}^{D_1}$ and $c_{lm}^{D_2}$):

$$\int_{\Omega} D_1(\theta,\phi)D_2(\theta,\phi)d\Omega = \sum_{l=0,even}^{\infty} \sum_{m=-l}^{l} c_{lm}^{D_1} c_{lm}^{D_2}. \tag{8}$$

Moreover, it can be shown that (see Appendix for derivations):

$$\int_{\Omega} D(\theta,\phi)d\Omega = 2\sqrt{\pi}c_{00}. \tag{9}$$

Therefore, sKL in Eq (5) can be expanded in terms of the SH series, as follows:

$$sKL(p,q) = \frac{1}{2}\left\{ \begin{aligned} &\frac{1}{c_{00}^{p}} \sum_{l=0,even}^{\infty} \sum_{m=-l}^{l} \left[c_{lm}^{p} d_{lm}^{p} - c_{lm}^{p} d_{lm}^{q}\right] \\ &+\frac{1}{c_{00}^{q}} \sum_{l=0,even}^{\infty} \sum_{m=-l}^{l} \left[c_{lm}^{q} d_{lm}^{q} - c_{lm}^{q} d_{lm}^{p}\right] \end{aligned} \right\}, \tag{10}$$

where $D_j = \sum_{l=0,even}^{\infty} \sum_{m=-l}^{l} c_{lm}^{j} Y_{lm}$, $\log(D_j) = \sum_{l=0,even}^{\infty} \sum_{m=-l}^{l} d_{lm}^{j} Y_{lm}$, and $j \in \{p, q\}$.

For numerical implementation, we use a truncated SH series with $l \le l_m$, where l_m is a positive even integer; the total length of the SH series is $n_b = (l_m+1)(l_m+2) / 2$. We follow the least-squares method [9, 10] to solve Eq (7), yielding the SH coefficients:

$$C = \left(B^T B\right)^{-1} B^T D. \tag{11}$$

Here $C = \left[c_0\, c_1\, ..\, c_{n_b-1}\right]^T$, and $D = \left[D(\theta_0,\phi_0)\; D(\theta_1,\phi_1)\; ..\; D(\theta_{n_s},\phi_{n_s})\right]^T$ which represents the diffusivity function measured in n_s gradient directions, and B is the matrix of basis functions, with elements $B_{ij} = Y_j(\theta_i,\phi_i)$. Here we map (c_{lm}, Y_{lm}) in Eq (7) to (c_j, Y_j), using the relationship $j = [(l^2+l) / 2] + m$. Usually $n_b << n_s$, so it is more cost-effective to compute sKL using the SH method (Eq (10)) rather than using Eq (5) directly.

2.2 Reorientation of Diffusivity Functions

Similar to diffusion tensors in DTI, the diffusivity functions in HARDI are oriented and their directions must be adjusted when the HARDI data are linearly or nonlinearly transformed. We adopt the "Preservation of Principal Directions (PPD)" method [15], which preserves the shape of the diffusivity function along the local principal fiber orientation. With DTI, given the local Jacobian matrix J of the image transformation, the PPD procedure yields a rotation matrix that rotates the first eigenvector $\mathbf{e}_1$ onto $J\mathbf{e}_1/|J\mathbf{e}_1|$ and the second eigenvector $\mathbf{e}_2$ onto the plane spanned by $J\mathbf{e}_1/|J\mathbf{e}_1|$ and $J\mathbf{e}_2/|J\mathbf{e}_2|$. In HARDI, however, a single diffusivity function may have multiple local maxima that are computationally expensive to determine [16], and thus not practical to perform at every iteration during image warping. Here we propose a fast algorithm to determine the principal direction of the diffusivity function, based on the principal component analysis (PCA) of its shape [17]. At each direction sampled by the diffusion gradient $g(\theta_i, \phi_i)$, $0 \leq i < n_s$, we define a point with distance to the origin $d_i = D(\theta_i, \phi_i)\, g(\theta_i, \phi_i) = (d_{i0}, d_{i1}, d_{i2})$, where the last term is the Cartesian coordinates of d_i. The mean and the covariance matrices, μ and Σ, of the point set $\{ d_i \}$ are given by

$$\mu_j = \frac{1}{n_s}\sum_{i=0}^{n_s-1} d_{ij}\,;\; \Sigma_{ij} = \frac{1}{n_s}\sum_{k=0}^{n_s-1}(d_{ki}-\mu_i)(d_{kj}-\mu_j),\; 0 \leq i,j < 3. \tag{12}$$

The principal direction of the diffusivity function is determined by the first eigenvector of Σ. The rotation matrix R, which adjusts the direction of the diffusivity function, is then obtained using the PPD procedure, and the new gradient directions $g(\theta'_i,\phi'_i) = R \cdot g(\theta_i,\phi_i)$.

However, it is advantageous to have values of the reoriented diffusivity function in the *original* directions (θ_i,ϕ_i), rather than the new ones (θ'_i,ϕ'_i), because (1) we do not need to keep track of new reoriented gradient directions at each iteration of image warping, and (2) sKL (or other cost functions) can be compared on diffusivity functions sampled at identical gradient directions for the target image (which is fixed) and the source (which is moving and in which the diffusivity functions are being reoriented). Because the gradient directions are only discretely sampled, the reoriented diffusivity functions are constructed by "pushing" the values sampled at the original directions to the new directions, so the values of the reoriented function at the original directions are not known. These new values can be computed from the SH series, as the basis functions Y_{lm} are continuous and defined at all spherical angles. If $(\Delta\theta_i,\Delta\phi_i) = (\theta'_i - \theta_i, \phi'_i - \phi_i)$, then the values of the reoriented diffusivity functions D' in the original directions (θ_i,ϕ_i) are given by

$$D'(\theta_i,\phi_i) = D(\theta_i - \Delta\theta_i, \phi_i - \Delta\phi_i) = \sum_{l=0,even}^{\infty}\sum_{m=-l}^{l} c_{lm} Y_{lm}(\theta_i - \Delta\theta_i, \phi_i - \Delta\phi_i), \tag{13}$$

where c_{lm} are the SH coefficients of the original diffusivity function D (see Eq (7)).

2.3 Interpolation of Diffusivity Functions

Diffusivity functions must be interpolated when the HARDI data is warped and the new voxel locations are not on lattice points. It is natural to interpolate diffusivity functions separately for each gradient direction (i.e., multichannel interpolation). We therefore performed linear interpolation of $D(\theta_i, \phi_i)$, $\log(D(\theta_i, \phi_i))$, and of the MR signals $S(\theta_i, \phi_i)$ in synthetic samples and compared the swelling effect (i.e., loss of anisotropy) of these three interpolation schemes.

3 Experiments and Results

Synthetic examples. We constructed a two-fiber diffusivity function using two orthogonal Gaussian tensors, T_0 and T_1, with typical eigenvalues for white-matter (WM) fibers [9, 10]. We set $T_0 = diag(200, 200, 1700) \times 10^{-6}$ (mm^2/s); T_1 was obtained by rotating T_0 90 degrees around the y-axis. We also generated an isotropic gray-matter

(GM) diffusivity function by setting $T_{iso} = diag(700, 700, 700) \times 10^{-6}$ (mm^2/s). Then the diffusivity function D is given by

$$D = -\frac{1}{b}\sum_{i=0}^{n-1} p_i \exp(-bg^T T_i g), \tag{14}$$

where n is the number of fibers. $p_0 = p_1 = 0.5$ for two-fiber structures and $p_0 = 1$ for the isotropic diffusivity function. The gradient direction vector g consisted of 162 sampled points determined using an electrostatic approach [18]. Different b values (500, 1500, 3000) s/mm^2 were tested. The order of the SH series (l_m) was set to 8.

HARDI data. The HARDI data was acquired from a healthy 22-year-old man imaged as part of a research study of twins on a 4T Bruker Medspec MRI scanner using an optimized diffusion tensor sequence [18]. Imaging parameters were: 21 axial slices (5 mm thick), FOV = 24 cm, TR/TE 6090/104.5 ms, 0.5 mm gap, with a 128x100 acquisition matrix and 30 images acquired at each location: 3 low ($b = 0$) and 27 high diffusion-weighted images in which the encoding gradient vectors were uniformly radially distributed in space ($b = 1100$ s/mm^2) using the electrostatic approach in [18]. The reconstruction matrix was 128x128, yielding a 1.875x1.875 mm^2 in-plane resolution. The total scan time was 3.09 minutes. We set $l_m = 4$ for the spherical harmonic analysis.

Fig. 1 shows that the principal directions determined from HARDI by the PCA method are compatible with those computed by DTI and persistent angle structures (PAS) fitting using the software Camino developed at University College, London [19], in major WM fiber structures. Fig. 2 compares the fiber directions when the HARDI data was rotated by 60 degrees around the inferior-superior axis passing through its center of mass, with and without reorientation of the diffusivity functions. As observed in [15, 20], our results show that the orientation of the diffusivity functions must be adjusted when the image is transformed, to maintain the spatial coherence

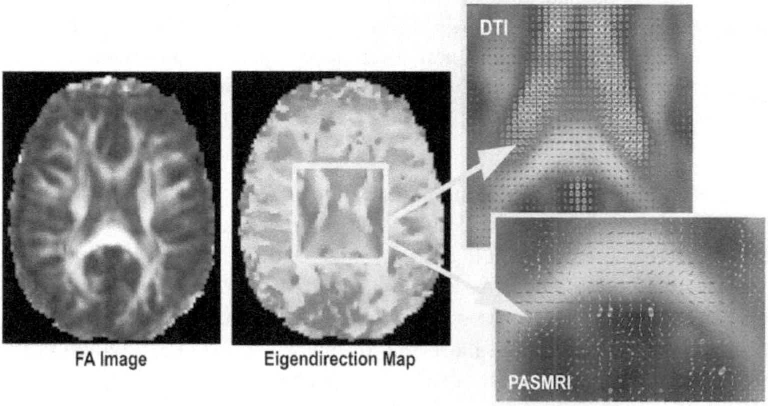

Fig. 1. The eigendirection map for the HARDI data, determined using the PCA method. Fibers with right-left orientation are shown in red, anterior-posterior in green, and inferior-superior in blue. The eigendirections correctly depict the orientations of major WM fiber structures, and are compatible with the tensor glyphs and PAS computed using the visualization software "Camino" [19]. FA: fractional anisotropy.

of the principal fiber directions. To do this, we used the PPD procedure, which is more accurate than other methods (e.g., Finite Strain [3, 15]) as it takes the original fiber directions into account. PCA determines one eigendirection, so it is appropriate for diffusivity functions with a single global maximum, or with a dominant local maximum relative to other small local maxima. In diffusivity functions with multiple local maxima, such as in regions where fibers cross (e.g. the synthetic samples in Fig. 3), the principal direction estimated by PCA becomes arbitrary, and the simple PPD procedure may not be applicable in these regions.

Fig. 3 shows diffusivity functions at intermediate positions $x = 0.1, 0.3, .. 0.9$, obtained by linear interpolation of the diffusivity function D, log(D), and MR signals S in each gradient direction, when the two-fiber synthetic function was placed at $x = 0$, and the isotropic one at $x = 1$.

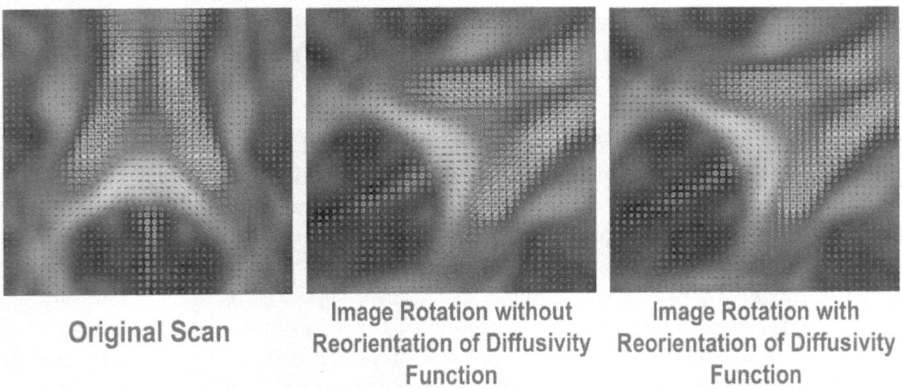

Fig. 2. The orientation-dependent diffusivity functions in the splenium of the corpus callosum are no longer consistent with the known directions of the underlying WM fibers when the image voxels are simply resampled to new locations by rotation but without reorientation of diffusivity functions. The PPD procedure corrects this, and the diffusivity functions remain aligned with the WM fibers that they represent.

Direct interpolation of the MR signals results in the least swelling, or loss of anisotropy, in the diffusivity function. Euclidean interpolation may also be more appropriate for the MR signals, which are physical entities. Linear interpolation using log(D) performs better than D (as least in terms of degrading the signal geometry). Computing log(D) may therefore be an acceptable alternative to computing S. Log(D) can be computed in the spherical harmonic domain (see Eq (10)), which is more economical in terms of memory than performing interpolation on S - this may be beneficial for HARDI registration.

We compared the symmetric KL-divergence (sKL) with other two cost functions, the inner product of diffusivity functions in Eq (8) with and without the linear ($l = 0$) term [3, 21], on synthetic examples that were noise-free, or with Rician noise added to MR signals S such that the signal-to-noise ratio (SNR) was 35 or 10 [22]. The inner product *without* the $l = 0$ term is designed to compare only the anisotropic part of the

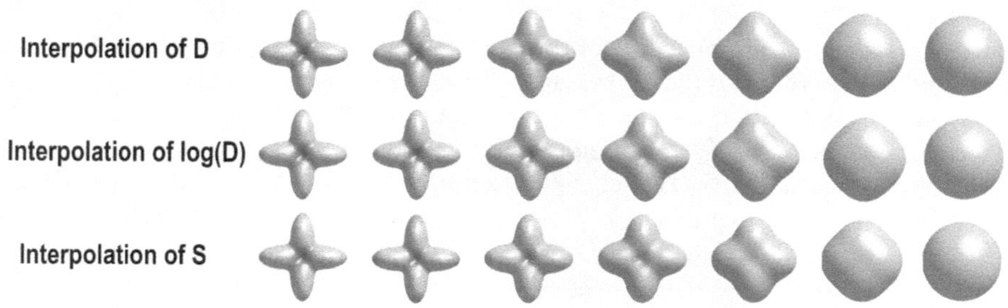

Fig. 3. Comparison of diffusivity functions obtained by linear interpolation of D, $\log(D)$ and S. Interpolation using the MR signal S best preserves the anisotropy of the diffusivity function.

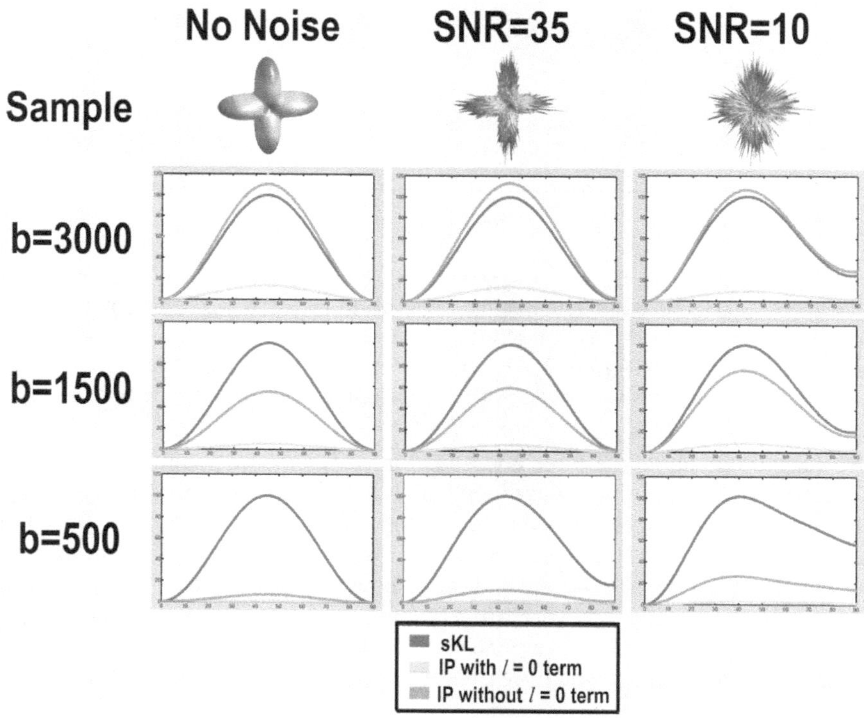

Fig. 4. Two identical synthetic diffusivity samples (no noise or with Rician noise added) were initially overlapped and rotated by $\varphi = 0$ to 90°. We compared the differences between the rotated and non-rotated samples with the symmetric KL-divergence (sKL) and inner product (IP) with/without $l = 0$ term. In noise-free samples, $\varphi = 45°$ gives the maximum sKL and minimum IP values. To facilitate comparisons, sKL and IP values have been normalized such that the *normalized* $sKL(\varphi) = 100 \times sKL(\varphi)/sKL(\varphi = 45°)$, and *normalized* $IP(\varphi) = 100 \times [1 - IP(\varphi)/IP(\varphi = 0°)]$.

diffusivity functions [3]. Two identical two-fiber synthetic diffusivity functions served as the source and the target objects, with the source object rotating from 0 (complete overlap) to 90 degrees. The three metrics were normalized for comparisons (as detailed in Fig. 4). Fig. 4 shows that at different noise levels, the sKL cost function detects angular discrepancies in diffusivity functions more sensitively than the inner product with/without the $l = 0$ term, in low b-settings. sKL is also still comparable in performance with the inner product without $l = 0$ term, at a high b-value. The performance of sKL is therefore stable under various diffusion weightings, and it is applicable in ordinary MRI/DTI acquisition settings, though a high b-value can detect higher-order angular structures in WM fibers, at the cost of a decreased SNR [1].

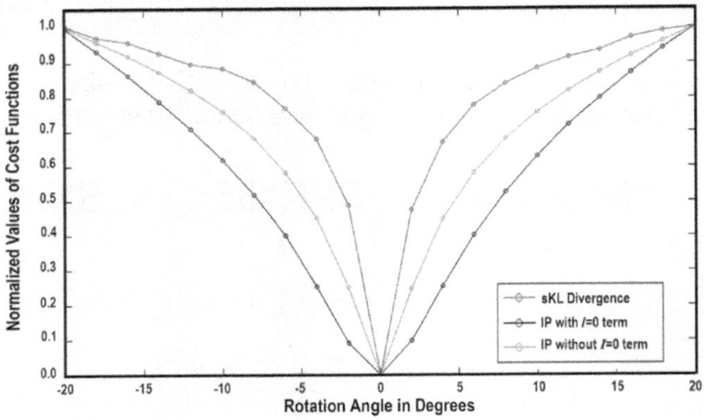

Fig. 5. Comparisons of the changes in symmetric KL-divergence (sKL) and inner product (IP) (with/without $l = 0$ term) at different rotation angles φ (from -20° to +20°, in increments of 2°) for two identical HARDI diffusion profiles. sKL and IP values have been normalized, with $normalized\,f(\varphi) = abs[(f(\varphi) - f(\varphi = 0°))/(f(\varphi = 20°) - f(\varphi = 0°))]$. The angular profile of sKL is very sharp, and can detect rotational deviations of the image, with a magnitude as small as 2°.

We further compared the three cost functions, which were summed over all voxels, in the 3D HARDI data. Two identical HARDI data was initially overlapped (rotation angle = 0 degree), and then one image was rotated (with diffusivity functions reoriented) up to ±20 degrees, with sKL and inner products (with/without $l = 0$ term) computed at every two degrees. Fig. 5 shows that sKL has very sharp gradient near the optimal solution, and is sensitive enough to detect 2-degree deviation of the images. The symmetric KL-divergence is therefore a good candidate cost function for registration of HARDI, which we expect to evaluate in the near future.

Acknowledgments. Funded by NIH grants (EB01651, RR019771, AG016570, NS049194 to PT, HD050735 to MW) and a Taiwan Government Fellowship (to MCC).

References

1. Tuch, D.S., et al.: High angular resolution diffusion imaging reveals intravoxel white matter fiber heterogeneity. Magn. Reson Med. 48(4), 577–582 (2002)
2. Cao, Y., et al.: Large deformation diffeomorphic metric mapping of vector fields. Medical Imaging, IEEE Transactions on 24, 1216–1230 (2005)

3. Zhang, H., et al.: Deformable registration of diffusion tensor MR images with explicit orientation optimization. Med. Image Anal. 10(5), 764–785 (2006)
4. Chiang, M.-C., et al.: Fluid registration of diffusion tensor images using information theory. IEEE Transactions on Medical Imaging (submitted) (2007)
5. Pollari, M., et al.: Comparative evaluation of voxel similarity measures for affine registration of diffusion tensor MR images in ISBI 2007, Arlington, Virginia (2007)
6. Chen, Y., et al.: Apparent Diffusion Coefficient Approximation and Diffusion Anisotropy Characterization in DWI, in Information Processing in Medical Imaging. 2005: Glenwood Springs, CO. pp. 246–257 (2005)
7. Rao, M., et al.: Cumulative residual entropy: a new measure of information. Information Theory. IEEE Transactions 50, 1220–1228 (2004)
8. Vemuri, B.C.: Variational Principles for Diffusion Weighted MRI Restoration and Segmentation. In: 2005 Computer and Robot Vision. In: Proceedings. The 2nd Canadian Conference on 2005, pp. xiv-xiv (2005)
9. Alexander, D.C., Barker, G.J., Arridge, S.R.: Detection and modeling of non-Gaussian apparent diffusion coefficient profiles in human brain data. Magn. Reson Med. 48(2), 331–340 (2002)
10. Descoteaux, M., et al.: Apparent Diffusion Coefficients from High Angular Resolution Diffusion Images: Estimation and Applications. Research Report No. 5681, 2005, INRIA Sophia Antipolis (2005)
11. McGraw, T., et al.: Denoising and visualization of HARDI data 2005, Tech. Report, Dept. CISE, U. Florida (2005)
12. Ozarslan, E., et al.: Fast orientation mapping from HARDI. In: Med Image Comput Comput Assist Interv (MICCAI), 2005. 8(Pt 1): p. 156–163 (2005)
13. Stejskal, E.O., Tanner, J.E.: Spin Diffusion Measurements: Spin Echoes in the Presence of a Time-Dependent Field Gradient. The Journal of Chemical Physics 42(1), 288–292 (1965)
14. Ozarslan, E., Vemuri, B.C., Mareci, T.H.: Generalized scalar measures for diffusion MRI using trace, variance, and entropy. Magn. Reson Med. 53(4), 866–876 (2005)
15. Alexander, D.C., et al.: Spatial transformations of diffusion tensor magnetic resonance. Medical Imaging, IEEE Transactions 20, 1131–1139 (2001)
16. Alexander, D.C.: Maximum Entropy Spherical Deconvolution for Diffusion MRI, in Information Processing in Medical Imaging 2005, Glenwood Springs, CO. pp. 76–87 (2005)
17. Fukunaga, K.: Introduction to statistical pattern recognition. In: Computer science and scientific computing, 2nd edn. vol. xiii, p. 591. Academic Press, Boston (1990)
18. Jones, D.K., Horsfield, M.A., Simmons, A.: Optimal strategies for measuring diffusion in anisotropic systems by magnetic resonance imaging. Magn. Reson Med. 42(3), 515–525 (1999)
19. Cook, P.A., et al.: Camino: Open-Source Diffusion-MRI Reconstruction and Processing, In: 14th Scientific Meeting of the International Society for Magnetic Resonance in Medicine 2006, Seattle, WA, p. 2759 (2006)
20. Xu, D., et al.: Spatial normalization of diffusion tensor fields. Magn. Reson Med. 50(1), 175–182 (2003)
21. Descoteaux, M., et al.: A fast and robust ODF estimation algorithm in Q-ball imaging, In: IEEE International Symposium on Biomedical Imaging: From Nano to Macro (ISBI) 2006, Arlington, Virginia (2006)
22. Sijbers, J., et al.: Estimation of the noise in magnitude MR images. Magn. Reson Imaging 16(1), 87–90 (1998)

Appendix

$$
\begin{aligned}
\int_{\Omega} D(\theta,\phi)d\Omega &= \int_{\theta=0}^{\pi}\int_{\phi=0}^{2\pi}\sum_{l=0,even}^{\infty}\sum_{m=-l}^{l} c_{lm}Y_{lm}(\theta,\phi)d\phi\sin\theta d\theta \\
&= \sum_{l=0,even}^{\infty} c_{l0}\int_0^{\pi}\int_0^{2\pi} Y_{l0}(\theta,\phi)d\phi\sin\theta d\theta \\
&+ \sum_{l=0,even}^{\infty}\sum_{m=-l,m\neq 0}^{l} c_{lm}\int_0^{\pi}\int_0^{2\pi} Y_{lm}(\theta,\phi)d\phi\sin\theta d\theta.
\end{aligned} \tag{A1}
$$

Given that

$$
\begin{aligned}
\int_0^{\pi}\int_0^{2\pi} Y_l^m(\theta,\phi)d\phi\sin\theta d\theta &= \sqrt{\frac{(2l+1)}{4\pi}\frac{(l-m)!}{(l+m)!}}\int_0^{\pi} P_l^m(\cos\theta)\sin\theta d\theta \\
&\cdot\left(\int_0^{2\pi} e^{im\phi}d\phi\right) \\
&= 0, \text{ if } m \neq 0,
\end{aligned} \tag{A2}
$$

since $\int_0^{2\pi} e^{im\phi}d\phi = 0$, if $m \neq 0$, we have

$$
\sum_{l=0,even}^{\infty}\sum_{m=-l,m\neq 0}^{l} c_{lm}\int_0^{\pi}\int_0^{2\pi} Y_{lm}(\theta,\phi)d\phi\sin\theta d\theta = 0. \tag{A3}
$$

Here we use the definition of Y_{lm} in Eq (7), where Y_{lm} comes from linear combinations of Y_l^m. Therefore, Eq (A1) becomes

$$
\begin{aligned}
\int_{\Omega} D(\theta,\phi)d\Omega &= \sum_{l=0,even}^{\infty} c_{l0}\int_0^{\pi}\int_0^{2\pi} Y_{l0}(\theta,\phi)d\phi\sin\theta d\theta \\
&= 2\pi\sum_{l=0,even}^{\infty}\sqrt{\frac{(2l+1)}{4\pi}}c_{l0}\int_0^{\pi} P_l^0(\cos\theta)\sin\theta d\theta \\
&= 2\pi\sum_{l=0,even}^{\infty}\sqrt{\frac{(2l+1)}{4\pi}}c_{l0}\int_{-1}^{1} P_l^0(x)dx.
\end{aligned} \tag{A4}
$$

As the associated Legendre polynomials are orthogonal, such that $\int_{-1}^{1} P_k^m P_l^m dx = \dfrac{2(l+m)!}{(2l+1)(l-m)!}\delta_{kl}$, where δ_{kl} is the Kronecker delta, we have

$$
\int_{-1}^{1} P_l^0(x)dx = \int_{-1}^{1} P_l^0(x)P_0^0(x)dx = 2\delta_{l0}, \tag{A5}
$$

where $P_0^0(x) = 1$. Therefore,

$$
\int_{\Omega} D(\theta,\phi)d\Omega = 4\pi\sum_{l=0,even}^{\infty}\sqrt{\frac{(2l+1)}{4\pi}}c_{l0}\delta_{l0} = 2\sqrt{\pi}c_{00}. \tag{A6}
$$

Segmentation of Sub-cortical Structures by the Graph-Shifts Algorithm

Jason J. Corso[1], Zhuowen Tu[1], Alan Yuille[2], and Arthur Toga[1]

[1] Center for Computational Biology
Laboratory of Neuro Imaging
[2] Department of Statistics
University of California, Los Angeles, USA
jcorso@ucla.edu

Abstract. We propose a novel algorithm called graph-shifts for performing image segmentation and labeling. This algorithm makes use of a dynamic hierarchical representation of the image. This representation allows each iteration of the algorithm to make both small and large changes in the segmentation, similar to PDE and split-and-merge methods, respectively. In particular, at each iteration we are able to rapidly compute and select the optimal change to be performed. We apply graph-shifts to the task of segmenting sub-cortical brain structures. First we formalize this task as energy function minimization where the energy terms are learned from a training set of labeled images. Then we apply the graph-shifts algorithm. We show that the labeling results are comparable in quantitative accuracy to other approaches but are obtained considerably faster: by orders of magnitude (roughly one minute). We also quantitatively demonstrate robustness to initialization and avoidance of local minima in which conventional boundary PDE methods fall.

1 Introduction

Segmenting an image into a number of labeled regions is a classic vision and medical imaging problem, see [1,2,3,4,5,6] for an introduction to the enormous literature. The problem is typically formulated in terms of minimizing an energy function or, equivalently, maximizing a posterior probability distribution. In this paper, we deal with a special case where the number of labels is fixed. Our specific application is to segment the sub-cortical structures of the brain, see section (2). The contribution of this paper is to provide a novel algorithm called *graph-shifts* which is extremely fast and effective for sub-cortical segmentation.

A variety of algorithms, reviewed in section (2), have been proposed to solve the energy minimization task for segmentation and labeling. For most of these algorithms, each iteration is restricted to small changes in the segmentation. For those methods which allow large changes, there is no procedure for rapidly calculating and selecting the change that most decreases the energy.

Graph-shifts is a novel algorithm that builds a dynamic hierarchical representation of the image. This representation enables the algorithm to make large

N. Karssemeijer and B. Lelieveldt (Eds.): IPMI 2007, LNCS 4584, pp. 183–197, 2007.
© Springer-Verlag Berlin Heidelberg 2007

changes in the segmentation which can be thought of as a combined split and merge (see [4] for recent work on split and merge). Moreover, the graph-shifts algorithm is able to exploit the hierarchy to rapidly calculate and select the best change to make at each iteration. This gives an extremely fast algorithm which also has the ability to avoid local minima that might trap algorithms which rely on small local changes to the segmentation.

The hierarchy is structured as a set of nodes at a series of layers, see figure (1). The nodes at the bottom layer form the image lattice. Each node is constrained to have a single parent. All nodes are assigned a model label which is required to be the same as its parent's label. There is a neighborhood structure defined at all layers of the graph. A *graph shift* alters the hierarchy by changing the parent of a node, which alters the model label of the node and of all its descendants. This is illustrated in figure (1), which shows three steps in a three layer graph coloring potential shifts that would change the energy black and others gray. The algorithm can be understood intuitively in terms of competing crime families as portrayed in films like the Godfather. There is a hierarchical organization where each node owes allegiance to its unique parent node (or boss) and, in turn, to its boss's boss. This gives families of nodes which share the same allegiance (i.e. have the same model label). Each node has a subfamily of descendants. The top level nodes are the "bosses of all bosses" of the families. The graph-shifts algorithm proceeds by selecting a node to switch allegiance (i.e. model label) to the boss of a neighboring node. This causes the subfamily of the node to also switch allegiance. The algorithm minimizes a global energy and at each iteration selects the change of allegiance that maximally decreases the energy.

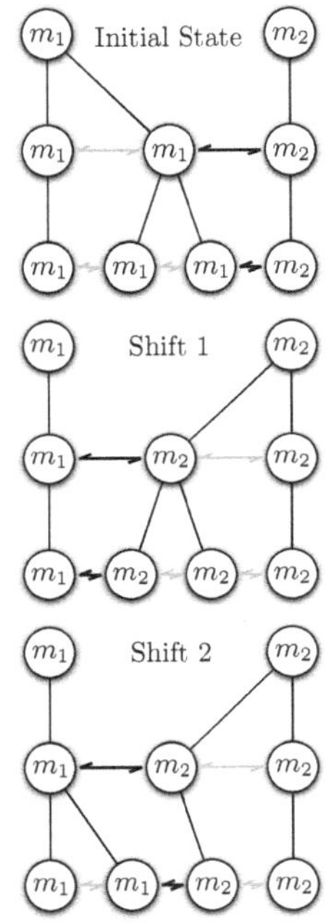

Fig. 1. Intuitive Graph-Shifts Example

The structure of this paper is as follows. In section (2) we give a brief background on segmentation. Section (3) describes the graph-shifts algorithm for a general class of segmentation problems. In section (4), we formulate the task of sub-cortical labeling in terms of energy function minimization and derive a graph-shifts algorithm. Section (5) gives experimental results and comparisons to other approaches.

2 Background

Many algorithms have been applied to segmentation, so we restrict our review to those methods most related to this paper. A common approach includes taking local gradients of the energy function at the region boundaries and thereby moving the boundaries. This region competition approach [2] can be successful when used with good initialization, but its local nature means that at each iteration step it can only make small changes to the segmentation. This can cause slowness and also risks getting stuck in local minima. See [7] for similar types of partial differential equations (PDE) algorithms using level sets and related methods. Graph cuts [3] is an alternative deterministic energy minimization algorithm that can take large leaps in the energy space, but it can only be applied to a restricted class of energy functions (and is only guaranteed to converge for a subset of these) [8]. Simulated annealing [1] can in theory converge to the optimal solution of any energy function but, in practice, is extremely slow. The data-driven Markov chain Monte Carlo method [4] can combine classic methods, including split and merge, to make large changes in the segmentation at each iteration, but remains comparatively slow.

There have been surprisingly few attempts to define segmentation algorithms based on dynamic hierarchical representations. But we are influenced by two recent papers. Segmentation by Weighted Aggregation (SWA) [9] is a remarkably fast algorithm that builds a hierarchical representation of an image, but does not attempt to minimize a global energy function. Instead it outputs a hierarchy of segments which satisfy certain homogeneity properties. Moreover, its hierarchy is fixed and not dynamic. The multiscale Swendson-Wang algorithm [10] does attempt to provide samples from a global probability distribution. But it has only limited hierarchy dynamics and its convergence rate is comparatively slow compared to SWA. A third related hierarchical segmentation approach is proposed in [11], where a *hyperstack*, a Gaussian scale-space representation of the image, is used to perform a probabilistic linking (similar to region growing) of voxels and partial volumes in the scale-space. Finally, Tu [12] proposed a related segmentation algorithm that was similarly capable of making both small-scale boundary adjustments and large-scale split-merge moves. In his approach, however, a fixed size hierarchy is used, and the split-merge moves are attempted by a stochastic algorithm, which requires the evaluation of (often difficult to compute) proposal distributions.

Our application is the important task of sub-cortical segmentation from three-dimensional medical images. Recent work on this task includes [5,6,13,14,15,16]. These approaches typically formulate the task in terms of probabilistic estimation or, equivalently, energy function minimization. The approaches differ by the form of the energy function that they use and the algorithm chosen to minimize it. The algorithms are usually similar to those described above and suffer similar limitations in terms of convergence rates. In this paper, we will use a comparatively simple energy function similar to conditional random fields [17], where the energy terms are learned from training examples by the probabilistic boosting tree (PBT) learning algorithm [18].

3 Graph-Shifts

This section describes the basic ideas of the graph-shifts algorithm. We first describe the class of energy models that it can be applied to in section (3.1). Next we describe the hierarchy in section (3.2), show how the energy can be computed recursively in section (3.3), and specify the general graph-shifts algorithm in section (3.4).

3.1 The Energy Models

The input image $\mathbf{I}$ is defined on a lattice D of pixels/voxels. For medical image applications this is a three-dimensional lattice. The lattice has the standard neighborhood structure and we define the notation $N(\mu, \nu) = 1$ if $\mu \in D$ and $\nu \in D$ are neighbors on the lattice, and $N(\mu, \nu) = 0$ otherwise. The task is to assign each voxel $\mu \in D$ to one of a fixed set of K models $m_\mu \in \{1, ..., K\}$. This assignment corresponds to a segmentation of the image into K, or more, connected regions.

We want the segmentation to minimize an energy function criterion:

$$E[\{m_\omega : \omega \in D\}] = \sum_{\nu \in D} E_1(\phi(\mathbf{I})(\nu), m_\nu) + \frac{1}{2} \sum_{\substack{\nu \in D, \mu \in D: \\ N(\nu,\mu)=1}} E_2(\mathbf{I}(\nu), \mathbf{I}(\mu), m_\nu, m_\mu). \tag{1}$$

In this paper, the second term E_2 is chosen to be a boundary term that pays a penalty only for neighboring pixels/voxels which have different model labels (i.e. $E_2(\mathbf{I}(\nu), \mathbf{I}(\mu), m_\nu, m_\mu) = 0$ if $m_\nu = m_\mu$). This penalty can either be a penalty for the length of the boundary, or may include a measure of the strength of local edge cues. It includes discretized versions of standard segmentation criteria such as boundary length $\int_{\delta R} ds$ and edge strength along boundary $\int_{\delta R} |\nabla \mathbf{I}|^2 ds$. (Here s denotes arc length, R denotes the regions with constant labels, and δR is their boundaries).

The first term E_1 gives local evidence that the pixel μ takes model m_μ, where $\phi(\mathbf{I})(\mu)$ denotes a nonlinear filter of the image evaluated at μ. In this paper, the nonlinear filter will give local context information and will be learned from training samples, as described in section (4.1). The model given in equation (1) includes a large class of existing models. It is restricted, however, by the requirement that the number of models is fixed and that the models have no unknown parameters.

3.2 The Hierarchy

We define a graph G to be a set of nodes $\mu \in \mathcal{U}$ and a set of edges. The graph is hierarchical and composed of multiple layers. The nodes at the lowest layer are the elements of the lattice D and the edges are defined to link neighbors on the lattice. The coarser layers are computed recursively, as will be described in section (4.2). Two nodes at a coarse layer are joined by an edge if any of their children are joined by an edge.

The nodes are constrained to have a single parent (except for the nodes at the top layer which have no parent) and every node has at least one child (except for nodes at the bottom layer). We use the notation $C(\mu)$ for the children of μ, and $A(\mu)$ for the parent. A node μ on the bottom layer (i.e. on the lattice) has no children, and hence $C(\mu) = \emptyset$. We use the notation $N(\mu, \nu) = 1$ to indicate that nodes μ, ν on the same layer are neighbors, with $N(\mu, \nu) = 0$ otherwise.

At the top of the hierarchy, we define a special *root* layer of nodes comprised of a single node for each of the K model labels. We write $\overline{\mu}_k$ for these root nodes and use the notation $m_{\overline{\mu}_k}$ to denote the model variable associated with it. Each node is assigned a label that is constrained to be the label of its parent. Since, by construction, all non-root nodes can trace their ancestry back to a single root node, an instance of the graph G is equivalent to a labeled segmentation $\{m_\mu : \mu \in D\}$ of the image, see equation (1).

3.3 Recursive Computation of Energy

This section shows that we can decompose the energy into terms that can be assigned to each node of the hierarchy and computed recursively. This will be exploited in section (3.4) to enable us to rapidly compute the changes in energy caused by different graph shifts.

The energy function consists of regional and edge parts. These depend on the node descendants and, for the edge part, on the descendants of the neighbors. The regional energy E_1 for assigning a model m_μ to a node μ is defined recursively by:

$$E_1(\mu, m_\mu) = \begin{cases} E_1\left(\phi(\mathbf{I})(\mu), m_\mu\right) & \text{if } C(\mu) = \emptyset \\ \sum_{\nu \in C(\mu)} E_1(\nu, m_\mu) & \text{otherwise} \end{cases} \tag{2}$$

where $E_1\left(\phi(\mathbf{I})(\mu), m_\mu\right)$ is the energy at the voxel from equation (1). The edge energy E_2 between nodes μ_1 and μ_2, with models m_{μ_1} and m_{μ_2} is defined recursively by:

$$E_2(\mu_1, \mu_2, m_{\mu_1}, m_{\mu_2}) = \begin{cases} E_2(\mathbf{I}(\mu_1), \mathbf{I}(\mu_2), m_{\mu_1}, m_{\mu_2}) & \text{if } C(\mu_1) = C(\mu_2) = \emptyset \\ \sum_{\substack{\nu_1 \in C(\mu_1),\ \nu_2 \in C(\mu_2)\ : \\ N(\nu_1, \nu_2) = 1}} E_2(\nu_1, \nu_2, m_{\mu_1}, m_{\mu_2}) & \text{otherwise} \end{cases} \tag{3}$$

where $E_2(\mathbf{I}(\mu_1), \mathbf{I}(\mu_2), m_{\mu_1}, m_{\mu_2})$ is the edge energy for pixels/voxels in equation (1).

The overall energy (1) was specified at the voxel layer, but it can be computed at any layer of the hierarchy. For example, it can be computed at the top layer by:

$$E\left(\{m_{\overline{\mu}_k} : k = 1, ..., K\}\right) = \sum_{k=1}^{K} E_1(\overline{\mu}_k, m_{\overline{\mu}_k}) + \frac{1}{2} \sum_{\substack{i,j:1,..,K \\ N(\overline{\mu}_i, \overline{\mu}_j) = 1}} E_2(\overline{\mu}_i, \overline{\mu}_j, m_{\overline{\mu}_i}, m_{\overline{\mu}_j}). \tag{4}$$

3.4 Graph-Shifts

The basic idea of the graph-shifts algorithm is to allow a node μ to change its parent to the parent $A(\nu)$ of a neighboring node ν, as shown in figure (1). We will represent this shift as $\mu \rightarrow \nu$.

This shift not have any effect on the labeling of nodes unless the new parent has a different label than the old one (i.e. when $m_{A(\mu)} \neq m_{A(\nu)}$, or equivalently, $m_\mu \neq m_\nu$). In this case, the change in parents will cause the node and its descendants to change their labels to that of the new parent. This will alter the labeling of the nodes on the image lattice and hence will change the energy.

Consequently, we only need consider shifts between neighbors which have different labels. We can compute the changes in energy, or *shift-gradient* caused by these shifts by using the energy functions assigned to the nodes, as described in section (3.3). For example, the shift from μ to ν corresponds to a shift-gradient $\Delta E(\mu \rightarrow \nu)$:

$$\Delta E(\mu \rightarrow \nu) = E_1(\mu, m_\nu) - E_1(\mu, m_\mu) + \sum_{\eta : N(\mu,\eta)=1} \left[E_2(\mu, \eta, m_\nu, m_\eta) - E_2(\mu, \eta, m_\mu, m_\eta) \right] . \qquad (5)$$

The graph-shifts algorithm begins by initializing the graph hierarchy (section 4.2). Then we calculate the shift-gradients of all the shifts using equations (2),(3), and (5). We exploit recursion to calculate these shift-gradients extremely rapidly, see section (4.3). In practice, very few of the neighbors in the hierarchy have different labels and so the shift-gradients only need be computed for a small fraction of the total nodes. We throw away all shift-gradients which are positive or zero, since these shifts do not decrease the energy. The remaining shift-gradients are stored in a sorted, or unsorted, *shift-gradient list*, denoted S in figure 2 (we discuss the tradeoffs in section 4.3).

Graph-shifts proceeds by selecting the steepest shift-gradient in the list and makes the corresponding shift in the hierarchy. This changes the labels in the part of the hierarchy where the shift occurs, but leaves the remainder of the hierarchy unchanged. The algorithm recomputes the shift-gradients in the changed part of the hierarchy and updates the weight list. We repeat the process until convergence, when the shift-gradient list is empty (i.e. all shift-gradients in the graph are positive or zero).

GRAPH-SHIFTS

Input: Volume **I** on lattice D.
Output: Label volume **L** on lattice D.

0 Initialize graph hierarchy (figure 3).
1 Compute exhaustive set of potential shifts S.
2 while S is not empty
3   $s \leftarrow$ the shift in S that best reduces the energy.
4   Apply shift s to the graph.
5   Update affected region and edge properties.
6   Recompute affected shifts on boundary and update S. (5 & 6 discussed in section 4)
7 Compute label volume **L** from final hierarchy.

Fig. 2. Graph-shifts pseudo-code

Each shift is chosen to maximally decrease the energy, and so the algorithm is guaranteed to converge to, at least, a local minimum of the energy function. The algorithm prefers to select shifts at the coarser layers of the hierarchy, because these typically alter the labels of many nodes on the lattice and cause large changes in energy. These large changes can ensure that the algorithm can escape from some bad local minima.

4 Segmentation of 3D Medical Images

Now we describe the specific application to sub-cortical structures. The specific energy function is given in section (4.1). Sections (4.2) and (4.3) describe the initialization and how the shifts are computed and selected for the graph-shifts algorithm.

4.1 The Energy

Our implementation uses eight models for sub-cortical structures together with a background model for everything else. The regional terms $E_1(\mu, m_\mu)$ in the energy function (1) contain local evidence that a voxel μ is assigned a label m_μ. This local evidence will depend on a small region surrounding the voxel and hence is influenced by the local image context. We learn this local evidence from training data where the labeling is given by an expert.

We apply the probabilistic boosting tree (PBT) algorithm [18] to output a probability distribution $P(m_\mu|\phi(\mathbf{I})(\mu))$ for the label m_μ at voxel $\mu \in D$ conditioned on the response of a nonlinear filter $\phi(\mathbf{I})(\mu)$. This filter depends on voxels within an $11 \times 11 \times 11$ window centered on μ, and hence takes local image context into account. The non-linear filter ϕ is learned by the PBT algorithm which is an extension of the AdaBoost algorithm [19], [20]. PBT builds the filter $\phi(.)$ by combining a large number of elementary image features. These are selected from a set of 5,000 features which include Haar basis functions and histograms of the intensity gradient. The features are combined using weights which are also learned by the training algorithm.

We define the regional energy term by:

$$E_1(\mu, m_\mu) = -\log P(m_\mu|\phi(\mathbf{I})(\mu)), \tag{6}$$

which can be thought of as a pseudolikelihood approximation [18].

The edge energy term can take two forms. We can use it to either penalize the length of the segmentation boundaries, or to penalize the intensity edge strength along the segmentation boundaries. This gives two alternatives:

$$E_2(\mathbf{I}(\nu), \mathbf{I}(\mu), m_\nu, m_\mu) = 1 - \delta_{m_\nu, m_\mu}, \tag{7}$$

$$E_2(\mathbf{I}(\nu), \mathbf{I}(\mu), m_\nu, m_\mu) = \{1 - \delta_{m_\nu, m_\mu}\}\psi(\mathbf{I}(\mu), \mathbf{I}(\nu)),. \tag{8}$$

where $\psi(\mathbf{I}(\mu), \mathbf{I}(\nu))$ is a statistical likelihood measure of an edge between μ and ν; a simple example of such a measure is given in equation (9).

4.2 Initializing the Hierarchy

We propose a stochastic algorithm to quickly initialize the graph hierarchy that will be used during the graph shifts process. The algorithm recursively coarsens the graph by activating some edges according to the intensity gradient in the volume and grouping the resulting connected components up to a single node in the coarser graph layer. The coarsening procedure begins by defining a binary edge activation variable $e_{\mu\nu}$ on each edge in the current graph layer G^t between neighboring nodes μ and ν (i.e., $N(\mu,\nu)=1$). The edge activation variables are then sampled according to

$$e_{\mu\nu} \sim \gamma\mathcal{U}(\{0,1\}) + (1-\gamma)\exp\left[-\alpha\left|\mathbf{I}(\mu)-\mathbf{I}(\nu)\right|\right] \tag{9}$$

where $\mathcal{U}$ is the uniform distribution on the binary set and γ is a relative weight between $\mathcal{U}$ and the conventional edge gradient affinity (right-hand side).

After the edge activation variables are sampled, a connected components algorithm is used to form node-groups based on the edge activation variables. The size of a connected component is constrained by a threshold τ, which governs the relative degree of coarsening between two graph layers. On the next graph layer, a node is created for each component. Following, edges in the new graph layer are induced by the connectivity on the current layer; i.e., two nodes in the coarse graph are connected if any two of their children are connected. The algorithm recursively executes this coarsening procedure until the size of the coarsened graph is within the range of the number of models, specified by a scalar β. Complete pseudo-code for this hierarchy initialization is given in figure 3.

Let G^T be the top layer of the graph hierarchy after initialization (example in figure 3(b)). Then, we append a model layer G^M on the hierarchy that contains a single node per model. Each node in G^T becomes the child of the node in G^M to which it has best fit, which is determined by evaluating the model fit $P(m|\mu)$ defined in section 4.1. One necessary constraint is that each node in G^M has at least one child in G^T, which is enforced by first linking each node in G^M to the node in G^T with highest probability to its model and the remaining links are created as described earlier.

HIERARCHY INITIALIZATION

Input: Volume $\mathbf{I}$ on lattice D.
Output: Graph hierarchy with layers $G^0, \dots, G^T$.
Initialize graph G^0 from lattice D.
$t \leftarrow 0$.
repeat
  Sample edge activation variables in G^t using (9).
  Label every node in G^t as OPEN.
  while OPEN nodes remain in G^t.
    Create new, empty connected component C.
    Put a random OPEN node into queue Q.
    while Q is not empty and $|C| < 1/\tau$.
      $\mu \leftarrow$ removed head of Q.
      Add ν to Q, s.t. $N(\mu,\nu)=1$ and $e_{\mu\nu}=1$.
      Add μ to C, label μ as CLOSED.
    Create G^{t+1} with a node for each C.
    Define $\mathbf{I}(C)$ as mean intensity of its children.
    Inherit connectivity in G^{t+1} from G^t.
    $t \leftarrow t+1$.
until $|G^t| < \beta * K$.

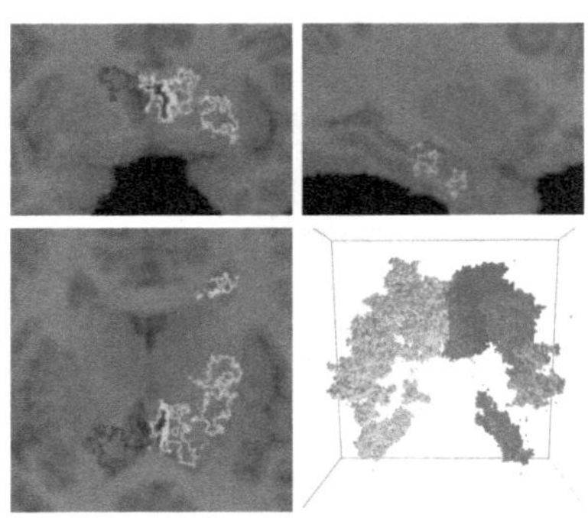

(b) Example initialization. Top-left is coronal, top-right is sagittal, bottom-left is axial, and bottom-right is a 3D view.

Fig. 3. Initialization pseudo-code (left) and example (right)

4.3 Computing and Selecting Graph-Shifts

The efficiency of the graph-shifts algorithm relies on fast computation of potential shifts and fast selection of the optimal shift every iteration. We now describe how to satisfy these two requirements. To quickly compute potential shifts, we use an energy caching strategy that evaluates the recursive energy formulas (2) and (3) for the entire graph hierarchy following its creation (section 4.2). At each node, we evaluate and store the energies, denoted $\hat{E}_1(\mu, m_\mu) \doteq E_1(\mu, m_\mu)$ and $\hat{E}_2(\mu, \nu, m_\mu, m_\nu) \doteq E_2(\mu, \nu, m_\mu, m_\nu)$ for all μ, ν: $N(\mu, \nu) = 1$. These are quickly calculated in a recursive fashion. The computational cost of initializing the energy cache is $O(n \log n)$.

Subsequently, we apply the cached energy to evaluate the shift-gradient (5) in the entire hierarchy; this computation is $O(1)$ with the cache. At each node, we store the shift with the steepest gradient (largest negative ΔE), and discard any shift with non-negative gradient. The remaining shifts are stored in the *potential shift list*, denoted S in figure 2. In the volumes we have been studying, this list is quite small: typically only about 2% of all edges numbering about 60,000 for volumes with 4 million voxels. The entire initialization including caching energies in the whole hierarchy takes 10 – 15 seconds on these volumes, which amounts to about 30% of the total execution time.

At step **??** in the graph-shifts algorithm (figure 2), we must find the optimal shift in the potential shift list. One can use a sorted or unsorted list to store the potential shifts, with tradeoffs to both; an unsorted list requires no initial computation, no extra computation to add to the list, but an $O(n)$ search at each iteration to find the best shift. The sorted list carries an initial $O(n \log n)$ cost, an $O(\log n)$ cost for adding, but is $O(1)$ for selecting the optimal shift. Since every shift will cause modifications to the potential shift list, and the size of the list decreases with time (as fewer potential shifts exist), we choose to store an unsorted list and expend the linear search at each iteration.

As the graph shifts are applied, it is necessary to dynamically keep the hierarchy in synch with the energy landscape. Recomputing the entire energy cache and potential shift set is prohibitively expensive. Fortunately, it is not necessary: by construction, a shift is a very local change to the solution and only affects nodes along the boundary of the recently shifted subgraph. The number of affected nodes is dependent on the node connectivity and the height of the graph (it is $O(\log n)$); the node connectivity is relatively small and constant since the coarsening is roughly isotropic, and the height of the graph is logarithmic in the number of input voxels.

First, we update the energy cache associated with each affected node. This amounts to propagating the energy change up the graph to the roots. Let $\mu \rightarrow \nu$ be the executed shift. The region energy update must remove the energy contribution to $A(\mu)$ and add it to $A(\nu)$, which is the new parent of μ after the shift. The update rule is

$$\hat{E}_1(A(\mu), m_\mu))' = \hat{E}_1(A(\mu), m_\mu) - \hat{E}_1(\mu, m_\mu) \quad (10)$$

$$\hat{E}_1(A(\nu), m_\nu))' = \hat{E}_1(A(\nu), m_\nu) + \hat{E}_1(\mu, m_\nu) \ , \quad (11)$$

and it must be applied recursively to each parent until the root layer. Due to limited space, we do not discuss the details of the similar but more complicated procedure to update the edge energy cache terms $\hat{E}_2$. Both procedures are also $O(\log n)$.

Second, we update the potential shifts given the change in the hierarchy. All nodes along the shift boundary both below and above the shift layer must be updated because the change in the energy could result in changes to the shift-gradients, new potential shifts, and expired potential shifts (between two now nodes with the same model). Generally, this remains a small set since the shifts are local moves. As before, at each of these nodes, we compute and store the shift with the steepest negative gradient using the cached energies and discard any shift with a non-negative gradient or between two nodes with the same model. There are $O(\log n)$ affected shifts.

5 Experimental Results

A dataset of 28 high-resolution 3D SPGR T1-weighted MR images was acquired on a GE Signa 1.5T scanner as series of 124 contiguous 1.5 mm coronal slices

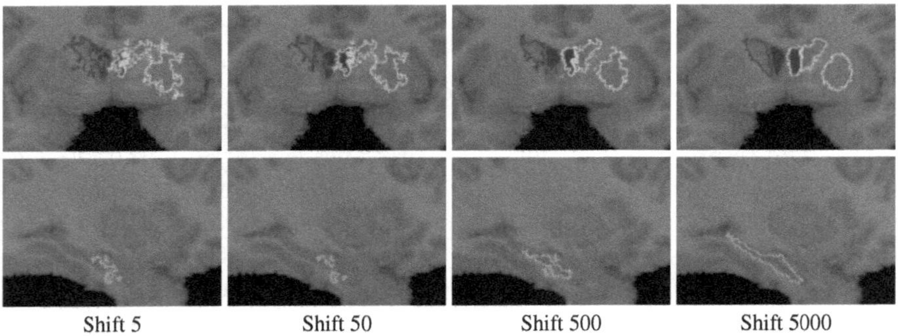

Fig. 4. Example of the graph-shifts process sampled during the minimization. Coronal and sagittal planes are shown, top and bottom respectively.

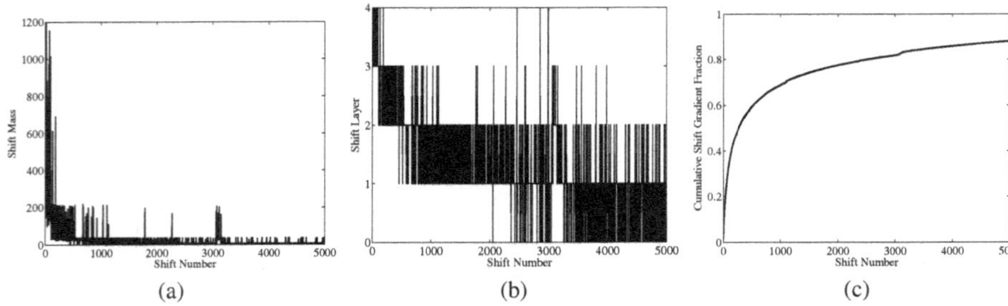

Fig. 5. (a) Graph shows the number of voxels (mass) that are moved per shift for 5000 shifts. (b) Graph shows the level in the hierarchy at which at shift occurs. (c) Graph shows the cumulative fraction of the total energy reduction that each shift effects.

(256x256 matrix; 20cm FOV). Brain volumes were roughly aligned and linearly scaled to perform 9 parameter registration. Four control points were manually given to perform this global registration. Expert neuro-anatomists manually labeled each volume into the following sub-cortical structures: hippocampus (LH, RH for left and right, resp. shown in green in figures), caudate (LC, RC in blue), putamen (LP, RP in purple), and ventricles (LV, RV, in red). We arbitrarily split the dataset in half and use 14 subjects for training and 14 for testing. The training volumes are used to learn the PBT region models and the boundary presence models. During the hierarchy initialization, we set the τ parameter to 0.15. We experimented with different values for τ, and found that varying it does not greatly affect the segmentation result.

The graph-shifts algorithm is very fast. We show an example process in figure 4 (this is the same volume as in figure 3(b)). Initialization, including the computation of the initial potential shift set, takes about 15 seconds. The remaining part of the graph shifts normally takes another 35 seconds to converge on a standard Linux PC workstation (2GB memory, 3Ghz cpu). Convergence occurs when no potential energy-reducing shift remains. Our speed is orders of magnitude faster than reported estimates on 3D medical segmentation: Yang et al. [13] is 120 minutes, FreeSurfer [5] is 30 minutes, Region Competition (PDE, obtained from a local implementation) is 5 minutes.

In figure 5-(c), we show the cumulative weight percentage of the same sequence of graph-shifts as figure 4. Here, we see that about 75% of the total energy reduction occurs within the first 1000 graph shifts. This large, early energy reduction corresponds to the shifts that occur at high layers in the hierarchy and have large masses as depicted in figure 5-(a) and (b). The mass of a shift is the number of voxels that are relabeled as a result of the operation. Yet, it is also clear from the plots that the graph-shifts at all levels at considered throughout the minimization process; recall, at any given time the potential shift list stores all energy reducing shifts and chooses the best one. Considering the majority of the energy reduction happens in the early stages of the graph-shift process, it is possible to stop the algorithm early when the shift gradient drops below a certain threshold.

In figure 6, we compare the total energy reduction of the dynamic hierarchical graph-shifts algorithm to the more conventional PDE-type energy minimization approach. To keep a fair comparison, we use the same structure and initial conditions in both cases. However, to approximate a PDE-type approach, we restrict the graph shifts to occur across single voxel boundaries (at the lowest layer in the hierarchy) only. As expected, the large-mass moves effect an exponential decrease in energy while the decrease from the single voxel moves is roughly linear.

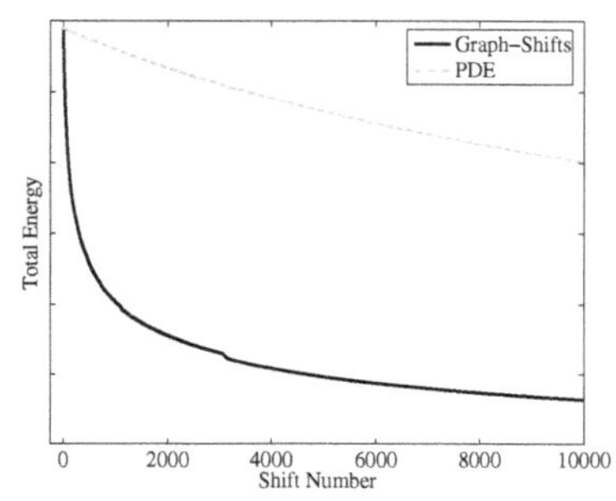

Fig. 6. Total energy reduction comparison of graph-shifts to a PDE method

Table 1. Segmentation accuracy using volume and surface measurements. A comparison to the FreeSurfer method run on the same data is included for the volume measurements in table 2.

	Training Set								Testing Set							
	LH	RH	LC	RC	LP	RP	LV	RV	LH	RH	LC	RC	LP	RP	LV	RV
Prec.	82%	70%	86%	86%	77%	81%	86%	86%	80%	58%	82%	84%	74%	74%	85%	85%
Rec.	60%	58%	82%	78%	72%	72%	88%	87%	61%	49%	81%	76%	67%	68%	87%	86%
Haus.	11.4	21.6	10.1	11.7	14.7	11.6	26.9	19.0	17.1	26.8	10.4	10.1	15.7	13.7	20.8	21.5
Mean	1.6	4.0	1.1	1.1	2.3	1.8	1.0	0.8	1.8	7.6	1.2	1.2	2.7	2.5	0.9	0.9
Med.	1.1	3.1	1.0	1.0	1.4	1.2	0.4	0.3	1.1	6.9	1.0	1.0	1.6	1.6	0.4	0.5

To quantify the accuracy of the segmentation, we use the standard volume (precision and recall), and surface distance (Hausdorff, mean and median) measurements. These are presented in table 1; in each case, the average over the set is given. In these experiments, we weighted the unary term four times as strong as the binary term; the power of the discriminative, context-sensitive models takes the majority of the energy while the binary term enforces local continuity and smoothness. Our accuracy is comparable or superior to the current state of the art in sub-cortical segmentation. To make a quantitative comparison, we computed the same scores using the FreeSurfer [5] method on the same data (results in table 2). We show a visual example of the segmentation in figure 7.

Table 2. FreeSurfer [5] accuracy

	LH	RH	LC	RC	LP	RP	LV	RV
Prec.	48%	51%	77%	78%	70%	76%	81%	69%
Rec.	67%	75%	78%	76%	83%	83%	76%	71%
Haus.	25.3	11.5	23.0	26.1	13.1	10.8	31.9	51.8
Mean	3.9	2.1	1.9	2.0	1.8	1.4	1.8	9.6
Med.	2.1	1.5	1.0	1.0	1.3	1.0	0.9	3.9

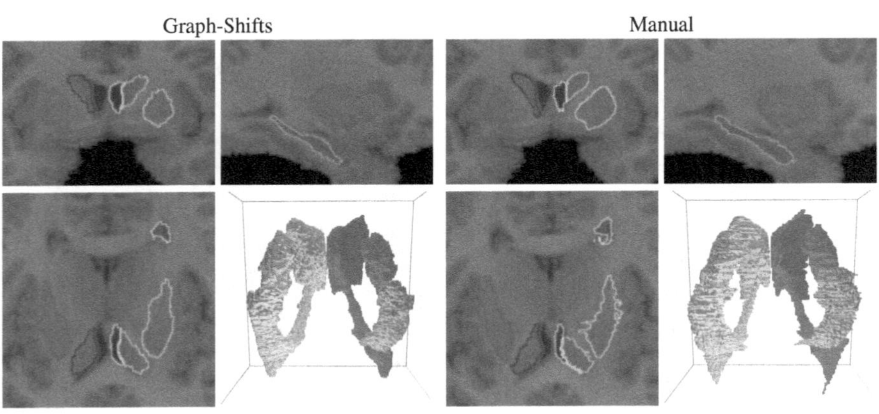

Fig. 7. An example of the sub-cortical structure segmentation result using the graph-shifts algorithm

Next, we show the graph-shifts algorithm is robust to initialization. We systematically perturbed the initial hierarchy by taking random shifts with positive gradient to increase the energy by 50%. Then, we started the graph-shifts from the degraded initial condition. In all cases, graph-shifts converged to (roughly) the same minimum; to quantify it, we calculated the standard deviation (SD) of the precision + recall score for over 100 instances. For all structures the SD is very small: LH: 0.0040, RH: 0.0011, LC: 0.0009, RC: 0.0013, LP: 0.0014, RP: 0.0013, LV: 0.0009, RV: 0.0014.

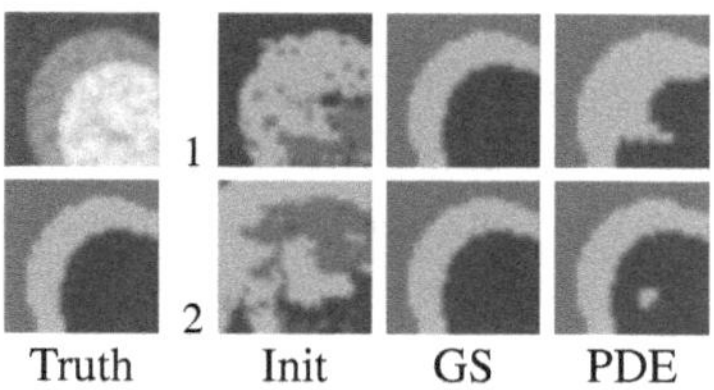

Fig. 8. Graph-shifts (GS) can avoid local minima. See text for details.

We now show that the large shifts provided by the hierarchical representation help avoid local minima in which PDE methods fall. We created a synthetic test image containing three separate i.i.d. Gaussian-distributed brightness models (depicted as red, green, and blue regions in figure 8). Following a similar perturbation as described above, we ran the graph-shifts algorithm as well as a PDE algorithm to compute the segmentation and reach a minimum. As expected, the graph-shifts method successfully avoids local minima that the PDE method falls into; in figure 8, we show two such cases. In the figure, the left column shows the input image and true labeling; the next three columns show the initial state, the graph-shifts result and the PDE result for two cases (rows 1 and 2).

6 Conclusion

We proposed graph-shifts, a novel energy minimization algorithm that manipulates a dynamic hierarchical decomposition of the image volume to rapidly and robustly minimize an energy function. We defined the class of energy functions it can minimize, and derived the recursive energy on the hierarchy. We discussed how the energy functions can include terms that are learned from labeled training data. The dynamic hierarchical representation makes it possible to make both large and small changes to the segmentation in a single operation, and the energy caching approach provides a deterministic way to rapidly compute and select the optimal move at each iteration.

We applied graph-shifts to the segmentation of sub-cortical brain structures in high-resolution MR 3D volumes. The quantified accuracy for both volume and surface distances is comparable or superior to the state-of-the-art for this problem, and the algorithm converges orders of magnitude faster than conventional minimization methods (about a minute). We demonstrated quantitative robustness to initialization and avoidance of local minima in which local boundary methods (e.g., PDE) fell.

In this paper, we considered the class of energies which used fixed model terms that were learned from training data. We are currently exploring extensions to the graph-shifts algorithm that would update the model parameters during the minimization. To further improve sub-cortical segmentation, we are investigating a more sophisticated shape model as well as additional sub-cortical structures. Finally, we are conducting more comprehensive experiments using a larger dataset and cross-validation.

Acknowledgements

This work was funded by the National Institutes of Health through the NIH Roadmap for Medical Research, Grant U54 RR021813 entitled Center for Computational Biology (CCB). Information on the National Centers for Biomedical Computing can be obtained from `http://nihroadmap.nih.gov/bioinformatics`

References

1. Geman, S., Geman, D.: Stochastic Relaxation, Gibbs Distributions, and Bayesian Restoration of Images. IEEE Trans. on Pattern Analysis and Machine Intelligence 6, 721–741 (1984)
2. Zhu, S.C., Yuille, A.: Region Competition. IEEE Trans. on Pattern Analysis and Machine Intelligence 18(9), 884–900 (1996)
3. Boykov, Y., Veksler, O., Zabih, R.: Fast Approximate Energy Minimization via Graph Cuts. IEEE Trans. on Pattern Analysis and Machine Intelligence 23(11), 1222–1239 (2001)
4. Tu, Z., Zhu, S.C.: Image Segmentation by Data-Driven Markov Chain Monte Carlo. IEEE Trans. on Pattern Analysis and Machine Intelligence 24(5), 657–673 (2002)
5. Fischl, B., Salat, D.H., et al.: Whole brain segmentation: Automated labeling of neuroanatomical structures in the human brain. Neuron 33, 341–355 (2002)
6. Pohl, K.M., Fisher, J., Kikinis, R., Grimson, W.E.L., Wells, W.M.: A Bayesian Model for Joint Segmentation and Registration. NeuroImage 31, 228–239 (2006)
7. Chan, T.F., Shen, J.: Image Processing and Analysis: Variational, PDE, Wavelet, and Stochastic Methods. Soc. for Industrial and Applied Mathematics (SIAM), Phil., PA (2005)
8. Kolmogorov, V., Zabih, R.: What Energy Functions Can Be Minimized via Graph Cuts? In: Heyden, A., Sparr, G., Nielsen, M., Johansen, P. (eds.) ECCV 2002. LNCS, vol. 2352, pp. 65–81. Springer, Heidelberg (2002)
9. Sharon, E., Brandt, A., Basri, R.: Fast Multiscale Image Segmentation. In: IEEE Conf. on Computer Vision and Pattern Recognition 2002, vol. I, pp. 70–77 (2000)
10. Barbu, A., Zhu, S.C.: Multigrid and Multi-level Swendsen-Wang Cuts for Hierarchic Graph Partitions. IEEE Computer Vision and Pattern Recognition, 731–738 (2004)
11. Vincken, K., Koster, A., Viergever, M.A.: Probabilistic Multiscale Image Segmentation. IEEE Trans. on Pattern Analysis and Machine Intelligence 19(2), 109–120 (1997)
12. Tu, Z.: An Integrated Framework for Image Segmentation and Perceptual Grouping. In: International Conference on Computer Vision 2005 (2005)
13. Yang, J., Staib, L.H., Duncan, J.S.: Neighbor-Constrained Segmentation with Level Set Based 3D Deformable Models. IEEE Trans. on Medical Imaging 23(8) (2004)

14. Pizer, S.M., Fletcher, P.T., et al.: Deformable m-reps for 3d medical image segmentation. International Journal of Computer Vision 55, 85–106 (2003)
15. Cocosco, C., Zijdenbos, A., Evans, A.: A Fully Automatic and Robust Brain MRI Tissue Classification Method. Medical Image Analysis 7, 513–527 (2003)
16. Wyatt, P.P., Noble, J.A.: MAP MRF joint segmentation and registration. In: Conference on Medical Image Computing and Computer-Assisted Intervention 2002, pp. 580–587 (2002)
17. Lafferty, J., McCallum, A., Pereira, F.: Conditional Random Fields: Probabilistic Models for Segmenting and Labeling Sequence Data. In: Int. Conference on Machine Learning 2001 (2001)
18. Tu, Z.: Probabilistic Boosting-Tree: Learning Discriminative Models for Classification, Recognition, and Clustering. In: International Conference on Computer Vision 2005 (2005)
19. Freund, Y., Schapire, R.E.: A Decision-Theoretic Generalization of On-line Learning and an Application to Boosting. Journal of Computer and System Science 55(1), 119–139 (1997)
20. Schapire, R.E., Singer, Y.: Improved Boosting Algorithms Using Confidence-Rated Predictions. Machine Learning 37(3), 297–336 (1999)

High-Quality Consistent Meshing of Multi-label Datasets

J.-P. Pons[1], F. Ségonne[1], J.-D. Boissonnat[2], L. Rineau[2], M. Yvinec[2], and R. Keriven[3]

[1] WILLOW, ENPC / ENS / INRIA, Paris, France
[2] GEOMETRICA, INRIA, Sophia-Antipolis, France
[3] ODYSSÉE, ENPC / ENS / INRIA, Paris, France

Abstract. In this paper, we extend some recent provably correct Delaunay-based meshing algorithms to the case of multi-label partitions, so that they can be applied to the generation of high-quality geometric models from labeled medical datasets. Our approach enforces watertight surface meshes free of self-intersections, and outputs surface and volume meshes of the different tissues which are consistent with each other, including at multiple junctions. Moreover, the abstraction of the tissue partition into an oracle that, given a point in space, answers which tissue it belongs to, makes our approach applicable to virtually any combination of data sources. Finally, our approach offers extensive control over the size and shape of mesh elements, through customizable quality criteria on triangular facets and on tetrahedra, which can be tuned independently for the different anatomical structures. Our numerical experiments demonstrate the effectiveness and flexibility of our approach for generating high-quality surface and volume meshes from real multi-label medical datasets.

1 Introduction

1.1 Motivation

The generation of realistic geometric patient models from high-resolution medical images is of great significance in many clinical and research applications. An increasing number of numerical simulations of physical or physiological processes (e.g. electroencephalography (EEG) and magnetoencephalography (MEG) [1,2], image-guided neurosurgery [3,4], electromagnetic modeling [5,6], ...) require geometrically-accurate and topologically-correct models. The latter consist either of surface meshes representing boundaries between different anatomical parts, or of volume meshes.

However, due to the lack of reliable fully-automated tools for the unstructured discretization of medical datasets, simplistic geometric models are still of wide use. For example, in electromagnetic modeling, such as specific absorption rate studies, for which finite element methods (FEM) on unstructured grids conforming to anatomical structures would be desirable [6], most numerical simulations have been conducted using finite difference methods on rectilinear grids, although the poor definition of tissue boundaries (stair-casing effect) strongly limits their accuracy. Similarly, in the EEG/MEG source localization problem using the boundary element method (BEM), as pointed out in [2], popular simplistic head models consisting of nested tissue layers may yield a significantly lower accuracy than realistic models featuring multiple junctions.

N. Karssemeijer and B. Lelieveldt (Eds.): IPMI 2007, LNCS 4584, pp. 198–210, 2007.
© Springer-Verlag Berlin Heidelberg 2007

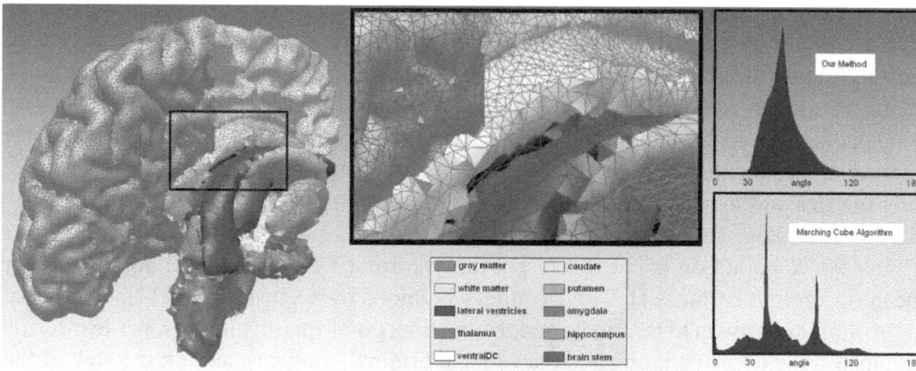

Fig. 1. Surface meshes. *Left:* Meshing the boundaries of brain tissues with a tissue-dependent resolution. We requested the cortical surface (colored in dark gray) to have a resolution twice higher than other tissues. As a result, output surface meshes of other anatomical structures have a coarse resolution except in *local* regions where they neighbor gray matter. This is apparent in the magnified view of the white matter mesh (in light gray), in which the gray matter interface has been partially removed for visualization purposes. *Right:* The quality of the obtained surface meshes is much higher than with the marching cubes algorithm.

In addition to accuracy, geometric patient models often have to fulfill several requirements in terms of smoothness, number, size and shape of mesh elements, sampling density, among others, in order to obtain acceptable results and make useful predictions, avoid instabilities in the simulations, or simply reduce the overall processing time. For instance, during image-guided neurosurgery, real-time constraints impose strong limitations on the complexity of the geometric brain model being dynamically registered onto the patient anatomy [3].

1.2 Previous Work

While different strategies can be used to obtain realistic geometric models from labeled medical datasets, few of them offer sufficient flexibility: handling of data coming from different sources, control over the density and quality of the mesh elements. Also, most existing approaches have been designed to extract surface meshes corresponding to boundaries between labeled anatomical structures, hence necessitating post-processing steps to generate volume meshes needed by finite element methods.

The most celebrated technique for producing surface meshes from sampled data is undoubtedly the *marching cubes* algorithm, introduced by Lorensen and Cline [7], and its variants (e.g. [8]). Given a scalar field sampled on a rectilinear grid, the marching cubes algorithm efficiently generates a triangular mesh of an isosurface by tessellating each cubic cell of the domain according to a case table constructed off-line.

Initially dedicated to binary classification, this method has been extended to non-binary volumes [9,10,11,12]. Unfortunately, these techniques produce unnecessarily large meshes (at least one triangle per boundary voxel) of very low quality (lots of skinny triangles). Frequently, the resulting meshes have to be regularized, optimized and decimated in order to obtain suitable representations, while simultaneously controlling the approximation accuracy and preserving some topological properties, such as the absence of self-intersections, which turns out to be a difficult task.

Delaunay-based meshing is recognized as one of the most powerful techniques for generating surface and volume meshes with guaranteed quality. It offers easy control over the size and shape of mesh elements, for instance through a (possibly non-uniform) sizing field.

Our work builds on some recent provably correct Delaunay-based algorithms for meshing smooth surfaces [13] and volumes bounded by such surfaces [14]. These two algorithms are proven to terminate and to construct good-quality meshes, while offering bounds on the approximation accuracy of the original boundary and on the size of the output mesh. The refinement process is controlled by highly customizable quality criteria on triangular facets and on tetrahedra. A notable feature of the method of Boissonnat and Oudot [13] is that the surface needs only to be known through an oracle that, given a line segment, detects whether the segment intersects the surface and, in the affirmative, returns an intersection point. This makes the algorithm useful in a wide variety of contexts and for a large class of surfaces. Very recently, Oudot, Rineau and Yvinec [14] have proposed to combine the latter Delaunay-based surface mesher with a Delaunay refinement volume mesher [15]. This algorithm has the particularity of sampling the interior and the boundary of the object at the same time.

However, the case of multi-label partitions is not addressed in these works, therefore restricting their applicability to real datasets. The contribution of our paper is to reformulate the two above methods in the non-binary perspective.

1.3 Novelty of Our Approach

Our work extends the method of Boissonnat and Oudot [13] and the method of Oudot, Rineau and Yvinec [14] to the case of multi-label partitions, so that they can be applied to the generation of high-quality geometric models from labeled medical datasets.

To that end, we define a *partition of Delaunay tetrahedra induced by a space subdivision*. It is related to the concept of *restricted Delaunay triangulation*, borrowed from computational geometry. In our approach, the subdivision of the domain of interest is approximated by a discrete partition of the Delaunay tetrahedralization of a point set: each Delaunay tetrahedron is labeled with one adequate tissue type. Output surface meshes are composed of the triangular facets adjacent to two tetrahedra having different labels. The point set is iteratively refined until it forms a "good" sample of the boundaries between the different anatomical structures, and, if a quality volume mesh is desired, a "good" sample of their interior.

Interestingly, our approach directly enforces watertight surface meshes free of self-intersections. Also, the consistency of surface meshes and volume meshes of the different tissues with each other is guaranteed by construction, including at multiple junctions.

Another notable feature of our approach is that the continuous partition need not to be represented explicitly. It is known only through a *labeling oracle* that, given a point in space, answers which tissue it belongs to. This makes our approach applicable to virtually any combination of data sources, including labeled 3D images, polyhedral surfaces, unstructured volume meshes, fuzzy membership functions, possibly having different resolutions and different coordinate systems. The different data sources may even be inconsistent with each other due to noise or discretization artefacts. In this case, the labeling oracle has the responsibility of resolving the conflicts using some user-defined rules. As a result, our meshing algorithm is not affected by the heterogeneity and possible inconsistency of the input datasets.

Finally, another major advantage of our approach is that the customizable quality criteria on boundary facets and/or on tetrahedra can be tuned independently for the different anatomical structures.

The remainder of this paper is organized as follows. Section 2 gives some background on the basic computational geometry concepts needed in our approach: Voronoi diagrams, Delaunay triangulations and restricted Delaunay triangulations. Our method is described in Sect. 3. In Sect. 4, we report on some numerical experiments which demonstrate the effectiveness and flexibility of our approach for generating high-quality surface and volume meshes from real multi-label medical datasets.

2 Background

2.1 Voronoi Diagram and Delaunay Triangulation

Voronoi diagrams are versatile structures which encode proximity relationships between objects. They are particularly relevant to perform nearest neighbor search and motion planning (e.g. in robotics), and to model growth processes (e.g. crystal growth in materials science). Delaunay triangulations, which are geometrically dual to Voronoi diagrams, are a classical tool in the field of mesh generation and mesh processing due to its optimality properties.

Most of the following definitions are taken from [13]. We also refer the interested reader to some computational geometry textbooks [16,17].

In the sequel, we call *k-simplex* the convex hull of $k+1$ affinely independent points. For example, a 0-simplex is a point, a 1-simplex is a line segment, a 2-simplex is a triangle and a 3-simplex is a tetrahedron.

Let $E = \{p_1, \ldots, p_n\}$ be set of points in $\mathbb{R}^d$. Note that in this work, we are mainly interested in $d = 3$. The *Voronoi region*, or *Voronoi cell*, denoted by $V(p_i)$, associated to a point p_i is the region of space that is closer from p_i than from all other points in E:

$$V(p_i) = \{p \in \mathbb{R}^d \ : \ \forall j, \ \|p - p_i\| \leq \|p - p_j\|\} \ . \tag{1}$$

$V(p_i)$ is the intersection of $n-1$ half-spaces bounded by the bisector planes of segments $[p_i p_j]$, $j \neq i$. $V(p_i)$ is therefore a convex polytope, possibly unbounded. The *Voronoi diagram* of E, denoted by $\text{Vor}(E)$, is the partition of space induced by the Voronoi cells $V(p_i)$.

See Fig. 2*(a)* for a two-dimensional example of a Voronoi diagram In two dimensions, the edges shared by two Voronoi cells are called *Voronoi edges* and the points shared by three Voronoi cells are called *Voronoi vertices*. Similarly, in three dimensions, we term *Voronoi facets, edges* and *vertices* the geometric objects shared by one, two and three Voronoi cells, respectively. The Voronoi diagram is the collection of all

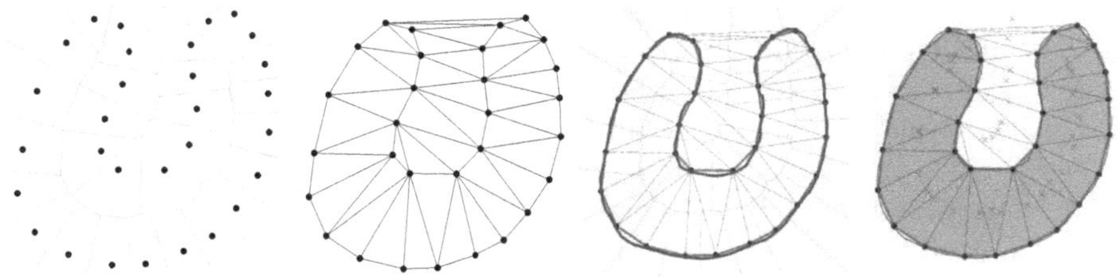

Fig. 2. *(a)* Voronoi diagram of a set ot points in the plane. *(b)* Its dual Delaunay triangulation. *(c)* The Delaunay triangulation restricted to the blue curve is plotted with a thick red line. *(d)* The Delaunay triangulation restricted to the region bounded by the blue curve is composed of the filled red triangles, whose circumcenters (blue crosses) are inside the region.

these k-dimensional objects, with $0 \leq k \leq d$, which we call *Voronoi objects*. In particular, note that Voronoi cells $V(p_i)$ correspond to d-dimensional Voronoi objects.

The *Delaunay triangulation* $\text{Del}(E)$ of E is defined as the geometric dual of the Voronoi diagram: there is an edge between two points p_i and p_j in the Delaunay triangulation if and only if their Voronoi cells $V(p_i)$ and $V(p_j)$ have a non-empty intersection. It yields a *triangulation* of E, that is to say a partition of the convex hull of E into d-dimensional simplices (i.e. into triangles in 2D, into tetrahedra in 3D and so on).

The fundamental property of the Delaunay triangulation is called the *empty circle* (resp. *empty sphere* in 3D) property: in 2D (resp. in 3D), a triangle (resp. tetrahedron) belongs to the Delaunay triangulation if and only if its circumcircle (resp. circumsphere) does not contain any other points of E in its interior.

The algorithmic complexity of the Delaunay triangulation of n points is $\mathcal{O}(n \log n)$ in 2D, and $\mathcal{O}(n^2)$ in 3D. Fortunately, as was recently proven in [18], the complexity in 3D drops to $\mathcal{O}(n \log n)$ when the points are distributed on a smooth surface, which is the case of interest here.

2.2 Restricted Delaunay Triangulation

Each k-simplex in the Delaunay triangulation is dual to a $(d-k)$-dimensional Voronoi object. In 3D, the dual of a Delaunay tetrahedron is the Voronoi vertex which coincides with the circumcenter of the tetrahedron, the dual of a Delaunay facet is a Voronoi edge, the dual of a Delaunay edge is a Voronoi facet, and the dual of a Delaunay vertex p_i is the Voronoi cell $V(p_i)$.

Given a subset $\Omega \in \mathbb{R}^d$, typically a manifold of dimension $k \leq d$, we call the *Delaunay triangulation of E restricted to Ω*, and we note $\text{Del}|_\Omega(E)$ the subcomplex of $\text{Del}(E)$ composed of the Delaunay simplices whose dual Voronoi objects intersect Ω. For example, in 2D, as illustrated in Fig. 2*(c)*, the Delaunay triangulation restricted to a curve C is composed of the Delaunay edges whose dual Voronoi edges intersect C. Similarly, as shown in Fig. 2*(d)*, the Delaunay triangulation restricted to a region R

is composed of the Delaunay triangles whose circumcenters are contained in R. The attentive reader may have noticed that in both cases the restricted Delaunay triangulation forms a good approximation of the object.

Actually, this is a general property of the restricted Delaunay triangulation. It can be shown that, under some assumptions, and especially if E is a "sufficiently dense" sample of Ω, in some sense defined in [19], $\mathrm{Del}|_{\Omega}(E)$ is a good approximation of Ω, both in a topological and in a geometric sense: as regards topology, $\mathrm{Del}|_{\Omega}(E)$ is homeomorphic to Ω; as regards geometry, the Hausdorff distance between $\mathrm{Del}|_{\Omega}(E)$ and Ω can be made arbitrarily small; normals and curvatures of Ω can be consistently approximated from $\mathrm{Del}|_{\Omega}(E)$.

Based on these approximation properties, a family of provably correct algorithms for mesh generation and mesh reconstruction from point clouds have been designed in the last decade. We refer the reader to [13] and references therein for more details.

3 Methods

3.1 Partition of Delaunay Tetrahedra

Let us consider $\mathcal{P} = \{\Omega_0, \Omega_1, \ldots, \Omega_n\}$ a partition of space into the background Ω_0 and n different tissues, i.e.

$$\mathbb{R}^3 = \sqcup_{i \in \{0,\ldots,n\}} \Omega_i \ , \tag{2}$$

and let Γ denote the boundaries of the partition:

$$\Gamma = \cup_i \delta\Omega_i \ . \tag{3}$$

Given a set of points E in $\mathbb{R}^3$, we define the *partition of Delaunay tetrahedra induced by* $\mathcal{P}$, denoted by $\mathrm{Del}|_{\mathcal{P}}(E)$, as the partition of the tetrahedra of $\mathrm{Del}(E)$ depending on the region containing their circumcenter. In other words,

$$\mathrm{Del}|_{\mathcal{P}}(E) = \{\mathrm{Del}|_{\Omega_0}(E), \ldots, \mathrm{Del}|_{\Omega_n}(E)\} \ ,$$

where $\mathrm{Del}|_{\Omega_i}(E)$ is the set of tetrahedra of $\mathrm{Del}(E)$ whose circumcenters are contained in Ω_i.

$\mathrm{Del}|_{\mathcal{P}}(E)$ induces mutually-consistent surface meshes and volume meshes of the different tissues. In particular, the surface meshes are composed of the triangular facets adjacent to two tetrahedra assigned to different tissues (i.e. belonging to different parts of $\mathrm{Del}|_{\mathcal{P}}(E)$) and of the convex hull facets adjacent to non-background tetrahedra. These facets are called *boundary facets* in the sequel.

It can be proven that the resulting surface and volume meshes form a good approximation of the original partition $\mathcal{P}$ as soon as E is a "sufficiently dense" sample of its boundaries, in some sense defined in [19]. The proof is omitted here due to space limitations. The outline of the proof is the same as in [13].

With this concept in hand, our meshing algorithm boils down to generating a point sample E which fulfills the above sampling condition as well as some additional user-defined quality criteria on boundary facets and tetrahedra.

3.2 Incremental Construction of the Point Sample

Our algorithm for generating E closely parallels the surface meshing algorithm of Boissonnat and Oudot [13]. The algorithm starts with a small initial point sample E_0 of Γ and, at each iteration, it inserts a new point of Γ into E and updates $\mathrm{Del}|_{\mathcal{P}}(E)$. Each point inserted into E is the intersection between Γ and the dual of a boundary facet (that is to say, a ray or a segment of the Voronoi diagram of E). We call *surface Delaunay ball* of a boundary facet the ball circumscribing the boundary facet and centered on the intersection point. Note that such an intersection always exists, by construction. In case there are several intersections, any of them can be chosen, without compromising the good continuation of the algorithm. The algorithm stops when there are no bad boundary facets left.

The surface is known only through a *labeling oracle* that, given a point in space, answers which tissue it belongs to. This oracle can be formulated as a *labeling function* $L_{\mathcal{P}} : \mathbb{R}^3 \rightarrow \{0, \ldots, n\}$ associated to the partition $\mathcal{P}$, such that $L_{\mathcal{P}}(p) = i$ if and only if $p \in \Omega_i$. Intersections of a segment or a line with Γ can be computed to the desired accuracy using a dichotomic search on $L_{\mathcal{P}}$.

When high-quality volume meshes are needed in addition to quality surface meshes, this procedure is complemented with the refinement of bad tetrahedra by insertion of their circumcenter in E. This technique, pioneered by Ruppert [15], is known as *Delaunay refinement*. Very recently, Oudot, Rineau and Yvinec [14,20] have described how to properly combine these two meshing levels (facet refinement and tetrahedron refinement) in the binary case.

Under these considerations, the overview of our algorithm is given below:

```
while there is a bad boundary facet or a bad tetrahedron do
  if there is a bad boundary facet then
    let f be the worst boundary facet
    let p be an intersection between Γ and the dual of f
    insert p in E
  else {there is a bad tetrahedron}
    let c be the circumcenter of the worst tetrahedron
    if there is a boundary facet f whose surface Delaunay ball contains c then
      let p be the center of the surface Delaunay ball
      insert p in E
    else
      insert c in E
    end if
  end if
  update Del|P(E)
end while
```

3.3 Quality Criteria

In the above algorithm, the determination of "good" and "bad" boundary facets and tetrahedra is devoted to some user-defined criteria, that are typically a combination of thresholds on the following elementary quality measures:

- **Boundary facets:** *aspect ratio* (minimum angle), *size* (circumradius of surface Delaunay ball), *curvature* (distance between facet circumcenter and center of surface Delaunay ball), *edge length*, ...
- **Tetrahedra:** *aspect ratio* (ratio between tetrahedron circumradius and shortest edge length), *size* (tetrahedron circumradius), *edge length*, *minimum angle*, ...

Note that these thresholds are possibly non-uniform over space, which allows to locally increase accuracy in a region of interest, while keeping the total size of the geometric model, and hence the computational and memory cost, sustainable. This capability is illustrated in Experiment 2 in Sect. 4.

Another important source of flexibility of our approach is that the quality criteria can be tuned independently for the different anatomical structures. Thus, a boundary facet must be tested against the criteria of its two adjacent tissues. It is classified as a good facet if it fulfills both criteria. For example, as illustrated in Experiment 3 in Sect. 4, if different resolutions are required for the two tissues adjoining the facet, the higher resolution is enforced.

3.4 Sliver Removal

While Delaunay refinement techniques can be proven to generate tetrahedra with a good *radius-edge ratio* (ratio between tetrahedron circumradius and shortest edge length), they cannot guarantee against badly-shaped tetrahedra of a special type called *slivers*. A sliver is a tetrahedron whose four vertices lie close to a plane and whose projection to that plane is a quadrilateral with no short edge. Such tetrahedra have a good radius-edge ratio but a very poor *radius-radius ratio* (ratio between circumradius and radius of largest contained sphere). Unfortunately, the latter measure typically influences the numerical conditioning of finite element methods.

In order to remove slivers from our volume meshes, we use a post processing step called *sliver exudation* [21]. This step does not include any new vertex in the mesh, nor does it move any of them. Simply each vertex is assigned a weight and the Delaunay triangulation is turned into a Delaunay weighted triangulation. The weights are carefully computed in such a way that no vertex nor any boundary facet disappear from the mesh. Within these constraints, the weight of each vertex is chosen in turn to maximize the minimum dihedral angles of tetrahedra incident to that vertex. Although the guaranteed theoretical bound on radius-radius ratio is known to be miserably low, this algorithm is efficient in practice and generates almost sliver-free meshes.

3.5 Implementation Aspects

By using *CGAL* (Computational Geometry Algorithms Library, homepage: www.cgal.org) [22], we have been able to implement our approach with only 1000 lines of C++ code. CGAL defines all the needed geometric primitives and provides an excellent algorithm to compute the Delaunay triangulation in 3D: it is robust to degenerate configurations and floating-point error, thanks to the use of exact geometric predicates, while being able to process millions of points per minute on a standard workstation.

Moreover, the incremental surface meshing algorithm of Boissonnat and Oudot [13] is now available as a CGAL package. Although this algorithm is dedicated to restricted Delaunay triangulations, the code can be modified to compute the partition of Delaunay tetrahedra induced by a partition. Although this is not optimal as regards computation time, we have chosen this option for our prototype. Also, our implementation of sliver pumping could be heavily optimized.

4 Experimental Results

In order to illustrate the wide applicability and the high flexibility of the proposed algorithm, we generated several meshes from real labeled medical datasets, under various parameter settings. The parameters (number of tissues and refinement criteria) and the quantitative results (number of vertices, of boundary facets and of tetrahedra; computation time) of our different experiments are gathered in Table 1.

Table 1. Parameters and quantitative results of our different numerical experiments

Experiment	1	2	3	4
# tissues	15	72	72	77
# vertices	11K	36K	112K	389K
# boundary facets	23K	79K	228K	536K
# tetrahedra	73K	231K	728K	2370K
Time (sec)	35	54	340	1363 + 5080 (sliver pumping)
Refinement criteria	minimum angle $> 30°$			
	size < 1mm	non-uniform size		cortex: size < 1mm others: size < 2mm
				tets: radius-edge ratio < 2 cortex tets: size < 1.5mm other tets: no size constraint

Experiment 1: Uniform surface meshing. In a first experiment (Fig. 3-*Left*), we meshed the interfaces of a labeled MR angiography of iliac veins and arteries ([23]) with a *uniform* boundary facet quality criterion: the output surface meshes are required not to contain any triangle greater than $1mm$. The resulting angle distribution illustrates the high-quality of the surface meshes that do not contain any badly-shaped triangles - no triangle forms an angle smaller than 30° (or larger than 120°). Note also that the angle distribution peaks around 60°.

Experiment 2: Non-uniform surface meshing. In the three following experiments, we use some segmented brain data which were automatically generated from a T1-weighted magnetic resonance (MR) image using FreeSurfer's Whole Brain Segmentation tool [24].

The second experiment demonstrates the ability of our algorithm to produce surface meshes with non-uniform resolution (Fig. 3-*Right*). The facet size criterion was chosen to be spatially-varying so that the occipital cortex would be more finely sampled than the frontal cortex. Although for clarity, only four surfaces are displayed (for each hemisphere, the cortical and cerebellum surfaces), a total number of 72 tissues were meshed using the aforementioned criteria.

Experiment 3: Surface meshing with tissue-dependent resolution. Figure 1 displays brain anatomical interfaces meshed with different sampling resolutions - different boundary facet quality criteria were assigned to different anatomical structures. The resulting meshes are consistent with each other (i.e. common anatomical interfaces share the same mesh representation) and interfaces are meshed with the finer density required for the neighboring anatomical structures.

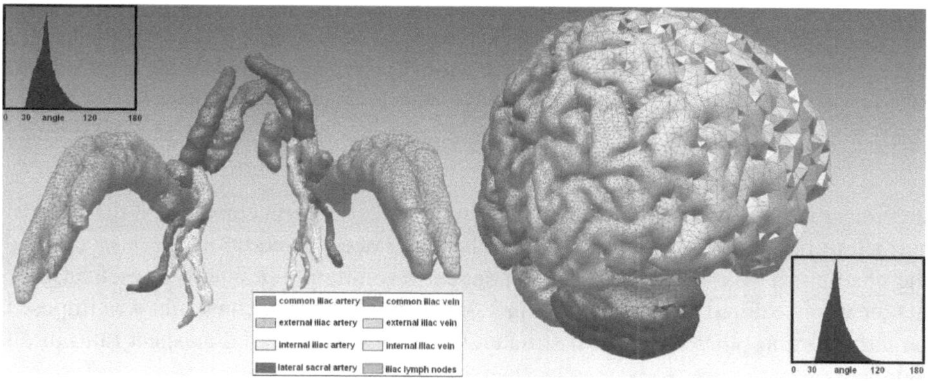

Fig. 3. Surface meshes. *Left:* Vascular mesh model, obtained by meshing uniformly 15 tissue interfaces. *Right:* Non-uniform surface meshing of brain tissues.

In this experiment, the cortical surface was required to have a finer resolution ($\leq 1mm$) than all other structures ($\leq 2mm$). Consequently, interfaces of anatomical structures other than cortical gray matter were meshed less densely, except for *local* regions where the structures were in contact with the cortex. This is clearly illustrated in the magnified region of Fig. 1, where the white matter interface is more densely meshed in regions that are in direct contact with gray matter.

In order to show the quality of the output surface meshes, we computed their angle distribution and compared it to the one of meshes extracted by a marching cubes algorithm [8]. Figure 1-*Right* shows both histograms. Contrarily to our method, which produces well-shaped triangles only, the MC algorithm yields meshes with lots of skinny triangles and whose angle distribution peaks around 45° and 90°.

Experiment 4: Surface and volume meshing with tissue-dependent resolution. The last experiment illustrates the ability of our method to generate high-quality consistent surface and volume meshes under elaborate tissue-dependent criteria. Similarly to the

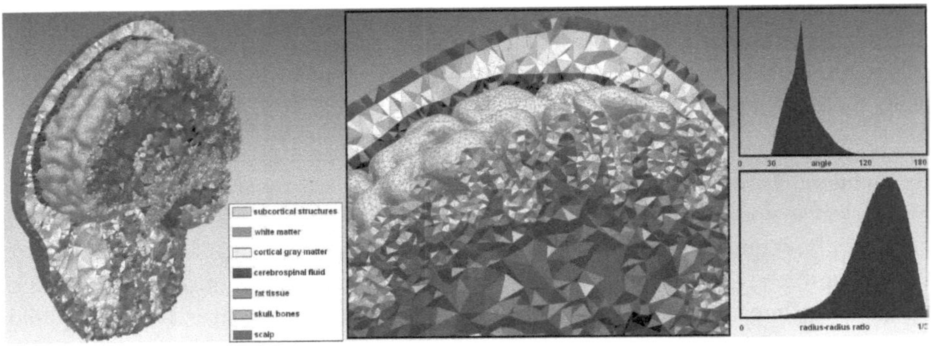

Fig. 4. Consistent tissue-dependent surface and volume meshes of head tissues. *Left:* The cortical surface and volume meshes (in yellow) both have a high resolution. Other anatomical structures have a coarser resolution except in regions adjacent to the cortex. *Center:* The magnified view exemplifies some consequences of tissue-dependent volume resolution: the unconstrained white matter tetrahedra (in red) become smaller as they approach the cortical surface. *Right:* Angle and radius-radius ratio distributions of surface meshes and volume meshes, respectively.

previous experiment, tissue-dependent boundary facet criteria constrained the cortical surface to be more finely meshed than other interfaces. In addition, we also meshed the anatomical volumes with tissue-dependent resolution. Tetrahedra in cortical gray matter were required to be smaller than $1.5mm$, while no size constraint was imposed on tetrahedra in other anatomical structures; on the other hand, the aspect ratio of all tetrahedra was required to be smaller than 2.

Figure 4 displays the resulting surface and volume meshes. Some cross-sections, obtained by cutting the models by different planes, reveal the high quality of tetrahedra. The surface meshes, which have tissue-dependent sampling densities, are consistent with the volume meshes. Note the size variation of white matter tetrahedra, which become very large as they get further from the cortical surface. The angle and radius-radius ratio distributions show that the obtained surface and volume meshes constitute high-quality geometric models of brain anatomical structures, well-adapted to numerical simulations.

5 Discussion and Conclusion

An increasing number of simulation tasks in clinical and research imaging necessitate more and more realistic geometric models (i.e. surface or volume meshes), whose elements (i.e. size, shape, number, ...) are often constrained by the numerical methods they are being designed for. The proposed approach has been designed to meet all these requirements, extensive control over the constructed meshes being achieved through two user-defined quality criteria on triangular facets and on tetrahedra (Sect. 3.3).

The produced models are watertight surface meshes, free of self-intersections and consistent with volume meshes of the different tissues. Contrarily to existing methods [14], the algorithm is not restricted to nested topologies and can handle multiple junctions. Our current implementation does not guarantee that each surface mesh constitutes a valid two-manifold when the resolution requested by the user is too low. A more elaborate refinement criterion automatically enforcing the manifold property is under development.

In conclusion, we have proposed a very flexible Delaunay-based technique for the generation of high-quality meshes from medical datasets. We plan to make our code available, and we hope that it will contribute to facilitate the creation of realistic geometric patient models.

References

1. Michel, C., Murray, M., Lantz, G., Gonzalez, S., Spinelli, L., de penalta, R.G: EEG source imaging. Clinical Neurophysiology 115(10), 2195–2222 (2004)
2. Kybic, J., Clerc, M., Faugeras, O., Keriven, R., Papadopoulo, T.: Generalized head models for MEG/EEG: boundary element method beyond nested volumes. Physics in Medicine and Biology 51, 1333–1346 (2006)
3. Warfield, S., Talos, F., Tei, A., Bharatha, A., Nabavi, A., Ferrant, M., Black, P., Ferenc, A., Kikinis, R.: Real-time registration of volumetric brain MRI by biomechanical simulation of deformation during image guided neurosurgery. Computing and Visualization in Science 5(1), 3–11 (2002)
4. Clatz, O., Litrico, S., Delingette, H., Ayache, N.: Dynamic model of communicating hydrocephalus for surgery simulation. IEEE Transactions on Biomedical Engineering (2006)
5. Angelone, L., Vasios, C., Wiggins, G., Purdon, P., Bonmassar, G.: On the effect of resistive EEG electrodes and leads during 7 Tesla MRI: simulation and temperature measurement studies. Magnetic Resonance Imaging 24, 801–812 (2006)
6. Scarella, G., Clatz, O., Lanteri, A., Beaume, G., Oudot, S., Pons, J.P., Piperno, S., Joly, P., Wiart, J.: Realistic numerical modelling of human head tissue exposure to electromagnetic waves from cellular phones. Comptes Rendus de l'Académie des Sciences - Physics 7(5), 501–508 (2006)
7. Lorensen, W., Cline, H.: Marching cubes: A high resolution 3d surface construction algorithm. ACM Computer Graphics 21(4), 163–170 (1987)
8. Natarajan, B.K.: On generating topologically consistent isosurfaces from uniform samples. The. Visual Computer 11(1), 52–62 (1994)
9. Bischoff, S., Kobbelt, L.: Extracting consistent and manifold interfaces from multi-valued volume data sets, (To appear) (2006)
10. Hege, H.C., Seebaß, M., Stalling, D., Zöckler, M.: A generalized marching cubes algorithm based on non-binary classifications. ZIB Preprint SC-97-05 (1997)
11. Reitinger, B., Bornik, A., Beichel, R.: Consistent mesh generation for non-binary medical datasets (2005)
12. Yamazaki, S., Kase, K., Ikeuchi, K.: Non-manifold implicit surfaces based on discontinuous implicitization and polygonization. Geometric Modeling and Processing, 138 (2002)
13. Boissonnat, J.D., Oudot, S.: Provably good sampling and meshing of surfaces. Graphical Models 67, 405–451 (2005)
14. Oudot, S., Rineau, L., Yvinec, M.: Meshing volumes bounded by smooth surfaces. In: International Meshing Roundtable 2005, 203–219 (2005)
15. Ruppert, J.: A Delaunay refinement algorithm for quality 2-dimensional mesh generation. Journal of Algorithms 18(3), 548–585 (1995)
16. Boissonnat, J.D., Yvinec, M.: Algorithmic Geometry. Cambridge University Press, Cambridge (1998)

17. de Berg, M., van Kreveld, M., Overmars, M., Schwarzkopf, O.: Computational Geometry, Algorithms and Applications. Springer, Heidelberg (1997)
18. Attali, D., Boissonnat, J.D., Lieutier, A.: Complexity of the Delaunay triangulation of points on surfaces: the smooth case. In: An Symp. on Comp. Geom 2003, pp. 201–210 (2003)
19. Amenta, N., Bern, M.: Surface reconstruction by Voronoi filtering. Discrete and Computational Geometry 22, 481–504 (1999)
20. Rineau, L., Yvinec, M.: A generic software design for Delaunay refinement meshing. Computational Geometry: Theory and Applications (To appear, 2007)
21. Cheng, S.W., Dey, T., Edelsbrunner, H., Facello, M., Teng, S.H.: Sliver exudation. Journal of the ACM 47(5), 883–904 (2000)
22. Boissonnat, J.D., Devillers, O., Teillaud, M., Yvinec, M.: Triangulations in CGAL. In: Annual Symposium on Computational Geometry, pp. 11–18 (2000)
23. Harisinghani, M., Weissleder, R.: Sensitive, non-invasive detection of lymph node metastases. PLOS-Medicine 1(3), 67 (2004)
24. Fischl, B., Salat, D., Busa, E., Albert, M., Dieterich, M., Haselgrove, C., Van der Kouwe, A., Killinay, R., Kennedy, D., Klaveness, S., Montillo, A., Makris, N., Rosen, B., Dale, A.: Whole Brain Segmentation: Automated labeling of neuroanatomical structures in the human brain. Neuron 33, 341–355 (2002)

Digital Homeomorphisms in Deformable Registration

Pierre-Louis Bazin, Lotta Maria Ellingsen, and Dzung L. Pham

Johns Hopkins University, Baltimore, USA

Abstract. A common goal in deformable registration applications is to produce a spatial transformation that is diffeomorphic, thereby preserving the topology of structures being transformed. Because this constraint is typically enforced only on the continuum, however, topological changes can still occur within discretely sampled images. This work discusses the notion of homeomorphisms in digital images, and how it differs from the diffeomorphic/homeomorphic concepts in continuous spaces commonly used in medical imaging. We review the differences and problems brought by considering functions defined on a discrete grid, and propose a practical criterion for enforcing digital homeomorphisms in the context of atlas-based segmentation.

1 Introduction

Deformable image registration has established itself as an important field of medical image analysis. It has been proposed as a computational framework for the study of anatomy [1,2], and is perhaps most prevalent in the neuroimaging literature, having been used for studying brain development, aging, and disease [3,4,5].

Among the desirable features of deformable registration methods, the ability to preserve the topological structure of the imaged anatomy while adapting to varying shapes has been a central issue. Topology is usually invariant in normal anatomy, and is an instrumental property for cortical unfolding and morphometric analysis. Starting with the work of Christensen et al. [6], many registration methods have sought to generate diffeomorphic deformations, which are bijective, smooth, and maintain the topology of the underlying space being deformed. Obtaining rigorous diffeomorphisms is far from trivial, and several competing approaches have been proposed, most based on constraining the Jacobian of the deformation [7,8,9,10,11,12]. Other approaches do not explicitly enforce the diffeomorphism constraint, and instead rely on simply regularizing the computed deformation field that, given appropriate parameter selection, should result in a diffeomorphism [13,14,15,16].

The problem with these methods is that they consider the images being transformed to be continuous functions. This becomes an issue particularly in atlas or template-based segmentation applications, where the image is made of a collection of solid objects. It can be shown that without proper care, the topology of the objects in a discretely sampled image is not guaranteed to be preserved after transformation, even when the Jacobian is constrained. Changes in topology can occur even in simple transformations, such as rotations. The main reason behind such a counter-intuitive result is the fact that topological properties of digital images can not be preserved based on constraining the transformation alone. One must consider the scale of the digital grid, its connectivity,

N. Karssemeijer and B. Lelieveldt (Eds.): IPMI 2007, LNCS 4584, pp. 211–222, 2007.
© Springer-Verlag Berlin Heidelberg 2007

as well as the geometry of the objects themselves. Therefore, the classical notions of diffeomorphism and homeomorphism, which are based on continuity properties, have to be carefully translated into the digital world.

In this paper, we describe a simple model of images as a set of continuous objects, and show how the topology of these objects, represented on a discrete grid either as binary objects or levelset functions, is affected by rigid and nonrigid deformations. Unlike the fully continuous case, the constraints required to make diffeomorphisms preserve the objects topology on the grid depend on the thickness of the deformed objects and may be impractical to compute. We propose an alternative approach to enforce topology preservation in spatial transformations based on the notion of simple point, which is well defined in digital topology [17,18]. We define such transformations as digital homeomorphisms, and derive a criterion that characterizes them for any number of objects in 2D and 3D images. We integrate this criterion into an approximation algorithm to build a digital homeomorphism from any transformation, and study how the objects interact with deformations encountered both in rigid and deformable registration.

2 Continuous Diffeomorphisms and Digital Homeomorphisms

Let Ω be a compact region of $\mathcal{R}^3$ of the form $[0, N_x] \times [0, N_y] \times [0, N_z]$, and $\{O_1, \ldots, O_K\}$ be the partition of Ω into K compact regions representing objects of interest. We assume that the objects fill the region such that $\Omega = \bigcup_{1,\ldots,k} O_k$, and that the objects do not overlap (formally, the intersection of any open sets inside O_k and O_l is empty, for all pairs k, l). If it exists, the boundary between two volumes k and l is a closed surface patch $S_{k,l} = O_k \cap O_l$. Note that because $S_{k,l}$ are compact, $\bigcup_l S_{k,l}$ is not the same as the closed surface bounding O_k, referred to as B_k. Where three objects meet, the common boundary is a line curve $L_{k,l,m} = O_k \cap O_l \cap O_m = S_{k,l} \cap S_{l,m} \cap S_{k,m}$ (see Fig. 1-b).

An image can be obtained from this partition by applying an observation model that associates intensity values or functions to a given object or set of objects. In medical images, the observation model includes noise, signal inhomogeneity, and many objects

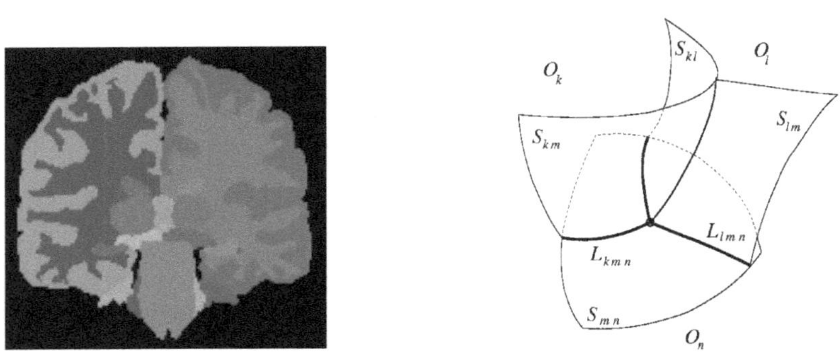

Fig. 1. Partition of an image into objects: a) the segmentation of a brain image into anatomical regions, b) the surface patches and line curves at the boundary between four objects

can have similar intensities. The topology of interest here is not the topology of the actual image, but of the underlying set of objects.

Given an image with a known partition into objects (the source), we seek to register it to a new image (the target) with a transformation that will preserve the topology of the partition. In the following, we consider the question of enforcing the preservation of topology for a given transformation.

2.1 Topology of Continuous and Discrete Objects

Although medical images represent a collection of objects in continuous space, these objects are nearly always represented discretely for computational reasons. The most common representation is the triangular surface mesh that approximates the continuous bounding surface of an object with arbitrary precision. Under this representation, the topology of the object can be characterized by the Euler characteristic of its bounding surface: $\chi(O_k) = V - E + F$ where V is the number of vertices, E the number of edges and F the number of faces in the mesh. The Euler characteristic describes the genus of the surface, which intuitively counts the number of handles in the object [19]. In case there are several disconnected parts or cavities in the object, the Euler characteristic of the object is the sum of Euler characteristics for each bounding surface.

If triangular surface meshes cannot be used directly, an alternative representation based on levelset functions has become the preferred approach for its ability to easily handle simple and complex geometries and the existence of efficient methods to solve partial difference equations on them [20]. Let Ω_D be a cubic grid that samples the region Ω along the x, y, z coordinates at a regular interval (set to 1 for simplicity). The sampling points are linked by edges along the x, y, z directions to form a cubic lattice (see Fig.2). Given the closed bounding surface B_k, a signed distance function can be constructed over each sampling point of Ω_D to build the levelset representation, and a surface mesh can be recovered by the marching cubes technique [21]. The recovered surface is a geometric approximation with the same topology as the original surface if the original surface cuts at most once through each edge between two neighboring

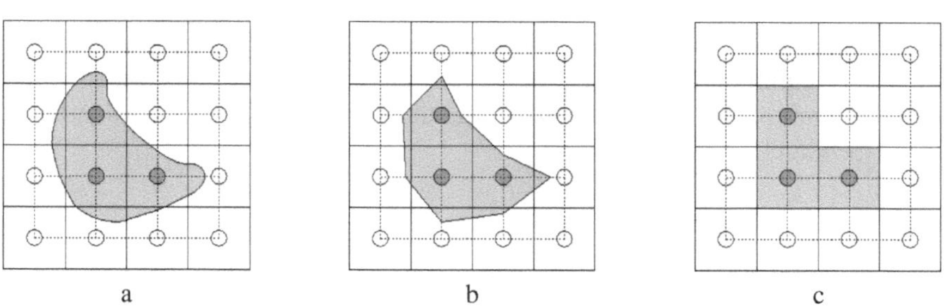

Fig. 2. Representation of an object on the digital grid: a) a continuous smooth surface, b) its approximation from a levelset function and marching cubes reconstruction, c) its approximation as a collection of voxels. Note that the voxel edges are different from the grid edges in this last case.

points and if its connectivity is consistent with a choice of digital connectivity on the grid [23]. Without loss of generality, we assume the segmentation has these two properties so that the continuous objects O_k are equivalent to the digital objects obtained by sampling them on Ω_D.

The marching cubes reconstruction performs only a trilinear interpolation of space, but more elaborate interpolation techniques introduce small perturbations on the distance function that may become topology artifacts and so the link between topological properties of the continuous and digital representations can be broken. The other interpolation method that will preserve topological properties is the nearest neighbor interpolation, which represents each sample point inside the object by a voxel. In either case, for matters of topology, the levelset representation can be replaced by a label image that associates the label k for each point inside O_k. For simplicity, we consider the voxel representation, though the following results apply identically to the levelset representation. The grid points are considered connected to their neighbors following usual connectivity rules: 6-connected points must share a voxel face, 18-connected points can share only a voxel edge, 26-connected points need only to share a voxel vertex.

2.2 Homeomorphisms and Diffeomorphisms in the Continuum

Two objects that have the same topology are called homeomorphic, and have the same Euler characteristic. By definition, two objects are homeomorphic if there exists a bijective transformation that maps one into the other and both the transformation and its inverse are continuous (the transformation is called a homeomorphism). The question of preserving topology is thus equivalent to finding a transformation that is a homeomorphism.

In the work of Christensen et al. [6], the topology preservation problems is reformulated into ensuring the transformation between two spaces is a diffeomorphism. A diffeomorphism is a bijective transformation that is differentiable and has invertible derivatives. To have invertible derivatives, it is necessary and sufficient that the transformation has a Jacobian strictly positive (or strictly negative) everywhere. In dimension 2 and 3, diffeomorphisms and homeomorphisms are strictly equivalent [22]. In practice, Christensen's method requires the Jacobian to be above 0.5, to avoid numerical singularities in solving the equations for computing the transformation. If it goes below that limit, the algorithm performs a regridding: the source image is transformed with the current diffeomorphism, and a new transformation is computed from this intermediary image to the target.

2.3 Diffeomorphisms on the Digital Grid

Continuous diffeomorphisms are not sufficient to prevent changes in the topology of objects represented on the digital grid. Let us take the simple example of an affine transformation: $\forall X \in \Omega, T(X) = AX + B$. The Jacobian is $J_T(X) = \|A\|$, which is a positive or negative constant provided that the transformation is not a projection. Yet, applying a rotation or scaling to the digital label or levelset image representing an object and then recovering the continuous surface will result in topological changes (see Fig. 3). In the case of a rotation, the connectivity of objects can change where the

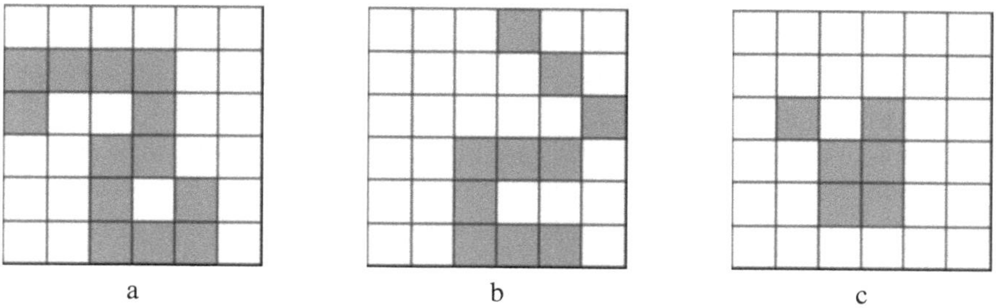

Fig. 3. Simple examples of transformations that affect topology on the digital grid: a) original object, b) after a rotation of 45 degrees, c) after a scaling of 2/3. Independently of the connectivity choice, the objects all have different topology.

distance between two boundaries is less than the largest distance between connected grid points ($\sqrt{3}$ in 3D, $\sqrt{2}$ in 2D). In the case of a scaling with a scale $s < 1$, all the details smaller than $1/s$ may disappear from the transformed object.

Combining both effects, we have the following property:

Theorem 1. *An affine transformation $T(X) = AX + B$ applied to an object O defined on a digital cubic grid Ω_D is guaranteed to preserve the topology of O if and only if the distance between any two points outside of O on the grid such that the line between them intersects O is strictly higher than $\sqrt{3}/\lambda$ in 3D or $\sqrt{2}/\lambda$ in 2D, where λ is the smallest eigenvalue of A.*

Full proof is a straightforward exercise in elementary geometry and omitted here. This constraint, unlike those for continuous homeomorphisms and diffeomorphisms, explicitly depends on the thickness of the object. It can be extended to any non-linear deformation by assuming that the transformation is locally affine at each grid point and computing the minimum thickness in that neighborhood of the object. In the case that the thickness requirement is not met, it is necessary either to change the deformation or to resample the object to a finer grid resolution. Compared to the previous requirements of regridding or imposing bounds on the transformation parameters, this is more complex. However, as we must now explicitly take into consideration the objects, we can utilize the simple points of digital topology instead.

2.4 Digital Homeomorphisms: Single Object

Let us consider the case of a single object O_1 and its bounding surface B_1. Implied here is a second object $O_2 = \Omega \backslash O_1$ representing the background, with $B_2 = B_1 = B$. In this case, it has been shown [24,25] that the boundary B can move over a grid point (changing it from object to background, or background to object) without changing its topology if and only if the grid point is a simple point. A point is simple if there is exactly one connected object region and one connected background region in the neighborhood of the point. The definition of connected region and neighborhood depends on the choice of connectivity: if the object is 26-connected, then the background is 6-connected and the neighborhood is the set of 26-connected neighbors of the point. In the case of an 18-connected object, the background is 6-connected and the neighborhood is the set of 18-connected neighbors. The other cases are obtained by swapping object and background in the definition.

By analogy with the continuous case, we define as *digital homeomorphism* a transformation of B that only exchanges simple points between O_1 and O_2. Any object deformation algorithm that preserves its topology implies a digital homeomorphism, from homotopic morphological operators [26,27] to topology-preserving levelset evolution [23]. In many cases, this homeomorphism is not explicitly computed, though topology-preserving levelset evolution could be directly integrated into levelset-based registration methods [15]. However, most image registration problems consider more than a single object, and an extension of this definition is needed for the general case.

2.5 Digital Homeomorphisms: Multiple Objects

The topological properties of a set of objects can be summarized by the Euler characteristic of all possible sub-groups of objects. By its definition, the Euler characteristic follows the inclusion-exclusion principle:

$$\chi(O_k \cup O_l) = \chi(O_k) + \chi(O_l) - \chi(O_k \cap O_l)$$

For a group of objects, this becomes:

$$\begin{aligned}\chi(\textstyle\bigcup_{k=1}^{K} O_k) = \sum_k \chi(O_k) - \sum_{k,l} \chi(O_k \cap O_l) + \sum_{k,l,m} \chi(O_k \cap O_l \cap O_m)\\ - \ldots + (-1)^{k-1}\chi(O_1 \cap \ldots \cap O_K)\end{aligned}$$

With our model, we have objects O_k, surface patches $S_{k,l} = O_k \cap O_l$, and lines $L_{k,l,m} = O_k \cap O_l \cap O_m$. Higher order intersections are either the empty set, disjoint sets of points, or coincide with an existing line. The intersection points cannot change their shape, and thus keep their (spherical) topology and have constant Euler characteristic. Points can appear and disappear as a byproduct of changes in the topology of the lines $L_{k,lm,}$ linking them, but this involves a change of topology for the lines themselves.

To ensure the topology of the set of objects is preserved, we have to find a transformation that maintains the Euler characteristic of all O_k, $S_{k,l}$ and $L_{k,l,m}$. Two objects can maintain their own topology and change the topology of their common boundary, and even when those are preserved, the surface patches can slide with regard to each other along the lines and affect their topology.

From the inclusion-exclusion principle, the Euler characteristic of $S_{k,l}$ and $L_{k,l,m}$ can be computed from the Euler characteristic of object groups:

$$\begin{aligned}\chi(S_{k,l}) &= \chi(O_k) + \chi(O_l) - \chi(O_k \cup O_l)\\ \chi(L_{k,l,m}) &= \chi(O_k) + \chi(O_l) + \chi(O_m) - \chi(O_k \cup O_l)\\ &\quad -\chi(O_l \cup O_m) - \chi(O_m \cup O_k) + \chi(O_k \cup O_l \cup O_m)\end{aligned}$$

Thus, the topology of the segmentation is preserved if the transformation preserves the topology of individual objects, object pairs and object triplets. Note that in the 2D case, we only need to preserve the topology of individual objects and pairs.

On the digital grid, this leads to a multi-object criterion for homeomorphisms:

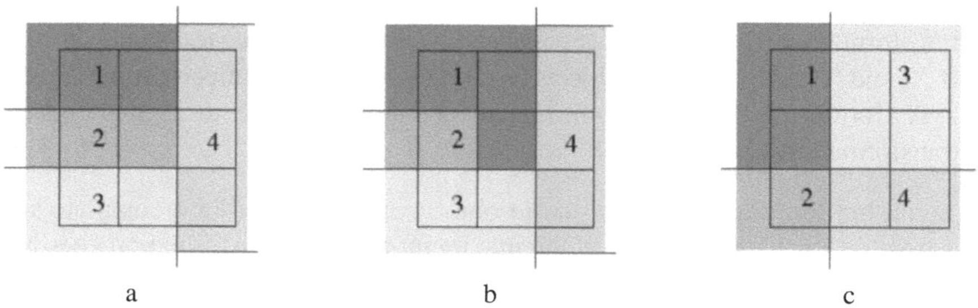

Fig. 4. Simple points for multiple objects: a) the central point can be exchanged between 2 and 4, but not 1 and 2 or 2 and 3 since these latter two cases would allow 1 and 3 to touch, b) the central point can swap from 1 to 3, but not 2 or 4, c) the central point is non-simple for any change if the objects are 6-connected, but can move from 3 to 2 if the objects are 26-connected (note that the groups 2-3 and 1-4 intersect each other in the latter case).

Theorem 2. (The Digital Homeomorphism Constraint) *A digital homeomorphism is a transformation that enforces, for a given partition of Ω, that any sample point $X \in \Omega_D$ may change from O_k to O_l if and only if X is a simple point for O_k, O_l, $\{O_k \cup O_m\}_{O_m \cap N_X \neq \emptyset, m \neq k,l}$, $\{O_l \cup O_m\}_{O_m \cap N_X \neq \emptyset, m \neq k,l}$, $\{O_k \cup O_m \cup O_n\}_{O_m, O_n \cap N_X \neq \emptyset, m,n \neq k,l}$, $\{O_l \cup O_m \cup O_n\}_{O_m, O_n \cap N_X \neq \emptyset, m,n \neq k,l}$, each considered as a single object.*

In other words, a point can change from O_k to O_l if it is a simple point for all groups of up to three objects including either O_k or O_l. The main difference with the single object case here is that simple points become object-dependent (see Fig. 4). In practice, the number of cases to test at each point is still low: two on most of the surfaces $S_{k,l}$, four at the lines $L_{k,l}$. More complex cases do appear when objects become one voxel thin, and when multiple objects meet, but such occurrences are very sparse in Ω.

All of these properties hold regardless of the choice of connectivity. In general, consistency would dictate that the connectivity be the same for all objects, but other choices are perfectly valid. Note, however, that having multiple objects with 18- or 26-connectivity means that objects may intersect each other. Having one connectivity for all objects is also more restrictive than the single object case, because both object and background would be required to be simple with the connectivity of the objects and its complement.

2.6 Homeomorphic Field Approximation

To study the impact of digital homeomorphisms as a constraint on registration, we developed an algorithm to approximate a given transformation with a digital homeomorphism. Given a transformation vector field such that $T(X) = X + \mathbf{u}$ and a partition $\{O_k\}$, we compute an approximation $\mathbf{u}'_i$ of the vector field for every point $X_i \in \Omega_D$ as follows:

1. Start from $\mathbf{u}'_i = 0$,
2. Find the closest 6-connected neighbor X_j along the direction $\mathbf{u}_i - \mathbf{u}'_i$,

3. If X_i and X_j are inside the same object, move from X_i to X_j and update the transformation $\mathbf{u}'_i = \mathbf{u}'_i + (X_j - X_i)$ and residual difference $\mathbf{u}_i - \mathbf{u}'_i$,
4. If X_i and X_j are in different objects O_k and O_l, check the homeomorphic constraint at X_j for O_k, O_l. If the constraint is satisfied move from X_i to X_j and update the transformation as above.

The algorithm terminates when no more objects can be moved in a complete sweep of the domain, or when the norm of the maximum residual transformation goes below one voxel. As the approximated deformation evolves smoothly from the identity to the given deformation, only one point is changed at a time and thus the topology can be preserved.

3 Experiments

3.1 Continuous Diffeomorphisms

First, let us assess how much the topology is affected by the digital grid in practical cases. We will consider four different partition images used in 3D brain segmentation: the automatically classified tissues obtained from a classification algorithm with no constraint on the topology (four classes, including the background), the manually

Table 1. Euler characteristics of segmented objects for different partitions and deformations. The connectivity is 6/26, although other choices yield similar results.

		Euler characteristics	
Automated tissue classification (AT)	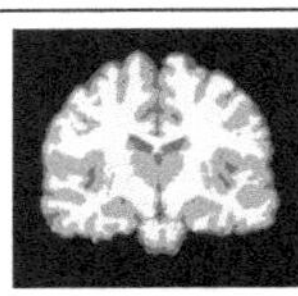	ORI	182, -6338, -3162, -110
		R05	204, -7042, -3386, -108
		S95	202, -6408, -3172, -152
		NRR1	560, -9616, -7918, -388
		NRR2	274, -11188, -4818, -342
Manual tissue classification (MT)	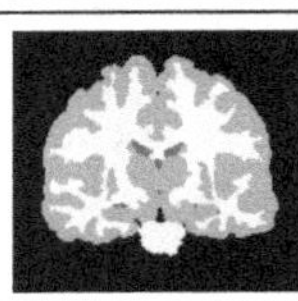	ORI	48, -14, -128, -448
		R05	64, -2, -148, -518
		S95	60, 2, -164, -470
		NRR1	442, 66, -1254, -732
		NRR2	134, 38, -634, -848
Manual region labeling (MR)	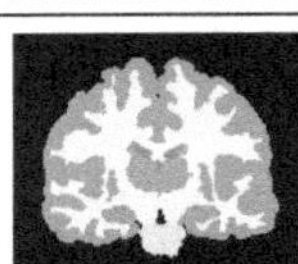	ORI	44, 4, -18, -18, -56, 2, 2, 2, 4, -22, -428
		R05	64, 4, -6, -22, -78, 4, 4, 0, -4, -36, -484
		S95	56, 4,- 2, -26, -86, 2, 2, 2, 4, -8, -464
		NRR1	396, 14, 52, 18, -1156, 34, 54, 18, 40, 6, -734
		NRR2	112, 4, 34, -32, -476, 14, 4, 4, 14, -38, -812
Topology corrected template (TT)	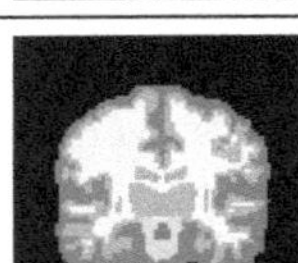	ORI	4, 2, 2, 2, 2, 4, 4, 4, 0, 4, -6
		R05	4, 2, 2, 2, 2, 4, 4, 4, 0, 4, -6
		S95	4, 2, 2, 2, 2, 4, 4, 4, 0, 4, -6
		NRR1	134, -1904, -30, 16, -9334, 4, 24, 38, 14, 10, -392
		NRR2	42, -508, 4, 6, -2500, 6, 2, 14, 16, 0, -228

labeled tissues for the same image as provided by an expert, an image with eleven manually labeled regions and finally a template image of the same regions each with corrected topology and a minimum thickness of 2 voxels. Both manual segmentations come from the Internet Brain Segmentation Repository (IBSR) [28] and the topologically corrected template was obtained from [29]. All images are 3D volumes with 1mm cubic resolution.

For all these images, we compare the Euler characteristic for all groups of up to four objects before (ORI) and after transformation with a rotation of 5 degrees (R05), a scaling with factor 0.95 (S95), and two deformations obtained from the registration of the IBSR image to another brain image within the IBSR dataset with a nonrigid registration algorithm [30] with low (NRR1) or high regularization constraints (NRR2). The second deformation is a continuous diffeomorphism for all but nine voxels of the image. The results for individual objects are summarized in Table 1. Groups of objects are omitted due to space limitations but yield similar numbers.

Both rotation and scaling significantly affect the topology, even though they are diffeomorphic and impose only small variations. The issue becomes even more important with a larger non-rigid deformation, diffeomorphic or not. The nature of the objects has also an influence on the results, as partitions with arbitrary topology (automated classification) vary most and manually edited images (with or without topology correction) have lower but similar variations in their Euler characteristics. The number of objects in an image increases the number of surface patches and line curves, while maintaining or lowering their complexity, and the transformations affect those similarly. Note that the topology-corrected template is not affected by the rotation or the scaling, because its minimum thickness is above $\sqrt{3}/\lambda$ in these cases.

3.2 Digital Homeomorphic Approximation

We now study the effect of imposing the digital homeomorphic constraint on the transformations themselves. The transformations described above are approximated with our homeomorphic approximation algorithm for the same four image partitions, and the original IBSR segmentation with 35 labels shown in Fig. 1. Table 2 quantifies the difference between original and approximated vector fields. During the approximation, the field is prevented to cross the image boundaries. As this correction amounts to an image boundary condition, we discarded in the measurements the corresponding differences

Table 2. Differences between original and approximated transformations: mean, standard deviation and maximum of the residual distance (in voxels) and percentage of changed vectors. Image acronyms are defined in Table 1.

	R05				S95				NRR1				NRR2			
image	mean	std	max	%	mean	std	max	%	mean	std	max	%	mean	std	max	%
AT	1.21E-2	0.198	7.3	0.504	8.60E-3	0.126	4.5	0.562	6.02E-2	0.621	24.9	1.493	4.38E-2	0.491	18.9	1.193
MT	6.40E-4	0.042	6.4	0.032	2.81E-3	0.060	4.2	0.230	6.24E-3	0.170	22.2	0.229	2.99E-3	0.112	16.2	0.115
MR	6.46E-4	0.042	6.4	0.032	2.81E-3	0.060	4.2	0.230	6.63E-3	0.176	22.2	0.240	3.12E-3	0.115	16.2	0.119
TT	4.03E-7	6.7E-4	1.4	3.7E-5	2.63E-3	0.057	2.8	0.218	5.11E-3	0.127	15.8	0.250	7.79E-4	0.040	10.4	5.2E-4
IBSR	7.05E-4	0.043	6.4	0.036	2.82E-3	0.060	4.2	0.232	7.31E-3	0.184	22.2	0.268	3.43E-3	0.119	16.2	0.134

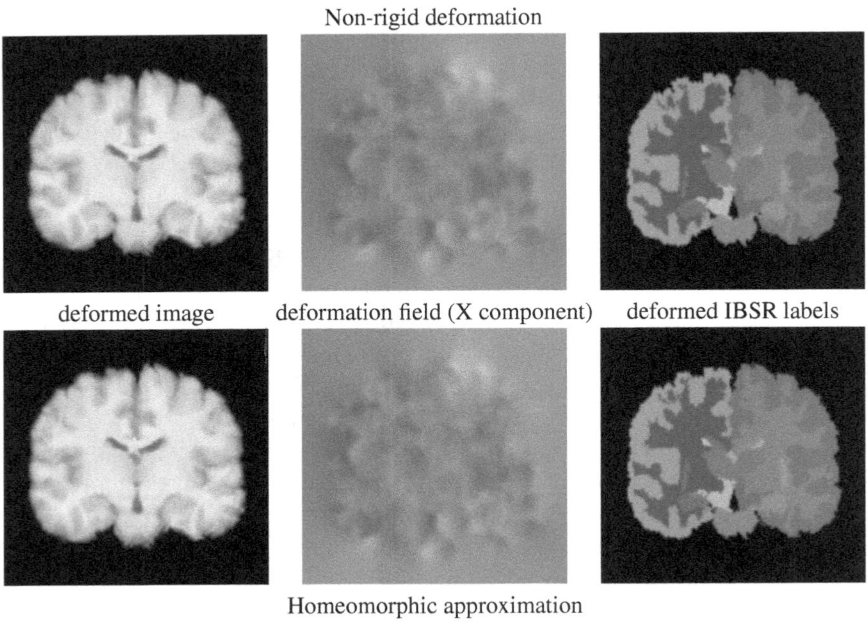

Fig. 5. Comparison of the non-rigid registration result NRR1 before (top) and after (bottom) applying the homeomorphic approximation. The mean Dice coefficient of overlap between the two transformed partition into the IBSR labels is 0.937.

which would otherwise mask the amount of change due to topology constraints at the objects boundary. The Euler characteristics for all transformed objects and groups of objects were computed and found identical to the originals in all cases.

The homeomorphic approximations are very close to the original transformations, in particular for partitions with simpler topology. In the case of large, non-rigid deformations, the template with corrected topology requires fewer changes than the manual labelings. The automated segmentation has an arbitrarily complex topology, and the homeomorphic approximation tends to prevent large deformations in such areas. When comparing the objects before and after the homeomorphic approximation, only small changes are noticeable and areas with a noisy aspect due to the lack of regularity in the deformation field are not smoothed (see Fig. 5). Thus, the homeomorphic approximation successfully transforms any diffeomorphic or irregular deformation into a digitally homeomorphic deformation with little impact on the deformation field or the transformed image, provided we have a labeling with simple topology.

4 Discussion

In this paper, we studied the impact of digital images on classical notions of topology. We demonstrated the limitations of continuous diffeomorphisms, which cannot guarantee to preserve the topology of segmented regions defined on the digital grid, unless additional constraints on the Jacobian and the regions of interest are taken into account. Using digital topology properties, we proposed an alternative, local criterion that enforces strict homeomorphisms for the digital images. The homeomorphic constraint is limited to the objects boundaries, instead of the entire 3D image space, and may provide more freedom for defining deformable transformations using flows or levelsets.

We proposed a field approximation technique based on this criterion, which creates homeomorphic transformations for images and the structures therein with little change from the original deformation field. Our experiments outlined the properties of different categories of image partitions into sets of objects, and indicated that corrected and simple object topology helps minimize the computed amount of approximation. The question of adequately modeling the topology of anatomical regions has been largely ignored up to now, yet it appears to have a significant impact on our ability to build homeomorphisms on the digital images.

We expect the homeomorphic criterion can be integrated directly into registration algorithms, complementing or replacing other regularization techniques. The shape and scale of the digital grid plays a key role in the issue, and multiscale representations might increase the flexibility of the grid [31]. Finally, even when preserving the topology of the digital segmentation is not required, continuous diffeomorphisms would benefit from integrating a topologically correct model of the anatomy to concentrate the computational effort at the boundary between the structures of interest.

References

1. Grenander, U., Miller, M.I.: Computational anatomy: an emerging discipline. Q. Appl. Math. LVI(4), 617–694 (1998)
2. Thompson, P.M., Toga, A.W.: A framework for computational anatomy. Computing and Visualization in Science 5, 1–12 (2002)
3. Resnick, S.M., Pham, D.L., Kraut, M.A., Zonderman, A.B., Davatzikos, C.: Longitudinal MRI studies of older adults: A shrinking brain. J. Neuroscience 23(8), 3295–3301 (2003)
4. Thompson, P., Hayashi, K., Sowell, E., Gogtay, N., Giedd, J., Rapoport, J., de Zubicaray, G., Janke, A., Rose, S., Semple, J., Doddrell, D., Wang, Y., van Erp, T., Cannon, T., Toga, A.: Mapping cortical change in Alzheimer's disease, brain development, and schizophrenia. NeuroImage, Special Issue on Mathematics in Brain Imaging (2004)
5. Gerig, G., Joshi, S., Fletcher, T., Gorczowski, K., Xu, S., Pizer, S., Styner, M.: Statistics of populations of images and its embedded objects: Driving applications in neuroimaging. In: Proc. IEEE Int. Symp. Biomedical Imaging, Arlington 2006 (2006)
6. Christensen, G.E.: Deformable shape models for anatomy. Electrical Engineering D.Sc. Dissertation, Washington University, St. Louis, Missouri (1994)
7. Christensen, G.E., Joshi, S.C., Miller, M.I.: Volumetric transformation of brain anatomy. IEEE Trans. Medical Imaging 16(6), 864–877 (1997)
8. Christensen, G.E., Johnson, H.J.: Consistent image registration. IEEE Trans. Medical Imaging 20(7), 568–582 (2001)
9. Rohde, G.K., Aldroubi, A., Dawant, B.M.: The adaptive bases algorithm for intensity-based nonrigid image registration. IEEE Trans. Medical Imaging 22(11), 1470–1479 (2003)
10. Avants, B.B., Gee, J.C.: Shape averaging with diffeomorphic flows for atlas creation. In: Proc. IEEE Int. Symp. Biomedical Imaging, pp. 595–598 (2004)

11. Narayanan, R., Fessler, J.A., Park, H., Meyer, C.H.: Diffeomorphic nonlinear transformations: a local parametric approach for image registration. In: Proc. Int. Conf. Information Processing in Medical Imaging, Glenwood Springs 2005 (2005)
12. Noblet, V., Heinrich, C., Heitz, F., Armspach, J.-P.: 3D deformable image registration: a topology preservation scheme based on hierarchical deformation models and interval analysis optimization. IEEE Trans. Image Processing 14(5), 553–566 (2005)
13. Rueckert, D., Sonoda, L., Hayes, C., Hill, D., Leach, M., Hawkes, D.: Non-rigid registration using free-form deformations: Application to breast MR images. IEEE Trans. Medical Imaging 18, 712–721 (1999)
14. Shen, D., Davatzikos, C.: Hammer: Hierarchical attribute matching mechanism for elastic registration. IEEE Trans. Medical Imaging 21(11) (2002)
15. Vemuri, B.C., Ye, J., Chen, Y., Leonard, C.M.: Image registration via level-set motion: Applications to atlas-based segmentation. Medical Image Analysis 20(1), 1–20 (2003)
16. Kybic, J., Unser, M.: Fast parametric elastic image registration. IEEE Trans. Image Processing 12(11), 1427–1442 (2003)
17. Kong, T.Y., Rosenfeld, A.: Digital topology: Introduction and survey. Computer Vision, Graphics, and Image Processing 48(3), 357–393 (1989)
18. Bertrand, G., Couprie, M.: A model for digital topology. In: Bertrand, G., Couprie, M., Perroton, L. (eds.) DGCI 1999. LNCS, vol. 1568, pp. 229–241. Springer, Heidelberg (1999)
19. Henle, M.: A Combinatorial Introduction to topology. W.H. Freeman and Company (1979)
20. Sethian, J.: Level Set Methods and Fast Marching Methods. Cambridge University Press, Cambridge (1999)
21. Lorensen, W.E., Cline, H.E.: Marching cubes: A high resolution 3D surface construction algorithm. In: Proc. SIGGRAPH'87 1987, vol. 21, pp. 163–169 (1987)
22. O'Neill, B.: Elementary Differential Geometry. Academic Press, San Diego (1997)
23. Han, X., Xu, C., Prince, J.L.: A topology preserving level set method for geometric deformable models. IEEE Trans. Pattern Analysis and Machine Intelligence 25(6), 755–768 (2003)
24. Malandain, G., Bertrand, G., Ayache, N.: Topological segmentation of discrete surfaces. Int. J. Computer Vision 10(2), 183–197 (1993)
25. Bertrand, G.: Simple points, topological numbers and geodesic neighborhood in cubic grids. Pattern Recognition Letters 15(10), 1003–1011 (1994)
26. Couprie, M., Bezerra, F., Bertrand, G.: Topological operators for grayscale image processing. J. Electronic Imaging 10(4), 1003–1015 (2001)
27. Mangin, J.F., Frouin, V., Bloch, I., Régis, J., López-Krahe, J.: From 3D magnetic resonance images to structural representations of the cortex topography using topology preserving deformations. J. Mathematical Imaging and Vision 5, 297–318 (1995)
28. Worth, A.: Internet brain seg mentation repository. (1996) `http://www.cma.mgh.harvard.edu/ibsr/`
29. Bazin, P.L., Pham, D.: Topology-preserving tissue classification of magnetic resonance brain images. In: IEEE Trans. Medical Imaging, Special Issue on Computational Neuroanatomy (in press) (2007)
30. Ellingsen, L.M., Prince, J.L.: Mjolnir: Deformable image registration using feature diffusion. In: Proc. SPIE Medical Imaging Conf., San Diego (2006)
31. Bai, Y., Prince, J.L.: Octree-based topology-preserving isosurface simplification. In: Proc. IEEE Int. Conf. Computer Vision and Pattern Recognition (CVPR'06), New York 2006 (2006)

Incorporating DTI Data as a Constraint in Deformation Tensor Morphometry Between T1 MR Images

Colin Studholme

Department of Radiology,
University of California San Francisco,
Northern California Institute for Research and Education,
VAMC San Francisco,
4150 Clement Street, San Francisco, U.S.A.
colin.studholme@ieee.org

Abstract. Deformation tensor morphometry provides a sensitive approach to detecting and mapping subtle volume changes in the brain from conventional high resolution T1W MRI data. However, it is limited in its ability to localize volume changes within sub-regions of uniform white matter in T1W MRI. In contrast, lower resolution DTI data provides valuable complementary microstructural information within white matter. An approach to incorporating information from DTI data into deformation tensor morphometry of conventional high resolution T1W imaging is described. A novel mutual information (MI) derived criteria is proposed, termed diffusion paired MI, using an approximation to collective many-channel MI between all images. This approximation avoids the evaluation of high dimensional joint probability distributions, but allows a combination of conventional and diffusion data in a single registration criteria. The local gradient of this measure is used to drive a viscous fluid registration between repeated DTI-MRI imaging studies. Results on example data from clinical studies of Alzheimer's disease illustrate the improved localization of tissue loss patterns within regions of white matter.

1 Introduction

Tracking of change in brain anatomy over time has emerged as a powerful tool in detecting and studying changes relating to disease diagnosis and progression in neurodegeneration and development. In particular, non-rigid registration based methods have been developed to map subtle geometric changes in brain anatomy over time, and separate true volume changes from tissue displacements [8,14,5]. Such methods have been almost entirely focused toward the analysis of conventional T1 weighted (T1W), T2 weighted (T2W) or proton density weighted (PDW) structural MRI data. These images provide basic contrast between gray matter, white matter and cerebro-spinal fluid, but are limited in their ability to spatially localize geometric change within regions of uniform tissue. In particular, current serial morphometry of MRI cannot probe within the bulk of

N. Karssemeijer and B. Lelieveldt (Eds.): IPMI 2007, LNCS 4584, pp. 223–232, 2007.
© Springer-Verlag Berlin Heidelberg 2007

white matter that holds the underlying connections between functional brain regions. White matter is known to be lost during normal aging [10] and many forms of dementia. These regions are critically important in relating structural changes occurring over time in different anatomical regions, in a range of neuro-degenerative conditions including Alzheimer's, Semantic and Fronto-Temporal Dementia, alcohol abuse and HIV.

DTI data [2] provides significant micro-structural information about tissues in the brain, which significantly compliments that provided by high resolution T1W imaging. There has been significant recent work on the alignment of DTI data to other DTI data, both within and between subjects. The alignment problem of DTI is more complex than the alignment of conventional scalar MRI values. This is because of the inherent local geometry of the diffusion measurements, which is modified by any spatial transformation of the data. DTI data itself, unlike T1W imaging, provides relatively calibrated measurements which are consistent between studies and this motivates the direct application of tensor metrics to evaluate their alignment. Recent work has seen the incorporation of these ideas into deformable DTI registration algorithms such as the elegant work of [4,3]. The work of [20] derives a novel method of incorporating this rotational information into an elastic registration scheme to align tensor orientations and locations simultaneously.

This paper examines a related but different problem: one of incorporating DTI alignment information within high resolution deformation morphometry of conventional T1W MRI data, in order to provide additional spatial constraints in deformation morphometry. T1W data is not directly compatible with the geometrically derived local diffusion measurements, but provides much greater spatial resolution in many areas of the brain (basic tissue boundaries and grey matter structure).

2 Method

Entropy based methods such as those using mutual information have been used to form a robust measure of image similarity between T1W images for accurate deformation morphometry, where, unlike the DTI tensor components, the intensity and contrast is essentially un-calibrated and can vary spatially within imaging studies. Given a pair of conventional T1 weighted images, with intensities $m^1(\mathbf{x})$ and $m^2(\mathbf{x})$ (superscripts denoting time point) in the same common space $\mathbf{x} \in X$, we can derive a measure of the mutual information between the sets of intensities M^1 and M^2 occurring together in the two images:

$$I(M^1; M^2) = H(M^1) + H(M^2) - H(H^1, M^2) \quad (1)$$

The local gradient of this criteria [9] can be used to drive a fluid registration allowing non-rigid alignment of images as in [7]. In this work we want to build on this by introducing information from DTI data.

If we assume that we additionally have sets of reconstructed diffusion tensor values over the same field of view of the T1 weighted MRI data at each time point $\mathbf{D}^1$ and $\mathbf{D}^2$, then we want to evaluate both MRI and DTI similarity simultaneously. In practice, here we will assume that the tensor contains six individual diffusion measures $\mathbf{D} = \{D_{xx}, D_{yy}, D_{xy}, D_{xz}, D_{yz}, D_{zz}\}$, but the methods can be extended to larger numbers of directions. For DTI data these calibrated tensor components can be related geometrically using methods such as [20,4,3] to derive a measure of similarity for DTI alignment. However, these measurements cannot be directly related conventional scalar image data. Ideally, a combined similarity measure is needed, which takes into account the changing relationship between the local orientation of the DTI data and the conventional structural data, as well as between the DTI information. A direct approach would be to evaluate the mutual information between all 7 image pairs (T1W intensity and the 6 diffusion tensor components) acquired for two imaging studies. This would make use of multi-channel mutual information methods previously proposed [15,17,11] to evaluate the collective mutual information between studies. For conventional matching where there is some shared information between image types, as illustrated in the upper part of figure 2, we can consider the shared information due to a combination of all the images. Given that the spatial relationships within studies is fixed [15], the registration similarity between studies can be evaluated from the mutual information between the two studies collectively:

$$I(M^1, \mathbf{D}^1; M^2, \mathbf{D}^2) = H(M^1, \mathbf{D}^1) + H(M^2, \mathbf{D}^2) - H(M^1, \mathbf{D}^1, M^2, \mathbf{D}^2) \quad (2)$$

where, $H(M^1, \mathbf{D}^1)$ is the collective information provided by the first study, $H(M^2, \mathbf{D}^2)$ is the collective information provided by the second study, and $H(M^1, \mathbf{D}^1, M^2, \mathbf{D}^2)$ is the information of the combined studies. However, both of these criteria would require, for six DTI directions, the estimation of the $(6+1) \times 2 = 14$ dimensional joint probability distribution for the joint entropy $H(M^1, \mathbf{D}^1, M^2, \mathbf{D}^2)$. i.e. we need to estimate the probability of co-occurrence of all possible combinations of 14 different values $(M^1, D^1_{xx}, \ldots M^2, D^2_{xx} \ldots D^2_{zz})$. This estimate would be extremely sparsely populated and require expensive computational methods to store and evaluate. One alternative approach is to simply ignore changes in shared information between different types of images and form a measure from a simple summation of MI between image pairs, each derived from the matching of one image type in one study to the same image type in the second study. This simplification however clearly ignores any influence that one image type may have in explaining the structure in the other image types.

An alternative formulation explored here is to use a simplification of the general case of equation (2). This simplification is based on the fact that the information provided by the different diffusion directions within a study is relatively un-correlated. For example: In conventional multi-channel MI based image registration, meaningful shared information between channels occurs when regions of a given intensity in one modality co-occur with intensities in a second modality (e.g. grey matter intensities in MRI co-occur with some fraction of a 'soft tissue' intensity range within CT). In DTI data complex curved tracts are exhibited as different combinations of diffusion strengths in each axis along its length. Thus, within a single DTI study, high values of diffusion components in the X axis D_{xx}

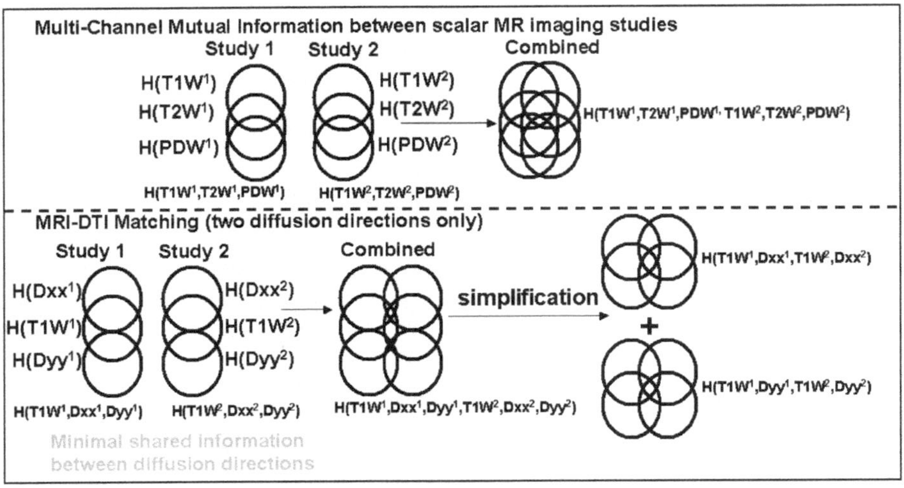

Fig. 1. An illustration of the derivation of different MI measures of similarity between multiple sets of images for conventional scalar images (top) and combined scalar and DTI data types (bottom). In conventional MRI data sets (T1W,PDW,T2W) there is appreciable shared information. For DTI data there is little shared information between individual diffusion direction maps. We can therefore consider the simplified relationship between DTI directional measurements separately paired with conventional MRI.

would not be expected to co-occur more frequently with a particular diffusion strength in the Y axis D_{yy}. (i.e. given a diffusion strength in direction X, we cannot guess what the diffusion strength in direction Y is going to be.) However, considering the pairing conventional MRI with diffusion measurements: within regions of white matter as seen in T1W MRI, there will be a certain fraction of voxels exhibiting a specific level of X axis diffusion D_{xx}, and a certain fraction exhibiting Y axis diffusion D_{yy}, reflecting for example anterior-posterior or inferior-superior connections within white matter. In addition, low MRI T1W intensities delineate regions of unreliable diffusion measurements in CSF and bone. Thus, the statistical co-occurrence of DTI diffusion components and conventional structural MRI intensity can provide a meaningful partitioning of diffusion information to clarify the alignment measure. In order to account for this shared structure, a criteria formed by combining mutual information measures evaluated between T1/Diffusion image pairs, say M^1, D^1_{xx}, at each time point can be considered. For each diffusion image, its match to the same diffusion direction at the later time point is evaluated, together with the high resolution T1W image intensities at each time point. Denoting this by $I(M^1, D^1_\phi; M^2, D^2_\phi)$, where $\phi \in \{xx, xy, yy, xz, yz, zz\}$ are the set of directions considered, the measure can be expressed as:

$$I\rho(M^1, \mathbf{D}^1; M^2, \mathbf{D}^2) = \sum_{\forall\phi} I(M^1, D^1_\phi; M^2, D^2_\phi) \tag{3}$$

where

$$I(M^1, D^1_\phi; M^2, D^2_\phi) = H(M^1, D^1_\phi) + H(M^2, D^2_\phi) - H(M^1, D^1_\phi, M^2, D^2_\phi). \quad (4)$$

This combined measure, termed diffusion paired MI, requires only 4 dimensional joint intensity distributions to be estimated, but takes into account the co-occurrence of structural and diffusion measures as image alignment is evaluated. The local gradient of this global measure, $\nabla I\rho(M^1, \mathbf{D}^1; M^2, \mathbf{D}^2)$, with respect to the local deformation at a given spatial location, can be derived from the sum of the gradients of each of the paired MI terms $I(M^1, D^1_\phi; M^2, D^2_\phi)$. These, in turn, can be derived using the approach of [9], to create a single force field driving the image sets into alignment.

2.1 Implementation

For these experiments in deformation tensor morphometry, a dense field image registration scheme is used, where the local voxel displacement mapping from one image to the other is given by a vector field such that:

$$\mathbf{x}_2 = \mathbf{x}_1 + \mathbf{u}(\mathbf{x}_1) \quad (5)$$

The registration force field $\mathbf{F}(\mathbf{x}) = \nabla I\rho(M^1, \mathbf{D}^1; M^2, \mathbf{D}^2)$ derived from the local gradient of the similarity measures with respect to the local displacement estimate is then used to drive a velocity based, viscous fluid deformation model to ensure topology preservation. The solution to the registration is formed by integrating steps along an instantaneous velocity field which is itself derived from a balance between the registration force field $\mathbf{F}(\mathbf{x})$ and the energy of a flowing viscous fluid. The instantaneous velocity vector $\mathbf{v}(\mathbf{x})$ of a point in the image is estimated such that:

$$\mu\nabla^2\mathbf{v}(\mathbf{x}) + (\mu + \lambda)\nabla(\nabla.\mathbf{v}(\mathbf{x})) = \mathbf{F}(\mathbf{x}), \quad (6)$$

where μ and λ are constants determining the relationships between stresses in the flow field. This is solved numerically in a similar way to [6] and [8], using Successive Over Relaxation [12]. From this velocity field estimate, a gradient ascent approach is used to refine the displacement estimate at each iteration. An iterative gradient ascent scheme is used to optimize the registration estimate. Although deformation will generally be small, larger changes can occur in serial studies. As a result we also include an updating of the local diffusion directions using the method of preserving the principal directions of diffusion [1], during the iterative registration.

At each step, the set of 6 4D joint probability distributions between the structural T1W MRI data paired each of the diffusion measurements at each time point is estimated. A discrete binned estimate, using 64 bins in each intensity range, is formed and smoothed using a recursive filter. From this probability distribution, a force field is estimated from the observed intensities and intensity gradients of the T1W and diffusion images. For the estimation of a given joint probability and its gradients with respect to intensity from this discrete binned histogram, a 4D Cubic B-Spline approximation [19] is used. As described by Thevenaz [18], the B-spline provides a positive function of data values essential for an interpolation model of probability estimates. Corresponding 2D histograms are formed for the marginal distributions and 2D Cubic B-Splines are used for approximation.

3 Results

3.1 Image Data

A subject with an initial clinical diagnosis of Alzheimer dementia was imaged on a 4T Siemens imaging system twice over a period of 9 months. Each imaging study included 3D T1 weighted MPRAGE acquisition with a resolution of $1 \times 1 \times 1mm$ (256×256 FOV with 256×256 matrix, 176 slices) acquired with a sagittal orientation with RF spoiling. The scan time is 5min 30sec. The phase encoding direction is anterior to posterior. The TR/TE/TI/flip angle=2300ms/3.37ms/950ms/7 degree. The acquisition was carried out using an 8 channel coil, using Grappa encoding and an acceleration factor of 2, with 50 reference lines of phase encoding. A diffusion tensor imaging protocol was then acquired consisting of a 2D double refocused spin-echo EPI sequence with a spatial resolution of 2x2x3mm with either 4 averages. The overall scan time was 3min with an axial acquisition of 40 slices without a gap between slices. The field of view $256 \times 224mm$ and the slice thickness is 3mm. The acquisition uses an interleaved scan with TR/TE=6sec/77ms and a Matrix size of 128x128. An 8 channel coil is used with Grappa reconstruction using 2 acceleration factors and 35 reference lines. For directional encoding of diffusion, two b-values (0 and 800 sec/cm^2) and 6 diffusion directions were used.

3.2 Data Pre-processing

The DTI data of each study was reconstructed into a rank 2 tensor and the b=0 image was rigidly and then non-rigidly aligned to the T1 MPRAGE data using a method derived from [13]. The non-rigid deformation estimate of the data was then applied to bring the diffusion tensors into the coordinate system and sampling resolution of the MPRAGE data (using cubic interpolation), taking into account the local change in geometry using the method of preservation of principal directions [1]. The initial rigid transformation mapping between the two MPRAGE images of the two studies was then estimated by maximization of normalized mutual information between scans [16].

3.3 Data and Registration Forces

Figure 2 shows a representation of the structural information being provided by the DTI dta and the MRI data together, in terms of the principal diffusion

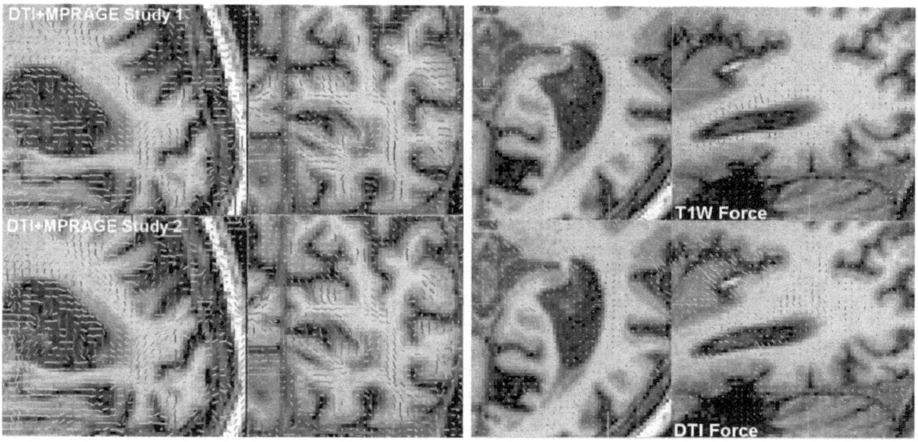

Fig. 2. Left: Sagittal and coronal slices though DTI and MRI data for the two studies of the subject analyzed in figure 3, showing the principal direction vectors (colour coded by direction) of the two DTI datasets overlayed onto the corresponding T1W MPRAGE studies. Right: Components of the force fields driving the studies into alignment, derived from conventional T1W MRI and DTI data. Note expanding ventricular boundary force in conventional MRI and additional forces within uniform regions of white matter from DTI data.

directions. This are displayed after initial rigid alignment, relative distortion correction and reorientation of the diffusion and MRI data (using the rview software tool http://rview.colin-studholme.net). In addition, a map of the components of the induced force field resulting from the conventional structural MRI and DTI data is shown, illustrating in particular, the alignment forces from DTI within bulk white matter.

3.4 Estimated Maps of Atrophy

The determinant of Jacobian matrix of the estimated deformation field was evaluated at each point in the first time point image and used to create a map of relative expansions and contractions required to force the anatomy at the first study to match the anatomy of the second. Results comparing the use of the proposed approach with conventional T1W deformation morphometry are shown in figure 3, for a subject diagnosed with Alzheimer's disease. The figure shows an improved localization of tissue contractions around the expanding ventricular space, when incorporating a measure of DTI alignment into the mapping process. Without DTI information, contractions of white matter around the expanding ventricle are significantly less constrained by the T1W imaging alone.

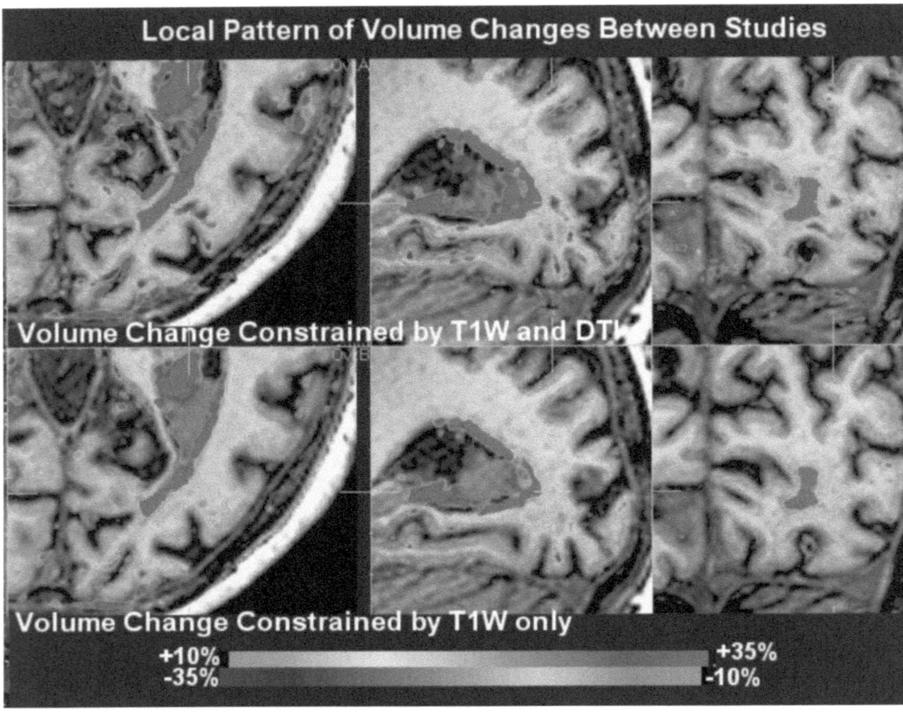

Fig. 3. A subject diagnosed with Alzheimer's Dementia scanned twice with an interval of 9 months (MMSE 25, Age 61.7), exhibiting tissue loss and ventricular expansion. The scan pairs were fluidly aligned using T1 only (bottom right) and T1 with the full diffusion tensor (top right). The incorporation of the additional structural information on the internal white matter structure provided by DTI assists in constraining the local volume changes mapped by the fluid registration within a more focal region of white matter.)

4 Discussion

This paper began be describing a new area of work in the general problem of deformation morphometry, that of using a combination of high resolution conventional scalar MRI data with diffusion tensor image data. The key motivation for this is the commonly observed loss of bulk white matter volume in conventional serial MRI of neurodegeneration. Without any structural features present within white matter in T1W MRI, this loss is simply distributed uniformly over large brain regions. By including information present within diffusion images, the aim is to provide improved localization of any volume losses in deformation morphometry studies, which may reveal characteristic losses related to cognitive decline.

An approach to solving this problem was described which makes use of an extension of mutual information based fluid registration techniques. The approach is aimed at making use of complimentary information provided by the modalities. Specifically, regions in brain diffusion images contain low or zero signal, particularly within fluid spaces, where they provide unreliable directional information. However, regions of low or high diffusion signal correspond to different intensities within the structural MRI data (dark CSF and bright tissue). At its simplest level, the use of the paired MI of values between structural and diffusion images can be seen as partitioning the DTI data into more and less useful regions of directional information. The conventional structural MRI data provides the majority of shared content between the two studies, since it has highest resolution and contrast to noise. However, in regions of uniform white matter, the gradient of the criteria will contain stronger contributions from the DTI data.

An alternative approach would have been to derive scalar, orientation independent measures of image values from the DTI data, and combine these with conventional image data. However, sub-structures in white matter are characterized by both rotationally invariant microstructural tissue integrity (FA, diffusivity) and the microstructural orientation. Neighboring regions of white matter may have identical integrity but differing orientation of tracts. This information is provided by the orientation components of the diffusion tensor, not FA or diffusivity. By using the diffusion values directly, but including their re-orientation during the warping process, we can use their relationship between studies to more fully constrain the deformation solution within white matter.

An interesting extension of this work is to look at optimal smoothing of the DTI data to help to maximize the complimentary registration information it provides to the higher resolution, lower noise T1W images. Methods for dealing with regional variations in tissue contrast arising from disease in conventional MRI data, as in [14], also need to be developed for the case of fusing MRI and DTI data. However, these preliminary results showing the basic step of combining image data are promising, and work is under way to evaluate this approach further using phantom imaging, and to examine its value in studying patterns of white matter and grey matter tissue loss in different forms of neurodegenerative condition.

Acknowledgements. This methods development work was primarily funded by grant NIH R01 NS 055064. This work would not have been possible without image data acquired as part of the NIH funded grants AG10897, P01 AG12435, NIA P01 AG19724, PO1 AA11493. The work would also not have been possible without additional imaging acquired by Dr Lara Stables and help from the faculty and staff of the center for imaging of neurodegenerative disease at the VA in San Francisco.

References

1. Alexander, D.C., Gee, J.C., Bajcsy, R.K.: Strategies for data reorientation during nonrigid warps of diffusion tensor image. In: Taylor, C., Colchester, A. (eds.) MICCAI'99. LNCS, vol. 1679, pp. 463–472. Springer, Heidelberg (1999)
2. Basser, P.J., Mattiello, J., Bihan, D.L.: Estimation of the effective self-diffusion tensor from the NMR spin echo. J. Mag. Res. 103, 247–254 (1994)

3. Cao, Y., Miller, M., Mori, S., Winslow, R., Younes, L.: Large deformation diffeomorphic metric mapping of fiber orientations. In: Proceedings of the International Conference on Computer Vision and Pattern Recognition, IEEE 2005 (2005)
4. Cao, Y., Miller, M., Mori, S., Winslow, R., Younes, L.: Diffeomoprphic matching of diffusion tensor images. In: Proceedings of the Computer Vision and Pattern Recognition Workshop (2006)
5. Cardenas, V.A., Studholme, C., Gazdzinski, S., Durazzo, T.C., Meyerhoff, D.J.: Deformation based morphometry of brain changes in alcohol dependence and abstinence. Neuroimage 34, 879–887 (2007)
6. Christensen, G.E., Miller, M.I., Vannier, M.W.: Individualizing neuroanatomical atlases using a massively parallel computer. Computer, pp. 32–38 (1996)
7. D'Agostino, E., Maes, F., Vandermeulen, D., Suetens, P.: A viscous fluid model for multimodal non-rigid image registration using mutual information. Medical Image Analysis 7, 565–575 (2003)
8. Freeborough, P.A., Fox, N.C.: Modeling brain deformations in Alzheimer's disease by fluid registration of serial 3D MR images. Journal of Computer Assisted Tomography 22(5), 838–843 (1998)
9. Hermosillo, G., Chefd'hotel, C., Faugeras, O.: Variational methods for multimodal image matching. International Journal of Computer Vision 50(3), 329–343 (2002)
10. Jernigan, T.L., Archibald, S.L., Fennema-Notestine, C., Gamst, A.C., Stout, J.C., Bonner, J., Hesselink, J.R.: Effects of age on tissues and regions of the cerebrum and cerebellum. Neurobiology of Aging 22(4), 581–591 (2001)
11. Pluim, J., Maintz, J.B., Viegever, M.A.: Mutual-information-based registration of medical images: A survey. IEEE Transactions on Medical Imaging 22(8), 986–1004 (2003)
12. Press, W.H., Flannery, B.P., Teukolsky, S.A., Vetterling, W.T.: Numerical Recipes in C. Cambridge University Press, Cambridge, England (1992)
13. Studholme, C., Constable, R.T., Duncan, J.S.: Accurate alignment of functional EPI data to anatomical MRI using a physics based distortion model. IEEE Transactions on Medical Imaging 19(11), 1115–1127 (2000)
14. Studholme, C., Drapaca, C., Iordanova, B., Cardenas, V.: Deformation based mapping of volume change from serial brain MRI in the presence of local tissue contrast change. IEEE transactions on Medical Imaging 25(5), 626–639 (2006)
15. Studholme, C., Hill, D.L.G., Hawkes, D.: Incorporating connected region labelling into automated image registration using mutual information. In: Proceedings of the IEEE Workshop on Mathematical Methods in Biomedical Image Analysis, pp. 23–31. IEEE Computer Society Press, Washington, DC, USA (1996)
16. Studholme, C., Hill, D.L.G., Hawkes, D.J.: An overlap invariant entropy measure of 3D medical image alignment. Pattern Recognition 32(1), 71–86 (1999)
17. Studholme, C., Hill, D.L.G., Maisey, M.N., Hawkes, D.: Registration measures for automated 3D alignment of PET and intensity distorted MR images. In: Proceedings in Image Fusion and Shape Variability Techniques, pp. 186–193. Leeds University Press (1996)
18. Thevenaz, P., Unser, M.: Optimization of mutual information for multiresolution image registration. IEEE Transactions on Image Processing 9(12), 2083–2099 (2000)
19. Wahba, G.: Spline Models for Observational Data. Society for Industrial and Applied Mathematics, Philadelphia (1990)
20. Zhang, H., Yushkevich, P.A., Alexander, D.C., Gee, J.C.: Deformable registration of diffusion tensor MR images with explicit orientation optimization. Medical Image Analysis 10(5), 764–785 (2000)

LV Segmentation Through the Analysis of Radio Frequency Ultrasonic Images

P. Yan, C.X. Jia, A. Sinusas, K. Thiele, M. O'Donnell, and J.S. Duncan

Yale University, University of Michigan, Philips Research, University of Washington

Abstract. LV segmentation is often an important part of many automated cardiac diagnosis strategies. However, the segmentation of echocardiograms is a difficult task because of poor image quality. In echocardiography, we note that radio-frequency (RF) signal is a rich source of information about the moving LV as well. In this paper, first, we will investigate currently used, important RF derived parameters: integrated backscatter coefficient(IBS), mean central frequency (MCF) and the maximum correlation coefficients (MCC) from speckle tracking. Second, we will develop a new segmentation algorithm for the segmentation of the LV boundary, which can avoid local minima and leaking through uncompleted boundary. Segmentations are carried out on the RF signal acquired from a Sonos7500 ultrasound system. The results are validated by comparing to manual segmentation results.

1 Introduction

The segmentation of the LV boundary is important for a variety of tasks related to the quantification of heart disease. Echocardiography continues to be one of the most promising noninvasive imaging modalities for quantifying this disease. However, the images can be difficult to interpret due to degradations in the B-mode (envelope detected) image data including intensity inhomogeneity, distortion, and speckle noise which cause most segmentation methods to fail.

The uncompressed RF signal from the ultrasound transducer carries a variety of useful information about the object being imaged. Thus, the RF ultrasonic signal is widely used in tissue characterization [1,2,3,4]. However, very little work has been dedicated to object segmentation based on the RF signal. The images usually used for segmentation are obtained by demodulating and interpolating the RF signal, and the spectral content is lost in this process.

Since echocardiography leads to very noisy images with low contrast differences between regions, most gray level-based segmentation methods are not suitable to find object boundaries. In some cases, the contrast between blood pool and myocardium is so low that even the manual segmentation is impossible. For these reasons, we set out to also extract information from RF signal in hope of using this additional information to help better segment the LV. Furthermore, we plan to exploit these parameters in a frame work based on fuzzy feature information and a Multilevel Free Form Deformation (MFFD) model defined active contour.

N. Karssemeijer and B. Lelieveldt (Eds.): IPMI 2007, LNCS 4584, pp. 233–244, 2007.
© Springer-Verlag Berlin Heidelberg 2007

This paper is organized as follows. Section 2 reviews the related work in the area. Section 3 introduces methods for deriving parameters from RF signal and the 3D segmentation method: Fuzzy-MFFD-Active Contour. Experiments are carried out on the B-mode image and the parametric images constructed from IBS, MCF and MCC. Quantitative evaluation is performed by comparing the results from our approach and other approaches with manual segmentation results. Finally, conclusions are drawn in section 5.

2 Related Work

As noted above, there are little efforts in the RF segmentation area to date. Recently, Boukerroui [5] used MCF and IBS as the parameters of their multi-parametric and multiresolution segmentation algorithm. In their approach, they estimate the parameters through a short-time Fourier analysis, which yields a well-known trade-off between spatial resolution and variance. Dydenko [6] introduced two types of RF-derived parameters: spectral autoregressive parameters and velocity-based parameters for their segmentation framework. The velocity-based parameters are based only on axial velocities along the RF line and this work assumes that the velocities in the muscle are relatively homogeneous, while the estimates in the blood approach random noise. The accuracy of these parameters are questionable. Davignon [7] proposed a parametric imaging approach for the segmentation of ultrasound data. They investigate the relevance of several parameters from both RF and B-mode image data computed from the envelope of the RF signal for the segmentation of ultrasonic data. This method was only tested on simulated data and using a gelatine-agar phantom.

Several approaches have been proposed to segment the B-mode image. Most of them are based on the pixel intensity and suffer from poor accuracy. In automatic segmentation approaches, a *priori* shape knowledge has been used to aid in accurate localization [8,9]. This shape knowledge is often learned via an off-line training process, which can require tedious human effort and is expertise-dependent. Tao [10] proposed an evolution strategy termed *tunneling descent* to avoid getting trapped in the spurious minima. In his model, the contour must be initialized totally outside or inside of the desired boundary and it leaks through incomplete boundary. Some groups introduce filtering methods to correct intensity inhomogeneity [11] and to reduce speckle noise in the ultrasound image [12]. It has been shown that the performance of image feature-based threshold methods will be improved after intensity correction and de-noising. But the evaluation of the effectiveness of these filtering methods still needs to be addressed.

3 Methods

3.1 RF Derived Parameters

Integrated Backscatter Coefficient. One of the most frequently used parameters for acoustical characterization is the integrated backscatter coefficient

(IBS) [13]. The IBS is an estimate of the backscattered energy, so it contains information about the number and the structure of the scatterers in the medium. It can be computed from an RF image using equation 1:

$$IBS = \sum_{BW} PSD(I(f)) \tag{1}$$

where PSD is the power spectral density and *I(f)* is the RF signal in the frequency domain *f*. The FFT and the auto regressive (AR) modeling are two popular techniques used for computing PSD, but they are limited by tradeoffs that must be made between spatial resolution and variance. Gorce proposed an AR model with spatial smoothing in a Bayesian approach for local spectral feature estimation [14]. In this work, we use the continuous wavelet transform (CWT) to derive the IBS from RF signal [15]. The CWT is more flexible and achieves a good tradeoff between time and frequency localization. The wavelet chosen in this work is the Morlet wavelet. In this work, the bandwidth(BW) is set as 0.6.

Mean Central Frequency (MCF). The MCF is another mostly used parameter for tissue characterization [14]. The MCF is related to the attenuation of the medium because of the dependence between attenuation and frequency. The attenuation increases with frequency and consequently modifies the frequency spectrum of a propagating acoustic wave. The MCF is given by 2:

$$MCF = \frac{\sum_{BW} f \cdot PSD(I(f))}{IBS} \tag{2}$$

The Maximum Correlation Coefficients (MCC) from Speckle Tracking. Speckle is not random in the same sense as noise. It is caused by constructive and destructive interference between the backscattered wavelets from the small scatters inside one ultrasound resolution cell. It is found that when an object is scanned twice under exactly the same conditions, one obtains identical speckle patterns [16]. Lubinski et al proposed the phase-sensitive method for speckle tracking [17].

A 3D motion vector (u, v, w) can be estimated at each position in a 3D image by performing a 3D correlation search on local speckles over successive volumetric frames as long as 3D speckle patterns remain correlated at the acquisition frame rate. The full-width, half maximum(FMHM) of the 3D autocorrelation function of the initial complex image defines the speckle size. This kernel is then cross-correlated with the complex frame following the initial one. Mathematically, 3D cross-correlation using phase-sensitive images can be generally formulated as:

$$\varsigma_1 = [\sum_i \sum_j \sum_h W_{ijh} |I_t(x+i, y+j, z+h)|^2]^{\frac{1}{2}} \tag{3}$$

$$\varsigma_2 = [\sum_i \sum_j \sum_h W_{ijh} |I_{t+1}(x+l_x+i, y+l_y+j, z+l_z+h)|^2]^{\frac{1}{2}} \tag{4}$$

$$\rho^{'} = \frac{\sum_i \sum_j \sum_h W_{ijh}[I_t(x+i, y+j, z+h) I^*_{t+1}(x+l_x+i, y+l_y+j, z+l_z+h)]}{\varsigma_1 \cdot \varsigma_2} \quad (5)$$

where $\rho^{'}$ is the unit-normalized, complex, resultant 3D correlation coefficient at pixel (x, y, z) as a function of lags (l_x, l_y, l_z), I_t and I_{t+1} are two successive complex images at time t and t+1, and W_{ijh} is a simple 3D weighting function over the 3D correlation kernel. The symbols i,j and h index every pixel within the 3D kernel. The 3D correlation coefficient is then filtered with a unity gain function ($\sum F_{ijh} = 1$) defined over a region of support (usually 2 times the speckle size [17]):

$$\rho_{xyz}(l_x, l_y, l_j) = \sum_i \sum_j \sum_h F_{ijh}[\rho^{'}_{x+i,y+j,z+h}(l_x, l_y, l_z)] \quad (6)$$

The MCC is the maximum correlation coefficient within the searching window. Since the motion of blood is irregular, the MCC in blood pool are relatively small (< 0.5). The MCC in myocardium are usually bigger than 0.7.

3.2 Fuzzy-MFFD-Active Contour

Here we describe an 'Active Contour' based on a Multilevel cubic B-Spline grid. The active contour moves to the boundary in the image by minimizing an energy function, which is defined by fuzzy feature information and a MFFD model. This method can avoid local minima and leaking through uncompleted boundary. The detail of the advantages of this method can be found in [18].

Energy Functions. The energy function for an active contour is defined as:

$$E = M \cdot \|\tau(C) - I\|^2 + T \sum \sum M log M \quad (7)$$

The C and the I represent the coordinates of contour and image pixels, respectively. The τ is defined as the transformation constrained by a MFFD model. Fuzzy theory provides a powerful mathematical tool for modeling the human ability to reach conclusions when the information is imprecise and incomplete. That is sometimes the case of segmenting medical images with noise, low contrast densities. The fuzzy matching matrix M is defined as:

$$M = \frac{1}{\sqrt{2\pi T^2}} e^{-\frac{\|\tau(C)-I\|^2}{T}} \cdot Q(e^{-\frac{1}{1+|\nabla G_\sigma * g(I)|^2}}) \quad (8)$$

The M shown in table 1 will be normalized in the range of [0,1] and the sums of rows and columns in M are equal to 1. S is the number of the points on boundary and N is the number of image pixels. G_σ is the Gaussian function with standard deviation σ. The $Q(*)$ is a threshold function. The g(I) is the gray level of I. The T is the annealing temperature which will gradually decrease during the iteration. The smaller the T, the bigger the impact of the points near the deforming active contour. In order to have fine control over the fuzziness, we use Deterministic Annealing(DA) technique [19]. It is done by adding an entropy term in the form of

$H = T\sum\sum MlogM$. The entropy term is minimized when all the elements in M are equal, i.e, the correspondence is most fuzzy. At higher temperatures, the entropy term dominates the energy function. As T is lowered, the influence of the entropy decreases and less fuzzy configurations of M are allowed. The new position of the contour measured by fuzzy feature information reads:

$$\tau(C) = \sum_{i=1}^{N} m_{ij}c_i / \sum_{i=1}^{N} m_{ij} \tag{9}$$

where N is the number of I. S is the number of points on the contour.

Table 1. Match table

m	I_1	I_2	...	I_{N-1}	I_N
C_1	m_{11}	m_{12}	...	$m_{1,N-1}$	$m_{1,N}$
C_2	m_{21}	m_{22}	...	$m_{2,N-1}$	$m_{2,N}$
...	...	...	...	...	...
C_{S-1}	$m_{S-1,1}$	$m_{S-1,2}$	...	$m_{S-1,N-1}$	$m_{S-1,N}$
C_S	$m_{S,1}$	$m_{S,2}$	...	$m_{S,N-1}$	$m_{S,N}$

3.3 Multilevel Free Form Deformation (MFFD)

MFFD is an extension to Free Form Deformation (FFD) [20]. The essence of the FFD is to deform an object by manipulating a regular control lattice overlaid on its volumetric embedding space. For example, the contour C is defined through a tensor product of Cubic B-spline:

$$C = \sum_{l=0}^{3}\sum_{m=0}^{3}\sum_{n=0}^{3} B_l(u)B_m(v)B_n(w)\Phi_{i+l,j+m,k+n} \tag{10}$$

where $i = \lfloor x \rfloor - 1$, $j = \lfloor y \rfloor - 1$, $k = \lfloor z \rfloor - 1$, $u = x - \lfloor x \rfloor$, $v = y - \lfloor y \rfloor$, $w = z - \lfloor z \rfloor$. $\lfloor * \rfloor$ denotes the largest integer smaller than *. The $B_l(u)$, $B_m(v)$ and $B_n(w)$ are the uniform cubic B-spline basis functions evaluated at u,v and w, defined as:

$$\begin{aligned} B_0(t) &= (1-t)^3/6, \\ B_1(t) &= (3t^3 - 6t^2 + 4)/6, \\ B_2(t) &= (-3t^3 + 3t^2 + 3t + 1)/6, \\ B_3(t) &= t^3/6 \end{aligned} \tag{11}$$

One can consider a deformation of this grid starting from an initial configuration Φ, and the deforming control lattice as $\Phi + \Delta\Phi$. Once a deformation has been applied, the new position of the contour is defined by:

$$\tau(C) = \sum_{l=0}^{3}\sum_{m=0}^{3}\sum_{n=0}^{3} B_l(u)B_m(v)B_n(w)(\Phi + \Delta\Phi) \tag{12}$$

From above equations, we know that the motion of any point on the contour relates to the motion of $4 \times 4 \times 4 = 64$ control points in its neighborhood. Thus, the spacing of control points will have an impact on the deformation of the active contour. In the MFFD, a hierarchy of control lattices, Φ_0, Φ_1, ..., Φ_k, are used to derive a sequence of deformation functions with the FFD manipulation. Let h_k be the space between control points on the initial configuration of lattice Φ_k. We assume that h_0 is given and that $h_{k+1} = \delta_h h_k$. δ_h is the decreasing rate for the space between control points. When the active contour C is deformed with a coarse control lattice, the positional constraints merge with each other and result in a smooth deformation, although they are not exactly satisfied. The remaining deviations between the deformed and specified positions will be handled by subsequent deformations with finer control lattices. In this method, the contour C is defined implicitly by the MFFD.

4 Experiments

4.1 RF Data Acquisition

The RF data is captured from a board termed Acoustic Frame Link (AFLink). It is an ultrasound RF signal capture system for the Sonos 7500 system that permits access to the beamformed RF acoustic data from the probe supported by the sonos system. In figure 2, we display a single line of Raw, Compressed and logged RF data, respectively.

4.2 Constructing Parametric Images

The raw-RF data is captured in the Frustum coordinate system as shown in figure 1. The data is saved as (R, θ, φ). We first calculate the parameters from the RF data in the Frustum coordinate system, then we reconstruct the image slice by slice as shown in figure 3. We display the RF data in the Frustum coordinate system in the left of figure 4 and a 2D image constructed in the new coordinate system in the right of figure 4. In the new coordinate system, the data is stored as (x, y, φ), where $x = R * \sin(\theta)$ and $y = R * \cos(\theta)$. A 2D slice of constructed B-mode image is shown in figure 5a. Figures 5b-c show the parametric images constructed by IBS, MCF and MCC. We find that the parametric image constructed from MCF has worse quality than the B-mode image, the parametric image constructed from IBS has a little better quality than the B-mode image and the parametric image constructed from MCC has the best quality. In this example, it is very hard to find the epicardium on the bottom from B-mode image because of the attenuation, but we can easily locate the epicardium on the parametric image constructed from MCC.

In order to get accurate speckle tracking estimates, we need to acquire images with a high frame rate. There is a trade-off between the high frame rate and the volume size for a Sonos 7500 imaging system. The frame rate is about 21-22Hz. In the experiments, we find only the images during the end diastole (ED) can get accurate speckle tracking estimates. We will improve the image acquisition

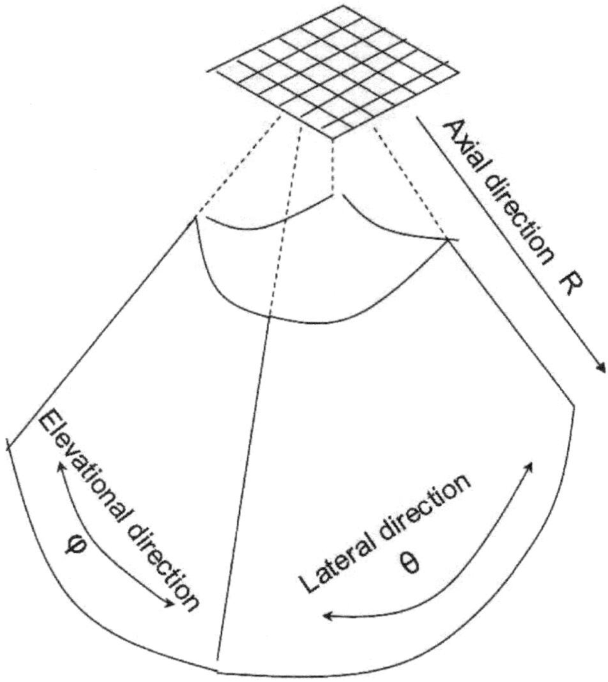

Fig. 1. The Frustum Coordinate System for X4 xMatrix transducer

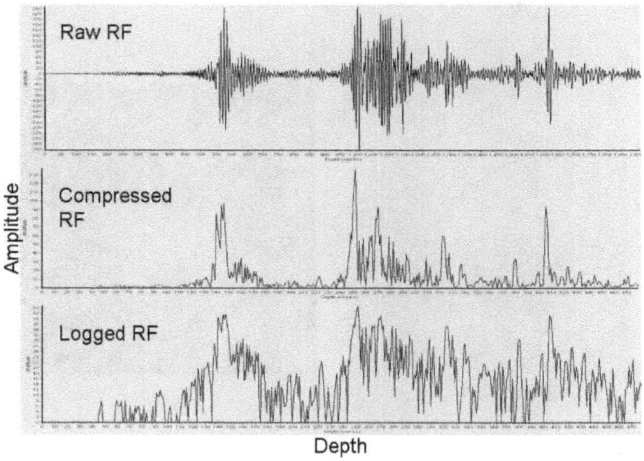

Fig. 2. A single line of Raw (**Top**), Compressed (**Middle**) and Logged (**Bottom**) RF data

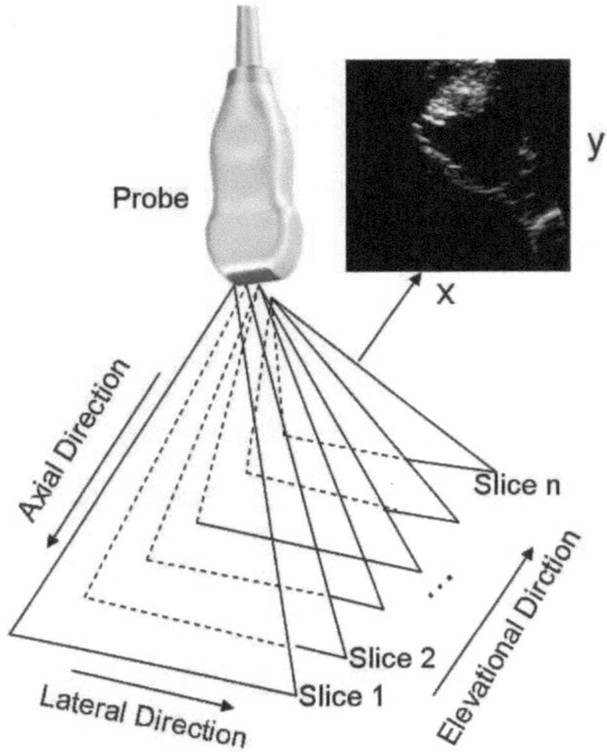

Fig. 3. The new Coordinate System RF image

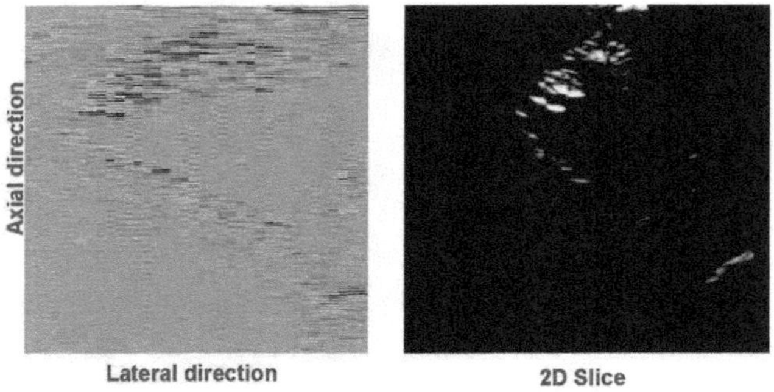

Fig. 4. Left: The RF image in the rectilinearly formatted Frustum coordinate system; **Right**: The B-mode image in the new coordinate system

method in the future, but it is not the importance of this paper. Thus, without special notice, in this paper, the images used are only from end diastole.

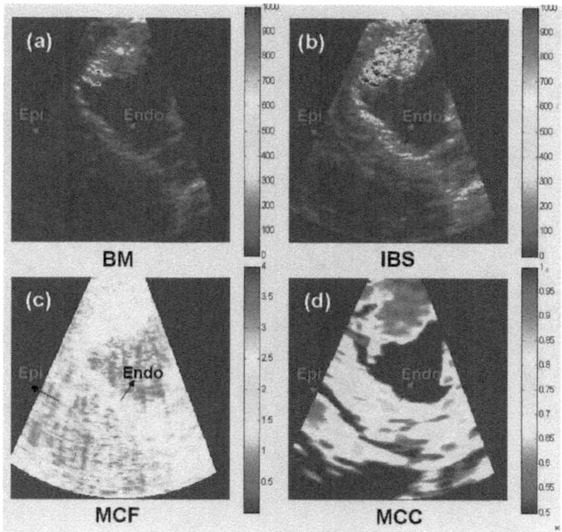

Fig. 5. A 2D slice of (a)B-mode image; parametric images constructed from (b)IBS; (c) MCF; (d) MCC

4.3 Segmentation

We apply the Fuzzy-MFFD-Active Contour algorithm on B-mode image and parametric images constructed from IBS, MCF and MCC, respectively. The results are shown in figure 6. Segmentation on the parametric image constructed from MCF failed because of the poor image quality. It is not realistic to track the boundary on such images. The segmentations are only carried out on the endocardium because most of epicardium is missing. While AFLink could not acquire full volume data at the time of these experiments. The full volume data will be available in the near future.

We then compared segmentation results from different approaches with manual segmentation results. Given two curves C_1 and C_2, we measured the extent of mismatch ratio of the surface as:

$$\epsilon = 1 - \frac{Area(\Omega_{C_1} \cap \Omega_{C_2})}{(Area(\Omega_{C_1}) + Area(\Omega_{C_2}))/2} \tag{13}$$

where Ω_C defines the region inside the contour C. In any given data, we measured mismatch ratios for the results from B-mode images and parametric images constructed from IBS and MCC, respectively, as shown in figure 7. The mismatch ratios for the results from the parametric images constructed from MCC are smaller than the results derived from the other images for all 10 studies. The parametric image constructed from MCC can improve the segmentation results. The parametric images constructed from IBS and MCF don't improve the segmentation results.

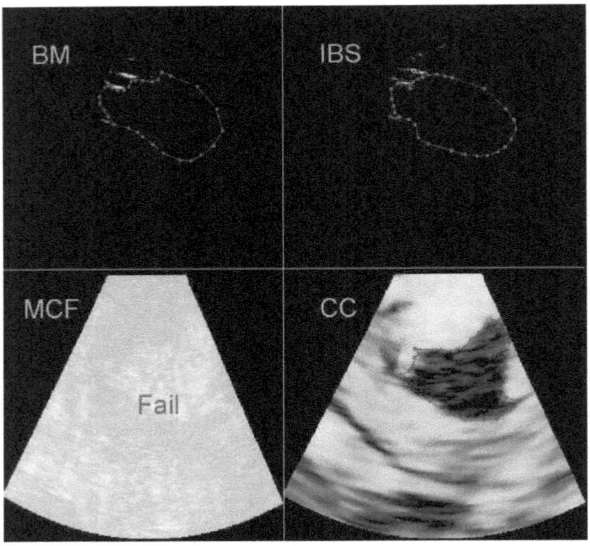

Fig. 6. The segmentation results of (a)B-mode image; parametric images constructed from (b)IBS; (c) MCF; (d) MCC

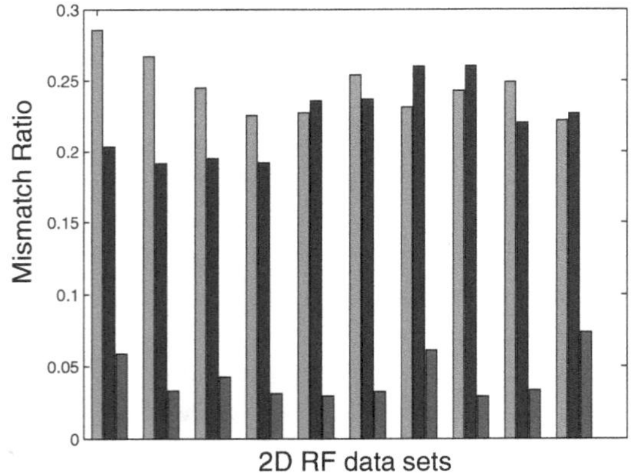

Fig. 7. Mismatch ratios of the endocardium segmentation results from B-mode image(**light gray**), parametric image constructed from IBS (**dark**), parametric image constructed from MCC (**dark gray**) on 10 2D RF images

5 Conclusions and Future Work

In this paper, we presented a new method for LV segmentation from RF data. RF data has rich information including not only the intensity, but also the spectrum and phase. The RF data used in this paper was acquired from the AFLink of Philips Sonos7500 imaging system.

We used the continuous wavelet transformation (CWT) to extract the parameters IBS and MCF from the RF signal. We also calculated the MCC using the phase-sensitive speckle tracking method on RF image sequences. The derived parameters IBS, MCF and MCC were used to construct parametric images. The parametric image constructed from MCC had the best quality and was the only useful one.

The Fuzzy-MFFD-Active Contour method can successfully avoid local minima and leaking through uncompleted boundary [18]. The method has been qualitatively compared against the approach with FFD and a level set approach. Further quantitative evaluation has been carried out by comparing the method generated boundaries against those drawn manually on four 3D echocardiographic images. The analysis shows that our method can successfully locate endocardial boundaries. When the image quality is very poor, this method still fails at finding the boundary. We use Fuzzy-MFFD-Active Contour method to find the boundaries on B-mode images and three different parametric images. The final results are compared to manual segmentation results. It shows that the results by using Fuzzy-MFFD-Active Contour on the parametric images constructed from MCC are the most accurate.

Currently, the AFLink system has the trade-off between image volume and frame rate. The phase sensitive speckle tracking method can only get accurate results when the deformation is small. Thus, our segmentation is only carried out on the image frames during end-diastole. In the near future, we will upgrade our AFLink system to get the RF data with full volume and high frame rate. We will extend this method to a 3D+T segmentation and tracking system.

References

1. Feleppa, E.J., Kalisz, A., Sokil-Melgar, J.B., Lizzi, F.L., Liu, T., Rosado, A.L., Shao, M.C., R, W., Wang, F.Y., Cookson, M.S., Reuter, V.E., Heston, W.D.W: Typing of prostate tissue by ultrasonic spectrum analysis. IEEE Trans. on Ultrasonics,Ferroelectrics, and Frequency Control 43, 609 (1996)
2. Schmitz, G., Ermert, H., Senge, T.: Tissue-characterization of the prostate using radio frequency ultrasonic signals. IEEE Trans. on Ultrasonics,Ferroelectrics, and Frequency Control 46, 126–138 (1999)
3. Georgiou, G., Cohen, F.S., Piccoli, C.W., Forsberg, F., Goldberg, B.B.: Tissue characterization using the continuous wavelet transform part ii: Application on breast rf data. IEEE Transactions on Ultrasonics, Ferroelectrics, and Frequency Control 48(2), 364–373 (2001)
4. Gefen, S., Tretiak, O., Piccoli, C., Donohue, K., Petropulu, A., Shankar, P., Dumane, V., Huang, L., Kutay, M., Genis, V., Forsberg, F., Reid, J.: Roc analysis of ultrasound tissue characterization classifiers for breast cancer diagnosis. IEEE Trans. Medical Imaging 22(2), 170–177 (2003)
5. Boukerroui, D., Basset, O., Baskurt, A., Gimenez, G.: A multiparametric and multiresolution segmentation algorithm of 3d ultrasonic data. IEEE Trans. on Ultrasonics,Ferroelectrics, and Frequency Control 48, 64–77 (2001)

6. Dydenko, I., Friboulet, D., Gorce, J.M., D'hooge, J., Bijnens, B., Magnin, I.E.: Towards ultrasound cardiac image segmentation based on the radiofrequency signal. Medical Image Analysis 7, 353–367 (2003)
7. Davignon, F., Deprez, J.F., Basset, O.: A parametric imaging approach for the segmentation of ultrasound data. Ultrasonics 43, 789–801 (2005)
8. Chen, Y., Thiruvenkadam, S., Tagare, H., Huang, F., Wilson, D., Geiser, E.: On the incorporation of shape priors into geometric active contours. In: IEEE Workshop on Variational and Level Set. Methods in Computer Vision, vol. 1, pp. 145–152 (2001)
9. Bosch, J., Mitchell, S., Lelieveldt, B., Nijland, F., Kamp, O., Sonka, M., Reiber, J.: Automatic segmentation of echocardiographic sequences by active appearance motion models. IEEE Trans. on Medical Imaging 21, 1374–1383 (2002)
10. Tao, Z., Jaffe, C.C., Tagare, H.D.: Tunneling descent: A new algorithm for active contour segmentation of ultrasound images. In: Taylor, C.J., Noble, J.A. (eds.) IPMI 2003. LNCS, vol. 2732, pp. 246–257. Springer, Heidelberg (2003)
11. Xiao, G., Brady, M., Noble, J., Zhang, Y.: Segmentation of ultrasound b-mode images with intensity inhomogeneity correction. IEEE Trans. Medical Imaging 21(1), 48–57 (2002)
12. Zong, X., Laine, A., Geiser, E.: Speckle reduction and contrast enhancement of echocardiograms via multiscale nonlinear processing. IEEE Trans. Medical Imaging 17(4), 532–540 (1998)
13. Rijsterborgh, H., Mastik, F., Lancee, C.T., Verdouw, P., Roelandt, J., Bom, N.: Ultrasound myocardial integrated backscatter signal processing:frequency domain versus time domain. Ultrasound Med. Biol. 19, 211–219 (1993)
14. Gorce, J., Friboulet, D., Dydenko, I., D'hooge, J., Bijnens, B., Magnin, I.: Processing radio frequency ultrasound images: A robust method for local spectral features estimation by a spatially constrained parametric approach. IEEE Transactions on Ultrasonics, Ferroelectrics, and Frequency Control 49(12), 1704–1719 (2002)
15. Hossen, A.: Power spectral density estimation via wavelet decomposition. Electroics Letters 40(17), 1055–1056 (2004)
16. Burckhardt, C.: speckle in ultrasound b-mode scans. IEEE transactions on sonics and ultrasonics 30(3), 156–163 (1983)
17. Lubinski, M., Emelianov, S., O'Donnell, M.: Speckle tracking methods for ultrasonic elasticity imaging using short time correlation. IEEE trans Ultrason Ferroelect Freq. Contr 46, 82–96 (1999)
18. Yan, P., Duncan, J.S., Sinusas, A.: Lv segmentation from 3d echocardiography using fuzzy features and a multilevel ffd model (2007)
19. Rangarajan, A., Chui, H., Mjolsness, E., Pappu, S., Davachi, L., Goldman-Rakic, P., Duncan, J.S.: A robust point matching algorithm for autoradiograph alignment. Medical Image Analysis 4(1), 379–398 (1997)
20. Lee, S., Wolberg, G., Chwa, K., Shin, S.: Image metamorphosis with scattered feature constraints. IEEE Trans. on Visualization and Computer Graphics 2(4), 337–354 (1996)

Chestwall Segmentation in 3D Breast Ultrasound Using a Deformable Volume Model

Henkjan Huisman and Nico Karssemeijer

Radboud University Medical Centre, Nijmegen, The Netherlands
H.Huisman@rad.umcn.nl

Abstract. A deformable volume segmentation method is proposed to detect the breast parenchyma in frontal scanned 3D whole breast ultrasound. Deformable volumes are a viable alternative to the deformable surface paradigm in noisy images with poorly defined object boundaries. A deformable ultrasound volume model was developed containing breast, rib, intercostal space and thoracic shadowing. Using prior knowledge about grey value statistics and shape the parameterized model deforms by optimization to match an ultrasound scan. Additionally a rib shadow enhancement filter was developed based on a Hessian sheet detector. An ROC chestwall detection study on 88 multi-center scans (20 non-visible chestwalls) showed a significant accuracy which improved strongly using the sheet detector. The results show the potential of our methodology to extract breast parenchyma which could help reduce false positives in subsequent computer aided lesion detection.

1 Introduction

Breast cancer screening with mammography is effective in women over 50. In younger women screening is controversial [1], because the high breast density in premenopausal women reduces the sensitivity of mammography and increases radiation risk. Screening below the age of 50 is desirable, in particular in women at risk due to genetic profile or family history. Ultrasound can be effective in this population and has been shown to detect cancers that are occult on dense mammograms and are not palpable [2]. Moreover, ultrasound does not involve ionizing radiation. The detection comes at the expense of an increased false positive (FP) rate, which is partly due to lack of experience of radiologists. More research is needed to develop ultrasound as a breast screening modality.

Conventional 2D, handheld ultrasound requires a skilled radiologist to examine both breasts. This renders ultrasound screening expensive, and also dependent on the operator. Recently, automated whole breast ultrasound scanning has become commercially available [3]. The scanner sweeps the breast with a 14.7 cm wide-aperture linear transducer during supine positioning. A technician using the scanner can acquire a bilateral breast exam in approximately 15 minutes. One such frontal scan covers an average whole breast. The digital 3D ultrasound exam is then read offline on a dedicated workstation by a skilled observer. Due to the large amount of data and the complexity of the images there is a large potential for using computer aided detection (CAD).

N. Karssemeijer and B. Lelieveldt (Eds.): IPMI 2007, LNCS 4584, pp. 245–256, 2007.
© Springer-Verlag Berlin Heidelberg 2007

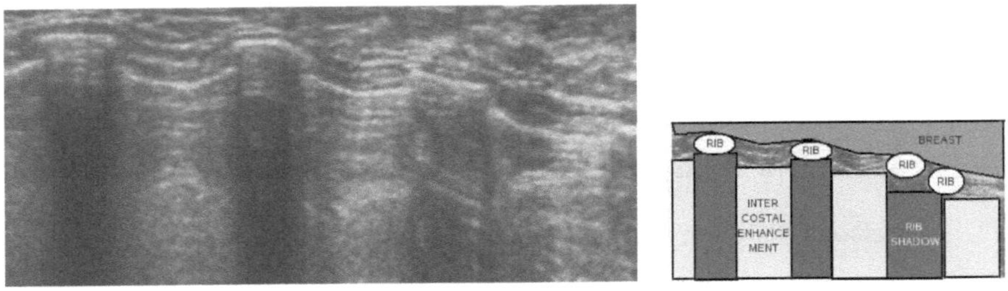

Fig. 1. Sagittal view of a frontal 3D breast ultrasound scan (left), schematic drawing on the right describes the visible structures. See text for detailed description.

CAD for ultrasound has received limited attention on 2D [4,5] and on localized 3D [6,7]. Actual testing of CAD was infeasible as no whole breast 3D ultrasound was available. We are developing and testing a CAD system to help radiologists with finding breast cancer in 3D whole breast ultrasound. The system consists of an initial detector that locates suspect areas based on a set of dedicated image features sensitive to echogenicity and spiculation. A whole image segmentation step automatically localizes the breast parenchyma which serves to masks out initially detected locations that are outside the breast. Each remaining suspicious location within the breast is then analyzed in more detail by segmenting the lesion it identifies. Additional features from within and below the lesion and from the segmented lesion topology are fed to a classifier which is trained to respond with the lesion malignancy likelihood.

In this paper we focus on a method to automatically detect and segment breast parenchyma in 3D ultrasound. During frontal scanning the transducer is scanned linearly over the flattened breast. Starting from the transducer surface and going downward the following tissues are visualized: skin, breast parenchyma, pectoral muscle, chestwall and thoracic volume. The image volume further exhibits near black areas (only electronic noise) where the transducer surface extended outside the breast tissue. It appears that the discrimination between breast parenchyma and chestwall is often very challenging, in particular in larger breasts where ribs are depicted less clear due to a larger distance to the transducer. Global information extracted from the image and prior knowledge is required to establish a reliable procedure for chestwall segmentation. Although many methods for ultrasound image segmentation exist [8] we will show that a deformable volume model is well suited for this task. In addition, we design a method to detect the presence of a chestwall, as in larger breasts it may be outside the imaged area.

2 Method

2.1 Overview

The thorax volume in a frontal 3D ultrasound scan is characterized by shadowing behind the ribs (see Figure 1). The presence of echoes from within the lung volume is due to an ultrasound artefact. The tissue-air interface reflects all ultrasound due to a large acoustic impedance mismatch between tissue and air. Strong reflective interfaces introduce mirror artefacts. Looking again at Figure 1 one can observe that ultrasound echoes appear to originate from within the lung volume that are actually mirror reflections of breast parenchyma scattering. This pattern depends strongly on the shape and orientation of the reflecting surface. The shadowing behind the rib is due to the lower reflectivity of the tissue-rib interface and strong attenuation within the rib resulting in a rapid decrease in the intensity of the mirror reflections. Because of the lower reflectivity at the rib surface, scattering from within the rib is present. In a coronal (or c-plane) view the ribs have a different texture compared to the surrounding tissue (see Figure 2). As ultrasound is a coherent imaging system we further have the common relatively high levels of so-called speckle noise. Finally, the presence of cysts or malignant lesions can it self introduce artefacts. Cysts are commonly diagnosed by the presence of a 'bright tail' due to the lower attenuation of the cysts content. Lesions accompanied by a dark tail are more often malignant which can be explained by the higher gross attenuation features of malignant tissue. In conclusion, segmenting the thorax in 3D breast ultrasound is a challenging task.

We chose to use a deformable volume to segment the thorax. Conventional thresholding and region growing paradigms are not suited because of a lack of homogeneity in the thorax area. Our idea is to use a physical chestwall model containing individual ribs. The model allows for inclusion of prior knowledge such as: expected rib size range and distance and shape characteristics. The model should also include rib shadow and inter costal tails as these allow for the positioning of the ribs such that they optimally describe the visible shadows. In doing so the whole volume of thorax is described and the remaining volume is the breast tissue volume of interest. A cost function is defined that maximizes when the ribs are at the correct location. The physical model can be defined either by a surface mesh or a set of volume elements. As the edge definition of the tails and other objects is rather poor, we feel that a deformable volume approach best fits this problem. We let the ribs define the whole model, and thus it is the deformation of the ribs that is of interest. We propose a multi-tubular rib model, where each tube's center line can be positioned. Internal shape constraints are imposed via the cost function. Furthermore, we limit the detail of tubes shapes by deriving local changes from a spline interpolated 3x3 deformation grid. This enforces smooth yet realistic rib cage shapes and a reasonable amount of parameters during optimization.

We have further developed a rib shadow detection feature that can serve as input to the deformable model detection and segmentation step. The feature comprises a Gaussian smoothed Laplacian filter followed by a Hessian operator. This is a well known technique where features can be derived from the eigen values of the Hessian matrix to be sensitive to blobs, lines or sheets. We have further restricted a sheet detection filter to be sensitive to vertical dark sheets

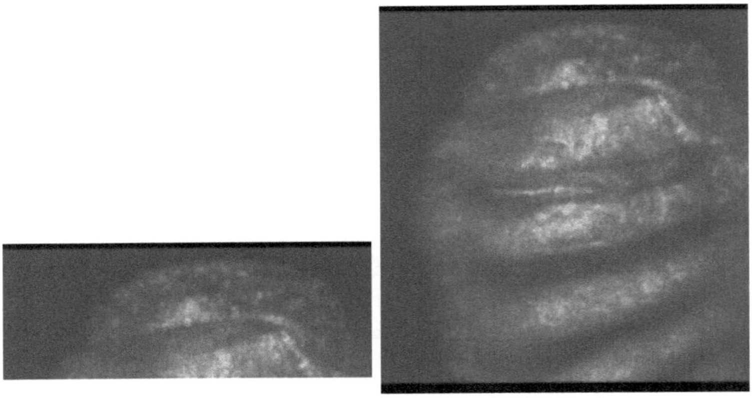

Fig. 2. A coronal (or c-plane) view of a frontal 3D breast scan. Rib size, shape, and distance form a pattern that help to identify individual rib shadows. As an example, all rib locations in the left image may not be obvious. Extending the image to include the other ribs (right image) allows to be more certain about the position of the same ribs in the left image.

only. We hypothesize that using the rib shadow detection feature will reduce artefacts in in vivo images and should thus improve the detection and segmentation performance.

2.2 Deformable Volume Model Definition

Each rib is modelled by a tube about a center line. Ribs are deformed by deforming the center line. A tube is divided into segments, represented by cuboids (rectangular box) with its center on the rib centerline. The cuboid axes are parallel to the image coordinate system (see figure 2.2). This cuboid orientation allows for fast computation of the cuboid's (and therefore a rib's) internal grey value statistics. The area below a rib segment extending to the bottom of the image defines a rib shadow segment. Although the rib cross-section is rectangular, the shadow projection can be quite smooth provided a sufficiently high number of segments (we use 60 per rib). The cuboid between two adjacent rib segments (with the same rib segment index) defines an intercostal segment. The area below an intercostal segment, similar to the rib segment, defines an inter costal 'shadow'. The area above a rib or intercostal segment extending to the top of the image is a breast segment. In this manner the whole image volume is divided into cuboids. Five sets (or compartments) of cuboids exist: Breast, Rib, Intercostal, Ribshadow, Intercostalshadow.

The previously defined volume model covers the whole image volume, and is defined only by the centerlines and rib size. The number of parameter needed to deform this model can be rather large. If we assume each rib comprises 60 segments and if we use 6 ribs and each segment is individually positioned, then

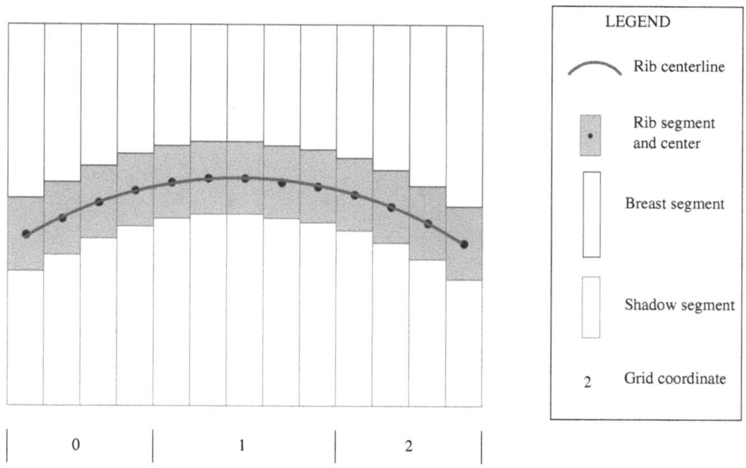

Fig. 3. Cross-section of the chestwall model showing one rib. Each rib is modelled by a series of segments (cuboids) centered about the centerline. The area below a rib segment that extents to the bottom of the image is a rib shadow segment, the area above the rib segment extending to the top of the image is the breast segment.

1080 parameters need to be optimized. This is too much and also redundant as the rib cage shape is rather smooth. Reducing the number of segments is not an option as that would degrade the model. Thus we reduced the number of model parameters by deriving the centerlines shape from a spline interpolated 3x3 grid. The 9 grid vertices contain displacement vectors that deform a basic flat equidistant set of centerlines by cubic B-spline interpolation. Moreover by creating ribs long enough to extent well outside the volume we need only deformations in two directions. This amounts to only 18 parameters that fully define the rib cage position and shape (see figure 4). Additional model parameters are: rib distance, length and number of ribs.

2.3 Deformable Volume Model Optimization

Segmentation with deformable volume models is to optimize the model parameters by minimizing a cost function. The deformable volume model is fully described by a reduced set of parameters: $p_{cw} = \{O, \theta_y, d, w, h, d_{i,j} : i = 1 \ldots 3, j = 1 \ldots 3\})$, where O is the position, θ_y is the rotation in the coronal plane, d the rib distance, w rib width, h rib height, $d_{i,j}$ the centerline displacement vector $(d_{i,j,x}, d_{i,j,z})$ in grid cell i,j, and assuming the usual x, y, z directions: left-right, ventral-dorsal, cranio-caudal. The optimal parameters $p_{cw,opt}$ are found by minimizing a cost function. Let $C_{ext}(p_{cw})$ and $C_{int}(p_{cw})$ be an external and internal cost function (to be defined later). Then the optimal parameters $p_{cw,opt}$ are found by minimizing the total cost:

$$p_{cw,opt} = \arg\min_{p_{cw}}\{C_{ext}(p_{cw}) + C_{int}(p_{cw})\}, \tag{1}$$

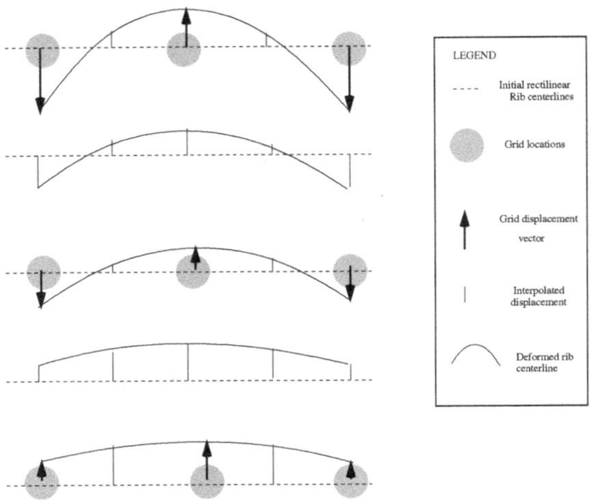

Fig. 4. Gridded rib deformation. The deformed rib centerlines start out as straight lines. At the grid locations a deformation vector is set. In between grid locations these deformation vectors are interpolated. Each rib centerline location is then displaced to finally form the deformed rib centerlines.

In our implementation the optimization is performed using the simplex method.

The optimization process is sub divided into three sequential stages each optimizing a part of the segmentation process:

- **Chest wall detection.** First the presence of a chest wall is detected. A small chestwall model at the bottom center of the volume is optimized only for position, and rib distance. No deformation takes place. A chestwall likelihood is defined and if above a certain threshold processing proceeds with the next step. Otherwise, processing stops as no chestwall is detected.
- **Chest wall shadow fit.** In the second stage the detected chest wall is further deformed in the z-direction (cranio-caudal) to match the shape of the ribs shadows. The optimization is restricted to: number of ribs, rib length and the z-deformation components of the grid displacement vectors.
- **Chest wall full fit.** The third and final segmentation step tries to find y-deformation (ventral-dorsal) components of the grid displacement vectors to match the visible rib cage. The ribs and intercostal segments and shadow segments then form the thorax volume. This thorax volume can be used as a mask to limit the detection search space in subsequent 3D breast ultrasound lesion detection methods.

Chest wall detection. The chestwall detection tries to find a characteristic chestwall shadow pattern (see Figure 2) at the dorsal end of the image volume. This detection step is again split up into two steps. First a single rib with small length (0.3 x available width in the x-direction) is initialized at the center bottom of the image and is rotated (θ) and translated (x, z) to match a single rib. The cost function is the average grey value of that rib:

$$C_{detect1} = v_{ribshadow}, \quad (2)$$

where $\overline{v}_X$ is the mean gray value of the voxels in model compartment X and s denotes standard deviation.

Secondly, the number of ribs is set to 3 and the search parameter list is extended with the rib distance. The rib width is set to half the rib distance during optimization. The optimizer then tries to find a combination of parameters that produce dark rib shadows and bright intercostal shadows. The cost function is defined as:

$$C_{detect2} = \frac{\overline{v}_{ribshadow} - \overline{v}_{intercostalshadow}}{s_{ribshadow}}, \quad (3)$$

The presence of a chestwall is detected by evaluating the value of the cost function after optimization $C_{detect2,opt}$. If below a preset threshold, then processing continues to chestwall segmentation stage 2, otherwise processing stops. In case of no chestwall detection the model parameters are set such that the whole image volume is labeled as breast tissue.

Chest wall shadow fit. In the second optimization stage the whole rib shadow area is detected by determining the length, total number and shape of the ribs in the z-direction. The chestwall parameters angle (θ) and position (O) are fixed.

The initially detected chestwall is deformed to fit the shadow area by minimizing the cost function using only the z-components of the 9 grid coordinates (d_z). The cost function now comprises an external and internal part. The external cost function is the same as during detection (Eq. 3) and favors dark rib shadows and bright intercostal shadows. The internal cost function constrains the shape such that local rib spacing is in between a minimum and maximum distance and imposes a maximum z-curvature constraint.

Final chest wall fit. The chest wall at this stage of the segmentation process covers the coronal plane and has the correct z-shape deformations. In this final stage the optimal deformation of the chestwall model in the y-direction is searched. To find the correct rib height in the y-direction the external cost function is based on the following concept. Each rib defines two curved sheets: the area above the rib should be breast parenchyma (ribbreast) and the area below the rib should be rib shadow. If the rib is too low, then the the ribbreast part will extend into the shadow area and consequently have an average grey value that is too low. On the other hand, if the rib is too high then the ribshadow extends into the breast parenchyma resulting in gray value that is too high. Simply maximizing the contrast between ribshadow and ribbreast leads to incorrect shapes as shadow and breast tissue area are rather inhomogeneous, and due to insufficient depth-gain compensation. An improvement resulted when incorporating information on the location of the rib. The local contrast between rib and intercostal grey values is high when the rib is within the rib shadow area, the contrast is less or even negative when in the breast area. This information is used construct a steerable cost function:

$$C_{final,ext,i,j} = (1 - w_{i,j})v_{ribshadow,i,j} - w_{i,j}v_{ribbreast,i,j} \tag{4}$$

where w is a weighting variable that switches between optimizing breast or shadow fit. The weight w is determined from the normalized difference between rib and intercostal mean value:

$$w_{i,j} = (v_{rib,i,j} - v_{intercostal,i,j})/s_{rib} \tag{5}$$

where w is limited to $0 < w < 1$. If the rib is in the rib shadow area, w is high and breast gray value should increase to decrease cost. If the rib is at the correct location the weight will be intermediate and the cost function thus has a smooth transition zone.

The internal cost function assigns costs to infeasible y-deformations. Local rib curvature and rib slopes are computed to construct a continuous assessment of the y-deformation shape cost of the rib cage. Each rib is required to be convex. Transducer - chestwall distance should increase in the caudal direction.

2.4 Rib Shadow Detection Feature

The deformable chestwall segmentation method is extended with a preprocessing step that helps to enhance the rib shadows and reduce noise. We used a sheet detector based on a smoothed second order derivative matrix (Hessian) [9,10,11,12]. The eigenvalues of the Hessian matrix $\lambda_1 < \lambda_2 < \lambda_3$ each identify the strength of a second order derivative in a perpendicular direction. Rib shadows are dark sheets or plate like structures. These should have only one strong eigenvalue. An operator sensitive for sheets is:

$$f_{sh} = \sigma^2 \lambda_3 * \exp(-\lambda_2^2 - \lambda_1^2), \tag{6}$$

which has positive maxima at dark sheet locations. The smoothing scale (σ) was set to 5mm.

The sheet detector (Eq. 6) in our 3D breast ultrasound is obviously also sensitive to the edges of the area in which the transducer had good contact with the breast. This could lead to erroneous chestwall detections and therefore we applied a mask to the Hessian sheet detector output blocking this breast-noise zone. The noise zone is well defined by image values below a certain threshold. The remaining 'valid' ultrasound zone was then eroded to form the sheeth detector mask. The result of which is shown in Fig. 5)

2.5 Experiment

The method was validated on a set of 88 3D ultrasound clinical breast scans. The scans are the first set of whole breast ultrasound exams of 25 women from

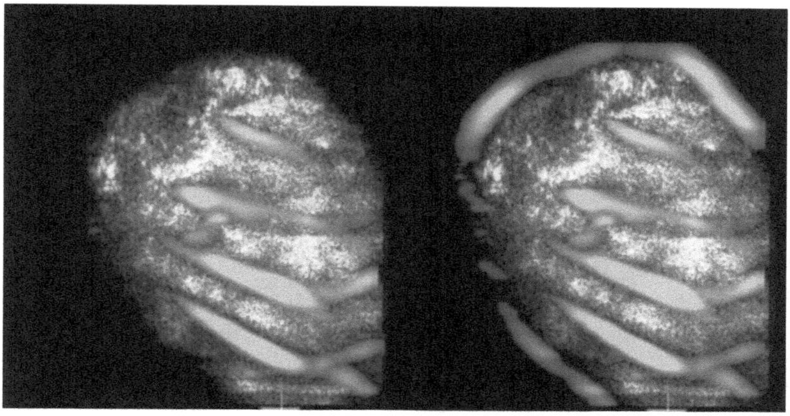

Fig. 5. The output of the rib shadow detector after (on the left) and before masking (right). Notice the removal of false rib locations at the edge of the valid ultrasound region.

3 imaging centers in the united states in the first quarter of 2006. The detection performance was estimated by performing an ROC study. For each scan the presence or absence of a chestwall was determined by visual assessment. For each scan the chestwall detection step of the segmentation method was applied to determine the likelihood that a chestwall is present. The detection was repeated for three settings: using the original grey value image, using the Hessian based sheet detector, and the same Hessian, but extended with a mask operator. Significance was determined using bootstrapping [13].

The data from the previous experiment was also used to determine a threshold of detection likehood above which the subsequent chestwall segmentation stages were carried out. Example segmentations will be shown.

3 Results

Annotation resulted in 20 scans that did not show and 68 that did show a chestwall. Figure 6 shows two results of the chestwall detection. The detected chestwall shadow pattern in a scan with a visible chestwall clearly matches the shadow pattern. In the scan with no visible chestwall the detected shadow pattern does not align with a shadow pattern. The calculated likelihood in the scan with chestwall present is higher. The general ability of the detection likelihood to separate chestwall presence and absence is visualized in the ROC curves shown in Figure 7. Three detection settings have been studied. Settings 1 and 2 (Hessian sheet detector) produce ROC curves that are indicative of a better detection performance over a wide range of thresholds compared to setting 0 (gray value based). However, differences between the methods were not statistically significant. Setting 2 was used for further processing and a threshold of detection

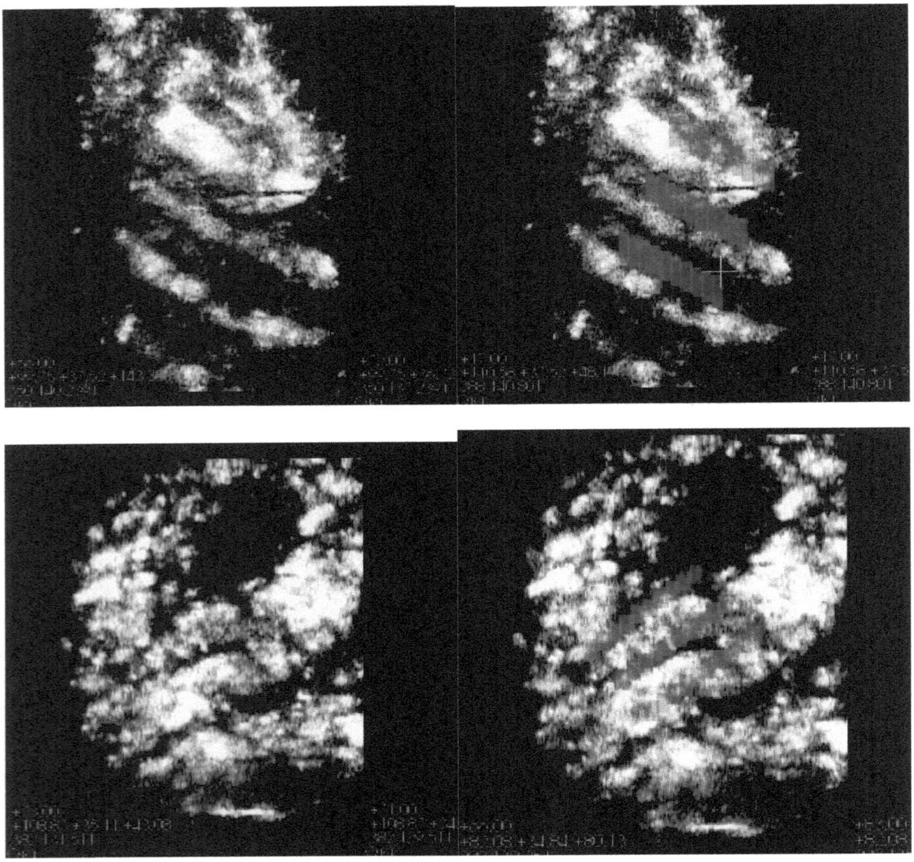

Fig. 6. Top row. Coronal slice of a scan with a visible chestwall (left). Detected chestwall rib shadows overlayed in red (Likelihood=0.91). Bottom row. Coronal slice of a scan with no visible chestwall (left). Detected chestwall rib shadows overlayed in red (Likelihood=0.27).

likelihood was then selected with a specificity of 100% (the 20/0 point on curve 2). At this setting only visible chestwalls are detected. Scans with a detection likelihood above this threshold were processed further with the following two chestwall segmentation steps. The segmented chestwall area in all these scans was at or below the actual chestwall. No breast tissue was incorrectly labeled as thorax.

4 Discussion

We have developed and tested a chestwall segmentation method that can operate on 3D whole breast ultrasound data. Using a Hessian based rib shadow

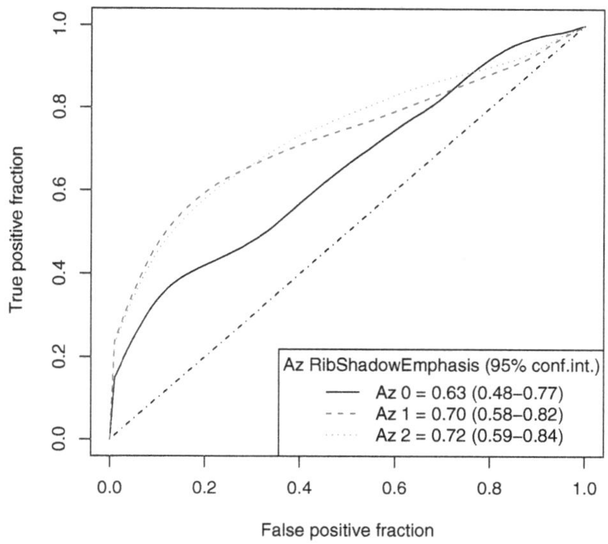

Fig. 7. Receiver operating curves summarising the diagnostic accuracy in detecting chestwall presence. Three settings for the detector were evaluated.

enhancement filter and a deformable volume model we were able to detect the presence of a visible chestwall with a reasonable accuracy. At a 100% specificity level a detection sensitivity of 20% was achieved. The subsequent full 3D segmentation of the actual chestwalls and thoracic volume did not include breast tissue. The proposed segmentation method can reduce the search space for a subsequent computer aided detection algorithm, and can thus reduce the number of false positives without missing lesions due to oversegmentation/detection.

The method in its current state is a first working prototype and it is obvious that the detection sensitivity needs to be increased to substantially decrease the number of false positives in a CAD system for actual use. Still, considering the challenging segmentation and detection task we feel that the deformable volume paradigm is good choice for this segmentation problem. The deformable volume method is appealing as it simulates real physical objects allowing for intuitive constraints (e.g. rib distance, shape). The volumetric definition enables fast computation of regional grey value properties. The deformable volume method in this application is not yet fully exploited and we expect further improvements.

The acquired data is a limited set of first series of a new 3D ultrasound machine for the acquisition of whole breast scans. The data quality can be expected to improve in future routine scanning. We need to further investigate scans with a missing chestwall as that may also lead to missing cancers. Preliminary results in this paper are a first step towards the development of a CAD system for detection of abnormalities in whole breast ultrasound. CAD can help reduce the level of required reading experience and reduce reading time and is already indicated by radiologists due to the overwhelming amount of data to be visualized.

References

1. Moss, S., Cuckle, H., Evans, A., Johns, L., Waller, M., Bobrow, L.: Effect of mammographic screening from age 40 years on breast cancer mortality at 10 years' follow-up: a randomised controlled trial. Lancet 368(9552), 2053–2060 (2006)
2. Kolb, T., Lichy, J., Newhouse, J.: Occult cancer in women with dense breasts: detection with screening US–diagnostic yield and tumor characteristics. Radiology 207(1), 191–199 (1998)
3. Destounis, S., Young, W., Murphy, P., Somerville, P., Seifert, P., Zuley, M.: Initial Experience of Automated Breast Ultrasound Screening Trial in the Setting of a Community Based Private Practice. RSNA (2006)
4. Drukker, K., Giger, M., Horsch, K., Kupinski, M., Vyborny, C., Mendelson, E.: Computerized lesion detection on breast ultrasound. Med. Phys. 29(7), 1438–1446 (2002)
5. Drukker, K., Giger, M., Metz, C.: Robustness of computerized lesion detection and classification scheme across different breast US platforms. Radiology 237(3), 834–840 (2005)
6. Sahiner, B., Chan, H., Roubidoux, M., Hadjiiski, L., Helvie, M., Paramagul, C., Bailey, J., Nees, A., Blane, C.: Malignant and Benign Breast Masses on 3D US Volumetric Images: Effect of Computer-aided Diagnosis on Radiologist Accuracy. Radiology (2007)
7. Sahiner, B., Chan, H., Roubidoux, M., Helvie, M., Hadjiiski, L., Ramachandran, A., Paramagul, C., LeCarpentier, G., Nees, A., Blane, C.: Computerized characterization of breast masses on three-dimensional ultrasound volumes. Med. Phys. 31(4), 744–754 (2004)
8. Noble, J., Boukerroui, D.: Ultrasound image segmentation: a survey. IEEE Trans Med. Imaging 25(8), 987–1010 (2006)
9. Sato, Y., Nakajima, S., Shiraga, N., Atsumi, H., Yoshida, S., Koller, T., Gerig, G., Kikinis, R.: Three-dimensional multi-scale line filter for segmentation and visualization of curvilinear structures in medical images. Med. Image Anal. 2(2), 143–168 (1998)
10. Frangi, A., Niessen, W., Hoogeveen, R., van Walsum, T., Viergever, M.: Model-based quantitation of 3-D magnetic resonance angiographic images. IEEE Trans Med. Imaging 18(10), 946–956 (1999)
11. Sato, Y., Westin, C., Kikinis, R.: Tissue classification based on 3D local intensity structures for volume rendering. IEEE Trans Vis. Comp. Graph 6(2), 160–180 (2000)
12. Ibanez, L., Schroeder, W.: The ITK software guide. Kitware Inc., (2005) `www.itk.org`
13. Rutter, C.: Bootstrap estimation of diagnostic accuracy with patient-clustered data. Acad. Radiol 7(6), 413–419 (2000)

Automatic Cortical Segmentation in the Developing Brain

Hui Xue[1,2], Latha Srinivasan[1], Shuzhou Jiang[1], Mary Rutherford[1], A David Edwards[1,3], Daniel Rueckert[2], and Jo V Hajnal[1]

[1] Imaging Sciences Department, Imperial College, London, Du cane Road, W12 0NN, UK
[2] Department of Computing, Imperial College, London, 180 Queen's Gate, SW7 2BZ, UK
[3] Department of Paediatrics, Imperial College, London, Du cane Road, W12 0NN, UK
{hui.xue,l.srinivasan,shuzhou.jiang,mary.rutherford, david.edwards,d.rueckert,jo.hajnal}@imperial.ac.uk

Abstract. The segmentation of neonatal cortex from magnetic resonance (MR) images is much more challenging than the segmentation of cortex in adults. The main reason is the inverted contrast between grey matter (GM) and white matter (WM) that occurs when myelination is incomplete. This causes mislabeled partial volume voxels, especially at the interface between GM and cerebrospinal fluid (CSF). We propose a fully automatic cortical segmentation algorithm, detecting these mislabeled voxels using a knowledge-based approach and correcting errors by adjusting local priors to favor the correct classification. Our results show that the proposed algorithm corrects errors in the segmentation of both GM and WM compared to the classic EM scheme. The segmentation algorithm has been tested on 25 neonates with the gestational ages ranging from ~27 to 45 weeks. Quantitative comparison to the manual segmentation demonstrates good performance of the method (mean Dice similarity: 0.758 ± 0.037 for GM and 0.794 ± 0.078 for WM).

1 Introduction

Clinical studies have shown delayed cortical folding, decreased thalamic volume and WM macro- and micro-structural changes in preterm infants at term equivalent age [1, 2]. By analyzing anatomically the development of the neonatal cortex, it is possible to detect these cerebral abnormalities in surviving preterm infants at term equivalent age. However, manual segmentations of the neonatal brains, particularly of the cortex are time-consuming, extremely tedious and have low inter-operator reproducibility. As a result, studies of cortical development involving multiple subjects are problematic. Note that a key requirement for any such developmental studies is the ability to automatically segment the cortex not only in normal term born infants, but also in preterm subjects.

An infant is usually referred to as term-born if its gestational age (the age from the beginning of pregnancy, GA) at birth is around 40 weeks. Infants who are born before 34 weeks are considered premature [3]. A key difference between the neonatal and adult brain is that the white matter (WM) / gray matter (GM) contrast on both T1 weighted (T1w) and T2 weighted (T2w) Magnetic Resonance (MR) images is usually

N. Karssemeijer and B. Lelieveldt (Eds.): IPMI 2007, LNCS 4584, pp. 257 – 269, 2007.
© Springer-Verlag Berlin Heidelberg 2007

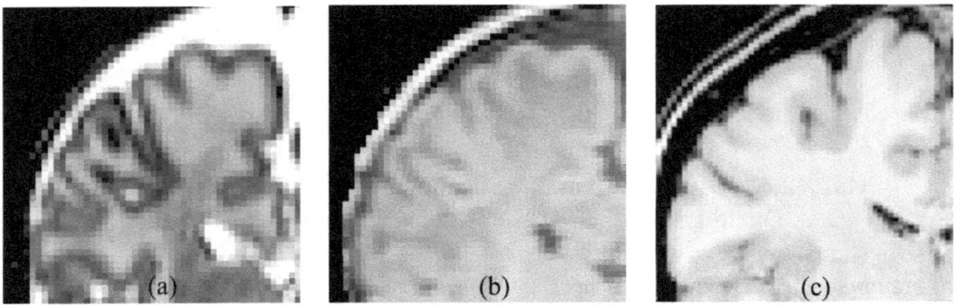

Fig. 1. Representative coronal MRI slices of neonates and adults show the different contrast patterns. (a) T2w and (b) T1w images for a neonate (GA at scan 39.86 weeks). Due to the inverted WM/GM contrast, many voxels on the CSF-GM boundary have the similar intensities to WM. If the brain is not properly extracted, the PVs will also appear between the non-brain tissues and CSF. For the purpose of comparison, an enlarged coronal T1w slice of an adult (male, 40 years) is shown in (c).

reversed. This is caused by the increased water content of all cerebral structures and the presence of unmyelinated WM. During the third trimester most of the WM is unmyelinated. The first structures to be covered with myelin are the WM tracts in the brain stem and mesencephalon (ca. 28 weeks GA). At full-term the posterior limb of internal capsule is myelinated. During the first two years of life various processes such as cortical organization and the myelination of all WM tracts cause dynamic changes in the T1 and T2 relaxation times. At the age of 2 years, the myelination process is nearly complete and the contrast is similar to that of adult brains. An excellent description of this brain development process can be found in [4]. For the sake of simplicity and since the majority of WM in neonatal brains is non-myelinated, we refer to non-myelinated WM in the remainder of the paper simply as WM.

Automatic segmentation of cortical GM in neonatal MRI is more challenging than segmentation of adult brains, which is mainly caused by the inverted WM/GM contrast. This leads to mislabeled voxels at the interface between the cerebrospinal fluid (CSF) and GM. Because CSF has the highest intensity in neonatal T2w images and the image resolution of neonatal MRI is limited, many voxels between CSF and GM will have similar intensities to WM which is brighter than GM and darker than CSF (Fig. 1a). These voxels can be incorrectly classified as WM by conventional intensity-based segmentation approaches (see Fig. 2). The same problem occurs in neonatal T1w images. In this case, CSF is the darkest and GM is the brightest; thus voxels at the interface between CSF and GM will have intensities similar to those of WM (Fig. 1b). In the following we refer to these voxels as mislabeled partial volume voxels (MLPVs) since the mislabeling is primarily a consequence of the mixing of tissues within voxels (partial volume). In T1w/T2w images of adult brains, partial volume effects also occur but these do not lead to similar MLPVs because the WM is fully myelinated and has the highest/lowest intensity.

Brain segmentation is usually preceded by brain extraction to exclude non-brain tissue. If brain extraction does not exclude all non-brain tissues, there will be another source of MLPVs at the CSF-non-brain tissue boundary. Because CSF has high signal intensity in T2w images and non-brain tissues generally have low signal intensity, there are voxels on the intermediate boundary having similar intensities to both GM and WM. In T1w images, CSF has low signal intensity and scalp has high signal intensity, so that similar MLPVs can appear. Please note that this kind of MLPVs can occur in adult images.

Besides the MLPV problem on the CSF/GM interface which is unique for neonatal MRI, there are some other issues which make the task of cortical segmentation more challenging. In particular, neonatal brain MRI shows substantial intra-class intensity variability, especially in WM. For preterm-born neonates, there are often diffuse high signal intensities in WM which are recognized as a common form of brain damage [5]. More issues include the lower signal-to-noise ratio in neonatal MRI caused by the shorter scanning time normally used to avoid motion artifacts, age dependent GM/WM contrast and rapid evolution of cortical morphometry.

Segmentation methods for neonates previously published [6, 7] are generally not optimal for the segmentation of the neonatal cortex. The MLPVs problem on the CSF-GM boundary has not been explicitly tackled in any of them. Thus, there are noticeable MLPVs left in their segmentation results, as shown in [6] and [7]. Also, previous methods use essentially spatially global intensity classification schemes, meaning that either parametric or non-parametric probability density estimators are used to estimate the distribution of tissue classes throughout the whole brain. However, in our experience the large intra-class intensity variability is also regionally different, especially in WM. This leads to a sub-optimal local segmentation of the cortical GM-WM boundary.

In this paper we develop a cortical segmentation algorithm addressing the difficulties of segmenting the developing neonatal cortex. Specifically, we propose a modified expectation-maximization (EM) scheme to perform the tissue classification in combination with a Markov Random Field (MRF) model to ensure spatial homogeneity in the tissue classification. The key contribution of our approach is the detection and removal of MLPVs using knowledge-based approach that identifies MLPVs after each EM iteration. In the proposed approach the corresponding MRF priors for MLPVs are adjusted to favor the correct classification classes. Once the modified EM algorithm converges most of the MLPVs are eliminated. To deal with the WM intensity variability, a brain splitting step is exploited after the global EM segmentation which refines the final segmentation.

2 Methods

2.1 Brain Extraction and Removal of Central Deep Tissues

As the first step in the segmentation process, we use a segmentation approach based on label propagation to achieve both brain extraction and removal of central deep tissues, since they are not relevant for the segmentation of the cortex and their signal intensities are similar to those of cortical GM. A template-based segmentation using label propagation was used (multiple templates were used here to favor the registration. see Section 3 for more details). Specifically, the GA range from 27wks to term was divided into 3 ranges and one subject from our study population from each age range was randomly selected to be used as a template. For each template, subcortical GM (including basal ganglia and thalamus), myelinated WM, corpus callosum and cerebellum were manually labeled by an expert observer. The template was non-rigidly aligned to all other subjects and the labels were propagated to new images. By performing the non-rigid registration between the template and new images, the brain extraction can also be achieved by propagating the brain mask of the template. The non-rigid registration algorithm we used is based on the maximization of normalized mutual information and free-form deformations (FFDs) [8].

2.2 Expectation-Maximization (EM) Algorithm for Tissue Classification

The EM algorithm is a general statistical technique to estimate missing information based on observed data. It has been widely used for the segmentation of brain MR images. Wells et al. [9] proposed an EM algorithm in which the PDF of every tissue class is modeled by a Gaussian distribution. This method was extended by introducing a probabilistic atlas to provide spatially varying prior probabilities at every voxel [10].

The EM algorithm consists of an Expectation step (E-step) which performs a classification and a Maximization step (M-step) which updates the Gaussian parameters. Given the initial parameters $\mu_k^{(0)}$ and $\sigma_k^{(0)}$, the algorithm iteratively maximizes the data likelihood and updates the tissue classification.

E-step: $$p(k|x_i) = \frac{p(x_i|k)prior(k)}{p(x_i)} \quad (1)$$

M-step: $$\mu_k^{(m+1)} = \frac{\sum_{i=1}^{N} p^{(m)}(k|x_i)x_i}{\sum_{i=1}^{N} p^{(m)}(k|x_i)} \qquad \left(\sigma_k^{(m+1)}\right)^2 = \frac{\sum_{i=1}^{N} p^{(m)}(k|x_i)(x_i - \mu_k)^2}{\sum_{i=1}^{N} p^{(m)}(k|x_i)}$$

Here x_i is the intensity of a voxel i and $prior(k)$ is the prior probability for every tissue component. $p(x_i|k)$ is the class likelihood probability which is a Gaussian distribution. The corresponding class posterior probabilities are computed in the E-step.

The EM algorithm requires an initial estimate of the probabilities at every voxel. Probabilistic atlases or templates are often used for this purpose. They act as the prior $p(k|x_i)$ to predict the probability of a voxel x_i belonging to the tissue class k and combine spatial distribution information of different tissues into the EM algorithm. However, the large anatomical changes that occur in the neonatal period preclude the use of a single standard atlas for the full age range in this study. To initialize the EM algorithm, we simply performed a k-means clustering on each individual to generate an initial segmentation. This initial segmentation is slightly blurred by a convolution with a Gaussian kernel ($\sigma = 1.5 \times voxelsize$) and normalized to simulate an atlas which is then used to initialize the M scheme. Pilot experiments showed there to be sufficient contrast between cortical GM and WM in T2w images of developing neonates for successful GM-WM segmentation to be obtained without a probabilistic atlas of the cerebral anatomy.

2.3 Mislabeled Partial Volume (MLPV) Voxel Detection and Removal

The EM algorithm in its original form will wrongly classify partial volume voxels on the CSF-GM boundary. An example illustrating this problem in a T2w image is shown in Fig. 2a-b: Many voxels on the CSF-GM boundary are incorrectly classified as WM. A similar problem occurs at the CSF-nonbrain tissue boundary because CSF has the highest signal intensity and non-brain background has the lowest signal intensity.

These undesired MLPVs are partly caused by the voxel-wise tissue classification used in the EM scheme, where every voxel is independently classified based on its signal intensity and prior probability. In many approaches Markov Random Fields (MRFs) are used to enforce spatial homogeneity of the tissue labeling [11, 12, 13].

Specifically, the tissue class k is assumed to be a realization of a random process and the Hammersley-Clifford theorem states that this random field can be described as a Gibbs Random Field [13]. Its configuration obeys the Gibbs distribution:

$$f(k|x_i,\boldsymbol{\Phi}) = Z(\boldsymbol{\Phi})^{-1} \exp(-U_{mrf}(k|x_i,\boldsymbol{\Phi})) \tag{2}$$

where $Z(\boldsymbol{\Phi}) = \sum_k \exp(-U_{mrf}(k|x_i,\boldsymbol{\Phi}))$ is the normalization constant and $U_{mrf}(k|x_i,\boldsymbol{\Phi})$ is the energy function and $\boldsymbol{\Phi}$ is the MRF parameters.

We exploit a first-order neighborhood system, i.e., only the six nearest neighbors on the 3D image grid are used. Given a voxel i, its neighborhood is defined by $N_i = \{i^n, i^s, i^w, i^e, i^t, i^b\}$ where i^n, i^s, i^w and i^e are four neighbors in the plane and i^t and i^b are top and bottom voxels out of the plane. Following the Potts model, the MRF energy function [12] at voxel i is:

$$U_{mrf}(k|i,\boldsymbol{\Phi}) = \boldsymbol{z}_i^t \boldsymbol{G} \boldsymbol{g}_i \tag{3}$$
$$\boldsymbol{z}_i = \boldsymbol{e}_k$$
$$\boldsymbol{g}_i = \boldsymbol{z}_{i^n} + \boldsymbol{z}_{i^s} + \boldsymbol{z}_{i^w} + \boldsymbol{z}_{i^e} + \boldsymbol{z}_{i^t} + \boldsymbol{z}_{i^b}$$

where $\boldsymbol{z}_i = \boldsymbol{e}_k$ is a unit vector with the kth component being one and $\boldsymbol{g}_i$ counts for every tissue class k the number of neighbor voxels belonging to k. The $K \times K$ matrix $\boldsymbol{G}$ is the so-called tissue class compatibility matrix. The (m,n) element in $\boldsymbol{G}$ denotes the contribution of a neighbor voxel belonging to class n to the energy function $U_{mrf}(m|i,\boldsymbol{\Phi})$.

Mean field theory is exploited to compute the optimal parameters for the MRF model [12]. The update equation (1) is kept unchanged while the posterior is now computed from both atlas prior $p_{atlas}(k|x_i)$ and MRF prior $p_{mrf}(k|x_i)$.

$$p(k|x_i) = \frac{p(x_i|k) \cdot prior(k|x_i)}{p(x_i)} \tag{4}$$

$$prior(k|x_i) = \frac{p_{atlas}(k|x_i) \cdot p_{mrf}(k|x_i)}{\sum_{j=1}^{K} (p_{atlas}(j|x_i) \cdot p_{mrf}(j|x_i))} \qquad p_{mrf}(k|x_i) = \frac{exp(-U_{mrf}(k|x_i, \Phi))}{\sum_{j=1}^{K} exp(-U_{mrf}(j|x_i, \Phi))}$$

Although isolated mislabeled partial volumes can be removed by the MRF approach, a large number of voxels on the CSF/GM boundary can be misclassified. If two voxels are misclassified and neighboring each other, one can prohibit the other from being correctly classified by contributing to its MRF energy function via the tissue class compatibility matrix (eq. 3). For example, if two WM MLPVs x_i and x_j are adjacent (x_i is a first-order neighbor of x_j), the prior $p_{mrf}(wm|x_i)$ will be positively influenced by x_j which is currently classified as WM. Therefore, to mostly favor the removal of MLPVs, we developed a knowledge based approach to enhance the EM-MRF scheme. We use the knowledge that WM MLPVs may appear on the CSF-GM boundary for neonatal T1w and T2w images. If a voxel is classified as WM and within its first-order neighborhood there are both CSF and GM voxels, this voxel is more likely to be a partial volume voxel. The same detection rule can be used for WM and GM MLPVs on the CSF-nonbrain tissue boundary in neonatal T2w images.

After each EM step we identify all candidate MLPVs. To avoid misclassifications that lead to MLPVs we adjust the MRF prior probabilities to enable more accurate tissue classes. For example, if a voxel x_i is likely to be incorrectly classified as WM on the CSF-GM boundary, the MRF prior probability $p_{mrf}(wm|x_i)$ should be decreased. Because the sum of prior probability of all tissue classes should always be one, the other possible tissue classes can be favored by increasing their prior probabilities. Specifically, the following rules are used to adjust $p_{mrf}(wm|x_i)$:

$$p_{mrf}r^{(m+1)}(wm|x_i) = \lambda p_{mrf}r^{(m)}(wm|x_i), \quad 0 < \lambda < 1 \tag{5}$$

$$p_{mrf}^{(m+1)}(CSF|x_i) = p_{mrf}^{(m)}(CSF|x_i)\left(1 + (1-\lambda)\frac{p_{mrf}r^{(m)}(wm|x_i)}{p_{mrf}^{(m)}(CSF|x_i) + p_{mrf}^{(m)}(gm|x_i)}\right)$$

$$p_{mrf}r^{(m+1)}(gm|x_i) = p_{mrf}r^{(m)}(gm|x_i)\left(1 + (1-\lambda)\frac{p_{mrf}r^{(m)}(wm|x_i)}{p_{mrf}r^{(m)}(CSF|x_i) + p_{mrf}^{(m)}(gm|x_i)}\right)$$

The idea behind these equations is that the decrease of $p_{mrf}(wm|x_i)$ is proportionally added to the prior probabilities of CSF and GM to keep the sum of all prior probabilities constant. The final classification of x_i will be determined by its prior and intensity value (influencing the class likelihood $p(x|k)$). As a result, the original two-step classification (EM-MRF) is extended into a three-step (EM-MRF-MLPVs) process. Fig. 2a-d indicates the segmentation results after the MLPVs removal step is integrated into the EM algorithm. The more iterations are preformed, the fewer misclassifications can be seen in the results. Finally, after the last iteration nearly all MLPVs are removed. The algorithm is stopped either when the parameters converge (the maximal change among all EM parameters is less than 0.01) or a maximal number of iterations is reached (in our experiments we found that 35 iterations are sufficient). Note that the only parameter that needs to be chosen in our algorithm is λ.

We have found that the segmentation results are insensitive to precise choices of λ, which mainly influences the speed of convergence. As a result we set λ to be 0.5 for all experiments.

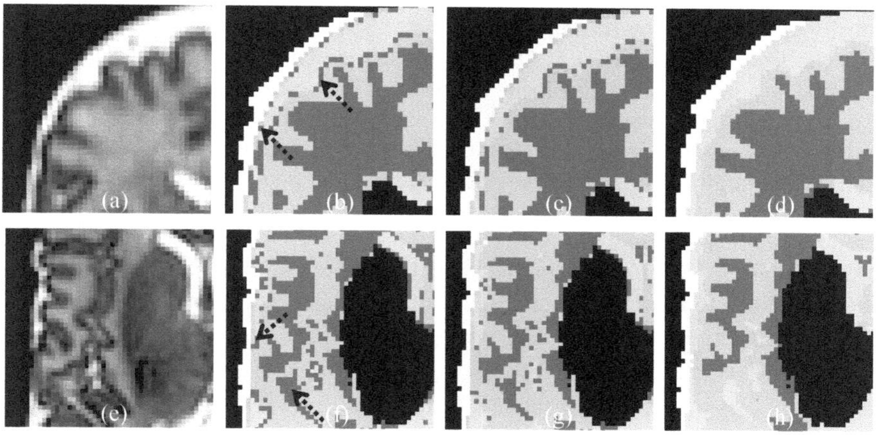

Fig. 2. An illustration of the three-step EM scheme with the PVs removal. (a) An enlarged neonatal T2w image; (b) Partial volume voxels (highlighted by arrows) on the CSF-GM and CSF-non-brain boundaries are incorrectly classified by the original EM method; (c) The segmentation results after the 4-th iteration of three-step EM method; (d) The final results after 14 iterations. Similarly, (e-f) shows that the CSF voxels in the sulci which are originally classified as WM due to partial volumes from adjacent GM are finally segmented properly. (g) Results after 8-th iteration; (h) Final results after 14-th iteration.

The MLPVs removal strategy can be extended to refine the classification of CSF voxels in sulci. Because of the limited image resolution, the CSF voxels in sulci are often mixed with the adjacent GM and have intensities similar to WM. As a result, they are often mislabeled as WM (Fig. 2e-f, arrows). We can detect these mislabeled CSF voxels and decrease their prior probability in a similar fashion. The prior of CSF is then increased to favor the correct tissue class and also keep the sum of priors constant. Mislabeled CSF voxels are detected by performing a connected component labeling on the WM volume after every iteration. Small unconnected components are identified if they are much smaller in volume than the largest component. The first-order neighborhood of every small component is checked. If the component is included within CSF or GM, it is suspected to be representing CSF voxels and the prior probabilities are then adjusted. Fig. 2g-h shows the detection and classification of CSF voxels in sulci. The misclassification is gradually corrected and the CSF voxels are properly segmented.

2.4 Local Segmentation by Brain Splitting

Neonatal brain MR images exhibit higher intra-tissue intensity variability than adult brain MR images mainly due to the immaturity of developing brain tissues. The effects of the innate intensity variations can not be totally eliminated by inhomogeneity correction. Therefore, its influence on the tissue classification cannot be ignored. On the other hand, the three-step EM method described in the previous section is essentially a global scheme, which means that a tissue class throughout the image is modeled by only one Gaussian distribution. The global scheme is not appropriate if the intensity variability is significant.

As the tissue boundaries are visible, a local segmentation should be able to improve the results. Because the local fluctuations of voxel intensities are small, the estimation of tissue-class PDF can be improved if the brain is split into multiple regions and a separate set of Gaussians is used for each region; that is, only voxels within in one region are used to estimate Gaussian parameters for this part. We have not found it necessary to use overlapping regions, to ensure reliable segmentation at region boundaries although this is an option.

A reasonable split of the brain should balance the ability to robustly estimate the PDF, the ability to tackle local intensity variability and the segmentation stability to noise. To perform the brain splitting, we assemble a 4D vector $\vec{d} = (x, y, z, I)$ from all GM and WM voxels which have been labeled by the global segmentation step, as these two tissues have the most intensity variability. (x, y, z) is the 3D coordinates of a voxel and I is its intensity. A k-means clustering is performed on the 4D vector and the coordinates of clustering centers are used to define a Voronoi tessellation on the brain space. We add the intensity I into the feature vector is to prevent the regions with consistent local intensity from being split. The k-means algorithm is initialized by the centroids of large voxel groups. To avoid the convergence to local minima, the clustering process is repeated 10 times with random perturbations of the initial cluster centers. The segmentation step is finally independently performed on every region of the Voronoi tessellation, and is initialized by the output of global segmentation.

To quantitatively evaluate the segmentation results, a human rater manually segmented three orthogonal slices for every subject. Manual segmentation of the whole cortex in 3D was not attempted due to the complexity of the structure and the large number of partial volume voxels which make this task prohibitively time consuming. The overlap rate between the automatic and manual segmentation is quantified by the Dice similarity coefficient (DSC). The Dice measure is normalized so that zero means the complete dissimilarity and one means perfect overlapping. Dice measures above 0.7 are usually regarded as a satisfactory level of agreement between two independent segmentations [16].

3 Results and Evaluation

We applied our method to 25 subjects selected from a large longitudinal MR study of cerebral development of term-born and premature neonates. The preterm infants were recruited from the Neonatal Intensive Care Unit at Hammersmith Hospital, and term born control infants were recruited from the postnatal wards.

MR images were acquired on a 3T Philips Intera system (Best, Holland) using a standard 6 head channel array coil. Preterm infants were sedated with chloral hydrate and term born controls were fed, swaddled and the examination was carried out in natural sleep. The MR sequence parameters were as follows: T2-weighted fast spin echo pseudo volumes: TR=1712/TE=160ms, FOV=220mm, matrix 224×224, flip angle 90°, voxel size of 0.86×0.86×2mm with the 50% slice overlapping, SENSE factor 1 with intensity normalized to a body coil image. All T2 weighted images were acquired in the transverse plane. Following acquisition, the T2 images were interpolated to isotropic $0.86mm^3$ voxels using cubic B-spline interpolation [14]. T1-weighted images were also acquired for all neonates. However, the contrast between cortical GM and WM/CSF is less pronounced on T1w images. Therefore, we have only used T2w images in this study. As RF inhomogeneity is more serious for high field MRI, a bias correction procedure is performed for all images using the N3 software [15] prior to application of our segmentation algorithm.

Since the brain development in neonates is rapid during the GA range from ~27 to 45 weeks, we divided the 25 neonates into three groups: ~27 – 34 weeks (simple brains, 9 subjects), 34 – 39 weeks (medium brains, 6 subjects) and 39 – 45 weeks (complex brains, 10 subjects). For each group one image was selected as a template and its subcortical GM, myelinated WM, corpus callosum and cerebellum were manually segmented. The template image was not used for evaluating the segmentation. The reason for this strategy is that choosing a template with a similar GA to the subject being segmented significantly simplifies the non-rigid registration. The resulting label propagation is effectively used to segment deep central tissues for new subjects.

Fig. 3 illustrates the improvements produced by the MLPVs removal step and local segmentation. A preterm neonate scanned at the term equivalent age, whose images showed WM intensity variability is presented in coronal view in Fig. 3a. When only the global Gaussian mixture model and two-step EM method is used, clear mislabeled partial volume voxels can be seen on the CSF-GM and CSF-non brain tissue boundaries (Fig. 3b). These voxels are assigned to the correct tissue class labels after the MLPVs removal step is integrated into the EM iteration (Fig. 3c). The segmentation of the inner cortical surface is refined after the brain splitting strategy is further used, as shown in Fig. 3d.

Results of the automatic segmentation of a number of neonates at different gestational ages are presented in Fig. 4. Visual inspection of these results shows that cortical GM is reasonably well segmented. Partial volume voxels on the CSF-GM and CSF-non brain boundaries are successfully removed. The CSF voxels in sulci are often correctly classified. Table 1 summarizes the results of comparison with the manual segmentation. The mean DSC values for cortical GM and WM for each GA group are presented. The WM results exclude the corpus callosum and any WM within the region of deep GM removed by the initial label propagation step.

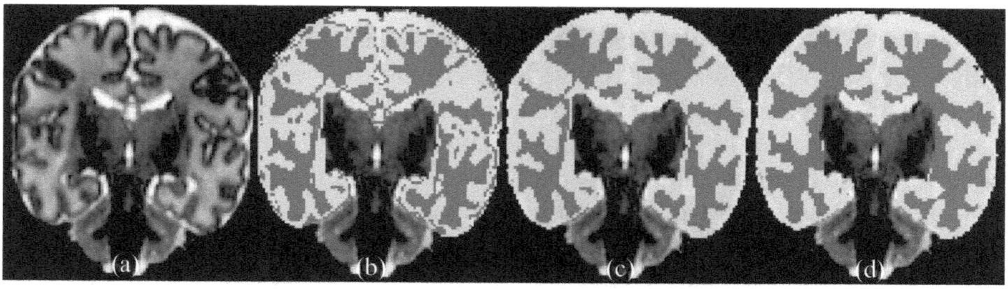

Fig. 3. An illustration to show the refined segmentation

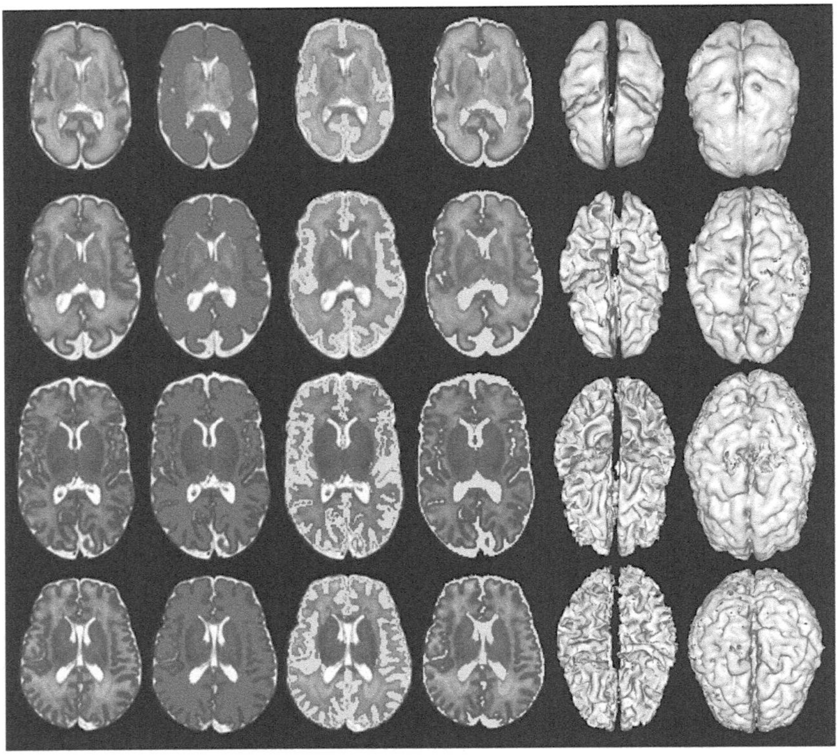

Fig. 4. 3D automatic brain segmentation results. From top to bottom, GAs are 30, 34, 40 and 44 weeks. From left to right, pictures listed are the transverse slice of T2w neonatal images, segmented WM, cortical GM and CSF respectively. The corpus callosum has been masked off by the label propagation. Last two columns show the 3D renderings of inner and outer cortical surfaces of the hard segmentation, where the visible imperfections, like holes and abruptions caused by image noises can be removed after the effective cortical reconstruction.

As a result, we draw the conclusion that the EM-MRF-MLPV scheme significantly improves the segmentation of cortical GM and WM compared to the EM-MRF method where no MLPV removal step is integrated (for GM: $t = 13.43$, $P < 0.0001$; for WM: $t = 4.90$, $P < 0.0001$; paired t-test). The performance of EM-MRF-MLPV scheme is further improved by combining the local segmentation (for GM: $t = 7.07$, $P < 0.0001$; for WM: $t = 5.35$, $P < 0.0001$). This improvement is more noticeable in preterm infants with non cystic WM disease who have diffuse excessive high signal intensity injury (DEHSI) on T2W images. Furthermore, for the simple brain group, as the intra-tissue class intensity variability is even more serious, we found that dividing the WM of these very premature infants into two tissue classes can improve the segmentation. A total of five classes (WM is modeled by two Gaussian distributions) were therefore used. The second row in Table 1 summarizes the corresponding DSC values. Compared to the results with four tissue classes (the first row in Table 1), the improvement for GM are significant (for GM: $t = 5.65$, $P = 0.0005$; for WM: $t = 2.34$, $P = 0.0472$).

Table 1. The Dice similarity values of cortical GM and WM for every GA groups

GA	GM			WM		
	Global	Global+PVs	Global+Local +PVs	Global	Global+PVs	Global+Local +PVs
27w–34w	0.665 ± 0.036	0.696 ± 0.038	0.708 ± 0.038	0.773 ± 0.019	0.810 ± 0.017	0.816 ± 0.016
27w–34w Five tissue classes	0.689 ± 0.034	0.716 ± 0.038	0.726 ± 0.032	0.765 ± 0.024	0.822 ± 0.012	0.824 ± 0.013
34w–39w	0.741 ± 0.026	0.763 ± 0.025	0.770 ± 0.022	0.748 ± 0.030	0.809 ± 0.019	0.813 ± 0.018
39w–45w	0.763 ± 0.019	0.781 ± 0.019	0.785 ± 0.016	0.711 ± 0.053	0.751 ± 0.113	0.757 ± 0.116

The current grouping according to gestational ages is, to some extent, empirical. To review the overall performance of automatic segmentation on developing neonates, the DSC values for all 25 subjects are computed. The mean DSC is 0.758 ± 0.037 for GM and 0.794 ± 0.078 for WM. The overall performance is good to excellent compared to the manual labeling as neonates become more mature. This supports the statement that from the very premature to term-equivalent age neonatal T2w MRI can consistently provide sufficient GM/WM contrast for intensity based segmentation.

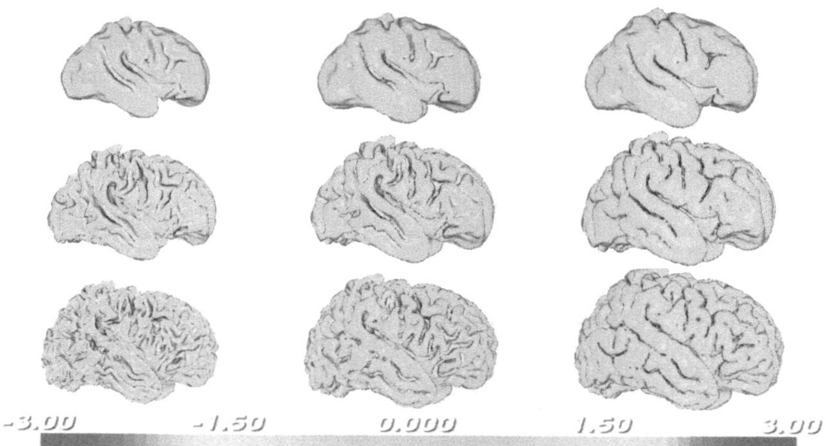

Fig. 5. 3D rendering of reconstructed central cortex surfaces for neonates. From left to right, the inner, central and outer surfaces are shown. From top to bottom, the GAs are 30w, 35w and 40w respectively. The mean curvature is used for color-coding.

After segmentation of the cortical GM and WM, an implicit cortical surface reconstruction algorithm [17] was applied to all subjects. We visually inspected the surface reconstructed by rendering the intersection contours on 2D slices as well as 3D surfaces to verify the performance of this method. Fig. 5 shows the reconstructed 3D surfaces of inner, central and outer cortical surfaces for neonates over a representative range of GA. The colors on the surfaces indicate the mean curvature.

4 Discussion and Conclusions

It is worth mentioning that only an atlas or template may not be sufficient to eliminate all MLPVs. First, the non-rigid registration between atlas and images may not be perfect throughout the images, especially in cortical regions. Second, the final posterior is determined by the combination of prior and class likelihood. The former is derived from the atlas while the latter is evaluated from the voxel intensity. As the MLPVs voxels on the GM-CSF boundary can have exactly the same intensity levels as the WM, even a prior from an atlas may not be sufficient to guarantee the accurate classification. Thus, the explicit MLPVs removal step is necessary.

Some authors have proposed different algorithms to address partial volumes in segmentation for adults T1w MRI [18, 19]. However, their applicability are based on the fact that the intensity levels of partial volumes in adult T1w do not largely overlap the characteristic intensity of any pure tissue class, which is not true for neonatal MRI due to the inverted gray-white matter contrast. As a result, these methods for adults may not work well in neonatal T2w MRI without sufficient spatial prior information.

By identifying the MLPVs problem associated with the specific signal properties of MR images of the brain for developing neonates at varying gestational ages during the third trimester, we have developed and evaluated segmentation methods designed specifically to extract the cortical GM. The resulting methods are effective for segmentation of cortical GM over a wide range of GA. The inner, central and outer cortical surfaces are then successfully reconstructed using the implicit surface evolution, which serves as a starting point for the longitudinal and cross-sectional studies of cortical morphometry for developing neonates.

References

1. Boardman, J.P., Serena, C.J., Rueckert, D., Kapellou, O., Bhatia, K.K., Aljabar, P., Hajnal, J., Allsop, J.M., Rutherford, M.A., Edwards, D.A.: Abnormal deep grey matter development following preterm birth detected using deformation-based morphometry. NeuroImage 32, 70–78 (2006)
2. McCormick, M.C., Workman-Daniels, K., Brooks-Gunn, J.: The behavioral and emotional well-being of school-age children with different birth weights. Pediatrics 97, 18–25 (1996)
3. Srinivasan, L., Allsop, J., Counsell, S.J., Boardman, J.P., Edwards, A.D., Rutherford, M.A.: Smaller cerebellar volumes in very preterm infants at term-equivalent age are associated with the presence of supratentorial lesions. AJNR Am J Neuroradiol. 27, 573–579 (2006)
4. Rutherford, M.A. (ed.): MRI of the Neonatal Brain. W.B.Saunders (2002)
5. Counsell, S.J., Allsop, J.M., Harrison, M.C., Larkman, D.J., Kennea, N.L., Kapellou, O., Cowan, F.M., Hajnal, J.V., Edwards, A.D., Rutherford, M.A.: Diffusion-weighted imaging of the brain in preterm infants with focal and diffuse white matter abnormality. Pediatrics 112, 1–7 (2003)
6. Prastawa, M., Gilmore, J.H., Lin, W.L., Gerig, G.: Automatic segmentation of MR images of the developing newborn brain. Medical Image Analysis 9, 457–466 (2005)
7. Weisenfeld, N. I., Mewes, A.U.J., Warfield, S.K.: Segmentation of newborn brain MRI. In: Proceedings of the 3rd IEEE International Symposium on Biomedical Imaging: Macro to Nano 2006, pp. 766–769 (2006)

8. Rueckert, D., Sonoda, L.I., Hayes, C., Hill, D.L., Leach, M.O., Hawkes, D.J.: Nonrigid registration using free-form deformations: application to breast MR images. IEEE Transactions on Medical Imaging 18, 712–721 (1999)
9. Wells, W.M., Kikinis, R., Grimson, W.E.L., Jolesz, F.: Adaptive segmentation of MRI data. IEEE Transactions of the Medical Imaging 15, 429–442 (1996)
10. Van Leemput, K., Maes, F., Vandermeulen, D., Suetens, P.: Automated Model-Based Bias Field Correction of MR Images of the Brain. IEEE Transactions of the Medical Imaging 18, 885–896 (1999)
11. Elfadel, I.M., Picard, R.W.: Gibbs Random Fields, Cooccurrences, and Texture Modeling. IEEE Transactions on Pattern Analysis and Machine Intelligence 16(1), 24–37 (1994)
12. Li, S.Z.: Markov Random Field Modeling in Computer Vision (Computer Science Workbench). Springer, Berlin, Germany (1995)
13. Van Leemput, K., Maes, F., Vandermeulen, D., Suetens, P.: Automated Model-Based Tissue Classification of MR Images of the Brain. IEEE Transactions on Medical Imaging 18(10), 897–908 (1999)
14. Unser, M.: Splines: a perfect fit for signal and Image processing. IEEE Signal Processing Magazine, 22–38 (1999)
15. Sled, J.G., Zijdenbos, A.E.A.: A nonparametric method for automatic correction of intensity nonuniformity in MRI data. IEEE Transactions on Medical Imaging 17(1), 87–97 (1998)
16. Zijdenbos, A.P., Dawant, B.M., Margolin, R.A., Palmer, A.C.: Morphometric analysis of white matter lesions in MR images: Method and validation. IEEE Transactions on Medical Imaging 13(4), 716–724 (1994)
17. Han, X., Pham, D.L., Tosun, D., Rettmann, M.E., Xu, C., Prince, J.L.: CRUISE: CRUISE: Cortical reconstruction using implicit surface evolution. NeuroImage 23, 997–1012 (2004)
18. Nocera, L., Gee, J.C.: Robust partial volume tissue classification of cerebral MRI scans. In: Proceedings of SPIE Medical Imaging 1997: Image Processing, vol. 3034, pp. 312–322 (1997)
19. Van Leemput, K., Maes, F., Vandermeulen, D., Suetens, P.: A Unifying Framework for Partial Volume Segmentation of Brain MR Images. IEEE Transactions on Medical Imaging 22(1), 105–119 (2003)

Comparing Pairwise and Simultaneous Joint Registrations of Decorrelating Interval Exams Using Entropic Graphs*

B. Ma[1], R. Narayanan[2], H. Park[1], A.O. Hero[2,3,4], P.H. Bland[1], and C.R. Meyer[1,2]

[1] Department of Radiology,
[2] Department of Biomedical Engineering,
[3] Department of Electrical Engineering and Computer Science,
[4] Department of Statistics,
University of Michigan, Ann Arbor, MI 48109, USA
{bingm,rnz,hyunjinp,hero,bland,cmeyer}@umich.edu

Abstract. The interest in registering a set of images has quickly risen in the field of medical image analysis. Mutual information (MI) based methods are well-established for pairwise registration but their extension to higher dimensions (multiple images) has encountered practical implementation difficulties. We extend the use of alpha mutual information (αMI) as the similarity measure to simultaneously register multiple images. αMI of a set of images can be directly estimated using entropic graphs spanning feature vectors extracted from the images, which is demonstrated to be practically feasible for joint registration.

In this paper we are specifically interested in monitoring malignant tumor changes using simultaneous registration of multiple interval MR or CT scans. Tumor scans are typically a decorrelating sequence due to the cycles of heterogeneous cell death and growth. The accuracy of joint and pairwise registration using entropic graph methods is evaluated by registering several sets of interval exams. We show that for the parameters we investigated simultaneous joint registration method yields lower average registration errors compared to pairwise. Different degrees of decorrelation in the serial scans are studied and registration performance suggests that an appropriate scanning interval can be determined for efficiently monitoring lesion changes. Different levels of observation noise are added to the image sequences and the experimental results show that entropic graph based methods are robust and can be used reliably for multiple image registration.

1 Introduction

Most malignant tumors are rapidly changing structures that threaten the life of the patient. Interval MR or CT scanning is often performed to follow these

* Work funded by USPHS DHHS NIH grants 1P01CA87634 and 1P01CA85878.

N. Karssemeijer and B. Lelieveldt (Eds.): IPMI 2007, LNCS 4584, pp. 270–282, 2007.
© Springer-Verlag Berlin Heidelberg 2007

changes. Quantification of such changes is important especially for early detection of response to therapy, or even more importantly as a means of validating mechanistic hypotheses regarding therapeutic action and cellular response. While segmentation of the interval exams is one method of quantifying response to therapy, since segmentation can be quite noisy, it is quite possible that such an approach is not capable of reliably detecting small changes. Another approach to quantifying tumor change is nonlinear registration of the serial interval exams followed by regional integration of the resulting Jacobian determinants [1]. Here the boundaries of the regional analysis need to be identified in only one of the interval exams as the registration will propagate those boundaries in a consistent manner to the remainder of the registered interval exams. Over the duration of interval imaging the tumor may morph significantly in a background of acquisition system related noise. For example, growing tumors generate heterogeneous regions of increased hypoxia and cellular density, as well as apoptosis and necrosis; likewise cells responding regionally to therapy die and necrose as well. Over the total span of interval imaging the tumor typically decorrelates with its initial appearance even with perfect registration due to cycles of heterogeneous cell death and growth.

There are typically two approaches to detecting these geometric deformations in serial interval exams – *pairwise* and *joint* registration. The *pairwise* registration method is to repeatedly perform pairwise registration over all the images in the set and settle for a transformation of all the images with a fixed reference frame based on a series of compositions. But this would not guarantee jointly optimal or unique results. On the other hand, *joint* registration achieves a consistent correspondence of pixels across all images and thus aligns them to a common spatial frame by optimizing an objective function that is calculated using all the images in the group. Recently several papers have discussed the importance of registering multiple images simultaneously and have shown improved registration accuracy compared to pairwise methods.

Bhatia et al. [2] binned all pairs of intensities, comprising the voxel intensity in the reference and the corresponding intensity in each image into a single histogram and computed normalized mutual information (NMI). This was applied to an atlas construction problem where the maximization of NMI was subjected to the condition that the total deformation onto the common spatial frame summed to zero. A minimum description length based framework was proposed in [3]. Groupwise registration was achieved by minimizing the length of the encoded messages consisting of the reference image, the reference frame, the transformation model and its parameters, and discrepancy images. Learned-Miller [4] discussed joint registration in the context of bias removal where entropy was computed at the same voxel across the image stack and summed over all voxels. Its applicability to small image sets (too few samples) may be limited by noisy entropy estimates.

All the above methods targeted same modality applications. A method of group alignment minimizing the summation of pairwise dissimilarity while improving inverse consistency and transitivity was discussed in [5]. Studholme and

Cardenas [6] estimated the joint density function of the image set and used a measure of self information to drive alignment. Zhang and Rangarajan [7] reported a study of several higher dimensional information theoretic measures for joint registration. In the last two methods joint densities are estimated and optimally stored. These methods are directly applicable to multi-modality registration.

Maximizing mutual information between images is one of the most broadly used methods for pairwise image registration [8,9,10]. Its primary advantage is the ability to accomplish reliable and accurate alignment between the image pairs although their intensities may be non-linearly related and thus it is the method of choice for multi-modality image registration. Even in isomodality registration applications such as interval MRI exams of tumors, the use of mutual information as an objective function can be beneficial over others such as cross-correlation, sum of square errors, etc. For example white matter tracts in the brain can change gray values for the same MR imaging sequence following initial tumor invasion without changes in associated morphology. In such cases the use of typical isomodality objective/cost functions would cause the white matter tracts to be mapped onto the wrong structures in the earlier interval exam due to the presence of simple intensity changes, while mutual information would recognize such changes as just another cluster in the joint density histogram to be optimized along with other clusters.

In mutual information based approach, probability densities are usually estimated using histogram or kernel techniques, which are well established for low-dimensional problems. While using histograms to compute mutual information for pairwise registration has been vastly studied and validated in registration literature, its extension to higher dimensions has encountered computational difficulties due to the sparse nature of the multi-dimensional histograms.

Neemuchwala et al. used alpha mutual information (αMI) – an extension of mutual information – as the similarity measure for image registration [11]. The introduction of entropic graphs enables the practical computation of the similarity measure in high dimensions. In this paper we extend the utilization of αMI to simultaneous registration of multiple images. With this unified similarity measure calculated based on all the images in the group we can maximize the joint correspondence through the optimization of a single objective function that measures the statistical dependency of all images simultaneously. Since this similarity measure is a mutual information it can be used for multi-modality registration. The alpha mutual information of a set of images is calculated through entropic graphs spanning the feature vectors extracted from the images. It eliminates the need to estimate joint densities of the feature vectors, which could become very computationally intensive for multiple image cases. Using k-nearest neighbor graphs we have demonstrated its computational feasibility by registering several images simultaneously.

While our effort is focused on following tumor shape change, clearly there are many other sources of serially decorrelating image sequences for which the following techniques and comparisons are applicable. In this paper we examine the relative registration accuracy of both pairwise and joint registration applied to 2D decorrelated image sequences; the 2D results can be generalized directly to 3D. Additionally entropic estimation of mutual information was implemented by extraction of wavelet feature vectors followed by entropic graph estimation of αMI [12]. Both joint and pairwise registration has been implemented and tested on the same data sets using the same initialization and geometric deformation model for performance comparison.

2 Methods

2.1 Alpha Mutual Information and Entropic Graphs

The alpha divergence between two densities f_1 and f_2 of fractional order $\alpha \in (0,1)$ is given by [13,14]

$$D_\alpha(f_1||f_2) = \frac{1}{\alpha-1}\log\int f_1^\alpha(z)\ f_2^{(1-\alpha)}(z)\ dz. \tag{1}$$

$D_\alpha(f_1||f_2)$ is a measure of dissimilarity between f_1 and f_2 and it converges to the Kullback-Liebler divergence $\int f_1(z)\log\frac{f_1(z)}{f_2(z)}dz$ as $\alpha \to 1$[13].

Let Z_1 and Z_2 be two random variables with marginal densities $f_1(z_1)$ and $f_2(z_2)$ and joint density $f_{1,2}(z_1,z_2)$. Similar to Shannon MI, the alpha mutual information between Z_1 and Z_2 is defined as the divergence between their joint density and the product of their marginal densities,

$$\begin{aligned}\alpha MI(Z_1,Z_2) &= D_\alpha\left(f_{1,2}(z_1,z_2)\,||\,f_1(z_1)f_2(z_2)\right)\\ &= \frac{1}{\alpha-1}\log\iint f_{1,2}^\alpha(z_1,z_2)\ \left[f_1(z_1)f_2(z_2)\right]^{1-\alpha}\ dz_1\,dz_2. \end{aligned}\tag{2}$$

If Z_1 and Z_2 are independent, we have $f_{1,2}(z_1,z_2) = f_1(z_1)f_2(z_2)$ and thus $\alpha\text{MI} = 0$, which means that the random variables do not provide any information about each other and thus agrees with their independence assumption. A limiting case of αMI when α approaches 1 is Shannon MI given by

$$MI(Z_1,Z_2) = \iint f_{1,2}(z_1,z_2)\log\frac{f_{1,2}(z_1,z_2)}{f_1(z_1)f_2(z_2)}\,dz_1\,dz_2. \tag{3}$$

The αMI among multiple random variables $Z_1,\ Z_2,\ \cdots,\ Z_M$ is a generalization of (2)

$$\begin{aligned}\alpha MI(Z_1,Z_2,\cdots,Z_M) = \frac{1}{\alpha-1}\log\int\cdots\int f_{1,2,\cdots,M}^\alpha(z_1,z_2,\cdots,z_M)\\ \cdot\left[f_1(z_1)\,f_2(z_2)\cdots f_M(z_M)\right]^{1-\alpha}\ dz_1\,dz_2\cdots dz_M\end{aligned}\tag{4}$$

The computational advantage of αMI relies on its direct estimation using entropic graphs (see [12] for details). Examples of entropic graphs are minimal spanning trees, Steiner trees, traveling salesman problems, k-nearest neighbor graphs, etc. By circumventing the intermediate estimation of the marginal and joint densities, entropic graph approaches to estimating αMI are suitable in multiple image registration.

2.2 Alpha Mutual Information as Similarity Measure for Image Registration

Since alpha mutual information is capable of capturing the information content across the whole set of images and it can be directly estimated using entropic graphs, we choose it as the similarity measure in simultaneous registration of multiple images.

The basic framework for entropic graph image registration is as follows. Given multiple images $I_1, I_2, \cdots, I_M$, let $\mathcal{X}$ represent the common coordinate space and $x \in \mathcal{X}$ is a spatial coordinate on which an image pixel is defined. To emphasize image dependence on the geometric space, we denote the images with explicit coordinates as $I_1(x), I_2(x), \cdots, I_M(x)$. For a geometric transformation set $T = \{T_1, T_2, \cdots, T_M\} \in \mathcal{T}$, the transformed images after interpolation are $I_1(T_1(x)), I_2(T_2(x)), \cdots, I_M(T_M(x))$, respectively. Notice that we have applied a transformation for each image which is not always required. If a certain image is selected as the reference, the transformation posed on it will be identity. We specify each transformation to show that if a common spatial frame other than any of the images is chosen as the reference, each image can be transformed to that common coordinate space. In such a framework, simultaneous multiple image registration can be solved by finding the optimal transformation set $\hat{T} \in \mathcal{T}$ such that the alpha mutual information is maximized:

$$\hat{T} = \arg\max_{T \in \mathcal{T}} \alpha MI \left(I_1(T_1(x)),\ I_2(T_2(x)),\ \cdots,\ I_M(T_M(x)) \right) \tag{5}$$

2.3 Feature Extraction

The αMI between a set of images is estimated using the entropic graphs spanning the feature vectors extracted from these images. Examples of feature vectors include: the intensity and spatial location of representative samples; the position and orientation of a randomly chosen edge; a vector of samples in a textured region; or the output vector of a spatial prediction filter. The choice of feature vectors is typically application dependent. The desirable feature vectors should be capable of thoroughly representing the images while keeping the number of feature vectors small since the construction of entropic graphs becomes more computationally expensive with the increase of the number of vectors.

To study the effect of different types of feature vectors on the estimation of αMI, we examine the estimated αMI as a function of transformation parameters. An axial MR T1 weighted slice (shown in Fig. 1(a)) is selected as the reference image and it is affine transformed to generate the floating image. We limit the geometric transformation to affine only since here our objective is to get a basic idea of the profile of this similarity measure. αMI between the reference and floating images is estimated using two types of features: (a) pixel intensity scalar and (b) concatenated wavelet coefficient vector.

Intensity value of a representative pixel is a straightforward choice for feature vector. In this case, the feature vector is in fact a scalar. In Fig. 1(b), αMI values

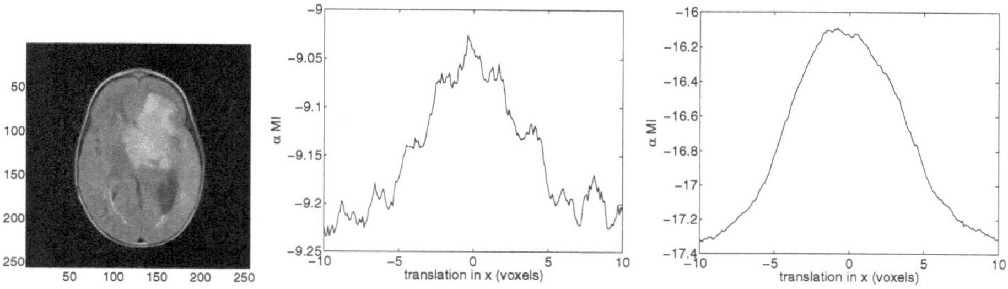

(a) brain MRI slice (b) feature: pixel intensity (c) feature: wavelet coefficients

Fig. 1. Profiles of αMI calculated based on different feature vectors: (a) An axial MR T1 weighted slice as the reference image; (b) intensity value of each pixel as the feature vector (scalar in this specific case); (c) concatenated wavelet coefficients except the high frequency component as the feature vector

are plotted with respect to the translation in the horizontal direction. The general trend of estimated αMI is as expected, i.e., peak at the center and tapering off from the center, but it suffers many local extrema due to high frequency noise in the MRI scan.

An immediate solution to this noisy objective function is to remove high frequency noise before estimating αMI. Over the past several years wavelet transforms have gained widespread acceptance in signal processing and image compression in particular with the establishment of the JPEG2000 standard [15]. They are capable of well representing an image using relatively small number of wavelet coefficients. We have taken advantage of the efficiency of wavelet transforms and used concatenated wavelet coefficients as feature vectors. The Daubechies wavelet transform with 4 coefficients is applied to the images and all coefficients except the high-frequency components are used to form the feature vector. Fig. 1(c) illustrates the objective function profile using the wavelet feature vectors. Note that the αMI curve is much smoother than its pixel intensity counterpart (Fig. 1(b)). Although calculating wavelet coefficients introduces some computational overhead, the much less noisy objective function not only leads to faster convergence, but is also less likely for the optimizer to get trapped in local optima. We used wavelet feature vectors in our experiments.

3 Experimental Results

In this paper we jointly register a series of decorrelating images using the proposed algorithm. While our effort is focused on following tumor shape change, the proposed joint registration algorithm applies to general multiple image registration as well since the derivation of the registration algorithm does not make any assumptions on the nature of the images.

3.1 Synthetic Decorrelating Image Sequences

Since our primary goal is to quantitatively compare the performance of joint and pairwise registration methods, it is necessary to know the ground truth. One way is to work on real image sequences and consult experts to manually draw the ground truth based on landmark correspondences. This is very time-consuming, labor-intensive and costly because a reasonably large number of experts are needed to provide reliable ground truth due to human subjectivity. An alternative is to use synthetic data via Monte Carlo simulations to demonstrate the statistical performance. We take the latter approach and systematically generate image sequences that mimic lesion changes.

1. Image Deformation and Decorrelation
During chemotherapy the lesion usually changes in the following fashion: some malignant cells die as a result of drug and/or radiation therapy; in the mean time some benign cells turn malignant due to the propagation of pathological cells. For a given patient during the monitoring period the existing lesion may change its shape and new lesion structure may be introduced as well. The lesion change can be modeled as a low order Markov chain due to the short temporal dependence between scans – simply put, in a series of exams, the lesion at a certain time point relies heavily on the previous Q exams (Q is a small integer). In our simulations, we choose first-order Markov model to generate the test image sequences.

Let $\mathcal{X}$ represent the coordinate space of the region we are interested. For $x \in \mathcal{X}$, $Y_i(x), i = 1, \cdots, N$, is the scene at x at the i-th scanning time point. The scenes are generated using the following rule:

$$Y_i(x) = \beta Y_{i-1}(T(x)) + (1-\beta)\, G_i(x), \quad i = 2, \cdots, N \tag{6}$$

where $Y_1(x)$ and $G_i(x)$, $i = 2, \cdots, N$ are Rayleigh random variables $\sqrt{v_1^2 + v_2^2}$, where v_1 and v_2 are lowpass filtered Gaussian random variables. A Gaussian filter of kernel size 23×23 was used in our experiments. T is a geometric deformation and $Y_{i-1}(T(x))$ is the interpolated scene after applying the deformation T. $Y_1(x)$ represents the structures that exist at the beginning of the imaging period while $G_i(x)$ includes new structures introduced along the imaging period.

$\beta \in (0, 1]$ is a constant which controls the correlation between adjacent image pairs assuming perfect registration. The smaller β is, the images are more decorrelated. In the trivial case of $\beta = 1$ the image sequence consists of deformations of existing structures only.

In the ideal noise-free case, the obtained images are exactly the scenes, i.e., $I_i = Y_i$. From the properties of first order Markov sequence, $MI(I_1, I_2, \ldots, I_N) = MI(I_1, I_N)$. Since the mutual information of the sequence is the same as the smallest mutual information between the image pairs, joint registration does not hold an advantage over pairwise.

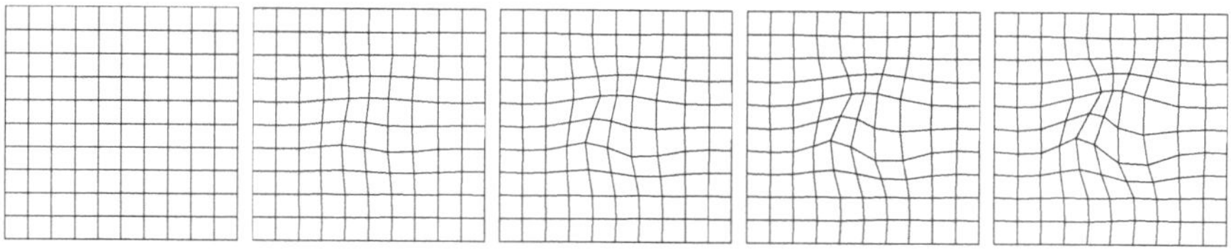

(a)

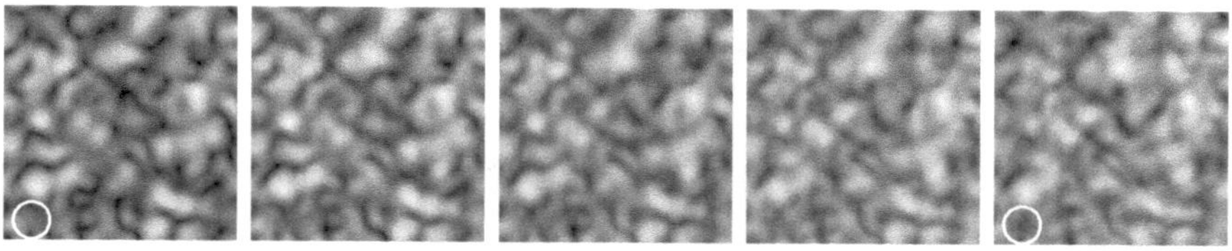

(b)

Fig. 2. Geometric deformations and generated images. (a) Consecutive TPS deformation; (b) An example of generated image sequence with $\beta = 0.8$.

However, during the image acquisition procedure random observation noise is inevitable and the images in the sequence are modeled as

$$I_i(x) = Y_i(x) + n_i(x), \quad i = 1, 2, \cdots, N \tag{7}$$

where $n_i(x)$ is a Rayleigh noise of the same characteristic as described above except that the lowpass Gaussian filter is of a much smaller kernel size (5×5 in our experiments).

The images for the simulations were generated serially based on (6) and (7). Each new image was obtained by first applying a geometric deformation (T) to the previous scene in the series and then adding Rayleigh noise and finally adding a random acquisition noise.

In our experiments, thin plate splines (TPS) model [16] is used as the geometric deformation T and thus the introduced deformation is a serially increasing TPS deformation shown in Fig. 2(a). An example of realizations of the Markov process for $\beta = 0.8$ is shown in Fig. 2(b), where both deformation of existing structures in the first image and introduction of new structures are included in the subsequent images. At the bottom left corner of the images (indicated by circles in white), there is a structure in the fifth image which has not shown in the first one. This is an example of new structures introduced during the Markov process since this area is out of the deformation field and thus the possibility that the structure is the result of geometric deformations is excluded.

2. Registration Results
To register a series of images, two approaches have been applied: sequentially pairwise registration and simultaneously joint registration of multiple images. In both approaches, αMI (5) is used as the similarity measure.

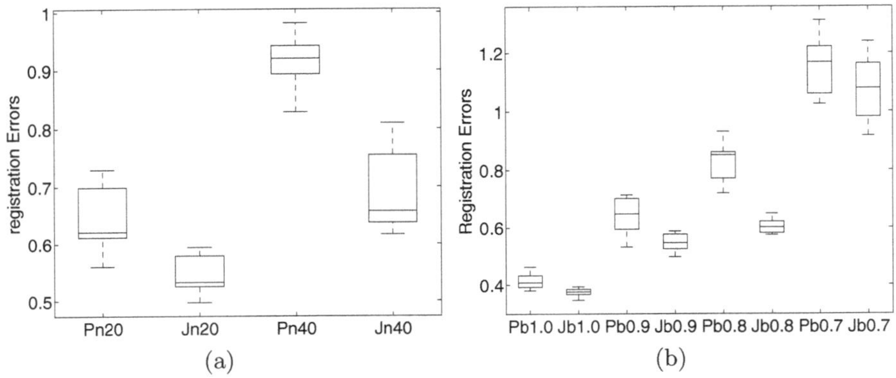

Fig. 3. Registration errors for both joint and pairwise registrations. (a) Average registration errors for different acquisition noise levels ($\beta = 0.9$); (b) Average registration errors for different β values (the acquisition noise level is 20%). The labels in the horizontal axis: 'P' and 'J' indicate pairwise and joint registration, respectively; the number following 'n' indicates the observation noise level, e.g., 'n20' means the noise level is 20% of the signal power; the number after 'b' is the value of β.

In all registration efforts TPS was employed as the deformation interpolant with 49 uniformly distributed control points placed on the nodes of a 7x7 rectangular grid spanning the deformed area in the image. k-nearest neighbor graphs were used to estimate αMI ($\alpha = 0.99$) due to their computational advantage.Optimization was implemented using Nelder-Mead simplex minimization [17] by moving the control points in the floating images. On a Pentium 4, 3.06 GHz with 4 Gb memory, it took approximately 12 minutes to register a pair of images and 4-5 hours for joint registration of five images.

The registration errors are illustrated with boxplots. In each boxplot, the bottom, middle, and upper lines of the box represent the 25th percentile, median, and 75th percentile of the errors. The whisker shows the extent of the rest of the data and the outliers are shown as "+". The performance comparison of pairwise and joint registration is shown in Fig. 3.

Fig. 3(a) shows the average registration errors for image sequences generated with $\beta = 0.9$. Joint registration outperforms its pairwise counterpart yielding lower registration errors. One common cause for pairwise registration errors is the propagation of errors along image pairs. This is due to the composition used to map all the floating images to a common reference. In joint registration, since every floating image is registered to the reference image simultaneously under the constraints of one unified objective function, this error propagation does not occur. Another reason for joint registration's better performance is that when all the images are registered simultaneously, they can provide additional information to other images. For example, with acquisition noise some structure is corrupted in an image, the other images may be able to provide supplemental information regarding the same structure and thus help the corrupted image to align with others.

Fig. 3(a) also shows the effects of additive acquisition noise on registration performance. Two noise levels have been tested: 20% and 40% of the signal power. At 40% noise level, the image quality is more deteriorated. As a result, the performance of both joint and pairwise registration methods is more adversely affected. For pairwise registration at such high noise levels, inaccurate registration is more likely to occur for some pair and the registration error will be carried over to the subsequent pairs. Therefore, although the observation noise is uncorrelated in each image, the noise in an image actually has affected the performance of registering the other images. On the other hand, for joint registration, even if every image in the sequence is severely corrupted, the uncorrelated observation noise will not affect the matching of other images. Therefore, the performance degradation is less severe for joint registration. So the higher the noise, the greater is the improvement observed for joint registration compared to pairwise.

β controls the weight of new structures in the whole signal component. The smaller the value of β, the more decorrelation and thus less mutual information between adjacent pairs of exams. For both joint and pairwise registration there must be adequate amount of mutual information between the images to achieve good registration accuracy. Therefore, β plays a crucial role in registration performance. The average errors for different values of β are shown in Fig. 3(b). The registration errors for both pairwise and joint methods increase as β decreases. With preliminary experimental results we observe that joint registration produces significantly lower average registration errors than pairwise when $\beta \geq 0.8$. When β is smaller than 0.8, the registration error increases significantly for both methods and there is no observable advantage of either method.

This study can be used to determine appropriate intervals for patient scanning to efficiently monitor lesion change. With small time interval between exams the adjacent exam pairs are highly correlated and registration results are expected to be excellent. However, imaging too frequently can be expensive and the difference between adjacent exams may be too trivial to track or analyze. On the other hand, long intervals render the registration problem intractable because of poorly correlated images with very different lesion structure. Clearly the sampling interval is an important consideration factor to monitor lesion change effectively.

3.2 Artificial Lesion Changes

With the promising results we have obtained above, we proceed to track lesion change in brain MRI scans. We choose a 256×256 brain MRI scan (the lower left image in Fig. 4) as the base image and introduce consecutive B-spline deformation to simulate a series of lesion changes. The introduced B-spline deformation is shown in the upper row of Fig. 4. The lower row shows an example of the image

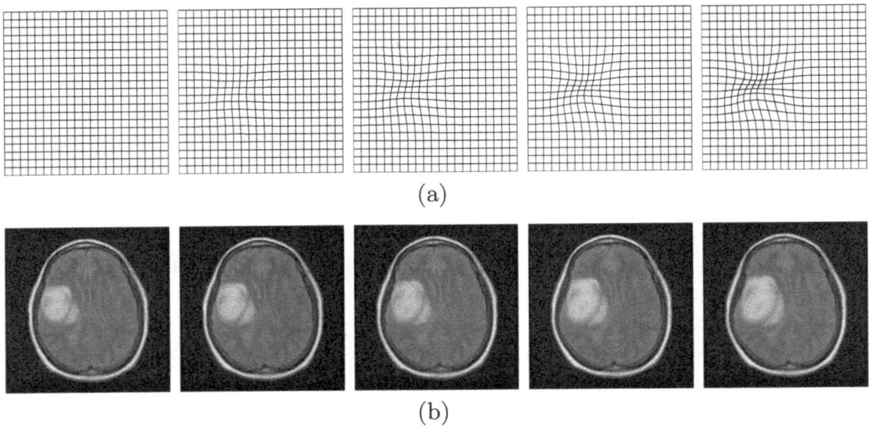

Fig. 4. Geometric deformations and corresponding brain images. (a) Consecutive B-spline geometric deformation; (b) Corresponding brain image sequence.

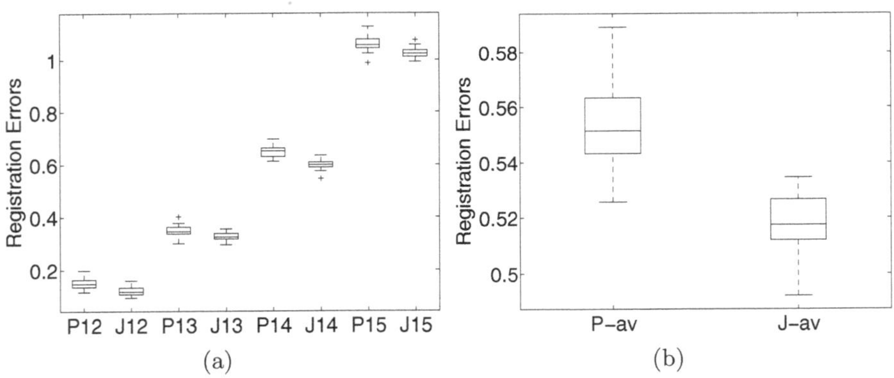

Fig. 5. Registration errors for both joint and pairwise registration of the brain sequences. (a) Registration errors between image pairs; (b) Average registration errors across the image sequence. The labels in the horizontal axis: 'P' and 'J' mean pairwise and joint registration, respectively; the two digits following 'P' or 'J' are the indices for an image pair, e.g., '14' means the alignment of I_4 to I_1; '-av' after 'P' or 'J' means average.

sequence generated with known deformation plus a random Rayleigh observation noise.

20 realizations of image sequences generated using the formula (6) and (7) with $\beta = 1$ underwent registration with both joint and pairwise approaches. Registration errors are calculated in the approximate area where the lesion is located. The registration errors plotted in Fig. 5 show that the joint method outperforms pairwise.

4 Conclusion

We have developed a joint registration algorithm using αMI as the similarity measure. We have implemented and tested the joint registration algorithm for multiple image registration on several sets of image data. For comparison, we have also registered the same data sets using the pairwise approach. The experimental results have affirmed that the joint method outperforms pairwise in registering noisy image sequences by yielding lower average registration errors. The high registration accuracy of αMI based joint registration shows that it can be used as a reliable means to simultaneously register multiple images.

We have studied the performance change of joint registration as correlation (β) decreases. In conclusion joint registration works well for sufficiently large β values (> 0.8) and this observation can help us pick the optimal scanning interval to efficiently and effectively monitor lesions.

References

1. Thirion, J.P., Calmon, G.: Deformation analysis to detect and quantify active lesions in 3D medical image sequences. IEEE Transactions on Medical Imaging 18, 429–441 (1999)
2. Bhatia, K., Hajnal, J., Puri, B., Edwards, A., Rueckert, D.: Consistent groupwise non-rigid registration for atlas construction. In: IEEE Symposium on Biomedical Imaging (ISBI) 2004, pp. 908–911 (2004)
3. Twining, C., Cootes, T., Marsland, S., Petrovic, V., Schestowitz, R., Taylor, C.: A unified information-theoretic approach to groupwise non-rigid registration and model building. In: Christensen, G.E., Sonka, M. (eds.) IPMI 2005. LNCS, vol. 3565, pp. 1–14. Springer, Heidelberg (2005)
4. Learned-Miller, E.: Data driven image models through continuous joint alignment. IEEE Transactions on PAMI 28(2) (2006)
5. Geng, X., Kumar, D., Christensen, G.: Transitive inverse-consistent manifold registration. In: Christensen, G.E., Sonka, M. (eds.) IPMI 2005. LNCS, vol. 3565, pp. 468–479. Springer, Heidelberg (2005)
6. Studholme, C., Cardenas, V.: A template free approach to volumetric spatial normalization of brain anatomy. Pattern Recognition Letters 25, 1191–1202 (2004)
7. Zhang, J., Rangarajan, A.: Multimodality image registration using an extensible information metric and high dimensional histogramming. In: Christensen, G.E., Sonka, M. (eds.) IPMI 2005. LNCS, vol. 3565, pp. 725–737. Springer, Heidelberg (2005)
8. Viola, P., Wells, W.M.: Alignment by maximization of mutual information. International Conference on Computer Vision (1995)
9. Collignon, A., Vandermeulen, D., Suetens, P., Marchal, G.: 3D multimodality medical image registration using feature space clustering. In: CVRMed, Nice. FR, pp. 829–837 (2003)
10. Meyer, C.R., Boes, J.L., Kim, B., Bland, P.H., Zasadny, K.R., Kison, P.V., Koral, K., Frey, K.A., Wahl, R.L.: Demonstration of accuracy and clinical versatility of mutual information for automatic multimodality image fusion using affine and thin-plate spline warped geometric deformations. Medical Image Analysis 1, 195–206 (1997)

11. Neemuchwala, H., Hero, A.O., Carson, P.L.: Image matching using alpha-entropy measures and entropic graphs. Signal Processing (Special Issue on Content-based Visual Information Retrieval) 85, 277–296 (2005)
12. Neemuchwala, H., Hero, A.O.: Entropic Graphs for Registration. In: Multi-Sensor Image Fusion and its Applications. CRC, 185–235 (2005)
13. Rényi, A.: On measures of entropy and information.In: Proc. 4th Berkeley Symp. Math. Stat. and Prob. vol. 1, pp. 547–561 (1961)
14. Csiszár, I.: Information-type measures of divergence of probability distributions and indirect observations. Studia Sci. Math. Hung. 2, 299–318 (1967)
15. JPEG 2000 `http://www.jpeg.org/jpeg2000/`
16. Bookstein, F.L.: Principal warps: thin-plate splines and the decomposition of deformations. IEEE Transactions on PAMI 11, 567–585 (1989)
17. Press, W.H., Flannery, B.P., Teukolsky, S.A., Vetterling, W.T.: Numerical Recipes in C: The Art of Scientific Computing. Cambridge University Press, Cambridge (1988)

Combining Radiometric and Spatial Structural Information in a New Metric for Minimal Surface Segmentation

Olivier Nempont, Jamal Atif, Elsa Angelini, and Isabelle Bloch

Ecole Nationale Supérieure des Télécommunications (GET - Télécom Paris)
CNRS UMR 5141 LTCI, Paris, France
{name}@enst.fr*

Abstract. Segmentation of anatomical structures via minimal surface extraction using gradient-based metrics is a popular approach, but exhibits some limits in the case of weak or missing contour information. We propose a new framework to define metrics, robust to missing image information. Given an object of interest we combine gray-level information and knowledge about the spatial organization of cerebral structures, into a fuzzy set which is guaranteed to include the object's boundaries. From this set we derive a metric which is used in a minimal surface segmentation framework. We show how this metric leads to improved segmentation of subcortical gray matter structures. Quantitative results on the segmentation of the caudate nucleus in T1 MRI are reported on 18 normal subjects and 6 pathological cases.

Index terms: minimal surface segmentation, level sets, spatial relations, fuzzy knowledge representation.

1 Introduction

Segmentation of structures expressed as a minimal surface extraction problem has been widely discussed in the medical imaging literature. Different optimization methods have been proposed in [1,2,3,4]. Minimal surface segmentation can be performed using geodesic deformable models involving an image-based metric computed from image gradients. An issue arises in the presence of noise and for low contrast structures, such as subcortical gray nuclei in brain magnetic resonance images (MRI), generating weak contour information. To overcome these limitations, some prior information can be incorporated in these methods. For instance, shape priors specific to the structures to segment were introduced in [5] as a non-geodesic additional term in the energy functional constraining the solution to correspond to an admissible shape. Another approach relies on the combination of region and edge information, as for instance in the geodesic active regions introduced in [6].

* This work has been partially funded by an INCA grant. J. Atif is now with Université des Antilles et de la Guyane, Guyane, France.

N. Karssemeijer and B. Lelieveldt (Eds.): IPMI 2007, LNCS 4584, pp. 283–295, 2007.
© Springer-Verlag Berlin Heidelberg 2007

In this paper, to preserve a strict geodesic formulation, we show how gray levels and structural spatial information can also be efficiently exploited in a metric, and we illustrate this idea on the segmentation of brain internal structures. Indeed, the spatial organization of brain structures is quite stable, and available as prior knowledge. Descriptions of this spatial organization through spatial relations between objects [7,8] were used in [9] to constrain a parametric deformable model, acting as an external force, to segment internal brain structures on normal brains. In [10], this approach was extended to level-set deformable models, in particular using a geodesic formulation. Although the combination of spatial relations information and edge information succeeded in constraining the segmentation to produce acceptable solutions, missing information in the image edge map was not explicitly balanced by the introduction of spatial priors.

We propose a new method to introduce structural information during the metric computation process, in order to obtain a map including complete object boundaries. We first summarize our approach for representing structural information as spatial fuzzy sets in Sect. 2. Our contribution for defining a metric taking into account such information is then detailed in Sect. 3. The integration of this metric into a level-set deformable model formulation is presented in Sect. 4 and applied to the segmentation of subcortical gray nuclei in normal and pathological brain MRI.

2 Representation of Structural Information Using Fuzzy Sets

Fuzzy sets constitute an appealing framework to represent spatial relations, modeling different types of imprecision, related to the imperfections of the image, and to the intrinsic vagueness of some relations [7]. The satisfaction of a given relation is then a matter of degree rather than a "true-or-false" fact. The semantics of spatial relations, which are imprecise but deterministic, is appropriately encoded using fuzzy representations, which then constitute better models than probabilistic ones. Given a relation with respect to a reference fuzzy object A, two types of questions can be formulated:

(i) compute to which degree a target object B fulfills this relation;
(ii) define the points in space where this relation is satisfied.

Formulations of the first type of question have been proposed for a wide range of relations including adjacency, distances, directions and symmetries. In this work, as in [9], we consider the second formulation, based on spatial representations of relations. We do not detail the definitions of the fuzzy sets representations of spatial relations here (see [7] for a review). A spatial relation SR with respect to some reference object is expressed as a fuzzy set in 3D space, with membership function denoted by μ_{SR} (i.e. $\mu_{SR}(x)$ denotes the degree to which a point x satisfies the relation). Most spatial relations can be computed using fuzzy mathematical morphology operations. When several relations are associated to describe the location of an object (as for the caudate nucleus as described below), the corresponding membership functions are combined using a fusion operator. In the following, μ_{SR} will be used to denote either one relation, or the fusion of several ones.

Spatial relations constitute an important part of the available knowledge about the spatial organization of the brain structures, as evidenced by usual anatomical descriptions, and they remain stable, even in the presence of tumors. In this paper, we rely on the following knowledge:

- for any structure A of the brain, the set $Adj(A)$ of adjacent structures O_i is known, and is assumed to completely surround A;
- the caudate nucleus (CN) is exterior to the lateral ventricle (LV) and close to it. We denote by $\mu_{SR_{CN}}$ the membership function of the spatial fuzzy set representing the fusion of these relations;
- the accumbens nucleus (AN) is located below the lateral ventricle and approximately equidistant from the ventricle and the brain surface; the fuzzy representation of these relations is denoted by $\mu_{SR_{AN}}$.

Note that the computation of $\mu_{SR_{CN}}$ and $\mu_{SR_{AN}}$ is based on a previous segmentation of the lateral ventricles and of the brain surface.

3 Metric Based on Gray-Levels and Spatial Information

Most approaches for minimal surface segmentation rely on low level features such as image gradient. In this section, we illustrate some limits of these approaches and propose to make use of structural knowledge. We derive a generic methodology to include both gray-level and spatial relations in the metric computation.

3.1 Fuzzy Map from Image Gradient

The simplest way to derive a fuzzy edge map μ_I from an image I is to apply an increasing function $g : \mathbb{R}^+ \rightarrow [0,1]$ to the norm of the image gradient. To reduce noise, a Gaussian filter G_σ can be applied, leading to: $\mu_I(x) = g(\|G_\sigma * \nabla I(x)\|)$. Various functions g can be used. As an illustrative example, we use a sigmoid function. This approach does not overcome classical problems related to weak gradients, for instance between the thalamus (Th) and the white matter (WM), as illustrated in Fig. 1 (b).

In [9] a method to enhance weak boundaries was proposed, using the radiometric mean and standard deviation of each type of tissue or structure:

$$\mu_I(x) = g(\|\nabla(p_A(I))(x)\|) = g(\|p'_A(I(x))\nabla(I)(x)\|) \tag{1}$$

where p_A is a Gaussian function defined for each individual structure A. This formula amounts to make g less sensitive to its parameters since it is applied to a contrast-independent representation. Figures 1 (c) and (f) illustrate this fuzzy gradient map for the caudate nucleus. The coronal view shows that there are still parts of the contour missing (cf. red frame).

3.2 Using Region Membership Functions

We propose an alternative method to reinforce the boundary map even in the absence of significant gradients, by using membership functions of the target object and all adjacent structures. Let A be a subset of the spatial domain Ω. The boundary of A may be defined by its morphological gradient: $\partial A = D(A, B_c) \setminus E(A, B_c)$ where D denotes the dilation operator, E the erosion operator, and B_c an elementary structuring element. This definition extends to the fuzzy case: let μ_A be a fuzzy subset of Ω representing object A. The *fuzzy morphological boundary of* A is defined as [11]: $\mu_{\partial A} = \top(D(\mu_A, B_c), D(c(\mu_A), B_c))$, where $\top$ is a t-norm (i.e. a fuzzy conjunction) and c a fuzzy complementation [12].

We can extend this definition to the *boundary between two objects* A *and* B, with membership functions μ_A and μ_B:

$$\mu_{\partial(A,B)} = \top(D(\mu_A, B_c), D(\mu_B, B_c)).$$

Note that this definition may lead to an empty set. On the other hand it may provide a large fuzzy subset if the objects intersect over a large area.

These definitions require the knowledge of the objects localization, i.e. prior segmentation results defining μ_A and μ_B, which are not yet available. However, from the available knowledge (gray levels, spatial relations...), we can easily obtain fuzzy subsets defining an approximate region of interest for A, denoted by μ_{Gl_A} in case of gray levels information, which is guaranteed to include A.

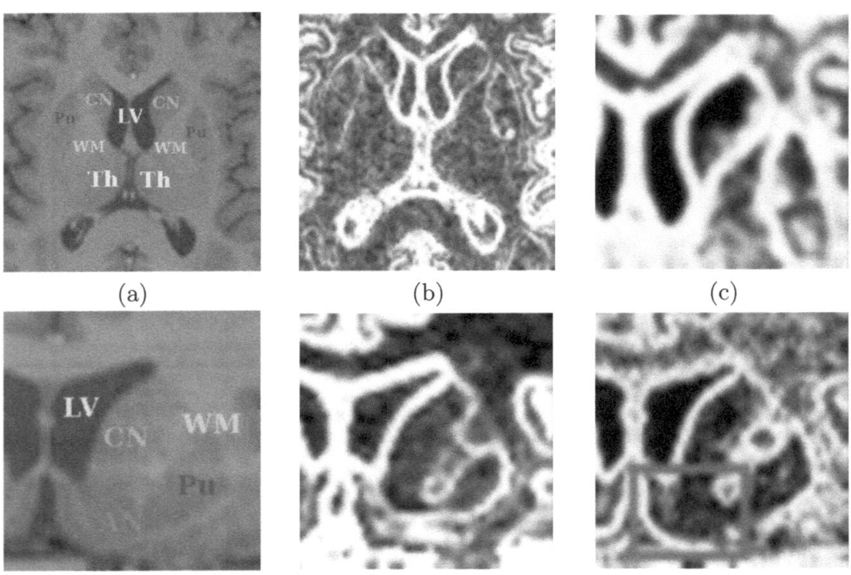

(a) (b) (c) (d) (e) (f)

Fig. 1. (a) One axial slice of a brain MRI volume. (b) $\|\nabla I\|$. (c) $g(\|\nabla(p_{CN}(I))\|)$ on an axial view. (d-f) Coronal views.

The fuzzy set μ_{Gl_A} is typically derived from a rough classification performed on the histogram. It does not need to be very accurate and only has to provide an overestimation so as to guarantee the inclusion property $\mu_A \subseteq \mu_{Gl_A}$. The following inclusion property also holds: $\mu_{\partial A} \subseteq D(\mu_{Gl_A}, B_c)$.

The fuzzy subset $D(\mu_{Gl_A}, B_c)$ contains both the object A and its boundaries, and therefore constitutes a poor representation of the object boundaries. To refine this estimation we propose to use prior knowledge about objects adjacent to A, i.e. in $Adj(A)$. Indeed, the boundary of an object A can be expressed as the union of its boundaries with adjacent objects. Since this set is exhaustive, we can write:

$$\mu_{\partial A} = \underset{i}{\perp}\, \mu_{\partial(A,O_i)} \ , \ O_i \in Adj(A),$$

where $\perp$ is a t-conorm (i.e. a fuzzy union operator). Since we also have $(\mu_A \subseteq \mu_{Gl_A}$ and $\mu_B \subseteq \mu_{Gl_B}) \Rightarrow \mu_{\partial(A,B)} \subseteq \top(D(\mu_{Gl_A}, B_c), D(\mu_{Gl_B}, B_c))$, we can derive the following inclusion:

$$\mu_{\partial A} \subseteq \underset{i}{\perp} \top(D(\mu_{Gl_A}, B_c), D(\mu_{Gl_{O_i}}, B_c)), O_i \in Adj(A). \tag{2}$$

This computational process is illustrated in Fig. 2. Our approach always provides a superset of the boundary, denoted by $\mu^*_{\partial A}$. From prior information on gray levels, we compute the fuzzy subsets $\mu_{Gl_{CN}}$ (b), $\mu_{Gl_{LV}}$ (c) and $\mu_{Gl_{WM}}$ (d) for other structures composed of white matter (WM), to guarantee $\mu_{LV} \subseteq \mu_{Gl_{LV}}$, $\mu_{CN} \subseteq \mu_{Gl_{CN}}$ and $\mu_{WM} \subseteq \mu_{Gl_{WM}}$. From these fuzzy sets we compute a fuzzy set ${\mu^*}_{\partial(CN,LV)}$ including the boundary $\mu_{\partial(CN,LV)}$ between caudate nucleus and

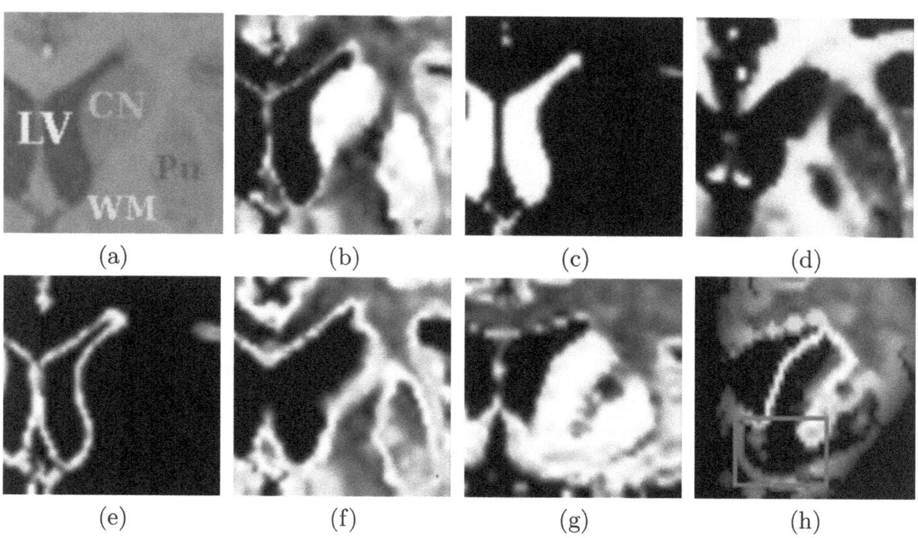

Fig. 2. (a) Zoom on one axial slice. (b) $\mu_{Gl_{CN}}$. (c) $\mu_{Gl_{LV}}$. (d) $\mu_{Gl_{WM}}$. (e) ${\mu^*}_{\partial(CN,LV)}$. (f) ${\mu^*}_{\partial(CN,WM)}$. On one coronal slice: (g) $\mu_{Gl_{CN}} = \mu_{Gl_{AN}}$. (h) $\perp({\mu^*}_{\partial(CN,LV)}, {\mu^*}_{\partial(CN,WM)})$.

lateral ventricle (e), and $\mu^*_{\partial(CN,WM)}$ including the boundary $\mu_{\partial(CN,WM)}$ between caudate nucleus and white matter (f).

While gray-level priors are sufficient to compute an accurate fuzzy subset including the boundary between the caudate nucleus and white matter or lateral ventricle, this is not the case for the accumbens nucleus. Since the caudate nucleus and the accumbens nucleus have similar biological compositions, they cannot be distinguished based on gray levels only (see Fig. 2 (g)). On the other hand considering only the boundary with white matter and lateral ventricle leads to a partial boundary detection, hence having similar drawbacks as gradient based methods (see ROI defined by the red frame in Fig. 2 (h)). Spatial information will allow us to overcome this problem.

3.3 Fusion of Fuzzy Edge Maps with Spatial Information

Prior information on the spatial arrangement of structures, as given in a medical knowledge database (see Sect. 2), is of great help to complete missing information in MRI images. In [10], spatial relations represented as fuzzy sets μ_{SR} were merged with boundary information computed by (1) in a conjunctive manner: $\top(\mu_I, \mu_{SR})$. However, as illustrated in Fig. 3, while this fusion operator removes some undesired boundaries, it cannot fill in missing information.

As an alternative approach, we propose to introduce spatial relations, formulated according to the methodology proposed above for fuzzy regions. Since the spatial relations defined for an object A are modeled as regions of interest μ_{SR_A} including the object to be segmented, we always have $\mu_A \subseteq \mu_{SR_A}$. A conjunctive fusion with the fuzzy set representation of gray-level priors is performed so that the property $\mu_A \subseteq \top(\mu_{SR_A}, \mu_{Gl_A})$ is fulfilled. A fuzzy subset including the object boundary is then computed using (2).

In our example this fusion defines a permitted region for the caudate nucleus $\mu^*_{CN} = \top(\mu_{Gl_{CN}}, \mu_{SR_{CN}})$ (Fig. 4 (c)) and one for the accumbens nucleus $\mu^*_{AN} = \top(\mu_{Gl_{AN}}, \mu_{SR_{AN}})$ (Fig. 4 (d)), which allows for a rough discrimination between the two structures. The boundary between the two structures is then computed (Fig. 4 (e)) and combined with the previous results to obtain a fuzzy subset $\mu^*_{\partial CN}$ (Fig. 4 (f)) including the whole boundaries of the caudate nucleus

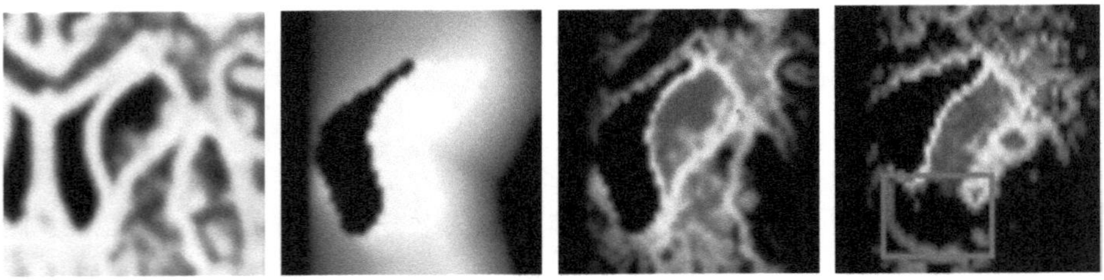

(a) (b) (c) (d)

Fig. 3. (a) μ_I computed from (1). (b) $\mu_{SR_{CN}}$. Fusion $\top(\mu_I, \mu_{SR_{CN}})$ on a axial view (c) and a coronal view (d).

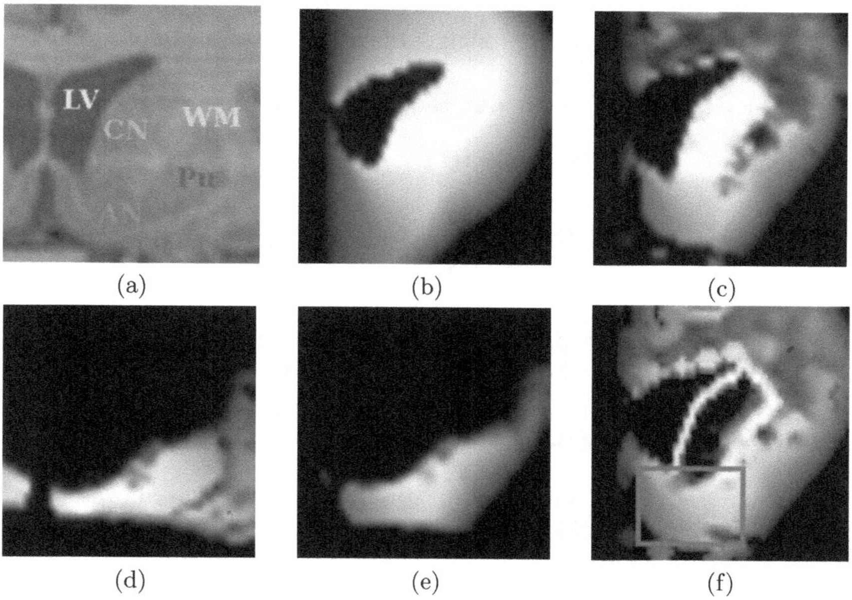

Fig. 4. (a) Zoom on one coronal slice. (b) $\mu_{SR_{CN}}$. (c) $\top(\mu_{SR_{CN}}, \mu_{Gl_{CN}})$. (d) $\top(\mu_{SR_{AN}}, \mu_{Gl_{AN}})$. (e) $\mu_{\partial(CN,AN)}$. (f) $\mu_{\partial CN}$.

$\mu_{\partial CN}$ ($\mu_{\partial CN} \subseteq \mu^*{}_{\partial CN}$), according to the following equation:

$$\mu^*{}_{\partial CN} = \perp(\mu^*{}_{\partial(CN,WM)}, \mu^*{}_{\partial(CN,LV)}, \mu^*{}_{\partial(CN,AN)}), \tag{3}$$

with $\mu^*{}_{\partial(CN,AN)} = \top(D(\mu^*{}_{CN}, B_c), D(\mu^*{}_{AN}, B_c))$. The comparison between Fig. 4 (f) and Fig. 3 (d) shows the improvement achieved by the proposed approach. The boundary is now somewhat wide where contour information is missing, but complete, and will be used to constrain the segmentation.

3.4 New Metric Definition

The minimal surface segmentation problem can be expressed as a minimization problem, of an integral formulation involving a metric f_A that should take low values on object boundaries and high values elsewhere. This approach is robust to noise in the sense that high metric values can be compensated by low ones in the integral. Therefore the result may include points corresponding to quite high metric values.

The complementary of the fuzzy set $\mu^*{}_{\partial A}$ defined by (3) takes low values on object boundaries and therefore could define a suitable metric ($f_A = c(\mu^*{}_{\partial A})$) to our minimal surface segmentation problem. However, as discussed above, this formulation may lead to solutions for object A whose boundaries contain low values of $\mu^*{}_{\partial A}$ and thus do not satisfy the key property 2: $\mu_{\partial A} \subseteq \mu^*{}_{\partial A}$, which ensures that $\mu^*{}_{\partial A}$ takes high values on all points of ∂A. In order to discard low values of $\mu^*{}_{\partial A}$ from the resulting surface, we propose to define the metric as: $f_A = -\log(\mu^*{}_{\partial A})$, which will strongly disfavor surfaces including points with low values of $\mu^*{}_{\partial A}$. For numerical purpose, we add an offset to $\mu^*{}_{\partial A}$, and we define the metric that will be used in the following as:

$$f_A = -\log((1-\varepsilon)\mu^*{}_{\partial A} + \varepsilon).$$

4 Level-Set Based Segmentation of Internal Structures of Normal and Pathological Brains

We now describe how the proposed metric can be incorporated in a minimal surface segmentation framework, using a level-set formulation.

4.1 Level-Set Formulation

From the superset of the boundary fuzzy set $\mu^*{}_{\partial A}$ described above, the minimal surface extraction problem is formulated in the level-set framework as the minimization of the following functional [13]:

$$E(\phi) = \int_{\Omega} f_A(x)\delta(\phi(x))|\nabla\phi(x)|dx, \tag{4}$$

where ϕ implicitly represents the surface as its zero level and is classically initialized using a signed distance function from an initial shape. The associated Euler-Lagrange equation given by:

$$\frac{\partial\phi}{\partial t} = \delta(\phi)\big(f_A \mathrm{div}\left(\frac{\nabla\phi}{\|\nabla\phi\|}\right) + <\nabla f_A, \nabla\phi>\big) \tag{5}$$

is used to find a local minimum of $E(\phi)$ from an initial surface. The result will thus be strongly dependent on the initial surface. To avoid a convergence towards the empty solution or a weak local minimum, a balloon force can be added.

4.2 Segmentation Protocol

We apply this segmentation method to subcortical gray matter nuclei on MRI brain data. We first extract the brain surface, the lateral ventricles and in pathological cases the tumor [14]. The used methods are robust enough to make the assumption that the resulting segmentations are correct. A Gaussian mixture estimation is performed to obtain gray level fuzzy subsets. Spatial relations are then computed and a boundary map is obtained using (3). This computational framework completely defines $E(\phi)$. The level-set based deformable surface evolution is driven by (5), from an initial shape. This initial shape is obtained automatically by combining spatial relation maps with gray level information. Due to lack of space we do not detail the procedure here but for instance the initialization of the segmentation of the caudate nucleus is based on the following relations: *closed to the body of lateral ventricle, strictly to its right.*

4.3 Data

Segmentation results are evaluated on the caudate nucleus for 18 healty subjects and 6 pathological cases.

The normal database is provided on the Internet Brain Segmentation Repository (IBSR) (http://www.cma.mgh.harvard.edu/ibsr). It contains 18 T1-weighted MR scans ($256 \times 256 \times 128$ volumes, with $1 \times 1 \times 1.5$ mm^3 resolution). A manual segmentation of 43 structures performed by an expert is also provided and is considered as the ground truth to evaluate our results.

The pathological database is composed of 6 cases illustrated in Fig. 6 affected by brain tumors. The tumors induce various degrees of deformation on the internal nuclei from weak to very large in case of subcortical tumors. The MR scans are $256 \times 256 \times 128$ axial volumes obtained by a SPGR sequence with $0.93 \times 0.93 \times 1.5$ mm^3 voxel size. Manual segmentation of 8 structures is considered as the ground truth.

4.4 Results

Some results are illustrated in Fig. 5 and 6. The influence of the spatial priors on the segmentation of the lower part of the caudate nucleus is clearly visible on these results. Segmentation accuracy is assessed through comparison with manual segmentations using the following measures:

(i) kappa coefficient: $\frac{2*|A \cap B|}{|A|+|B|}$, which measures agreement between A and B,
(ii) average distance between the surfaces of A (reference) and B (our result),
(iii) Hausdorff distance between A and B.

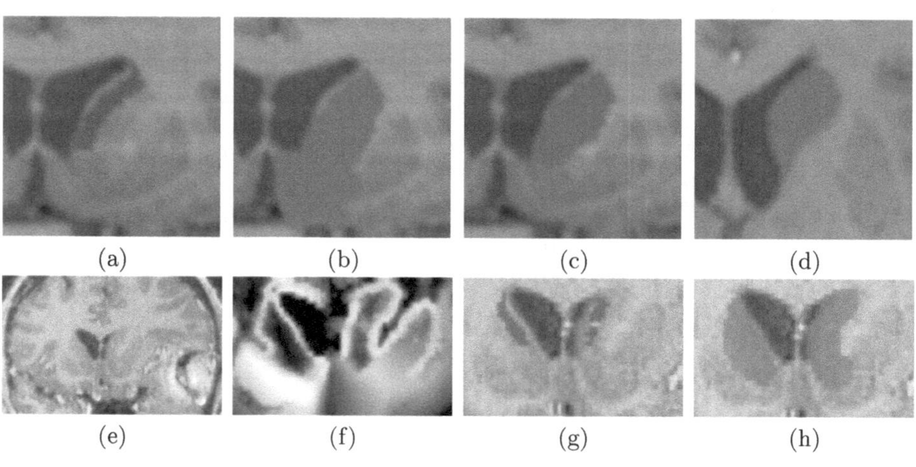

Fig. 5. Segmentation of the caudate nuclei on a normal case. (a) Initialization. (b) Segmentation result without spatial priors. (c, d) Segmentation with spatial priors on a coronal slice and on an axial slice. (e) Coronal slice of a pathological case. (f) $\mu^*_{\partial CN}$. (g) Initialization. (h) Segmentation with spatial priors.

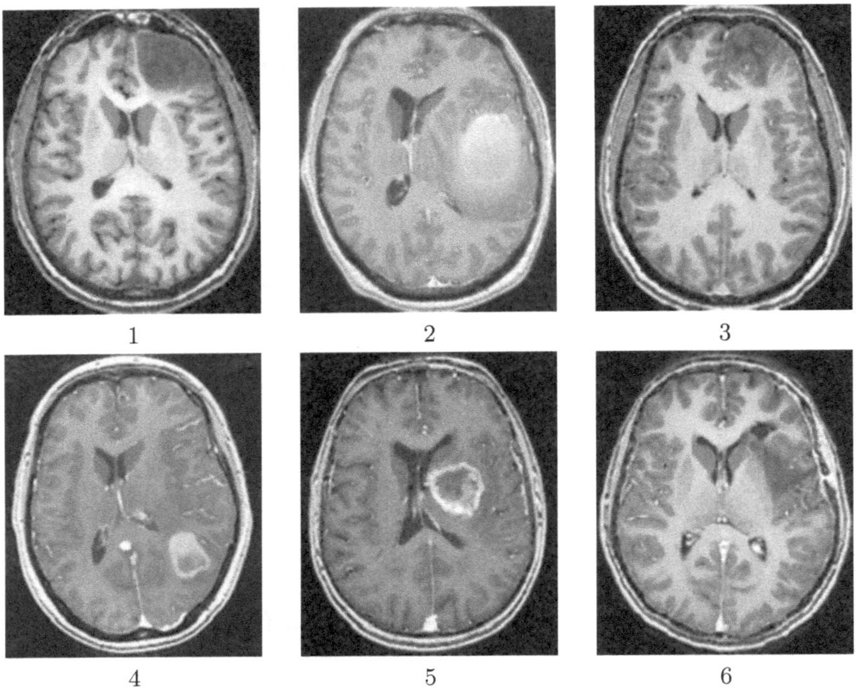

Fig. 6. Axial views of 6 pathological cases. Segmentation results are overlayed in red.

Table 1. Evaluation of the segmentation of the caudate nuclei on IBSR database

Case	Kappa		Average (mm)		Hausdorff (mm)		Case	Kappa		Average (mm)		Hausdorff (mm)	
	left	right	left	right	left	right		left	right	left	right	left	right
1	0.86	0.82	0.68	0.63	6.78	5.74	10	0.82	0.82	0.66	0.57	5.83	5.10
2	0.81	0.85	0.62	0.43	4.90	3.46	11	0.78	0.86	0.61	0.42	5.74	3.46
3	0.80	0.74	0.75	0.81	9.89	4.24	12	0.83	0.84	0.59	0.52	4.90	4.12
4	0.78	0.78	0.77	0.67	5.48	5.48	13	0.82	0.84	0.78	0.59	9.43	5.48
5	0.85	0.85	0.47	0.47	3.00	3.16	14	0.84	0.85	0.50	0.54	3.74	3.74
6	0.83	0.78	0.63	0.96	5.10	7.07	15	0.85	0.85	0.43	0.57	3.00	6.16
7	0.81	0.79	0.50	0.52	4.58	3.61	16	0.83	0.84	0.57	0.69	3.74	5.66
8	0.74	0.74	0.77	0.65	8.54	8.54	17	0.83	0.86	0.77	0.59	6.40	5.74
9	0.82	0.83	0.57	0.52	5.39	6.56	18	0.75	0.75	0.99	1.23	5.48	8.60
							Mean	0.81		0.64		5.50	

Results on normal cases are summarized in Table 1. As an example, results can be compared to those reported in [15] for the same database (where a mean kappa of 0.65 and average distance of $1.71mm$ are reported), or in [16] and [17]

Table 2. Evaluation of the segmentation of the caudate nuclei on pathological cases

Case	Kappa		Average (mm)		Hausdorff (mm)		Case	Kappa		Average (mm)		Hausdorff (mm)	
	left	right	left	right	left	right		left	right	left	right	left	right
1	0.84	0.83	0.67	0.55	10.95	5.83	4	0.75	0.75	0.67	0.72	5.20	9.00
2	0.78	0.85	0.77	0.55	8.06	6.32	5	0.72	0.82	1.58	0.70	19.41	9.11
3	0.80	0.82	0.69	0.55	6.78	5.00	6	0.82	0.85	0.66	0.93	6.17	7.68
							Mean	0.80		0.75		8.29	

for other databases (respectively average distances of $1.60mm$ and $0.60mm$). We can note that the average distance is less than the voxel size (generally $1{\times}1{\times}1.5\,mm^3$), and kappa coefficients over 0.7 indicate high agreements between the segmentations [18]. The Hausdorff distance, which corresponds to the worst point, is much more variable, due to imprecise delineation between CN and AN, leading to an arbitrary cut in both manual and automatic segmentations, and thinness of the tail (and also the end of the body) for which minimal surface segmentation is not suited. Results for pathological cases are summarized in Table 2. Among the 12 segmentations, 11 show similar accuracy as in the normal cases. Despite the deformations, spatial knowledge and thus our segmentation framework remain stable. Concerning subject 5, the tumor is adjacent to the left caudate nucleus and induces very large deformations. Improving the results in such cases could rely on an adaptation of the spatial relations, as proposed in [19].

5 Conclusion

The main contribution of this paper is to define a new metric for minimal surface segmentation, incorporating, in a original way, radiometric and structural information. We have shown that missing contour information can be compensated for by exploiting spatial information, based on region gray levels and spatial relations, and how to integrate all these pieces of information in a fuzzy set framework to define metrics for minimal surface extraction. Our approach has been applied, in a geodesic level-set framework, to the segmentation of the caudate nuclei in normal and pathological brain MRI with promising results. Future work aims at extending this approach to other brain structures: while the approach is general, including fuzzy sets have to be specified according to spatial relations specific to each structure.

Acknowledgements. The data have been acquired at the Pitié-Salpétriére, Val-de-Grâce and Sainte-Anne hospitals in Paris. We would like also to thank Hassan Khotanlou for the segmentation of the tumors.

References

1. Caselles, V., Kimmel, R., Sapiro, G.: Geodesic active contours. In: IEEE International Conference on Computer Vision, ICCV 1995, pp. 694–699 (1995)
2. Boykov, Y., Kolmogorov, V.: Computing geodesics and minimal surfaces via graph cuts. In: IEEE International Conference on Computer Vision, ICCV 2003. pp. 26–33 (2003)
3. Cohen, L., Kimmel, R.: Global Minimum for Active Contour Models: A Minimal Path Approach. International Journal of Computer Vision 24(1), 57–78 (1997)
4. Grady, L.: Computing exact discrete minimal surfaces: Extending and solving the shortest path problem in 3D with application to segmentation. In: IEEE Conference on Computer Vision and Pattern Recognition, CVPR 2006. vol. 1, pp. 69–78 (2006)
5. Leventon, M., Grimson, W., Faugeras, O.: Statistical shape influence in geodesic active contours. In: IEEE Conference on Computer Vision and Pattern Recognition, CVPR 2000. vol. 1, pp. 316–323 (2000)
6. Paragios, N., Deriche, R.: Geodesic active regions: A new framework to deal with frame partition problems in computer vision. Journal of Visual Communication and Image Representation 13(1), 249–268 (2002)
7. Bloch, I.: Fuzzy Spatial Relationships for Image Processing and Interpretation: A Review. Image and Vision Computing 23(2), 89–110 (2005)
8. Bloch, I., Géraud, T., Maître, H.: Representation and Fusion of Heterogeneous Fuzzy Information in the 3D Space for Model-Based Structural Recognition - Application to 3D Brain Imaging. Artificial Intelligence 148, 141–175 (2003)
9. Colliot, O., Camara, O., Bloch, I.: Integration of Fuzzy Spatial Relations in Deformable Models - Application to Brain MRI Segmentation. Pattern Recognition 39, 1401–1414 (2006)
10. Atif, J., Nempont, O., Colliot, O., Angelini, E., Bloch, I.: Level Set Deformable Models Constrained by Fuzzy Spatial Relation. In: Information Processing and Management of Uncertainty in Knowledge-Based Systems, IPMU 2006, pp. 1534–1541 (2006)
11. Bloch, I., Maître, H., Anvari, M.: Fuzzy Adjacency between Image Objects. International Journal of Uncertainty, Fuzziness and Knowledge-Based Systems 5(6), 615–653 (1997)
12. Dubois, D., Prade, H.: Fuzzy Sets and Systems: Theory and Applications. Academic Press, New-York (1980)
13. Gout, C., Le Guyader, C., Vese, L.: Segmentation under geometrical conditions using geodesic active contours and interpolation using level set methods. Numerical Algorithms 39(1), 155–173 (2005)
14. Khotanlou, H., Colliot, O., Bloch, I.: Automatic Brain Tumor Segmentation using Symmetry Analysis and Deformable Models. In: International Conference on Advances in Pattern Recognition, ICAPR 2007, pp. 198–202 (2007)
15. Ciofolo, C., Barillot, C.: Brain Segmentation with Competitive Level Sets and Fuzzy Control. In: Christensen, G.E., Sonka, M. (eds.) IPMI 2005. LNCS, vol. 3565, pp. 333–344. Springer, Heidelberg (2005)
16. Pitiot, A., Delingette, H., Thompson, P., Ayache, N.: Expert knowledge-guided segmentation system for brain MRI. Neuroimage 23(1), 85–96 (2004)
17. Xue, J., Ruan, S., Moretti, B., Revenu, M., Bloyet, D.: Knowledge-based segmentation and labeling of brain structures from MRI images. Pattern Recognition Letters 22(3), 395–405 (2001)

18. Zijdenbos, A., Dawant, B., Margolin, R.: Morphometric analysis of white matter lesions in MR images: method and validation. IEEE Transactions on Medical Imaging 13(4), 716–724 (1994)
19. Atif, J., Hudelot, C., Fouquier, G., Bloch, I., Angelini, E.: From Generic Knowledge to Specific Reasoning for Medical Image Interpretation using Graph-based Representations. In: International Joint Conference on Artificial Intelligence, IJCAI 2007, pp. 224–229 (2007)

A Fuzzy, Nonparametric Segmentation Framework for DTI and MRI Analysis

Suyash P. Awate and James C. Gee

Department of Radiology, University of Pennsylvania, Philadelphia, PA 19104, USA
{awate,gee}@mail.med.upenn.edu

Abstract. This paper presents a novel statistical fuzzy-segmentation method for diffusion tensor (DT) images and magnetic resonance (MR) images. Typical fuzzy-segmentation schemes, e.g. those based on fuzzy-C-means (FCM), incorporate Gaussian class models which are inherently biased towards ellipsoidal clusters. Fiber bundles in DT images, however, comprise tensors that can inherently lie on more-complex manifolds. Unlike FCM-based schemes, the proposed method relies on *modeling the manifolds* underlying the classes by incorporating nonparametric data-driven statistical models. It produces an optimal fuzzy segmentation by maximizing a novel information-theoretic energy in a Markov-random-field framework. For DT images, the paper describes a consistent statistical technique for nonparametric modeling in Riemannian DT spaces that incorporates two very recent works. In this way, the proposed method provides *uncertainties* in the segmentation decisions, which stem from imaging artifacts including noise, partial voluming, and inhomogeneity. The paper shows results on synthetic and real, DT as well as MR images.

1 Introduction

Diffusion tensor (DT) magnetic resonance (MR) imaging has become exceedingly popular because of its ability to measure the anisotropic diffusion of water in structured biological tissue. It allows us to differentiate between the anatomical structures of cerebral white/gray matter, that was previously impossible with MR imaging (MRI), *in vivo* and noninvasively. The segmentation of fiber tracts in the brain, such as the corpus callosum or the lateral corticospinal tract, is of key interest in several clinical applications [1,2]. DT imaging also helps to noninvasively differentiate between thalamic nuclei based on the DT characteristic in each nucleus [3]. The study of thalamic changes holds importance in the study of schizophrenia and Parkinson's disease. Hippocampus analysis is important in the diagnosis of several diseases such as Alzheimer's disease and schizophrenia. The hippocampal substructures, which can not be easily differentiated in MR data, might be separable using DT images [4].

DT imaging is a relatively new modality and is persistently plagued by the presence of artifacts such as noise, partial voluming, and inhomogeneity in images. Typically, these artifacts reduce the efficacy and utility of post-processing methods on DT images. Such methods include classic segmentation methods

N. Karssemeijer and B. Lelieveldt (Eds.): IPMI 2007, LNCS 4584, pp. 296–307, 2007.
© Springer-Verlag Berlin Heidelberg 2007

and tractography methods that exclusively label each voxel to one or the other classes/structures. For instance, tractography methods that typically incorporate thresholds on the fractional anisotropy and fiber curvature to terminate tracing, can consistently underestimate the size of the fiber bundles [5]. The problem, with tractography, is exacerbated for thin tracts undergoing sharp changes in orientation. One way of accounting for the noise/partial-voluming artifacts is by *not* assigning voxels exclusively to one class or the other, but rather to estimate the *membership* of each voxel in the classes. The membership values effectively provide information about the *uncertainties* in delineating tracts/structures. This necessitates the formulation of a statistical fuzzy-segmentation framework for DT images. Advantages of fuzzy segmentation of MR tissue intensities are well known [6]. For DT images, we can use such fuzzy-membership information to: (a) increase the reliability and accuracy of tract extraction associated with clinical studies, (b) improve the accuracy of DT processing methods such as tractography, (c) aid experts in reliably labeling fiber bundles for constructing tract-based atlases, etc.

Many previous works in DT-image segmentation [2,1] employ Gaussian models, in Riemannian spaces, to model the DT statistics in specific structures of interest. These Gaussian models, however, may not effectively model the DT statistics because they are inherently biased towards ellipsoidal clusters [7]. The fundamental anatomical characteristics of fiber bundles are such that the *fibers can change their orientation* significantly—they bend—as they connect different brain structures. Thus, tensors in fiber bundles inherently lie on manifolds that do not conform to Gaussian models that are characterized by the mean. For instance, tensors in U-shaped bundles, where the tensors start and end at the similar orientations, must lie on a *closed manifold* in the tensor space.

This paper makes several contributions. It proposes a novel fuzzy-segmentation approach in the nonparametric-statistical framework that does not impose strong parametric models on the data. Rather, it provides the power to model and adapt to arbitrary (but smooth) probability density functions (PDFs) via data-driven strategies. Such nonparametric PDFs capture the manifold(s) underlying the classes as well as the variability of the data around the manifold(s). Recent work have clearly demonstrated the advantages of nonparametric-statistical modeling for general image segmentation [8] as well as MR-image tissue classification [9]. We employ a kernel-based approach for the nonparametric modeling [10]. We combine results from two very recent works—one describing a generic (tensor-metric independent) Riemannian kernel PDF estimation scheme [11] and the other describing the Log-Euclidean Riemannian metric [12]—to propose a statistically *consistent* nonparametric PDF estimation scheme for DT data. Subsequently, we propose a novel information-theoretic generalization of the fuzzy-C-means (FCM) framework [13] that replaces the classic ellipsoidal models/clusters for classes by generic manifold-based models. In this way, the proposed method provides the uncertainties in the segmentation decisions, which are caused by artifacts including noise, partial voluming, and inhomogeneity. We show results on synthetic and real data, including DT and MR images.

2 Related Work

Early work on DT segmentation [14] relied on a simplified feature space of an invariant anisotropy measure. It employed a level-set framework to differentiate between the anisotropic and isotropic regions in the brain. Such anisotropy measures, however, make it impossible to distinguish between fiber bundles with different orientations. Wiegell *et al.* [3] and Rousson *et al.* [15] use the Euclidean Frobenius norm between tensors during the segmentation. Lenglet *et al.* [1] present a Riemannian distance measure between tensors and model each class by a single Gaussian in the Riemannian space. The proposed method extends their modeling approach by incorporating a generic nonparametric model for each class that is able to accurately model tensor statistics in fiber bundles. Wang and Vemuri [2] propose an affine-invariant distance measure based on the J-divergence of two Gaussians corresponding to two diffusion tensors. They employ a piecewise-smooth Mumford-Shah segmentation framework to capture the tensor statistics. The proposed method, however, relies on a nonparametric statistical approach in the Markov-random-field framework. Furthermore, it provides fuzzy segmentations by optimizing an information-theoretic energy.

The utility of Riemannian tensor metrics for processing DT images is well established in the literature [16,12,1,17]—Euclidean metrics lead to averages that cause artificial *tensor swelling*, where the determinant, and thus dispersion, of the average tensor can be larger than the individual tensors. The proposed kernel-based PDF estimation scheme also relies on a weighted-averaging scheme that incorporates contributions from several tensors to measure the probability at a particular point in tensor space. Riemannian metrics avoid such swelling effects and, therefore, we employ such a metric in this paper.

FCM relies on representing each class by *only a single point* in the feature space, namely, the class mean [13]. In this way, FCM measures class membership based on the Euclidean or Mahalanobis distance to the class mean. Modeling each class by a *single Gaussian* extends the FCM scheme into a probabilistic scheme popularly known as the Gaussian-mixture PDF modeling [18] that has been widely used for MR image segmentation [19]. Such a scheme, however, continues to measure class membership based on the Mahalanobis distance to the Gaussian mean. We propose a method that generalizes the representation of a class—instead of a single point (mean) in the feature space—to the *manifold* underlying the class in order to measure class membership based on the distance from the manifold that accurately represents the class.

Pham and Prince [6] employ the FCM method for fuzzy tissue classification of MR images by iteratively adapting to the intensity homogeneity. The proposed method, on the other hand, extends FCM by generalizing the underlying representation of the classes to an arbitrary manifold. This generic approach also retains the efficacy of the method for inhomogeneity-corrupted images. Kim *et al.* [8] and Awate *et al.* [9] employ nonparametric models for texture segmentation and MR-image segmentation, respectively. This paper proposes a different objective function that produces fuzzy segmentations and extends the resulting scheme for DT images. O'Donnell *et al.* [20] present a scheme for interface detection in DT data, based on a generalized local structure tensor, as a step towards segmentation, registration, and automatic detection of the visually-elusive fiber-bundle interfaces in DT images. The proposed fuzzy-segmentation method also fits in this context; voxels having significant memberships to more than one class indicate the presence of an interface. On the other hand, the proposed method is more general—giving a membership value at each voxel—and performs this in a mathematically-sound statistical framework.

3 Nonparametric Tensor Statistics

This section describes the statistical formulation underlying the proposed nonparametric modeling technique. It starts by describing a generic kernel-based modeling scheme, that is independent of the particular metric associated with the Riemannian space. It then presents an appropriate tensor metric that considerably simplifies the scheme, from a practical point of view, while maintaining the mathematical soundness of the framework.

The statistics literature presents several methods for nonparametric modeling of the data based on Fourier expansions, splines, kernels, etc. We propose to use the kernel-based PDF approach known as Parzen-window PDF estimation [10] that essentially performs scattered-data interpolation by superposing kernel functions placed at each datum. For DT data, the kernel functions are smooth functions of the Riemannian geodesic distance on the tensor manifold. The mathematical expression for the Parzen-window tensor-PDF estimate is consistent with the expression of the usual kernel-PDF estimate in Euclidean spaces. For instance, it also relies on the intuitive notion of a kernel function that has the highest value at the datum and monotonically-decreasing values with increasing distance from the datum. In the Riemannian case, each datum is the intrinsic mean of the associated kernel provided for sufficiently small bandwidths.

3.1 Kernels in Riemannian Spaces

This section first describes the mathematical expression for the Parzen-window estimate on generic Riemannian manifolds from the very recent work by Pelletier [11]. We start by providing the associated notation.

Let $\mathcal{M}$ be a compact Riemannian manifold without boundary, of dimension D, with an associated metric-tensor g. The metric tensor induces an inner product on the manifold, that in turn leads to the notion of the geodesic distance function $d_g(\cdot,\cdot)$ between two entities on $\mathcal{M}$. Let Z be a random variable on the probability space $(\Omega, \mathcal{A}, P)$ that takes values in $(M, \mathcal{B})$ where $\mathcal{B}$ denotes the Borel sigma-field of $\mathcal{M}$. Assume that the image of the probability measure P, under the map Z, is continuous with respect to the volume measure on $\mathcal{M}$. Let $\{z_1, z_2, \ldots, z_n\}$, where each $z_i \in \mathcal{M}$, be an independently-drawn and identically-distributed random sample derived from the PDF $P(Z)$. Let $K(\cdot)$ be a nonnegative and sufficiently-smooth kernel function.

In order to make sure that the PDF $P(Z)$ on $\mathcal{M}$ integrates to one, we need to set up a framework that allows us to perform the integration. This entails computing the ratio of the volume measures on the Riemannian manifold $\mathcal{M}$ and its tangent space $T_a(\mathcal{M})$ at each point a. If a and b be two points on $\mathcal{M}$, then the volume density function on $\mathcal{M}$ is

$$\theta_a(b) = \frac{\mu_{\exp_a^* g}}{\mu_{g_a}} \left(\exp_a^{-1}(b)\right), \tag{1}$$

which is the quotient of the canonical measure of the Riemannian metric $\exp_a^* g$ on $T_a(\mathcal{M})$ (pullback of the metric-tensor g by the exponential-map $\exp_a$) by the Lebesgue measure of the Euclidean structure g_a on $T_a(\mathcal{M})$. This is the same as the square root of the determinant of the metric-tensor g expressed in the geodesic normal coordinates at a and evaluated at $\exp_a^{-1}(b)$. This also gives an indication of the curvature of the Riemannian space. For the special case where $\mathcal{M}$ is the Euclidean space $\Re^D$, $\theta_a(b) = 1$. Thus, the PDF estimate is

$$\hat{P}(z) = \frac{1}{N} \sum_{i=1}^{N} \frac{1}{\theta_{z_i}(z)} \frac{1}{\sigma^D} K\left(\frac{d_g(z, z_i)}{\sigma}\right), \tag{2}$$

where σ is the bandwidth of the associated kernel. Pelletier [11] recently proved the asymptotic (as $N \to \infty$) consistency of the estimator with respect to the true PDF $P(Z)$ with an L^2 rate of convergence. In this paper, we define $K(\cdot)$ to be the standard-Normal PDF: $K(\beta) = (1/(2\pi)^{D/2}) \exp(-\beta^2/2)$.

To evaluate the probability at any one point z we need to, in general, compute $\theta_{z_i}(z)$ separately for all the points z_i in the Parzen-window sample. Evaluating Parzen-window probabilities in this framework can become cumbersome, depending on the particular Riemannian tensor metric employed. For Gaussians using the affine-invariant Riemannian metric [17], Lenglet *et al.* [1] give the first-order Taylor-series approximation of the square root of the metric tensor in the case of small bandwidth σ. The next section employs the Log-Euclidean Riemannian metric to eliminate this issue altogether.

3.2 Riemannian Kernels with Log-Euclidean Metrics

Recently, Arsigny *et al.* [12] proposed a Riemannian tensor metric, namely the Log-Euclidean metric. In contrast to the affine-invariant Riemannian metric in [16,1,17], the Log-Euclidean metric induces a Riemannian space having zero curvature. The Log-Euclidean framework defines a mapping where the DT space of 3×3 symmetric positive definite matrices is isomorphic, diffeomorphic, and *isometric* to the associated *Euclidean vector space* of 3×3 symmetric matrices. This mapping is precisely the matrix logarithm, namely Log .

The isometry property equates geodesic distances in the Riemannian space to Euclidean distances in the vector space, i.e.

$$d_g(z, z_i) = \| \operatorname{Log}(z) - \operatorname{Log}(z_i) \|_{\text{Frobenius}} . \tag{3}$$

Isometry also implies that the determinant of the metric tensor is unity everywhere [21]. Indeed, the Log-Euclidean metric defines a Euclidean structure on the tensor space. This simplifies $\theta_{z_i}(z)$ to evaluate to unity. The Parzen-window PDF estimate simplifies to

$$\hat{P}(z) = \frac{1}{N} \sum_{i=1}^{N} G(z; z_i, \sigma), \text{ where} \quad (4)$$

$$G(z; z_i, \sigma) = \frac{1}{(2\pi)^{D/2}} \frac{1}{\sigma^D} \exp\left(\frac{- \| \operatorname{Log}(z) - \operatorname{Log}(z_i) \|^2_{\text{Frobenius}}}{2\sigma^2} \right) \quad (5)$$

is the Riemannian analogue (with the Log-Euclidean metric) for the Euclidean Gaussian kernel. In practice, this allows us to map the diffusion tensors, through the matrix logarithm, to a Euclidean space and, in turn, compute probabilities from standard Parzen-window PDF estimation in the Euclidean space.

4 Fuzzy Segmentation with Manifold-Based Models

This section proposes a novel extension to the FCM fuzzy segmentation framework. Specifically, we generalize FCM's representation of classes in feature-space by the manifolds underlying the classes and, subsequently, measure class memberships based on the distances from these manifolds. For DT images, we achieve this by employing the accurate and practical Parzen-window PDF estimation scheme proposed in the previous section. This section first describes a fuzzy segmentation framework by formulating an information-theoretic objective function relying on the nonparametric class models. It then proposes an iterative optimization strategy and presents the segmentation algorithm.

To have a generic framework, we consider a Markov random field (MRF) image model. Assume that the tensor image is derived from an underlying MRF $\mathbf{X} = \{X_t\}_{t \in \mathcal{T}}$, where $\mathcal{T}$ is the set of voxels on the Cartesian grid and the random variable X_t, at each voxel t, is defined on the sample-space Ω. Denote the tensor values in the image by x_t that lie in the Riemannian space $\mathcal{M}$. Let $\mathcal{N} = \{\mathcal{N}_t\}_{t \in \mathcal{T}}$ be the neighborhood system associated with the MRF for the voxel set $\mathcal{T}$. Define random vectors $\mathbf{Y}_t = \{X_t\}_{t \in \mathcal{N}_t}$—note that $t \notin \mathcal{N}_t$—and $\mathbf{Z}_t = (X_t, \mathbf{Y}_t)$. The PDF $P(\mathbf{Z}_t)$ is the joint PDF of the tensors in DT-image neighborhoods.

4.1 Information-Theoretic Objective Function

Our goal is to segment the image into C different classes ($c = 1, 2, \ldots, C$) which are distinguished by their respective PDFs $\{P_c(\cdot)\}_{c=1,2,\ldots,C}$. The segmentation problem is, in a way, equivalent to that of deducing these PDFs. Voxels in a fuzzy-segmentation framework can be *members* of more than one class. This is a standard notion in fuzzy set theory that does *not* constrain entities to belong to one set alone. We incorporate this notion using the fuzzy-membership functions that we define next. Consider C random variables $\{F_c\}_{c \in C}$ where, for each c, the random variable $F_c : \mathcal{M} \to \Re$ gives a class-membership value for each element $\mathbf{z} \in \mathcal{M}$ belonging to class c. The constrains on the membership values are:

$$\forall t \in \mathcal{T}, \forall c = 1, \ldots, C : 0 \leq F_c(\mathbf{z}_t) \leq 1, \text{ and} \quad (6)$$

$$\forall t \in \mathcal{T} : \sum_{c=1}^{C} F_c(\mathbf{z}_t) = 1. \tag{7}$$

Typical hard (non-fuzzy) segmentation approaches capture the homogeneity of classes using the Shannon's entropy of the classes. To achieve fuzzy segmentation, we replace the Shannon's entropy for the class c by the following function:

$$h_c(\mathbf{Z}) = -\int_{\mathcal{M}} F_c(\mathbf{z}) P_c(\mathbf{z}) \,\mathrm{Log}\; P_c(\mathbf{z}) d\mathbf{z}. \tag{8}$$

In this way, each observation $\mathbf{z} \in \mathcal{M}$ contributes an amount to the newly-defined "entropy" of class c that is proportional to its membership in class c. This modification alone, however, is insufficient and the optimization defaults to zero/one values for $F_c(\mathbf{z})$, thereby implying a hard segmentation. To overcome this problem, we must also, simultaneously, maximize the entropy of the fuzzy-membership function. Thus, we define the optimal fuzzy segmentation as:

$$\underset{\{F_c(\cdot)\}_{c=1}^{C}}{\mathrm{argmax}} \sum_{c=1}^{C} \left(\int_{\mathcal{M}} F_c(\mathbf{z}) P_c(\mathbf{z}) \,\mathrm{Log}\; P_c(\mathbf{z}) d\mathbf{z} - \alpha \int_{\mathcal{M}} F_c(\mathbf{z}) \,\mathrm{Log}\; F_c(\mathbf{z}) d\mathbf{z} \right), \tag{9}$$

under the constraints on the membership function given in (6) and (7). Here, α is a user-controlled parameter that controls the degree of fuzziness imposed on the segmentation. Setting $\alpha \leftarrow 0$ gives a hard segmentation, while $\alpha \rightarrow \infty$ gives a completely-fuzzy segmentation, i.e. where $F_c(\mathbf{z}) = 1/C, \forall t \in \mathcal{T}, \forall c = 1, 2, \ldots, C$.

We now simplify the formulation in (9) by rewriting it as:

$$\underset{\{F_c(\cdot)\}_{c=1}^{C}}{\mathrm{argmax}} \sum_{c=1}^{C} \left(E_{P(\mathbf{Z})} \left[F_c(\mathbf{Z}) \,\mathrm{Log}\; P_c(\mathbf{Z}) \right] - \alpha \int_{\mathcal{M}} F_c(\mathbf{z}) \,\mathrm{Log}\; F_c(\mathbf{z}) d\mathbf{z} \right) \tag{10}$$

$$\approx \underset{\{F_c(\cdot)\}_{c=1}^{C}}{\mathrm{argmax}} \sum_{c=1}^{C} \sum_{t \in \mathcal{T}} \left[F_c(\mathbf{z}_t) \,\mathrm{Log}\; P_c(\mathbf{z}_t) - \alpha F_c(\mathbf{z}_t) \,\mathrm{Log}\; F_c(\mathbf{z}_t) \right], \tag{11}$$

where $E_{P(\mathbf{Z})}[\cdot]$ denotes an expectation over the PDF $P(\mathbf{Z})$. The approximation for the first term comes from an ergodicity assumption on the MRF X—this (asymptotically) equates ensemble averages to spatial averages.

4.2 Constrained Optimization Using Lagrange Multipliers

This section describes the optimization strategy to maximize the proposed objective function in (10) and presents the associated algorithm. We employ the method of Lagrange multipliers to solve the constrained optimization problem—the constraints are given in (6 and (7). Using the short-hand terms F_{ct} and P_{ct} for the terms $F_c(\mathbf{z}_t)$ and $P_c(\mathbf{z}_t)$ respectively—the objective function becomes

$$\mathcal{J} = \sum_{c=1}^{C} \sum_{t \in \mathcal{T}} \left[F_{ct} \,\mathrm{Log}\; P_{ct} - \alpha F_{ct} \,\mathrm{Log}\; F_{ct} \right] + \sum_{t \in \mathcal{T}} \lambda_t \left[\sum_{c=1}^{C} F_{ct} - 1 \right], \tag{12}$$

where $\{\lambda_t\}_{t \in \mathcal{T}}$ is the set of Lagrange multipliers and the probabilities P_{ct} are

$$P_{ct} = \frac{1}{|\mathcal{S}_c|} \sum_{s \in \mathcal{S}_c} G(\mathbf{z}_t; \mu_{cs}, \sigma_c), \tag{13}$$

where the tensors $\{\mu_{cs}\}_{s \in \mathcal{S}_c}$ and the bandwidth σ_c together model class c. This PDF captures both: the manifold(s) underlying the data in class c as well as the variability of the data around the manifold(s).

We need to maximize $\mathcal{J}$ with respect to F_{ct}, μ_{cs}, and λ_t. Solving the Karush-Kuhn-Tucker (KKT) necessary conditions for optimality gives the update for the fuzzy memberships as:

$$\forall t \in \mathcal{T}, \forall c = 1, 2, \ldots, C : F_{ct} = \frac{(P_{ct})^{\frac{1}{\alpha}}}{\sum_{c=1}^{C} (P_{ct})^{\frac{1}{\alpha}}}. \tag{14}$$

Observe that, as expected, a large probability P_{ct} for voxel t to be in class c produces a correspondingly larger membership value F_{ct} of that voxel in class c. As $\alpha \to \infty$, we see that $F_{ct} \to 1/|C|$ and we get a completely fuzzy segmentation. As $\alpha \to 0$, we see that $F_{ct} \to 1$ if class c with the largest P_{ct}; otherwise $F_{ct} \to 0$.

Solving the KKT conditions gives the update for the class parameter μ_{cs} as:

$$\forall s \in \mathcal{S}_c, \forall c = 1, 2, \ldots, C : \mu_{cs} = \frac{\sum_{t \in \mathcal{T}} F_{ct} \frac{G(\mathbf{z}_t; \mu_{cs}, \sigma_c)}{P_{ct}} \mathbf{z}_t}{\sum_{t \in \mathcal{T}} F_{ct} \frac{G(\mathbf{z}_t; \mu_{cs}, \sigma_c)}{P_{ct}}}, \tag{15}$$

where the updated parameter μ_{cs} is a weighted average of the data $\mathbf{z}_t$. Observe that the weights take values between 0 and 1. Moreover, one need not worry about numerical-stability issues during implementation because, by construction, $0 \leq F_{ct} \leq 1$ and $0 \leq \frac{G(\mathbf{z}_t - \mu_{cs}; \sigma_c)}{P_{ct}} \leq 1$. Furthermore, the limiting case of $|\mathcal{S}_c| \to 1$ implies that $G(\mathbf{z}_t; \mu_{cs}, \sigma_c) = P_{ct}$ that causes the updates to default to the FCM updates using Mahalanobis distances.

Given an initial segmentation, the proposed algorithm iterates as follows:

1. For each class, assign the bandwidth $\sigma_c \leftarrow \sigma_{\mathrm{ML}}$, where σ_{ML} is a penalized maximum-likelihood estimate for the entire image $\mathbf{z}_{t \in \mathcal{T}}$ [22].
2. Select a fraction of voxels γ from the initialized classes to produce feature vectors $\{\mu_{cs}\}_{s \in \mathcal{S}_c}$. Selecting too many voxels entails estimating too many parameters from the given (finite) data. Too few parameters reduce the capability of the model to accurately represent the PDF, or the manifold underlying, the class. Results in this paper use $\gamma = 0.5$.
3. Use (14) to update F_{ct} for $c = 1, \ldots, C, \forall t \in \mathcal{T}$.
4. Use (15) to update the class models μ_{cs} for all $c = 1, \ldots, C, \forall s \in \mathcal{S}_c$.
5. Repeat steps 3 and 4 until convergence.

5 Results, Discussion, and Conclusion

This section gives the results on real and synthetic DT images as well as MR images. For synthetic DT images, we simulate noise using the method described

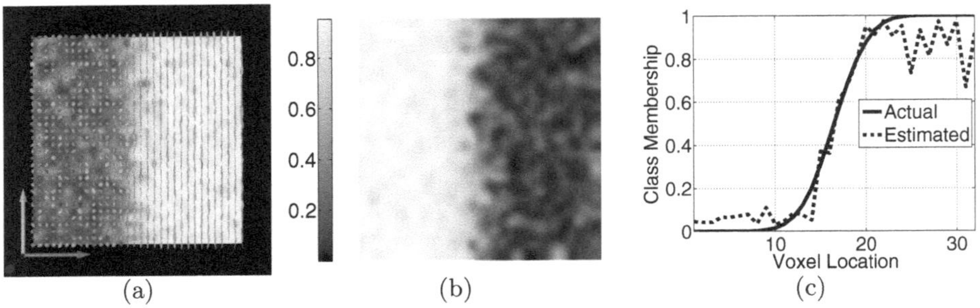

Fig. 1. (a) Synthetic DT image with 2 classes ($C = 2$) (tensor orientations encoded in glyph colors, finite anisotropy encoded in the grayscale background) showing noise and partial voluming near the interface. (b) Fuzzy-membership values for one of the classes (without any Markov model): blue (red) implies low (high) membership values. (c) Comparing membership functions for a specific horizontal scanline: estimated and the true (obtained from the image without noise and partial voluming).

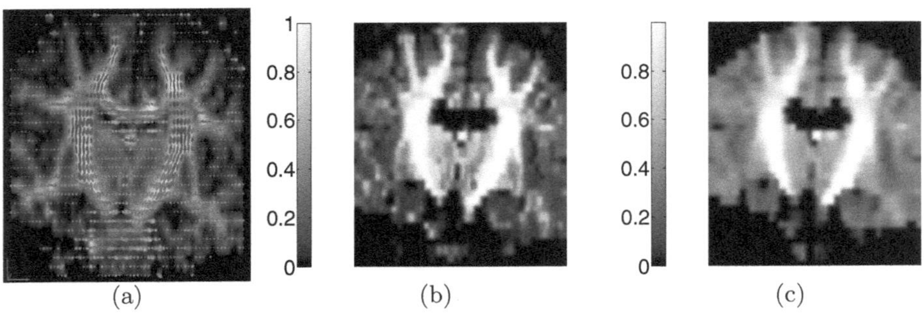

Fig. 2. (a) Real DT image (coronal slice) showing the lateral corticospinal tract. Fuzzy segmentations ($\alpha = 1, C = 2$): (b) without a Markov model and (c) with a 3×3 Markov neighborhood.

in [2]. We simulate partial voluming by spatially averaging (Gaussian smoothing) the tensors in the Riemannian space using a Log-Euclidean metric. We initialize the segmentation based on thresholding the fractional-anisotropy values and tensor orientations to approximately obtain the tract of interest. Figure 1(a) shows a DT image with 2 classes with partial voluming and noise. The one on the right (left) has anisotropic (isotropic) tensors. Figure 1(b) gives the fuzzy membership values (no Markov model used) for the anisotropic-tensor class that indicates uncertainties in the segmentation near the interface and in excessively noisy regions. Figure 1(c) plots the estimated membership function for one scanline of the noisy image and compares it with the actual membership function obtained from the noiseless image—the latter shows the amount of averaging.

Figure 2 gives fuzzy segmentations (2 class) on one slice of real DT image that shows the lateral corticospinal tract. It shows the effects of partial voluming,

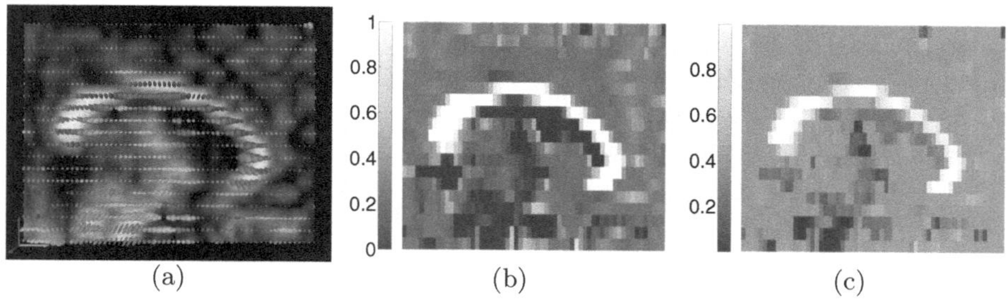

Fig. 3. (a) Real DT image (sagittal slice) showing the corpus callosum. Fuzzy-segmentations ($C = 2$, no Markov model) with a degree of fuzziness of: (b) $\alpha = 1$, and (c) $\alpha = 2$ (more fuzzy).

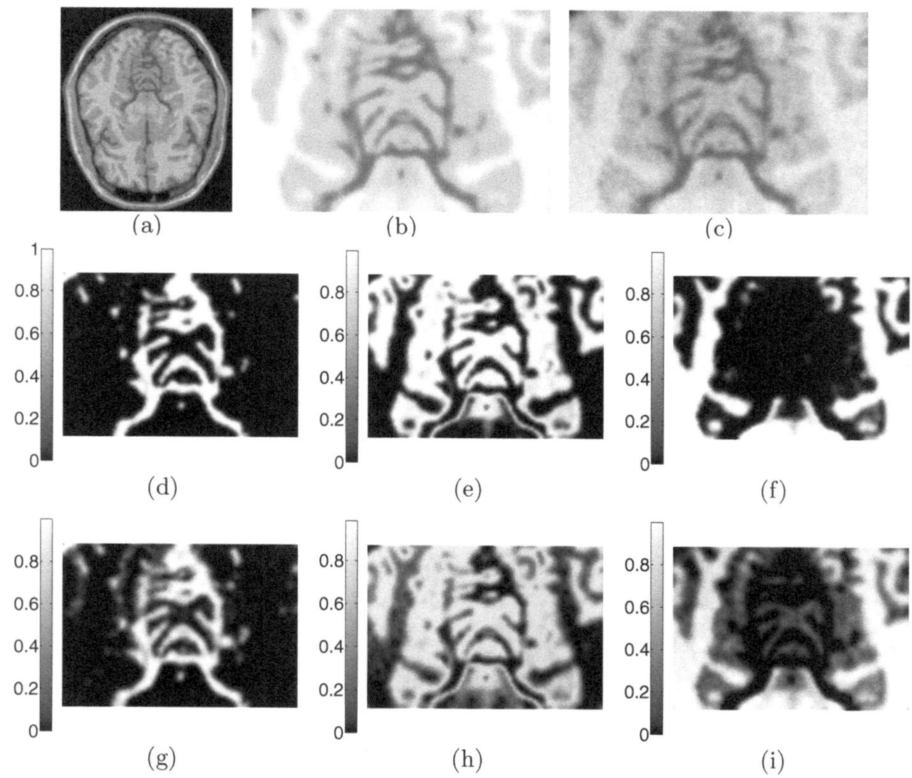

Fig. 4. (a) Uncorrupted simulated BrainWeb [23] T1-weighted MR image, (b) its zoomed inset, and (c) its corrupted version with 5% noise and a 40% inhomogeneity field. Note: intensities in each image have been scaled to use the entire grayscale range in order to provide maximum contrast. Fuzzy-segmentations ($C = 3$) with a 3×3 Markov neighborhood and $\alpha = 1$ for: (d) cerebrospinal fluid (CSF), (e) gray matter (GM), and (f) white matter (WM). Fuzzy-segmentations ($C = 3$) with a 3×3 Markov neighborhood and $\alpha = 3$ for: (g) CSF, (h) GM, and (i) WM.

especially as the tracts reach closer to the cortex. This is where the fibers from this tract come close to those emerging from the corpus callosum. Figure 2(c) demonstrates the regularizing effect of Markov statistical modeling on the tensor image relative to the result in Figure 2(b). Figure 3 gives the results for a sagittal view of the corpus callosum. It demonstrates the effect of varying the parameter α that controls the degree of fuzziness in the segmentation (Section 4.2).

Figure 4 gives results on T1-weighted simulated BrainWeb [23] MR image (5% noise and 40% inhomogeneity field) that employ 3×3 Markov neighborhoods with two different degrees of fuzziness: $\alpha = 1$ and $\alpha = 3$. The figures clearly indicate the partial voluming at the interfaces of tissue classes, especially those of the cerebrospinal fluid. The nonparametric scheme does well in spite of the significant inhomogeneity field present in the image.

To summarize, the paper presents a statistical framework for fuzzy segmentation using nonparametric PDF models. Such models capture the manifold(s) underlying the classes as well as the variability of the data around the manifold(s). The paper generalizes the FCM framework by replacing the classic ellipsoidal models/clusters for classes by generic manifold-based models and computing an optimal segmentation by maximizing a information-theoretic energy in a Markov-random-field framework. Furthermore, the proposed fuzzy-classification framework extends in a straightforward manner to multimodal MR images and data from Q-ball imaging. Future work includes application of the proposed method for tract extraction in DT images and validation for MR images.

Acknowledgments

This work was supported by the NIH under grants HD042974, HD046159, NS045839, and EB06266. Thanks to Hui Zhang for providing the DT-visualization software.

References

1. Lenglet, C., Rousson, M., Deriche, R., Faugeras, O., Lehericy, S., Ugurbil, K.: A Riemannian approach to diffusion tensor image segmentation. Proc. Info. Proc. Med. Imag, 591–602 (2005)
2. Wang, Z., Vemuri, B.: DTI segmentation using an information theoretic tensor dissimilarity measure. IEEE Trans. Med. Imag. 24(10), 1267–1277 (2005)
3. Wiegell, M., Tuch, D., Larsson, H., Wedeen, V.: Automatic segmentation of thalamic nuclei from diffusion tensor magnetic resonance imaging. Neuroimage 19(2), 391–401 (2003)
4. Zhang, J., van Zijl, P., Mori, S.: Three-dimensional diffusion tensor magnetic resonance microimaging of adult mouse brain and hippocampus. Neuroimage 15(4), 892–901 (2002)
5. Kinoshita, M., Yamada, K., Hashimoto, N., Kato, A., Izumoto, S., Baba, T., Maruno, M., Nishimura, T., Yoshimine, T.: Fiber tracking does not accurately estimate size of fiber bundles in pathological conditions: initial neurosurgical experience using neuronavigation and subcortical white matter stimulation. NeuroImage 25(2), 424–429 (2005)

6. Pham, D., Prince, J.: An adaptive fuzzy segmentation algorithm for three-dimensional magnetic resonance images. In: Proc. Info. Proc. Med. Imag, pp. 140–153 (1999)
7. Ziyan, U., Tuch, D., Westin, C.F.: Segmentation of thalamic nuclei from DTI using spectral clustering. In: Proc. Med. Image Comput. and Comp. Assisted Intervention, 807–814 (2006)
8. Kim, J., Fisher, J.W., Yezzi, A.J., Cetin, M., Willsky, A.S.: A nonparametric statistical method for image segmentation using information theory and curve evolution. IEEE Trans. Image Processing 14(10), 1486–1502 (2005)
9. Awate, S.P., Tasdizen, T., Foster, N.L., Whitaker, R.T.: Adaptive, nonparametric markov modeling for unsupervised, MRI brain-tissue classification. Medical Image Analysis 10(5), 726–739 (2006)
10. Wand, M., Jones, M.: Kernel Smoothing. Chapman and Hall (1995)
11. Pelletier, B.: Kernel density estimation on Riemannian manifolds. Stat. and Prob. Letters 73, 297–304 (2005)
12. Arsigny, V., Fillard, P., Pennec, X., Ayache, N.: Geometric means in a novel vector space structure on symmetric positive-definite matrices. SIAM J. Matrix Analysis and Applications (In press) (2006)
13. Bezdek, J.: Pattern Recognition with Fuzzy Objective Function Algorithms. Kluwer Academic Publishers, Dordrecht (1981)
14. Zhukov, L., Museth, K., Breen, D., Whitaker, R., Barr, A.: Level set modeling and segmentation of DT-MRI brain data. J. Electronic Imaging 12(1), 125–133 (2003)
15. Rousson, M., Lenglet, C., Deriche, R.: Level set and region based surface propagation for diffusion tensor MRI segmentation. In: ECCV Workshops CVAMIA and MMBIA, pp. 123–134 (2004)
16. Fletcher, P.T., Joshi, S.C.: Principal geodesic analysis on symmetric spaces: Statistics of diffusion tensors. In: ECCV Workshops CVAMIA and MMBIA, pp. 87–98 (2004)
17. Pennec, X., Fillard, P., Ayache, N.: A Riemannian framework for tensor computing. Int. J. Comput. Vision 66(1), 41–66 (2006)
18. Zhuang, X., Huang, Y., Palaniappan, K., Zhao, Y.: Gaussian mixture density modeling, decomposition, and applications. IEEE Trans. Image Proc. 5(9), 1293–1302 (1996)
19. Wells, W.M., Grimson, W.E.L., Kikinis, R., Jolesz, F.A.: Adaptive segmentation of MRI data. IEEE Tr. Med. Imaging 15(4), 429–443 (1996)
20. O'Donnell, L., Grimson, E., Westin, C.F.: Interface detection in diffusion tensor MRI. In: Proc. Med. Imag. Comput. Comp. Assist. Inter, 360–367 (2004)
21. Boothby, W.: An Introduction to Differentiable Manifolds and Riemannian Geometry. Academic Press, London (2002)
22. Chow, Y., Geman, S., Wu, L.: Consistant cross-validated density estimation. Annals of Statistics 11(1), 25–38 (1983)
23. Collins, D.L., Zijdenbos, A.P., Kollokian, V., Sled, J.G., Kabani, N.J., Holmes, C.J., Evans, A.C.: Design and construction of a realistic digital brain phantom. IEEE Trans. Med. Imag. 17(3), 463–468 (1998)

Symmetric Positive 4th Order Tensors & Their Estimation from Diffusion Weighted MRI*

Angelos Barmpoutis[1], Bing Jian[1], Baba C. Vemuri[1], and Timothy M. Shepherd[2]

[1] Computer and Information Science and Engineering, University of Florida, Gainesville FL 32611, USA,
{abarmpou, bjian, vemuri}@cise.ufl.edu
[2] Department of Neuroscience, University of Florida, Gainesville FL 32611, USA,
tms@mbi.ufl.edu

Abstract. In Diffusion Weighted Magnetic Resonance Image (DW-MRI) processing a 2nd order tensor has been commonly used to approximate the diffusivity function at each lattice point of the DW-MRI data. It is now well known that this 2nd-order approximation fails to approximate complex local tissue structures, such as fibers crossings. In this paper we employ a 4th order symmetric positive semi-definite (PSD) tensor approximation to represent the diffusivity function and present a novel technique to estimate these tensors from the DW-MRI data guaranteeing the PSD property. There have been several published articles in literature on higher order tensor approximations of the diffusivity function but none of them guarantee the positive semi-definite constraint, which is a fundamental constraint since negative values of the diffusivity coefficients are not meaningful. In our methods, we parameterize the 4th order tensors as a sum of squares of quadratic forms by using the so called Gram matrix method from linear algebra and its relation to the Hilbert's theorem on ternary quartics. This parametric representation is then used in a nonlinear-least squares formulation to estimate the PSD tensors of order 4 from the data. We define a metric for the higher-order tensors and employ it for regularization across the lattice. Finally, performance of this model is depicted on synthetic data as well as real DW-MRI from an isolated rat hippocampus.

1 Introduction

Data processing and analysis of matrix-valued image data is becoming quite common as imaging sensor technology advances allow for the collection of matrix-valued data sets. In medical imaging, during the last decade, it has become possible to collect magnetic resonance image (MRI) data that measures the apparent diffusivity of water in tissue *in vivo*. A 2nd order tensor has commonly

* This research was in part funded by the NIH grants NS42075 & EB007082 to BCV, and in part by the University of Florida Alumni Fellowship to AB.

N. Karssemeijer and B. Lelieveldt (Eds.): IPMI 2007, LNCS 4584, pp. 308–319, 2007.
© Springer-Verlag Berlin Heidelberg 2007

been used to approximate the diffusivity profile at each image lattice point in a DW-MRI [3]. The approximated diffusivity function is given by

$$d(\mathbf{g}) = \mathbf{g}^T \mathbf{D} \mathbf{g} \tag{1}$$

where $\mathbf{g} = [g_1 \; g_2 \; g_3]^T$ is the magnetic field gradient direction and $\mathbf{D}$ is the estimated 2nd-order tensor. This approximation yields a diffusion tensor (DT-MRI) data set $\mathbf{D}_i$, which is a 3D matrix-valued image, where subscript i denotes location on a 3D lattice. These tensors $\mathbf{D}_i$ are elements of the space of 3×3 symmetric positive-definite matrices. Mathematically, these tensors belong to a Riemannian symmetric space, where a Riemannian metric assigns an inner product to each point of this space. Using this metric, one can perform various computations, e.g. interpolation, geodesics, geodesic PCA [2,7,12].

Use of higher order tensors was proposed in [9] to represent more complex diffusivity profiles which better approximate the diffusivity of the local tissue geometry. *To date however, none of the methods reported in literature for the estimation of the coefficients of higher order tensors preserve the positive definiteness of the diffusivity function.*

The use of a 4th-order covariance tensor was proposed by Basser and Pajevic in [4]. This covariance tensor is employed in defining a Normal distribution of 2nd order diffusion tensors. This distribution function has been employed in [5] for higher-order multivariate statistical analysis of DT-MRI datasets using spectral decomposition of the 4th-order covariance matrix into eigenvalues and eigentensors (2nd order). However, 2nd order tensors are used to approximate the diffusivity of each lattice point of a MR dataset, failing to approximate complex local tissue structures, such as fiber crossings.

In this paper we approximate the diffusivity profile using 4th-order tensors. We propose a novel parametrization of these positive-definite higher order tensors as a sum of squares of quadratic (2nd-order) forms. This parametrization is enforced by employing the Gram matrix method in conjunction with the Hilbert's theorem on ternary quartics [8]. We present an efficient algorithm which estimates 4th-order symmetric positive semi-definite diffusion tensors from diffusion weighted MR images. We also propose a distance measure for the space of higher-order tensors that can be computed in closed form, and employ it to regularize the estimated data across the lattice. Finally, we present experimental results using real diffusion-weighted MR data from an isolated rat hippocampus. The motivation for processing and analyzing the hippocampus lies in its important role in semantic and episodic formation, which is particularly vulnerable to acute or chronic injury [1,16]. Based on knowledge of hippocampal anatomy, complex local tissue structures such as fiber crossings are commonly present at the anatomical regions of stratum lacunosum-moleculare, hilus, molecular layer (see fig. 3(d) region 4) and stratum lucidum (fig. 3(d) region 5). The techniques being developed here can approximate accurately such crossings and complex fiber structures and thus could prove useful in improving the sensitivity and specificity of diffusion MRI for detecting and monitoring hippocampal diseases.

The rest of the paper is organized as follows: In section 2, we present a novel parametrization of the 4th-order tensors that is used to enforce the positivity semi-definiteness of the estimated tensors. In section 2.1, we present a method to estimate 4th-order tensors from diffusion-weighted MR images. Furthermore, in section 2.2 we propose a distance measure for the space of 4th-order tensors, and we employ it for regularization of the estimated tensor field. Section 3 contains the experimental results and comparisons with other methods using simulated diffusion MRI data and real MR data from an isolated rat hippocampus. In section 4 we conclude.

2 Diffusion Tensors of 4th Order

The diffusivity function can be modeled by Eq. (1) using a 2nd-order tensor. Studies have shown that this approximation fails to model complex local structures of the diffusivity in real tissues [10] and a higher-order approximation must be employed instead. A 4th-order tensor can be employed in the following diffusivity function

$$d(\mathbf{g}) = \sum_{i+j+k=4} D_{i,j,k} g_1^i g_2^j g_3^k \tag{2}$$

where $\mathbf{g} = [g_1\ g_2\ g_3]^T$ is the magnetic field gradient direction. It should be noted that in the case of 4th-order symmetric tensors there are 15 unique coefficients $D_{i,j,k}$, while in the case of 2nd-order tensors we only have 6.

In DW-MRI the diffusivity of the water is a positive quantity. This property is essential since negative diffusion coefficients are nonphysical. However there is no guarantee that the estimated coefficients $D_{i,j,k}$ by the above process, will form a positive semi-definite tensor. Therefore, we need to develop a new parametrization of the 4th-order tensor, which enforces the positive semi-definite property of the estimated tensor.

Regarding g_i in (2) as variables, the equivalence between symmetric tensors and homogeneous polynomials is straightforward. Moreover if a symmetric tensor is PSD, then its corresponding polynomial must be nonnegative for all real-valued variables. Hence here we are concerned with the positive definiteness of homogenous polynomials of degree 4 in 3 variables, or the so called *ternary quartics.* In this work we propose a novel parametrization of the symmetric 4th-order PSD tensors, using the Hilbert's theorem on positive ternary quartics, was first proved by Hilbert in 1888 (see [14] for modern exposition):

Theorem 1. *Every positive real ternary quartic is a sum of three squares of quadratic forms.*

Assuming the most general case, a PSD ternary quartic can be expressed as a sum of N squares of quadratic forms as.

$$d(\mathbf{g}) = (\mathbf{v}^T\mathbf{q}_1)^2 + ... + (\mathbf{v}^T\mathbf{q}_N)^2 = \mathbf{v}^T\mathbf{Q}\mathbf{Q}^T\mathbf{v} = \mathbf{v}^T\mathbf{G}\mathbf{v} \tag{3}$$

where $\mathbf{v}$ is a properly chosen vector of monomials, (e.g. $[g_1^2\ g_2^2\ g_3^2\ g_1g_2\ g_1g_3\ g_2g_3]^T$), $\mathbf{Q} = [\mathbf{q}_1|...|\mathbf{q}_N]$ is a $6 \times N$ matrix by stacking the 6 coefficient vectors $\mathbf{q}_i$ and $\mathbf{G} = \mathbf{Q}\mathbf{Q}^T$ is the so called *Gram matrix.*

Using this Gram matrix $\mathbf{G}$ expression, Eq. (2) can be written as $d(\mathbf{g}) = \mathbf{v}^T\mathbf{G}\mathbf{v}$, and the correspondence between the 4th-order tensor coefficients $D_{i,j,k}$ of Eq. (2) and the Gram matrix $\mathbf{G}$ can be established as follows:

$$\mathbf{G} = \begin{pmatrix} D_{4,0,0} & a & b & \frac{1}{2}D_{3,1,0} & \frac{1}{2}D_{3,0,1} & d \\ a & D_{0,4,0} & c & \frac{1}{2}D_{1,3,0} & e & \frac{1}{2}D_{0,3,1} \\ b & c & D_{0,0,4} & f & \frac{1}{2}D_{1,0,3} & \frac{1}{2}D_{0,1,3} \\ \frac{1}{2}D_{3,1,0} & \frac{1}{2}D_{1,3,0} & f & D_{2,2,0}-2a & \frac{1}{2}D_{2,1,1}-d & \frac{1}{2}D_{1,2,1}-e \\ \frac{1}{2}D_{3,0,1} & e & \frac{1}{2}D_{1,0,3} & \frac{1}{2}D_{2,1,1}-d & D_{2,0,2}-2b & \frac{1}{2}D_{1,1,2}-f \\ d & \frac{1}{2}D_{0,3,1} & \frac{1}{2}D_{0,1,3} & \frac{1}{2}D_{1,2,1}-e & \frac{1}{2}D_{1,1,2}-f & D_{0,2,2}-2c \end{pmatrix} \quad (4)$$

where a, b, c, d, e, f are free parameters, i.e for any choice of those parameters the obtained Gram matrix represents the same 4th-order tensor [13]. According to Theorem 1, if $N = 3$ (i.e. Gram matrix $\mathbf{G}$ has rank 3) then the whole space of PSD ternary quartics is spanned. For some specific choices of the parameters a, b, c, d, e, f of Eq. (4), the rank of matrix $\mathbf{G}$ becomes 3 [13]. Powers and Reznick in [13] worked on finding fundamentally different choices of those parameters that yield the same given PSD ternary quartic, i.e. in how many different ways can a ternary quartic be expressed as a sum of squares of three quadratic forms. However, given a Gram matrix $\mathbf{G}$ we can uniquely compute the coefficients $D_{i,j,k}$ of the tensor (see Eq. (4)). Therefore, we can employ the Gram matrix method for the estimation of the coefficients $D_{i,j,k}$ of the diffusion tensor from MR images using the following two steps: 1) first we estimate a Gram matrix $\mathbf{G}$ from the MR signal of the given images, and then 2) we uniquely compute the coefficients $D_{i,j,k}$ of the 4th-order tensor by using formulas obtained from Eq. (4). Note that although the estimated matrix $\mathbf{G}$ is not unique, the coefficients $D_{i,j,k}$ are uniquely determined.

In the following section we will employ this Gram matrix method to enforce the positive semi-definite property of the estimated diffusion tensors from the diffusion weighted MR images.

2.1 Estimation from DWI

The coefficients $D_{i,j,k}$ of a 4th order diffusion tensor can be estimated from diffusion-weighted MR images by minimizing the following cost function:

$$E(\mathbf{Q}, S_0) = \sum_{i=1}^{M}(S_i - S_0 e^{-b_i \mathbf{v}_i^T \mathbf{Q}\mathbf{Q}^T \mathbf{v}_i})^2 \quad (5)$$

where M is the number of the diffusion weighted images associated with gradient vectors $\mathbf{g}_i$ and b-values b_i; S_i is the corresponding acquired signal and S_0 is the zero gradient signal. Using the magnetic field gradient directions $\mathbf{g}_i$ we construct the 6-dimensional vectors $\mathbf{v}_i = [g_{i1}^2\ g_{i2}^2\ g_{i3}^2\ g_{i1}g_{i2}\ g_{i1}g_{i3}\ g_{i2}g_{i3}]^T$. In Eq. (5), the 4th order diffusion tensor is parameterized using the Gram matrix $\mathbf{G} = \mathbf{Q}\mathbf{Q}^T$, where $\mathbf{Q}$ is a $6 \times N$ matrix and $N \geq 3$ is a predefined constant. In our experiments we used $N = 3$, which is justified by Theorem 1. Having estimated the matrix

$\mathbf{Q}$ that minimizes Eq. (5), the coefficients $D_{i,j,k}$ can be computed directly from the Gram matrix using the relation described by the matrix of Eq. (4). S_0 can either be assumed to be known or estimated simultaneously with the coefficients $D_{i,j,k}$ by minimizing Eq. (5).

Starting with an initial guess for S_0 and $\mathbf{Q}$, we can use any optimization method in order to minimize Eq. (5). For the optimization schemes that employ the gradients of Eq. (5) with respect to the unknown coefficients of $\mathbf{Q}$, the gradient is given by the following equation

$$\nabla_{\mathbf{Q}} E(\mathbf{Q}, S_0) = 4 \sum_{i=1}^{M} b_i S_0 e^{-b_i \mathbf{v}_i^T \mathbf{Q}\mathbf{Q}^T \mathbf{v}_i} (S_i - S_0 e^{-b_i \mathbf{v}_i^T \mathbf{Q}\mathbf{Q}^T \mathbf{v}_i}) \mathbf{v}_i^T \mathbf{v}_i \mathbf{Q} \quad (6)$$

Now given $\mathbf{Q}$ at each iteration of the optimization algorithm we can update S_0 by again minimizing Eq. (5). The derivative of this equation with respect to the unknown S_0 is

$$\nabla_{S_0} E(\mathbf{Q}, S_0) = -2 \sum_{i=1}^{M} (S_i - S_0 e^{-b_i \mathbf{v}_i^T \mathbf{Q}\mathbf{Q}^T \mathbf{v}_i}) e^{-b_i \mathbf{v}_i^T \mathbf{Q}\mathbf{Q}^T \mathbf{v}_i} \quad (7)$$

By setting Eq. (7) equal to zero, we derive the following update formula for S_0

$$S_0 = \sum_{i=1}^{M} S_i e^{-b_i \mathbf{v}_i^T \mathbf{Q}\mathbf{Q}^T \mathbf{v}_i} / \sum_{i=1}^{M} e^{-2b_i \mathbf{v}_i^T \mathbf{Q}\mathbf{Q}^T \mathbf{v}_i} \quad (8)$$

In our experiments we used the well known Lavenberg-Marquardt (LM) nonlinear least-squares method, which has advantages over other optimization methods, in terms of stability and computational burden.

As pointed out earlier, although the coefficients $D_{i,j,k}$ are uniquely estimated, the Gram matrix parametrization $\mathbf{G} = \mathbf{Q}\mathbf{Q}^T$ is not unique, i.e. there exist different matrices $\mathbf{Q}$ which parameterize the same Gram matrix. For example there are infinitely many matrices $\mathbf{Q}$ that yield the same $\mathbf{G}$, due to the orthogonality property ($\mathbf{R}\mathbf{R}^T = \mathbf{I}$) of the rotation matrices $\mathbf{R}$, where $\mathbf{I}$ is the identity matrix. Thus, in the case that $\mathbf{Q}$ is of size 6×3, for any 3×3 orthogonal matrix $\mathbf{R}$ we have $(\mathbf{QR})(\mathbf{QR})^T = \mathbf{Q}\mathbf{Q}^T$. In order to reduce this infinite solution space to a finite set of solutions, which theoretically can be handled by the optimization techniques, we use the well known QR decomposition of real square matrices to uniquely decompose any given 6×3 matrix $\mathbf{Q}$ in the form $\mathbf{Q} = \begin{bmatrix} \mathbf{TR} \\ \mathbf{A} \end{bmatrix}$, where all matrices are of size 3×3 and specifically $\mathbf{T}$ is lower triangular, and $\mathbf{R}$ is an orthogonal matrix. Then by setting $\mathbf{R} = \mathbf{I}$ we reformulate $\mathbf{Q}$ as $\mathbf{Q} = \begin{bmatrix} \mathbf{T} \\ \mathbf{A} \end{bmatrix}$ and thus the infinitely non-unique issue is replaced by a countably non-uniqueness issue, which can be handled by the optimization algorithm. Note that using this formulation there are only 15 unknown parameters in matrix $\mathbf{Q}$, which is equal to the number of the unknown coefficients $D_{i,j,k}$ of the estimated tensor.

2.2 Distance Measure

In the previous section we discussed about estimating PSD 4th-order tensors from DW-MRI data. After having estimated the tensor coefficients $D_{i,j,k}$, we can perform tensor regularization across the lattice. The regularization can be performed by a functional minimization method using the following regularization term

$$\sum_j \sum_{i \in \eta_j} dist(\mathbf{D}_j, \mathbf{D}_i)^2 \tag{9}$$

where η_j is the set of lattice indices whose distance from lattice index 'j' is 1. In the regularization term defined in Eq. (9) we need to employ an appropriate distance measure between the tensors $\mathbf{D}_i$ and $\mathbf{D}_j$. Here we use the notation $\mathbf{D}$ in order to denote the set of 15 unique coefficients $D_{i,j,k}$ of a 4th-order tensor.

We can define a distance measure between the 4th-order diffusion tensors $\mathbf{D}_1$ and $\mathbf{D}_2$ by computing the normalized L_2 distance between the corresponding diffusivity functions $d_1(\mathbf{g})$ and $d_2(\mathbf{g})$ leading to the equation,

$$dist(\mathbf{D}_1, \mathbf{D}_2)^2 = \frac{1}{4\pi} \int_{S^2} [d_1(\mathbf{g}) - d_2(\mathbf{g})]^2 d\mathbf{g} \tag{10}$$

$$\begin{aligned}
= \frac{1}{315}[(&\Delta_{4,0,0} + \Delta_{0,4,0} + \Delta_{0,0,4} + \Delta_{2,2,0} + \Delta_{0,2,2} + \Delta_{2,0,2})^2 + \\
&4[(\Delta_{4,0,0} + \Delta_{2,2,0})^2 + (\Delta_{4,0,0} + \Delta_{2,0,2})^2 + (\Delta_{0,4,0} + \Delta_{2,2,0})^2 + \\
&(\Delta_{0,4,0} + \Delta_{0,2,2})^2 + (\Delta_{0,0,4} + \Delta_{0,2,2})^2 + (\Delta_{0,0,4} + \Delta_{2,0,2})^2] + \\
&23(\Delta_{4,0,0}^2 + \Delta_{0,4,0}^2 + \Delta_{0,0,4}^2) - 6(\Delta_{2,2,0}^2 + \Delta_{0,2,2}^2 + \Delta_{2,0,2}^2) + \\
&2(\Delta_{4,0,0} + \Delta_{0,4,0} + \Delta_{0,0,4})^2 + (\Delta_{2,1,1} + \Delta_{0,3,1} + \Delta_{0,1,3})^2 + \\
&(\Delta_{1,2,1} + \Delta_{3,0,1} + \Delta_{1,0,3})^2 + (\Delta_{1,1,2} + \Delta_{3,1,0} + \Delta_{1,3,0})^2 + \\
&2\left[(\Delta_{3,1,0} + \Delta_{1,3,0})^2 + (\Delta_{3,0,1} + \Delta_{1,0,3})^2 + (\Delta_{0,3,1} + \Delta_{0,1,3})^2\right] + \\
&2(\Delta_{3,1,0}^2 + \Delta_{3,0,1}^2 + \Delta_{1,3,0}^2 + \Delta_{0,3,1}^2 + \Delta_{1,0,3}^2 + \Delta_{0,1,3}^2)]
\end{aligned}$$

where, the integral of Eq. (10) is over all unit vectors $\mathbf{g}$, i.e., the unit sphere S^2 and the coefficients $\Delta_{i,j,k}$ are computed by subtracting the coefficients of the tensor $\mathbf{D}_1$ from the corresponding coefficients of the tensor $\mathbf{D}_2$.

As shown above, the integral of Eq. (10) can be computed analytically and the result can be expressed as a sum of squares of the terms $\Delta_{i,j,k}$. In this simple form, this distance measure between 4th-order tensors can be implemented very efficiently. Note that this distance measure is invariant to rotations in 3-dimensional space since it was defined as an integral over all directions $\mathbf{g}$.

Another property of the above distance measure is that the average element (mean tensor) $\hat{\mathbf{D}}$ of a set of N tensors $\mathbf{D}_i$, $i = 1 \ldots N$ is defined as the Euclidean average of the corresponding coefficients of the tensors. This property can be proved by verifying that $\hat{\mathbf{D}}$ minimizes the sum of squares of distances $\sum dist(\mathbf{D}, \mathbf{D}_i)^2$. Similarly, it can be shown that geodesics (shortest paths) between 4th-order tensors are defined as Euclidean geodesics.

3 Experimental Results

In this section we present experimental results on our method applied to simulated DW-MRI data as well as real DW-MRI data from an isolated rat hippocampus.

In order to motivate the need of the PSD constraint in the 4th-order estimation process, we performed the following experiment using a synthetic dataset. The synthetic data was generated by simulating the MR signal from a single fiber using the realistic diffusion MR simulation model in [15]. Then, we added different amounts of Riccian noise to the simulated dataset and we estimated the 4th-order tensors from the noisy data by: a) minimizing $\sum_{i=1}^{M}(S_i - S_0 exp(-b_i d(\mathbf{g}_i)))^2$ without using the proposed parametrization to enforce PSD constraint, by employing the method in [11] and b) our method, which guarantees the PSD property of the tensors. (S_i is the MR signal of the ith image and S_0 is the zero-gradient signal).

It is known that the estimated 4th-order tensors represent more complex diffusivity profiles with multiple fiber orientations which better approximate the diffusivity of the local tissue geometry compared to the traditional 2nd-order tensors [9]. Studies on estimating fiber orientations from the diffusivity profile have shown that the peaks of the diffusivity profile do not necessarily yield the orientations of the distinct fiber bundles [10]. One should instead employ the displacement probability profiles . The displacement probability $P(\mathbf{R})$ is given by the Fourier integral $P(\mathbf{R}) = \int E(\mathbf{q})exp(-2\pi i\mathbf{q}\cdot\mathbf{R})d\mathbf{q}$ where $\mathbf{q}$ is the reciprocal space vector, $E(\mathbf{q})$ is the signal value associated with vector $\mathbf{q}$ divided by the zero gradient signal and $\mathbf{R}$ is the displacement vector. In our experiments, we numerically estimated the displacement probability profiles from the 4th-order tensors.

Then, we computed the displacement probability profiles of the 4th-order tensors estimated earlier with the two different methods, and we computed the fiber orientations from the maxima of the probability profiles. The error angles (mean

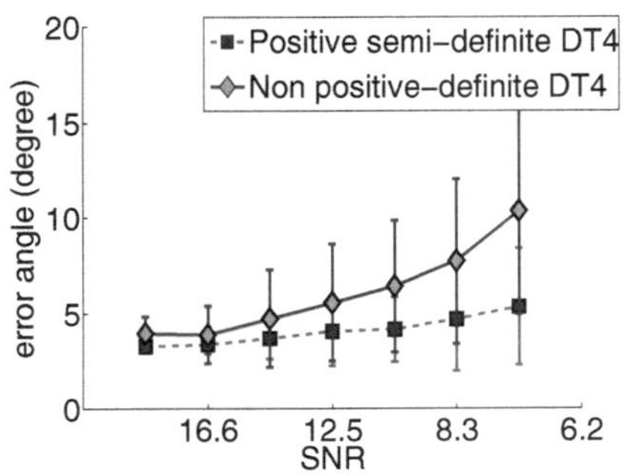

Fig. 1. Comparison of the fiber orientation errors for different amount of noise in the data, obtained by using: a) our parametrization to enforce positivity and b) without enforcing positivity of the estimated tensors

and standard deviation) of the two methods for different amount of noise in the data are plotted in Fig. 1. As expected, our method yields smaller errors in comparison with the method that does not enforces the PSD property of the tensors. When we increase the amount of noise in the data, the errors observed by the later method are significantly increased, while our proposed method shows clearly much smaller errors. This conclusively demonstrates the need for enforcing the PSD property of the estimated tensors and validates the accuracy of our proposed method.

Furthermore, in order to compare our proposed method with other existing techniques that do not employ 4th-order tensors, we performed an other experiment using synthetic data. The data were generated for different amounts of noise by following the same method as previously using the simulated MR signal of a 2-fiber crossing (see Fig. 2(a)) . We estimated 4th-order tensors from the corrupted simulated MR signal using our method and then we computed the fiber orientations from the corresponding probability profiles. For comparison we also estimated the fiber orientations using the DOT method described in [10] and the ODF method presented in [6]. For all three methods we computed the estimated fiber orientation errors for different amount of noise in the data (shown in Fig. 2(b)). The results conclusively demonstrate the accuracy of our method, showing small fiber orientation errors ($\sim 6^o$) for typical amount of noise with signal to noise ratios (SNR): 12.5-16.6. Furthermore, by observing the plot, we also conclude that the accuracy of our proposed method is very close to that of the DOT method and is significantly better than the ODF method.

In the following experiments, we used MR data from an isolated rat hippocampus. The diffusion weighted MR images of this dataset were acquired using the following protocol. This protocol included acquisition of 22 images using a pulsed gradient spin echo pulse sequence with repetition time (TR) = 1.5 s, echo time

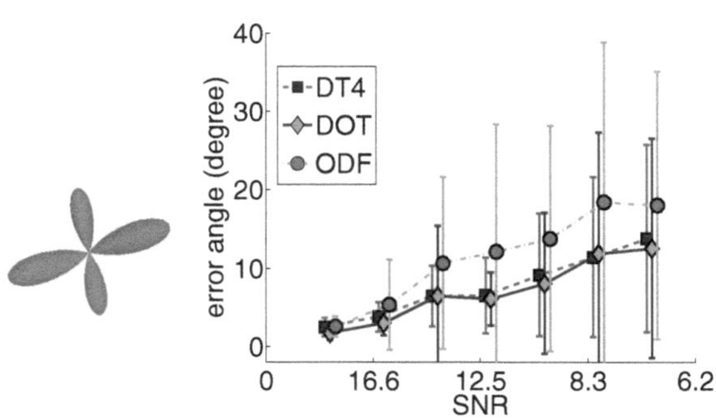

(a) (b)

Fig. 2. Fiber orientation errors for different SNR in the data using our method for the estimation of positive 4th-order tensors and two other existing methods: 1) DOT and 2) ODF. In the experiment we used simulated MR signal of a 2-fiber crossing, whose probability profile is shown in (a).

(TE) = 28.3 ms, bandwidth = 35 kHz, field-of-view (FOV) = 4.5 × 4.5 mm, matrix = 90 × 90 with 56 continuous 200-μm-thick axial slices (oriented transverse to the septo-temporal axis of the isolated hippocampus). After the first image set was collected without diffusion weighting (b $\sim$ 0 s/mm^2), 21 diffusion-weighted image sets with gradient strength (G) = 415 mT/m, gradient duration (δ) = 2.4 ms, gradient separation (Δ) = 17.8 ms and diffusion time (T_δ) = 17 ms were collected. Each of these image sets used different diffusion gradients (with approximate b values of 1250 s/mm^2) whose orientations were determined from the 2nd order tessellation of an icosahedron projected onto the surface of a unit hemisphere. The image without diffusion weighting had 36 signal averages (time = 81 min), and each diffusion-weighted image had 12 averages (time = 27 min per diffusion gradient orientation) to give a total imaging time of 10.8 h per hippocampus. Temperature was maintained at 20 ± 0.2°C throughout the experiments using the temperature control unit of the magnet previously calibrated by methanol spectroscopy. Figures 3(a) and 3(b) show the S_0 image and the FA map respectively of a slice extracted from the 3D volume of the above dataset.

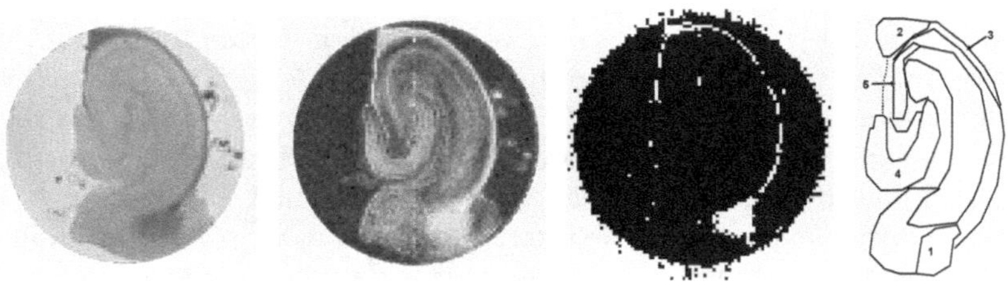

(a) (b) (c) (d)

Fig. 3. Isolated rat hipppocampus. a) S_0, b) FA, c) White pixels indicate locations where the estimated 4th-order tensor was not positive-definite, d) Manually labeled image based on knowledge of hippocampal anatomy. The index of the labels is: 1) dorsal hippocampal commissure, 2) fimbria, 3) alveus, 4) molecular layer, 5) mixture of CA3 stratum pyramidale and stratum lucidum.

First, we estimated a 4th-order diffusion tensor field from this dataset by minimizing $\sum_{i=1}^{M}(S_i - S_0 exp(-b_i d(\mathbf{g}_i)))^2$ without using the proposed parametrization to enforce positivity [11]. As expected, some of the estimated tensors were not positive. In Fig. 3(c) we show in white color the locations where those non-positive-definite tensors were estimated. These tensors are mainly located in the regions "dorsal hippocampal commissure", "fimbria" and "alevus", which correspond to the regions 1, 2 and 3 respectively, shown in Fig. 3(d). Based on knowledge of hippocampal anatomy, those regions are highly anisotropic with FA $\sim$ 0.9. Therefore, from the experimental results (Fig. 3(c)) we conclude that highly anisotropic diffusivities are most likely to be inaccurately approximated by a non-positive semi-definite tensor. Thus one needs to employ a method that guarantees the PSD property.

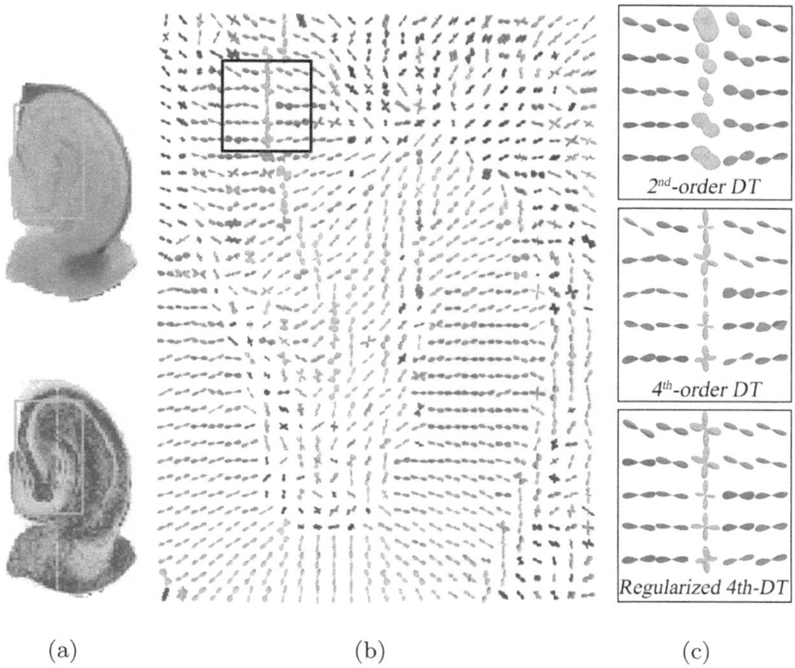

Fig. 4. The estimated 4th-order tensor field from an isolated rat hippocampus dataset using our method. (a) top:S_0 and bottom:FA, (b) the estimated displacement probability profiles of the 4th-order tensor field in the region of interest (ROI) indicated by a green rectangle in (a). (c)Comparison of the estimated 2nd-order tensors (top)and the estimated probability profiles of the 4th-order tensors without (middle) and with regularization (bottom) in a ROI indicated by a black rectangle in (b).

We computed the displacement probability profiles from: a) the 4th-order tensor field estimated previously without the positive-definite constraint, and b) the 4th-order tensor field estimated by our proposed method. In order to compare the results of the above algorithms, in Fig. 5 we plot the corresponding probability profiles from a region of interest in the "dorsal hippocampal commissure". By observing this figure, we can say that the field of probability profiles is noisy if we do not enforce the PSD constraint (Fig. 5 middle). On the other hand the profiles obtained by our method (Fig. 5 right) are more coherent and smooth. Note that this is a result of enforcing the PSD constraint, since in this experiment we did not use any regularization. This demonstrates the superior performance of our algorithm and motivates the use of the proposed PSD constraint.

Finally Fig. 4(b) shows displacement probability profiles computed from the estimated (by our method) 4th-order tensor field in another region of hippocampus. This tensor field corresponds to the region of interest denoted by a green rectangle in S_0 and FA map shown in Fig. 4a. The X, Y, Z components of the dominant orientation of each profile are assigned to R, G, B (red, green, blue)

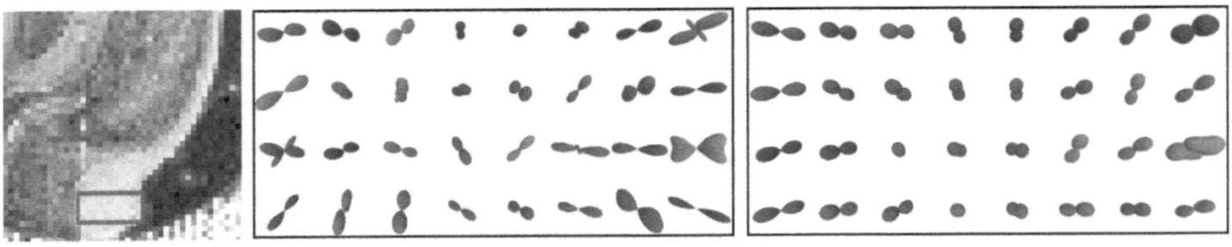

Fig. 5. Left: The region of interest from the "dorsal hippocampal commissure", which is magnified in the next plates of this figure. Comparison between the displacement probability profiles computed from non-PSD 4th-order tensors (middle) and PSD tensors estimated by our method (right).

components of the color of each surface. By observing Fig. 4(b) we can see several fiber crossings in different regions of the rat hippocampus. One of those regions is marked by a black rectangle and it is presented enlarged in Fig. 4(c). This region is consisted of a mixture of CA3 stratum pyramidale and stratum lucidum, and it is most likely to contain fiber-crossings. As expected, in the center of this region there are profiles presenting fiber crossings. These fiber crossings cannot be resolved by using 2nd-order diffusion tensors estimated from the same dataset (shown on the top of Fig. 4(c)). Finally in the bottom plate of Fig. 4(c), we show an example using the regularization term defined in section 2.2. By comparing the probability profiles shown in this image with those of the middle plate of Fig. 4(c) we can see that the regularization of the estimated data removes some of the noise in the dataset, and as a consequence some of the crossings are observed more clearly (see at the center of the image).

4 Conclusions

In diffusion weighted MR imaging 2nd-order tensors have commonly been used to approximate the diffusivity profile. 4th-order tensors were employed in this work, showing better approximation capabilities compared to the 2nd-order case. We presented a method for estimating the coefficients of 4th-order tensors from diffusion-weighted MR images. Our technique guarantees the positive semi-definite property of the estimated tensors, which is the main contribution of our work. This property is essential since non-PSD diffusivity profiles are not meaningful from the point of view of physics of diffusion. To date, there is no other reported work in literature which handles this constraint for rank-4 tensors. We applied our proposed algorithm to a real MR dataset from an isolated rat hippocampus. The superior performance of our method in the experimental results demonstrates the need for employing the constraint and motivates the use of our technique. The accuracy of our model was validated by using simulated MR data of fiber crossings, and compared to other existing methods. In our future work we plan to employ the methods proposed here to extend various techniques used for the 2nd-order tensor fields such as segmentation, registration and fiber-tracking, to the space of higher-order tensors.

References

1. Amaral, D., Witter, M.: Hippocampal formation. In The Rat Nervous System, pp. 443–493. Academic Press, San Diego (1995)
2. Barmpoutis, A., Vemuri, B.C., Forder, J.R.: Robust tensor splines for approximation of Diffusion Tensor MRI data. In: Proceedings of MMBIA06, pp. 86–86, 17-18 June 2006 (2006)
3. Basser, P.J., Mattiello, J., Lebihan, D.: Estimation of the Effective Self-Diffusion Tensor from the NMR Spin Echo. J. Magn. Reson. B 103, 247–254 (1994)
4. Basser, P.J., Pajevic, S.: A normal distribution for tensor-valued random variables: Applications to diffusion tensor MRI. IEEE Trans. on Medical Imaging 22, 785–794 (2003)
5. Basser, P.J., Pajevic, S.: Spectral decomposition of a 4th-order covariance tensor: Applications to diffusion tensor MRI. Signal Processing 87, 220–236 (2007)
6. Descoteaux, M., Angelino, E., Fitzgibbons, S., Deriche, R.: A fast and robust odf estimation algorithm in q-ball imaging. In: International Symposium on Biomedical Imaging: From Nano to Macro 2006, pp. 81–84 (2006)
7. Fletcher, P., Joshi, S.: Principal geodesic analysis on symmetric spaces: Statistics of diffusion tensors. In: Proc. of CVAMIA 2004, pp. 87–98 (2004)
8. Hilbert, D.: Über die darstellung definiter formen als summe von formenquadraten. Math. Ann. 32, 342–350 (1888)
9. Özarslan, E., Mareci, T.H.: Generalized diffusion tensor imaging and analytical relationships between diffusion tensor imaging and high angular resolution diffusion imaging. Magn. Reson. Med. 50(5), 955–965 (2003)
10. Özarslan, E., Shepherd, T.M., Vemuri, B.C., Blackband, S.J., Mareci, T.H.: Resolution of complex tissue microarchitecture using the diffusion orientation transform (DOT). NeuroImage 31, 1086–1103 (2006)
11. Özarslan, E., Vemuri, B.C., Mareci, T.: Fiber orientation mapping using generalized diffusion tensor imaging. In: ISBI, pp. 1036–1038 (2004)
12. Pennec, X., Fillard, P., Ayache, N.: A Riemannian framework for tensor computing. International Journal of Computer Vision, 65 (2005)
13. Powers, V., Reznick, B.: Notes towards a constructive proof of Hilbert's theorem on ternary quartics. In: Quadratic Forms and Their Applications (Dublin, 1999), Contemp. Math. 272, Am. Math. Soc., Providence, RI, pp. 209–227 (2000)
14. Rudin, W.: Sums of squares of polynomials. Am. Math. Monthly 107, 813–821 (2000)
15. Söderman, O., Jönsson, B.: Restricted diffusion in cylindrical geometry. J. Magn. Reson., A 117, 94–97 (1995)
16. Squire, L., Stark, C., Clark, R.: The medial temporal lobe. Annu. Rev. Neurosci. 27, 279–306 (2004)

Atlas-to-Image Non-rigid Registration by Minimization of Conditional Local Entropy

Emiliano D'Agostino, Frederik Maes, Dirk Vandermeulen, and Paul Suetens

Katholieke Universiteit Leuven, Faculties of Medicine and Engineering, Medical Imaging Center (Radiology - ESAT/PSI), University Hospital Gasthuisberg, Herestraat 49, B-3000 Leuven, Belgium
Emiliano.DAgostino@esat.kuleuven.be

Abstract. In this paper an algorithm for atlas-to-image non-rigid registration based on regional entropy minimization is presented. Tissue class probabilities in the atlas are registered with the intensities in the target image. The novel aspect of the paper consists in using tissue class probability maps that include the three main regions (for the brain, white matter, gray matter and csf) and a further partitioning thereof. For example, gray matter is further subdivided into basal ganglia (each of them defining its own class) and the rest (of gray matter). This guarantees a regional entropy minimization instead of just a global one.In other words, the local labels in the atlas will be adjusted in order to obtain the best explanation for the intensity distribution in the corresponding subregion of the target image.

1 Introduction

In medical image analysis, object segmentation is complicated by the complex nature of the 3-D image data and the ambiguity about object boundaries induced by noise, poor local contrast and all kinds of image artefacts. Traditional low-level segmentation approaches are therefore in general not sufficient and model-based approaches are required that incorporate prior knowledge of the shape and the photometric appearance of the objects in the scene. A powerful approach for model-based image segmentation is to represent such prior knowledge as an iconic template or atlas, that is matched to the image under study by a 3-D deformation field obtained by local non-rigid image registration, such that object labels annotated in the atlas are correctly projected onto the anatomically corresponding structures in the study image. Non-rigid image registration within the context of atlas-based segmentation involves the optimization of a suitable registration criterion or similarity measure of the atlas and study images, constrained by an appropriate regularization to ensure that the resulting deformation field is physically valid and well behaved depending on the application (e.g. one-to-one, locally smooth or volume preserving, elastic, viscous, ...).

A popular choice for the registration criterion is maximization of mutual information (MI) [1]. MI measures the statistical dependence between corresponding voxel intensities, which is assumed to be maximal when the images are properly

N. Karssemeijer and B. Lelieveldt (Eds.): IPMI 2007, LNCS 4584, pp. 320–332, 2007.
© Springer-Verlag Berlin Heidelberg 2007

aligned. The fact that MI is histogram-based rather than intensity-based (the co-occurrence of intensity values is evaluated, rather than differences between these values) makes the approach applicable to multimodal registration applications and more robust against intensity degradations and artifacts in case of unimodal registration. MI has been shown to yield subvoxel registration accuracy for rigid body registration of CT, MR and PET brain images [1]. Its extension to non-rigid registration is an active area of research in the field and several approaches using different schemes for histogram estimation and spatial regularization of the deformation field have been proposed [2,3,4] (just to name a few).

The use of mutual information of corresponding voxel intensities as a similarity measure for non-rigid registration in the context of atlas-based segmentation has some important drawbacks. First of all, it assumes that the atlas contains a grayscale image template whose intensities are similar (i.e. statistically related) to the intensities in the study image. This is typically obtained by intensity averaging of a training set of images of different subjects, all co-registered to the same reference space. Such a template will hence be necessarily biased by the choice of the reference space and affected by residual geometric (e.g. topological) and intensity differences between the registered images, which will induce local ambiguity in the atlas and in the atlas-to-image registration process itself. Moreover, with highly constrained rigid body or affine registration using MI, evidence about local intensity similarity is combined from all over the image domain in order to find the registration solution that can be expected to correspond to globally optimal object alignment in the images to be registered. With intensity-based non-rigid registration, however, local deformations will be optimized as to maximize local intensity similarity without guarantee that this indeed also aligns the underlying objects, as the relation between image intensities and object labels is in general not one to one.

In previous work [5], we introduced a novel information-theoretic registration criterion that matches probabilistic voxel label information in the atlas directly to the image intensities in the target image without need for an intensity-averaged atlas template. The algorithm minimizes the class conditional image intensity entropy, i.e. the uncertainty about a voxel's intensity in the study image given its object class derived from the atlas, weighted over all classes. This is akin to deforming the atlas to match the study image in such a way that the intensity variance within each class is minimized, however without assuming that the intensity within each class is normally distributed. The algorithm was applied and evaluated in the context of atlas-based MR brain image registration and segmentation, using 4 different atlas classes, namely white matter (WM), gray matter (GM), cerebrospinal fluid (CSF) and other (OTHER), and a viscous fluid deformation model for regularization, allowing for large deformations that are assured to be one to one everywhere [5].

The WM, GM, CSF and OTHER classes relate to a limited number of objects that are fairly globally distributed over the entire registration domain (in casu the brain). Hence, intensity information from all over the image domain pertaining to a single class is combined in a single distribution, which is assumed to be spatially stationary. However, the presence of spatial intensity inhomogeneity in the image data is not unlikely in case of MR data, which introduces artificial uncertainty that is not related to the quality of the non-rigid registration, but to the fact that a single global similarity measure is used where in fact a more local similarity measure may be more appropriate. Also, when the atlas-based segmentation is intended to target subcortical structures such as the basal ganglia, ventricles or corpus callosum, it makes sense to include these objects specifically in the registration process, rather than only the global tissue classes (GM, CSF and WM respectively) which they belong to.

In this work, we extend the approach of [5] to include more extensive voxel label information consisting of a probabilistic atlas with prior spatial distributions of global tissue classes L_1 (WM, GM, CSF, OTHER) and of different local subregions L_2 (basal ganglia, corpus callosum, brain stem, ...). Atlases L_1 and L_2 are co-registered with each other by construction, but are otherwise independent. In our case, atlas L_1 was obtained by inter-subject averaging of the WM, GM, CSF and OTHER segmentation maps of a training set of MR brain images obtained by automated model-based pixel classification using the algorithm of [6], while atlas L_2 was obtained by applying the same averaging process on manual expert delineations of subcortical structures in these same images, as described in [7]. Hence, each tissue L_1 is divided in anatomical subregions L_2. Likewise, each anatomical region L_2 may consist of different tissue classes L_1. Our method assume that the image intensities in the study image should have minimal entropy (i.e. be maximally clustered) within each subregion $r \in L_1 \times L_2$.

Encoding the labels L_1 and L_2 on a same axis (therefore in a 2D histogram), would first require a remapping of all labels onto L_k, where k represents the combination of all possible regions i, in labels L_1 and j in labels L_2. However this wouldn't imply any computational simplification and would furthermore yield a less easy generalizable model when dealing with more than 2 label sets.

2 Material and Methods

2.1 Joint Histogram Definition

In a previous work [5], we introduced a registration algorithm where probabilistic atlas labels, for white matter, gray matter and csf, where registered with intensities in a target image. The joint histogram defined there, was characterized by a number of columns equal to number of intensity bins used to represent the histogram of the target image and a number of rows corresponding to the number of prior classes coming with atlas (four classes: white and gray matter, csf and the rest class).In this work, we extend such approach by using ulterior atlas knowledge. In fact, we have at our disposal not only prior distributions for the main brain regions (already mentioned) but also for different subregions. This gives us the possibility to further partition each main region into different relevant structures. For example, the gray matter prior is subdivided into basal ganglia and cortex.

This new prior information is used to build a 3D joint histogram h, where the third dimension has a number of entries equal to the total number of subregions used. In our experiments we had 25 different subregions, including nucleus caudate (left and right), hippocampus (left and right), ventricles (different horns, left and right) and corpus callosum, just to name a few. These regions were selected because of their particular clinical interest. Figure 1 shows a schematic representation of the histogram.

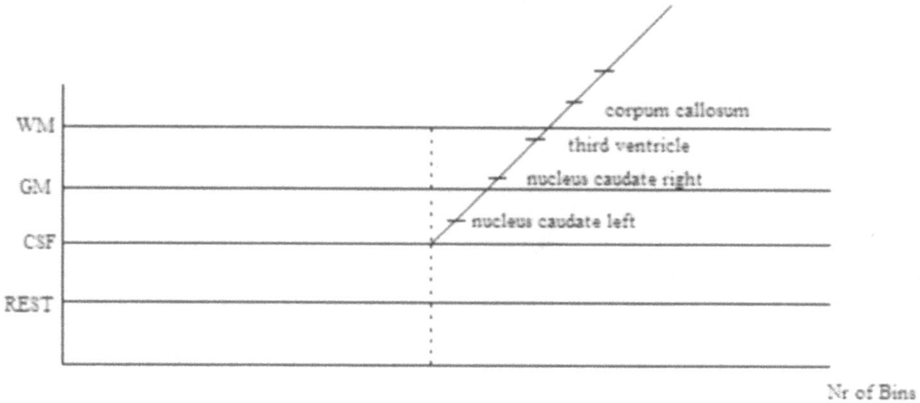

Fig. 1. Sketch of the 3D joint histogram

The joint histogram h has the following expression:

$$h(r, l_1, l_2) = \sum_{i=1}^{N} \sum_{n=1}^{8} w_{i,j_n(i)} . \delta(r - r_i) . c_{j_n(i),l_1} . c_{j_n(i),l_2} \tag{1}$$

with $w_{i,j_n(i)}$ the trilinear interpolation weights of y_i with respect to the its eight nearest neighbors $j_n(i)$, $n = 1, ...8$, on the grid of the template (atlas) image, $c_{j_n(i),l_1}$ the probability for label l_1 (main region) at voxel j in the atlas, $c_{j_n(i),l_2}$ the probability for label l_2 (sub-partition) and $\delta(r - r_i) = 1$ if $r = r_i$, zero otherwise. Furthermore the following holds:

$$\sum_{l_1} c_{j_n(i),l_1} = 1 ,$$

$$\sum_{l_2} c_{j_n(i),l_2} = 1$$

As it can be seen from the previous formula, given a contribution to a particular main class with label l_1, this contribution will be further divided into different labels l_2.

Figure 2 shows the atlas used in the registration algorithm. The main prior distributions (white matter etc,) and (some of) the substructures, are shown.

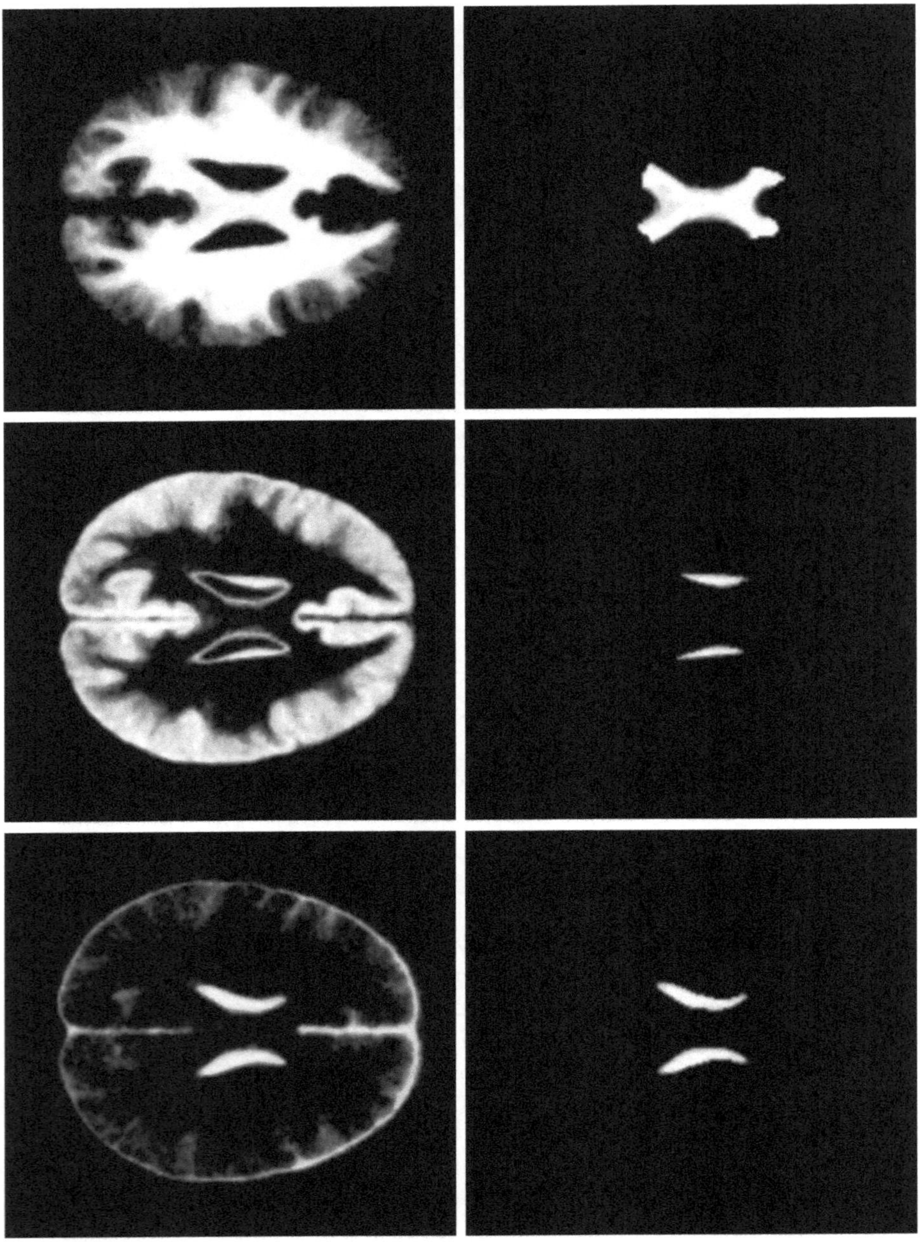

Fig. 2. Representation of the atlas priors for the main regions (left column) and for the substructures (right column). Top: white matter and corpus callosum; middle: gray matter and caudate nuclea; bottom: csf and lateral ventricles.

2.2 Similarity Measure and Its Derivative

In the algorithm we discuss in this paper, minimization of local entropy is used as similarity measure for the registration. The entropy is defined as follows:

$$H = \sum_{l_1} \sum_{l_2} H(r|l_1, l_2) p(l_1, l_2) \tag{2}$$

where l_1 and l_2 represent the two sets of labels (the main and the sub partition). $H(r|l_1, l_2)$ is the conditional entropy of having a certain intensity i, given the labels l_1 and l_2. In the following we will recompute the expression of the entropy as a function of the histogram, as it was defined in the previous section.

The conditional entropy can be written as:

$$H(r|l_1, l_2) = -\sum_{r} p(r|l_1, l_2) log_2 p(r|l_1, l_2) \tag{3}$$

where we introduced the conditional probability $p(r|l_1, l_2)$ of having intensity r, given the labels l_1 and l_2. This probability can be written as function of the joint histogram as follows:

$$p(r|l_1, l_2) = \frac{p(r, l_1, l_2)}{p(l_1, l_2)} \tag{4}$$

where the following holds:

$$p(r, l_1, l_2) = \frac{h(r, l_1, l_2)}{N}$$

and

$$p(l_1, l_2) = \frac{\sum_r h(r, l_1, l_2)}{N}$$

h being, as already mentioned, the joint histogram and N the total number of voxels, also obtained from h:

$$N = \sum_{r} \sum_{l_1} \sum_{l_2} h(r, l_1, l_2)$$

We can now rewrite the entropy as a function of the joint histogram:

$$\begin{aligned} H &= -\sum_{r} \sum_{l_1} \sum_{l_2} \frac{p(r, l_1, l_2)}{p(l_1, l_2)} log_2 \frac{p(r, l_1.l_2)}{p(l_1, l_2)} p(l_1, l_2) \\ &= -\sum_{r} \sum_{l_1} \sum_{l_2} p(r, l_1, l_2) log_2 \frac{p(r, l_1.l_2)}{p(l_1, l_2)} \\ &= \sum_{r} \sum_{l_1} \sum_{l_2} p(r, l_1, l_2) log_2 \frac{p(l_1.l_2)}{p(r, l_1, l_2)} \end{aligned} \tag{5}$$

Last we can introduce h explicitly:

$$H = \frac{1}{N}\sum_r \sum_{l_1} \sum_{l_2} h(r,l_1,l_2) log_2 \frac{\sum_r h(r,l_1,l_2)}{h(r,l_1,l_2)} \tag{6}$$

Starting from this last expression, we can compute the variation of the entropy for a small spatial displacement u_i:

$$\frac{\partial H}{\partial u_i} = \frac{\partial H}{\partial h}\frac{\partial h}{\partial u_i} \tag{7}$$

We start computing the first term. We have:

$$\frac{\partial H}{\partial h} = \frac{1}{N} log_2 \frac{h(l_1,l_2)}{h(r,l_1,l_2)} - \frac{1}{N}\frac{h(r,l_1,l_2)}{h(l_1,l_2)}\frac{h(l_1,l_2)}{h(i,l_1,l_2)} + \frac{\partial H}{\partial N}\frac{\partial N}{\partial h} + \frac{\partial H}{\partial h(l_1,l_2)}\frac{\partial h(l_1 m l_2)}{\partial h}$$

where, for sake of generality, we assumed that the number of voxels can change during the registration. The second term can be rewritten as:

$$\frac{\partial H}{\partial N}\frac{\partial N}{\partial h} = -\frac{H}{N}$$

where we exploited the fact that
$N = \sum_r \sum_{l_1} \sum_{l_2} h(r,l_1,l_2)$ and therefore $\frac{\partial N}{\partial h} = 1$.
The last term in equation 9 can be reformulated as:

$$\frac{\partial H}{\partial h(l_1,l_2)}\frac{\partial h(l_1,l_2)}{\partial h} = \frac{1}{N}\frac{\sum_r h(r,l_1,l_2)}{h(l_1,l_2)}$$

where in this case we used the fact that $h(l_1,l_2) = \sum_r h(r,l_1,l_2)$ and also $\frac{\partial h(l_1,l_2)}{\partial h} = 1$.

The term $\frac{\partial h}{\partial u_i}$ is easily computed. If we use trilinear interpolation to compute the joint histogram, we obtain:

$$\frac{\partial h}{\partial u_i} = \sum_{i=1}^{N}\sum_{n=1}^{8} \frac{\delta w_{i,j_n(i)}}{\partial u_i}.\delta(r - r_i).c_{j_n(i),l_1}.c_{j_n(i),l_2} \tag{8}$$

which is still a joint histogram with the trilinear weights given by the spatial derivatives of the original weights.

2.3 Viscous Fluid Regularization

Allowing each voxel i to be displaced independently of all others by u_i is likely to yield deformation fields that are physically not acceptable, such that some form of regularization is required to impose local smoothness. We adopt the free-form registration approach of [5] and use the force fields F as derived in the previous section (as the derivative of the similarity measure) to drive a viscous fluid regularizer by iteratively solving its simplified Navier-Stokes governing equation:

$$\nabla^2 v + \nabla (\nabla . v) + F(x, u) = 0 \tag{9}$$

with $v(x, t)$ the deformation velocity experienced by a particle at position x and time point t. An approximate solution of (9) is obtained by convolution with a spatial Gaussian kernel ψ_σ characterized by a (spatially isotropic) variance σ:

$$v = \psi_\sigma \star F \tag{10}$$

The deformation field $u^{(k+1)}$ at iteration $(k + 1)$ is found by integration over time:

$$R^{(k)} = v^{(k)} - \sum_{i=1}^{3} v_i^{(k)} \left[\frac{\partial u^{(k)}}{\partial x_i} \right] \tag{11}$$

$$u^{(k+1)} = u^{(k)} + R^{(k)}.\Delta t \tag{12}$$

The time step Δt is constrained by $\Delta t \leq \max(\|R\|).\Delta u$, with Δu the maximal voxel displacement that is allowed in one iteration. Regridding and template propagation are used to preserve topology.

2.4 Image Database

The set of 20 high-resolution normal brain MR images (10 females, 10 males, median age 31 years) used in this study for atlas construction and validation was

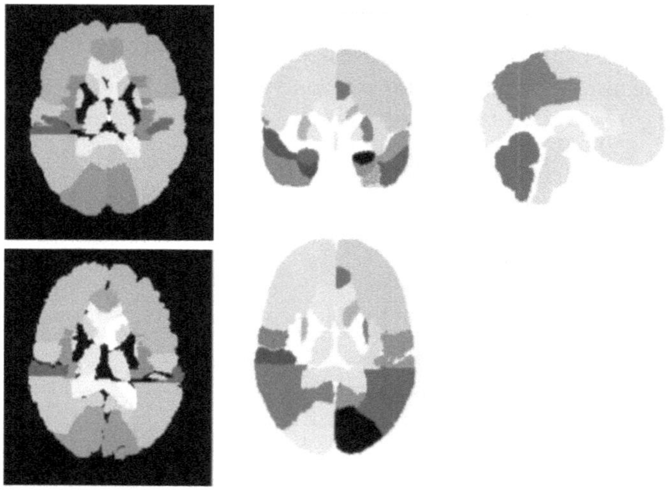

(a) (b)

Fig. 3. (a) Manual segmentation for two images in the database; (b) Maximum probability label image of the AT3 atlas constructed from statistical probabilistic anatomical maps of 49 regions computed from the 20 segmentations in the database acquired at Hammersmith Hospital, Imperial College London, UK [8]. All images have voxel sizes around 0.937 mm^3 and image dimensions of $[165-195] \times [198-199] \times [155-175]$. Each brain was manually segmented into 49 sub-structures as illustrated in figure 3. These include major brain structures such as the ventricles, cerebellum or corpus callosum, as well as the major lobes and gyri and the deep gray matter structures such as hippocampus, putamen, caudate nucleus and thalamus.

The images are first globally aligned by affine registration of each image to our own T1-weighted MR template (atlas) using maximization of mutual information [1].

In a second step our T1-weighted MR template was registered to the 20 images, using the algorithm discussed here.

2.5 First Results

In this section we will show some first results of the new algorithm and especially try to show the effect of local entropy minimization, in different brain substructures. In all our experiments white matter, gray matter, csf and 'rest',were used as main classes and the following substructures (in total 25) were included to define the third dimension of the joint histogram:

-Brain stem
-Corpus callosum
-Hippocampus (left and right apart)
-Amygdala (left and right apart)
-Basal ganglia (left and right apart)
-Ventricles (left and right and frontal/temporal apart)

Along with these substructures the respective complementary structures were also used (for example, white matter was partitioned in brain stem, corpus callosum and the rest of white matter as complementary region). At each voxel

Table 1. Overlap coefficients, averaged over 20 registrations, after affine (left column), IC non-rigid (second column) registration and ICC registration. Significance values (issued from a t-test) are also shown.

	Affine registration	IC registration	ICC registration	t-test p value
Hippocampus	69.98	76.81	78.07	0.016
Amygdala	72.81	78.56	76.89	0.058
Brain Stem	87.38	92.87	91.98	0.003
Caudate Nucleus	75.98	81.10	83.80	0.000
Nucleus Accumbens	57.38	63.11	62.50	0.691
Putamen	75.55	72.25	76.41	0.006
Thalamus	82.97	81.98	88.15	0.000
Globus Pallidum	70.22	66.77	74.44	0.000
Corpus Callosum	74.20	84.07	83.88	0.669
Ventricles	56.24	70.78	72.23	0.000

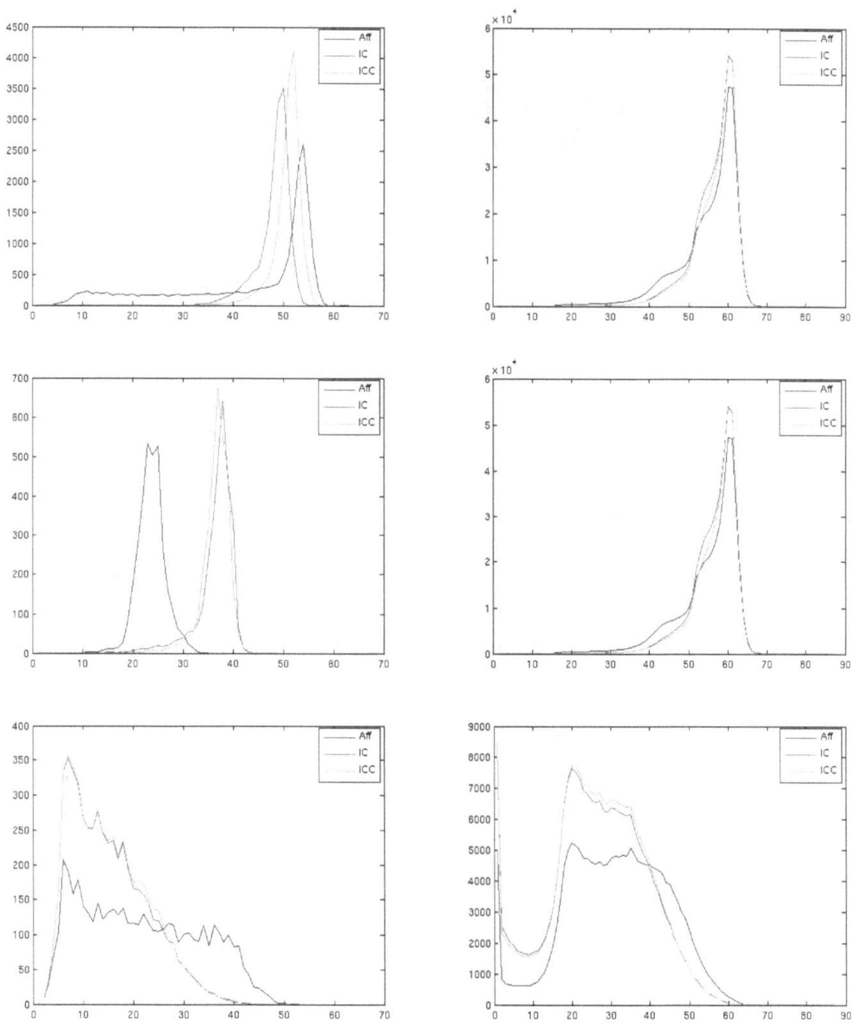

Fig. 4. Conditional histograms for white matter, gray matter, csf (right column) and three of their substructures (left column). Top: corpus callosum and white matter; middle: caudate nucleus and gray matter; bottom: lateral ventricle and csf.

the sum over all substructures was equal to one such that the probability of the main regions, at that place, was preserved.

Figure 4 shows the change in entropy for two different substructures, after affine and non-rigid registration. As it can be seen (especially in the white matter and csf substructures), the presented algorithm determines an important re-clustering of the intensity profiles for different substructures. This is equivalent to a local minimization of the conditional entropy of the intensities, given the labels. This effect is less evident in the caudate nucleus (although still present) because of the smaller number of voxels included in this region.

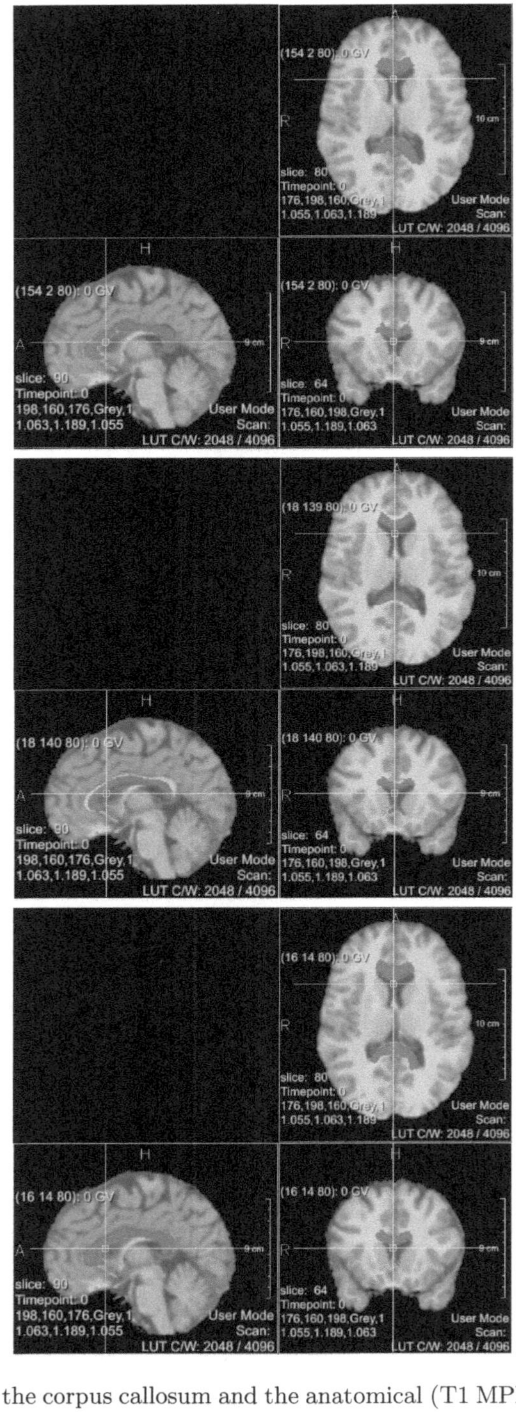

Fig. 5. Overlay of the corpus callosum and the anatomical (T1 MPRAGE) image. Top: ground truth (manual delineation); middle: result after affine registration; bottom: result after non-rigid registration.

Table 1 shows the overlap coefficient, for different registration algorithms. In particular, we considered affine registration, IC registration and ICC registration, averaged over 20 experiments. The IC algorithm was introduced in a previous work of our group and uses what we called hybrid mutual information, as similarity measure (IC stands for intensities vs class probabilities). Atlas priors are registered onto intensity histogram of the study image. The ICC algorithm is the one introduced in this paper.

In figure 5 we show the segmentation of the corpus callosum overlaid on top of the the anatomical image, after affine and non-rigid registration.

3 Discussion and Conclusion

In this paper we presented a novel non-rigid registration similarity measure based on minimization of regional conditional entropy. With respect to other methods where heuristic rules are used to determine the extension of the neighborhoods where the entropy is minimized, we propose here a global measure that implicitly minimizes entropy in different anatomical related substructures. The minimization of conditional entropy approach presented in this work, is equivalent to maximization of mutual information between the reference image intensities, on one side, and the atlas labels, on the other one.

The advantages of this approach are twofold: on the one hand the optimization is, as told, global, which should ensure an increased robustness of the method; on the other hand only anatomical relevant substructures are taken into account in the registration process, instead of fictitious partitions (i.e. not anatomy related) of the image. We can enforce local (i.e. anatomy related) entropy minimization in cortical subregions along with entropy minimization in the more global regions (such as, in our experiments, WM, GM and CSF). This is not possible when using standard mutual information, where only a single joint histogram is used for the entire image.

Moreover, our approach yields a segmentation of the study image in both global tissue classes as well as in subcortical regions (nucleus caudate, corpus callosum, etc. in our application). The potential thereof for atlas-based segmentation will be investigated in further work, along with an extended comparison with state-of-the-art algorithms, such as HAMMER [9].

References

1. Maes, F., Collignon, A., Vandermeulen, D., Marchal, G., Suetens, P.: Multi-modality image registration by maximization of mutual information. IEEE Transactions on Medical Imaging 16(2), 187–198 (1997)
2. Rueckert, D., Sonoda, L.I., Hayes, C., Hill, D.L.G., Leach, M.O., Hawkes, D.J.: Non-rigid registration using free-form deformations: Application to breast mr images. IEEE Transactions on Medical Imaging 18(8) (1999)
3. D'Agostino, E., Maes, F., Vandermeulen, D., Suetens, P.: A viscous fluid model for multimodal non-rigid image registration using mutual information. Medical image analysis 7(4), 565–575 (2003)

4. Loeckx, D., Maes, F., Vandermeulen, D., Suetens, P.: Temporal subtraction of thorax cr images using a statistical deformation model. IEEE Transactions on Medical Imaging (2003)
5. D'Agostino, E., Maes, F., Vandermeulen, D., Suetens, P.: An information theoretic approach for non-rigid image registration using voxel class probabilities. Medical Image Analysis 10(3), 413–431 (2006)
6. Van Leemput, K., Maes, F., Vandermeulen, D., Suetens, P.: Automated model-based tissue classification of MR images of the brain. IEEE Transactions on Medical Imaging 18(10), 897–908 (1999)
7. Wang, Q., Seghers, D., D' Agostino, E.: Construction and validation of mean shape atlas templates for atlas-based brain image segmentation. In: Staib, L. (ed.) IPMI 2005. LNCS, vol. 3565, pp. 689–700. Springer, Heidelberg (2005)
8. Hammers, A., Koep, M.J., Free, S.L., Brett, M., Richardson, M.P., Labbé, C., Cunningham, V.J., Brooks, D.J., Duncan, J.: Implementation and application of a brain template for multiple volumes of interest. Human Brain Mapping 15(3), 165–174 (2002)
9. Shen, D., Davatzikos, C.: Hammer: Hierarchical attribute matching mechanism for elastic registration. IEEE Transactions on Medical Imaging 21, 1421–1439 (2002)

Shape Modeling and Analysis with Entropy-Based Particle Systems

Joshua Cates[1], P. Thomas Fletcher[1], Martin Styner[2], Martha Shenton[3], and Ross Whitaker[1]

[1] School of Computing, University of Utah, Salt Lake City UT, USA
[2] Departments of Computer Science and Psychiatry, University of North Carolina at Chapel Hill, Chapel Hill NC, USA
[3] Psychiatry Neuroimaging Laboratory, Brigham and Women's Hospital, Harvard Medical School; and Laboratory of Neuroscience, VA Boston Healthcare System, Brockton MA, USA

Abstract. This paper presents a new method for constructing compact statistical point-based models of ensembles of similar shapes that does not rely on any specific surface parameterization. The method requires very little preprocessing or parameter tuning, and is applicable to a wider range of problems than existing methods, including nonmanifold surfaces and objects of arbitrary topology. The proposed method is to construct a point-based sampling of the shape ensemble that simultaneously maximizes both the geometric accuracy and the statistical simplicity of the model. Surface point samples, which also define the shape-to-shape correspondences, are modeled as sets of dynamic particles that are constrained to lie on a set of implicit surfaces. Sample positions are optimized by gradient descent on an energy function that balances the negative entropy of the distribution on each shape with the positive entropy of the ensemble of shapes. We also extend the method with a curvature-adaptive sampling strategy in order to better approximate the geometry of the objects. This paper presents the formulation; several synthetic examples in two and three dimensions; and an application to the statistical shape analysis of the caudate and hippocampus brain structures from two clinical studies.

1 Introduction

Statistical analysis of sets of similar shapes requires quantification of shape differences, which is a fundamentally difficult problem. One widely used strategy for computing shape differences is to compare the positions of corresponding points among sets of shapes, often with the goal of producing a statistical model of the set that describes a mean and modes of variation. Medical or biological shapes, however, are typically derived from the interfaces between organs or tissue types, and usually defined implicitly in the form of *segmented volumes*, rather than explicit parameterizations or surface point samples. Thus, no a priori relationship is defined between points across surfaces, and correspondences

N. Karssemeijer and B. Lelieveldt (Eds.): IPMI 2007, LNCS 4584, pp. 333–345, 2007.
© Springer-Verlag Berlin Heidelberg 2007

must be inferred from the shapes themselves, which is a difficult and ill-posed problem.

Until recently, correspondences for shape statistics were established manually by choosing small sets of anatomically significant landmarks on organs or regions of interest, which would then serve as the basis for shape analysis. The demand for more detailed analyses on ever larger populations of subjects has rendered this approach unsatisfactory. Brechbühler et al. pioneered the use of spherical parameterizations for shape analysis that can be used to implicitly establish relatively dense sets of correspondences over an ensemble of shape surfaces [1]. Their methods, however, are purely geometric and seek only consistently regular parameterizations, not optimal correspondences. Davies et al. [2] present methods for optimizing correspondences among point sets that are based on the information content of the set, but these methods still rely on mappings between fixed spherical surface parameterizations. Most shapes in medicine or biology are not derived parametrically, so the reliance on a parameterization presents some significant drawbacks. Automatic selection of correspondences for nonparametric, point-based shape models has been explored in the context of surface registration [3], but because such methods are typically limited to pairwise correspondences and assume a fixed set of surface point samples, they are not sufficient for the analysis of sets of segmented volumes. Several methods have been proposed that warp a set of images to a reference image, establishing correspondence among images through the deformations [4,5]. These methods are purely image based, however, and do not deal with the problem of selecting surface landmarks for correspondence or establishing geometrically accurate surface samplings.

This paper presents a new method for extracting dense sets of correspondences that also optimally describes ensembles of similar shapes. The proposed method is *nonparametric*, and borrows technology from the computer graphics literature by representing surfaces as discrete point sets. The method iteratively distributes sets of dynamic particles across an ensemble of surfaces so that their positions optimize the information content of the system. This strategy is motivated by a recognition of the inherent tradeoff between geometric accuracy (a good sampling) and statistical simplicity (a compact model). Our assertion is that units of information associated with the model implied by the correspondence positions should be balanced against units of information associated with the individual surface samplings. This approach provides a natural equivalence of information content and reduces the dependency on ad-hoc regularization strategies and free parameters. Since the points are not tied to a specific parameterization, the method operates directly on volumetric data, extends easily to higher dimensions or arbitrary shapes, and provides a more homogeneous geometric sampling as well as more compact statistical representations. The method draws a clear distinction between the objective function and the minimization process, and thus can more readily incorporate additional information such as high-order geometric information for adaptive sampling.

2 Related Work

The strategy of finding parameterizations that minimize information content across an ensemble was first proposed by Kotcheff and Taylor [6], who represent each two-dimensional contour as a set of N samples taken at equal intervals from a parameterization. Each shape is treated as a point in a $2N$-dimensional space, with associated covariance Σ and cost function, $\sum_k \log(\lambda_k + \alpha)$, where λ_k are the eigenvalues of Σ, and α is a regularization parameter that prevents the very *thinnest* modes (smallest eigenvalues) from dominating the process. This is the same as minimizing $\log |\Sigma + \alpha I|$, where I is the identity matrix, and $|\cdot|$ denotes the matrix determinant.

Davies et al. [2] propose a cost function for 2D shapes based on *minimum description length* (MDL). They use quantization arguments to limit the effects of thin modes and to determine the optimal number of components that should influence the process. They propose a piecewise linear reparameterization and a hierarchical minimization scheme. In [7] they describe a 3D extension to the MDL method, which relies on spherical parameterizations and subdivisions of an octahedral base shape, with smoothed updates that are represented as Cauchy kernels. The parameterization must be obtained through another process such as [1], which relaxes a spherical parameterization onto an input mesh. The overall procedure requires significant data preprocessing, including a sequence of optimizations—first to establish the parameterization and then on the correspondences—each of which entails a set of free parameters or inputs in addition to the segmented volumes. A significant concern with the basic MDL formulation is that the optimal solution is often one in which the correspondences all collapse to points where all the shapes in the ensemble happen to be near (e.g., crossings of many shapes). Several solutions have been proposed [7,8], but they entail additional free parameters and assumptions about the quality of the initial parameterizations.

The MDL formulation is mathematically related to the min-log $|\Sigma + \alpha I|$ approach, as noted by Thodberg[8]. Styner et al. [9] describe an empirical study that shows ensemble-based statistics improve correspondences relative to pure geometric regularization, and that MDL performance is virtually the same as that of min-log $|\Sigma + \alpha I|$. This last observation is consistent with the well-known result from information theory: MDL is, in general, equivalent to minimum entropy [10].

Another body of relevant work is the recent trend in computer graphics towards representing surfaces as scattered collections of points. The advantage of so-called *point-set surfaces* is that they do not require a specific parameterization and do not impose topological limitations; surfaces can be locally reconstructed or subdivided as needed [11]. A related technology in the graphics literature is the work on particle systems, which can be used to manipulate or sample [12] implicit surfaces. A particle system manipulates large sets of particles constrained to a surface using a gradient descent on radial energies that typically fall off with distance. The proposed method uses a set of interacting particle systems, one for each shape in the ensemble, to produce optimal sets of surface correspondences.

3 Methods

3.1 Entropy-Based Surface Sampling

We treat a surface as a subset of $\Re^d$, where $d = 2$ or $d = 3$ depending whether we are processing curves in the plane or surfaces in a volume, respectively. The method we describe here deals with smooth, closed manifolds of codimension one, and we will refer to such manifolds as *surfaces*. We will discuss the extension to nonmanifold curves and surfaces in Section 5. We sample a surface $\mathcal{S} \subset \Re^d$ using a discrete set of N points that are considered random variables $Z = (X_1, X_2, \ldots, X_N)$ drawn from a probability density function (PDF), $p(X)$. We denote a realization of this PDF with lower case, and thus we have $z = (x_1, x_2, \ldots, x_N)$, where $z \in \mathcal{S}^N$. The probability of a realization x is $p(X = x)$, which we denote simply as $p(x)$.

The amount of information contained in such a random sampling is, in the limit, the differential entropy of the PDF, which is $H[X] = -\int_S p(x) \log p(x) dx = -E\{\log p(X)\}$, where $E\{\cdot\}$ is the expectation. When we have a sufficient number of points sampled from p, we can approximate the expectation by the sample mean [10], which gives $H[X] \approx -(1/N) \sum_i \log p(x_i)$. We must also estimate $p(x_i)$. Density functions on surfaces can be quite complex, and so we use a nonparametric, Parzen windowing estimation of this density using the particles themselves. Thus we have

$$p(x_i) \approx \frac{1}{N(N-1)} \sum_{j=1, j \neq i}^{N} G(x_i - x_j, \sigma_i) \tag{1}$$

where $G(x_i - x_j, \sigma_i)$ is a d-dimensional, isotropic Gaussian with standard deviation σ_i. The cost function C, is therefore an approximation of (negative) entropy: $-H[X] \approx C(x_1, \ldots, x_N) = \sum_i \log \frac{1}{N(N-1)} \sum_{j \neq i} G(x_i - x_j, \sigma_i)$,

In this paper, we use a gradient-descent optimization strategy to manipulate particle positions. The optimization problem is given by:

$$\hat{z} = \arg\min_z E(z) \text{ s.t. } x_1, \ldots, x_N \in \mathcal{S}. \tag{2}$$

The negated gradient of C is

$$-\frac{\partial C}{\partial x_i} = \frac{1}{\sigma_i^2} \frac{\sum_{j \neq i}^{N} (x_i - x_j) G(x_i - x_j, \sigma_i)}{\sum_{j \neq i}^{N} G(x_i - x_j, \sigma_i)} = \sigma_i^{-2} \sum_{j \neq i}^{N} (x_i - x_j) w_{ij}, \tag{3}$$

where $\sum_j w_{ij} = 1$. Thus to minimize C, the surface points (which we will call *particles*) must move away from each other, and we have a set of particles moving under a repulsive force and constrained to lie on the surface. The motion of each particle is away from all of the other particles, but the forces are weighted by a Gaussian function of inter-particle distance. Interactions are therefore local for sufficiently small σ. We use a Jacobi update with forward differences, and thus each particle moves with a *time* parameter and positional update $x_i \leftarrow x_i - \gamma \frac{\partial C}{\partial x_i}$, where γ is a time step and $\gamma < \sigma^2$ for stability.

The preceding minimization produces a *uniform* sampling of a surface. For some applications, a strategy that samples adaptively in response to higher order shape information is more effective. From a numerical point of view, the minimization strategy relies on a degree of regularity in the tangent planes between adjacent particles, which argues for sampling more densely in high curvature regions. High-curvature features are also considered more interesting than flat regions as important landmarks for biological shapes. To this end, we extend the above uniform sampling method to adaptively oversample high-curvature regions by modifying the Parzen windowing in Eqn. 1 as follows

$$\tilde{p}(x_i) \approx \frac{1}{N(N-1)} \sum_{j=1, j \neq i}^{N} G\left(\frac{1}{k_j}(x_i - x_j), \sigma_i\right) \tag{4}$$

where k_j is a scaling term proportional to the curvature magnitude computed at each neighbor particle j. The effect of this scaling is to warp space in response to local curvature. A uniform sampling based on maximum entropy in the warped space translates into an adaptive sampling in unwarped space, where points pack more densely in higher curvature regions. The extension of Eqn 3 to incorporate the curvature-adaptive Parzen windowing is straightforward to compute since k_j is not a function of x_i, and is omitted here for brevity.

There are many possible choices for the scaling term k. Meyer, et al. [13] describe an adaptive surface sampling that uses the scaling $k_i = \frac{1+\rho\kappa_i(\frac{s}{2\pi})}{\frac{1}{2}s\cos(\pi/6)}$, where κ_i is the root sum-of-squares of the principal curvatures at surface location x_i. The user-defined variables s and ρ specify the ideal distance between particles on a planar surface, and the ideal density of particles per unit angle on a curved surface, respectively. Note that the scaling term in this formulation could easily be modified to include surface properties other than curvature.

The surface constraint in both the uniform and adaptive optimizations is specified by the zero set of a scalar function $F(x)$. This constraint is maintained, as described in several papers [12], by projecting the gradient of the cost function onto the tangent plane of the surface (as prescribed by the method of Lagrange multipliers), followed by iterative reprojection of the particle onto the nearest root of F by the method of Newton-Raphson. Principal curvatures are computed analytically from the implicit function as described in [14]. Another aspect of this particle formulation is that it computes Euclidean distance between particles, rather than the geodesic distance on the surface. Thus, we assume sufficiently dense samples so that nearby particles lie in the tangent planes of the zero sets of F. This is an important consideration; in cases where this assumption is not valid, such as highly convoluted surfaces, the distribution of particles may be affected by neighbors that are outside of the true manifold neighborhood. Limiting the influence of neighbors whose normals differ by some threshold value (e.g. 90 degrees) does limit these effects. The question of particle interactions with more general distance measures remains for future work.

Finally, we must choose a σ for each particle, which we do automatically, before the positional update, using the same optimality criterion described above. The contribution to C of the ith particle is simply the probability of that particle position, and optimizing that quantity with respect to σ gives a maximum likelihood estimate of σ for the current particle configuration. We use Newton-Raphson to find σ such that $\partial p(x_i, \sigma)/\partial\sigma = 0$, which typically converges to machine precision in several iterations. For the adaptive sampling case, we find σ such that $\partial\tilde{p}(x_i, \sigma)/\partial\sigma = 0$, so that the optimal σ is scaled locally based on the curvature.

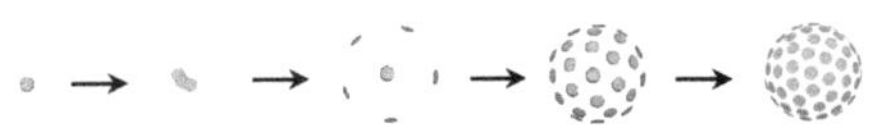

Fig. 1. A system of 100 particles on a sphere, produced by particle splitting

There are a few important numerical considerations. We must truncate the Gaussian kernels, and so we use $G(x, \sigma) = 0$ for $|x| > 3\sigma$. This means that each particle has a finite radius of influence, and we can use a spatial binning structure to reduce the computational burden associated with particle interactions. If σ for a particle is too small, a particle will not interact with its neighbors at all, and we cannot compute updates of σ or position. In this case, we update the kernel size using $\sigma \leftarrow 2 \times \sigma$, until σ is large enough for the particle to interact with its neighbors. Another numerical consideration is that the system must include bounds σ_{min} and σ_{max} to account for anomalies such as bad initial conditions, too few particles, etc. These are not critical parameters. As long as they are set to include the minimum and maximum resolutions, the system operates reliably.

The mechanism described in this section is, therefore, a self tuning system of particles that distribute themselves using repulsive forces to achieve optimal distributions, and may optionally adjust their sampling frequency locally in response to surface curvature. For this paper we initialize the system with a single particle that finds the nearest zero of F, then splits (producing a new, nearby particle) at regular intervals until a specific number of particles are produced and reach a steady state. Figure 1 shows this process on a sphere.

3.2 The Entropy of the Ensemble

An ensemble $\mathcal{E}$ is a collection of M surfaces, each with their own set of particles, i.e. $\mathcal{E} = z^1, \ldots, z^M$. The ordering of the particles on each shape implies a correspondence among shapes, and thus we have a matrix of particle positions $P = x_j^k$, with particle positions along the rows and shapes across the columns. We model $z^k \in \Re^{Nd}$ as an instance of a random variable Z, and propose to minimize the combined ensemble and shape cost function

$$Q = H(Z) - \sum_k H(P^k), \tag{5}$$

which favors a compact ensemble representation balanced against a uniform distribution of particles on each surface. The different entropies are commensurate so there is no need for ad-hoc weighting of the two function terms.

For this discussion we assume that the complexity of each shape is greater than the number of examples, and so we would normally choose $N > M$. Given the low number of examples relative to the dimensionality of the space, we must impose some conditions in order to perform the density estimation. For this work we assume a normal distribution and model $p(Z)$ parametrically using a Gaussian with covariance Σ. The entropy is then given by

$$H(Z) \approx \frac{1}{2} \log |\Sigma| = \frac{1}{2} \sum_{j=1}^{Nd} \log \lambda_j, \tag{6}$$

where $\lambda_1, ..., \lambda_{Nd}$ are the eigenvalues of Σ.

In practice, Σ will not have full rank, in which case the entropy is not finite. We must therefore regularize the problem with the addition of a diagonal matrix αI to introduce a lower bound on the eigenvalues. We estimate the covariance from the data, letting Y denote the matrix of points minus the sample mean for the ensemble, which gives $\Sigma = (1/(M-1))YY^T$. Because $N > M$, we perform the computations on the dual space (dimension M), knowing that the determinant is the same up to a constant factor of α. Thus, we have the cost function G associated with the ensemble entropy:

$$\log |\Sigma| \approx G(P) = \log \left| \frac{1}{M-1} Y^T Y, \right| \text{ and } -\frac{\partial G}{\partial P} = Y(Y^T Y + \alpha I)^{-1}. \tag{7}$$

We now see that α is a regularization on the inverse of $Y^T Y$ to account for the possibility of a diminishing determinant. The negative gradient $-\partial G/\partial P$ gives a vector of updates for the entire system, which is recomputed once per system update. This term is added to the shape-based updates described in the previous section to give the update of each particle:

$$x_j^k \leftarrow \gamma \left[-\partial G/\partial x_j^k + \partial E^k/\partial x_j^k \right]. \tag{8}$$

The stability of this update places an additional restriction on the time steps, requiring γ to be less than the reciprocal of the maximum eigenvalue of $(Y^T Y + \alpha I)^{-1}$, which is bounded by α. Thus, we have $\gamma < \alpha$, and note that α has the practical effect of preventing the system from slowing too much as it tries to reduce the thinnest dimensions of the ensemble distribution. This also suggests an annealing approach for computational efficiency (which we have used in this paper) in which α starts off somewhat large (e.g., the size of the shapes) and is incrementally reduced as the system iterates.

The choice of a Gaussian model for $p(Z = z)$ is not critical for the proposed method. The framework easily incorporates either nonparametric, or alternate parametric models. In this case, the Gaussian model allows us to make direct comparisons with the MDL method, which contains the same assumptions. Research into alternative models for Z is outside the scope of this paper and remains of interest for future work.

3.3 A Shape Modeling Pipeline

The particle method outlined in the preceding sections may be applied directly to binary segmentation volumes, which are often the output of a manual or automated segmentation process. A binary segmentation contains an implicit shape surface at the interface of the labeled pixels and the background. Any suitably accurate distance transform from that interface may be used to form the implicit surface necessary for the particle optimization. Typically, we use a fast-marching algorithm [15], followed by a slight Gaussian blurring to remove the high-frequency artifacts that can occur as a result of numerical approximations.

A collection of shape segmentations must often be aligned in a common coordinate frame for modeling and analysis. We first align the segmentations with respect to their centers of mass and the orientation of their first principal eigenvectors. Then, during the optimization, we further align shapes with respect to rotation and translation using a Procrustes algorithm [16], applied at regular intervals after particle updates. Because the proposed method is completely generalizable to higher dimensions, we are able to process shapes in 2D and 3D using the same *C++* software implementation, which is templated by dimension. For all the experiments described in this paper, the numerical parameter $\sigma_{\min}$ is set to machine precision and $\sigma_{\max}$ is set to the size of the domain. For the annealing parameter α, we use a starting value roughly equal to the diameter of an average shape and reduce it to machine precision over several hundred iterations. Particles are initialized on each shape using the splitting procedure described in Section 3.1, but are distributed under the full correspondence optimization to keep corresponding points in alignment. We have found these default settings to produce reliably good results that are very robust to the initialization. Processing time on a 2GHz desktop machine scales linearly with the number of particles in the system and ranges from 20 minutes for a 2D system of a few thousand particles to several hours for a 3D system of tens of thousands of particles.

4 Results

This section details several experiments designed to validate the proposed method. First, we compare models generated using the particle method with models generated using MDL for two synthetic 2D datasets. Next, a simple experiment on tori illustrates the applicability of the method to nonspherical topologies. Finally, we apply the method to a full statistical shape analysis of several 3D neuroanatomical structures from published clinical datasets.

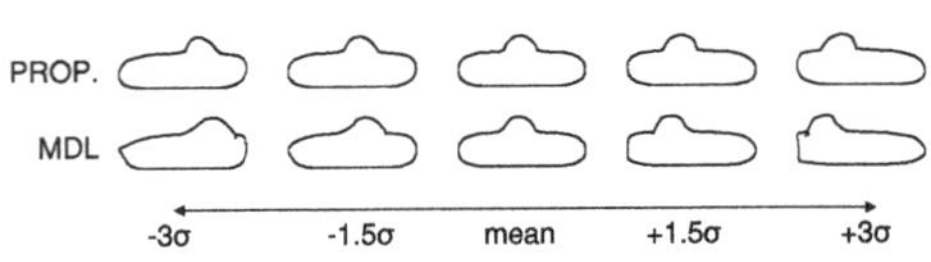

Fig. 2. The *box-bump* experiment

We begin with two experiments on closed curves in a 2D plane and a comparison with the 2D open-source Matlab MDL implementation given by Thodberg [8]. In the first experiment, we used the proposed, particle method to optimize 100 particles per shape under uniform sampling on 24

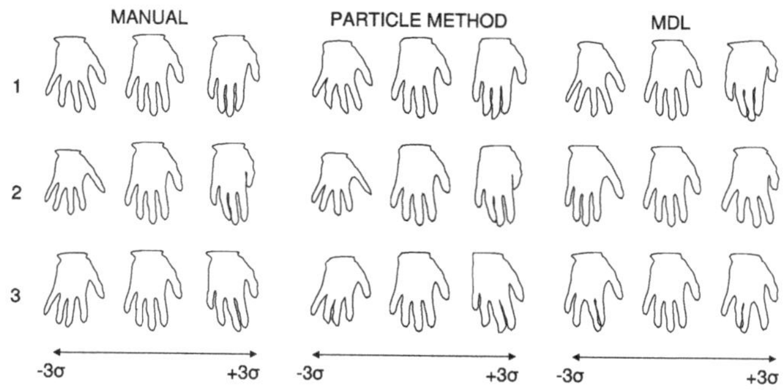

Fig. 3. The mean and ±3 std. deviations of the top 3 modes of the hand models.

box-bump shapes, similar to those described in [8]. Each shape was constructed as a fast-marching distance transform from a set of boundary points using cubic b-splines with the same rectangle of control, but with a bump added at a random location along the top of its curve. This example is interesting because we would, in principle, expect a correspondence algorithm that is minimizing information content to discover this single mode of variability in the ensemble.

MDL correspondences were computed using 128 nodes and *mode 2* of the Matlab software, with all other parameters set to their defaults (see [8] for details). Principal component analysis identified a single dominant mode of variation for each method, but with different degrees of leakage into orthogonal modes. MDL lost 0.34% of the total variation from the single mode, while the proposed method lost only 0.0015%. Figure 2 illustrates the mean and three standard deviations of the first mode of the two different models. Shapes from the particle method remain more faithful to those described by the original training set, even out to three standard deviations where the MDL description breaks down. A striking observation from this experiment is how the relatively small amount of variation left in the minor modes of the MDL case produce such a significant effect on the results of shape deformations along the major mode.

The second experiment was conducted on the set of 18 hand shape contours described in [2], again applying both the particle method and MDL using the same parameters as described above. Distance transforms from from spline-based contour models again form the inputs. In this case, we also compared results with a set of *ideal*, manually selected correspondences, which introduce anatomical knowledge of the digits. Figure 3 compares the three resulting models in the top three modes of variation to ±3 standard deviations. A detailed analysis of the principal components showed that the proposed particle method and the manually selected points both produce very similar models, while MDL differed significantly, particularly in first three modes.

Non-spherical Topologies. Existing 3D MDL implementations rely on spherical parameterizations, and are therefore only capable of analyzing shapes topologically equivalent to a sphere. The particle-based method does not have this limitation. As a demonstration of this, we applied the proposed method to a set

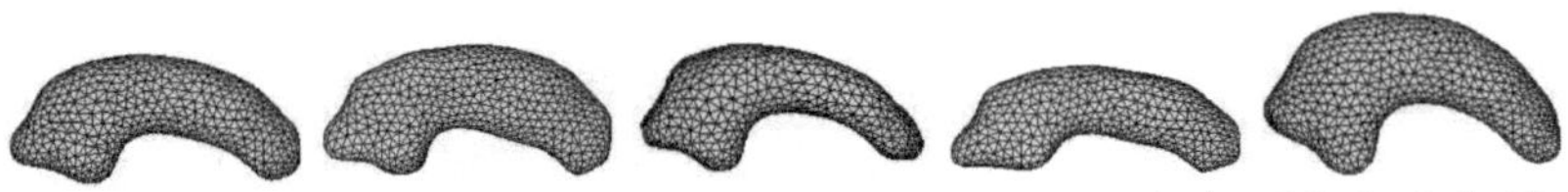

Fig. 4. Right hippocampus model mean and ±3 standard deviations in two modes

of 25 randomly chosen tori, drawn from a 2D, normal distribution parameterized by the small radius r and the large radius R. Tori were chosen from a distribution with mean $r = 1, R = 2$ and $\sigma_r = 0.15, \sigma_R = 0.30$, with a rejection policy that excluded invalid tori (e.g., $r > R$). We optimized the correspondences using a uniform sampling and 250 particles on each shape. An analysis of the resulting model showed that the particle system method discovered the two pure modes of variation, with only 0.08% leakage into smaller modes.

Shape Analysis of Neuroanatomical Structures. As a further validation of the particle method, we performed hypothesis testing of group shape differences on data from two published clinical studies. The first study addresses the shape of the hippocampus in patients with schizophrenia. The data consists of left and right hippocampus shapes from 56 male adult patients versus 26 healthy adult male controls, segmented from MRI using a template-based semi-automated method [17]. The second study addresses the shape of the caudate in males with schizo-typal personality disorder. The data consists of left and right caudate shapes from 15 patients and 14 matched, healthy controls, and was manually segmented from MRI brain scans of the study subjects by clinical experts [18]. All data is normalized with respect to intercranial volume.

For each study, we aligned and processed the raw binary segmentations as described in Section 3.3, including Procrustes registration. Models were optimized with 1024 correspondence points per shape and the curvature-adaptive sampling strategy, which proved more effective than uniform sampling. Separate models were created for left and right structures using the *combined* data from patient and normal populations. Models were generated without knowledge of the shape classifications so as not to bias the correspondences to one class or the other. On inspection, all of the resulting models appear to be of good quality; each major mode of variation describes some plausible pattern of variation observed in the training data. As an example, Figure 4 shows several surface meshes of shapes generated from the pointsets of the right hippocampus model.

After computing the models, we applied statistical tests for group differences at every surface point location. The method used is a nonparametric permutation test of the Hotelling T^2 metric with false-discovery-rate (FDR) correction, and is described in [19]. We used the open-source implementation of the algorithm [19], with 20,000 permutations among groups and an FDR bound set to 5%. The null hypothesis for these tests is that the distributions of the locations of corresponding sample points are the same regardless of group.

Figure 5 shows the raw and FDR-corrected p-values for the left and right hippocampi from the schizophrenia study. Areas of significant group differences

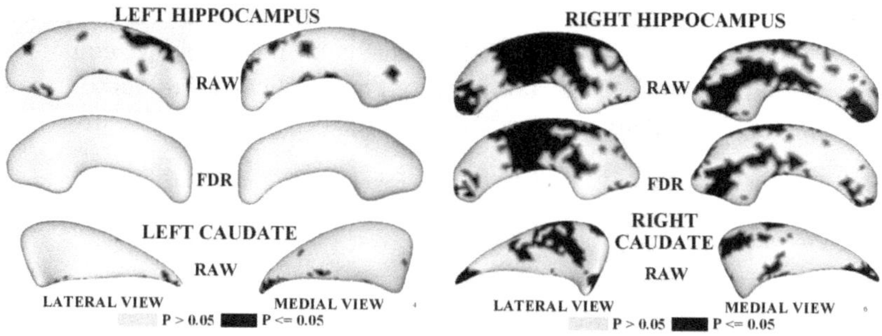

Fig. 5. P-value maps for the hippocampus and caudate shape analyses, shown on the mean shape. Red (dark in grayscale) indicates significant group differences ($p <= .05$).

($p <= 0.05$) are shown in red. Areas with insignificant group differences ($p > 0.05$) are shown in blue. The right hippocampus shows significant differences in the mid-region and the tail, even after FDR-correction. The left hippocampus appears to exhibit few group differences, with none detected after FDR correction. Differences in the tail, especially on the right side were also observed by Styner et al. in [9]. Our results also correlate with those reported for the spherical harmonics method (SPHARM) [17] and spherical wavelet analysis [20].

Raw p-values for the caudate analysis are shown at the bottom of Fig 5. No significant differences on either shape were found after FDR correction. The raw p-values, however, suggest that both structures may exhibit group differences in the tail, and that the right caudate contains more group differences than the left, an observation that agrees with results given in [19], [18], [17], and [20]. The current formulation of the particle method optimizes point correspondences under the assumption of a Gaussian model with a *single* mean, and may introduce a conservative bias that reduces group differences. We are investigating methods, such as nonparametric density estimation, for addressing this issue.

5 Conclusions

We have presented a new method for constructing statistical representations of ensembles of similar shapes that relies on an optimal distribution of a large set of surface point correspondences, rather than the manipulation of a specific surface parameterization. The proposed method produces results that compare favorably with the state of the art, and statistical analysis of several clinical datasets shows the particle-based method yields results consistent with those seen in the literature. The method works directly on volumes, requires very little parameter tuning, and generalizes easily to accommodate alternate sampling strategies such as curvature adaptivity. The method can extend to other kinds of geometric objects by modeling those objects as intersections of various constraints. For instance, the nonmanifold boundaries that result from interfaces of three or more tissue types can be represented through combinations of distance functions to the individual tissue types. Curves can be represented as the intersection of the zero sets of two scalar fields or where three different scalar fields achieve equality (such as the curves where three materials meet). The application of these extensions to joint modeling of multiple connected objects is currently under investigation.

Acknowledgments

The authors wish to thank Hans Henrik Thodberg for the use of his open source MDL Matlab code and Tim Cootes for the hand data.

This work is funded by the Center for Integrative Biomedical Computing, National Institutes of Health (NIH) NCRR Project 2-P41-RR12553-07. This work is also part of the National Alliance for Medical Image Computing (NAMIC), funded by the NIH through the NIH Roadmap for Medical Research, Grant U54 EB005149. The hippocampus data is from a study funded by the Stanley Foundation and UNC-MHNCRC (MH33127). The caudate data is from a study funded by NIMH R01 MH 50740 (Shenton), NIH K05 MH 01110 (Shenton), NIMH R01 MH 52807 (McCarley), and a VA Merit Award (Shenton).

References

1. Brechbühler, C., Gerig, G., Kübler, O.: Parametrization of closed surfaces for 3-d shape description. Computer Vision Image Understanding 61, 154–170 (1995)
2. Davies, R.H., Twining, C.J., Cootes, T.F., Waterton, J.C., Taylor, C.J.: A minimum description length approach to statistical shape modeling. IEEE Trans. Med. Imaging 21(5), 525–537 (2002)
3. Audette, M., Ferrie, F., Peters, T.: An algorithmic overview of surface registration techniques for medical imaging. Medical Image Analysis 4, 201–217 (2000)
4. Frangi, A., Rueckert, D., Schnabel, J., Niessen, W.: Automatic construction of multiple-object three-dimensional statistical shape models: Application to cardiac modeling. IEEE Trans. Med. Imaging 21(9), 1151–1166 (2002)
5. Twining, C.J., Cootes, T.F., Marsland, S., Petrovic, V.S., Schestowitz, R., Taylor, C.J.: A unified information-theoretic approach to groupwise non-rigid registration and model building. In: IPMI 2005, pp.1–14 (2005)
6. Kotcheff, A., Taylor, C.: Automatic Construction of Eigenshape Models by Direct Optimization. Medical Image Analysis 2, 303–314 (1998)
7. Davies, R.H., Twining, C.J., Cootes, T.F., Waterton, J.C., Taylor, C.J.: 3d statistical shape models using direct optimisation of description length. In: Heyden, A., Sparr, G., Nielsen, M., Johansen, P. (eds.) ECCV 2002. LNCS, vol. 2352, pp. 3–20. Springer, Heidelberg (2002)
8. Thodberg, H.H.: Minimum description length shape and appearance models. In: IPMI, pp. 51–62 (2003)
9. Styner, M., Lieberman, J., Gerig, G.: Boundary and medial shape analysis of the hippocampus in schizophrenia. In: Ellis, R.E., Peters, T.M. (eds.) MICCAI 2003. LNCS, vol. 2879, pp. 464–471. Springer, Heidelberg (2003)
10. Cover, T., Thomas, J.: Elements of Information Theory. Wiley, Chichester (1991)
11. Boissonnat, J.D., Oudot, S.: Provably good sampling and meshing of surfaces. Graphical Models 67, 405–451 (2005)

12. Meyer, M.D., Georgel, P., Whitaker, R.T.: Robust particle systems for curvature dependent sampling of implicit surfaces. In: Proceedings of the International Conference on Shape Modeling and Applications 2005, pp. 124–133 (2005)
13. Meyer, M.D., Nelson, B., Kirby, R.M., Whitaker, R.: Particle systems for efficient and accurate high-order finite element visualization. IEEE Transactions on Visualization and Computer Graphics (Under Review)
14. Kindlmann, G., Whitaker, R., Tasdizen, T., Moller, T.: Curvature-based transfer functions for direct volume rendering. In: Proceedings of IEEE Visualization, pp. 512–520 (2003)
15. Sethian, J.: Level Set Methods and Fast Marching Methods. Cambridge University Press, Cambridge (1996)
16. Goodall, C.: Procrustes methods in the statistical analysis of shape. J. R. Statistical Society B 53, 285–339 (1991)
17. Styner, M., Xu, S., El-SSayed, M., Gerig, G.: Correspondence evaluation in local shape analysis and structural subdivision. In: IEEE Symposium on Biomedical Imaging ISBI 2007, in print (2007)
18. Levitt, J., Westin, C.F., Nestor, P., Estepar, R., Dickey, C., Voglmaier, M., Seidman, L., Kikinis, R., Jolesz, F., McCarley, R., Shenton, M.: Shape of caudate nucleus and its cognitive correlates in neuroleptic-naive schizotypal personality disorder. Biol. Psychiatry 55, 177–184 (2004)
19. Styner, M., Oguz, I., Xu, S., Brechbühler, C., Pantazis, D., Levitt, J., Shenton, M., Gerig, G.: Framework for the statistical shape analysis of brain structures using SPHARM-PDM. The Insight Journal (2006)
20. Nain, D., Niethammer, M., Levitt, J., Shenton, M., Gerig, G., Bobick, A., Tannenbaum, A.: Statistical shape analysis of brain structures using spherical wavelets. In: IEEE Symposium on Biomedical Imaging ISBI 2007, in print

A Volumetric Approach to Quantifying Region-to-Region White Matter Connectivity in Diffusion Tensor MRI

P. Thomas Fletcher, Ran Tao, Won-Ki Jeong, and Ross T. Whitaker

School of Computing, University of Utah, Salt Lake City, UT, USA

Abstract. In this paper we present a volumetric approach for quantitatively studying white matter connectivity from diffusion tensor magnetic resonance imaging (DT-MRI). The proposed method is based on a minimization of path cost between two regions, defined as the integral of local costs that are derived from the full tensor data along the path. We solve the minimal path problem using a Hamilton-Jacobi formulation of the problem and a new, fast iterative method that computes updates on the propagating front of the cost function at every point. The solutions for the fronts emanating from the two initial regions are combined, giving a voxel-wise connectivity measurement of the optimal paths between the regions that pass through those voxels. The resulting high-connectivity voxels provide a volumetric representation of the white matter pathway between the terminal regions. We quantify the tensor data along these pathways using nonparametric regression of the tensors and of derived measures as a function of path length. In this way we can obtain volumetric measures on white-matter tracts between regions without any explicit integration of tracts. We demonstrate the proposed method on several fiber tracts from DT-MRI data of the normal human brain.

1 Introduction

Diffusion tensor magnetic resonance imaging (DT-MRI) has the ability to reveal *in vivo* properties of white matter tissue in the human brain. As such, DT-MRI is becoming a powerful technique for clinical studies of white matter abnormalities in neurological disorders as well as studies of normal brain development. The usefullness of diffusion imaging relies on the fact that the motion of water is impeded in directions that are not parallel to the axons. In DT-MRI a diffusion tensor at each voxel gives an estimated model of the pattern of water diffusion aggregated over a point-spread function of the measurements. The neural fiber orientation is typically inferred from the principal eigenvector of the diffusion tensor, which is the direction of highest probability of water motion.

Clinical studies have been mostly limited to analysis of white matter properties in a region of interest (ROI) [1,2]. Typically, statistics are computed on derived tensor measurements, such as fractional anisotropy (FA) or mean diffusivity (MD). This analysis is done either on a voxel-by-voxel basis or as an

N. Karssemeijer and B. Lelieveldt (Eds.): IPMI 2007, LNCS 4584, pp. 346–358, 2007.
© Springer-Verlag Berlin Heidelberg 2007

aggregate measurement within the ROI. Because of the complexity of the diffusion tensor data, registration of images to a common atlas for voxelwise statistics is particularly problematic. Recent work has explored statistical analysis of derived measures [3,4] and also of the entire tensors [5] along fiber pathways.

Much of the work in DT-MRI connectivity focuses on fiber tractography [6], in which streamlines are computed, by forward integration from a seed point, of the field of vectors defined by the principal eigenvector of the tensor at each point (interpolated between voxels), and where the twofold ambiguity of eigenvector directions is resolved by the continuity of paths. While tractography is an excellent tool for visualization of white matter pathways, it is not ideal for quantitative analysis for several reasons. First, imaging noise can cause fiber tracts to stray due to accumulating errors in the integration. The second issue is partial voluming. The finite size of a voxel measurement at fiber crossings (combined with sensor noise) can cause the direction of the major eigenvector to be ambiguous, further misleading the streamlines. This problem is aggravated by the fact that streamlines are often computed, displayed, and analyzed at subvoxel resolution—suggesting a level of precision that is not warranted by the data. Finally, region-to-region analysis with conventional tractography is challenging, because there is no way to steer tracts from a seed point toward a particular target region. To address these problems, several researchers propose tractography algorithms that rely on a stochastic integration, in which flow vector are chosen from a distribution around the principal eigenvector. These stochastic techniques can be combined with Monte-Carlo simulations, which may include tens of thousands of paths from a single seed, of which only a small fraction will typically reach the target [7,8,9,10].

Several Hamilton-Jacobi (H-J) methods for white matter connectivity have been proposed to overcome some of the difficulties arising in tractography. These methods compute the cost of the shortest path from a seed region to every pixel in the volume (usually a white-matter mask). This cost function consists of an integral that depends on path position and orientation, and typically penalizes paths that do not agree with the tensors. These H-J formulations result in first-order partial differential equations (PDEs) which model evolving fronts whose speeds are determined by information from the diffusion tensor. These methods are inherently more robust to noise in the diffusion weighted measurements than standard tractography. Parker et al. [11] evolve a front with speed related to the inner product of the front normal with the principal eigenvector of the tensor. O'Donnell et al. [12] propose using the diffusion tensor as a Riemannian metric in the image domain and compute a front representing arrival time of geodesics beginning at a single seed point. Connectivity to that point is defined as a ratio of Euclidean path length to Riemannian distance. Jackowski et al. [13] use a speed derived as a function of the diffusivity magnitude in the front normal direction. They solve this Hamiltonian equation using a Lax-Friedrichs scheme, also beginning with an intial seed point. Pichon et al. [14] define a directionally dependent local cost function that extends the H-J framework to high-angular diffusion data. In all of these works, the end result is either a dense field of connectivities to regions or a set of optimal paths emanating from a seed region, which are determined by integrating the characteristics of the PDEs.

In this paper we present a new method for quantifying white matter connectivity based on a H-J formulation, which we solve with a front propagating method. However, unlike previous H-J methods, which solve for the minimal cost of paths emanating from a single region, we formulate a cost for a very large number of paths *between* two regions. This results in a measure of region-to-region connectivity as well as a volumetric representation of the pathway between the two regions, without any explicit integration of individual paths. This approach is targeted to the study of white matter circuits between functional regions of the grey matter. We demonstrate the quantification of white matter properties, including both full tensor and derived measurements, along fiber pathways using nonparametric regression.

2 Region-to-Region Connectivity

Our formulation of region-to-region connectivity is based on the principle of minimal cost paths. Using information from the entire diffusion tensor, we construct a local cost function based the current position and directionality of a path. This leads to a first-order nonlinear PDE that computes the minimal cost from a starting region to each point in the image. Unlike previous front-propagation methods for DT-MRI, we then solve for minimal cost from a second target region. The two solutions are then combined, giving the minimal cost through each voxel of paths restricted to travel between the two target regions.

2.1 Minimum Cost Paths

Given a path $c : [a, b] \to \Omega$, where Ω is a compact image domain, we define the total cost of c as

$$E(c) = \int_a^b \psi(c(t), T(t))dt, \tag{1}$$

where $T(t) = c'(t)/\|c'(t)\|$ is the unit tangent vector of c. The total cost is defined as the integral of a *local cost function*, $\psi : \Omega \times S^1 \to \mathbb{R}$, where $\psi(x, v)$ gives the cost of moving in the unit direction $v \in S^1$ from the point $x \in \Omega$. We require that the local cost be symmetric, $\psi(x, v) = \psi(x, -v)$, which is generally consistent with the model of diffusion through passive media.

This metric in (1) allows for a wide range of cost functions ψ that incorporate tangents. Pichon et al. [14] describe the properties of this metric, the choices of ψ for high-angular diffusion data, and the relationship between this cost function and the corresponding *speed* that controls the motion of the wavefront in the H-J formulation. In this work we use a quadratic (bilinear) local cost function, with the understanding that all of the results in this paper generalize to high-angular data using the methods described in [14]. Thus we have

$$\psi(x, v) = v^T M^{-1}(x)v, \tag{2}$$

where $M(x)$ is a symmetric, positive-definite matrix defined at each point $x \in \Omega$.

The relationship between the measured diffusion tensor and M must be considered carefully. For instance, several researchers [12,15] use as their cost, the bilinear product with the inverse of the diffusion tensor itself. However, even in ideal situations (straight bundles of healthy axons) [16], the tensors are not be perfectly anisotropic, because of some degree of diffusion between or through cells. Thus, good measurements of tissue with relatively high FA, such as in the corpus collosum, might have values as low as 0.7, which would not offer sufficient penality for paths that cross the principal eigen directions. Because of this, the paths are relatively unconstrained by the diffusion tensors themselves, and solutions tend toward the shortest paths in the Euclidean sense, rather than following the white matter tracts. The same is true if we use the tensors directly in a second order PDE and model the diffusion of water from the tensors [12]—the resulting connectivities spread too easily outside of the paths defined by the principal eigenvectors, which limits their usefulness. On the other extreme, we could construct tensors from the principal eigenvectors that produce a virtually infinite penalty (zero speed) for all other directions. This, however, would ignore any meaningful differences between different tensor shapes, including the case of oblate tensors which are thought to represent fiber crossings and provide virtually equal evidence for all directions spanned by the first two eigenvectors.

One middle ground between these two extremes is to *sharpen* the tensor, which is done by raising it to a power α. This must be combined with a normalization, and for this work we normalize by the tensor volume. If we consider the sharpened tensor to be speed (in the H-J formulation), which gives low cost along the principal eigen directions, the cost is the inverse, and we have

$$M(x) = |D(x)|^{\frac{1}{3}} \left(\frac{D(x)}{|D(x)|^{\frac{1}{3}}} \right)^{\alpha}, \tag{3}$$

where $\alpha > 1$ is a constant and $|D(x)|$ denotes the determinant of $D(x)$. The sharpened tensor field M has the following properties:

1. If $D(x)$ has eigenvalues $\lambda_i(x)$, then $M(x)$ has eigenvalues $\lambda_i(x)^{\alpha}|D(x)|^{\frac{1-\alpha}{3}}$.
2. $|M(x)| = |D(x)|$ for all $x \in \Omega$, i.e., tensor volume is preserved.
3. If $D(x) = aI$, then $M(x) = D(x)$, in other words, isotropic tensors are left unchanged.

We can consider all paths emanating from a region $R_1 \subset \Omega$. Let $u_1(x)$ denote the minimal cost as defined by (1) over all paths beginning in the region R_1 and terminating at the point x. Then u_1 satisfies the first-order equation

$$\|\nabla u_1(x)\| = \psi\left(x, \nabla u / \|\nabla u\|\right), \tag{4}$$

with initial conditions $u_1(R_1) = 0$.

2.2 Costs Between Regions

While u_1 gives us a measure of the connectivity from the region R_1 to any point in the image, we would like to assess the specific connectivity to a second target

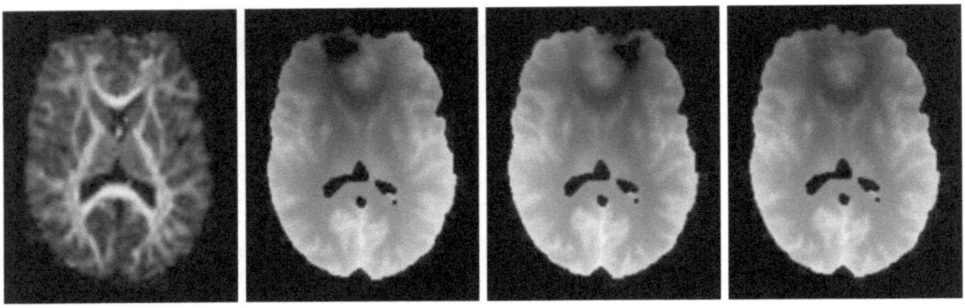

Fig. 1. An axial slice from the FA image with regions R_1 and R_2 highlighted (left). The cost functions u_1 and u_2 (middle two). The total cost function $u = u_1 + u_2$ (right).

region. To do this, we define a second region $R_2 \subset \Omega$ and corresponding minimal cost function u_2 also satisfying (4). Consider all paths beginning in the region R_1 and terminating in R_2. Now we define the *total cost function* for regions R_1 and R_2 to be $u(x) = u_1(x) + u_2(x)$. The value of $u(x)$ is the minimal cost of all paths between R_1 and R_2 *that are constrained to pass through* x. This is formalized in the following theorem.

Theorem 1. *Let $x \in \Omega$, and let Γ be the space of all paths $\gamma : [a_\gamma, b_\gamma] \to \Omega$ such that $\gamma(a_\gamma) \in R_1$ and $\gamma(b_\gamma) \in R_2$ and $\gamma(t) = x$ for some $t \in [a_\gamma, b_\gamma]$, then $u(x)$ satisfies*

$$u(x) = \min_{\gamma \in \Gamma} E(\gamma).$$

Proof. By definition of the path space Γ, we can break any path $\gamma \in \Gamma$ into a path γ_1 from R_1 to the point x and a path γ_2 from the point x to the region R_2. We thus have $E(\gamma) = E(\gamma_1) + E(\gamma_2)$. Because $u_1(x)$ minimizes the cost $E(\gamma_1)$ and $u_2(x)$ minimizes the cost $E(\gamma_2)$, $u(x) = u_1(x) + u_2(x)$ must also minimize the cost $E(\gamma)$. □

Thus, the function u assigns to each point x in the image the cost of that point being included in a pathway between regions R_1 and R_2. The construction of the total cost function u is demonstrated in Figure 1, showing a tract through the genu of the corpus callosum in DT-MRI data from a normal brain. If we assume a compact image domain Ω, then u must have a minimum value in Ω. As the next theorem shows, this minimal value is in fact achieved everywhere along the minimal cost path connecting the two regions.

Theorem 2. *Let $\gamma : [a, b] \to \Omega$ be the minimal total cost path with $\gamma(a) \in R_1$ and $\gamma(b) \in R_2$. Then u is constant along γ with $u(\gamma(t)) = E(\gamma)$ for all $t \in [a, b]$. Furthermore, $u(\gamma(t)) = \min_x u(x)$.*

Proof. Let $T(t) = \gamma'(t)/\|\gamma'(t)\|$ be the unit tangent vector of γ. Given any point $t_0 \in [a, b]$, we have $E(\gamma) = \int_a^{t_0} \psi(\gamma(t), T(t))dt + \int_{t_0}^b \psi(\gamma(t), T(t))dt$. Due to the symmetry of the local cost, $\psi(x, v) = \psi(x, -v)$, this implies that $E(\gamma) =$

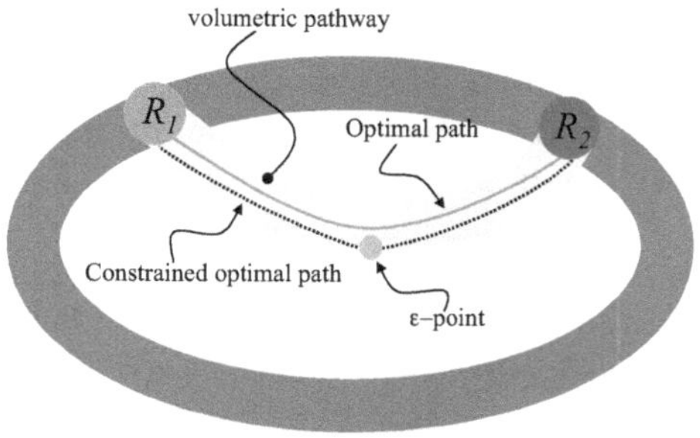

Fig. 2. Diagram of the volumetric connectivity framework

$\int_a^{t_0} \psi(\gamma(t), T(t))dt + \int_b^{t_0} \psi(\gamma(s), -T(s))ds = u_1(\gamma(t_0)) + u_2(\gamma(t_0)) = u(\gamma(t_0))$. Finally, if $u(\gamma(t)) \neq \min_x u(x)$, then there is a point $y \in \Omega$ with $u(y) < u(\gamma(t))$. However, by Theorem 1 this would mean there is a path from R_1 to R_2 with lower cost than γ, which is a contradiction. □

The properties described in Theorems 1 and 2 all generalize to the high-angular form of (1) so long as the solutions are symmetric, which is guaranteed by $\psi(x, T(x)) = \psi(x, -T(x))$.

2.3 Volumetric Connectivity

Here we define the framework for volumetric connectivity. Let γ be the minimal total cost path, and fix a threshold $\epsilon > 0$, which is the tolerance of paths relative to the optimum. We define an *ϵ-point* as a point whose constrained minimum cost is less than $(1 + \epsilon)E(\gamma)$. The set of all such ϵ-points defines a *volumetric pathway* between R_1 and R_2. This region is the set of voxels that belong to the fiber connection between R_1 and R_2. By definition, a volumetric pathway must contain γ for any value of $\epsilon > 0$. Figure 2 gives a pictoral representation of a volumetric pathway.

The total cost u along a pathway is obviously affected by the Euclidean length of that path. We wish to define a connectivity measure that is independent of the length of a path. Let c_x be the minimal total cost path constrained to pass through the point $x \in \Omega$. By definition, this path has total cost $E(c_x) = u(x)$. As described in Section 3.1, we can solve for $g(x)$, the Euclidean arclength of c_x using a first-order PDE. This allows us to define a *normalized cost* function, $\tilde{u}$, in a volumetric pathway as $\tilde{u}(x) = u(x)/g(x)$. The integral over the ϵ-region of the normalized cost in a volumetric pathway gives a length-invariant measure of the total connectivity of the represented pathway.

2.4 Numerical Implementation

We do not consider the problem of numerical solutions to (4) to be a significant aspect of this paper. However, in the analysis of circuits between large sets of cortical regions, the speed of solutions is a consideration, and the availability of the efficient numerical algorithms will be important.

Several options exist to solve (4) for the cost functions u_1, u_2. For instance, the Lax-Friedrichs method used in [13] is stable but excessively diffusive. Tsai et al. [17] propose a Gudonov approximation for the Hamiltonian, which includes one-sided deratives, and a sweeping method for iteratively updating the solution. In this case, the number of sweeps depends on the complexity of the data. We solve (4) using a new numerical method, the Fast Iterative Method (FIM), which solves the general static Hamilton-Jacobi equation using the Gudonov approximation, which gives an explicit solution for the characteristic direction, and thereby does not require differentiating the cost to obtain path lengths. The FIM updates a list of points whose solutions depend on updated points but are not yet final. This list of points is maintained by removing or adding points based on the convergence of the solution and their dependencies on solved points. The method iteratively updates solutions of the points until the list becomes empty. For full details of the FIM algorithm and implementation, see [18]. Because we are only interested in connectivity in the white matter, we use a white matter mask in which to compute the cost function solutions. For improved numerical accuracy we compute the solution on a grid supersampled by two from the original data. Supersampling is done on the original DWI measurements.

3 Nonparametric Regression of Path Data

Identifying white matter fiber connections as volumetric pathways leaves us with a collection of unparameterized voxels, defined on the original DTI grid, each of which contains information on the tensor, path cost, path length, and path orientation. This collection of raw voxel data offers several possibilities for quantification of the tensor data along these paths. One interesting possibility is the set of integral properties such as average FA, connectivity, etc. In this section we describe a nonparametric regression method for generating a compact statistical description of diffusion tensor data as a function of position along a fiber pathway. The first step is to compute a parameter s for each voxel in the pathway, which is the Euclidean arclength along the minimal cost curves. This arclength will serve as the independent variate in a nonparametric regression of the tensor data along the pathway. Using this regression, we compute mean and variance statistics along fiber pathways of the full diffusion tensor data as well as derived measurements, without any explicit integration of paths.

3.1 Solving for Distance Along Paths

For a given pathway we wish to find the Euclidean arclength along the constrained minimum cost paths between regions R_1 and R_2. We do this by solving a first-order, linear PDE that results in distance along the minimal path to individual targets. If $g_1(x)$ denotes Euclidean arclength along a minimal cost path from R_1 to the point x, it satisfies the advection equation

$$\nabla g_1 \cdot T_1 = 1, \tag{5}$$

where T_1 is the unit length tangent vector to the minimal path connecting each point in Ω to R_1. Likewise for g_2, T_2, R_2, and u_2. There are two possible strategies for evaluating the tangents, T_1. One strategy is the use the characteristics of u_1, which are given by $T_1 = M^{-1}\nabla u_1$, where ∇u_1 is approximated with finite differences, as described in [13]. Alternatively, the Gudonov approximation given in [17], which we use for this paper, requires an explicit calculation of the characteristic direction at each iteration. For this work, we save these vectors, after the solution has converged, and use them for T_1 in Eq. 5.

To solve (5), we use an iterative, fixed point strategy with an up-wind approximation of the gradient of g_1. The initial solution for g_1 is set to a Manhattan distance computed on the set of points for which the speed function is nonzero. It typically converges in several dozen iterations.

In this way, we can also compute the Euclidean arclength, $g_2(x)$, of the minimial cost path from R_2 to the point x. Summing these two distances, g_1 and g_2, we get the total arclength of the minimal cost path from R_1 to R_2 that is constrained to pass through the point x. We denote this total arclength as $g = g_1 + g_2$. The parameter that we use for the dependent variable in our regression is $s = g_1/g$, the percentage of arclength along the minimal cost path from R_1 to R_2. As such, the parameter s takes values in $[0, 1]$.

3.2 Path Regression

Let P be a volumetric pathway, and let $\{x_i\}_{i=1}^N$ be the collection of voxel locations within P. Each voxel has an associated parameter $s_i = s(x_i)$, as defined abovve. Denote by f_i a data value at the location x_i. This data may be a diffusion weighted value, a full diffusion tensor, or a derived measure, such as FA or MD. We compute a continuous description of the data as a function of s using a Nadaraya-Watson nonparametric regression [19,20] with a Gaussian kernel.

$$f(s) = \frac{\sum_{i=1}^N f_i G(s - s_i, \sigma)}{\sum_{i=1}^N G(s - s_i, \sigma)}, \tag{6}$$

where $G(\mu, \sigma)$ denotes a Gaussian with mean μ and standard deviation σ. We choose the kernel width σ used in the regression equation automatically, by minimizing the sum-of-squares cross-validation error. We solve this optimization using a Golden Ratio search. Typical values for the optimal σ are 1–4% of the path length. The function f defined above gives a continuous average of the data along the pathway. Given this mean function, we can use the same regression to estimate the variance of the data along the path:

$$\sigma_f^2(s) = \frac{\sum_{i=1}^N (f_i - f(s))^2 G(s - s_i, \sigma)}{\sum_{i=1}^N G(s - s_i, \sigma)}. \tag{7}$$

In addition to computing diffusion properties along a pathway, it is also possible to statistically quantify the geometry of the path in a similar fashion. Using

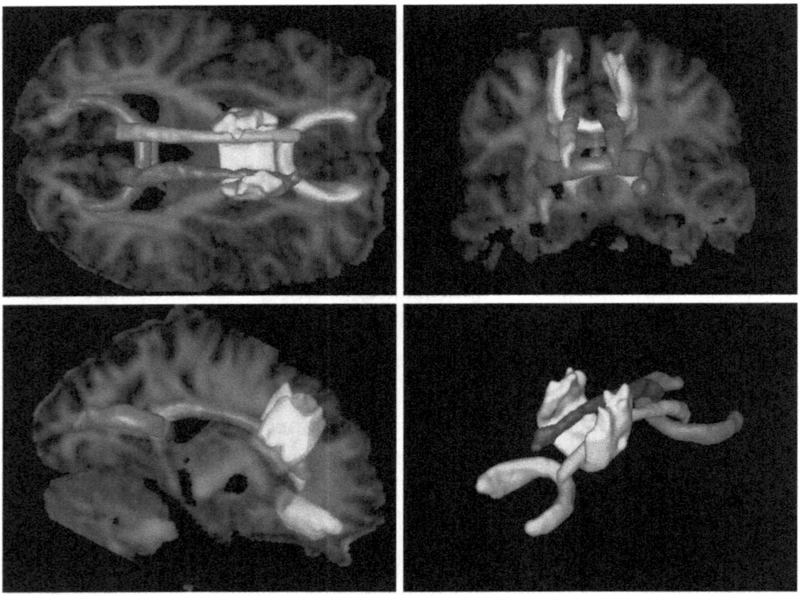

Fig. 3. Volumetric pathways for the GCC (cyan), BCC (yellow), SCC (red), LCG (green) and RCG (blue). Axial, coronal and sagittal views are shown against FA slices.

(6), we can compute the average voxel position along a pathway as a function of s. This results in an curve $(x(s), y(s), z(s))$, which represents the average geometry of the fibers in the connection. Once again, the σ is determined through optimality of the cross validation.

4 Results

We apply our quantitative DTI connectivity analysis to a single high-resolution ($2 \times 2 \times 2.5\text{mm}^3$) 3T image from a database of healthy controls. We selected five tracts for analysis: three bundles through the genu (GCC), splenium (SCC), and body (BCC) of the corpus callosum, and the left (LCG) and right (RCG) cingulum bundles. Using the FA image, we outlined the terminal regions R_1 and R_2 at the white/grey matter interface for each tract. An example of the segmented regions is shown in Figure 1.

For each of the five tracts, we solved for the total cost function u as described in Section 2.3. We chose an ϵ value of 0.10, i.e., we included voxels in the volumetric pathway within $\pm 10\%$ of the optimal total cost curve. Figure 3 shows the resulting volumetric pathways for the five tracts. Next we quantified the FA along each pathway using the nonparametric regression analysis. Figure 4 shows the original raw FA data from all the voxels included in the GCC volumetric pathway and also the mean and standard deviation result from the regression. The regression analysis for the FA of the other four tracts is shown in Figure 5.

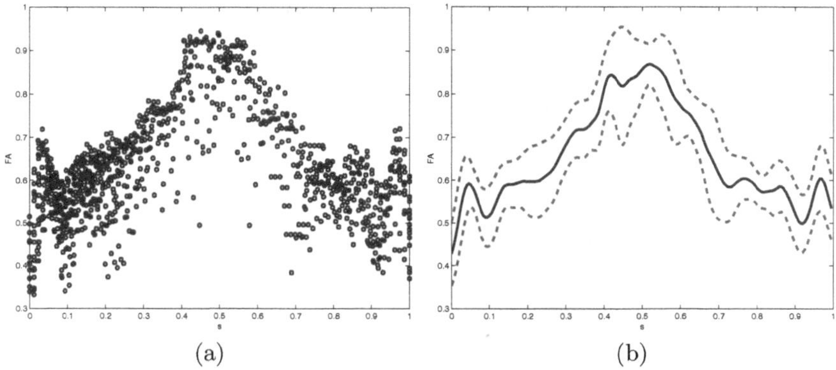

Fig. 4. FA along the GCC: (a) scatterplot of raw data, and (b) nonparametric regression. The solid curve shows average FA, and dashed curves show standard deviation.

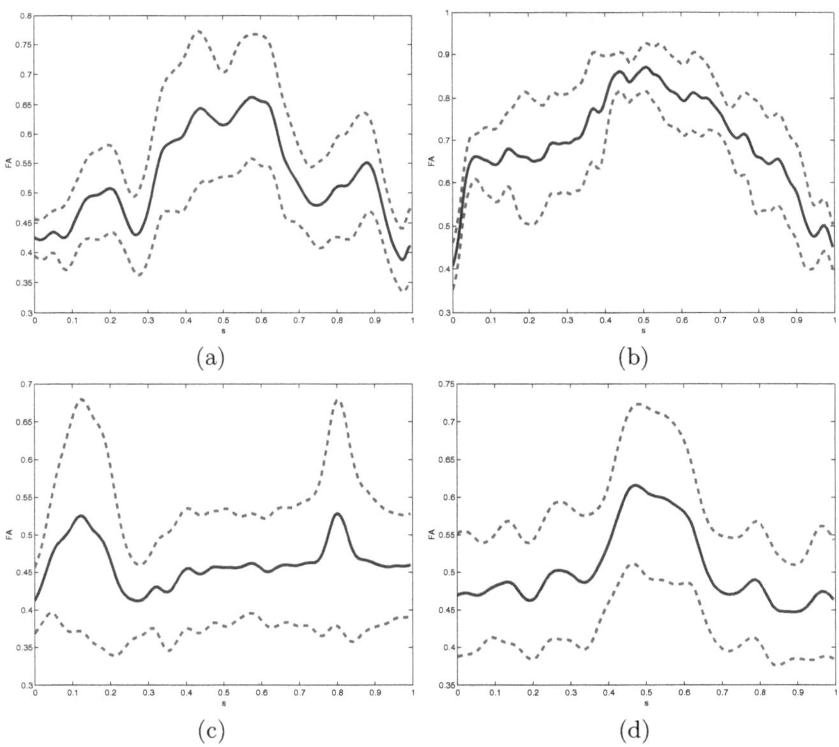

Fig. 5. Nonparametric regression of FA along the (a) BCC, (b) SCC, (c) LCG, and (d) RCG

Notice the similar pattern in each of the corpus callosum pathways, where the FA increases as it passes through the tightly packed fibers of the corpus callosum. In Table 1 we show the aggregate connectivity measurements for each tract,

Table 1. Mean connectivity metrics, normalized cost and alignment, for the five tracts

Measure	GCC	BCC	SCC	LCG	RCG
Norm. Cost	10.8	16.1	7.5	22.8	18.6
Alignment	0.797	0.789	0.708	0.611	0.788

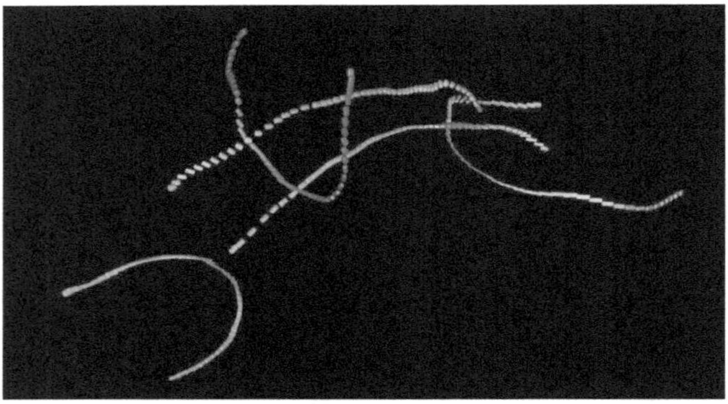

Fig. 6. Average diffusion tensors along the pathways displayed on the average fiber geometries. Rendered using superquadric glyphs [21].

including the average normalized cost $\tilde{u}$, and the average alignment, i.e., dot product, of the major tensor eigenvector and the tangent of the optimal curve at each voxel. Notice that the tracts through the corpus callosum, which have higher anisotropy, also have lower normalized cost (higher connectivity) than the cingulum tracts. The connectivity of the cingulum tracts is also reduced due to partial voluming with the adjacent corpus callosum tensors. Finally, we computed the average positions and average diffusion tensors along each tract, resulting in compact average fiber descriptions, shown in Figure 6.

Acknowledgement

This work is part of the National Alliance for Medical Image Computing (NAMIC), funded by the National Institutes of Health through the NIH Roadmap for Medical Research, Grant U54 EB005149. This work was made possible in part by software from the NIH/NCRR Center for Integrative Biomedical Computing, P41-RR12553-07. Additional funding was provided by Exxon-Mobil Upstream Research and Development. We thank Dr. Janet Lainhart, Dr. Andrew Alexander, Dr. Erin Bigler, and Molly DuBray, of NICHD U19 HD35476 (Neuroimaging component) and the Collaborative Program of Excellence in Autism for their practical support. We thank Dave Weinstein for help in creating visualizations using SCIRun [22], which was used in Figures 3 and 6.

References

1. Kubicki, M., Westin, C.F., Maier, S.E., Mamata, H., Frumin, M., Ernst-Hirshefeld, H., Kikinis, R., Jolesz, F.A., McCarley, R.W., Shenton, M.E.: Diffusion tensor imaging and its application to neuropsychiatric disorders. Harvard Review of Psychiatry 10, 234–336 (2002)
2. Lim, K., Helpern, J.: Neuropsychiatric applications of DTI—a review. NMR in Biomedicine 15, 587–593 (2002)
3. Ding, Z., Gore, J., Anderson, A.: Classification and quantification of neuronal fiber pathways using diffusion tensor MRI. Magnetic Resonance in Medicine 49, 716–721 (2003)
4. Jones, D., Catani, M., Pierpaoli, C., Reeves, S., Shergill, S., O'Sullivan, M., Golesworthy, P., McGuire, P., Horsfield, M., Simmons, A., Williams, S., Howard, R.: Age effects on diffusion tensor magnetic resonance imaging tractography measures of frontal cortex connections in schizophrenia. Human Brain Mapping 27, 230–238 (2006)
5. Corouge, I., Fletcher, P.T., Joshi, S., Gouttard, S., Gerig, G.: Fiber tract-oriented statistics for quantitative diffusion tensor MRI analysis. Medical Image Analysis 10(5), 786–798 (2006)
6. Basser, P.J., Pajevic, S., Pierpaoli, C., Duda, J., Aldroubi, A.: In-vivo fiber tractography using DT-MRI data. Magnetic Resonance in Medicine 44, 625–632 (2000)
7. Koch, M.A., Norris, D.G., M, H.G.: An investigation of functional and anatomical connectivity using magnetic resonance imaging. NeuroImage 16, 241–250 (2002)
8. Behrens, T., Woolrich, M., Jenkinson, M., Johansen-Berg, H., Nunes, R., Clare, S., Matthews, P., Brady, J., Smith, S.: Characterization and propagation of uncertainty in diffusion-weighted MR imaging. Magnetic Resonance in Medicine 50, 1077–1088 (2003)
9. Parker, G.J.M., Haroon, H.A., Wheeler-Kingshott, C.A.M.: A framework for a streamline-based probabilistic index of connectivity (PICo) using a structural interpretation of MRI diffusion measurements. Journal of Magnetic Resonance Imaging 18, 242–254 (2003)
10. Lazar, M., Alexander, A.L.: Bootstrap white matter tractography (BOOT-TRAC). NeuroImage 24, 524–532 (2005)
11. Parker, G., Wheeler-Kingshott, C., Barker, G.: Estimating distributed anatomical connectivity using fast marching methods and diffusion tensor imaging. Transactions on Medical Imaging 21, 505–512 (2002)
12. O'Donnell, L., Haker, S., Westin, C.F.: New approaches to estimation of white matter connectivity in diffusion tensor MRI: elliptic PDEs and geodesics in a tensor-warped space. In: MICCAI 2002, pp. 459–466 (2002)
13. Jackowski, M., Kao, C.Y., Qiu, M., Constable, R.T., Staib, L.H.: Estimation of anatomical connectivity by anisotropic front propagation and diffusion tensor imaging. In: MICCAI 2004, pp. 663–667 (2004)
14. Pichon, E., Westin, C.F., Tannenbaum, A.: A Hamilton-Jacobi-Bellman approach to high angular resolution diffusion tractography. In: MICCAI. 2005 180–187 (2005)
15. Lenglet, C., Deriche, R., Faugeras, O.: Inferring white matter geometry from diffusion tensor MRI: application to connectivity mapping. In: ECCV 2004 (2004)
16. Beaulieu, C.: The basis of anisotropic water diffusion in the nervous system – a technical review. NMR in Biomedicine 15, 435–455 (2002)
17. Tsai, Y., Cheng, L., Osher, S., Zhao, H.: Fast sweeping methods for a class of hamilton-jacobi equations. SIAM Journal of Numerical Analysis 41, 673–694 (2003)

18. Jeong, W.K., Whitaker, R.: A fast iterative method for eikonal equations. Technical report, Scientific Computing and Imaging Institute, University of Utah (2007)
19. Nadaraya, E.A.: On non-parametric estimates of density functions and regression curves. Theory of Probability and its Applications 10, 186–190 (1965)
20. Watson, G.S.: Smooth regression analysis. Sankhy'a Ser. A 26, 101–116 (1964)
21. Kindlmann, G.: Superquadric tensor glyphs. In: Proceedings of IEEE TVCG/EG Symposium on Visualization 2004, pp. 147–154 (2004)
22. SCIRun: A scientific computing problem solving environment, Scientific Computing and Imaging Institute (SCI), `http://software.sci.utah.edu/scirun.html`

Brain Image Registration Using Cortically Constrained Harmonic Mappings

Anand Joshi[1], David Shattuck[2], Paul Thompson[2], and Richard Leahy[1]

[1] Signal and Image Processing Institute,
University of Southern California, Los Angeles 90089, USA
ajoshi@sipi.usc.edu, leahy@sipi.usc.edu
[2] Laboratory of Neuro Imaging,
UCLA school of Medicine, Los Angeles, CA 90095, USA
shattuck@loni.ucla.edu, thompson@loni.ucla.edu

Abstract. Volumetric registration of brains is required for inter-subject studies of functional and anatomical data. Intensity-driven registration typically results in some degree of misalignment of cortical and gyral folds. Increased statistical power in group studies may be achieved through improved alignment of cortical areas by using sulcal landmarks. In this paper we describe a new volumetric registration method in which cortical surfaces and sulcal landmarks are accurately aligned. We first compute a one-to-one map between the two cortical surfaces constrained by a set of user identified sulcal curves. We then extrapolate this mapping from the cortical surface to the entire brain volume using a harmonic mapping procedure. Finally, this volumetric mapping is refined using an intensity driven linear elastic registration. The resulting maps retain the one-to-one correspondence between cortical surfaces while also aligning volumetric features via the intensity-driven registration. We evaluate performance of this method in comparison to other volumetric registration methods.

1 Introduction

Morphometric and functional studies of human brain require that neuroanatomical data from a population be normalized to a common template. The goal of registration methods is to find a map that assigns a correspondence from every point in a subject brain to a corresponding point in the template brain. Since cytoarchitectural and functional parcellation of the cortex is intimately related to the folding of the cortex, it is important when comparing cortical anatomy and function in two or more subjects that the cortical surfaces are accurately aligned. However, it is a non-trivial problem to find a map from a subject brain to a template brain which maps grey matter, cortical surface and white matter to the corresponding regions in the template brain.

Volumetric brain image registration methods [1,2,3,4,5,6,7,8] find a deformation field that aligns one volume to another using intensity values, ideally to establish a diffeomorphism between the two brain image volumes. Using intensity only typically results in accurate registration of subcortical structures,

N. Karssemeijer and B. Lelieveldt (Eds.): IPMI 2007, LNCS 4584, pp. 359–371, 2007.
© Springer-Verlag Berlin Heidelberg 2007

but poorer alignment of cortical features. Information such as landmark points, curves and surfaces can be incorporated as additional constraints in an intensity-based warping method to improve alignment of the cortical surface [9,10,11,12,13,14,15]. For example, landmarks, curves [13] and image matching [12] can be applied in a hierarchical manner in a large deformation framework to ensure generation of diffeomorphisms [16,17]. Hybrid methods such as HAMMER [18] implicitly incorporate surface as well as volume information in the alignment.

An alternative approach for studying the cortex is to use a surface based analysis. A number of surface-based techniques have been developed for inter-subject registration of cortices. These techniques involve flattening the two cortical surfaces to a plane [19,20] or to a sphere [21,22] and then registering the two surfaces in the intermediate flat space [23,21] or in the intrinsic surface geometry via covariant derivatives [24,25]. These approaches can be automatic [26,23], or semi-automatic using sulcal landmarks [24,25]. Although progress has been made towards automatic surface registration [26,23], accurate fully automatic registration remains a challenge.

The main advantage of a purely surface based method is that the cortical surface can be modeled at high resolution, producing a precise point correspondence between cortical surfaces such that sulcal landmarks are aligned. However, these methods do not define a volumetric correspondence, so one is restricted to analyzing only cortical effects. The goal of this paper is to develop a registration method in which we retain the advantage of accurate cortical and sulcal alignment within a fully 3D volumetric registration. This approach takes advantage of strengths of both types of methods: the ability of surface based methods to accurately align complicated folding patterns and the ability of volumetric intensity based methods to align internal subcortical structures.

The algorithm we develop consists of three steps: (i) extraction, labelling and alignment of the cortical surfaces, (ii) extrapolation of the surface mapping to the volume using harmonic maps, and (iii) refinement of the volumetric map using an intensity driven linear elastic warp. We describe the cortical surface extraction and alignment procedure in Section 3. The result of this alignment is a 2D parameterization of the two cortical surfaces in which sulcal landmarks are aligned. The extrapolation of these parameterizations to three dimensions is then computed using harmonic mapping, an approach which we review below. Finally, we use an intensity-driven linear elastic warp as described in Section 5.

A number of existence, uniqueness, and regularity results have been proven for harmonic maps [27,28,29]. Harmonic maps and their generalized counterparts, p-harmonic maps [30], have been used for various applications such as surface parameterization and registration [31,32], [20] and image smoothing [33]. Wang, et al. [34] describe a method for volumetric mapping of the brain to the unit ball $B(0,1)$. In recent papers, Joshi, et al. [35][36] described a method for combined surface and volume registration that used a similar three step procedure. In that case, the harmonic mapping used an intermediate unit ball representation which has the advantage of allowing the cortical surfaces to flow within each other. The distortion introduced in the intermediate space was corrected by associating a Riemannian metric with that representation. The limitation of this approach is that by using the map to the unit ball, the method is restricted to mapping only the cerebral volume contained within the cortical surface. Here we avoid this restriction by computing the harmonic map directly in Euclidean space so that the entire brain volume can be registered. We do this by fixing the correspondence between all points on the cortical surface rather than just the sulcal curves as in [35][36]. Since the map between the cortical surfaces is fixed, there is no longer a need for the intermediate spherical representation. While this approach places a more restrictive constraint on the mapping of the surface, in practice we see little difference between the two methods in the mapping of the interior of the cerebrum.

2 Problem Statement and Formulation

The registration problem is formulated in the following manner. We start by aligning the cortical surfaces, semi-automatically, using sulcal landmarks. We then use harmonic maps to extrapolate this surface mapping to the entire cortex. It is nontrivial to extend the surface map to the full 3D volumetric map due to large inter-subject variability in sulcal structures and the complicated folding pattern of the sulci. For example, the widely used linear elastic or thin-plate spline registration methods based on landmarks are not useful for this extrapolation due to their tendency to generate folds [37]. Harmonic maps, on the other hand, are particularly suitable for this task since they tend to be bijective provided that the boundary (the cortical surface in this case) is mapped bijectively [38,34]. The volumetric point correspondence obtained from these harmonic maps is then refined further using volumetric registration based on image intensity.

Given two 3D manifolds M and N representing brain volumes, with ∂M_1, ∂M_2 and ∂N_1, ∂N_2 representing surfaces corresponding to cortical grey/white matter and grey/CSF boundaries, we want to find a map from M to N such that (i) ∂M_1, the grey/white matter surface of M, maps to ∂N_1, the grey/white matter surface of N; (ii) ∂M_2, the grey/CSF surface of M, maps to ∂N_2, the grey matter/CSF surface of N; and (iii) the intensities of the images in the interior of M and N are matched. The surfaces, $\partial M_1, \partial M_2$ and $\partial N_1, \partial N_2$, are assumed to have a spherical topology. We solve the mapping problem in three steps:

1. Surface matching which computes maps between surface pairs - the cortical surfaces and the grey matter/csf surfaces of the two brains, with sulcal alignment constraints (Section 3);
2. extrapolation of the surface map to the entire cortical volume. This is done by computing a harmonic map between M and N subject to a surface matching constraint (Section 4), and
3. Refinement of the harmonic map on the interiors of M and N to improve intensity alignment of subcortical structures (Section 5).

3 Surface Registration

Assuming as input two T1-weighted MRI volumes corresponding to the subject and the template, cortical surfaces are extracted using the BrainSuite software [39]. BrainSuite includes a six stage cortical modeling sequence. First the brain is extracted from the surrounding skull and scalp tissues using a combination of edge detection and mathematical morphology. Next the intensities of the MRI are corrected for shading artifacts. Each voxel in the corrected image is labeled according to tissue type using a statistical classifier. Co-registration to a standard atlas is then used to automatically identify the white matter volume, fill ventricular spaces and remove the brain stem and cerebellum, leaving a volume whose surface represents the outer white-matter surface of the cerebral cortex. It is likely that the tessellation of this volume will produce surfaces with topological handles. Prior to tessellation, these handles are identified and removed automatically using a graph based approach. A tessellated isosurface of the resulting mask is then extracted to produce a genus zero surface which is subsequently split into two cortical hemispheres. These extracted surfaces are hand labeled with 23 major sulci on each cortical hemisphere according to a sulcal labeling protocol with established intra- and inter-rater reliability [39]. Grey

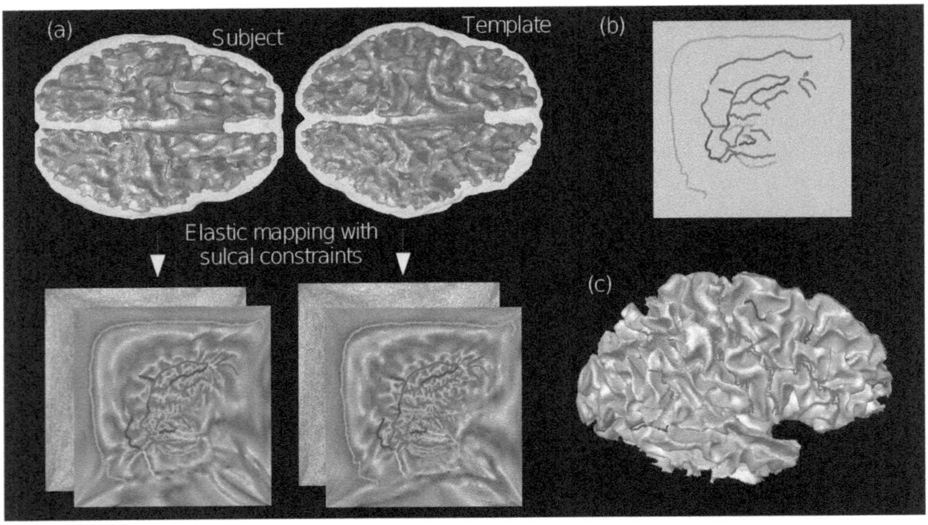

Fig. 1. (a) Our surface registration method involves simultaneous flattening and sulcal landmark alignment of the two cortical surfaces, which produces accurate sulcal mapping from one cortex to another. The outer grey matter/CSF surface is shown in semi-transparent grey color and the inner grey/CSF surface is opaque. Shown below are flat maps of a single hemisphere for the inner cortical surface of the two brains. (b) Mapping of the aligned sulci in the flat space and (c) sulci mapped back to the inner cortical surface of the template.

matter/CSF surfaces are extracted similarly except that topology correction was done manually by morphological operation tools in BrainSuite.

One method for alignment of surfaces with sulcal constraints is based on intrinsic thin-plate spline registration [25]. In that method, a deformation field is found in the intrinsic geometry of the cortical surface, which results in the required sulcal alignment. Covariant derivatives with the metric for the flat coordinates are used in order to make the deformation independent of the flat representation. The method requires the surfaces to be re-sampled on a regular or semi-regular grid in the flat space for discretization of the covariant derivatives. In addition to the loss of resolution, this leads to an added computational cost of interpolations for the re-sampling brain surface in the flat space. To overcome this problem, we follow a registration method described in [40] which registers surfaces by simultaneously parameterizing and aligning homologous sulcal landmarks. In order to generate such a parameterization with prealigned landmarks, we model the cortical surface as an elastic sheet by solving the linear elastic equilibrium equation in the geometry of the cortical surface using the form:

$$\mu \Delta \phi + (\mu + \lambda) \nabla (\nabla \cdot \phi) = 0, \tag{1}$$

where μ and λ are Lamé's coefficients and ϕ denotes 2D coordinates assigned to each point on the surface. The operators Δ and ∇ represent the Laplace-Beltrami and covariant gradient operators, respectively, with respect to the surface geometry. The solution of this equation can be obtained variationally by minimizing the integral on the cortical surface [41]:

$$E(\phi) = \int_S \frac{\lambda}{4} (\mathrm{Tr}\,((D\phi)^T + D\phi))^2 + \frac{\mu}{2} \mathrm{Tr}\,(((D\phi)^T + D\phi)^2) dS, \tag{2}$$

where $D\phi$ is the covariant derivative of the coordinate vector field ϕ. The integral $E(\phi)$ is the total *strain energy.* Though the elastic equilibrium equation models only small deformations, in practice we have found that it is always possible to get a flat map of the cortex by setting the parameters $\mu = 10$ and $\lambda = 1$.

Let ϕ_M and ϕ_N denote the 2D coordinates to be assigned to corresponding hemispheres of M and N brains respectively. We then define the Lagrangian cost function $C(\phi_M, \phi_N)$ as

$$C(\phi_M, \phi_N) = E(\phi_M) + E(\phi_N) + \sigma^2 \sum_{k=1}^{K} (\phi_M(x_k) - \phi_N(y_k))^2, \tag{3}$$

where $\phi_M(x_k)$ and $\phi_N(y_k)$ denote the coordinates assigned to the set of K sulcal landmarks $x_k \in M$, $y_k \in N$ and σ^2 is a Lagrange multiplier. The cost function is then discretized in the intrinsic surface geometry by finite elements as described in [40] and minimized by conjugate gradients. This procedure is applied to both the inner and outer pairs of cortical surfaces $\partial M_1, \partial N_1$ and $\partial M_2, \partial N_2$ to achieve a bijective point correspondence between each pair. This surface alignment and parameterization procedure is illustrated for the inner grey/white cortical boundary in Fig. 1.

4 Harmonic Mapping

The surface registration procedure described in Section 3 sets up a point to point correspondence between the pairs of surfaces $\partial M_1, \partial M_2$ and $\partial N_1, \partial N_2$. As noted earlier, treating these surfaces as landmarks is not helpful since they are highly convoluted and finding a volumetric diffeomorphism consistent with the surface map is non-trivial. One approach that can achieve such a diffeomorphism is to compute a harmonic map. A harmonic map $u = (u^1, u^2, u^3)$ from 3D manifold M to 3D manifold N is defined as the minimizer of the harmonic energy [29],

$$E_h(u) = \frac{1}{2}\int_M \sum_{i=1}^{3}\sum_{\alpha=1}^{3}\left(\frac{\partial u^\alpha(x)}{\partial x^i}\right)^2 dV. \qquad (4)$$

Note that (4) is quadratic in u^α and that the summands are decoupled with respect to α. Consequently the harmonic energy $E_h(u)$ can be separately minimized with respect to each component u^α, $\alpha \in \{1, 2, 3\}$.

We compute the minimizer of $E_h(u)$ using a conjugate gradient method with Jacobi preconditioner. The mapping of the two surfaces computed in the previous sections act as constraints such that ∂M_1 maps to ∂N_1 and ∂M_2 maps to ∂N_2. This harmonic mapping extrapolates the surface mappings to the entire volume such that the surface alignments are retained.

5 Volumetric Intensity Registration

The previous harmonic mapping step matches inner and outer cortical boundaries by computing a large deformation of the template brain to obtain a constrained bijective mapping between the two brain volumes. However, this map uses only the shape and not the MRI intensity values. Consequently we need a final small scale deformation to refine the mappings so that subcortial and extra-cerebral structures are also aligned. To compute this refinement we use a linear elastic registration method [6] as described below. We impose the constraint that cortical boundaries remain stationary during this refinement so that the cortical correspondence is retained.

Let $f_M(x)$ denote the MRI intensity value at location $x = (x_1, x_2, x_3)^t$ for the brain M and let $f_N(x)$ denote the MRI intensity value at location $x = (x_1, x_2, x_3)^t$ for the brain N. In order to find a smooth deformation field $d = (d_1, d_2, d_3)^t$ such that the mean squared error between MRI intensity values of the two brains $f_M(x+d)$ and $f_N(x)$ is minimized, we minimize the cost function

$$C(d) = \|Ld\|^2 + \alpha\|f_M(x+d) - f_N(x)\|^2 \qquad (5)$$
$$\text{subject to } d(s) = 0 \text{ for } s \in \partial M_1, \partial M_2$$

where $L = \nabla^2 + \mu\nabla(\nabla\cdot)$ denotes the Cauchy-Navier elasticity operator in M. By imposing the constraint (6) on the deformation field, we ensure that the surface alignment is not affected. Assuming that the deformation d is small compared

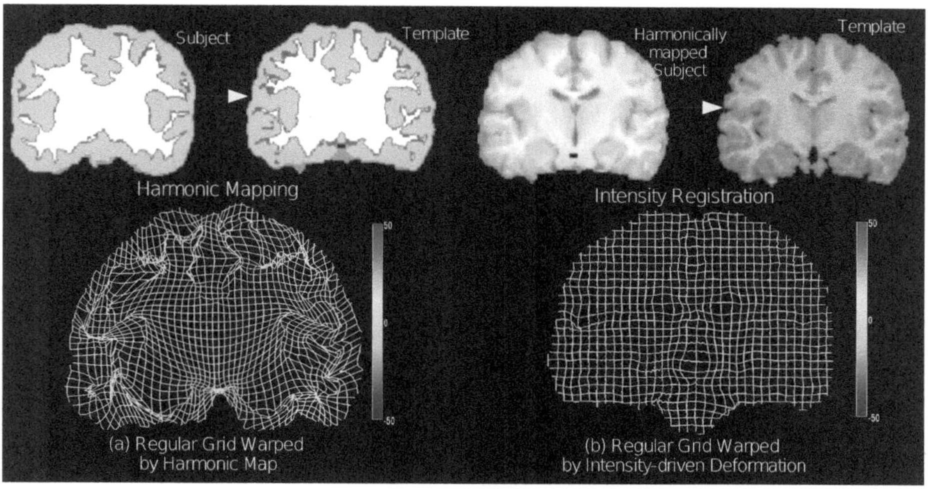

Fig. 2. (a) Illustration of the extrapolation of the surface mapping to the 3D volume by harmonic mapping. The pairs of surfaces are shown in red and green. The deformation field is represented by placing a regular grid in the central coronal slice of the brain and deforming it according to the harmonic map. The projection of this deformation onto a 2D plane is shown with the in-plane value encoded according to the adjacent color bar. (b) The result of harmonic mapping and linear elastic refinement of the subject brain to the template brain. Note that the inner and outer cortical surfaces, by constraint, are exactly matched. The linear elastic refinement produces an approximate match between subcortical structures. The deformation field here shows the result of cortically constrained intensity-driven refinement. Note that the deformations are zero at the boundary and nonzero in the vicinity of the ventricles, thalamus and other subcortical structures.

to the rate of change of f_M, then using a Taylor series approximation, we have $f_M(x+d) \approx f_M(x) + \nabla f_M(x) \cdot d$. Substituting this approximation in (5) and (6), we get

$$C(d) \approx \|Ld\|^2 + \alpha \|\nabla f_M(x) \cdot d(x) + f_M(x) - f_N(x)\|^2 \quad \text{subject to } d(s) = 0 \text{ for } s \in \partial M_1, \partial M_2 \tag{6}$$

Note that this is a quadratic cost function and can again be minimized by the conjugate gradient method. We use a preconditioned conjugate gradient method with Jacobi preconditioner.

This final refinement completes the surface-constrained registration procedure. While there are several steps required to complete the registration, each step can be reduced to either a surface or a volume mapping cast as an energy minimization problem with constraints, and can be effectively computed using a preconditioned conjugate gradient method. Thus, the entire procedure can be completed efficiently.

6 Results

In this section we demonstrate the application of the surface constrained registration procedure to T1-weighted MR brain images. We took the genus zero cortical mask, the tessellated cortical surface, the sulcal labels, and the original image intensities for two brains and applied our alignment procedure as described above. Shown in Fig. 3 are three orthogonal views of a subject before and after alignment to the template image. Note that before alignment the surfaces of the subject and template are clearly different, while after matching the subject surface almost exactly matches the morphology of that of the template. However, since at this point we do not take the image intensities into account, the interior structures are somewhat different. Following the final intensity-based alignment procedure the interior structures, such as the subject ventricles, are better matched to those of the template. There is no gold standard for evaluating the performance of registration algorithms such as the one presented here. However, there are several properties that are desirable for any such surface

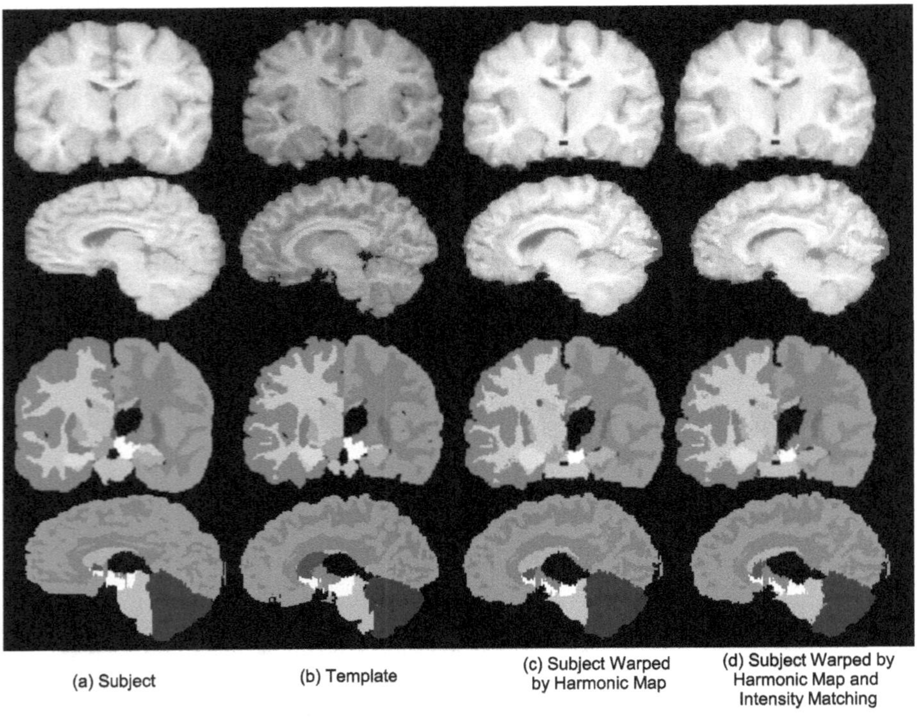

Fig. 3. Examples of surface constrained volumetric registration. (a) Original subject volume; (b) template; (c) registration of subject to template using surface constrained harmonic mapping, note that the cortical surface matches that of the template; (d) intensity-based refinement of the harmonic map of subject to template.

and volume registration algorithm. Our method for evaluating the quality of our registration results is based on the following two desirable properties:

1. Alignment of the cortical surface and sulcal landmarks. We expect the sulcal landmarks to be accurately aligned after registration and for the two surfaces to coincide.
2. Alignment of subcortical structures. We also expect the boundary of subcortical structures (thalamus, lateral ventricles, corpus callosum) to be better aligned after coregistration than before.

For evaluating performance with respect to the first property, we compared the RMS error in sulcal landmark registration for pair-wise registration of a total of five brain volumes. We performed a leave-one-out validation in which we removed one sulcus from the set of curves to be aligned and then computed the RMS error in alignment for that sulcus; the procedure was repeated for each sulcus in turn. The mean squared distance (misalignment) between the respective sulcal landmarks was $11mm$ using a 5th order intensity-only registration with AIR [3] and $11.5mm$ for the HAMMER algorithm [18,42], which uses a feature vector based on a set of geometric invariants. The RMS error for our approach was $2.4mm$. The difference reflects the fact that our approach explicitly constrains these sulcal features to match, which AIR and HAMMER do not.

For the second property, we used manually labeled brain data from the IBSR database at the Center for Morphometric Analysis at Massachusetts General Hospital. These data include volumetric MRI data and hand segmented and labeled structures. We first traced the 23 sulci for each brain. We then applied the HAMMER software and our method using the sulcal landmarks as additional constraints. To evaluate accuracy, we computed the Dice coefficients for each structure, where the structure names and boundaries were taken from the IBSR database. The Dice coefficient measures overlap between any two sets representing regions S_1 and S_2, and is defined as $\frac{2|S_1 \cap S_2|}{|S_1|+|S_2|}$ where $|\cdot|$ denotes size of the region [43]. A comparison of the Dice coefficients is shown in Table 6, where we show Dice coefficients for our method before and after application of the final intensity-based alignment step.

These results show superior alignment of cortical grey matter while HAMMER achieves superior alignment of subcortical structures. These results appear reasonable since HAMMER uses boundary information throughout the volume as part of the feature vector and thus can produce superior alignment of subcortical boundaries than our method which is based solely on image intensity. Conversely, the more specific cortical information in our approach leads to superior results in the cortical grey matter. Based on these preliminary observations, we believe that the approach described here could be appropriate for use in applications where cortical alignment may be of particular importance such as morphometric studies of cortical thinning, fMRI studies and analysis of DTI fiber tract data.

Table 1. Comparison of Dice coefficients and RMS errors in sulci

Subcortical Structure	AIR	HAMMER	Harmonic	Harmonic with intensity
Left Thalamus	0.7943	0.7365	0.6852	0.7163
Left Caudate	0.3122	0.5820	0.5036	0.6212
Left Putamen	0.6136	0.5186	0.4040	0.4700
Left Hippocampus	0.3057	0.6837	0.5661	0.5918
Right Thalamus	0.7749	0.8719	0.6645	0.7291
Right Caudate	0.3232	0.8107	0.4607	0.5474
Right Putamen	0.5370	0.6759	0.5229	0.5862
Right Hippocampus	0.3373	0.5974	0.5877	0.6988
Left Cerebral WM	0.5826	0.7858	0.9029	0.9118
Left Cerbral GM	0.6233	0.8388	0.9094	0.9117
Left Cerebellum WM	0.4092	0.6170	0.5333	0.6793
Left Cerebellum GM	0.5246	0.8597	0.7857	0.8227
Right Cerebral WM	0.5897	0.7938	0.9014	0.9113
Right Cerbral GM	0.6048	0.7208	0.9022	0.9050
Left Cerebellum WM	0.3686	0.5763	0.6474	0.6721
Left Cerebellum GM	0.5252	0.8535	0.8303	0.8604
RMS Error in Sulci	$11mm$	$11.5mm$	$2.4mm$	$2.4mm$

Acknowledgment

The authors would like to thank the Center for Morphometric Analysis at Massachusetts General Hospital for providing the MRI brain data sets and their manual segmentations. The MRI and segmentation data sets are available at `http://www.cma.mgh.harvard.edu/ibsr/`

References

1. Talairach, J., Tournoux, P.: Co-planar Stereotaxic Atlas of the Human Brain: 3-Dimensional Proportional System - an Approach to Cerebral Imaging. Thieme Medical Publishers, New York, NY (1988)
2. Ashburner, J., Friston, K.: Spatial normalization. In: Toga, A. (ed.) Brain Warping, pp. 27–44. Academic Press, London (1999)
3. Woods, R.P., Grafton, S.T., Holmes, C.J., Cherry, S.R., Mazziotta, J.C.: Automated image registration: I. General methods and intrasubject, intramodality validation. Journal of Computer Assisted Tomography 22, 139–152 (1998)
4. Hill, D.L.G., Batchelor, P.G., Holden, M., Hawkes, D.J.: Medical image registration. Phys. Med. Biol. 46(4), R1–R45 (2001)
5. Christensen, G.E., Rabbitt, R.D., Miller, M.I., Joshi, S.C., Grenander, U., Coogan, T.A., Essen, D.C.V.: Topological properties of smooth anatomic maps. In: IPMI 1995, 101–112 (1995)
6. Christensen, G.E., Rabbit, R.D., Miller, M.I.: Deformable templates using large deformation kinematics. IEEE Transactions on Image Processing 5(10), 1435–1447 (1996)

7. Glaunès, J., Vaillant, M., Miller, M.I.: Landmark matching via large deformation diffeomorphisms on the sphere. J. Math. Imaging Vis. 20(1-2), 179–200 (2004)
8. Avants, B.B., Gee, J.C.: Shape averaging with diffeomorphic flows for atlas creation. In: ISBI 2004, pp. 324–327 (2004)
9. Thompson, P.M., Toga, A.W.: A surface-based technique for warping 3-dimensional brain. IEEE Transactions on Medical Imaging 15(4), 1–16 (1996)
10. Downs, J.H., Lancaster, J.L., Fox, P.T.: Surface based spatial normalization using convex hulls. In: Brain Warping, Academic Press, San Diego, CA (1999)
11. Hartkens, T., Hill, D., Castellano-Smith, A.D., Hawkes, D., Maurer, C., Martin, A., Hall, W.H., Liu, C.T.: Using points and surfaces to improve voxel-based nonrigid registration. In: Dohi, T., Kikinis, R. (eds.) MICCAI 2002. LNCS, vol. 2489, pp. 565–572. Springer, Heidelberg (2002)
12. Davatzikos, C., Prince, J., Bryan, R.: Image registration based on boundary mapping. IEEE Transactions on Medical Imaging 15(1), 112–115 (1996)
13. Davatzikos, C., Prince, J.: Brain image registration based on curve mapping. In: IEEE Workshop Biomedical Image Anal, pp. 245–254 (1994)
14. Collins, D.L., Goualher, G.L., Evans, A.C.: Non-linear cerebral registration with sulcal constraints. In: Wells, W.M., Colchester, A.C.F., Delp, S.L. (eds.) MICCAI 1998. LNCS, vol. 1496, pp. 974–984. Springer, Heidelberg (1998)
15. Cachier, P., Mangin, J.F., Pennec, X., Rivière, D., Papadopoulos-Orfanos, D., Régis, J., Ayache, N.: Multisubject non-rigid registration of brain mri using intensity and geometric features. In: Niessen, W.J., Viergever, M.A. (eds.) MICCAI 2001. LNCS, vol. 2208, pp. 734–742. Springer, Heidelberg (2001)
16. Joshi, S.C., Miller, M.I.: Landmark matching via large deformation diffeomorphisms. IEEE Transactions on Image Processing 9(8), 1357–1370 (2000)
17. Gerig, G., Joshi, S., Fletcher, T., Gorczowski, K., Xu, S., Pizer, S.M., Styner, M.: Statistics of population of images and its embedded objects: Driving applications in neuroimaging. In: ISBI April 2006, pp. 1120–1123 (2006)
18. Liu, T., Shen, D., Davatzikos, C.: Deformable registration of cortical structures via hybrid volumetric and surface warping. NeuroImage 22(4), 1790–1801 (2004)
19. Hurdal, M.K., Stephenson, K., Bowers, P.L., Sumners, D.W.L., Rottenberg, D.A.: Coordinate system for conformal cerebellar flat maps. NeuroImage 11, S467 (2000)
20. Joshi, A.A., Leahy, R.M., Thompson, P.M., Shattuck, D.W.: Cortical surface parameterization by p-harmonic energy minimization. In: ISBI 2004, pp. 428–431 (2004)
21. Fischl, B., Sereno, M.I., Tootell, R.B.H., Dale, A.M.: High-resolution inter-subject averaging and a coordinate system for the cortical surface. Human Brain Mapping 8, 272–284 (1998)
22. Bakircioglu, M., Grenander, U., Khaneja, N., Miller, M.I.: Curve matching on brain surfaces using frenet distances. Human Brain Mapping 6, 329–333 (1998)
23. Tosun, D., Rettmann, M.E., Prince, J.L.: Mapping techniques for aligning sulci across multiple brains. Medical Image Analysis 8(3), 295–309 (2005)
24. Thompson, P.M., Wood, R.P., Mega, M.S., Toga, A.W.: Mathematical/computational challenges in creating deformable and probabilistic atlases of the human brain (invited paper). Human Brain Mapping 9(2), 81–92 (2000)
25. Joshi, A.A., Shattuck, D.W., Thompson, P.M., Leahy, R.M.: A framework for registration, statistical characterization and classification of cortically constrained functional imaging data. In: Christensen, G.E., Sonka, M. (eds.) IPMI 2005. LNCS, vol. 3565, pp. 186–196. Springer, Heidelberg (2005)

26. Wang, Y., Chiang, M.C., Thompson, P.M.: Automated surface matching using mutual information applied to Riemann surface structures. In: Duncan, J.S., Gerig, G. (eds.) MICCAI 2005. LNCS, vol. 3750, pp. 666–674. Springer, Heidelberg (2005)
27. Eells, J., Sampson, J.H.: Harmonic mappings of Riemannian manifolds. Ann. J. Math., 109–160 (1964)
28. Hamilton, R.: Harmonic maps of manifolds with boundary. In: Lecture Notes in Mathematics. 471, Springer, Heidelberg (1975)
29. Jost, J.: Riemannian geometry and geometric analysis. Springer Verlag, Heidelberg (2002)
30. Fardoun, A., Regbaoui, R.: Heat flow for p-harmonic maps between compact Riemannian manifolds. Indiana Univ. Math. J. 51, 1305–1320 (2002)
31. Angenent, S., Haker, S., Tannenbaum, A., Kikinis, R.: Laplace-Beltrami operator and brain surface flattening. IEEE Transactions on Medical Imaging 18, 700–711 (1999)
32. Kanai, T., Suzuki, H., Kimura, F.: Three-dimensional geometric metamorphosis based on harmonic maps. The Visual Computer 14(4), 166–176 (1998)
33. Tang, B., Sapiro, G., Caselles, V.: Diffusion of general data on non-flat manifolds via harmonic maps theory: The direction diffusion case. International Journal of Computer Vision 36(2), 149–161 (2000)
34. Wang, Y., Gu, X., Yau, S.T.: Volumetric harmonic map. Communications in Information and Systems 3(3), 191–202 (2004)
35. Joshi, A.A., Shattuck, D.W., Thompson, P.M., Leahy, R.M.: Simultaneous surface and volumetric registration using harmonic maps. In: Proceedings of SPIE Feb 2007 (2007)
36. Joshi, A., Shattuck, D., Thompson, P., Leahy, R.: Simultaneous surface and volumetric brain registration using harmonic mappings. IEEE TMI (submitted)
37. Eriksson, A.P., Åström, K.: On the bijectivity of thin plate transforms. In: Swedish Symposium on Image Analysis 2005, pp. 53–56 (2005)
38. Jost, J., Schoen, R.: On the existence of harmonic diffeomorphisms between surfaces. Invent. math. 66, 353–359 (1982)
39. Shattuck, D.W., Leahy, R.M.: BrainSuite: An automated cortical surface identification tool. Medical Image Analysis 8(2), 129–142 (2002)
40. Joshi, A., Shattuck, D., Thompson, P., Leahy, R.: A finite element method for elastic parameterization and alignment of cortical surfaces using sulcal constraints. In: Proc. of ISBI 2007 (2007)
41. Hermosillo, G., Chefd'hotel, C., Faugeras, O.: Variational methods for multimodal image matching. International Journal of Computer Vision 50(3), 329–343 (2002)
42. Shen, D., Davatzikos, C.: HAMMER: Hierarchical attribute matching mechanism for elastic registration. IEEE Trans. on Med. Imag. 21(11), 1421–1439 (2002)
43. Zijdenbos, A.P., Dawant, B.M., Margolin, R.A., Palmer, A.: Morphometric analysis of white matter lesions in mr images. IEEE TMI 13, 716–724 (1994)
44. Leow, A., Thompson, P.M., Protas, H., Huang, S.C.: Brain warping with implicit representations. In: ISBI, IEEE 2004, pp. 603–606 (2004)
45. Mémoli, F., Sapiro, G., Thompson, P.: Implicit brain imaging. NeuroImage 23(1), S179–S188 (2004)
46. Camion, V., Younes, L.: Geodesic interpolating splines. Lecture Notes in Computer Science, pp. 513–527 (2001)
47. Ge, Y., Fitzpatrick, J.M., Kessler, R.M., Jeske-Janicka, M., Margolin, R.A.: Intersubject brain image registration using both cortical and subcortical landmarks. In: Proc. SPIE May 1995, vol. 2434, pp. 81–95 (1995)

48. Christensen, G.E.: Consistent linear-elastic transformations for image matching. In: Kuba, A., Sámal, M., Todd-Pokropek, A. (eds.) IPMI 1999. LNCS, vol. 1613, pp. 224–237. Springer, Heidelberg (1999)
49. Mémoli, F., Sapiro, G., Osher, S.: Solving variational problems and partial differential equations mapping into general target manifolds. J. Comput. Phys. 195(1), 263–292 (2004)
50. Christensen, G.E., Joshi, S.C., Miller, M.I.: Volumetric transformation of brain anatomy. IEEE TMI 16(6), 864–877 (1997)

Probabilistic Clustering and Quantitative Analysis of White Matter Fiber Tracts

Mahnaz Maddah[1,2], William M. Wells III[1,2], Simon K. Warfield[3], Carl-Fredrik Westin[2], and W. Eric L. Grimson[1]

[1] Computer Science and Artificial Intelligence Laboratory, Massachusetts Institute of Technology, Cambridge, MA 02139, USA
[2] Surgical Planning Laboratory, Brigham and Women's Hospital, Harvard Medical School, Boston, MA 02115, USA
[3] Computational Radiology Laboratory, Children's Hospital, Harvard Medical School, Boston, MA 02115, USA*
mmaddah@mit.edu

Abstract. A novel framework for joint clustering and point-by-point mapping of white matter fiber pathways is presented. Accurate clustering of the trajectories into fiber bundles requires point correspondence determined along the fiber pathways. This knowledge is also crucial for any tract-oriented quantitative analysis. We employ an expectation-maximization (EM) algorithm to cluster the trajectories in a Gamma mixture model context. The result of clustering is the probabilistic assignment of the fiber trajectories to each cluster, an estimate of the cluster parameters, and point correspondences along the trajectories. Point-by-point correspondence of the trajectories within a bundle is obtained by constructing a distance map and a label map from each cluster center at every iteration of the EM algorithm. This offers a time-efficient alternative to pairwise curve matching of all trajectories with respect to each cluster center. Probabilistic assignment of the trajectories to clusters is controlled by imposing a minimum threshold on the membership probabilities, to remove outliers in a principled way. The presented results confirm the efficiency and effectiveness of the proposed framework for quantitative analysis of diffusion tensor MRI.

1 Introduction

In recent years, a significant amount of work has been devoted to extracting information from diffusion tensor images to study brain changes related to development, aging, and different pathologies. Developing tools to perform accurate and comprehensive quantitative analysis is thus of great interest [1]. However,

* The authors would like to thank A. Khakifirooz. Tensor estimation was performed with the unu tool, part of the Teem toolkit, available at http://teem.sourceforge.net. This work is supported in part by NIH grants P41 RR013218, U54 EB005149, U41 RR019703, P30 HD018655, R01 RR021885, R03 CA126466, and R21 MH067054 and by NSF ITR 0426558 from CIMIT, and grant RG 3478A2/2 from the NMSS.

N. Karssemeijer and B. Lelieveldt (Eds.): IPMI 2007, LNCS 4584, pp. 372–383, 2007.
© Springer-Verlag Berlin Heidelberg 2007

most clinical studies performed to date are limited to the analysis of local parameters, such as fractional anisotropy, measured in a manually defined region of interest (ROI) and averaged over groups of healthy and patient cases. Such methods are sensitive to the accuracy of specifying the ROIs and are prone to user errors. Others have performed a voxel-based analysis of a registered DTI dataset, which requires non-linear warping of the tensor field [2], which in turn needs re-orientation of the tensors [3,4].

An alternative approach is to compute the quantitative parameters of interest along the trajectories [1,5] which makes more sense as the underlying anatomical unit in DTI is a fiber tract, not a voxel. Such analysis is valuable especially if performed on a group of trajectories that correspond to an anatomical bundle of a fiber tract. To accomplish this goal, algorithms are required to segment the trajectories into bundles and to obtain correspondence between points on trajectories within a bundle.

Several papers have addressed the issue of grouping the trajectories into bundles [6,7,8] but without going further into quantitative analysis. The outcome of these methods is a set of labeled trajectories, each assigned to a cluster. Point-by-point correspondence between the trajectories of each cluster, however, is not determined rigorously. In one of the early works on DT-MRI analysis, Ding *et al.* [9] tackled the issue of quantification of tracts by finding the corresponding segments, which they defined as the portion of a trajectory that has point-wise correspondence to a portion of another trajectory. They assumed that the seed points of two trajectories to be compared correspond to each other, which is not the case unless all trajectories are seeded from a small ROI. The algorithm is thus inadequate for whole brain fiber analysis. Batchelor *et al.* [10] proposed different tools to quantify the shape of fiber tracts. They noted the problem of point correspondence but made the assumption that it is approximately achieved by proper choice of the seed point and regularly sampling the arc-length. With point correspondence roughly known, they applied the Procrustes algorithm to register the trajectories. There is also a series of work by Gerig *et al.* (see for example [1]), which described methods and applications for tract-oriented quantitative analysis. They dealt with the issue of correspondence by letting the user define a common origin for the set of trajectories in each cluster based on geometric criteria or based on anatomical landmarks. In their latest work [11], they also proposed the Procrustes algorithm for the registration of the trajectories to compute the average tensor. Although these methods provide some valuable information about the fibers, they suffer from a number of issues. They need manual setting of the common start points for all the trajectories in a cluster. Also, they assume the trajectories in a cluster have the same length, which is a reasonable assumption only if a small ROI is considered as the tractography seed points and the tractography algorithm gives full-length trajectories. Otherwise a thorough preprocessing is required. In our earlier work [12], we used a string matching algorithm to align all extracted trajectories with each cluster center at each iteration of our expectation-maximization (EM) clustering. The accuracy of this approach was limited by the simple curve matching algorithm used.

More sophisticated three-dimensional (3-D) curve matching methods could be performed but at the expense of increased computational effort [10].

This paper presents a clustering method that aims to facilitate quantitative analysis as the next step in the study of DT images. A statistical model of the fiber bundles is calculated as the mean and standard deviation of a parametric representation of the trajectories. Using this model representation, expectation-maximization (EM) is performed to cluster the trajectories in a mixture model framework. We obtain correspondence between points on trajectories within a bundle by building distance maps for each cluster center. The proposed method can potentially benefit from an atlas for the initialization step and as the prior map in the EM algorithm. All these tasks are done in a unified framework and the results are soft assignment of trajectories to labels and the point-by-point correspondence to each cluster center.

2 Similarity Measure

Determining the point correspondence between a pair of trajectories is not trivial [9,7] but if achieved, it not only makes the computation of their similarity, needed for clustering, straightforward but also makes it possible to measure the quantitative parameters within a bundle. Although many authors acknowledge that point-by-point correspondence of the trajectories should be defined by a curve matching algorithm for accurate clustering and quantitative analysis [1,10,9], to our knowledge this problem has not been solved to date. The difficulty lies in the fact that the number of trajectories is usually very large, especially when tractography is performed on the whole brain. This makes it computationally very inefficient, if not impossible, to perform a rigorous curve matching algorithm on every pair of trajectories. Here, we propose a novel approach for measuring the similarity of 3-D curves in a large dataset that includes the whole information of the curve for more accurate clustering and further quantitative analysis.

We treat each trajectory as a 3-D curve, i.e., an ordered set of points, $\mathbf{r}_i = \{\mathbf{r}_{ij}\}$. The set of trajectories is clustered into a number of subsets by assigning a membership probability p_{ik} to each trajectory, $\mathbf{r}_i$, to denote its membership in the kth cluster ($\forall i$, $\sum_k p_{ik} = 1$). For each cluster, a 3-D curve, $\boldsymbol{\mu}_k = \{\boldsymbol{\mu}_{kj}\}$, is defined as the cluster center where each point, $\boldsymbol{\mu}_{kj}$, is obtained as the average of all of its corresponding points on the trajectories: $\boldsymbol{\mu}_k = \sum_i p_{ik}\mathbf{r}_i^{(k)}$, where $\mathbf{r}_i^{(k)}$ is the trajectory $\mathbf{r}_i$, re-parametrized to have point correspondence to cluster k, and the summation is performed over all trajectories.

Our space includes a set of 3-D curves and a number of cluster centers. From each center, $\boldsymbol{\mu}_k$, we construct an Euclidean distance map:

$$\mathcal{D}_k(\mathbf{x}) = \min_j d(\mathbf{x}, \boldsymbol{\mu}_{kj}) \tag{1}$$

and the nearest-neighbor transform, $\mathcal{L}_k$:

$$\mathcal{L}_k(\mathbf{x}) = \arg\min_j d(\mathbf{x}, \boldsymbol{\mu}_{kj}) \tag{2}$$

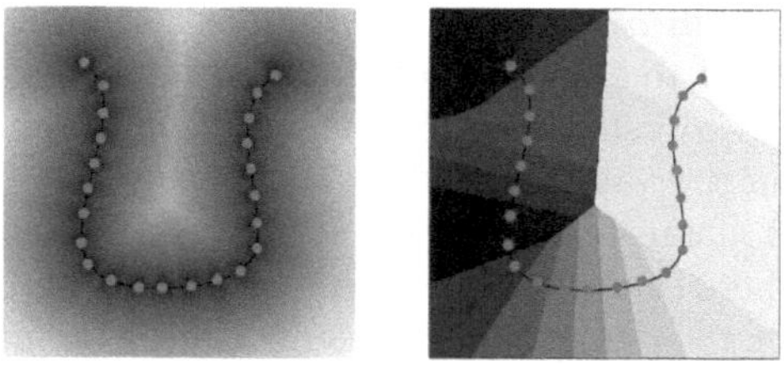

(a) (b)

Fig. 1. (a) Distance map from sample points on a cluster center and (b) the point correspondence label map with the center overlaid. Each region in the label map, displayed by a different color, consists of all of the points in the space that have the minimum distance to a specific point on the cluster center. Therefore, projecting any curve onto this label map determines the point correspondence of each of its samples to the center based on which region that sample is located.

where $d(\mathbf{x}, \boldsymbol{\mu}_{kj})$ is the Euclidean distance from the point $\mathbf{x}$ in the space to the jth point on the kth center. Each element of $\mathcal{L}_k$ will thus contain the linear index of the nearest point of the center $\boldsymbol{\mu}_k$. Fig. 1 shows the distance map and label map constructed from a sample 2-D curve. The label map partitions the space into Voronoi cells that each correspond to a point of the center. Now, for every curve, $\mathbf{r}_i = \{\mathbf{r}_{ij}\}$ in the space, the distance to the center $\boldsymbol{\mu}_k$ can be measured simply as:

$$d_E(\mathbf{r}_i, \boldsymbol{\mu}_k) = \sum_j \mathcal{D}_k(\mathbf{r}_{ij}), \tag{3}$$

and by projecting it onto the label map, its point correspondence to the center is readily achieved.

A spatial distance by itself does not encode enough information for measuring the pair-wise similarity. One obvious issue is the variable lengths of the trajectories. Another issue is whether the trajectory has one-to-one point correspondence to the cluster center, which is the case when they are similar in shape. Thus, any repeated or missing match represents shape dissimilarity. A penalty is therefore added if there are multiple points on the trajectory that correspond to a single point on the cluster center. We add the penalty term, d_{penalty} to the Euclidean distance and normalize it to the length of the fiber trajectory, L_i, to obtain the adjusted distance, $d_a(\mathbf{r}_i, \boldsymbol{\mu}_k)$:

$$d_{ik} = d_a(\mathbf{r}_i, \boldsymbol{\mu}_k) = \frac{d_E(\mathbf{r}_i, \boldsymbol{\mu}_k) + d_{\text{penalty}}(\mathbf{r}_i, \boldsymbol{\mu}_k)}{L_i}. \tag{4}$$

3 Mixture Model

In the previous section, we mapped our variable-length 3-D curves to a distance matrix, $\mathbf{d}_a = \{d_{ik}\}_{N \times K}$ where N is the number of curves and K is the number of clusters. Note that d_{ik}'s depend on the cluster centers, $\boldsymbol{\mu}_k$'s, which evolve during the EM algorithm as will be discussed in the next section. In other words, the trajectories are mapped to the distance space through the cluster centers. The goal of this section is to estimate the likelihood membership of each curve to each cluster based on the values of the d_{ik}'s.

In mixture-model clustering, the data set is modeled by a finite number of density functions, where each cluster is represented by a parametric distribution. A common choice for the density functions of the data points, d_{ik}'s here, is the Gaussian distribution. However, a Gaussian distribution does not accurately represent the nature of the 3-D distance of the trajectories from the cluster centers. In the simplest form, the number of possible trajectories with a given distance from the center grows linearly with the distance, while the probability that they belong to that cluster decays exponentially. Among the well-known distributions, the Gamma distribution well models this combined trend. Furthermore, this distribution belongs to the exponential family of distribution functions for which the convergence of the EM algorithm is guaranteed. Given that the d_{ik}'s are non-negative, we assume that distance metrics for each cluster follow a Gamma distribution with shape and scale parameters α_k and β_k, respectively:

$$\text{Gamma}(d|\alpha_k, \beta_k) = d^{\alpha_k - 1} \frac{\beta_k^{\alpha_k} e^{-\beta_k d}}{\Gamma(\alpha_k)} \quad \text{for } d \in [0, \infty) \tag{5}$$

where $\Gamma(.)$ is the gamma function. The mixture model then takes the following form:

$$p(\mathbf{r}_i|\Theta) = p(\mathbf{d}_i|\{\theta_k, w_k\}) = \sum_k w_k \text{Gamma}(d_{ik}|\theta_k), \tag{6}$$

where $\mathbf{r}_i$ represents a trajectory which is mapped to a vector of distance metrics, $\mathbf{d}_i = [d_{i1}, ..., d_{iK}]$ as described in the previous section, w_k's are mixing weights, and Θ is the collection of cluster parameters, $\theta_k = \{\alpha_k,\ \beta_k\}$, and the mapping parameter, $\boldsymbol{\mu}_k$. The goal is to infer Θ from a set of data points, $\mathbf{r}_i$'s, assumed to be samples of distributions with density given by Equ. 6:

$$\hat{\Theta} = \arg\max_{\Theta}\{\log p(\mathbf{r}|\Theta)\} \tag{7}$$

which gives a *maximum likelihood* (ML) estimation of the parameters. Since this estimation cannot be found analytically, the usual approach is to incorporate the *Expectation-Maximization* (EM) approach, which finds the local maximum of the likelihood function. Details are presented in the next section.

Cluster "no-match" (Outliers) – In mixture-model clustering, it is assumed that each data point is modeled by the mixture of a finite number of density components. However, in our case, there might be trajectories generated by the tractography that do not resemble any of the user- or atlas-initialized cluster centers or are not valid at all due to errors in the tractography stage. One way to deal with this issue is to allow the variance of densities to increase to accommodate these data. This would result in producing very spread bundles or even instability of the algorithm. A more practical alternative is to set a threshold so that if the membership likelihood of a particular trajectory in all clusters were less than that value, that trajectory would be removed from the processing data. In fact, with this threshold, the heterogeneity of the trajectories within each cluster is controlled. The larger the threshold is, the more compact are the resulting bundles, and consequently the greater is the number of unclustered trajectories. Handling outliers in such a principled way is not straightforward in previously proposed clustering schemes [7,8,12]. Unlike those methods, we allow the distribution of each cluster to have a different set of parameters (α_k's, β_k's), all inferred from the data by using the EM algorithm, and hence the user needs to set only the mentioned threshold to effectively remove the outliers.

4 Expectation Maximization Clustering

The EM algorithm produces a sequence of estimates of the parameters, Θ, and the hidden data, p_{ik}'s, in two consecutive steps:

Membership assignments(E-Step)– Assuming that the parameters of the clusters are known, the probability that the trajectory $\mathbf{r}_i$ belongs to cluster k is

$$p_{ik} = \Pr(k|\mathbf{r}_i, \Theta) = \frac{w_k p(\mathbf{r}_i|\theta_k)}{\sum_k w_k p(\mathbf{r}_i|\theta_k)}, \tag{8}$$

where $p(\mathbf{r}_i|\theta_k) = \text{Gamma}(d_{ik}|\alpha_k, \beta_k)$.

Updating model parameters(M-Step)– The updated mixing weights are calculated as

$$w_k = \frac{1}{N}\sum_{i=1}^{N} p_{ik}. \tag{9}$$

Unlike the Gaussian mixture model, there is no closed form to update the ML estimate of the shape parameter of the Gamma distribution. A good approximation can be made as [13]:

$$\alpha_k \approx \frac{3 - x + \sqrt{(x-3)^2 + 24x}}{12x}, \tag{10}$$

where

$$x = \log\left(\frac{\sum_i p_{ik} d_{ik}}{\sum_i p_{ik}}\right) - \frac{\sum_i p_{ik}\log(d_{ik})}{\sum_i p_{ik}}. \tag{11}$$

The ML estimate of the scale parameter is then updated by:

$$\beta_k = \alpha_k \sum_i p_{ik} / \sum_i p_{ik} d_{ik}. \tag{12}$$

With the point correspondence between each trajectory and cluster centers determined, the mapping parameter for each cluster is readily updated at each stage as:

$$\boldsymbol{\mu}_k = \frac{\sum_i p_{ik}\mathbf{r}_i^{(k)}}{\sum_i p_{ik}} \tag{13}$$

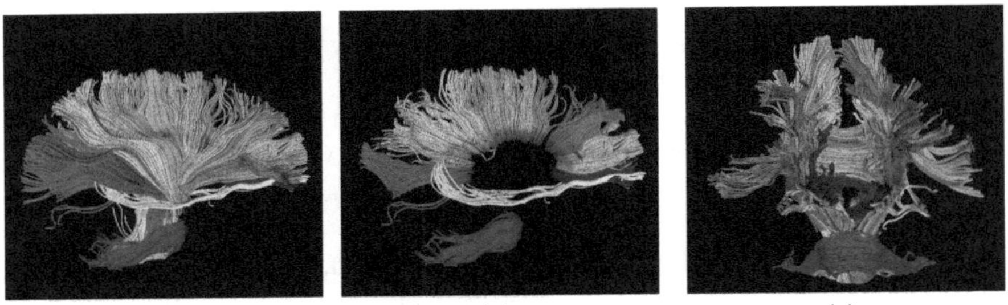

(a) (b) (c)

Fig. 2. About 3000 trajectories clustered to 25 user-initialized bundles. Clusters include different segments of the corpus callosum, tapetum, middle cerebellar peduncle, corticobulbar and corticospinal tracts, and different portions of thalamic radiation.

Initialization – We set the shape parameter of the Gamma distribution equal to one to have an exponential distribution which favors those trajectories most similar to the initial center. The scale parameter is then initialized to the mean values of data points of each cluster. The centers of clusters can be initialized manually by selecting a set of trajectories with different shapes from the data. Dependency of the algorithm on the initial centers will be discussed in Section 5. As an alternative, the initial cluster centers can be supplied by an atlas of fiber tracts, if available, such that the mean trajectories of the atlas clusters are employed after registering of the case to the atlas.

5 Results and Discussion

We applied our method on 3T DT-MR images with a spatial resolution of $1.054 \times 1.054 \times 2$ mm, acquired from healthy volunteers. The streamline tractography [14] was used to reconstruct the trajectories from 3-D diffusion tensor data. The stopping criteria was reaching a point with fractional anisotropy (FA) less than 0.15 or a change of direction greater than 45°. As a three-dimensional curve, we represent each trajectory with an equally-spaced sequence of points. In our implementation, the distance between the successive samples is 5 mm, so the number of samples are different for each trajectory.

Fig. 2 shows the results of clustering roughly 3000 trajectories from corpus callosum, middle cerebellar peduncle, corticobulbar, and corticospinal tracts into 25 bundles. As the initial centers, 25 trajectories from the data were selected manually, each representing an expected cluster. The membership probability of the trajectories to each cluster is obtained using the EM algorithm as described in Section 4. The trajectories in Fig. 2 are colored based on their maximum membership probabilities. One of the difficult bundles of fiber tracts to cluster is the cingulum. Even starting tractography from a user-defined ROI results in a set of disordered trajectories, mostly short in length because of low FA. Also, due to its adjacency to the corpus callosum, many callosal trajectories are included

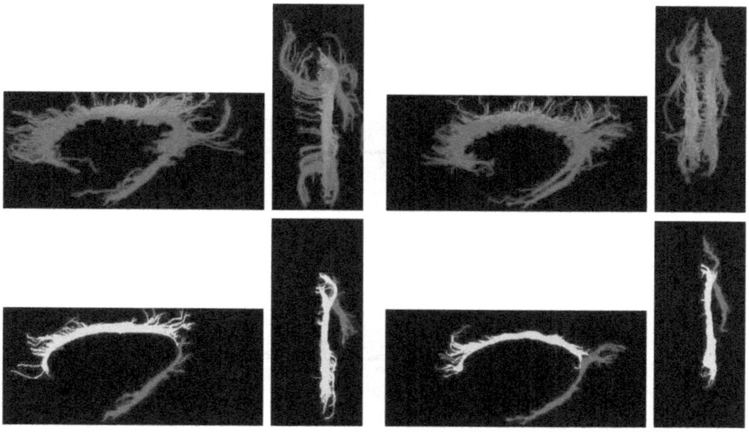

Fig. 3. Clustering of cingulum trajectories (top) into 2 bundles (bottom) for two healthy subjects. Saggital and axial views are shown for each case. Two arbitrary trajectories from the superior and inferior parts of the left cingulum were selected as the initial centers.

that adversely affect any further analysis of the bundle. As shown in Fig. 3 for two subjects, our method is well capable of clustering these trajectories into the desired bundles. Two arbitrary trajectories, one from the the superior and one from the posterior part of the cingulum were selected as the initial cluster centers. Knowledge of the point correspondence and hence rigorous calculation of the similarity measure is essential for clustering of such a disordered set of trajectories. Fig. 4 illustrates the evolution of the Gamma distribution for the clusters of the first case shown the Fig. 3. Convergence is achieved just after a few iterations of the EM algorithm. The Gamma distribution was initialized with $\alpha = 1$, corresponding to a exponential distribution, to value those trajectories that have no distance to the initial cluster center. However, as the algorithm proceeds, the Gamma distribution evolves from a very broad distribution to a narrow distribution with small but non-zero mode.

A spatial model of the fiber bundles represented by the mean trajectory and its spatial variation is also obtained. This is shown in Fig. 5 in which the abstract models of five fiber bundles are visualized by their spatial mean and isosurfaces corresponding to the mean plus three standard deviations (3σ) of the 3-D coordinates along the cluster center. Such an abstract spatial model for fiber bundles could be used for neurosurgery applications. It enables one to easily visualize the extent of the fiber tracts adjacent to the brain lesions to minimize the damage to the bundles when removing the lesion. Moreover, having the mean trajectory for each bundle of fiber tract allows us to study the shape of the bundle. As an example, the curvature versus the normalized arc length of the cluster centers are plotted in Fig. 6 for each cluster shown in Fig. 5.

To investigate the sensitivity of the clustering to the initial centers, we randomly selected different sets of trajectories from each cluster shown in Fig. 5.

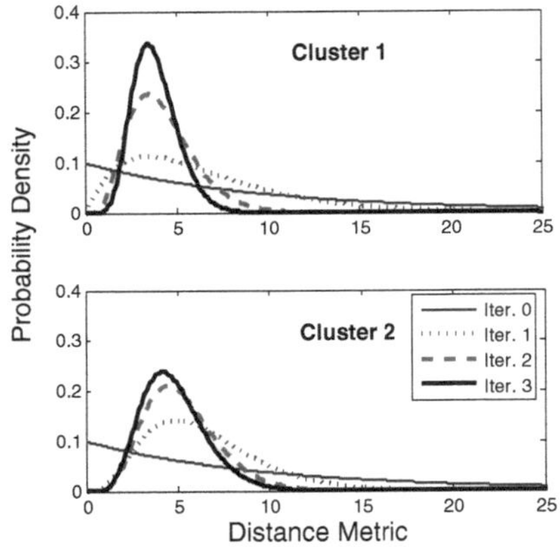

Fig. 4. Evolution of the Gamma distributions that describe the normalized distance metric for the two clusters shown on the left in Fig. 3. After just a few iterations, the distribution converges to a narrow distribution with small but non-zero mode.

At each run with one of the sets as the initial centers, the final centers obtained by the clustering algorithm are almost identical as shown in Fig. 7. This demonstrates the robustness of the algorithm with respect to the variations in the initial centers within each cluster. To demonstrate the suitability of our framework for tract-oriented quantitative analysis, we compute the mean and variation of the anisotropy parameters along the trajectories for clusters shown in Fig. 5. If any anisotropy measure, such as fractional anisotropy (FA) or the eigenvalues, or any of the local shape descriptors, such as curvature and torsion, are available along the trajectories, calculation of the mean and standard deviation of that parameter is quite straightforward. In fact, with the point correspondence obtained using the distance map described in Section 2, no further alignment of the quantitative parameters is necessary. Thus, similar to the computation of spatial mean and covariance of the clusters, performed in the M-stage of the EM algorithm, the mean and standard deviation of the parameters are obtained considering the membership probabilities of trajectories. Fig. 8 shows the mean and standard deviation of FA values along the normalized arc length of the cluster centers for each of the bundles in Fig. 5. To highlight the accuracy of our approach in aligning the fiber trajectories, the FA values along the aligned versions of all trajectories are also plotted (blue curves). These plots reveal the pattern of the FA values in the examined bundles.

Being able to perform such an analysis is valuable since it enables us to study the local changes of quantitative parameters along the fibers. This is especially interesting for study of temporal changes of fiber tracts during brain development and also opens new possibilities to compare normal and pathological subjects. The unavailability of efficient tools for tract-oriented quantitative analysis has limited most clinical studies to date to evaluation of scalar averages of parameters over an ROI. Local variations that provide significant information about brain development [15] and pathologies [16] are thus lost in the course of study.

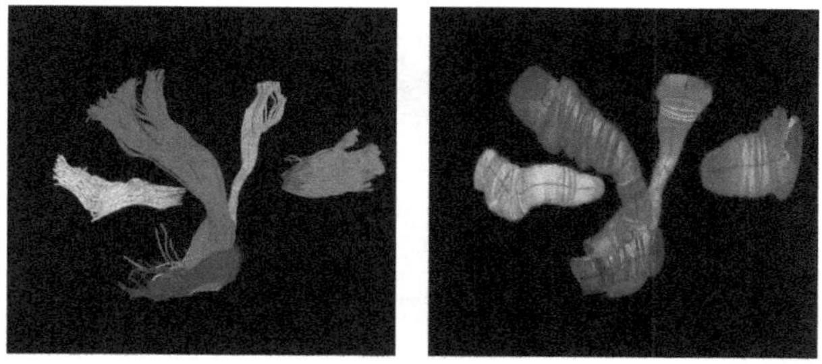

(a) (b)

Fig. 5. (a) Trajectories of 5 different clusters used for quantitative analysis: splenium (yellow), corticospinal (red), corticobulbar (green), middle cerebellar peduncle (blue), and genu (magenta). (b) A model representation of the bundles as the mean trajectory and the isosurfaces corresponding to spatial variation of the clusters.

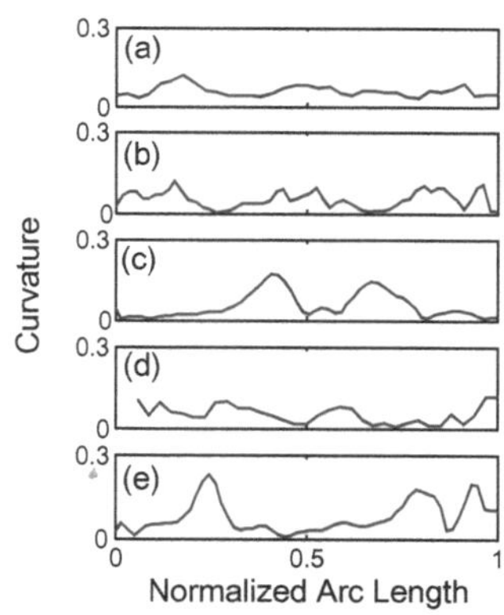

Fig. 6. Curvature of the cluster center along its normalized arc length for fiber bundles shown in Fig. 5: (a) splenium, (b) genu, (c) middle cerebellar peduncle, (d) corticospinal, and (e) corticobulbar fiber tracts.

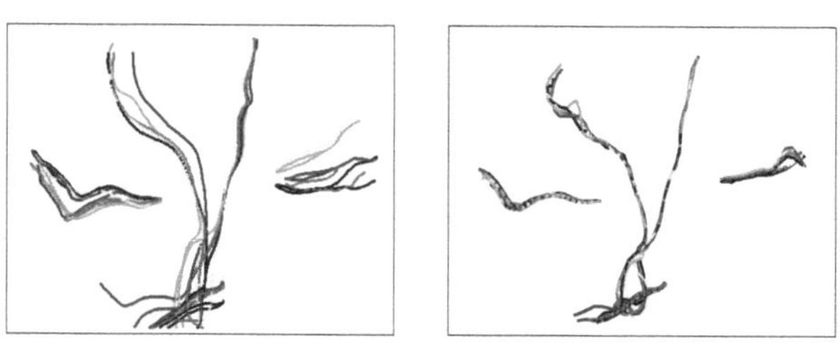

(a) (b)

Fig. 7. Robustness of the EM algorithm with respect to the initial cluster centers. The algorithm was run 5 times with different initial centers (a) to cluster the trajectories in Fig. 5. Final cluster centers collected in (b) show little dependence on initial centers.

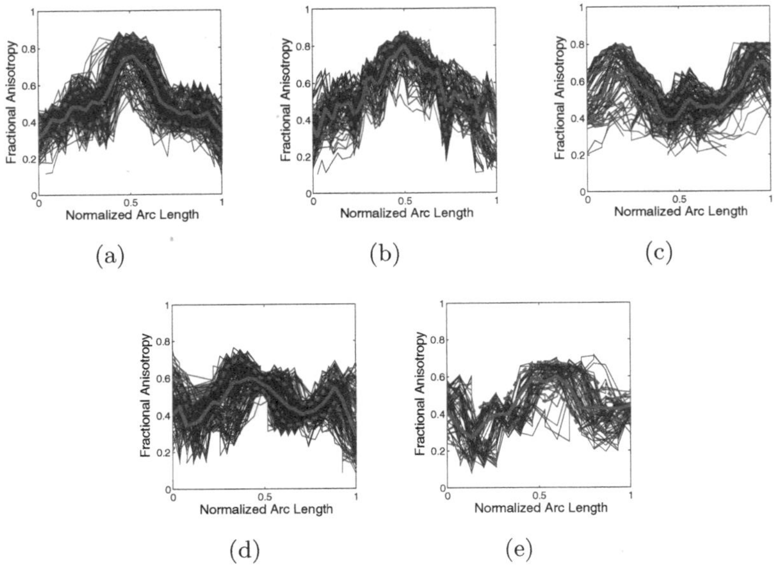

Fig. 8. Fractional anisotropy vs. normalized arc length for fiber bundles in Fig. 5: (a) splenium, (b) genu, (c) middle cerebellar peduncle, (d) corticospinal, and (e) corticobulbar fiber tracts

6 Conclusion

We demonstrated joint clustering and point-by-point mapping of white matter fiber trajectories using an EM algorithm in a Gamma mixture model context. The Gamma distribution enabled us to effectively model the normalized distance of the trajectories from each cluster center. Point correspondence of trajectories was obtained by constructing a distance map from each cluster centers at every EM iteration. This provides a time-efficient alternative to pairwise curve matching of all trajectories with respect to each cluster center. Probabilistic assignment of the trajectories to clusters was controlled with a minimum threshold on the membership posteriors, to offer flexibility in trading off between the robustness of the clusters and the number of outliers. Point correspondence calculated in our algorithm is an essential requirement of the tract-orientated quantitative analysis which is overlooked in previous works.

References

1. Gerig, G., Gouttard, S., Corouge, I.: Analysis of brain white matter via fiber tract modeling. In: Proc. IEEE Int. Conf. EMBS 2004 (2004)
2. Ruiz-Alzola, J., Westin, C.F., Warfield, S.K., Nabavi, A., Kikinis, R.: Nonrigid registration of 3D scalar, vector and tensor medical data. In: Delp, S.L., DiGoia, A.M., Jaramaz, B. (eds.) MICCAI 2000. LNCS, vol. 1935, pp. 541–550. Springer, Heidelberg (2000)

3. Alexander, D.C., Pierpaoli, C., Basser, P.J., Gee, J.C.: Spatial transformations of diffusion tensor magnetic resonance images. IEEE Trans. Med. Imag. 20, 1131–1139 (2001)
4. Park, H.J., Kubicki, M., Shenton, M.E., Guimond, A., McCarley, R.W., Maier, S., Kikinis, R., Jolesz, F.A., Westin, C.F.: Spatial normalization of diffusion tensor MRI using multiple channels. NeuroImage 20(4), 1995–2009 (2003)
5. Fillard, P., Gerig, G.: Analysis tool for diffusion tensor MRI. In: Ellis, R.E., Peters, T.M. (eds.) MICCAI 2003. LNCS, vol. 2879, pp. 967–968. Springer, Heidelberg (2003)
6. Shimony, J.S., Snyder, A.Z., Lori, N., Conturo, T.E.: Automated fuzzy clustering of neuronal pathways in diffusion tensor tracking. In: Proc. Int. Soc. Mag. Reson. Med, 10 (2002)
7. Brun, A., Knutsson, H., Park, H.J., Shenton, M.E., Westin, C.F.: Clustering fiber tracts using normalized cuts. In: Barillot, C., Haynor, D.R., Hellier, P. (eds.) MICCAI 2004. LNCS, vol. 3216, pp. 368–375. Springer, Heidelberg (2004)
8. O'Donnell, L., Westin, C.F.: White matter tract clustering and correspondence in populations. In: Duncan, J.S., Gerig, G. (eds.) MICCAI 2005. LNCS, vol. 3749, pp. 140–147. Springer, Heidelberg (2005)
9. Ding, Z., Gore, J.C., Anderson, A.W.: Classification and quantification of neuronal fiber pathways using diffusion tensor MRI. Mag. Reson. Med. 49, 716–721 (2003)
10. Batchelor, P., Calamante, F., Tournier, J.D., Atkinson, D., Hill, D.L., Connelly, A.: Quantification of the shape of fiber tracts. Magn. Reson. Med. 55, 894–903 (2006)
11. Corouge, I., Fletcher, P.T., Joshi, S., Gouttard, S., Gerig, G.: Fiber tract-oriented statistics for quantitative diffusion tensor MRI analysis. Med. Image Anal. 10 (2006)
12. Maddah, M., Grimson, W.E.L., Warfield, S.K.: Statistical modeling and EM clustering of white matter fiber tracts. In: IEEE Int. Symp. Biomedical Imaging 2006, pp. 53–56 (2006)
13. Hogg, R.V., Craig, A.T.: Introduction to Mathematical Statistics, 4th edn. Macmillan, New York (1978)
14. Basser, P., Pajevic, S., Pierpaoli, C., Duda, J., Aldroubi, A.: In vivo fiber tractography using DT-MRI data. Magn. Reson. Med. 44, 625–632 (2000)
15. Berman, J.I., Mukherjee, P., Partridge, S.C., Miller, S.P., Ferriero, D.M., Barkovich, A.J., Vigneron, D.B., Henry, R.G.: Quantitative diffusion tensor MRI fiber tractography of sensorimotor white matter development in premature infants. NeuroImage 27, 862–871 (2005)
16. Goldberg-Zimring, D., Mewes, A.U.J., Maddah, M., Warfield, S.K.: Diffusion tensor magnetic resonance imaging in multiple sclerosis. J. Neuroimaging 15, 68S–81S (2005)

Multi-fiber Reconstruction from Diffusion MRI Using Mixture of Wisharts and Sparse Deconvolution

Bing Jian and Baba C. Vemuri

Department of Computer and Information Science and Engineering
University of Florida, Gainesville, FL 32611, USA*
{bjian,vemuri}@cise.ufl.edu

Abstract. In this paper, we present a novel continuous mixture of diffusion tensors model for the diffusion-weighted MR signal attenuation. The relationship between the mixing distribution and the MR signal attenuation is shown to be given by the Laplace transform defined on the space of positive definite diffusion tensors. The mixing distribution when parameterized by a mixture of Wishart distributions (MOW) is shown to possess a closed form expression for its Laplace transform, called the Rigaut-type function, which provides an alternative to the Stejskal-Tanner model for the MR signal decay. Our model naturally leads to a deconvolution formulation for multi-fiber reconstruction. This deconvolution formulation requires the solution to an ill-conditioned linear system. We present several deconvolution methods and show that the nonnegative least squares method outperforms all others in achieving accurate and sparse solutions in the presence of noise. The performance of our multi-fiber reconstruction method using the MOW model is demonstrated on both synthetic and real data along with comparisons with state-of-the-art techniques.

1 Introduction

As the only noninvasive and in vivo imaging method available today which allows neural tissue architecture to be probed at a microscopic scale, diffusion-weighted magnetic resonance imaging (DW-MRI) provides unique clues to the microstructure of tissues and to changes associated with various physiological and pathological states. By producing quantitative data of water molecule motion that naturally occurs in brain tissues as part of the physical diffusion process, DW-MRI has also been used to map the fiber orientation in the brain white matter tracks. This valuable information can be further exploited for neuronal connectivity inference and brain developmental studies [1].

Assuming a displacement probability characterized by an oriented Gaussian probability distribution function, diffusion tensor MRI (DT-MRI) [2] provides a relatively simple way of quantifying diffusional anisotropy as well as predicting the local fiber direction within the tissue from multidirectional DW-MRI data. However, the major drawback of diffusion tensor MRI is that it can only reveal a single fiber orientation in

* This research was in part supported by NIH EB007082, NIH NS42075.We thank Dr. Evren Özarslan for many technical discussions. The MRI data were obtained at the Advanced Magnetic Resonance Imaging and Spectroscopy (AMRIS) facility in the McKnight Brain Institute at the University of Florida.

N. Karssemeijer and B. Lelieveldt (Eds.): IPMI 2007, LNCS 4584, pp. 384–395, 2007.
© Springer-Verlag Berlin Heidelberg 2007

each voxel and fails in voxels with orientational heterogeneity [3], which makes DT-MRI an inappropriate model for use in the presence of multiple fibers within a voxel.

This limitation of diffusion tensor model has prompted interest in the development of both improved image acquisition strategies and more sophisticated reconstruction methods. Both spherical harmonic expansion [4] and the equivalent higher order tensor model [5] have been used to represent the diffusivity profile based on the Stejskal-Tanner mono-exponential attenuation model. Knowing that the peaks of the diffusivity profile do not necessarily yield the orientations of the distinct fiber populations, a number of model-independent approaches attempt to transform the multi-directional signals into a probability function describing the probability of water molecular displacement. The q-ball imaging (QBI) method approximates the radial integral of the displacement probability distribution function (PDF) by the spherical Funk-Radon transform [6]. More recent studies have expressed QBI's Funk-Radon transform in a spherical harmonic basis [7, 8, 9]. Diffusion spectrum imaging (DSI) can measure the microscopic diffusion function directly based on the Fourier relation between the diffusion signal and the diffusion function, but is limited by the time-intensive q-space sampling burden [10]. The diffusion orientation transform (DOT) transforms the diffusivity profiles into probability profiles by explicitly expressing the Fourier relation in spherical coordinates and evaluating the radial part of the integral analytically [11].

Some multi-compartmental models have also been used to model the diffusion-attenuated MR signal using a finite mixture of Gaussians [3, 12, 13]. A continuous extension of the finite discrete mixture model is the spherical deconvolution method [14]. Compared to the multi-compartment models, the spherical deconvolution framework has two significant advantages. *First*, it is not required to specify the number of underlying fiber populations before deconvolution while this number has to be known in order to build the multi-compartment models. *Second*, the spherical deconvolution methods often yield a linear system which can be solved efficiently while the multi-compartment models usually involve the expensive nonlinear fitting. Recognizing these merits of the spherical deconvolution framework, recently many researchers have proposed a number of variants of spherical deconvolution approaches [7, 15, 16] with different choices of basis functions, deconvolution kernels and regularization schemes.

In this paper, we present a novel probabilistic model that significantly generalizes the traditional diffusion tensor model [2]. First, we assume that each voxel is associated with an underlying probability distribution defined on the space of diffusion tensors (the manifold of 3×3 positive-definite matrices). Conceptually, our model can be viewed as a natural extension of the multiple-compartment models [3, 13]. Moreover, this extension relates the continuous mixture model to MR signal attenuation through a Laplace transform defined for matrix-variate functions. It is worth noting that the Laplace transform can be evaluated in closed form for Wishart distributions and the resulting closed form leads to a Rigaut-type function which has been used in the past to explain the MR signal decay [17]. Our model naturally leads to a deconvolution formulation of the multi-fiber reconstruction problem, where the deconvolution kernel is the Laplace transform kernel and the basis functions are Wishart distributions. We develop an efficient and robust scheme for reconstructing the multiple fiber bundles using the proposed model and show several comparisons with other state-of-the-art methods.

2 Theory

By generalizing the discrete Gaussian mixture model to the continuous case, we postulate that at each voxel there is an underlying probability measure associated with the manifold of $n \times n$ symmetric positive-definite matrices, $\mathcal{P}_n$ (by default $\mathcal{P}_3$). Let $f(\mathsf{D})$ be its density function with respect to some carrier measure $\mathrm{d}\mathsf{D}$ on $\mathcal{P}_n$. Then the diffusion weighted MR signal $S(\boldsymbol{q})$ can be modeled as:

$$S(\boldsymbol{q})/S_0 = \int_{\mathcal{P}_n} f(\mathsf{D}) \exp[-b\boldsymbol{g}^T \mathsf{D}\boldsymbol{g}] \, \mathrm{d}\mathsf{D} \,, \tag{1}$$

where S_0 is the signal in the absence of diffusion weighting gradient, $\boldsymbol{q}$ encodes the magnitude (G) and direction ($\boldsymbol{g}$) of the diffusion sensitizing gradients, and b is the diffusion weighting factor depending on the strength as well as the effective time of diffusion. Note that Eq. (1) implies a continuous form of mixture model with $f(\mathsf{D})$ being a mixing density over the components in the mixture. Clearly, our model simplifies to the diffusion tensor model when the underlying probability measure is the Dirac measure.

Since $b\boldsymbol{g}^T \mathsf{D}\boldsymbol{g}$ in Eq.(1) can be replaced by $\mathrm{trace}(\mathsf{BD})$ where $\mathsf{B} = b\boldsymbol{g}\boldsymbol{g}^T$, the equation (1) can be expressed as the Laplace transform (matrix variable case) [18]:

$$S(\boldsymbol{q})/S_0 = \int_{\mathcal{P}_n} \exp(-\mathrm{trace}(\mathsf{BD}))\, f(\mathsf{D})\mathrm{d}\mathsf{D} = (\mathscr{L}_f)(\mathsf{B}) \,, \tag{2}$$

where $\mathscr{L}_f$ denotes the Laplace transform of a function f which takes its argument as symmetric positive definite matrices from $\mathcal{P}_n$.

This expression naturally leads to an inverse problem: recovering of a distribution defined on $\mathcal{P}_n$ that best explains the observed diffusion signal $S(\boldsymbol{q})$. This is an ill-posed problem and in general is intractable without prior knowledge of the probabilistic structure. In conventional DT-MRI, the diffusion tensor is usually estimated by solving a linear or nonlinear least squares problem, which amounts to applying the maximum likelihood estimator. Instead our approach views the diffusion tensor as random variable (matrix) belonging to some known distribution family, which allows us to model the uncertainty in the diffusion tensor estimation. Note that in DT-MRI, the diffusion tensor can be interpreted as the concentration matrix (inverse of the covariance matrix) of the Gaussian distribution in the q-space. It is a common practice to put a Wishart distribution (see definition below) prior, on the concentration matrix in multivariate analysis. Moreover, in the case of a Wishart distribution, a closed form expression for the Laplace transform exists and leads to a Rigaut-type asymptotic fractal law for the MR signal decay behavior which has been observed in the past (see explanation below).

Definition 1. *[18] For $\Sigma \in \mathcal{P}_n$ and for p in $\left(\frac{n-1}{2}, \infty\right)$, the Wishart distribution $\gamma_{p,\Sigma}$ with scale parameter Σ and shape parameter p is defined as* [1]

$$\mathrm{d}\gamma_{p,\Sigma}(\mathsf{Y}) = \Gamma_n(p)^{-1} \,|\mathsf{Y}|^{p-(n+1)/2}\, |\Sigma|^{-p}\, e^{-\mathrm{trace}(\Sigma^{-1}\mathsf{Y})}\, \mathrm{d}\mathsf{Y}, \tag{3}$$

where Γ_n is the multivariate gamma function and $|\cdot|$ is the matrix determinant.

[1] Note that the correspondence between this definition and the conventional Wishart distribution $W_n(p, \Sigma)$ is given simply by $\gamma_{p/2,2\Sigma} = W_n(p, \Sigma)$.

The Wishart distribution $\gamma_{p,\Sigma}$ is known to have the closed-form Laplace transform:

$$\int e^{-\mathrm{trace}(\Theta \mathsf{Y})}\, \mathrm{d}\gamma_{p,\Sigma}(\mathsf{Y}) = (1+\mathrm{trace}(\Theta\Sigma))^{-p} \quad \text{where } (\Theta + \Sigma^{-1}) \in \mathcal{P}_n. \tag{4}$$

Let f in (2) be the density function of $\gamma_{p,\Sigma}$ with the expected value $\hat{\mathsf{D}} = p\Sigma$. We have

$$S(\boldsymbol{q}) = S_0 \left(1 + (b\,\boldsymbol{g}^T \hat{\mathsf{D}} \boldsymbol{g})/p\right)^{-p}. \tag{5}$$

This is a familiar Rigaut-type asymptotic fractal expression [19] implying a signal decay characterized by a power-law which is the expected asymptotic behavior for the MR signal attenuation in porous media. Note that although this form of a signal attenuation curve had been phenomenologically fitted to the diffusion-weighted MR data before [17], until now, there was no rigorous derivation of the Rigaut-type expression used to explain the MR signal behavior as a function of b-value. Therefore, this derivation may be useful in understanding the apparent fractal-like behavior of the neural tissue in diffusion-weighted MR experiments. Also note when p tends to infinity, we have $S(\boldsymbol{q}) \to S_0 \exp(-b\boldsymbol{g}^T \hat{\mathsf{D}} \boldsymbol{g})$, which implies that the mono-exponential model can be viewed as a limiting case ($p \to \infty$) of our model.

The single Wishart distribution model has a drawback in that it can not resolve the intra-voxel orientational heterogeneity due to the single mode of the Wishart distribution. Hence it is natural to use a discrete mixture of Wishart distribution model where the mixing distribution in Eq.(2) is expressed as $\mathrm{d}F = \sum_{i=1}^{N} w_i \mathrm{d}\gamma_{p_i,\Sigma_i}$. In order to make the problem tractable, several simplifying assumptions are made as follows. First, in this model (p_i, Σ_i) are treated as the basis and will be fixed as described below. This leaves us with the weights, $\boldsymbol{w} = (w_i)$, as the unknowns to be estimated. Note that the number of components in mixture, N, only reflects the resolution of the discretization and should not be interpreted as the expected number of fiber bundles. We assume that all the p_i take the same value, $p_i = p = 2$, based on the analogy between the Eq.(5) and Debye-Porod law of diffraction [20] in 3D space. Since the fibers have an approximately cylindrical geometry, it is reasonable to assume that the two smaller eigenvalues of diffusion tensors are equal. In practice, we fix the eigenvalues of $\mathsf{D}_i = p\Sigma_i$ to specified values $(\lambda_1, \lambda_2, \lambda_3) = (1.5, 0.4, 0.4)\mu^2/ms$ consistent with the values commonly observed in the white-matter tracts [3]. This rotational symmetry leads to a tessellation where N unit vectors evenly distributed on the unit sphere are chosen as the principal directions of Σ_i. For K measurements with $\boldsymbol{q}_j$, the signal model equation:

$$S(\boldsymbol{q}) = S_0 \sum_{i=1}^{N} w_i (1 + \mathrm{trace}(\mathsf{B}\Sigma_i))^{-p} \tag{6}$$

leads to a linear system $\mathsf{A}\boldsymbol{w} = \boldsymbol{s}$, where $\boldsymbol{s} = (S(\boldsymbol{q})/S_0)$ contains the normalized measurements, A is the matrix with $A_{ji} = (1 + \mathrm{trace}(\mathsf{B}_j \Sigma_i))^{-p}$, and $\boldsymbol{w} = (w_i)$ is the weight vector to be estimated.

Like many existing reconstruction methods, our method can be cast into a unified convolution framework as follows:

$$S(\boldsymbol{q})/S_0 = \int_{\mathcal{M}} R(\boldsymbol{q}, x) f(x) \mathrm{d}x \tag{7}$$

In Eq. (7), the signal is expressed as the convolution of a probability density function and a kernel function. The integration is over a manifold $\mathcal{M}$ whose elements x contain the useful information like orientation and anisotropy. The convolution kernel, $R(\boldsymbol{q}, x) : \mathbb{R}^3 \times \mathcal{M} \mapsto \mathbb{R}$ represents the response derived from a single fiber. In order to handle the intra-voxel orientational heterogeneity, the volume fractions are represented by a continuous function $f(x) : \mathcal{M} \mapsto \mathbb{R}$. The deconvolution problem is to estimate the $f(x)$ given the specified $R(\boldsymbol{q}, x)$ and measurements $S(\boldsymbol{q})/S_0$. In literature, $f(x)$ is usually expressed as a linear combination of N basis functions: $f(x) = \sum w_j f_j(x)$. The choices of convolution kernels and basis functions are related to the underlying manifold $\mathcal{M}$. A simple example is to set $\mathcal{M}$ to the unit sphere, which leads to the spherical deconvolution problem [15]. Though involving the manifold of diffusion tensors, several other approaches still reduce to the sphere deconvolution problem since only rotationally symmetric tensors are considered. [14, 13, 7].

The types of basis functions include radial basis functions [15], spherical harmonics [14, 7]. Like in [14, 13, 7], our method uses the standard diffusion tensor kernel. However, it is the Wishart basis function that distinguishes our method from these related methods. It is worth noting that the Wishart basis reduces to the Dirac function on $\mathcal{P}_n$ when $p = \infty$ and thus leading to the tensor basis function method introduced in [13]. The fiber orientation estimated using the continuous axially symmetric tensors (FORECAST) method proposed in [7] also resembles (very closely) our method with the basis function being chosen as the spherical harmonics.

3 Stable, Sparse and Positive Deconvolution

The deconvolution problem can be formulated in a general form of as,

$$\mathsf{A}\boldsymbol{w} = \boldsymbol{s} + \eta, \tag{8}$$

where $\boldsymbol{s}$ contains K measurements $S(\boldsymbol{q})/S_0$, the $K \times N$ matrix $\mathsf{A} = \{A_{ij}\}$ is given by $A_{ij} = \int_M R(\boldsymbol{q}_i, x) f_j(x) \mathrm{d}x$ and η represents certain noise model. Note that the integral to compute the entries of A may have an analytical solution as in our model and others that use the tensor kernel [14,13,7], or needs to be numerically approximated as in [15]. But, once the response kernel $R(\boldsymbol{q}, x)$ and the basis function are specified, the matrix A can be fully computed (or approximated) and only $\boldsymbol{w}$, a column vector containing K unknown coefficients, remains to be estimated.

Under the assumption that the measurement errors η are i.i.d. and normally distributed, the maximum likelihood estimate of $\boldsymbol{w}$ naturally leads to the L_2 norm as a measure of goodness of the fit. Without inequality constraints, the corresponding quadratic programming (QP) problem minimizing the residual sum of squares

$$(P_1) \qquad \min \|\mathsf{A}\boldsymbol{w} - \boldsymbol{s}\|^2 \tag{9}$$

can be efficiently solved by solving a linear system using for instance, direct methods when the size of the linear system in Eq. (9) is not large as in our application. The solution in the least squares sense is given by $\boldsymbol{w} = \mathsf{A}^+\boldsymbol{s}$ where $\mathsf{A}^+ = (\mathsf{A}^T\mathsf{A})^{-1}\mathsf{A}^T$ is the pseudoinverse of the A. The advantage of applying the pseudoinverse is in its light computational burden since the matrix A is identical in each voxel and its pseudoinverse only

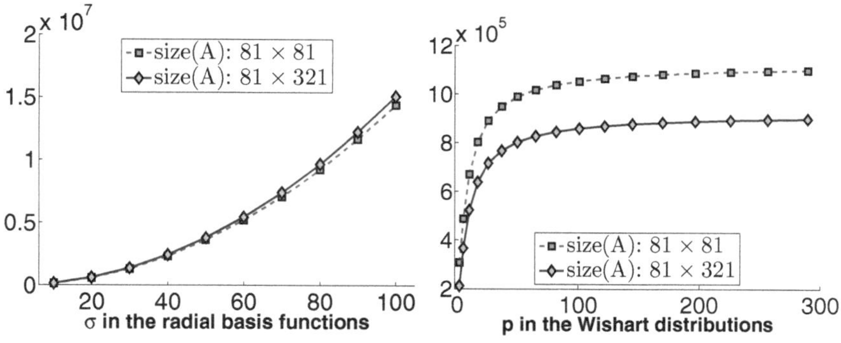

Fig. 1. Left plot shows the case where the A matrices are constructed from the radial basis function and the tensor kernel model as in [15]. Right plot shows the case with a standard diffusion tensor kernel weighted by a mixture of Wisharts. Both assume 81 diffusion gradient directions and two tessellation schemes (81 and 321 directions) are considered for each model.

needs to be computed once. However, this simplicity and efficiency comes at the cost of higher susceptibility to noise, due to the fact that the matrix A is usually ill-conditioned in our application as illustrated in Fig. 1. Efforts at reliable multi-fiber reconstruction in the presence of noise have included low-pass filtering [14], the maximum entropy principle [15] and Tikhonov regularization [16]. In the Tikhonov regularization framework, the problem in Eq. (8) can be formulated as:

$$(P_2) \qquad \min \|\mathsf{A}\boldsymbol{w} - \boldsymbol{s}\|^2 + \alpha\|\mathsf{T}\boldsymbol{w}\|^2 \tag{10}$$

where α is a regularization parameter and T is a regularization operator. In order to penalize the magnitude of the estimates, (P_2) in (10) with T being the identity operator I is often used and yields the relation: $\boldsymbol{w} = (\mathsf{A}^T\mathsf{A} + \alpha\mathsf{I})^{-1}\mathsf{A}^T\boldsymbol{s}$. Recently, a Damped Singular Value Decomposition was used to regularize the fiber orientation distribution [21] where the damping factor α is determined by minimizing the Generalized Cross Validation (GCV) criterion, which provides a simple and objective method, though not really optimal, for choosing the regularization parameter.

In practice, the number of diffusion MR image acquisition sequence, K, is rarely greater than 100. On the other hand, a high resolution tessellation with $N > 100$ is usually taken to obtain an accurate reconstruction. This under-determined linear system has infinite solutions in the least squares sense and usually produces the $\boldsymbol{w}$ with many negative-valued components which are not physically meaningful. Another issue related to this configuration is the sparsity constraint. Since the number of significant spikes in $\boldsymbol{w}$ is indicative of the number of maxima in the displacement probability surfaces, $\boldsymbol{w}$ is expected to have a sparse support. Recently a series of significant research articles have been published by Candés and collaborators (see [22] and references therein) on a theory of signal recovery from highly incomplete information. The central result relevant to us here, states that a sparse vector $\boldsymbol{w} \in \mathbb{R}^N$ can be recovered from a small number of linear measurements $\boldsymbol{s} = \mathsf{A}\boldsymbol{w} \in \mathbb{R}^K$, $K \ll N$ (or $\boldsymbol{s} = \mathsf{A}\boldsymbol{w} + \eta$ when there is measurement noise) by solving a convex program. Among the several problems they have discussed, we are particularly interested in the following two problems: (1) Min-L_1 with equality constraints:

$$(P_3) \quad \min \|\boldsymbol{w}\|_1 \quad \text{subject to} \quad \mathsf{A}\boldsymbol{w} = \boldsymbol{s} \tag{11}$$

and (2) Min-L_1 with quadratic constraints:

$$(P_4) \quad \min \|\boldsymbol{w}\|_1 \quad \text{subject to} \quad \|\mathsf{A}\boldsymbol{w} - \boldsymbol{s}\|_2 \leq \epsilon \tag{12}$$

where ϵ is a user specified parameter. Both problems (P_3) and (P_4) find the vector with smallest L_1 norm ($\|\boldsymbol{w}\|_1 = \sum_i |w_i|$) that best explains the observation $\boldsymbol{s}$. (P_3) can be recast as an linear-programming (LP) problem while (P_4) can be recast as a second order cone programming (SOCP) problem (see [22, 23] and references therein for details). We will report the results of implementation of these methods for the sake of comparisons in the next section.

However, (P_3) and (P_4) do not explicitly enforce the nonnegative constraints. The straight forward solution is to incorporate a nonnegative constraint while minimizing the least-squares criterion:

$$(P_5) \quad \min \|\mathsf{A}\boldsymbol{w} - \boldsymbol{s}\|^2 \quad \text{subject to} \quad \boldsymbol{w} \geq 0. \tag{13}$$

This non-negative least squares (NNLS) minimization is precisely a quadratic programming problem: Find the minimum point of a concave quadratic function in a linearly bounded convex feasible hyperspace. The most used algorithm for NNLS was developed in [24, Ch. 23], which treats the linear inequality constraints using an *active set strategy*. Though the sparsity constraint is not explicitly imposed, the active set strategy tends to find the sparse solution quickly if there exists such one. Additionally, unlike other iterative methods mentioned above, this algorithm requires no arbitrary cutoff parameter and hence the output is not susceptible to mis-tuning of the input parameters. More comparisons of these methods on simulation data are shown in Section 4.

After $\boldsymbol{w}$ is estimated, the displacement probabilities can be approximated by the Fourier transform $P(\boldsymbol{r}) = \int (S(\boldsymbol{q})/S_0) \exp(-i\boldsymbol{q} \cdot \boldsymbol{r})\, \mathrm{d}\boldsymbol{q}$ where $\boldsymbol{r}$ is the displacement vector. Assuming a continuous diffusion tensor model (1) with mixing distribution $F(\mathsf{D}) = \sum_{i=1}^{N} w_i \mathrm{d}\gamma_{p_i,\Sigma_i}$, we have

$$P(\boldsymbol{r}) = \int_{R^3} \int_{\mathcal{P}_n} e^{-\boldsymbol{q}^T \mathsf{D} \boldsymbol{q} t} \mathrm{d}F(\mathsf{D}) e^{-i\boldsymbol{q}\cdot\boldsymbol{r}} \mathrm{d}\boldsymbol{q} \approx \sum_{i=1}^{N} \frac{w_i}{\sqrt{(4\pi t)^3 |\hat{\mathsf{D}_i}|}} \exp\left(\frac{-\boldsymbol{r}^T \hat{\mathsf{D}_i}^{-1} \boldsymbol{r}}{4t}\right) \tag{14}$$

where $\hat{\mathsf{D}_i} = p\Sigma_i$ are the expected values of γ_{p,Σ_i}. Note that the end result is expressed as a mixture of oriented Gaussians. Due to its good analytic properties, many of the quantities produced by other methods including the radial integral of $P(\boldsymbol{r})$ in QBI [6] and the integral of $P(\boldsymbol{r})\boldsymbol{r}^2$ in DSI [10] are analytically computable using our technique.

4 Experimental Results

4.1 Numerical Simulations

Prior to performing the experiments on real diffusion MRI data, we first test the performance of the methods described in the previous section on the HARDI simulations of 1-,2- and 3-fiber geometries with known fiber orientations as shown in Fig. 2. The diffusion MR signals were realistically simulated by using the formulas from the cylindrical boundary restricted diffusion model in [25] with the same parameter settings as in [11]. In order to compare the performance of the five deconvolution methods described in Section 3, we first apply all of them on the noiseless 1-fiber HARDI simulation data and the results of $\boldsymbol{w}$ obtained from these methods are plotted in Fig. 3. We observe that the least squares solution to (P_1) contains a large portion of negative weights and has relatively large magnitude. A zeroth-order Tikhonov regularization (P_2) is able to reduce the magnitude significantly but does not help achieve the sparsity and non-negativity. By minimizing the L_1 norm with equality constraints, (P_3) yields relative sparse solution but the magnitude and the negative values are not controlled. The result produced by (P_4) has better sparsity and non-negativity. Evidently, the best result is obtained by solving (P_5) using NNLS. Among the 321 components, there are only two nonzero and significant spikes which both lie in the neighborhood of true fiber orientation $(30°, 90°)$. It is important to note that (1) the true fiber orientations do not necessarily occur at the maximum of the discrete $\boldsymbol{w}$ vector; and (2) although all of these different results for $\boldsymbol{w}$ actually lead to a very good approximation of the true displacement probability function $P(\boldsymbol{r})$ after taking the Fourier transforms, a sparse positive representation of $\boldsymbol{w}$ obviously offers a great advantage in setting the initial guess in the optimization procedure used to find the fiber orientations by estimating the extrema of $P(\boldsymbol{r})$. Considering the additional computational overhead for solving (P_3), (P_4) and (P_5) due to the iterative optimization, (P_5) is slightly slower than (P_3) (LP) but significantly faster than (P_4) (SOCP). It only takes MATLAB's built-in *lsqnonneg* around 20-200ms to solve a problem of size 81×321. Fig. 4 further shows the results of using NNLS on the noisy simulated data. Clearly, NNLS is still able to produce quite accurate solutions which also are sparse representations.

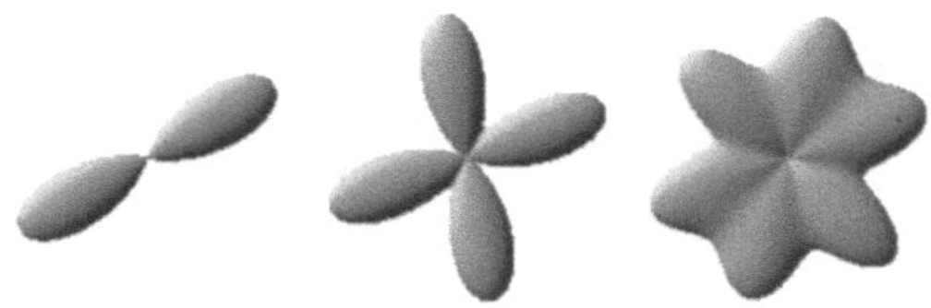

Fig. 2. HARDI simulations of 1-, 2- and 3-fibers ($b = 1500s/mm^2$) visualized in QBI ODF surfaces using [7, Eq.(21)]. Orientation configurations: azimuthal angles: $\phi_1 = 30°, \phi_2 = \{20°, 100°\}, \phi_3 = \{20°, 75°, 135°\}$; polar angles are all 90°.

Finally, as a conclusion to our experiments on the simulated data, we compare the proposed method mixture of Wisharts (MOW) model with two model-free methods, namely, the Q-ball ODF [6] and the DOT [11]. In order to provide a quantitative comparison, all the resulting $P(\boldsymbol{r})$ surfaces were represented by spherical harmonics coefficients up to order $l = 6$. As before, the Q-ball ODF is computed using the formula in [7, Eq.(21)]. First, to gain a global assessment of these methods in terms of stability,

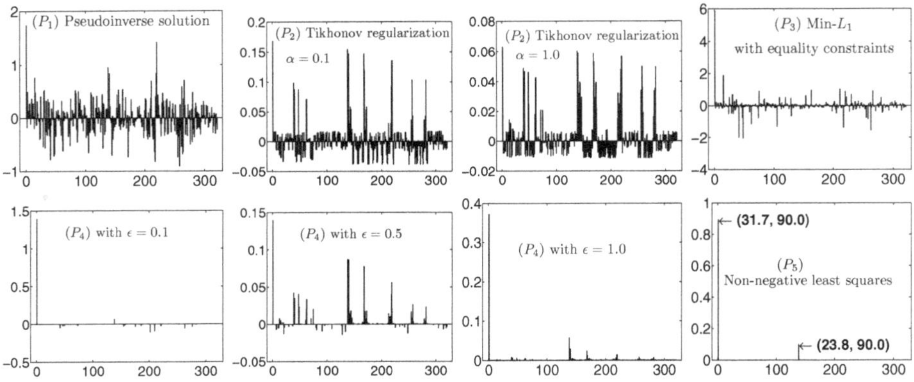

Fig. 3. Deconvolution-based computation of $\boldsymbol{w}$ in the 1-fiber HARDI simulation. The matrix A is of size 81×321 and is built from the Wishart model but with $p = \infty$. The Min-L_1 algorithms are solved using the package developed in [23]. The NNLS solver is the MATLAB built-in *lsqnonneg* function based on Lawson and Hanson's algorithm [24].

we calculated the similarity between each noisy $P(\boldsymbol{r})$ and the corresponding noiseless $P(\boldsymbol{r})$ using the angular correlation coefficient formula given in [7, Eq.(71)]. The angular correlation ranges from 0 to 1 where 1 implies identical probability profiles. Then, we estimated the fiber orientations of each system by numerically finding the maxima of the probability surfaces with a Quasi-Newton algorithm and computed the deviation angles between the estimated and the true fiber orientations. Figure 5 shows the mean and standard deviation of the angular correlation coefficients, and error angles, respectively, for the two-fiber simulation. Note that among the three methods examined, only MOW results in small error angles and high correlation coefficients in presence of relatively large noise. This trend also holds for the 1-fiber and the 3-fiber simulations. This can be explained by noting that NNLS is able to locate the sparse spikes quite accurately even in the presence of large noise.

4.2 Real Data Experiments

The rat optic chiasm provides an excellent "platform" to experimentally validate our approach due to its distinct myelinated structure with both parallel and descussating (crossing) optic nerve fibers. Decussating fibers carry information from the temporal visual fields to the geniculate body. A HARDI data set was acquired from a perfusion-fixed excised rat optic chiasm at 14.1T using a Bruker Avance imaging system with a diffusion-weighted spin echo pulse sequence. DW-MRI data were collected using 46 directions with a b-value of $1250s/mm^2$ and a single image with $b \approx 0s/mm^2$. Echo time and repetition time were $23ms$ and $0.5s$ respectively; Δ and δ values were set to $12.4ms$ and $1.2ms$ respectively; bandwidth was set to $35kHz$; signal average was 10; a matrix size of $128 \times 128 \times 5$ and a resolution of $33.6 \times 33.6 \times 200\mu m^3$ was used. The optic chiasm images were signal averaged to $67.2 \times 67.2 \times 200\mu m^3$ resolution prior to computation of the water molecule displacement probability field.

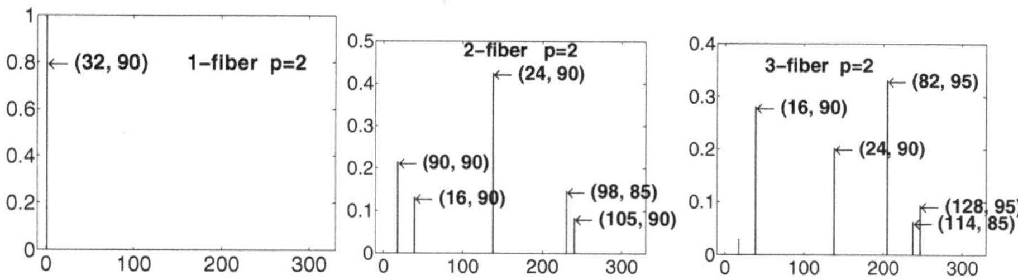

Fig. 4. Deconvolution-based computation of w using NNLS on simulated data in presence of Riccian noise with $\sigma = .06$. The matrix A is constructed by using the Wishart model with $p = 2$ and the tessellation of size $N = 321$. From left to right are the 1-fiber, 2-fiber and 3-fiber simulations, respectively. The spikes in each resulting w are marked with the corresponding azimuthal and polar angles in degrees. Note all the spikes detected are close to the ground truth orientations specified in Figure 2.

Three methods are used to generate the displacement probability functions for the optic chiasm image. The results on a region of interest are shown in Figure 6. The corresponding S_0 image is also shown in the upper left corner as a reference. As seen from the figure, the fiber-crossings in the optic chiasm region is not identifiable in Figure 6 (c). Note that both the DOT method and the MOW method are able to demonstrate the distinct fiber orientations in the central region of the optic chiasm where ipsilateral myelinated axons from the two optic nerves cross and form the contralateral optic tracts. However, it is evident from the figure that compared to all other solutions, the MOW scheme yields significantly sharper displacement probability surfaces. This is particularly borne out in the central location of the figure labeled, the optic chiasm. One of the reasons for the blurred appearance of these probability surfaces in the QBI and DOT models is due to the fact that neither of them yield the actual displacement probability surfaces but a corrupted $P(\boldsymbol{r})$ where the corrupting factor is a a zeroth order Bessel function in the QBI method and a function that does not have an analytic form in the

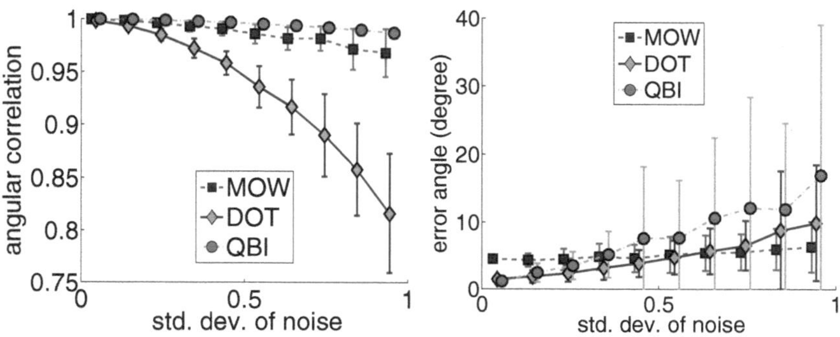

Fig. 5. Mean and standard deviation of (a) angular correlation coefficient and (b) error angles for the two-fiber simulation. The displayed values for error angles are averaged over the two fibers.

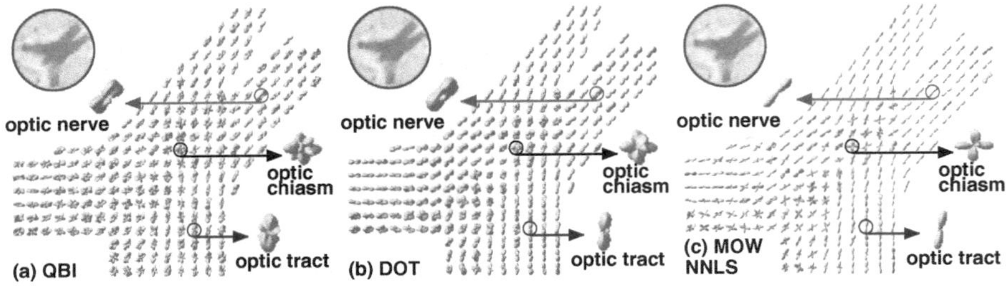

Fig. 6. Probability surfaces computed from a rat optic chiasm image using three methods. Note the decussation of myelinated axons from the two optic nerves at the center of the optic chiasm.

case of DOT. This corruption effects the accuracy of the reconstructed fiber orientations as evidenced in the simulated data case where ground truth was known.

5 Conclusions

In this paper, we present a novel mathematical model which relates the diffusion MR signals and probability distributions for positive definite matrix-valued random variables through Laplace transforms. We further show that the closed form expression for the Laplace transform of Wishart distributions leads to Rigaut-type asymptotic fractal law for the MR signal decay behavior which has been observed experimentally in the past [17]. Moreover in this case, the traditional diffusion tensor model is the limiting case of the expected signal attenuation. We further develop a spherical deconvolution method for resolving multiple fiber orientations using the mixture of Wisharts (MOW) model. To address the numerical issues and sparsity constraints raised in solving this deconvolution problem, we investigate a number of deconvolution techniques and demonstrate that the classic non-negative least squares (NNLS) algorithm developed in [24] is most suitable for our deconvolution problem in achieving sparseness and robustness. Experimental results on both synthetic and real data sets have also shown that the proposed MOW model combined with NNLS deconvolution provides better overall performance than other state-of-the-art techniques for multi-fiber reconstruction.

References

[1] Bihan, D.L.: Looking into the functional architecture of the brain with diffusion MRI. Nat Rev Neurosci. 4, 469–480 (2003)
[2] Basser, P.J., Mattiello, J., Bihan, D.L.: MR diffusion tensor spectroscopy and imaging. Biophys. J. 66, 259–267 (1994)
[3] Tuch, D.S., Reese, T.G., Wiegell, M.R., Makris, N., Belliveau, J.W., Wedeen, V.J.: High angular resolution diffusion imaging reveals intravoxel white matter fiber heterogeneity. Magn. Reson. Med. 48, 577–582 (2002)
[4] Frank, L.: Characterization of anisotropy in high angular resolution diffusion weighted MRI. Magn. Reson. Med. 47, 1083–1099 (2002)

[5] Özarslan, E., Mareci, T.H.: Generalized diffusion tensor imaging and analytical relationships between diffusion tensor imaging and high angular resolution diffusion imaging. Magn. Reson. Med. 50, 955–965 (2003)

[6] Tuch, D.S.: Q-ball imaging. Magn. Reson. Med. 52, 1358–1372 (2004)

[7] Anderson, A.W.: Measurement of fiber orientation distributions using high angular resolution diffusion imaging. Magn. Reson. Med. 54, 1194–1206 (2005)

[8] Hess, C.P., Mukherjee, P., Han, E.T., Xu, D., Vigneron, D.B.: Q-ball reconstruction of multimodal fiber orientations using the spherical harmonic basis. Magn. Reson. Med. 56, 104–117 (2006)

[9] Descoteaux, M., Angelino, E., Fitzgibbons, S., Deriche, R.: A fast and robust ODF estimation algorithm in q-ball imaging. In: ISBI 2006, pp. 81–84 (2006)

[10] Wedeen, V.J., Hagmann, P., Tseng, W.Y.I., Reese, T.G., Weisskoff, R.M.: Mapping complex tissue architecture with diffusion spectrum magnetic resonance imaging. Magn. Reson. Med. 54, 1377–1386 (2005)

[11] Özarslan, E., Shepherd, T.M., Vemuri, B.C., Blackband, S.J., Mareci, T.H.: Resolution of complex tissue microarchitecture using the diffusion orientation transform (DOT). NeuroImage 31, 1086–1103 (2006)

[12] Behrens, T., Woolrich, M., Jenkinson, M., Johansen-Berg, H., Nunes, R., Clare, S., Matthews, P., Brady, J., Smith, S.: Characterization and propagation of uncertainty in diffusion-weighted MR imaging. Magn. Reson. Med. 50, 1077–1088 (2003)

[13] Ramirez-Manzanares, A., Rivera, M., Vemuri, B.C., Mareci, T.H.: Basis functions for estimating intra-voxel structure in DW-MRI. In: Proc. IEEE Medical Imaging Conference, Roma, Italy 2004, pp. 4207–4211 (2004)

[14] Tournier, J.D., Calamante, F., Gadian, D.G., Connelly, A.: Direct estimation of the fiber orientation density function from diffusion-weighted MRI data using spherical deconvolution. NeuroImage 23, 1176–1185 (2004)

[15] Alexander, D.C.: Maximum entropy spherical deconvolution for diffusion MRI. In: IPMI 2005, pp. 76–87 (2005)

[16] Tournier, J.D., Calamente, F., Connelly, A.: Improved characterisation of crossing fibres: spherical deconvolution combined with Tikhonov regularization. In: ISMRM 2006 (2006)

[17] Köpf, M., Metzler, R., Haferkamp, O., Nonnenmacher, T.F.: NMR studies of anomalous diffusion in biological tissues: Experimental observation of Lévy stable processes. Fractals in Biology and Medicine. 2, 354–364 (1998)

[18] Mathai, A.M.: Jacobians of Matrix Transformations and Functions of Matrix Argument. World Scientific, Singapore (1997)

[19] Rigaut, J.P.: An empirical formulation relating boundary lengths to resolution in specimens showing 'non-ideally fractal dimensions. J Microsc 133, 41–54 (1984)

[20] Sen, P.N., Hürlimann, M.D., de Swiet, T.M.: Debye-Porod law of diffraction for diffusion in porous media. Phys Rev B 51, 601–604 (1995)

[21] Sakaie, K.E., Lowe, M.J.: An objective method for regularization of fiber orientation distribution derived from diffusion-weighed MRI. NeuroImage 34, 169–176 (2007)

[22] Candès, E.J., Romberg, J.K., Tao, T.: Robust uncertainty principles: exact signal reconstruction from highly incomplete frequency information. IEEE Trans. Info. Theory 52, 489–509 (2006)

[23] Candés, E., Romberg, J.: l_1-MAGIC (2006) //www.l1-magic.org

[24] Lawson, C., Hanson, R.J.: Solving Least Squares Problems. Prentice-Hall, Englewood Cliffs (1974)

[25] Söderman, O., Jönsson, B.: Restricted diffusion in cylindirical geometry. J. Magn. Reson. B 117, 94–97 (1995)

A Hamiltonian Particle Method for Diffeomorphic Image Registration

Stephen Marsland and Robert McLachlan

Massey University, Private Bag 11-222
Palmerston North, New Zealand
{s.r.marsland,r.mchlachlan}@massey.ac.nz

Abstract. Diffeomorphic image registration, where images are aligned using diffeomorphic warps, is a popular subject for research in medical image analysis. We introduce a novel algorithm for computing diffeomorphic warps that solves the Euler equations on the diffeomorphism group explicitly, based on a discretisation of the Hamiltonian, rather than using an optimiser. The result is an algorithm that is many times faster than those considered previously.

1 Introduction

Image registration has received much research over the past few years, not least because of its many applications in medicine. For example, it is useful for removing motion artefacts caused by patient breathing, heartbeat, and patient movement [1], aligning to an atlas [2], monitoring disease progression [3], assisting in disease diagnosis [4], and measuring anatomical variability between subjects [5]. For further details about these applications see [5]. A more general survey of image registration, highlighting its uses in synthetic aperture radar and other applications is given in [6].

For applications in disease diagnosis and measuring anatomical variability, some form of measurement on the space of images is essential, to allow statistical analysis of the image warps. This generally requires using diffeomorphic image registration, where the choice of image warps that can be used to solve the registration problem are constrained to be diffeomorphisms, i.e., smooth functions that have smooth inverses. There has therefore been recent interest in the use of diffeomorphic deformations (warps) to align medical images.

In 1966 Arnold made the profound discovery that the Euler equations for a perfect fluid are geodesic equations on the group of volume-preserving diffeomorphisms with respect to a group-invariant metric defined by the kinetic energy of the fluid [7]. This point of view allowed stability and existence results [8] that have not been bettered today. For diffeomorphic image warping, it is the group of *all* diffeomorphisms that is considered, and the warp ϕ is constructed as a geodesic (shortest path) between two images, leading to a right-invariant Riemannian metric. This diffeomorphism has typically been computed as an optimisation problem; see [9,4] for an overview.

N. Karssemeijer and B. Lelieveldt (Eds.): IPMI 2007, LNCS 4584, pp. 396–407, 2007.
© Springer-Verlag Berlin Heidelberg 2007

In this paper we introduce a novel formulation of the problem that is based on solving the partial differential equations that govern the motion. These PDEs are the Euler equations for the full diffeomorphism group, given by equations (1) and (2) below; for derivations, following [7], see [9,10]. We introduce a particle method that enables us to solve for the diffeomorphism directly, resulting in an algorithm that is orders of magnitude faster than previous ones. We demonstrate the algorithm using standard forward-Euler and Runge-Kutta integrators, and discuss the benefits of using a symplectic integrator.

1.1 Problem Formulation

The aim of diffeomorphic image registration is to find a diffeomorphism ϕ that takes a free image F to a reference image R, i.e., $R = F\circ\phi$. The diffeomorphism ϕ is defined on some domain $\Omega \in \mathbb{R}^2$ or $\mathbb{R}^3$, and the images are typically greyscale, so that $R, F : \mathbb{R}^2 \to \mathbb{R}$ or $R, F : \mathbb{R}^3 \to \mathbb{R}$. The method used to find the desired ϕ is generally optimisation of some norm $\|R - F \circ \phi\|$. Typical choices include the L^2 norm (sum-of-squares error) and mutual information [11,12], although there are other alternatives, including the correlation ratio [13] and the normalised gradient-based method [14].

In this paper, we describe a novel method of constructing the diffeomorphisms. The standard approach is to use an energy minimisation, which produces the diffeomorphism as a geodesic [4,17,15,16]. Instead, we compute the Hamiltonian of the Euler equations on the diffeomorphism group, discretise them and integrate them explicitly. For the case of the full diffeomorphism group, $\mathfrak{G} = \mathrm{Diff}(\mathbb{R}^n)$, that we consider here, the Euler equations are (see [18,19] for further details):

$$\dot{m} + u \cdot \nabla m + \nabla u^T \cdot m + m(\mathrm{div}\ u) = 0, \tag{1}$$

where $\dot{m}$ denotes differentiation with respect to time, $u(x,t)$ $(u, x \in \mathbb{R}^n,\ t \in \mathbb{R})$ is a velocity field, and $m(x,t)$ its associated momentum. The velocity u and momentum m are related by:

$$m = \mathcal{A}u, \tag{2}$$

where $\mathcal{A}$ is an elliptic operator (e.g., $\mathcal{A} = (1 - \nabla^2)^k$) called the inertia operator. The inverse of $\mathcal{A}$ is given by convolution with the Green's function $\mathbf{G}$ of $\mathcal{A}$, i.e., $u = \mathbf{G}{*}m$, where $*$ denotes convolution and $\mathcal{A}\mathbf{G}(x,x') = \delta(x-x')$ for $x, x' \in \mathbb{R}^n$.

A striking feature of Euler equations on diffeomorphism groups is that they admit (formally, at least) exact solutions in which the momentum is concentrated at a finite set of points. For fluid equations these are point vortices, which are widely studied both in their own right and as a means of approximating the evolution of smooth or other vorticities [20,21]. In analogy with the point vortices of fluid dynamics, we call the image registration equivalents *point particles.*

2 A Particle Method for Image Registration

We are considering the deformation of an image Ω, with the deformation defined by a set of points i (some subset of the pixels of the image) with position and momentum $(q^i(t), p^i(t))$, where $p_i = \dot{q}_i$ as they move from their initial state (q_0^i, p_0^i) to their endpoints at $t = 1$. Starting from the Euler equations on the diffeomorphism group ((1) and (2)) we compute the Hamiltonian (see [22] for a derivation of the Hamiltonian from the Lagrangian via the Legendre transform), which is the kinetic energy, and then discretise it by introducing the particle ansatz $m(x,t) = \sum_{j=1}^{N} p_j(t)\delta(x - q_j(t))$, where $\delta(\cdot)$ is Kronecker delta function.The evolution of the particles is then given by the Hamiltonian:

$$H = \frac{1}{2}\sum_{i,j} p_i \cdot p_j G(q_i - q_j), \tag{3}$$

where $G(\cdot)$ is the Green's function corresponding to the chosen metric on Diff(Ω). The most common choice in image registration, and the one that we will use in this paper is the H^∞ metric, which corresponds to using a Gaussian Green's function $G(r) = \frac{1}{\epsilon^2}\exp(-r^2/\epsilon^2)$, where ϵ is the length-scale in the metric. Other choices include the thin-plate and clamped-plate splines – see [4] for a review.

Solutions to (1) of this form obey Hamilton's equations for (3), in which the components of q_i and p_i are canonically conjugate variables (see [23] for further details). Here $q_1, \ldots, q_N$ represent the positions of the N particles that define the deformation, and $p_1, \ldots, p_N$ their momenta. The equations of motion of the point particles are:

$$\dot{q}_i = \sum_{j=1}^{N} G(\|q_i - q_j\|)p_j, \tag{4}$$

$$\dot{p}_i = -\sum_{j}(p_i \cdot p_j)G'(\|q_i - q_j\|)\frac{q_i - q_j}{\|q_i - q_j\|}. \tag{5}$$

Computing the diffeomorphism defined by q_i and p_i is then simply a case of integrating the motion forward in time using (4) and (5), and then interpolating the motion of the rest of the image in some way. The integration requires fewer timesteps than the optimisation methods, enables the accuracy of the method to be computed explicitly, and is computationally significantly faster. This leads us to a description of our complete algorithm for image registration, following which we discuss several important implementation details.

Our Image Registration Algorithm

- Choose point particle positions q on image T
- Initialise the particle momenta p randomly
- Optimise $\|R - T \circ \phi\|$ over p:
  - For current p, integrate point particles forward in time
  - Integrate positions of the test particles
  - Interpolate between the test particles
  - Compute $\|R - T \circ \phi\|$ for chosen distance measure
- Add more point particles and iterate

Position of point particles. There are several possible choices for placing the point particles, such as placing them in a grid, positioning them on points of interest in the image (such as edges and corners), or using the discrepancy image [24] to select places where the two images do not match. In line with [24], for registration of brains, we initially place some points around the skull of head images and, after optimising them, place more points using the discrepancy image method. For the hand images shown in the next section, we use a uniform grid.

Initialisation of point momenta. In the current implementation, the momenta of the point particles are initialised with a uniform random direction, and with a small uniform random magnitude for the warp. One option that improves the results, although at a moderate computational cost, is to perform a coarse search over this relatively small number of parameters (2 for each of the point particles, of which there may be 10-20 on the initial pass).

Choice of integrator. The primary component of our method is the computation of the current geodesic, based on q and the current p. This is calculated by numerically integrating the particle dynamics forward in time using (4) and (5). We can choose a timestep for the integration, and the method of numerical integration. The standard choices would generally be Euler's method, or a second-order improvement, such as second-order Runge-Kutta.

The factors that affect the computation of the diffeomorphism are the number of point particles and test particles, the number of timesteps, and the order of the integrator (how errors accumulate during the integration). In consideration of the last two of these points, in section 5 we discuss the possible benefits and disadvantages of using a symplectic integrator, together with a possible reduction in the computational complexity of the algorithm.

Test particles and interpolation. We can induce the value of the actual diffeomorphism $\phi(x)$ by the current geodesic on each pixel by placing test particles with zero momentum (so $q(0) = x, p(0) = 0$) on the pixels, and computing their trajectories under the induced velocity field (i.e., solving the ODE $\dot{q} = f(q,t)$). Assuming that the deformation is not too large ($\|T\phi - 1\|$ is small), we can make some computational savings by placing a test particle every k pixels, and interpolating ϕ between them. This saves a factor of k^2 computations, but changes the computed diffeomorphism from the exact one that relates to the flow (it may actually stop the warp being diffeomorphic, although this does not seem to be a problem in general). We have found that using $k = 4$ and bi-linear interpolation has negligible effect on the accuracy in real registrations, as is demonstrated in the table on the left of Fig. 3.

Choice of metric. Inherent in the choice of Green's function $G(r)$ is a choice of the metric under which the particle dynamics occur. There is complete freedom of choice over this metric. By far the most common choice to date for image registration has been to use a Gaussian metric, i.e., Green's function $G(r) = \frac{1}{\epsilon^2}\exp(-r^2/\epsilon^2)$, where ϵ is the length-scale in the metric. The role of this length-scale is important. If it is set too small (say smaller than the pixel spacing) then the kernels will not overlap, and the movement of each particle will be entirely independent of the rest of the image. This will require the number of point particles to tend to infinity to represent an arbitrary diffeomorphism. We do not consider how to choose the length-scale in this paper, but it may be that starting with a large value of ϵ and allowing it to shrink is a useful method of iteratively refining the solution.

The Gaussian is by no means the only possible choice of metric. One fairly general formulation, which includes the Gaussian as the limit as $k \to \infty$, are the H^k metrics, $(1 - \epsilon^2\nabla^2)^k$; see [25] for a discussion of these. Finally, it may well be useful to choose the metric so that it vanishes on some set of motions that are not important. Examples could be affine or rigid motions.

Optimisation method. The choice of a suitable optimiser is obviously crucial, together with the choice of objective function for the image matching. In the current implementation we are using the sum-of-squares distance measure, which leads fairly naturally to a least-squares non-linear optimiser. We use the `lsqnonlin` function in Matlab 7.1, which is a subspace trust region method based on the interior-reflective Newton method. Experimentation has found that allowing 100 iterations is usually more than sufficient for the algorithm to converge, although further work will investigate this more thoroughly.

Adding more points. In our implementation we position new point particles for further levels of optimisation using the discrepancy image. This uses the objective function (here the sum-of-squares error) to find regions where the two images do not match, and then places new point particles there. We tested initialising the momenta of these particles as either zero, or small random numbers, and found that the first was the most effective. This is not surprising, because points with zero momentum are carried along with the flow, which is a reasonable initial guess for how they should behave, and the optimiser then improves on this.

3 Experiments

We present four main experiments in this paper. In all of them, the image is scaled into $[-1, 1]^2$ and a value of $\epsilon = 1$ was used. The first experiment considers how far apart the spacing should be between the test particles – the wider apart, the faster the implementation, but the less accurate the approximation to the true diffeomorphism. In order to decide a suitable spacing, we took a series of 10 registrations of hands, as used for the registration shown in Fig. 2 and described below, and tested out different spacings between the test particles for two different numbers of point particles (with the initial values for the momenta of the point particles fixed between the runs). The average results over the 10 registrations are shown in the table on the left of Fig. 1, and show that a spacing of 4 between test particles provides a reasonable compromise between computational time and final function value, hence we have used a spacing of 4 for all the computations used in this paper.

For the second experiment, we investigated how the performance of the integrators change as the number of timesteps is varied. The right of Fig.1 shows

Spacing	Time (s)	Final function value
9 point particles		
12	39.13	7.78e7
8	43.13	7.43e7
4	47.71	7.08e7
1	112.6	6.95e7
25 point particles		
12	123.17	1.06e8
8	133.95	9.82e7
4	163.05	9.37e7
1	944.72	8.85e7

Timesteps	1	2	4	8
Small perturbation, initial error 60.2%				
Integrator				
Euler	5.2%	3.6%	2.9%	2.5%
RK2	4.3%	2.2%	2.2%	2.2%
Large perturbation, initial error 84%				
Euler	16.3%	10.3%	8.6%	8.1%
RK2	4.3%	5.9%	6.4%	6.7%

Fig. 1. *Left:* Comparison of changing the spacing between the test particles. Results are the average of 10 values. A spacing of 4 appears to give a reasonable compromise between computational cost and the final diffeomorphism. *Right:* The effect of changing the number of timesteps (errors relative to reference image). For RK2 the integration error is far below other sources, but for Euler it is significant for large perturbations.

the results for registrations with 9 point particles using the `peaks(40)` function in Matlab to make the reference image, with the free image being the same image with a rotation applied. The second-order method needs fewer timesteps than the first-order forward-Euler. Indeed, adding more timesteps can make the second-order results worse. The reason for this is currently under investigation.

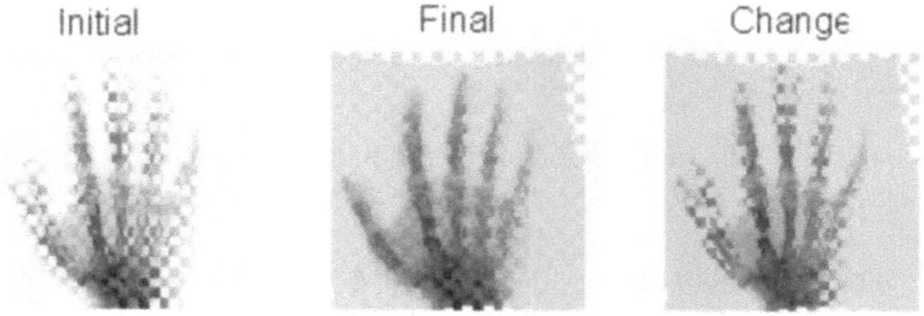

Fig. 2. Chequer-board plots showing the difference between the initial images of the hands (left), the final images (centre), and the change between the initial and final versions of the free image (right).

We now present two different image registrations. The first is of a pair of hand images, while the second are two 2D T1-weighted MR scans of the human brain. The hand results shown in Fig. 2 were computed using 9 knotpoints, positioned in a 3×3 grid on the image. The optimiser ran for 40 iterations before converging, and then an additional 7 points were added to the image using the discrepancy image. It can be seen that even after this relatively small amount of computation, the registration is very good. Computing this registration took 251.4 seconds on a 1.8GHz G5 Apple Macintosh. Another 37 iterations were then performed by

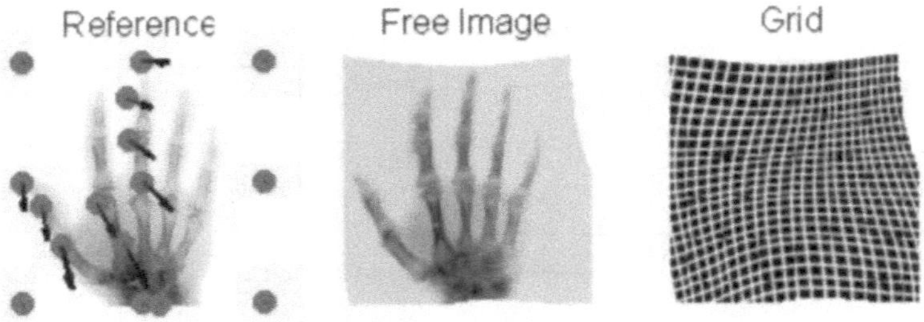

Fig. 3. The registration of the two hands. The reference image, together with the positions of the particles and their momenta are shown on the left, the final result is shown in the middle, and the effect of the warp on a grid is shown on the right.

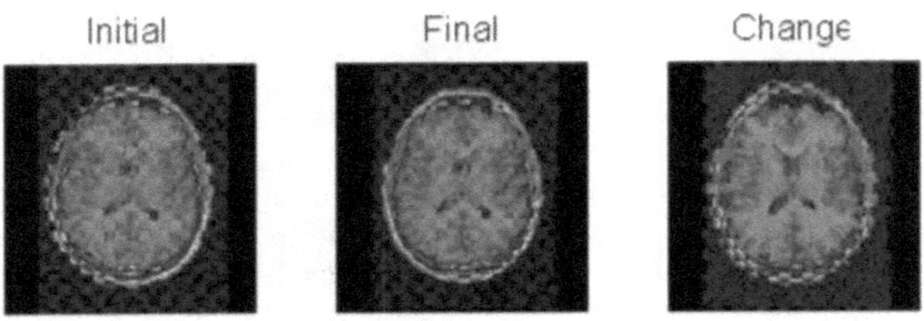

Fig. 4. Chequer-board plots showing the different between the initial images of the T1-weighted brains(left), the final images (centre), and the change between the initial and final versions of the free image (right). The registration has lined up the skulls and the major structures within the brain, but there is still more fine-scale work to be done.

the optimiser, with the final result being that shown. Fig. 3 shows the positions of the points and the initial momenta on the reference image, the final output, and the effect of the warp on a regular grid.

Fig. 4 show a sample registration of 2 brains. A set of 10 points were positioned evenly around the skull, and the result optimised for 20 iterations. Following this, an additional set of 11 knotpoints were added, with 50 iterations of optimisation then being performed. This registration took under 7 minutes on the same computer, and it can be see that the final result is not bad. There is still work to be done on the interior (and further optimisations do indeed correct this), but the skull and major structures have all been brought into alignment.

These results are much faster than using an optimisation method for finding the diffeomorphism – the method described in [4] took just under 2 hours to perform the brain registration described above. One of the main reasons for this is that those optimisation methods take many more timesteps to find the diffeomorphism, usually 20 timesteps are used to guarantee a diffeomorphism. With our current method, for relatively small deformations, only 1-4 timesteps are needed.

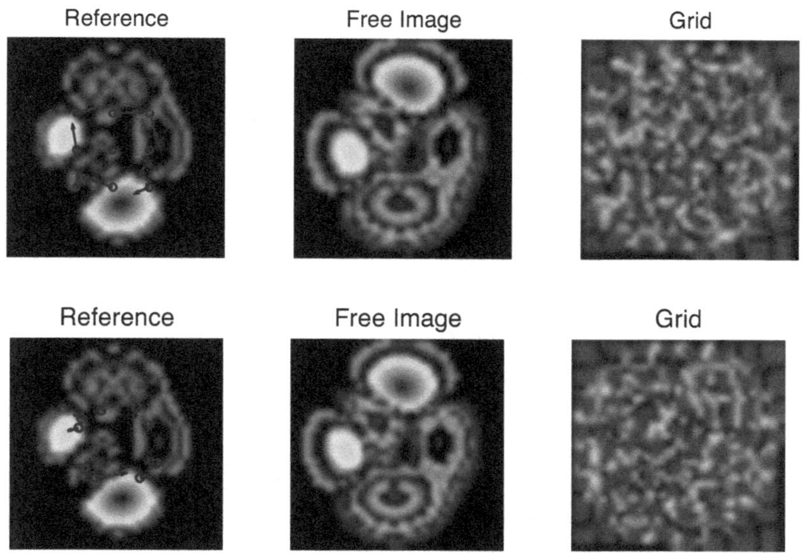

Fig. 5. Two regimes of optimisation. *Top:* Optimatisation of particle momenta only. *Bottom:* Simultaneous optimisation of both particle locations and momenta. The particles form into a ring showing the rotation that occurred.

4 Optimising Positions and Momenta

In the experiments described above we chose locations for the point particles, and then optimised their momenta. However, there is no reason why one cannot optimise the point locations as well as their momenta. We have performed some initial experiments with this based on the images produced by the `peaks(40)` function in Matlab. A typical result is shown in Fig. 5. The free image is a rotated version of the reference image (note that no affine registration is performed). The top line shows the optimisation if only the momenta of the particles are optimised, not their positions, while the bottom line shows the results when both are optimised, starting from the points being arranged on the uniform grid. It can be seen that the particle locations move to form a circle that reflects the rotation that was applied. Averaged over registrations of 10 random rotations, the final objective function value after 20 optimisation iterations was 5.85 for the momenta-only optimisations, and 1.59 for the full optimisation (the initial objective function value is around 2000).

The problem is that the method becomes more prone to becoming stuck in poor local minimas as the complexity of the image grows, since the dimensionality of the optimisation is so large. When it works it does very well, and resolves smaller image features, but for medical images it is only successful about half of the time. Finding suitable implementation methods to get around this problem, possibly using multiple scales of resolution, is a current area of research.

5 Use of Symplectic Integrators

The equations of motion (4, 5) are Hamiltonian and their flow is therefore symplectic [26]. In long-time simulations of Hamiltonian systems (in celestial and molecular mechanics, for example) it has been found extremely advantageous to use symplectic integrators, which preserve the symplectic structure. This leads to good energy behaviour and a lack of dissipation. Therefore, it is natural to consider their use here; it is also in accord with the 'Discrete Mechanics and Optimal Control' philosophy in which both the cost function and dynamics are discretized in a parallel, Hamiltonian way [27]. In fact, some implementations of image registration by diffeomorphisms have used symplectic integrators, because calculating geodesics by minimizing a discrete path length gives such an integrator [4]. However, the diffeomorphism itself, calculated from the motion of the test particles, has never been done symplectically. We give a preliminary analysis of the cost and benefits of using a symplectic integrator in image registration.

At first sight, the cost is a problem. The cheapest, explicit symplectic integrators apply to separable Hamiltonians of the form $T(p) + V(q)$; Eq. (3) is not separable, so only implicit symplectic integrators, notably the Gaussian Runge-Kuttas [26], are available; these methods have unconditional stability for linear problems, which allows larger time-steps to be used. These involve solving a set of equations for s internal stages; when $s = 1$, we have the midpoint rule

$$x_{k+1} = x_k + \Delta t f(\bar{x}_k), \quad \bar{x}_k = (x_k + x_{k+1})/2.$$

Moreover, to ensure exact symplecticity and that the solution varies smoothly with respect to the initial conditions, the equations must be solved extremely accurately, generally down to round-off error. In most situations, it is best to simply solve the equations by iteration

$$x_{k+1}^{l+1} = x_k + \Delta t f((x_k + x_{k+1}^l)/2), \quad l = 0, 1, 2, \ldots$$

after choosing some initial guess x_{k+1}^0. If m iterations are required then the cost per time step is ms times the cost of Euler's method. In initial value problems with a large time step, as we want to use here, m can be quite large, say 5–15.

However, this cost penalty for initial value problems vanishes for optimization problems, in which we want to repeatedly solve the same initial value problem for a sequence of nearby initial values. We simply store the internal stage values as part of the orbit segment and use this as initial guesses (e.g. x_{k+1}^0 for the midpoint rule) when the initial conditions are changed. Most optimization algorithms estimate the derivatives of the objective function using finite differences, which requires repeatedly altering the initial conditions by about 10^{-6}; for these evaluations we can solve the implicit equations in a *single* iteration. The error constants of the Gaussian Runge-Kutta methods are extremely small so we expect that this method could be superior both for cost and accuracy.

For the point particles, the simple iteration (5) can be improved using the $4N \times 4N$ Jacobian derivative matrices of f; calculating these is essentially cost-free, because the entries are simply related to the Green's functions, which have already been evaluated. Newton's method would cost $\mathcal{O}(N^3)$, which is presumably prohibitive, but the modifed iteration

$$\bar{x}^l = (x_k + x^l_{k+1})/2, \; w^l = x_k + \Delta t f(\bar{x}^l) \tag{6}$$

$$x^{l+1}_k = w^l + \frac{1}{2}\Delta t f'(\bar{x}^l)(w^l - x^l_k) \tag{7}$$

converges much more quickly than (5) and still costs only $\mathcal{O}(N^2)$. Moreover, the derivatives of the stage values with respect to the initial momenta can be approximated in a similar way, giving excellent initial guesses. Experiments will determine whether this cost is justified.

For very large numbers of point particles, the cost $\mathcal{O}(N^2 + NM)$ of evaluating the vector field may be too expensive. The cost can be reduced to $\mathcal{O}(N + M)$ using the marker-and-cell method [28], while still using symplectic integrators for the particle paths [29]. A regular grid with $\mathcal{O}(N)$ grid points is laid over the domain and the particle momenta interpolated to the grid. Then the velocity field induced by the momentum field is calculated on the grid using a fast algorithm, such as multigrid ($\mathcal{O}(N)$) or Fourier transform ($\mathcal{O}(N \log N)$). This velocity field is interpolated back to the particle positions, which are then updated. This algorithm has been implemented with enormous numbers (more than 1 million) particles in an initial value problem in atmospheric dynamics [29]. However, very large numbers of point particles, which may well be required for convergence to an arbitrary diffeomorphism, will introduce new difficulties for the optimization has the problem has now become ill-posed. Some degree of regularization, enforcing smoothness of the initial momentum field, will be required.

6 Conclusions and Open Questions

We have presented a method of performing diffeomorphic image registration that has links to the methods of discrete mechanics and optimal control. The implementation described in this paper has been demonstrated to perform high quality registrations in reasonably short computational time – orders of magnitude less than using energy minimisation methods. While they are not necessary for all image registration tasks, for applications where it is *variation* that is of interest, for example in disease diagnosis or measurement of anatomical variability, the access to a right-invariant Riemannian metric on the diffeomorphism group makes diffeomorphic registration methods essential.

There are a great many unanswered questions and areas for future research. We are particularly interested in the dynamical behaviour of the Euler equations on the diffeomorphism group, and how it relates to point vortices in fluid dynamics, which act on the volume-preserving subgroups. Some of our work on these topics is available in [25,30].

However, with regard to using the method for image registration, there are also several areas for further work. Firstly, we are currently investigating the use of the midpoint rule symplectic integrator and the marker-and-cell method, as discussed in section 5, and a second question that we highlighted earlier in the paper is that of a suitable choice of metric and corresponding length-scale.

Acknowledgements

We are grateful to Jan Modersitzki for the use of the hand images and to the Royal Society of New Zealand Marsden fund and NZIMA for their financial support.

References

1. Rueckert, D., Sonoda, L.I., Hayes, C., Hill, D.L.G., Leach, M.O., Hawkes, D.J.: Non-rigid registration using free-form deformations: Application to breast MR images. IEEE Transactions on Medical Imaging 18(8), 712–721 (1999)
2. Gee, J., Reivich, M., Bajcsy, R.: Elastically deforming 3D atlas to match anatomical brain images. Journal of Computer Assisted Tomography 17(2), 225–236 (1993)
3. Thompson, P., Hayashi, K.M., Sowell, E.R., Gogtay, N., Giedd, J.N., Rapoport, J.L., de Zubricara, C., Janke, G.A.L., Rose, S.E., Semple, J., Doddrell, D.M., Wang, Y., van Erp, T.G., Cannon, T.D., Toga, A.W.: Mapping cortical change in alzheimer's disease, brain development, and schizophrenia. NeuroImage 23, S2–S18 (2004)
4. Marsland, S., Twining, C.: Constructing diffeomorphic representations for the groupwise analysis of non-rigid registrations of medical images. IEEE Transactions on Medical Imaging 23(8), 1006–1020 (2004)
5. Toga, A.W.: Brain Warping. Academic Press, San Diego (1999)
6. Zitová, B., Flusser, J.: Image registration methods: A survey. Image and Vision Computing 21, 977–1000 (2003)
7. Arnold, V.I.: Sur la géométrie différentielle des groupes de Lie de dimension infinie et ses applications hydrodynamique des fluides parfaits. Annales de L'Institut Fourier (Grenoble) 16(1), 319–361 (1966)
8. Ebin, D.G., Marsden, J.E.: Groups of diffeomorphisms and the motion of an incompressible fluid. Annals of Mathematics 92, 102–163 (1970)
9. Miller, M., Trouvé, A., Younes, L.: On metrics and the Euler-Lagrange equations of computational anatomy. Annual Reviews in Biomedical Eng. 4, 375–405 (2002)
10. Holm, D.D., Ratnanather, J.T., Trouvé, A., Younes, L.: Soliton dynamics in computational anatomy. NeuroImage 23(Suppl. 1), S170–S178 (2004)
11. Viola, P., Wells III, W.M.: Alignment by maximization of mutual information. International Journal of Computer Vision 24(2), 137–154 (1997)
12. Maes, F., Collignon, A., Vandermeulun, D., Marchal, G., Suetens, P.: Multimodality image registration by maximization of mutual information. IEEE Transactions on Medical Imaging 16(2), 187–198 (1997)
13. Roche, A., Malandain, G., Pennec, X., Ayache, N.: The correlation ratio as a new similarity measure for multimodal image registration. In: Wells, W.M., Colchester, A.C.F., Delp, S.L. (eds.) MICCAI 1998. LNCS, vol. 1496, pp. 1115–1124. Springer, Heidelberg (1998)
14. Haber, E., Modersitzki, J.: Beyond mutual information: A simple and robust alternative. In: Bildverarbeitung für die Medizin, Springer, Heidelberg (2005)
15. Joshi, S.C., Miller, M.M.: Landmark matching via large deformation diffeomorphisms. IEEE Transactions on Image Processing 9(8), 1357–1370 (2000)
16. Beg, M.F., Miller, M.I., Trouv'e, A., Younes, L.: Computing large deformation metric mappings via geodesic flows of diffeomorphisms. International Journal of Computer Vision 61(2), 139–157 (2005)

17. Camion, V., Younes, L.: Geodesic interpolating splines. In: Figueiredo, M., Zerubia, J., Jain, A.K. (eds.) EMMCVPR 2001. LNCS, vol. 2134, pp. 513–527. Springer, Heidelberg (2001)
18. Holm, D.D., Marsden, J.E., Ratiu, T.S.: The Euler-Poincaré equations and semidirect products, with applications to continuum theories. Advances in Mathematics 137(1), 1–81 (1998)
19. Mumford, D.: Pattern theory and vision. In: Questions Mathématiques En Traitement Du Signal et de L'Image. Institute Henri Poincaré, Paris, pp. 7–13 (1998)
20. Leonard, A.: Vortex methods for flow simulation. Journal of Computational Physics 37, 289–305 (1980)
21. Beale, J.T., Majda, A.: Vortex methods. II: Higher order accuracy in two and three dimensions. Mathematics of Computation 39(159), 29–52 (1982)
22. Mills, A., Marsland, S., Shardlow, T.: Computing the geodesic interpolating spline. In: Pluim, J.P.W., Likar, B., Gerritsen, F.A. (eds.) WBIR 2006. LNCS, vol. 4057, pp. 169–177. Springer, Heidelberg (2006)
23. Marsden, J., Ratiu, T.: Introduction to Mechanics and Symmetry: A Basic Exposition of Classical Mechanical Systems, 2nd edn. Springer, Berlin (1999)
24. Marsland, S., Twining, C.: Constructing data-driven optimal representations for iterative pairwise non-rigid registration. In: Gee, J.C., Maintz, J.B.A., Vannier, M.W. (eds.) WBIR 2003. LNCS, vol. 2717, pp. 50–60. Springer, Heidelberg (2003)
25. McLachlan, R.I., Marsland, S.: N-particle dynamics of the Euler equations for planar diffeomorphisms. Dynamical Systems. (In press) (2007)
26. Hairer, E., Lubich, C., Wanner, G.: Geometric Numerical Integration: Structure-Preserving Algorithms for Ordinary Differential Equations. Springer, Berlin (2002)
27. Junge, O., Marsden, J.E., Ober-Blbaum, S.: Discrete mechanics and optimal control. In: Proceedings of International Federation of Automatic Control Conference 2005 (2005)
28. Harlow, F.H., Welsh, J.E.: Numerical calculation of time-dependent viscous incompressible flow of fluid with free surface. Physics of Fluids 8, 2182–2189 (1965)
29. Frank, J., Gottwald, G., Reich, S.: A Hamiltonian particle-mesh method for the rotating shallow-water equations. In: Siefkes, D. (ed.) Meshfree methods for partial differential equations. Lecture Notes in Computer Science Engineering, vol. 26, pp. 131–142. Springer, Berlin (2003)
30. McLachlan, R.I., Marsland, S.: The Kelvin-Helmholtz instability of momentum sheets in the Euler equations for planar diffeomorphisms. SIAM Journal on Applied Dynamical Systems 5(4), 726–758 (2006)

Inter and Intra-modal Deformable Registration: Continuous Deformations Meet Efficient Optimal Linear Programming

Ben Glocker[1,2], Nikos Komodakis[1,3]
Nikos Paragios[1], Georgios Tziritas[3], and Nassir Navab[2]

[1] GALEN Group, Laboratoire de Mathématiques Appliquées aux Systèmes
Ecole Centrale de Paris
{nikos.paragios}@ecp.fr
[2] Chair for Computer Aided Medical Procedures & Augmented Reality
Technische Universität München
{glocker, navab}@in.tum.de
[3] Computer Science Department, University of Crete
{komod,tziritas}@csd.uoc.gr

Abstract. In this paper we propose a novel non-rigid volume registration based on discrete labeling and linear programming. The proposed framework reformulates registration as a minimal path extraction in a weighted graph. The space of solutions is represented using a set of a labels which are assigned to predefined displacements. The graph topology corresponds to a superimposed regular grid onto the volume. Links between neighborhood control points introduce smoothness, while links between the graph nodes and the labels (end-nodes) measure the cost induced to the objective function through the selection of a particular deformation for a given control point once projected to the entire volume domain. Higher order polynomials are used to express the volume deformation from the ones of the control points. Efficient linear programming that can guarantee the optimal solution up to (a user-defined) bound is considered to recover the optimal registration parameters. Therefore, the method is gradient free, can encode various similarity metrics (simple changes on the graph construction), can guarantee a globally sub-optimal solution and is computational tractable. Experimental validation using simulated data with known deformation, as well as manually segmented data demonstrate the extreme potentials of our approach.

Keywords: Discrete Optimization, Deformable Registration, Linear Programming.

1 Introduction

Deformable registration is one of the most challenging problems in medical imaging. The problem consists of recovering a local transformation that aligns two signals that have a non-linear relationship often unknown. Several methods exist in the literature where specific metrics are designed to account for this non-linearity and optimize the transformation that brings together these two signals. This optimization is often sub-optimal due the non convexity of the designed cost functions. The aim of our approach

N. Karssemeijer and B. Lelieveldt (Eds.): IPMI 2007, LNCS 4584, pp. 408–420, 2007.
© Springer-Verlag Berlin Heidelberg 2007

is to overcome both limitations present in all registration methods. Dependency on the similarity metric selection, as well as to the initial conditions.

Local image alignment is often performed according to geometric or photometric criteria. Landmark-based methods [1] are a classic example of geometric-driven registration. In such a setting, a number of anatomical key points [2]/structures (segmented values) are identified both in the source and the target image and a transformation that aims to minimize the Euclidean distance between these structures is to be recovered. The main limitation of these methods related to the selection and extraction of landmarks, while their main strength is the simplicity of the optimization process.

Iconic registration methods seek for "visual" correspondences between the source and the target image. Such a problem is tractable when one seeks registration for images from the same modality due to an explicit photometric correspondence of the image intensities. Sum of squared differences [3], sum of absolute differences [3], cross correlation [3] or distances on subspaces that involve both appearance and geometry (intensities, curvature, higher order image moments) [4] have been considered. On the other hand it becomes more challenging when seeking transformations between different modalities where a non-linear transformation often relates them. Non-linear metrics have often been used [5] like normalized mutual information [6], kulback-leiber divergence [7] and correlation ratio [8] are some of the metrics used to define similarity between different modalities.

In this paper we propose a novel technique that can either be used for inter or intra modal image registration. Towards satisfying smoothness of the deformation field and reducing the dimensionality of the problem we represent deformation through Free Form Deformations. Our method reformulates registration as an MRF optimization where a set of labels is associated with a set of deformations, and one seeks to attribute a label to each control point such that once the corresponding deformation has been applied, the similarity metric between the source and the target is maximal for all voxels. The optimization procedure is independent from the graph construction, and therefore any similarity metric can be used.

The reminder of this paper is organized as follows; In section 2 we introduce the proposed registration framework, while in section 3 we discuss the optimization aspects. Implementation and experimental validation are part of section 4. The last section concludes our paper.

2 Deformable Registration in a Discrete Setting

In order to introduce the concept of our approach, we consider (without loss of generality) the 2D image domain. Let us consider a source $f : [1,N] \times [1,M] \rightarrow \mathcal{R}^n$ and a target image g. In general, these images are related with a non linear transformation as well as a non-linear relation between intensities, that is

$$g(\mathbf{x}) = h \circ f(\mathcal{T}(\mathbf{x})) \tag{1}$$

where $\mathcal{T}$ is the transformation and h is a non-linear operator explaining the changes of appearance between them. The most common way to formulate the registration problem, is through the definition of a distance between the source and the target image that is to be minimized in the entire domain Ω, or

$$E(\mathcal{T}) = \iint_{\Omega} \rho(g(\mathbf{x}), h \circ f(\mathcal{T}(\mathbf{x}))d\mathbf{x} \tag{2}$$

where ρ is a similarity metric used to determine meaningful correspondence. Since in most of the cases the non-linear transformation relating the two images is not known, the selection of similarity metric ρ explicitly or implicitly accounts for this non-linearity, or

$$E(\mathcal{T}) = \iint_{\Omega} \rho_h(g(\mathbf{x}), f(\mathcal{T}(\mathbf{x}))d\mathbf{x} \tag{3}$$

2.1 Continuous Domain

Since we are interested in local registration, let us introduce a deformation grid $\mathcal{G} : [1,K] \times [1,L]$ (usually $K \ll M$ and $L \ll N$) super-imposed to the image (no particular assumption is made on the grid resolution). The central idea of our approach is to deform the grid (with a 2D displacement vector $\mathbf{d}_p$ for each control point) such that the underlying image structures are perfectly aligned. Without loss of generality one can assume that the transformation of an image pixel $\mathbf{x}$ can be expressed using a linear or non-linear combination of the grid points, or

$$\mathcal{T}(\mathbf{x}) = \mathbf{x} + \mathcal{D}(\mathbf{x}) \quad \text{with} \quad \mathcal{D}(\mathbf{x}) = \sum_{p \in \mathcal{G}} \eta(|\mathbf{x} - \mathbf{p}|)\, \mathbf{d}_p \tag{4}$$

where $\eta(\cdot)$ is the weighting function measuring the contribution of the control point p to the displacement field $\mathcal{D}$. The position of point p is denoted as $\mathbf{p}$. In such a theoretical setting without loss of generality we consider Free Form Deformations (FFD) based on cubic B-splines as a transformation model. FFD are successfully applied in non-rigid image registration [9,10]. Deformation of an object is achieved by manipulating an underlying mesh of uniformly spaced control points. The displacement field for a two-dimensional FFD based on cubic B-Splines is defined as

$$\mathcal{D}(\mathbf{x}) = \sum_{l=0}^{3} \sum_{m=0}^{3} B_l(u) B_m(v)\, \mathbf{d}_{i+l,j+m} \tag{5}$$

where $i = \lfloor x/K \rfloor - 1$, $j = \lfloor y/L \rfloor - 1$, $u = x/K - \lfloor x/K \rfloor$, and $v = y/L - \lfloor y/L \rfloor$ and where B_l represents the lth basis function of the B-Spline. The three-dimensional version is defined straightforward.

By defining the registration problem based on such a deformation model we can now rewrite the criterion earlier introduced,

$$E_{\text{data}}(\mathcal{T}) = \sum_{p \in \mathcal{G}} \iint_{\Omega} \eta^{-1}(|\mathbf{x} - \mathbf{p}|) \cdot \rho_h(g(\mathbf{x}), f(\mathcal{T}(\mathbf{x})))d\mathbf{x}. \tag{6}$$

where $\eta^{-1}(\cdot)$ is the inverse projection for the contribution to the objective of the image pixel $\mathbf{x}$ according to the influence of the control point p.

Such a term will guarantee photometric correspondence between the two images. Hence, this term is also called the data term. The transformation due to the interpolation inherits some implicit smoothness properties. However, in order to avoid folding of the deformation grid, one can consider a smoothness term on the grid domain, or

$$E_{\text{smooth}}(\mathcal{T}) = \sum_{p \in \mathcal{G}} \phi(|\nabla_{\mathcal{G}} \mathbf{d}_p|) \tag{7}$$

with ϕ being a smoothness penalty function for instance penalizing the first derivatives of the grid deformation. The complete term associated with the registration problem is then defined as the sum of the data and smoothness term, or

$$E_{\text{total}} = E_{\text{data}} + E_{\text{smooth}}. \tag{8}$$

The most common way to obtain the transformation parameters is through the use of a gradient-descent method in an iterative approach. Thus given an initial guess, one updates the estimate according to the following formula $\left[\mathcal{T}^m = \mathcal{T}^{m-1} - \delta t \frac{E_{\text{total}}}{\partial T}\right]$. Such a process involves the derivative of the similarity metric with respect to the transformation parameters and therefore it is model and criterion dependent. Slight modifications on the cost function could lead to a different derivative and require novel numerical approximation methods.

2.2 Discrete Domain

Let us now consider a discrete set of labels $\mathcal{L} = \{u^1, ..., u^i\}$ corresponding to a quantized version of the deformation space $\times = \{\mathbf{d}^1, ..., \mathbf{d}^i\}$. A label assignment u_p to a grid node p is associated with displacing the node by the corresponding vector $\mathbf{d}^{u_p}$. The image transformation associated with a certain discrete labeling u becomes

$$\mathcal{D}(\mathbf{x}) = \sum_{p \in \mathcal{G}} \eta(|\mathbf{x} - \mathbf{p}|)\, \mathbf{d}^{u_p}. \tag{9}$$

One can reformulate the registration as a discrete optimization problem, that is assign individual labels u_p to the grid nodes such that

$$E_{\text{data}}(u) = \sum_{p \in \mathcal{G}} \iint_{\Omega} \eta^{-1}(|\mathbf{x} - \mathbf{p}|)\rho_h(g(\mathbf{x}), f(\mathcal{T}(\mathbf{x})))d\mathbf{x} \approx \sum_{p \in \mathcal{G}} V_p(u_p) \tag{10}$$

where $V_p(\cdot)$ represents a local similarity metric. There is a main issue coming along when using MRF-based optimization methods for our proposed setting. Here, the singleton potential functions $V_p(\cdot)$ are not independent, thus the defined data term can only be approximated. Hence, we pre-compute the $|\mathcal{L}| \times |\mathcal{G}|$ data term look-up table for a given image pair by simple shift operators. The entry for node p and labels u_p is determined by

$$V_p(u_p) = \iint_{\Omega} \eta^{-1}(|\mathbf{x} - \mathbf{p}|)\rho_h(g(\mathbf{x}), f(\mathbf{x} + \mathbf{d}^{u_p}))d\mathbf{x}. \tag{11}$$

The computation of such functions is very fast and straightforward. Any similarity metric can be simply plugged in this formulation without any changes or adaptations. Since the metrics are only considered on the image domain and no further analytical differentiation is needed, our approach is extremely flexible. Due to the approximation of the data term we allow to improve the estimation by successive optimizations resulting in a series of cost functions, or

$$E^t_{\text{data}}(u) = \sum_{p \in \mathcal{G}} \iint_{\Omega} \eta^{-1}(|\mathbf{x}-\mathbf{p}|)\rho_h(g(\mathbf{x}), f(\mathcal{T}^{t-1}(\mathbf{x}) + \mathbf{d}^{u_p}))d\mathbf{x}. \tag{12}$$

We should note, that from the optimization point of view we achieve (quasi) optimal solutions for the discrete labeling in every cycle. However, we can achieve a higher accuracy by successive cycles using the previous transformation $\mathcal{T}^{t-1}$.

The number of labels and their range play a significant role to the registration process. It is clear that setting the number of labels to infinity will converge to the continuous formulation which though it is intractable from computational perspective. However, the fact that we perform several cycles to improve the accuracy of the deformation allows us to keep the set of labels quite small.

The next aspect to be addressed, is the definition of the smoothness term in the label domain. One can express distances between the deformation vectors using difference between labels if a ranking has been considered within the definition of the label set, or

$$E_{\text{smooth}}(u) = \sum_{p,q \in \mathcal{E}} V_{pq}(u_p, u_q) \tag{13}$$

where $\mathcal{E}$ represents the neighborhood system associated with the deformation grid $\mathcal{G}$. For the distance $V_{pq}(\cdot,\cdot)$ we consider a simple piecewise smoothness truncated term based on the euclidean geometric distances between the deformations corresponding to the assigned labels:

$$V_{pq}(u_p, u_q) = \lambda_{pq} \min\left(|\mathbf{d}^{u_p} - \mathbf{d}^{u_q}|, T\right) \tag{14}$$

with T being the maximum penalty and λ_{pq} being a (spacial varying) weighting to control the influence of the prior term. Basically, this is a discrete approximation of the smoothness term defined in equation 7 extended by the piecewise property. Such a smoothness term together with the data term allows to convert the problem of image registration into the form of a Markov Random Field (MRF) [11] in a discrete domain, or

$$E_{\text{total}}(u) = \sum_{p \in \mathcal{G}} V_p(u_p) + \sum_{p,q \in \mathcal{E}} V_{pq}(u_p, u_q). \tag{15}$$

3 MRF Optimization Based on Linear Programming

For optimizing the resulting MRF, we seek to assign a label $u_p \in \mathcal{L}$ to each node $p \in \mathcal{G}$, so that the MRF energy in (15) is minimized. To this end, a recently proposed method, called Fast-PD, will be used [12]. This is an optimization technique, which builds upon principles drawn from the duality theory of linear programming in order to efficiently derive almost optimal solutions for a very wide class of NP-hard MRFs. When applied to the image registration task, this technique thus offers a series of important advantages compared to prior art (see section 3.2).

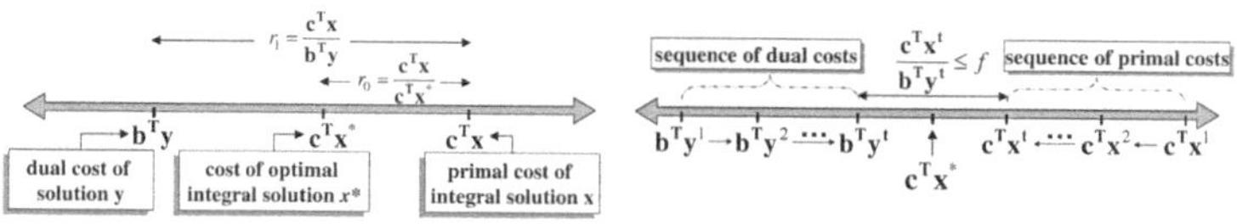

(a) The primal-dual principle (b) The primal-dual schema

Fig. 1. **(a)** By weak duality, the optimal cost $\mathbf{c}^T\mathbf{x}^*$ will lie between the costs $\mathbf{b}^T\mathbf{y}$ and $\mathbf{c}^T\mathbf{x}$ of any pair $(\mathbf{x},\mathbf{y})$ of integral-primal and dual feasible solutions. Therefore, if $\mathbf{b}^T\mathbf{y}$ and $\mathbf{c}^T\mathbf{x}$ are close enough (e.g. their ratio r_1 is $\leq f$), so are $\mathbf{c}^T\mathbf{x}^*$ and $\mathbf{c}^T\mathbf{x}$ (e.g. their ratio r_0 is $\leq f$ as well), thus proving that $\mathbf{x}$ is an f-approximation to $\mathbf{x}^*$. **(b)** According to the primal-dual schema, dual and integral-primal feasible solutions make local improvements to each other, until the final costs $\mathbf{b}^T\mathbf{y}^t$, $\mathbf{c}^T\mathbf{x}^t$ are close enough (e.g. their ratio is $\leq f$). We can then apply the primal-dual principle (as in Fig. (a)) and thus conclude that $\mathbf{x}^t$ is an f-approximation to $\mathbf{x}^*$.

For more details about the Fast-PD algorithm, the reader is referred to [12,13]. Here, we will just provide a brief, high level description of the basic driving force behind that algorithm. This driving force will consist of the *primal-dual schema*, which is a well-known technique in the Linear Programming literature.

3.1 The Primal-Dual Schema for MRF Optimization

To understand how the primal-dual schema works in general, we will need to consider the following pair of primal and dual Linear Programs (LPs):

$$\begin{array}{llll} \text{PRIMAL:} & \min \mathbf{c}^T\mathbf{x} & \quad \text{DUAL:} & \max \mathbf{b}^T\mathbf{y} \\ & \text{s.t. } \mathbf{A}\mathbf{x} = \mathbf{b}, \mathbf{x} \geq \mathbf{0} & & \text{s.t. } \mathbf{A}^T\mathbf{y} \leq \mathbf{c} \end{array} \tag{16}$$

Here $\mathbf{A}$ represents a coefficient matrix, while $\mathbf{b},\mathbf{c}$ are coefficient vectors. Also, $\mathbf{x}$, $\mathbf{y}$ represent the vectors of primal and dual variables respectively. We seek an optimal solution to the primal program, but with the extra constraint of $\mathbf{x}$ being integral. Due to this integrality requirement, this problem is in general NP-hard and so we need to settle with estimating approximate solutions. A primal-dual f-approximation algorithm achieves that by use of the following principle (illustrated also in Fig. 1(a)):

Primal-Dual Principle 1. *If* $\mathbf{x}$ *and* $\mathbf{y}$ *are integral-primal and dual feasible solutions having a primal-dual gap less than* f*, i.e.:*

$$\mathbf{c}^T\mathbf{x} \leq f \cdot \mathbf{b}^T\mathbf{y}, \tag{17}$$

then $\mathbf{x}$ *is an* f*-approximation to the optimal integral solution* $\mathbf{x}^*$*, i.e.* $\mathbf{c}^T\mathbf{x}^* \leq \mathbf{c}^T\mathbf{x} \leq f \cdot \mathbf{c}^T\mathbf{x}^*$

Based on the above principle, that lies at the heart of any primal-dual technique, the following iterative schema can be used for deriving an f-approximate solution (this schema is also illustrated graphically in Fig. 1(b)):

Primal-Dual Schema 1. *Keep generating pairs of integral-primal, dual solutions* $\{(\mathbf{x}^k, \mathbf{y}^k)\}_{k=1}^t$, *until the elements* $\mathbf{x}^t$, $\mathbf{y}^t$ *of the last pair are both feasible and have a primal-dual gap which is less than* f, *i.e. condition* (17) *holds true.*

In order to apply the above schema to MRF optimization, it suffices that we cast the MRF optimization problem as an equivalent integer program. To this end, the following integer programming formulation of (15) has been used as the primal problem:

$$\min \sum_{p \in \mathcal{G}} \sum_{l \in \mathcal{L}} V_p(l) x_p(l) + \sum_{(p,q) \in \mathcal{E}} \sum_{l,l' \in \mathcal{L}} V_{pq}(l,l') x_{pq}(l,l') \tag{18}$$

$$\text{s.t.} \sum\nolimits_l x_p(l) = 1 \qquad \forall\, p \in \mathcal{G} \tag{19}$$

$$\sum\nolimits_l x_{pq}(l,l') = x_q(l') \qquad \forall\, l' \in \mathcal{L},\ (p,q) \in \mathcal{E} \tag{20}$$

$$\sum\nolimits_{l'} x_{pq}(l,l') = x_p(l) \qquad \forall\, l \in \mathcal{L},\ (p,q) \in \mathcal{E} \tag{21}$$

$$x_p(\cdot),\ x_{pq}(\cdot,\cdot) \in \{0,1\}$$

Here, in order to linearize the MRF energy, we have replaced the discrete variables u_p with the binary variables $x_p(\cdot)$ and $x_{pq}(\cdot,\cdot)$. More specifically, the $\{0,1\}$-variable $x_p(l)$ indicates that node p is assigned label l (i.e., $u_p = l$), while the $\{0,1\}$-variable $x_{pq}(l,l')$ indicates that vertices p,q are assigned labels l,l' respectively (i.e., $u_p = l,\ u_q = l'$). Furthermore, the constraints in (19) simply express the fact that each node must receive exactly one label, while constraints (20), (21) maintain consistency between variables $x_p(\cdot), x_q(\cdot)$ and variables $x_{pq}(\cdot,\cdot)$, in the sense that if $x_p(l) = 1$ and $x_q(l') = 1$ holds true, then these constraints force $x_{pq}(l,l') = 1$ to hold true as well (as desired).

The linear programming relaxation of the above integer program is then taken (by relaxing the binary constraints to $x_p(\cdot) \geq 0, x_{pq}(\cdot,\cdot) \geq 0$), and the dual of the resulting LP is used as our dual problem. The Fast-PD algorithm is then derived by applying the primal-dual schema to this pair of primal-dual LPs, while using $f = 2\frac{d_{\max}}{d_{\min}}$[1] as the approximation factor in (17).

3.2 Advantages of the Primal-Dual Approach

Fast-PD has many nice properties, which makes it a perfect candidate for our image registration task. In particular, it offers the following advantages: **1) Generality:** Fast-PD can handle a very wide class of MRFs, since it merely requires $V_{pq}(\cdot,\cdot) \geq 0$. Hence, by using Fast-PD, our image registration framework can automatically incorporate any similarity metric, as well as a very wide class of smoothness penalty functions. **2) Optimality:** Furthermore, Fast-PD can always guarantee that the generated solution will be an f-approximation to the true optimum (where $f = 2\frac{d_{\max}}{d_{\min}}$). **3) Per-instance approximation factors:** In fact, besides the above worst-case approximation factor, Fast-PD can also continuously update a *per-instance* approximation factor during its execution. In practice, this factor drops to 1 very quickly, thus allowing the global optimum to be found up to a user/application bound. **4) Speed:** Finally, Fast-PD provides great computational efficiency, since it can reach an almost optimal solution very fast and in an efficient manner.

[1] $d_{\max} \equiv \max_{a \neq b} d(a,b)$, $d_{\min} \equiv \min_{a \neq b} d(a,b)$.

4 Implementation Details and Validation

4.1 Implementation Details

In order to prove our concept, we implemented a non-rigid image registration framework based on discrete optimization. We are using multi-level free-form deformations [14] together with a pyramidal image representation. The deformations are computed on each level in a course-to-fine manner. We define the set of labels for the finest pyramid by setting a minimum and maximum displacement and the number steps. Additionally, the displacements are scaled for the coarser levels to recover a larger deformations. In general, before running our algorithm, we rescale the image intensities of the source and target image to values between 0 and 1. Thus, the weighting of the prior term is less sensitive. In all experiments, we use an empirically determined $\lambda_{pq} = 0.0001$ equally for all grid nodes. In order to demonstrate the flexibility of our framework, we implemented a range of well-known similarity metrics, namely the Sum of Absolute Differences (SAD) [3], the Sum of Squared Differences (SSD) [3], the Normalized Cross Correlation (NCC) [3], the Normalized Mutual Information (NMI) [6], the Correlation Ratio (CR) [8], and the Sum of Absolute Differences plus image gradient information (SADG). The SADG metric involves an intensity-based and a geometric-based term. An additional weighting factor γ is used to control the influence of these two terms. The SADG metric is defined as

$$\begin{aligned}\rho(g(\mathbf{x}), f(\mathcal{T}(\mathbf{x}))) &= (1-\gamma)|g(\mathbf{x}) - f(\mathcal{T}(\mathbf{x}))| + \\ &+ \gamma \arccos\left(\frac{\nabla g(\mathbf{x})}{|\nabla g(\mathbf{x})|} \cdot \frac{\nabla f(\mathcal{T}(\mathbf{x}))}{|\nabla f(\mathcal{T}(\mathbf{x}))|}\right).\end{aligned} \tag{22}$$

4.2 Validation Using Known and Unknown Deformations

In order to evaluate our framework we test our method on several data sets. In general, the evaluation and thus, validation of non-rigid image registration methods is a difficult task. Usually, ground truth data for real deformations, especially, in medical applications is not available. Therefore, we performed several experiments hopefully illustrating the great potentials of our approach.

Realistic Synthetic Registration. The first two experiments are concerning the nature of the free choice of similarity metrics inherent in our framework. In order to evaluate the efficiency of different metrics we test our method on simulated realistic data. The target image is generated from the 2D MRI source image by randomly displaced deformation grid. Additionally, we added uniformly distributed noise up to 15 percent of the original target intensities. For the multi-modal experiment we use the inverse target image and squared intensities. The image resolution is 256x256. The registration is performed using a three-level image and grid pyramid. The range of the set of labels is from 0.25 to 5 pixels in 5 steps for the finest pyramid level defined on the 8 main

Table 1. Angular error (in degrees) and magnitude of difference error (in pixels) for the realistic synthetic image registration using different similarity metrics

Metric	AE Mean	AE Median	AE Std	MOD Mean	MOD Median	MOD Std
SSD	2.290	1.143	2.854	0.242	0.139	0.297
SADG $\gamma = 1.0$	1.957	1.077	2.350	0.227	0.136	0.349
SAD	1.220	0.675	1.653	0.123	0.071	0.194
SADG $\gamma = 0.75$	1.129	0.709	1.313	0.122	0.082	0.169
SADG $\gamma = 0.25$	1.046	0.603	1.307	0.104	0.067	0.142
SADG $\gamma = 0.5$	1.036	0.589	1.292	0.111	0.066	0.159
NMI	0.999	0.629	1.060	0.099	0.079	0.080
CR	0.927	0.536	1.116	0.089	0.068	0.092
NCC	0.765	0.402	1.082	0.070	0.047	0.076
CR	2.244	1.039	3.465	0.234	0.110	0.373
NMI	0.846	0.607	0.826	0.086	0.071	0.070

directions (horizontal, vertical, and diagonal) leading to 41 labels in total (including the zero displacement). We perform 3 optimization cycles per pyramid level. The initial grid resolution is 6x6 increased to 11x11 and finally 21x21. One registration takes between 5-30 seconds depending on the similarity metric. The results are shown in Table 1. For the evaluation, two error metrics are considered, namely the angular error (AE) [15] and the magnitude of difference (MOD). We only consider the deformation field within a region of interest which is determined by the image mask shown in Fig. 2(d).

Automatic Cartilage Segmentation. Our third experiment is aiming at the registration accuracy. The medical application is similar to the one described in [16]. An automatic segmentation of the cartilage should be performed. Assuming that manual segmentations are available, one may create statistical models for an atlas-based segmentation procedure.

Table 2. Results for the cartilage segmentation experiment

Image	OR	SD In	SD Out	HD
1	0.922	0.079	0.632	1.398
2	0.914	0.068	1.280	3.064
3	0.876	0.089	1.626	3.250
4	0.884	0.081	1.469	3.250
5	0.873	0.099	1.434	3.064
6	0.905	0.070	0.641	1.976

In our experiment, 7 data sets (256x256x20), all manually segmented by medical experts, are available. The MRI data was acquired for a follow-up experiment. Due to the intra-subject property and the limited number of data sets we simply selected one of it as a template segmentation. By deforming the template to the six other data sets and warping the corresponding segmentations, we are able to achieve a fully automatic segmentation in less than 80 seconds. We use a three-level pyramid, the SAD metric and a set of labels from 0.25 to 5 pixels in 5 steps in the six main directions ($\pm$x, $\pm$y, and $\pm$z) leading to 31 labels in total. We perform 5 optimization cycles per pyramid level. The segmentation results are then compared to the manual segmentations. With our method we achieve an average overlap ratio (OR) of 0.90($\pm$0.02), an average surface distance inside (SD In) of 0.08($\pm$0.01)mm, average surface distance outside (SD Out) of 1.18($\pm$0.44)mm, and an average Haussdorf distance (HD) of 2.67($\pm$0.79)mm (which is less than the slice thickness of 3mm). (see also Table 2 and Fig. 3). The comparison of the segmentations is done using the tool[2] described in [17].

[2] Available on http://www.ia.unc.edu/dev/download/valmet/

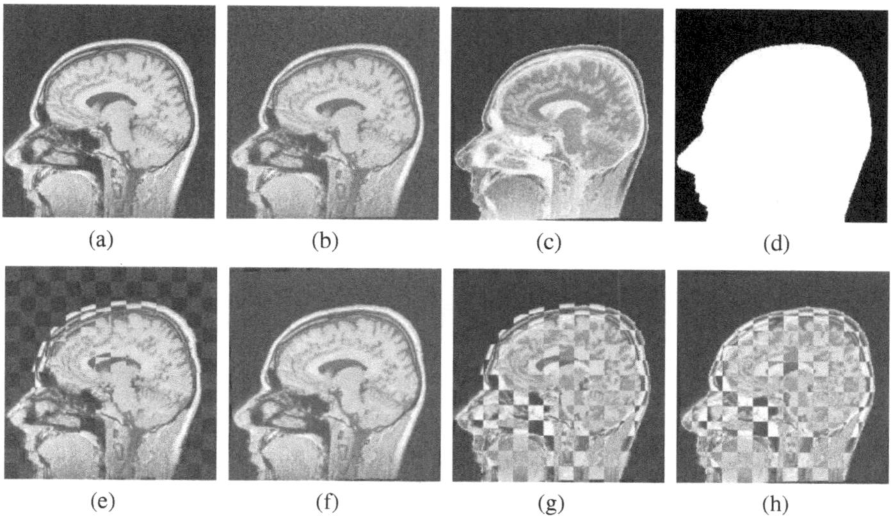

Fig. 2. Realistic synthetic data. **(a)** The source image, and **(b)** target image of the first (mono-modal) experiment. **(c)** Target image of the second (multi-modal) experiment. **(d)** Image mask used for error evaluation. **(e)** Checkerboard visualization before and **(f)** after registration using NCC for the mono-modal experiment. **(g)** Checkerboard visualization before and **(h)** after registration using NMI for the multi-modal experiment.

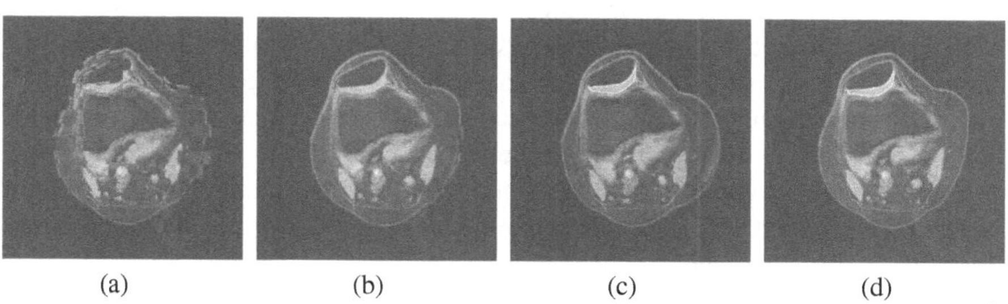

Fig. 3. Results for the cartilage segmentation of the first image. **(a)** Checkerboard visualization before and **(b)** after registration. **(c)** Template segmentation. **(d)** Warped template on top of the target image.

Comparison to State-of-the-art. Schnabel et al. [10] propose a non-rigid image registration method[3] based on B-Spline FFD together with a gradient-descent optimization. In order to obtain meaningful comparable results we try to set the registration parameters as similar as possible. Both algorithms are using the same deformation model and the SSD metric. We use a set of labels from 0.1 to 2 pixels in 5 steps and allow 20 optimization cycles. The test data are two CT volumes showing the heart of a pig. The image resolution is 128x128x88 with a voxel size of 0.848x0.848x1.25mm. Due

[3] Available on http://wwwhomes.doc.ic.ac.uk/~dr/software/

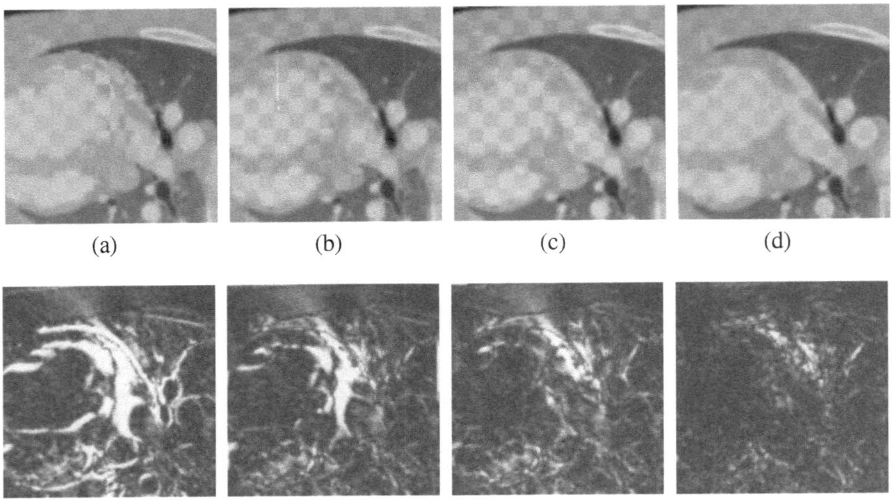

Fig. 4. (**a**) Checkerboard visualization before registration, (**b**) after registration using the method in [10], and (**c**) after registration using our method (**d**) After registration using our approach with pyramidal settings. Same order for the difference images in (**e**)-(**h**).

to the heart beat a deformation of the shape is clearly visible. We run both methods on a deformation grid with 10mm control point spacing. Within the region of interest enclosing the heart and an average SSD error of 12278 before registration, we achieve an average SSD error of 3180, where the other method converges to a value of 3402. Also, by visual perception of the difference images we can achieve better results (see Fig. 4). Last but not least, the running time of our algorithm is less than 2 minutes in contrast to a running time of more than 2 hours for the other method (AMD Athlon64 2.21 GHz). We should note, that this experiment was not performed to obtain the best registration of the two data sets, but rather to compare the two algorithms. With our standard pyramidal approach we obtain a SSD error of 1233 by same running time of about 2 minutes.

5 Discussion

In this paper we have proposed a novel framework to deformable image registration that bridges the gap between continuous deformations and optimal discrete optimization. Our method reformulates registration using a MRF definition, and recovers the optimal solution to the designed objective function through efficient linear programming. Towards capturing important deformations, we propose an incremental estimation of the deformation component. These objectives are met through a min cut problem defined over a graph with two terminal links. Graph edges introduce smoothness on the deformation field, while edges with the terminal links encode the image support for a given deformation hypothesis versus another. Therefore, the method is gradient free, can encode any similarity metric and can recover the optimal solution up to a bound.

In several applications, building anatomical atlases and models of variations between training examples is feasible. In such a context, one can consider a partial graph where connections, as well as t-links hypotheses are determined according to the density of expected deformations. Such a direction will introduce prior knowledge in the registration process and will make the optimization step more efficient. Moreover, the use of shape and appearance models can be considered to perform segmentation through registration. Assuming a prior model that involves both geometry and texture, and given a new volume one can define/recover segmentation through the deformation of the model to the image that is a natural registration problem which can be optimally addressed from the proposed framework.

References

1. Hellier, P., Barillot, C.: Coupling dense and landmark-based approaches for nonrigid registration. IEEE Medical Imaging 22(2) (2003)
2. Pennec, X., Ayache, N., Thirion, J.P.: Landmark-based registration using features identified through differential geometry. In: Handbook of medical imaging, pp. 499–513 (2000)
3. Hajnal, J., Hill, D.L.G., Hawkes, D.J. (eds.): Medical Image Registration. CRC Press, Boca Raton, FL (2001)
4. Davatzikos, C., Prince, J., Bryan, R.: Image registration based on boundary mapping (1996)
5. Hermosillo, G., Chefd'hotel, C., Faugeras, O.: Variational methods for multimodal image matching. Int. J. Comput. Vision 50(3), 329–343 (2002)
6. Maes, F., Collignon, A., Vandermeulen, D., Marchal, G., Suetens, P.: Multimodality image registration by maximization of mutual information. IEEE Medical Imaging 16(2), 187–198 (1997)
7. Zollei, L., Fisher, J., Wells, W.: An Introduction to Statistical Methods of Medical Image Registration. In: Handbook of Mathematical Models in Computer Vision, Springer, Heidelberg (2005)
8. Roche, A., Malandain, G., Pennec, X., Ayache, N.: The correlation ratio as a new similarity measure for multimodal image registration. In: Wells, W.M., Colchester, A.C.F., Delp, S.L. (eds.) MICCAI 1998. LNCS, vol. 1496, pp. 1115–1124. Springer, Heidelberg (1998)
9. Rohlfing, T., Maurer, C.R.J., Bluemke, D., Jacobs, M.: Volume-preserving nonrigid registration of mr breast images using free-form deformation with an incompressibility constraint. IEEE Medical Imaging 22(6) (2003)
10. Schnabel, J.A., Rueckert, D., Quist, M., Blackall, J.M., Castellano-Smith, A.D., Hartkens, T., Penney, G.P., Hall, W.A., Liu, H., Truwit, C.L., Gerritsen, F.A., Hill, D.L.G., Hawkes, D.J.: A generic framework for non-rigid registration based on non-uniform multi-level free-form deformations. In: Niessen, W.J., Viergever, M.A. (eds.) MICCAI 2001. LNCS, vol. 2208, pp. 573–581. Springer, Heidelberg (2001)
11. Li, S.Z.: Markov random field modeling in image analysis. Springer-Verlag, New York (2001)
12. Komodakis, N., Tziritas, G., Paragios, N.: Fast, approximately optimal solutions for single and dynamic mrfs. In: Computer Vision and Pattern Recognition (2007)
13. Komodakis, N., Tziritas, G.: A new framework for approximate labeling via graph cuts. In: IEEE International Conference on Computer Vision (2005)
14. Forsey, D.R., Bartels, R.H.: Hierarchical b-spline refinement. SIGGRAPH Comput. Graph. 22(4), 205–212 (1988)

15. Fleet, D.J.: Measurement of Image Velocity. Kluwer Academic Publishers, Norwell, MA, USA (1992)
16. Folkesson, J., Dam, E., Olsen, O.F., Pettersen, P., Christiansen, C.: Automatic segmentation of the articular cartilage in knee mri using a hierarchical multi-class classification scheme. In: Duncan, J.S., Gerig, G. (eds.) MICCAI 2005. LNCS, vol. 3749, pp. 327–334. Springer, Heidelberg (2005)
17. Gerig, G., Jomier, M., Chakos, M.: Valmet: A new validation tool for assessing and improving 3d object segmentations. In: Niessen, W.J., Viergever, M.A. (eds.) MICCAI 2001. LNCS, vol. 2208, Springer, Heidelberg (2001)

Tracer Kinetics Guided Dynamic PET Reconstruction

Shan Tong[1] and Pengcheng Shi[1,2]

[1] Department of Electronic and Computer Engineering, Hong Kong University of Science and Technology, Hong Kong
[2] School of Biomedical Engineering, Southern Medical University, China*

Abstract. Dynamic PET reconstruction is a challenging issue due to the spatio-temporal nature and the complexity of the data. Conventional frame-by-frame approaches fail to explore the temporal information of dynamic PET data, and may lead to inaccurate results due to the low SNR of data. Due to the ill-conditioning of image reconstruction, proper prior knowledge should be incorporated to constrain the reconstruction. In this paper, we propose a tracer kinetics guided reconstruction framework for dynamic PET imaging. The dynamic reconstruction problem is formulated in a state-space representation, where compartment model serves as a continuous-time system equation to describe the tracer kinetic processes, and the imaging data is expressed as discrete sampling of the system states in a measurement equation. The reconstruction problem has therefore become a state estimation problem in a continuous-discrete hybrid paradigm, and sampled-data H_∞ filtering is applied to for the estimation. As H_∞ filtering makes no assumptions on the system and measurement statistics, robust reconstruction results can be obtained for dynamic PET imaging where the statistical properties of measurement data and system uncertainty are not available *a priori*.

1 Introduction

Dynamic positron emission tomography (PET) imaging can provide measurements of the spatial distribution and kinetics of radiotracer-labeled biological substrates in living tissue [1]. The spatio-temporal nature and the complexity of the data, however, makes the reconstruction of dynamic PET a challenging issue. The conventional approach is to reconstruct a sequence of activity images *independently* at each of the measurement times, using analytical or statistical methods from static image reconstruction [2,3]. These frame-by-frame strategies, however, fail to explore the temporal information of dynamic PET data, and may lead to inaccurate results due to the low signal-to-noise ratio (SNR) of data (SNR is sacrificed for temporal resolution in dynamic imaging). Moreover, although statistical methods have produced much superior performance, and

* Thanks to IBM PhD fellowship for supporting Shan Tong. This work was supported in part by the National Basic Research Program of China (2003CB716104) and by the Hong Kong Research Grants Council (CERG HKUST6151/03E).

N. Karssemeijer and B. Lelieveldt (Eds.): IPMI 2007, LNCS 4584, pp. 421–433, 2007.
© Springer-Verlag Berlin Heidelberg 2007

there have been numerous attempts on object function design and optimization for their improvement [2], it remains true that all statistical methods are based on specific assumptions on the measurement distribution (Poisson or Shifted Poisson [4]). In practice, however, PET data has complicated statistics due to various sources of uncertainties [1], and such assumptions may not capture the statistics well, especially for low SNR cases in dynamic imaging. As a result, the quality of the reconstruction will be subject to limits imposed by the statistical quality of data in these statistical approaches.

Due to the ill-conditioning of image reconstruction, the importance of incorporating prior knowledge into statistical reconstruction is well appreciated [2]. For static reconstruction, such efforts can be largely classified as mathematical regularization with various smoothness constrains [5], and anatomy-constrained reconstruction with shape priors [6], all of which attempt to capture the spatially structured properties of images. There have also been attempts to incorporate temporal priors in dynamic reconstruction via signal sub-spaces or splines [7,8]. While such works can improve the SNR, their temporal models have only explored the temporal correlation of the data, and the underlying physiological processes that generate the PET data are not taken into account.

From the above analysis, the reconstruction problem of dynamic PET need to be addressed with proper consideration of the following issues: the temporal kinetics of underlying physiological processes, the need for proper priors, and the complicated statistics and noisy nature of data.

Tracer kinetic studies aim to understand the physiology and pathophysiology of the metabolism of substances in a biological system. The kinetics of a substance are its spatial and temporal distributions in the system, which result from complex physiological events including circulatory dynamics, transport and utilization [9]. Various models have been proposed to convert the radiotracer concentrations reconstructed from PET data into measures of the physiological processes, which can be classified as noncompartmental, compartmental, and distributive models [1]. As these models provide quantitative description of the kinetic processes that generate the PET measurements, it is natural to incorporate tracer kinetic modeling as prior information in dynamic PET reconstruction.

In this paper, we propose a tracer kinetics guided reconstruction framework for dynamic PET imaging. The dynamic reconstruction problem is formulated in a state-space representation, where compartment model serves as a continuous-time system equation to describe the tracer kinetic processes, and the imaging data is expressed as discrete sampling of the system states in a measurement equation. The reconstruction problem has therefore become a state estimation problem in a continuous-discrete hybrid paradigm, and sampled-data H_∞ filtering is applied to achieve robust estimation. The main contribution of our work lies in the following aspects. Firstly, as tracer kinetics is adopted to guide the reconstruction, information of the underlying physiological processes is included, and physiologically more meaningful results can thus be expected. Secondly, instead of using a frame-by-frame approach, the temporal information of the data is fully explored. Thirdly, since H_∞ filtering makes no assumptions on the system and measurement statistics, it is particular suited for PET imaging where the statistical properties of measurement data and system uncertainty remain difficult to acquire. Finally, our work provides a general framework for incorporating prior knowledge to guide reconstruction. Anatomical priors or mathematical regularization can be integrated with tracer kinetics in the state equation, so that the spatio-temporal nature of the data can be exploited to assist reconstruction.

2 Methodology

2.1 Two-Tissue Compartmental Modeling of PET Tracer Kinetics

Due to their simple implementation and biological plausibility, compartment models have been widely employed to quantitatively describe regional tracer kinetics in PET imaging [1], where one need to postulate a linear or nonlinear structure in a number of compartments and their interconnections, and resolve them from the measurement data [9]. A compartment is a mathematical abstraction which represents a particular form or location of tracer that behaves in a kinetically equivalent manner, while the interconnections represent fluxes of material and biochemical conversions.

In this paper, a two-tissue compartment model is adopted to describe the radiotracer kinetic processes, so that the model can serve as physiologically meaningful priors to guide the dynamic PET reconstruction. This model is commonly used to describe the uptake and retention of an analog of glucose, 2-deoxy-2-$[^{18}F]$ fluoro-D-glucose (FDG). The structure of the model is illustrated in Fig.1, where C_P is the arterial concentration of nonmetabolized tracer in plasma, C_E is the concentration of nonmetabolized tracer in tissue, C_M is the concentration of the radioisotope-labeled metabolic products in tissue, and the kinetic parameters k_1, k_2, k_3, k_4 (min^{-1}) are first-order rate constants specifying the the tracer exchange rates between compartments. While our reconstruction framework will be derived under this particular model, the framework itself is very general *per se*, and compartment models of other forms or in higher complexities can also be incorporated without fundamental changes.

By applying the model in Fig.1 to all voxels and assuming a space-invariant tracer delivery C_P, the kinetic process for any voxel i ($i = 1, ..., N$) is governed by the following differential equation [9]:

$$\begin{bmatrix} \dot{C}_{Ei}(t) \\ \dot{C}_{Mi}(t) \end{bmatrix} = \begin{bmatrix} -(k_{2i}+k_{3i}) & k_{4i} \\ k_{3i} & -k_{4i} \end{bmatrix} \begin{bmatrix} C_{Ei}(t) \\ C_{Mi}(t) \end{bmatrix} + \begin{bmatrix} k_{1i} \\ 0 \end{bmatrix} C_P(t) \quad (1)$$

with the subscript i denoting different voxel locations. The above kinetic equation can be expressed in a compact notation as:

$$\dot{x}_i(t) = a_i x_i(t) + b_i C_P(t) \quad (2)$$

where $x_i(t) = [C_{Ei}(t) \;\; C_{Mi}(t)]^T$, $a_i = \begin{bmatrix} -(k_{2i}+k_{3i}) & k_{4i} \\ k_{3i} & -k_{4i} \end{bmatrix}$, $b_i = [k_1 \;\; 0]^T$. The input $C_P(t)$ is assumed known here, which in practice can be measured directly

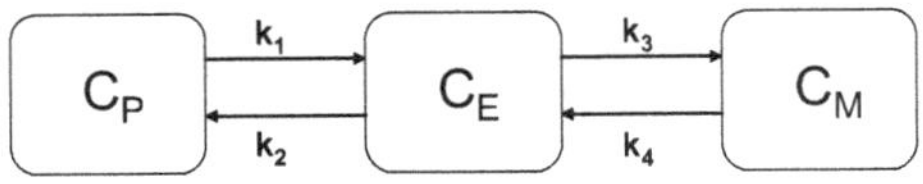

Fig. 1. Two-tissue compartment model with four kinetic parameters

from arterial plasma samples during the imaging procedure [1], or estimated from imaged volumes that consist primarily of blood [10]. The total concentration of radioactivity in tissue $C_{Ti}(t)$, which directly generates the PET measurements through positron emission, can be expressed as:

$$C_{Ti}(t) = (1 - V_{Bi})[C_{Ei}(t) + C_{Mi}(t)] + V_{Bi}C_{WB}(t) \tag{3}$$

where V_{Bi} is the vascular volume fraction at voxel i, and $C_{WB}(t)$ is the radioactivity concentration in whole blood. In practice, V_{Bi} can be obtained from vessel segmentation in MR angiography (MRA), followed by registration of PET and MRA images. For computational simplicity and without losing generality [9,11], $C_{Ti}(t)$ is simplified in this paper as the sum of the concentrations of nonmetabolized and metabolized tracer at that voxel location:

$$C_{Ti}(t) = C_{Ei}(t) + C_{Mi}(t) = [1 \;\; 1]x_i(t) \tag{4}$$

Our emphasis here is to illustrate the rationales of the tracer kinetics guided reconstruction framework, while Eq.(3) can also be adopted without fundamental changes ($V_{Bi}C_{WB}(t)$ can be considered as a known input).

2.2 Imaging Model for Dynamic PET Data

Dynamic PET imaging involves a sequence of contiguous acquisition with different temporal resolutions, and a time series of activity images need to be reconstructed from the measurement data. For voxel i ($i = 1, ..., N$), the kth scan ($k = 1, ..., K$) attempts to measure the accumulation of the total concentration of radioactivity on the scanning time interval $[t_{k-1}, t_k]$, so the measured activity in scan k for voxel i is expressed as:

$$\lambda_{ik} = \int_{t_{k-1}}^{t_k} C_{Ti}(t)dt = \int_{t_{k-1}}^{t_k} [1 \;\; 1]x_i(t)dt \tag{5}$$

with the subscript k denoting the scan index. The activity image of the kth scan Λ_k is obtained by lexicographic ordering of the integrated radioactivity at different voxels λ_{ik}, i.e. $\Lambda_k = [\lambda_{1k}, \lambda_{2k}, ..., \lambda_{Nk}]^T$.

In PET imaging, the true coincidences are contaminated by the accidental coincidence (AC) and the scattered coincidence (SC) events, so the the raw emission data $y_k^{(p)}$ is usually pre-corrected for AC events to produce the corrected measurements y_k. The raw data is measured by coincidence detection using a prompt time window with mean $E[y_k^{(p)}] = D\Lambda_k + r_k + s_k$, where D is the imaging matrix, r_k is mean of the AC events, and s_k is mean of the SC events. The AC events are estimated in a delayed window with mean $E[y_k^{(d)}] = r_k$. The corrected measurements $y_k = y_k^{(p)} - y_k^{(d)}$ are thus with mean $E[y_k] = D\Lambda_k + s_k$, and can be further expressed in a measurement equation as:

$$y_k = D\Lambda_k + g_k \tag{6}$$

where y_k is an $M \times 1$ vector with M being the number of the detector bins, and the measurement noise g_k is to account for all the unknown measurement errors (including the SC events) during the imaging. The imaging matrix $D = [d_{ji}]_{M\times N}$ contain the probabilities of detecting an emission from voxel site i at detector pair j, and depends on various factors: the geometry of the detection system, detector efficiency, attenuation effects, dead time correction factors, the extent of scattering between source and detector, etc. Due to the AC correction, y_k is not Poisson-distributed, violating the assumption in most statistical reconstruction methods. Consequently, other models like the Shifted-Poisson model have been proposed for the AC-corrected data [4]. In practice, however, y_k has very complicated statistics due to SC events, scanner sensitivity and dead time, making it difficult to well capture its distribution with one certain model *a priori*. As this problem become more severe for dynamic PET imaging where the data has low SNR, we propose to formulate the dynamic reconstruction as a filtering problem in a state-space setting.

2.3 State-Space Formulation for Dynamic PET Reconstruction

Eq.(2) and (6) form a state-space-like representation for the dynamic PET reconstruction problem, with (2) describing the tracer kinetics and (6) expressing the measurement model. However, the intermediate step in Eq.(5) makes the problem in a nonstandard state-space formulation, and thus hinders direct application of filtering strategies to the activity reconstruction. The integration of activity in Eq.(5) also leads to difficulty in other statistical reconstruction approaches, and is often simplified with direct sampling of $C_{Ti}(t)$ at the midpoint of the scan interval or assuming $C_{Ti}(t)$ piece-wise constant during each scan [11]. These approximations become very crude for long scan intervals or fast changing kinetics, and we believe an accurate integration model is necessary for proper dynamic reconstruction. In our work, several transforms are performed to convert the problem into a more standard state-space representation.

Constructing the state equation via time integration. Let $f_i(t) = \int_0^t x_i(\tau)d\tau$, Eq.(2) can then be integrated to generate an equivalent form as:

$$\dot{f}_i(t) = a_i f_i(t) + b_i \tilde{C}_P(t) \tag{7}$$

with $\tilde{C}_P(t) = \int_0^t C_P(\tau)d\tau$, and the measured activity in Eq.(5) can be written as:

$$\lambda_{ik} = [1 \;\; 1][f_i(t_k) - f_i(t_{k-1})] \tag{8}$$

Defining the state vector $F(t) = [f_1(t)^T, f_2(t)^T, ..., f_N(t)^T]^T$ (a $2N \times 1$ vector), and also introducing a system noise term $\tilde{v}(t)$, the system kinetic equation for all voxels can be constructed from Eq.(7) as:

$$\dot{F}(t) = AF(t) + B\tilde{C}_P(t) + \tilde{v}(t) \tag{9}$$

where the system matrix A is a $2N \times 2N$ block diagonal matrix with blocks a_i, the input gain B is of size $2N \times 1$ as $B = [b_1^T, b_2^T, ..., b_N^T]^T$, and $\tilde{v}(t)$ is to account for the uncertainties in tracer kinetics coming from input disturbances and modeling errors. The activity image Λ_k can then be expressed as:

$$\Lambda_k = T_r[F(t_k) - F(t_{k-1})] \tag{10}$$

where the $N \times 2N$ transformation matrix T_r is block diagonal with each block being $[1 \;\; 1]$.

The reason why we introduce tracer kinetic modeling into the reconstruction problem can be understood more clearly here. With Eq.(9) describing the radiotracer kinetic process, we are able to incorporate prior knowledge of physiological meaningfulness to guide our reconstruction.

Deriving the measurement equation. Defining the new measurements $z_k = \sum_{l=1}^{k} y_l$, the new measurement equation can be derived from Eq.(6) and (10) as

$$z_k = DT_rF(t_k) + e_k = CF(t_k) + e_k \tag{11}$$

where $C = DT_r$ is the measurement matrix, and e_k is the measurement noise after the transform with $e_k = \sum_{l=1}^{k} g_l$.

Eq.(9)(11) have formed a standard state-space representation for dynamic PET reconstruction, where (9) describes the *continuous-time* radiotracer kinetics, and (11) models the transformed PET data as *discrete sampling* of the continuous system states. Given the sampled measurements z_k, our goal is to estimate the state of the continuous kinetic process $F(t)$, and to obtain the reconstructed activity images Λ_k using Eq.(10). In consequence, the dynamic PET reconstruction problem can be formulated as a state estimation problem in such a *continuous-discrete hybrid paradigm* of Eq.(9) and (11), and a sampled-data H_∞ filtering strategy is proposed in Sec.2.4 for estimation in the hybrid paradigm.

2.4 Sampled-Data H_∞ Filtering Framework for Dynamic PET Reconstruction

As mentioned in Sec.2.2, the PET data after AC correction is not Poisson-distributed, and has highly complicated statistics due to SC events, scanner sensitivity and dead time. Instead of imposing certain distribution (Poisson or Shifted Poisson) on the data, the mini-max H_∞ estimation criterion is adopted in our filtering framework, which minimizes the worst possible effects of the disturbances on the state estimation errors, and requires no *a priori* knowledge of noise statistics, making it an appropriate choice for PET reconstruction where the noise statistics is complicated. The mini-max H_∞ criterion has been applied in [12] for static PET reconstruction, which has a similar spirit to our motivation here to achieve robustness in the estimation. Despite this similarity, our work formulates *dynamic* PET reconstruction in a *hybrid* paradigm of Eq.(9) and (11) based on tracer kinetic modeling, so a *sampled-data* filtering solution is needed for the estimation due to the incompatibility of system and measurements(continuous kinetics, discrete measurements).

The performance of the sampled-data H_∞ filter is measured by the value of the estimation error relative to the values of the process noise, the measurement noise, and the uncertainty in the initial state, defined as the following:

$$J = \frac{\|F(t) - \hat{F}(t)\|^2_{S(t)}}{\|\tilde{v}(t)\|^2_{Q(t)^{-1}} + \|e(k)\|^2_{V(t)^{-1}} + \|F_o - \hat{F}_o\|^2_{P_0^{-1}}} \tag{12}$$

with $\hat{F}(t)$ denoting the estimate of $F(t)$. The notation $\|x\|^2_G$ is defined as the square of the weighted (by G) L_2 norm of x, i.e. $\|x\|^2_G = x^T Gx$. Here, $S(t), Q(t)$, $V(t)$ and P_0 are the weighting matrices for the estimation error, the process noise, the measurement noise, and the initial estimate, respectively, and $\hat{F}_o$ is the initial state estimate. The denominator of J can thus be regarded as "mixed L_2/l_2" norm [13] on the uncertain disturbances affecting the system. The performance measure of the sampled-data H_∞ filter is defined directly in terms of the continuous-time system state $F(t)$ and disturbance $\tilde{v}(t)$, and inter-sample behavior of the system(i.e. kinetics between samples) is thus taken into account.

Given a prescribed noise attenuation level $\gamma > 0$, the sampled-data H_∞ filter will search $\hat{F}(t)$ such that the optimal estimate of $F(t)$ should satisfy

$$\sup J \leq \gamma^2 \tag{13}$$

where the supremum is taken over all possible disturbances and initial states. The sampled-data H_∞ filter can be interpreted as a *mini-max* problem where the estimator strategy plays against the exogenous disturbances $\tilde{v}(t)$, $e(k)$ and the uncertainty in the initial state F_o. The problem formulation in equation (13) guarantees the bounded estimation error over all possible disturbances of finite energy, regardless of the noise statistics. As a result, the filter achieves greater robustness to disturbance variations and is well suited to such real-world problems as in PET reconstruction, where system disturbances and data uncertainties have highly complicated statistics and can not be well modeled *a priori*.

The sampled-data H_∞ filtering algorithm for our hybrid paradigm of dynamic PET reconstruction described by Eq.(9) and (11) is given as follows [13]:

$$\dot{\hat{F}}(t) = A\hat{F}(t) + B\tilde{C}_P(t) \tag{14}$$

$$\hat{F}(t_k) = \hat{F}(t_k^-) + P(t_k)C^T V(t)^{-1}[z_k - C\hat{F}(t_k^-)] \tag{15}$$

where $\hat{F}(t_k^-) = \lim_{\varepsilon\to 0} \hat{F}(t_k - \varepsilon)$, and $P(t_k)$ is the stabilizing solution to the following Riccati equation with jumps:

Table 1. Kinetic parameters for different tissue regions in Zubal thorax phantom

Region	$k_1(min^{-1})$	$k_2(min^{-1})$	$k_3(min^{-1})$	$k_4(min^{-1})$
ROI a	0.55951	2.75288	0.44793	0.01101
ROI b	0.37811	1.04746	0.13483	0.00857
ROI c	0.78364	1.15641	0.11200	0.02706

$$\dot{P}(t) = AP(t) + P(t)A^T + \frac{P(t)S(t)P(t)}{\gamma^2} + Q(t) \tag{16}$$

$$P(t_k) = P(t_k^-)[I + C^T V(t)^{-1} CP(t_k^-)]^{-1} \tag{17}$$

with the initial condition $P(0) = P_0$.

The filter given above is a linear system with finite jumps at discrete instants of time, which also has an intuitively appealing structure. Between the sampling instants when the PET data is collected, the state estimate evolves according to the continuous-time system kinetics, and the predicted state $\hat{F}(t_k^-)$ is obtained by solving equation (14) on the time interval $[t_{k-1}, t_k]$, with the previous state estimate $\hat{F}(t_{k-1})$ as the initial condition of the differential equation. Then at the observation time $t = t_k$, the new measurement z_k is used to update the estimate with the filter gain being $P(t_k)C^T V(t)^{-1}$. $P(t_k^-)$ is also obtained by solving the differential equation (16) with $P(t_{k-1})$ as the initial condition.

Numerical integration is usually required for solving Riccati differential equation (16), and its property of movable singularities usually leads to stability problems when Runge-Kutta routines are applied. The Möbius schemes proposed in [14] are based on viewing the Riccati equation in its natural geometric setting, as a flow on the Grassmannian of the vector space. Since there are no singularities in the associated flow, the schemes are able to deal with numerical instability and pass accurately through the singularities. Thus we adopt Möbius schemes in our implementation, and the detailed algorithm can be found in [14].

3 Experiments and Discussions

3.1 Simulation Experiments on Phantom

Simulation experiments have been conducted to illustrate the accuracy and robustness of the sampled-data H_∞ filtering strategy. Fig.2(a) shows a schematic representation of the Zubal thorax phantom, which has 4 regions including the background. The phantom is digitized at 32×32 pixels. The kinetic parameters of different regions are obtained from tracer kinetic study of glucose utilization [15], and are given in Table.1, with their corresponding time activity curves shown in Fig.2(b). The two-tissue compartment model is simulated with these parameters, and time frames of activity images are generated via accumulation of total activity concentration on each scan interval according to Eq.(5). The

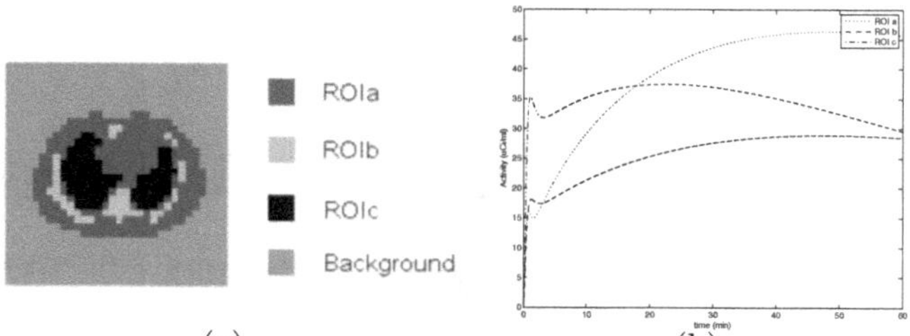

(a) (b)

Fig. 2. (a): Zubal thorax phantom with multiple tissue regions indicated by different colors. (b): Time activity curves for three distinct tissue regions in Zubal thorax phantom.

total scan time is $60min$, divided into 18 time frames with $4 \times 0.5min$, $4 \times 2min$, and $10 \times 5min$. The plasma function $C_P(t)$ is generated using [10]:

$$C_P(t) = (A_1 t - A_2 - A_3)e^{\alpha t} + A_2 e^{\beta t} + A_3 e^{\gamma t} \tag{18}$$

with $A_1 = 851.1225\mu Ci/mL/min$, $A_2 = 20.8113\mu Ci/mL$, $A_3 = 21.8798\mu Ci/mL$, $\alpha = -4.133859min^{-1}$, $\beta = -0.01043449min^{-1}$, and $\gamma = -0.1190996min^{-1}$. The decay of FDG tracer is also included with a decay constant of $0.0063min^{-1}$.

The 18 frames of activity images obtained from the above compartment model simulation are projected into sinograms using a Poisson model to generate the raw data $y_k^{(p)}$. The imaging matrix is modeled using the MATLAB toolbox developed by Prof. Jeff Fessler. Poisson-distributed AC events are then generated for each frame to simulate $y_k^{(d)}$, and the corrected measurements y_k are produced through subtraction. The AC events rate is assumed to be constant throughout each sinogram, and two fractions: 30% and 50%, of the total counts per scan are used to simulate low and high noise levels respectively. The effect of different counts is also simulated, where the low count case has 10^5 counts for the entire dynamic data set (divided among the 18 sinograms in accordance with the time behavior), and the high count case has 10^7 counts.

Given the above data sets with different counts and noise levels, our task is to reconstruct the 18 activity images based on tracer kinetic models. Ideally, if we have perfect prior knowledge of the model, the reconstruction can be performed with very high accuracy. In practice, however, the kinetic parameters of the model are usually not known *a prior* for a specific subject or tissue region, so information from previous studies has to be used instead. To simulate this model mismatch, we perform two kinds of recovery, denoted as the "perfect model" and "disturbed model" cases. In the first case, the parameters in recovery are the same as those in forward data generation, while in the second one a disturbed model is used in data generation with 10% noise added to the parameters. For each case of recovery, the statistical method maximum likelihood-expectation maximization(ML-EM) is also implemented for comparison.

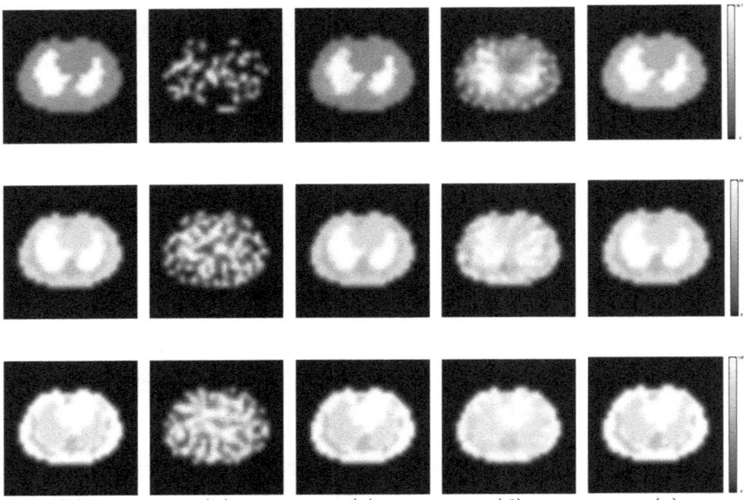

(a) (b) (c) (d) (e)

Fig. 3. Reconstructed activity images with perfect model from low noise data at frames #4, #8, #12 (top to bottom). (a): ground truth. (b): ML-EM results for low counts. (c): H_∞ results for low counts. (d): ML-EM results for high counts. (e): H_∞ results for high counts and color scale.

Fig.3 shows the ground truth and estimated activity images at frames #4, #8, #12 for the "perfect model" case, where all the reconstructions in this figure are performed on data with 30% noise level. The purpose here is to compare the strategies (ML-EM and H_∞ filter) at different counts. While ML-EM can give reasonable estimates for high counts in Fig.3(d), it fails for low count case (Fig.3(b)) where the SNR is sacrificed for the temporal resolution. In contrast, with the guidance of the compartment model, our filtering strategy generates significantly better results (Fig.3(c)(e)), illustrating the advantages of introducing physiologically meaningful priors into reconstruction. Moreover, as the mini-max H_∞ criterion guarantees bounded estimation error for all disturbances of finite energy, regardless of types and levels of noises, the filtering performance is still very satisfying even for the low count case in Fig.3(c). This has important implications for small animal imaging and drug discovery, where the low tracer dosage produces data of very low counts.

The ground truth and reconstructed activity images for the "disturbed model" case are shown in Fig.4, where all the recoveries are from low counts data. Not surprisingly, ML-EM fail for all low count cases due to the low SNR and violation of Poisson assumption. In contrast, although the kinetic model used for reconstruction here is not the same as the one for data generation (10% disturbance on parameters), the sampled-data H_∞ filter can still reliably and accurately estimate the activity images from the noisy measurements. These results

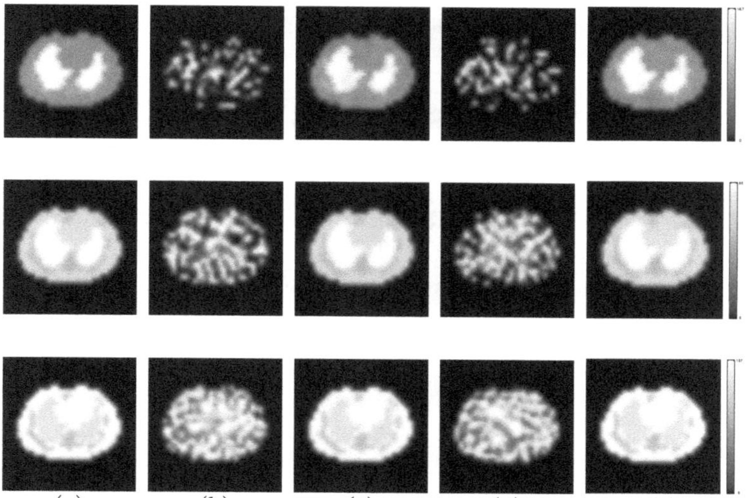

(a) (b) (c) (d) (e)

Fig. 4. Reconstructed activity images with disturbed model from low counts data at frames #4, #8, #12 (top to bottom). (a): ground truth. (b): ML-EM results for low noise. (c): H_∞ results for low noise. (d): ML-EM results for high noise. (e): H_∞ results for high noise and color scale.

further validate the necessity and importance of incorporating kinetic models (*even not perfect ones*) into reconstruction.

Table.2 provides a quantitative comparison of the strategies for different data sets (different counts, different noise levels) and different prior models (perfect model and disturbed model), where the reconstruction results are evaluated using absolute bias and variance defined as $bias = \frac{1}{N}\sum_{i=1}^{N}|\lambda_{ik} - \hat{\lambda}_{ik}|/\lambda_{ik}$, $variance = \frac{1}{N-1}\sum_{i=1}^{N}(|\lambda_{ik} - \hat{\lambda}_{ik}|/\lambda_{ik})^2$. The error bias and variance are averaged over the 18 frames of reconstruction to give the estimates $E[bias]$ and $E[variance]$. From Table.2, we can see that the sampled-data H_∞ filter provides stable and accurate reconstruction results for different counts and noise levels, demonstrating its desired robustness for dynamic PET reconstruction, where the data has complicated statistics and can not be well modeled *a priori*.

3.2 Discussions on Future Works

We have developed a tracer kinetics guided reconstruction framework for dynamic PET imaging, where sampled-data H_∞ filtering is applied to provide physiologically meaningful and robust reconstruction results. Other prior knowledge can also be incorporated into our framework, such as shape priors from anatomy, and attenuation information from CT-PET imaging, which can help to build more accurate kinetic models for different tissues. Parametric reconstruction can also be naturally dealt with in our framework.

Table 2. Quantitative analysis of estimated activity images for different data sets and different prior models, with *var* denoting *variance*

	Low Counts				High Counts			
	30%*noise*		50%*noise*		30%*noise*		50%*noise*	
	bias	*var*	*bias*	*var*	*bias*	*var*	*bias*	*var*
H_∞(perfect model)	0.0346	0.0255	0.0367	0.0264	0.0410	0.0351	0.0421	0.0372
ML-EM(perfect model)	0.9303	2.3751	0.9722	2.6883	0.1745	0.0831	0.1837	0.0934
H_∞(disturbed model)	0.0450	0.0025	0.0445	0.0025	0.1284	0.1030	0.1499	0.1163
ML-EM(disturbed model)	0.9416	2.6547	0.9464	2.6459	0.1748	0.0850	0.1813	0.0892

Currently, we are trying to apply the framework to real dynamic PET data. Efforts on Monte Carlo simulations and algorithm speedup are also underway.

References

1. Phelps, M.E.: PET: molecular imaging and its biological applications. Springer, New York (2004)
2. Leahy, R.M., Qi, J.: Statistical approaches in quantitative positron emission tomography. Statistics and Computing 10(2), 147–165 (2000)
3. Lewitt, R.M., Matej, S.: Overview of methods for image reconstruction from projections in emission computed tomography. Proceedings of the IEEE, 91 pp. 1588–1611 (2003)
4. Yavuz, M., Fessler, J.: Statistical image reconstruction methods for randoms-precorrected PET scans. Medical Image Analysis 2(4), 369–378 (1998)
5. Green, P.: Bayesian reconstructions from emission tomography data using a modified EM algorithm. IEEE Transactions on Medical Imaging 9(1), 84–93 (1990)
6. Bowsher, J.E., Johnson, V.E., Turkington, T.G., Jaszczak, R.J., Floyd, C.E., Coleman, R.E.: Bayesian reconstruction and use of anatomical a priori information for emission tomography. IEEE Transactions on Medical Imaging 15, 673–686 (1996)
7. Wernick, M.N., Infusino, E.J., Milosevic, M.: Fast spatio-temporal image reconstruction for dynamic PET. IEEE Transactions on Medical Imaging 18, 185–195 (1999)
8. Nichols, T.E., Qi, J., Asma, E., Leahy, R.M.: Spatiotemporal reconstruction of list-mode PET data. IEEE Transactions on Medical Imaging 21, 396–404 (2002)
9. Cobelli, C., Foster, D., Toffolo, G.: Tracer Kinetics in Biomedical Research. Kluwer Academic/Plenum Publishers, New York (2000)
10. Wong, K., Feng, D., Meikle, S., Fulham, M.: Simultaneous estimation of physiological parameters and the input function - in vivo PET data. IEEE Transactions on Information Technology In: Biomedcine. 5, 67–76 (2001)
11. Kamasak, M.E., Bouman, C.A., Morris, E.D., Sauer, K.: Direct reconstruction of kinetic parameter images from dynamic PET data. IEEE Transactions on Medical Imaging 24(5), 636–650 (2005)
12. Liu, H., Tian, Y., Shi, P.: Pet image reconstruction: A robust state space approach. In: Information Processing in Medical Imaging, 197–209 (2005)

13. Sun, W., Nagpal, K.M., Khargonekar, P.: H ∞ control and filtering for sampled-data systems. IEEE Transactions on Automatic Control 38, 1162–1175 (1993)
14. Schiff, J., Shnider, S.: A natural approach to the numerical integration of Riccati differential equations. SIAM Journal on Numerical Analysis 36, 1392–1413 (1996)
15. Li, X., Feng, D., Lin, K., Huang, S.: Estimation of myocardial glucose utilization with PET using the left ventricular time-activity curve as a noninvasive input function. Medical and Biological Engineering and Computing 36, 112–117 (1998)

Maximum Likelihood Estimators in Magnetic Resonance Imaging

M. Dylan Tisdall[1], M. Stella Atkins[1], and R.A. Lockhart[2]

[1] School of Computing Science, Simon Fraser University, Burnaby BC V5A 1S6
[2] Department of Statistics & Actuarial Science, Simon Fraser University, Burnaby BC V5A 1S6

Abstract. Images of the MRI signal intensity are normally constructed by taking the magnitude of the complex-valued data. This results in a biased estimate of the true signal intensity. We consider this as a problem of parameter estimation with a nuisance parameter. Using several standard techniques for this type of problem, we derive a variety of estimators for the MRI signal, some previously published and some novel. Using Monte Carlo experiments we compare the estimators we derive with others previously published. Our results suggest that one of the novel estimators we derive may strike a desirable trade-off between bias and mean squared error.

1 Introduction

Greyscale MR images are normally produced by taking the pixel-wise magnitude of a complex-valued image with zero-mean complex additive white noise. The magnitude operation performed on this data produces an image with a Rician noise distribution [1,2]. This distribution has a spatially varying bias that is inversely related to signal strength, and thus reduces image contrast. In order to reduce the bias of this signal estimate, a variety of approaches have been presented in the literature. The first major group assumes pixels are independent, and attempts to construct a less-biased estimator for the signal value using only information recorded at a single location[1,3,4,5,6,7,8]. The second group assumes that pixels are related either in signal or phase values and uses inference between neighbouring pixels in order to estimate pixel values [9,10,11,12,13,14,15,16].

In this work, we will focus on the first group. In particular, we are interested in how the notion of a nuisance parameter can be used to construct a variety of different estimators from the established model of the MRI data. As we will see, in the majority of MR imaging situations, only one of the two parameters is of interest. The choice of how these parameters' effects are separated is fundamental in determining what sort of estimator will be produced. However, despite the rich statistical literature on estimation with nuisance parameters, the notion does not seem common in the literature on MRI signal magnitude estimation [17,18,19,20]. In this work, we will attempt to employ some of the variety of techniques available for maximum likelihood estimation with a nuisance parameter.

N. Karssemeijer and B. Lelieveldt (Eds.): IPMI 2007, LNCS 4584, pp. 434–445, 2007.
© Springer-Verlag Berlin Heidelberg 2007

In doing so, we will derive some estimators that are previously published as well as new estimators.

To begin, in section 2 we introduce the model we will use for the MRI data. In section 3 we proceed to derive a variety of estimators using the maximum likelihood framework. In section 4 we describe some other estimators for this problem that have been presented in the MRI literature but do no arise from the maximum likelihood estimator. Finally, in section 5 we compare all of the estimators. Since closed form expressions for the bias and mean squared error (MSE) are not available for all of the estimators we derive, our comparison is based on Monte Carlo experiments using clinically realistic parameters.

2 MRI Data

For many clinically useful pulse sequences, the recorded MRI data f can be well described at each pixel as a complex-valued signal with magnitude s and phase ϕ, summed with two independent noises q_r and q_i which are both drawn from the zero-mean normal distribution $\mathcal{N}(0, \sigma)$ with σ fixed for all pixels. The two noises are aligned in the complex plane such that q_r is noise in the real direction and q_i is noise in the imaginary direction. Thus, for a given pixel we have [3]

$$f = s \exp(\mathrm{i}\phi) + q_r + \mathrm{i}q_i \,. \tag{1}$$

Since we are assuming that each pixel is independent and that the values of s and ϕ and unrelated between pixels, we can model each pixel independently with $f = a + ib$ and the multinormal distribution

$$p(a, b; s, \phi, \sigma) = \frac{1}{2\pi\sigma^2} \exp\left(-\frac{(a - s\cos(\phi))^2 + (b - s\sin(\phi))^2}{2\sigma^2} \right) . \tag{2}$$

Converting this to polar coordinates $f = r\exp(\mathrm{i}\theta)$, where we will find most of our work more natural, we get

$$p(r, \theta; s, \phi, \sigma) = \frac{r}{2\pi\sigma^2} \exp\left(-\frac{s^2 + r^2 - 2sr\cos(\theta - \phi)}{2\sigma^2} \right) . \tag{3}$$

Since multiple excitations are often used in order to repeat measurements, we will use a_i and b_i to represent the measurements from the ith excitation and $\boldsymbol{a}$ and $\boldsymbol{b}$ to represent the vectors of real and imaginary measurements at a given location. Similarly, we will use r_i and θ_i for the ith excitation and $\boldsymbol{r}$ and $\boldsymbol{\theta}$ to represent the vectors of polar measurements. Finally, we will simplify notation in some places by using $A = \sum_{i=1}^{n} a_i$ and $B = \sum_{i=1}^{n} b_i$.

In the majority of clinical imaging cases, we desire to display a greyscale image where the intensities represent the value of s. This leaves ϕ, a nuisance parameter required to complete the model but not of interest in producing our images. We will be given n replicated samples from each pixel and asked to produce an estimate of s from these values.

Note that for the purposes of this paper, we will assume that σ is known. In practice σ will usually be estimated either from a region of air where it is known that $s = 0$ or from the aggregate of image pixels. In the latter case, we take advantage of the fact that, for the pulse sequences we will consider, σ is the same for all pixels in the image and so it is relatively easy to estimate given more than one replication at each pixel.

3 Maximum Likelihood Estimators with Nuisance Parameters

If we desire to estimate $s \cos \phi$ and/or $s \sin \phi$, then the MLE is a good approach. To find this estimate given the likelihood function $L(s, \phi; \boldsymbol{a}, \boldsymbol{b})$, we set the score function with respect to each parameter equal to zero, substitute in the measured values of $\boldsymbol{a}$ and $\boldsymbol{b}$, and then solve the system

$$\frac{\partial}{\partial(s \cos \phi)} \log L(s, \phi; \boldsymbol{a}, \boldsymbol{b}) = 0 \tag{4}$$

$$\frac{\partial}{\partial(s \sin \phi)} \log L(s, \phi; \boldsymbol{a}, \boldsymbol{b}) = 0 \,. \tag{5}$$

This produces an unbiased estimate of $(s \cos \phi, s \sin \phi)$. However, unbiasedness does not apply when we attempt to estimate s alone. Due to the nonlinear change of parameters between $(s \cos \phi, s \sin \phi)$ and (s, ϕ), there is not one estimator of s that can be easily justified theoretically. In this section we will consider several different approaches to estimating s without ϕ. Some of the estimators derived are previously published, while some are new to the MRI literature.

3.1 Maximum Likelihood Estimate

Let $(\hat{s}_{\mathrm{ML}}, \hat{\phi}_{\mathrm{ML}})$ be the MLE of (s, ϕ) computed by solving

$$\frac{\partial}{\partial s} \log L(s, \phi; \boldsymbol{r}, \boldsymbol{\theta}) = 0 \tag{6}$$

$$\frac{\partial}{\partial \phi} \log L(s, \phi; \boldsymbol{r}, \boldsymbol{\theta}) = 0 \,. \tag{7}$$

If we take $\hat{s}_{\mathrm{ML}}$ as our estimate of s alone, this is also called the maximum likelihood estimate. This is the same as substituting $\hat{\phi}_{\mathrm{ML}}$ into the score function for s, and then solving the equation

$$\frac{\mathrm{d}}{\mathrm{d}s} \log L(s; \hat{\phi}_{\mathrm{ML}}, \boldsymbol{r}, \boldsymbol{\theta}) = 0 \,. \tag{8}$$

Noting that $\hat{s}_{\mathrm{ML}}$ is just the magnitude image computed at each pixel from the average of the excitations, one should not be surprised to find this estimator is biased since it has a Rician distribution as discussed in section 1. The bias and MSE of this estimator are

$$E[\hat{s}_{\mathrm{ML}} - s] = \frac{\sqrt{2\pi}\sigma}{2\sqrt{n}} {}_1\mathrm{F}_1\left(-\frac{1}{2}; 1; -\frac{ns^2}{2\sigma^2}\right) - s \tag{9}$$

$$E[(\hat{s}_{\mathrm{ML}} - s)^2] = 2(s^2 + \sigma^2/n) - \frac{s\sqrt{2\pi}\sigma}{\sqrt{n}} {}_1\mathrm{F}_1\left(-\frac{1}{2}; 1; -\frac{ns^2}{2\sigma^2}\right), \tag{10}$$

with ${}_1\mathrm{F}_1$ being the confluent hypergeometric function. Despite the non-zero bias, this is the most prevalent form of MR signal estimate, being commonly known as the 'magnitude image' in MRI.

For this problem, we also find that the maximum profile likelihood estimate is the same as the maximum likelihood estimate [18]. The profile likelihood for s is defined as

$$L_p(s; \boldsymbol{r}, \boldsymbol{\theta}) = \max_{\phi} L(s, \phi; \boldsymbol{r}, \boldsymbol{\theta}) \tag{11}$$

We find that $\hat{s}_{\mathrm{ML}} = \max_{s} L_p(s; \boldsymbol{r}, \boldsymbol{\theta})$ by noting the maximum value of $L(s, \phi; \boldsymbol{r}, \boldsymbol{\theta})$ with s fixed is independent of the choice of s. Thus, for the problem of estimating the MRI signal, the $\hat{s}_{\mathrm{ML}}$ can be thought of as either the maximum likelihood estimate or the maximum profile likelihood estimate.

3.2 Maximum Marginal Likelihood Estimate

We note that equation (3) can be marginalized with respect to θ to produce

$$\begin{aligned} p(r; s, \phi) &= \int_{-\pi}^{\pi} p(r, \theta; s, \phi, \sigma)\, \mathrm{d}\theta \\ &= \frac{r}{2\pi\sigma^2} \exp\left(-\frac{s^2 + r^2}{2\sigma^2}\right) \int_{-\pi}^{\pi} \exp\left(\frac{sr\cos(\theta - \phi)}{\sigma^2}\right) \mathrm{d}\theta\,. \end{aligned} \tag{12}$$

Using the identity $\int_{-\pi}^{\pi} \exp\left(z\cos(\theta)\right) \mathrm{d}\phi = \frac{1}{2\pi} \mathrm{I}_0(z)$, where $\mathrm{I}_0(z)$ is the zeroth-order modified Bessel function, we can rewrite this as

$$p(r; s, \phi) = \frac{r}{\sigma^2} \exp\left(-\frac{s^2 + r^2}{2\sigma^2}\right) \mathrm{I}_0\left(\frac{sr}{\sigma^2}\right). \tag{13}$$

We can see that by performing this marginalization we have removed the dependence on ϕ since it does not appear anywhere on the right side of the equation. Thus, if we measure only the magnitude and not the phase (or simply ignore the measured phase) then ϕ has no effect on our magnitude measurement. We can use this probability to produce a marginal likelihood function, which can then be maximized to produce an estimate of s [18].

This procedure is exactly the one employed by Sijbers *et al.*, although in this previous work the justification for discarding the phase was the assumption that bias correction was being performed given only a magnitude image [6]. Regardless of how we justify the marginalization, given that we have n independent measurements of this value, we can follow a similar derivation and write

$$\begin{aligned} p(\boldsymbol{r}; s) &= \prod_{i=1}^{n} p(r_i; s) \\ &= \prod_{i=1}^{n} \frac{r_i}{\sigma^2} \exp\left(-\frac{s^2 + r_i^2}{2\sigma^2}\right) \mathrm{I}_0\left(\frac{s r_i}{\sigma^2}\right) . \end{aligned} \tag{14}$$

From this we can find

$$\frac{\mathrm{d}}{\mathrm{d}s} \log L(s; \boldsymbol{r}) = \frac{1}{\sigma^2} \left(\sum_{i=1}^{m} r_i \frac{\mathrm{I}_1\left(\frac{s r_i}{\sigma^2}\right)}{\mathrm{I}_0\left(\frac{s r_i}{\sigma^2}\right)} - ns \right) . \tag{15}$$

Setting this equal to zero produces an equation whose solutions have been studied previously using catastrophe theory [6]. The basic result of this previous work is that the maximum marginal likelihood estimate of s is 0 when $\sum_{i=1}^{n} r_i^2 \leq 2n\sigma^2$. Otherwise, there is one positive maximum which can be found numerically.

3.3 Maximum Integrated Likelihood Estimate

A very similar result to the above is produced if, instead of marginalizing out $\boldsymbol{\theta}$, we choose a uniform distribution on the range $(-\pi, \pi]$ as a prior for ϕ. The choice of a uniform prior in this case can be supported with two arguments. First, for a variable with a restricted range like ϕ, a uniform prior is often considered non-informative in Bayesian terms [21]. Second, although it is known experimentally that ϕ is likely to have a low-curvature structure [9,10,16], the estimators we are considering assume that each pixel's parameters are independent. With this restriction, based on experimental results it is approximately equally likely that a single pixel chosen at random could have any value for ϕ in the valid range.

Proceeding with the uniform prior, we can then write

$$p(\boldsymbol{r}, \boldsymbol{\theta}; s) = \int_{-\pi}^{\pi} p(\boldsymbol{r}, \boldsymbol{\theta}; s, \phi) p(\phi) \, \mathrm{d}\phi . \tag{16}$$

We first note that

$$p(\boldsymbol{r}, \boldsymbol{\theta}; s, \phi) p(\phi) = \frac{1}{2\pi} \prod_{i=1}^{n} \frac{r_i}{2\pi\sigma^2} \exp\left(-\frac{s^2 + r_i^2 - 2 s r_i \cos(\theta_i - \phi)}{2\sigma^2}\right) . \tag{17}$$

Then we can substitute this in and simplify to produce

$$\begin{aligned} p(\boldsymbol{r}, \boldsymbol{\theta}; s) &= \frac{1}{2\pi} \int_{-\pi}^{\pi} \prod_{i=1}^{n} \frac{r_i}{2\pi\sigma^2} \exp\left(-\frac{s^2 + r_i^2 - 2 s r_i \cos(\theta_i - \phi)}{2\sigma^2}\right) \mathrm{d}\phi \\ &= \exp\left(-\frac{n s^2}{2\sigma^2}\right) \left(\prod_{i=1}^{n} \frac{r_i}{2\pi\sigma^2} \exp\left(-\frac{r_i^2}{2\sigma^2}\right) \right) \mathrm{I}_0\left(\frac{s\sqrt{A^2 + B^2}}{\sigma^2}\right) . \end{aligned} \tag{18}$$

We can then write the score function as

$$\frac{\mathrm{d}}{\mathrm{d}s} \log L(s; \boldsymbol{r}, \boldsymbol{\theta}) = \frac{1}{\sigma^2} \left(\sqrt{A^2 + B^2} \frac{\mathrm{I}_1\left(\frac{s\sqrt{A^2+B^2}}{\sigma^2}\right)}{\mathrm{I}_0\left(\frac{s\sqrt{A^2+B^2}}{\sigma^2}\right)} - ns \right) . \tag{19}$$

This can be set equal to zero and solved for s using the same approach as in the previous section. The only difference between this new estimator and the one in the previous section is that this approach first averages the measurements together before applying the previous estimator.

3.4 Maximum Profile Likelihood Estimate with Saddlepoint Correction

In section 3.1 we saw that the maximum profile likelihood estimate is $\hat{s}_{\mathrm{ML}} = \frac{1}{n}\sqrt{A^2 + B^2}$. One approach to removing the bias from this estimate involves a form of a technique called saddlepoint correction [19]. Using this approach, we compute a correction to the score function, equation (8), and then set the corrected score to zero and solve for our estimate. In our problem, the correction suggested by Levin *et al.* is given by [19]

$$\frac{\mathrm{d}}{\mathrm{d}s} \log L(s; \hat{\phi}_{\mathrm{ML}}, \boldsymbol{r}, \boldsymbol{\theta}) + B = 0 . \tag{20}$$

with

$$\begin{aligned} B &= -\frac{\sigma^2}{2ns^2} E\left(\frac{\partial}{\partial s}\frac{\partial^2}{\partial \phi^2} \log p(\boldsymbol{r}, \boldsymbol{\theta}\,;\, s, \phi)\right) \\ &= -\frac{1}{2s} . \end{aligned} \tag{21}$$

Setting the corrected profile score function to zero and solving for s gives the maximum corrected profile likelihood estimate

$$\hat{s}_{\mathrm{Corr}} = \frac{\hat{s}_{\mathrm{ML}} + \sqrt{\hat{s}^2_{\mathrm{ML}} - 2\sigma^2/n}}{2} , \tag{22}$$

where $\hat{s}_{\mathrm{ML}}$ is the uncorrected profile likelihood estimate as defined in section 3.1. This corrected estimator raises a difficulty when $\hat{s}^2_{\mathrm{ML}} < 2\sigma^2/n$ as our estimate becomes complex valued. We will resolve this by taking the real part as the estimate.

4 Other Published Estimators

In addition to the estimators derived above, there are several others that are significant in the MRI literature. A variety of previous approaches to reducing bias in magnitude MRI images are all based on noting that [1,3,4,5,8]

$$E[r_i^2] = s^2 + 2\sigma^2 . \tag{23}$$

The estimator proposed independently by McGibney *et al.* and Miller *et al.* was created by replacing $E[r_i^2]$ with r_i^2 in this equation, and then solving for s, giving (in the general case with n measurements) [4,5]

$$\hat{s}_{\mathrm{MM}} = \sqrt{\frac{1}{n}\sum_{i=1}^{n} r_i^2 - 2\sigma^2}\,. \tag{24}$$

As with the corrected profile likelihood estimate, we take the real component of equation (24) as the estimated value. Practically, this means setting $\hat{s}_{\mathrm{MM}} = 0$ whenever $\frac{1}{n}\sum_{i=1}^{n} r_i^2 < 2\sigma^2$.

The estimator proposed by Gudbjartsson *et al.* is quite similar. Starting with just the Rician-distributed magnitude measurements, they propose to make the resulting estimator's distribution closer to Gaussian by using [1]

$$\tilde{s}_{\mathrm{G}} = \sqrt{\left|\frac{1}{n}\sum_{i=1}^{n} r_i^2 - \sigma^2\right|}\,. \tag{25}$$

With the introduction of the absolute value inside the square root, we are guaranteed a real-valued estimate.

Lastly, the estimator due to Koay *et al.* was designed for the situation where σ is unknown and may vary between pixels [8]. Since, for the purposes of our experiment, we assume that σ is known or can be estimated well and further that it is fixed for all pixels, we will not consider this estimator further.

5 Comparison of Estimators

5.1 Methods

It is hypothesized that the spatially varying bias of magnitude MRI images causes difficulties for observers [12,22]. This is assumed to be due to the reduction in image contrast. Bright image regions have essentially zero bias in magnitude images while dark regions are biased positively. Experiments involving human observers looking at biased and unbiased MRI images indicates that bias may hamper detection of dim features against a dark background (e.g., weak edges) [23]. Additionally, we assume that the variance of an estimator likely has some impact on detectability as well. Noting this, we will compare estimators both in terms of bias and MSE.

To perform these comparisons, we used Monte Carlo experiments under a series of realistic conditions, similar to those presented by Sijbers *et al.*[6,7] since we do not have analytic forms for the MSE and bias of the estimators. The one exception to this was the MLE, where the bias and MSE are given in equations (9) and (10) and so are simply evaluated directly. The experiments were conducted with signals between 0 and 4 at intervals of 0.25 with noise fixed at $\sigma = 1$. We tried each signal value with one, two, and four simulated excitations. In order to ensure a low error in our experiment, we ran 20,000 iterations of each condition for use in computing the relevant statistics.

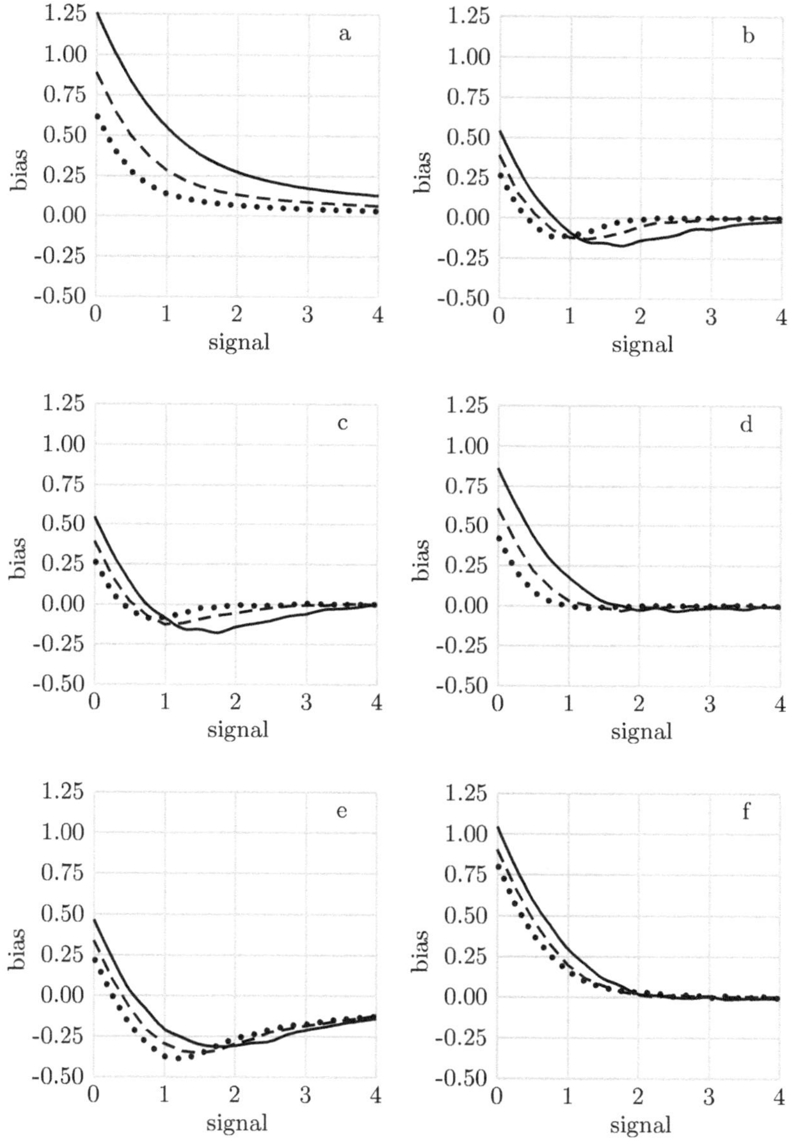

Fig. 1. Biases of the estimators. Each plot displays the bias of one estimator (a: maximum likelihood, b: maximum marginal likelihood, c: maximum integrated likelihood, d: maximum saddlepoint corrected profile likelihood, e: McGibney *et al.* and Miller *et al.*, f: Gudbjartsson *et al.*). The x-axis is the true signal value, and the y-axis is the mean bias of the estimate either computed directly or via the Monte Carlo experiments. The three lines in each plot correspond to $n = 1$ (solid), $n = 2$ (dashed), and $n = 4$ (dotted).

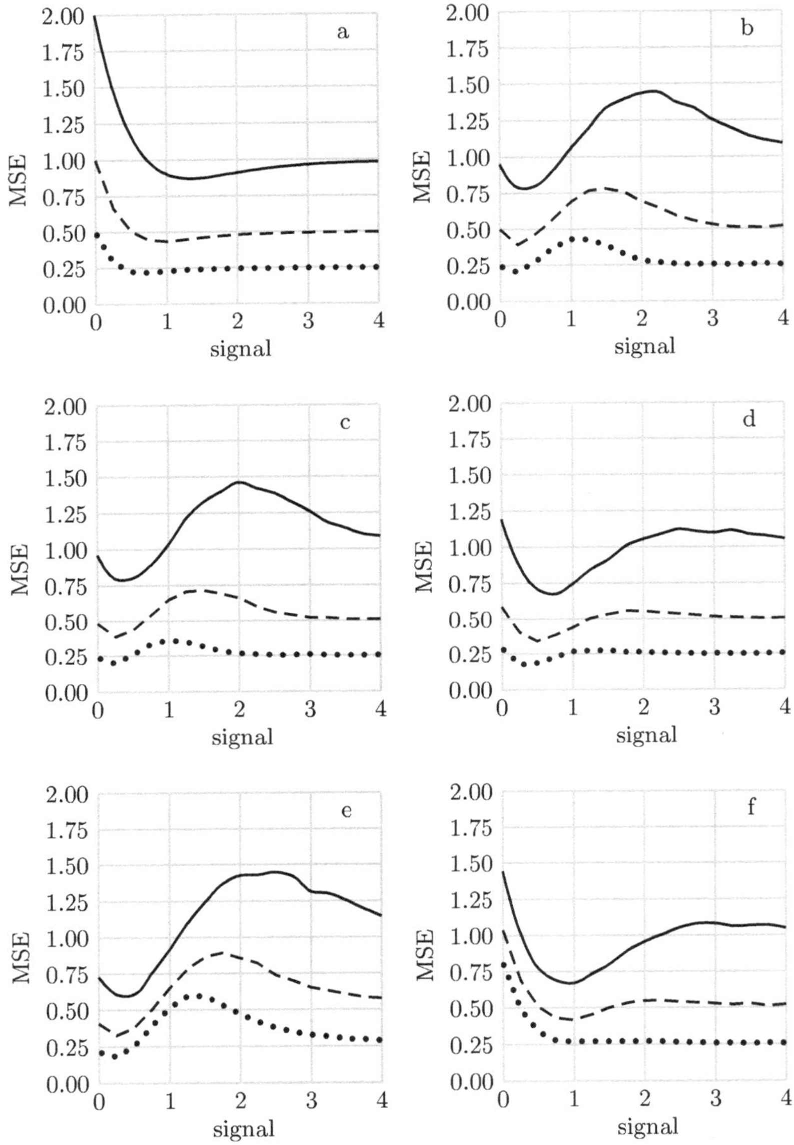

Fig. 2. MSEs of the estimators. Each plot displays the MSE of one estimator (a: maximum likelihood, b: maximum marginal likelihood, c: maximum integrated likelihood, d: maximum saddlepoint corrected profile likelihood, e: McGibney *et al.* and Miller *et al.*, f: Gudbjartsson *et al.*). The x-axis is the true signal value, and the y-axis is the MSE of the estimate either computed directly or via the Monte Carlo experiments. The three lines in each plot correspond to $n = 1$ (solid), $n = 2$ (dashed), and $n = 4$ (dotted).

5.2 Results and Discussion

In figure 1, we show the bias results. We can see that the McGibney *et al.* and Miller *et al.* estimate (e), along with the integrated and marginal likelihood estimators (b, c) are the least biased when the signal is 0. However, the corrected profile likelihood (d) is the most quick to converge to having no bias as the true signal increases. We note as the number of excitations increases the integrated likelihood estimate improves more rapidly than the marginal likelihood estimate. However, the corrected profile likelihood estimate converges to zero bias more quickly than the others with one, two, or four excitations.

In figure 2, we show the MSE results. The maximum likelihood estimate (a) produces the lowest MSE once $s > 1.5$. The next closest estimators are the corrected profile likelihood (d) and the Gudbjartsson *et al.* estimator (f). For signal values approaching 0, the McGibney *et al.* and Miller *et al.* estimator has the lowest MSE, followed by the integrated and marginal likelihood estimators (b, c). Again we note that the MSE of the integrated likelihood estimate improves more rapidly than the marginal likelihood estimate. Additionally, we find that the corrected profile likelihood estimate becomes increasingly competitive with the integrated and marginal likelihood estimates in terms of MSE as the number of excitations increases.

Considering these results together, our experiments suggest that the corrected profile likelihood estimate (d) provides less bias than the maximum likelihood estimate while trading a lower MSE at $s < 1.5$ for a slightly higher MSE at $s > 1.5$. These results seem to indicate that this new estimator offers a competitive alternative to those already published.

One practical consideration is the computational costs of these estimators. The marginal and integrated likelihood estimates both require several steps of some optimization algorithm. Although an efficient optimization algorithm for this problem has been previously presented [6], they are still substantially more expensive to compute than the the maximum corrected profile likelihood, McGibney *et al.* and Miller *et al.*, or Gudbjartsson *et al.* estimators. As such, we suspect that in a practical setting, the benefits achieved by applying the maximum corrected profile likelihood estimator could be sufficient to offset the minimal computational cost required for every image.

6 Conclusions

We have demonstrated that a variety of estimators for MRI, both previously published and new, can be generated by applying some of the statistical approaches to maximum likelihood estimation in the presence of nuisance parameters. Our results suggest that the rich literature on this type of problem in statistics offers useful tools that can be applied to signal estimation in MRI.

As there is no clear theoretical grounds for choosing one of these estimators, we have used Monte Carlo experiments to compare the estimators. We have shown that a novel MRI signal estimator, the maximum corrected profile likelihood, offers a decrease in bias compared to the magnitude image, in exchange for a slight increase in variance. Additionally, our results suggest that in situations with multiple excitations there can be substantial advantage to using this new estimator. Due to the limitations of the metrics being used for the evaluations, the results can only be considered to suggest further work. Experiments with humans observing estimated images are necessary to determine if any of these estimators provide a practical improvement in MR images.

Acknowledgments

The authors would like the Natural Sciences and Engineering Research Council of Canada for their support of this work.

References

1. Gudbjartsson, H., Patz, S.: The Rician distribution of noisy MRI data. Magn. Reson. Med. 34, 910–914 (1995)
2. Macovski, A.: Noise in MRI. Magn. Reson. Med. 36, 494–497 (1996)
3. Henkelman, R.M.: Measurement of signal intensities in the presence of noise in MR images. Med. Phys. 12(2), 232–233 (1985)
4. McGibney, G., Smith, M.R.: An unbiased signal-to-noise ratio measure for magnetic resonance images. Med. Phys. 20(4), 1077–1078 (1993)
5. Miller, A.J., Joseph, P.M.: The use of power images to perform quantitative analysis on low SNR MR images. Magn. Reson. Imaging 11, 1051–1056 (1993)
6. Sijbers, J., den Dekker, A.J., Scheunders, P., Dyck, D.V.: Maximum-likelihood estimation of Rician distribution parameters. IEEE Trans. Med. Imag. 17(3), 357–361 (1998)
7. Sijbers, J., den Dekker, A.J.: Maximum likelihood estimation of signal amplitude and noise variance from mr data. Magn. Reson. Med. 51, 586–594 (2004)
8. Koay, C.G., Basser, P.J.: Analytically exact correction scheme for signal extraction from noisy magnitude MR signals. J. Magn. Reson. 179, 317–322 (2006)
9. Ahn, C.B., Cho, Z.H.: A new phase correction method in NMR imaging based on autocorrelation and histogram analysis. IEEE Transactions on Medical Imaging 6(1), 32–36 (1987)
10. Bernstein, M.A., Perman, W.H.: Least-squares algorithm for phasing MR images. In: Book of Abstracts vol. 2, p. 801. In: Sixth Annual Meeting of SMRM, Society of Magnetic Resonance in Medicine August 1987 (1987)
11. Noll, D., Nishimura, D., Macovski, A.: Homodyne detection in magnetic resonance imaging. IEEE Trans. Med. Imag. 10, 154–163 (1991)
12. Nowak, R.D.: Wavelet-based Rician noise removal for magnetic resonance imaging. IEEE Trans. Image Processing 8(10), 1408–1418 (1999)
13. Alexander, M.E., Baumgartner, R., Summers, A.R., Windischberger, C., Klarhoefer, M., Moser, E., Somorjai, R.L.: A wavelet-based method for improving signal-to-noise ratio and contrast in MR images. Magn. Reson. Imaging 18, 169–180 (2000)
14. Bao, P., Zhang, L.: Noise reduction for magnetic resonance images via adaptive multiscale products thresholding. IEEE Trans. Med. Imag. 22(9), 1089–1099 (2003)
15. Tisdall, M.D., Atkins, M.S.: MRI denoising via phase error estimation. In: Proc. SPIE. vol. 5747, pp. 646–654 (2005)

16. Chang, Z., Xiang, Q.S.: Nonlinear phase correction with an extended statistical algorithm. IEEE Trans. Med. Imag. 24(6), 791–798 (2005)
17. Bartlett, M.S.: Approximate confidence intervals: III a bias correction. Biometrika 42(1/2), 201–204 (1955)
18. Kalbfleisch, J.D., Sprott, D.A.: Application of likelihood methods to models involving large numbers of parameters. Journal of the Royal Statistical Society B 32(2), 175–208 (1970)
19. Levin, B., Kong, F.: Bartlett's bias correction to the profile score function is a saddlepoint correction. Biometrika 77(1), 219–221 (1990)
20. Liang, K.Y., Zeger, S.L.: Inference based on estimating functions in the presence of nuisance parameters. Statistical Science 10(2), 158–173 (1995)
21. Jeffreys, H.: Theory of Probability, 3rd edn. Claredon Press (1961)
22. Bernstein, M.A., Thomasson, D.M., Perman, W.: Improved detectability in low signal-to-noise ratio magnetic resonance images by means of a phase-corrected real reconstruction. Med. Phys. 16, pp. 813–817 (1989)
23. Tisdall, M.D., Atkins, M.S.: Perception of dim targets on dark backgrounds in MRI.In: SPIE Medical Imaging 2007, Proceedings of 2007 (2007)

Quantifying Metabolic Asymmetry Modulo Structure in Alzheimer's Disease

P. Thomas Fletcher[1], Stephanie Powell[2], Norman L. Foster[3], and Sarang C. Joshi[2]

[1] School of Computing, University of Utah, Salt Lake City, UT, USA
[2] Department of Bioengineering, University of Utah, Salt Lake City, UT, USA
[3] Department of Neurology, University of Utah, Salt Lake City, UT, USA

Abstract. In this paper we describe a new method for quantifying metabolic asymmetry modulo structural hemispheric differences. The study of metabolic asymmetry in Alzheimer's disease (AD) serves as a driving application. The approach is based on anatomical atlas construction by large deformation diffeomorphic metric mapping (LDDMM) first introduced in [1]. Using invariance properties of the LDDMM, we define a structurally symmetric coordinate frame in which metabolic asymmetries between the left and the right hemispheres can be studied. This structurally symmetric coordinate system of each subject provides the correspondence between left and right hemispheric structures in an individual brain. These correspondences are used for measuring metabolic asymmetry modulo structural asymmetry. Again using the atlas construction framework, we build a common symmetric coordinate system of a entire population. The metabolic asymmetry maps of individuals in a population under study are mapped into the common structurally symmetric coordinate frame, allowing for a statistical description of the populations metabolic asymmetry. In this paper we prove certain invariance properties of the LDDMM atlas construction framework that make the definition of structurally symmetric coordinate systems possible. We present results from applying the methodology to images from the Alzheimer's Disease Neuroimaging Initiative (ADNI)[2].

1 Introduction: Metabolic Asymmetry in Alzheimer's Disease

Glucose metabolism in normal elderly individuals is, on average, symmetric. Individual patients with dementia, however, can have remarkable asymmetry. Some of the earliest studies of FDG-PET in AD noticed that patients sometimes had predominant left or right hemisphere hypometabolism and that this metabolic asymmetry corresponded to individual differences in symptoms and cognitive deficits [3,4,5] While metabolic asymmetry has been frequently reported, its cause is still unknown.

An understanding of why AD causes asymmetric glucose hypometabolism in some patients would provide new insights into the disease mechanisms that could

N. Karssemeijer and B. Lelieveldt (Eds.): IPMI 2007, LNCS 4584, pp. 446–457, 2007.
© Springer-Verlag Berlin Heidelberg 2007

be exploited to develop novel approaches to diagnosis and treatment. The lack of progress in understanding the origin of metabolic asymmetry is largely because most research has been conducted using grouped, rather than individual data for analyses. Explanatory studies focused on typical or average changes in different diseases or clinical correlations and were not concerned with individual variations. Different kinds of analyses are needed to account for individual heterogeneity. Recently, as FDG-PET has become widely available as a diagnostic test for dementia, it has become even more important to recognize the normal range of individual metabolic asymmetry and its possible variation with dementing diseases. This has spurred a reconsideration of asymmetry and its underlying cause.

Despite significant advances in image analysis methods, little that is new to evaluate metabolic asymmetry has been developed since the 1980s when ratios of volume or metabolic rates were calculated in corresponding left and right anatomic regions of interest. Although deformable image registration techniques have been applied in the past to study structural asymmetry [6,7,8], they have not been applied to the study of metabolic asymmetry. Clinical brain scans almost always are interpreted using only visual inspection. The eye can detect subtle asymmetries and this is exploited to identify disease clinically. However, it is easy to misinterpret asymmetries and difficult to judge accurately when it is pathologic. Tilting of the patient's head can make symmetric structures appear asymmetric or exaggerate differences. Furthermore, the structure and function of the normal brain is not truly symmetric, and some variation in right and left glucose metabolism is expected.

In this paper we present a new quantitative method based on large deformation diffeomorphic atlas construction for the analysis of metabolic asymmetry. Our method builds a symmetric structural MRI for each individual, in which asymmetries in that subject's PET data can be quantified without artifacts due to structural asymmetry. We also build a symmetric, normative structural MRI atlas along with the associated atlas of metabolic asymmetry. By mapping an individual's data to this atlas, the method highlights metabolic asymmetry anywhere in the brain and identifies the statistical significance of the asymmetry in comparison to a normal control population.

2 Methods

One of the most confounding factors in measuring metabolic asymmetry is the inherent structural asymmetry associated with the normal brain. Shown in the top row of Figure 1 are midaxial MRI slices from four representative normal control subjects from the ADNI database [2]. Following the ADNI protocol, all the images were corrected for intensity inhomogeneity and oriented in to a standard coordinate system based on the AC-PC. Notice the structural asymmetry as well as the individual structural variability in all the subjects.

The method presented herein, based on large deformation diffeomorphic metric mapping (LDDMM) accommodates structural asymmetry and is able to

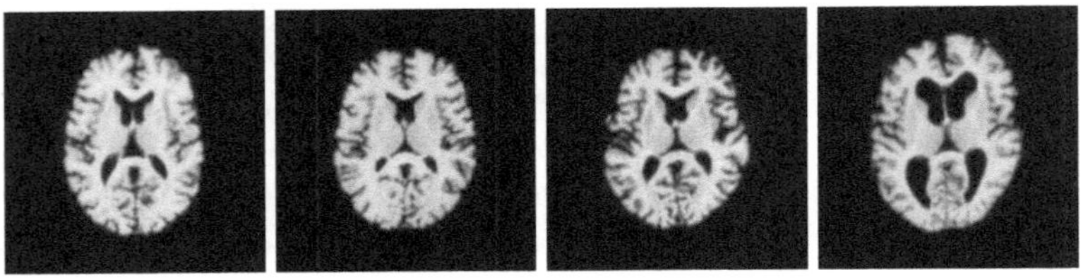

Fig. 1. Midaxial slices from 4 representative normal control subjects from the ADNI database

quantify the metabolic asymmetry *volumetrically* modulo the structural asymmetry. The process involves the following general steps:

1. Quantifying individual structural asymmetry by
   - Estimating the plane of structural symmetry for each subject.
   - Building large deformation diffeomorphic transformations characterizing structural asymmetry.
2. Quantifying individual metabolic asymmetry modulo structural asymmetry.
3. Building statistical cross-sectional normal metabolic asymmetry atlas.
4. Statistically testing individual asymmetry against the cross-sectional asymmetry atlas.

Underlying the above process is the methodology for the construction of an unbiased atlas from a collection of brain images. Although the atlas construction methodology has been previously published[1], we briefly review it here as the invariance properties of the atlas construction process, proved here for the first time, allow us to precisely study metabolic asymmetry.

2.1 Large Deformation Diffeomorphic Atlas Construction and Its Invariance Properties

The study of anatomical shape is inherently related to the construction of transformations of the underlying coordinate space, which map one anatomy to another. Recent work has suggested that representing the geometry of shapes or images in *flat spaces* undermines our ability to represent natural variability in populations [9,10]. Several researchers have proposed the use of nonlinear spaces defined as *groups*, in which each point in the space is related to another via the transformation. These groups vary in dimensionality from simple global translations and rigid rotations to the infinite-dimensional group of diffeomorphisms (denoted $\mathcal{H}$) [11].

We rely on the theory of large deformation diffeomorphisms [12,13], in which the dense field of image displacements, $h \in \mathcal{H}$, are integrals of smooth vector fields $v(x,t)$, defined on an image domain Ω and varying with time $t \in [0,1]$. The diffeomorphic property is important as it provides us with the ability to transform points between atlases and subjects and back without the loss of structure or information. Furthermore, the space of diffeomorphisms has an associated metric induced by a *function space norm* (Sobolov norm) via a partial differential operator L on the velocity fields v. The metric is defined via the squared distance, $d(e,h)^2$, between a transformation h and the identity transformation e as

$$d(e,h)^2 = \min_v \int_0^1 \int_\Omega \|Lv(x,t)\|^2 \, dx \, dt, \text{ subject to : } h(x) = \int_0^1 v(h(x,t),t) \, dt. \tag{1}$$

The differential operator L ensures smoothness, which guarantees that when we integrate v, the resulting displacements, h, will be diffeomorphic. Thus, a right invariant metric between any two diffeomorphisms, which satisfies all of the properties of a metric [14], is given by $d(h_1,h_2) = d(e, h_2 \circ h_1^{-1})$. As we will see, this property will play a crucial role in our study of asymmetry.

Averages in metric spaces: In a vector space with addition and scalar multiplication well defined, an average representation of the training set can be computed as the arithmetic average. Linear averaging cannot be directly applied to the space of diffeomorphisms because it is not a vector space and is not closed under addition. The space of diffeomorphisms is a nonlinear infinite-dimensional group. We do, however, have a metric for diffeomorphisms, and thus use the approach presented in [1], which applies the statistical method of averaging in general metric spaces proposed by Fréchet [15]. For a metric space M with a distance $d : M \times M \to R$, the *intrinsic mean* for a collection of data points $x_i \in M$ is the minimizer of the sum-of-squared distances to each of the data points. That is, $\mu = \arg\min_{x \in M} \sum_{i=1}^N d(x,x_i)^2$.

The input data for the construction of an MRI brain template or atlas is a collection of N structural MRIs. For such a collection the challenging variability is not that of the noise of the imaging modality, but the inherent biological variability of the geometry or shape of the underlying anatomy. The Fréchet mean estimation problem for atlas construction is formulated using the metric on the space of diffeomorphisms combined with a squared-error dissimilarity measure on the image intensities. The template image $\hat{I}$ that is the best representative for a population of N anatomical images $\{I_i\}_{i=1}^N$, is the image that on average minimizes the sum-of-squared distances between it and each I_i. That is,

$$\begin{aligned} \hat{I} &= \text{Atlas}(\{I_1, \ldots, I_N\}) \\ &= \arg\min_{h_i, I} \sum_{i=1}^N \int_\Omega \left(I_i \circ h_i^{-1}(x) - I(x)\right)^2 dx + d(e,h_i)^2. \end{aligned} \tag{2}$$

This involves a minimization procedure that considers all the images at once. The procedure is unbiased and not dependent on the order of processing of the images.

Invariance Properties of LDDMM Atlas Construction: We now prove some invariance properties of the above atlas construction process that form the basis of its application to the study of metabolic asymmetry. We first prove the following general invariance lemma:

Lemma 1. *Let ϕ be an isometry of Ω. Let $\hat{I}$ be the LDDMM atlas of images I_i, $i = 1, \ldots, N$. Assuming the operator L in (1) is invariant to isometries, then the LDDMM atlas of images $I_i^{'} = I_i \circ \phi^{-1}$ is given by $\hat{I}' = \hat{I} \circ \phi^{-1}$.*

Proof. Since L is invariant to isometries, we have $d(e, h) = d(e, \phi h \phi^{-1})$. From (2), using the change of variables $g_i = \phi h_i \phi^{-1}$ and $y = \phi^{-1}(x)$, we get

$$\begin{aligned}
\text{Atlas}(\{I_i^{'}\}) &= \arg\min_{g_i, I} \sum_{i=1}^{N} \int_{\Omega} \left(I_i^{'} \circ g_i^{-1} - I\right)^2 dx + d(e, g_i)^2 \\
&= \arg\min_{h_i, I} \sum_{i=1}^{N} \int_{\Omega} \left((I_i \circ \phi^{-1}) \circ (\phi h_i^{-1} \phi^{-1}) - I\right)^2 dx + d(e, \phi h_i \phi^{-1})^2 \\
&= \arg\min_{h_i, I} \sum_{i=1}^{N} \int_{\Omega} \left(I_i \circ (h_i^{-1} \phi^{-1}) - I\right)^2 dx + d(e, h_i)^2 \\
&= \arg\min_{h_i, I} \sum_{i=1}^{N} \int_{\Omega} \left(I_i \circ h_i^{-1} - I \circ \phi\right)^2 dy + d(e, h_i)^2 \\
&= \text{Atlas}(\{I_i\}) \circ \phi^{-1}.
\end{aligned}$$

□

Using the above lemma, we now prove the following two important symmetry properties of the LDDMM atlas formation methodology, which will enable us to study asymmetry in brain images.

Theorem 1. *Let H_p be a reflection about the plane p, and let $I_2 = I_1 \circ H_p$. Then the unbiased diffeomorphic average, $\hat{I}$, of I_1, I_2 is symmetric about p, i.e., $\hat{I} = \hat{I} \circ H_p$.*

Proof. This follows directly from Lemma 1 and using the fact that H_p is idempotent. Since H_p is idempotent, we get the equality $\text{Atlas}(I_1, I_2) = \text{Atlas}(I_2 \circ H_p, I_1 \circ H_p)$. Now using the fact that H_p is an isometry, we get the identity $\text{Atlas}(I_2 \circ H_p, I_1 \circ H_p) = \text{Atlas}(I_2, I_1) \circ H_p$. □

Theorem 2. *Let H_p be a reflection about the plane p. Given N symmetric images about the plane p, that is, $I_i = I_i \circ H_p$, $i = 1, \ldots, N$, then the diffeomorphic average, $\hat{I} = \text{Atlas}(\{I_1, \ldots, I_N\})$ is symmetric about p, i.e., $\hat{I} = \hat{I} \circ H_p$.*

Proof. This again directly follows from applying the Lemma 1. As each of the images are symmetric about the plane p, $\text{Atlas}(\{I_1, \ldots, I_N\}) = \text{Atlas}(\{I_1 \circ H_p, \ldots, I_N \circ H_p\})$. Now by Lemma 1, we have $\text{Atlas}(\{I_1 \circ H_p, \ldots, I_N \circ H_p\}) = \text{Atlas}(\{I_1, \ldots, I_N\}) \circ H_p$, implying that $\hat{I} = \hat{I} \circ H_p$. □

2.2 Quantifying Individual Structural Asymmetry

The application of the above theorems allows us to effectively employ the LD-DMM atlas building technology to quantify structural asymmetry. We first build a structurally symmetric image from an individual MRI and quantify structural asymmetry as the deviation from this symmetric image. A symmetric structural image also acts as an anatomical coordinate system in which metabolic asymmetry can be quantified. Quantifying individual structural asymmetry involves the following steps:

1. **Estimating the Plane of Symmetry:** Given a scalar 3D MR image, $I_1(x)$, we begin by estimating the plane of symmetry, based on the approach developed in [8]. The method here uses the equivalent, but somewhat simpler, computations over rigid transformations rather than affine. We define the *plane of symmetry* as the plane about which a reflection of the image results in maximal similarity (least difference) with the original. If H_p denotes reflection about the plane p, the plane of symmetry is defined formally as

$$\hat{p} = \arg\min_{p} \int_{\Omega} \|I_1(x) - I(H_p(x))\|^2 dx.$$

   The symmetry plane is found by first reflecting the image I_1 about the midsagittal plane, p_0, which forms the initialization, and then rigidly registering the reflected image $I_1 \circ H_{p_0}$ to the image I_1 through iterative updates using a gradient descent. If (R, v) is the resulting rotation and translation, then the plane of symmetry, $\hat{p}$, is given by rotating the midsagittal plane p_0 by half the amount, $R^{1/2}$, and translating it by $(1/2)R^{1/2}v$. This process is illustrated in Figure 2.
2. **Characterizing Structural Asymmetry:** Let $I_2 = I_1 \circ H_{\hat{p}}$ denote the image I_1 reflected about its plane of symmetry. The symmetric structural image is defined as the unbiased average, $\hat{I} = \text{Atlas}(\{I_1, I_2\})$. By Theorem 1 the average image is guaranteed to be symmetric. Intuitively, $\hat{I}$ is the symmetric image that requires minimal deformation to both I_1 and its reflection I_2. Figure 3 illustrates the construction of the symmetric structural image. The magnitude of the diffeomorphism h_1 captures the degree of structural asymmetry, which is the minimal amount of deformation needed to symmetrize the structural image.

2.3 Quantifying Individual Metabolic Asymmetry

Having quantified the structural asymmetry of a brain, we can study the metabolic asymmetry modulo the structural asymmetry by transforming the PET data into this symmetric image space. We begin by rigidly aligning the PET data to the original MRI image, I_1, using mutual information and a gradient descent algorithm. A reflected version of the PET data is also aligned to the reflected MR image, I_2, in the same manner. This results in a PET image P_1, aligned with the

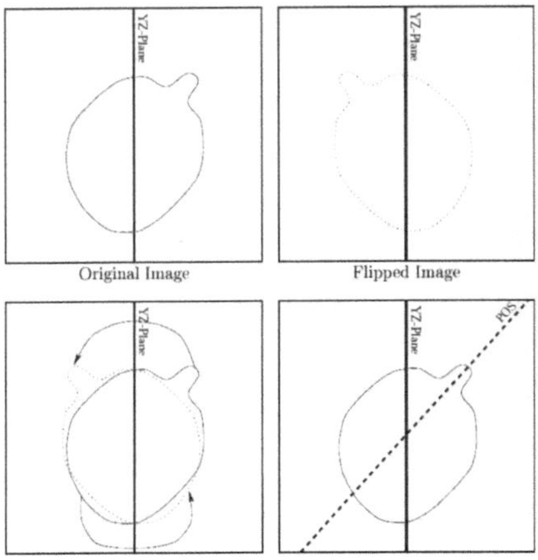

Fig. 2. Calculation of the structural symmetry plane

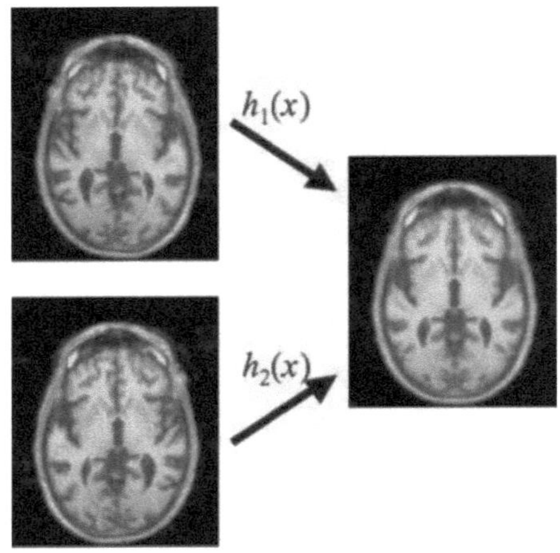

Fig. 3. Illustration of the construction of the symmetric structural image via diffeomorphic averaging

structural image, I_1, and a reflected PET image P_2, aligned with the reflected MR image, I_2. The PET images P_1 and P_2 are then mapped into the symmetric structural image space by applying the mappings h_1 and h_2, respectively. The resulting images, $\hat{P}_1 = P_1 \circ h_1$ and $\hat{P}_2 = P_2 \circ h_2$, are now in the same structurally symmetric image space and can be directly compared. Given a point x in the structurally symmetric image space, the PET response at this point is given by $P_1(h_1(x))$. The PET response at the corresponding point on the opposite hemisphere of the brain is given by $P_2(h_2(x))$. Therefore, metabolic asymmetry may be now quantified via the difference image, $P_{\text{asym}}(x) = (P_1(h_1(x)) - P_2(h_2(x)))$.

Because we have removed any variations in the PET signal due to structural asymmetry, P_{asym} measures only metabolic asymmetry, i.e., the differences in PET response between corresponding structures in the left and right hemisphere. Shown in Figure 4(d) is the result of applying this procedure to a representative data set.

2.4 Statistical Quantification of Metabolic Asymmetry

To study normative cross-sectional asymmetry we build an aggregate symmetric structural atlas from the individual symmetric structural images. Given a collection of symmetric structural images $\{\hat{I}_i\}$, computed as described above, symmetric structural atlas is built from this collection as the unbiased diffeomorphic average of these images. By Theorem 2 the resulting atlas image is also symmetric about the yz-plane.

Shown in Figure 5(a) are the symmetric structural images associated with four of the 10 normal subjects that were used to build a normative symmetric atlas. Figure 5(b) shows the resulting symmetric atlas.

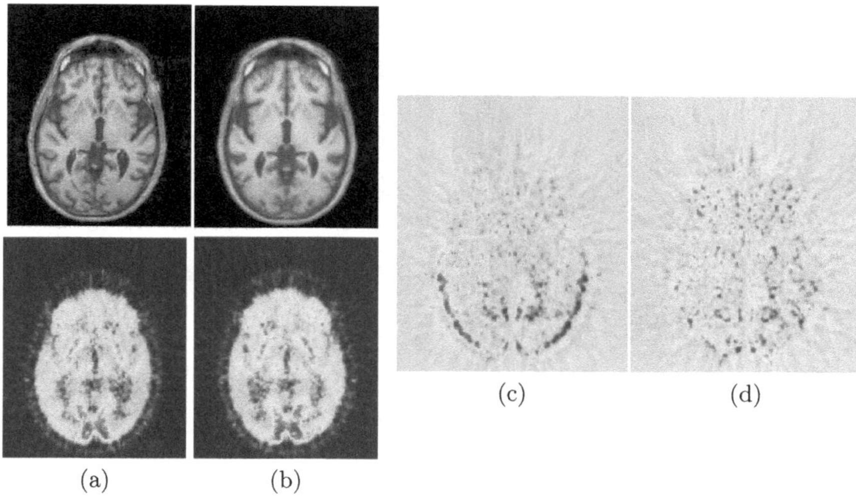

Fig. 4. a) Axial slice of original MR image and the associated PET image. b) The symmetric structural image constructed using unbiased diffeomorphic averaging and the associated PET image transformed. c) Difference in the PET image and its reflection about the structural plane of symmetry. d) Metabolic asymmetry image modulo structural asymmetry, i.e., difference in the PET image and its reflection after mapping to the symmetric structural image space. Notice the reduction in the asymmetry signal due to removal of the structural asymmetry from the PET image. (See electronic version for color images.)

The symmetric structural atlas for a group serves as a coordinate system for quantifying the metabolic asymmetry of that group. Each individual's metabolic asymmetry image, P_{asym}, is mapped into the symmetric structural atlas using the structural diffeomorphism that maps that subject's symmetric structural image to the atlas. In this way the asymmetry of every individual in the group is represented in a common reference frame.

3 Results

We now present results from a pilot study of quantifying metabolic asymmetry from 10 normal subjects from the ADNI database. For each of the subjects we begin with co-registered PET and the MRI scans rigidly aligned to the AC-PC coordinate system. Following methods outlined above, for each subject a structural symmetric image was constructed. Shown in Figure 5(a) are examples of four such structurally symmetric images. A symmetric structural atlas from these 10 structurally symmetric images was also constructed and is shown in Figure 5(b). Using the transformation computed during the atlas construction process, all the PET images were transformed into this coordinate system for quantifying the metabolic asymmetry of the group modulo structure. Shown in

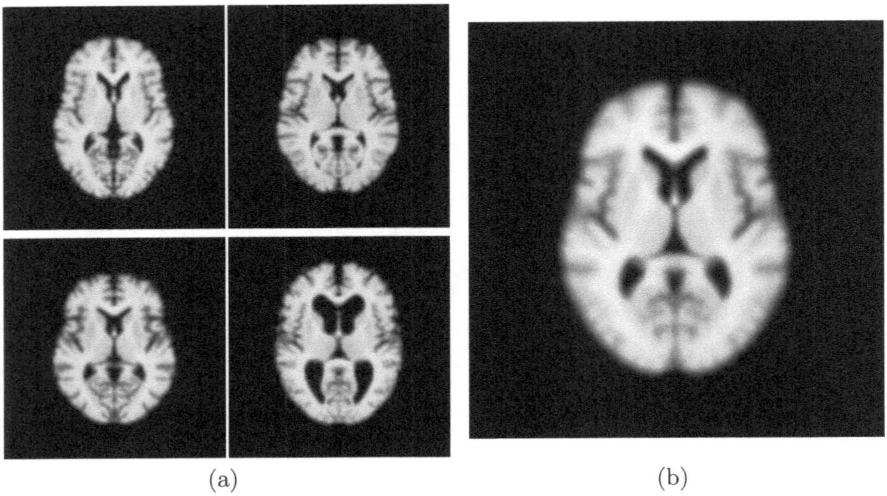

Fig. 5. (a) Axial slices through four of the individual structurally symmetric images that were used to build the symmetric atlas, shown in (b)

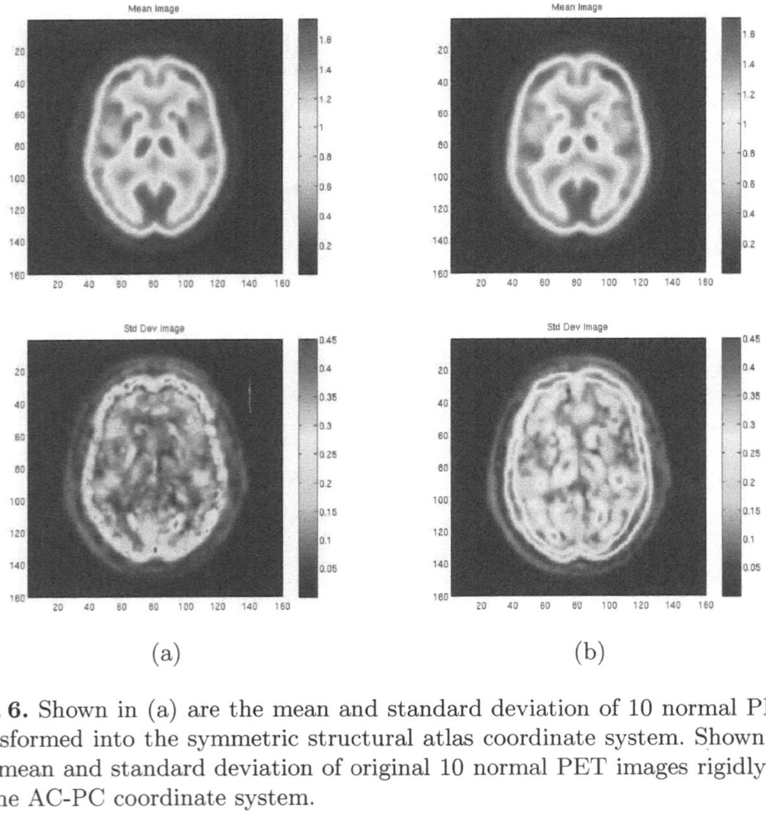

Fig. 6. Shown in (a) are the mean and standard deviation of 10 normal PET images transformed into the symmetric structural atlas coordinate system. Shown in (b) are the mean and standard deviation of original 10 normal PET images rigidly registered to the AC-PC coordinate system.

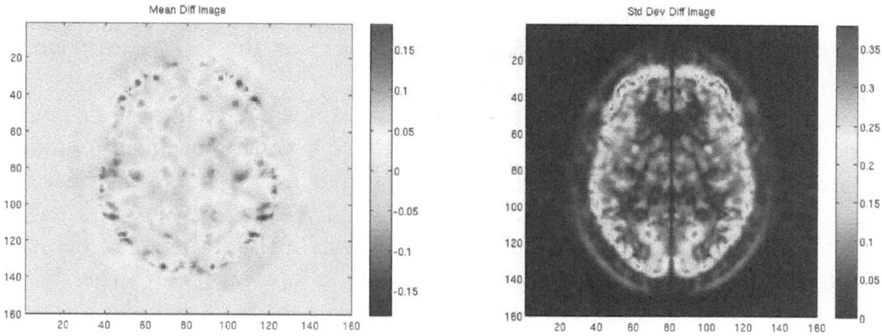

Fig. 7. The mean and standard deviation of the metabolic asymmetry of the 10 normal subjects transformed to the symmetric structural atlas coordinate system

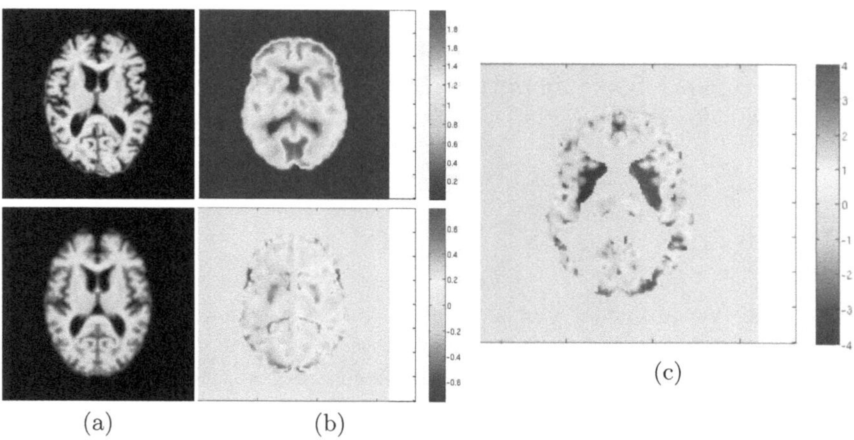

Fig. 8. Shown in (a) are original MRI scan (top) and the associated structurally symmetric image (bottom) of a subject with AD. Shown in (b) top is the subjects PET scan. Shown in the (b) bottom is the metabolic asymmetry image mapped in to the atlas space. Shown in (c) is the image of the statistical significance of metabolic asymmetry as compared to the normative atlas.

Figure 6(a) are the means and the standard deviation of the PET images of the 10 normal subjects transformed to the symmetric structural atlas coordinate system. For comparison, shown in Figure 6(b) are the mean and standard deviations of original 10 PET images rigidly registered to the AC-PC coordinate system. Notice the reduction in variance accomplished by the atlas construction process.

For studying asymmetry across the population, each individual metabolic asymmetry image was also transformed to atlas space using the corresponding structural transformation. Shown in Figure 7 are the mean and the standard deviations of the difference images statistically capturing the metabolic asymmetry of the normal population.

Having constructed a statistical description of normative metabolic asymmetry modulo structure, we now present results of quantifying an individual AD patient's asymmetry. Shown in top row of Figure 8 are MRI and associated PET scans of an AD patient as part of the ADNI study. After close inspection of the PET image, subtle asymmetries in the metabolism of the subject can be noticed. The left hemisphere appears to be hypometabolic as compared to the right. We now statistically quantify this observation. To quantify metabolic asymmetry modulo structure of the subject, a structurally symmetric image of the subject was constructed. Shown in Figure 8(a bottom) is the structurally symmetric MRI image of the patient. To statistical quantify the asymmetry as compared to the normal population, the individual structural symmetric image was mapped to the normative atlas. Shown in panel (b) bottom is the metabolic asymmetry in the structurally symmetric atlas space. Using the mean and the standard deviation of the metabolic asymmetry of the normal population, a voxel-wise z-score was computed. Shown in right panel of Figure 8 are the significant z-scores ($\text{abs}(z) > 2.0$) for the subject. The asymmetric metabolic areas can be clearly identified.

4 Discussion

In this paper we present a new framework for the statistical quantification of metabolic asymmetry modulo inter-hemispheric structural differences. Although the results presented herein are from a pilot study consisting of only 10 normative subjects, the ADNI initiative aims to longitudinally follow 800 subjects, 200 patients diagnosed with AD, 400 with MCI, and 200 normal controls. As the ADNI data becomes available, we plan to execute a large scale study on the entire ADNI database and correlate the degree of metabolic asymmetry of patients diagnosed with AD to clinical symptoms and hope to gain new insights into the disease mechanisms that could be exploited to develop novel approaches to diagnosis and treatment.

Acknowledgement

This research, including data collection and sharing, was funded by the Alzheimer's Disease Neuroimaging Initiative, NIH grant U01 AG024904. This work is also part of the National Alliance for Medical Image Computing (NAMIC), funded by the National Institutes of Health through the NIH Roadmap for Medical Research, Grant U54 EB005149. We thank Ross Whitaker and Tolga Tasdizen for insightful discussions.

References

1. Joshi, S., Davis, B., Jomier, M., Gerig, G.: Unbiased diffeomorphic atlas construction for computational anatomy. NeuroImage 23(Suppl.1), S151–S160 (2004)
2. Mueller, S.G., Weiner, M.W., Thal, L.J., Petersen, R.C., Jack, C., Jagust, W., Trojanowski, J.Q., Toga, A.W., Beckett, L.: The Alzheimer's disease neuroimaging initiative. Neuroimaging Clin N Am 15, pp. 869–877 (2005)
3. Foster, N.L., Chase, T.N., Fedio, P., Patronas, N.J., Brooks, R.A., Chiro, G.D.: Alzheimer's disease: focal cortical changes shown by positron emission tomography. Neurology 33(8), 961–965 (1983)
4. Martin, A., Brouwers, P., Lalonde, F., Cox, C., Teleska, P., Fedio, P., Foster, N.L., Chase, T.N.: Towards a behavioral typology of Alzheimer's patients. J Clin. Exp. Neuropsychol 8(5), 594–610 (1986)
5. Koss, E., Friedland, R.P., Ober, B.A., Jagust, W.J.: Differences in lateral hemispheric asymmetries of glucose utilization between early- and late-onset Alzheimer-type dementia. Am. J Psychiatry 142(5), 638–640 (1985)
6. Thompson, P.M., Moussai, J., Zohoori, S., Goldkorn, A., Khan, A.A., Mega, M.S., Small, G.W., Cummings, J.L., Toga, A.W.: Cortical variability and asymmetry in normal aging and alzheimer's disease. Cerebral Cortex 8, 492–509 (1998)
7. Thirion, J.-P., Prima, S., Subsol, G., Roberts, N.: Statistical analysis of normal and abnormal dissymmetry in volumetric medical images. In: IEEE Workshop on Biomedical Image Analysis 1998, pp. 74–83 (1998)
8. Joshi, S., Lorenzen, P., Gerig, G., Bullitt, E.: Structural and radiometric asymmetry in brain images. Medical Image Analysis 7, 155–170 (2003)
9. Grenander, U., Miller, M.I.: Computational anatomy: An emerging discipline. Quarterly of Applied Mathematics 56, 617–694 (1998)
10. Fletcher, P., Lu, C., Pizer, S., Joshi, S.: Principal geodesic analysis for the study of nonlinear statistics of shape. IEEE Transactions on Medical Imaging 23, 995–1005 (2004)
11. Miller, M., Younes, L.: Group actions, homeomorphisms, and matching: A general framework. International Journal of Computer Vision, 61, 61–84 (2001)
12. Joshi, S.C., Miller, M.I.: Landmark matching via large deformation diffeomorphisms. IEEE Transactions On Image Processing 9, 1357–1370 (2000)
13. Beg, M.F., Miller, M.I., Trouvé, A., Younes, L.: Computing large deformation metric mappings via geodesic flows of diffeomorphisms. International Journal of Computer Vision 61(2), 139–157 (2005)
14. Miller, M.I., Trouve, A., Younes, L.: On the metrics and euler-lagrange equations of computational anatomy. Annual Review of Biomedical Engineering 4, 375–405 (2002)
15. Fréchet, M.: Les éléments aléatoires de nature quelconque dans un espace distancié. Ann. Inst. H. Poincaré 10, 215–310 (1948)

Adaptive Time-Frequency Models for Single-Trial M/EEG Analysis

Christian Bénar[1], Maureen Clerc[2], and Théodore Papadopoulo[2]

[1] INSERM U751, La Timone, Marseille, 13006 France
[2] INRIA/ENPC/ENS Odyssée Laboratory, INRIA Sophia-Antipolis, 06902 France

Abstract. A new method is introduced for estimating single-trial magneto- or electro-encephalography (M/EEG), based on a non-linear fit of time-frequency atoms. The method can be applied for transient activity (e.g. event-related potentials) as well as for oscillatory activity (e.g. gamma bursts), and for both evoked or induced activity. In order to benefit from all the structure present in the data, the method accounts for (i) spatial structure of the data via multivariate decomposition, (ii) time-frequency structure via atomic decomposition and (iii) reproducibility across trials via a constraint on parameter dispersion. Moreover, a novel iterative method is introduced for estimating the initial time-frequency atoms used in the non-linear fit. Numerical experiments show that the method is robust to low signal-to-noise conditions, and that the introduction of the constraint on parameter dispersion significantly improves the quality of the fit.

1 Introduction

A classical method for analyzing brain electric and magnetic waves in humans consists in averaging many EEG or MEG trials, obtained in similar conditions, in order to improve the signal to noise ratio (SNR).

When the waves are sufficiently time-locked with respect to the reference time (usually the time of stimulation), the average can be performed directly in the time-domain ("event-related potentials", ERPs, in EEG and "event-related fields", ERFs, in MEG). For activity with higher time dispersion with respect to one wave period, the resulting variation of phase across trials can cause the waves to cancel out in the average signal. This is particularly relevant for high-frequency activity (above 20 Hz), where a small time delay can cause a large phase difference. This cancellation can be circumvented by averaging the power of the signal in the time-frequency or time-scale plane. Several methods have been introduced for evaluating the average increase of energy in given frequency band, whether time-locked ("evoked" energy) or not ("induced" energy) (e.g. [1]).

For both ERPs and oscillations, the averaging procedure relies on the assumption of similarity of the activity of interest across trials. However, there is often significant variability in shape and latency from one trial to another, even when measuring responses to repetitions of the exact same stimulus. This variability can arise from habituation effects, fluctuations in the level of attention and arousal, or different response strategies.

N. Karssemeijer and B. Lelieveldt (Eds.): IPMI 2007, LNCS 4584, pp. 458–469, 2007.
© Springer-Verlag Berlin Heidelberg 2007

Inter-trial variations are problematic when averaging. In particular, fluctuations in latency result in a blurring of the average signal, producing a false impression of events lasting longer than their actual duration. Moreover, comparing the amplitude of averages between conditions (for example, response to rare events versus response to frequent events), as done routinely in event-related potentials, does not permit to distinguish between an actual amplitude effect across conditions or a higher dispersion in latencies within one condition.

Nevertheless, variability can also be a source of information. For example, Jung and colleagues have demonstrated different trial-to-trial behaviors of event-related waves measured on ICA components, some being phased-locked to the stimulus and others to the subjects' responses [2]. Recently, studies have demonstrated correlations between the fluctuations of energy in the gamma band and the phase of theta oscillations, indicating an interaction between activities at different frequencies [3]. Variability between trials can also be used to measure relations between brain regions, or relations between different modalities recorded simultaneously, such as EEG and functional MRI [4].

Many different classes of methods have been introduced for detecting trial-to-trial variations in event-related potentials (ERPs) or event-related fields (ERFs). These include spline models, autoregressive models, template matching, neural networks and other multivariate classification methods, Bayesian analysis, non-linear analysis.

A promising class of methods is based on time-scale (i.e. wavelet) analysis and on time-frequency analysis. These methods permit to adapt the analyzing functions to the signals of interest, based on prior shape information. Quian Quiroga and colleagues have proposed to estimate single-trial ERPs by building fixed wavelet filters based on the average signal [5]. Estimating the wavelet filters from the average signal is subject to the difficulties mentioned above, i.e. that the average may not be fully representative of the single trials. The wavelet basis used is orthogonal, which allows fast decomposition and reconstruction of filtered signals, but is not translation-invariant and therefore ill-suited to represent latency jitters. Finally, the inter-trial fluctuations in latency or scale may necessitate the selection of a large number of coefficients in the time-scale plane, independently of the trial under consideration, which can be sensitive to noise. Some of these drawbacks have been addressed by Benkherrat and colleagues [6], who consider the average energy of the wavelet transforms of single trials instead of the transform of the average, and by [7] who use translation-invariant wavelet transforms. Statistical issues in the detection of activity have been studied in the work of Durka and colleagues, who use the matching pursuit approach and bootstrap resampling [8].

Up to now, most effort in single-trial analysis has been directed to slow-varying ERPs (in the range of 1-20Hz). Less attention has been given to the estimation of single-trial oscillatory activity, for example gamma activity around 40 Hz. Such oscillatory activity has been hypothesized to play a major role in the communication between different brain areas, for example in feature binding or matching stimuli to a target stored in memory (reviews in [9], [10]).

Another important aspect is the use of the full range of structure contained in the data, i.e. not only according to its the temporal structure, but also to its spatial structure (obtained directly across sensors or via estimated brain sources) [11], [2] and its time-frequency signature.

The new method presented here is designed to track fluctuations in brain electromagnetic activity, for any given set of frequency bands. Our method has several original features. First, we introduce a methodology for defining a reference set of Gabor time-frequency atoms, or "template", that is capable of modelling both low frequency event-related potentials and high frequency oscillations. Second, the template is deformed across trials with nonlinear optimization, which permits to follow accurately the fluctuations of the actual signal and obtain a sparse final representation of the data. Third, the deformations for each trial are constrained using information arising from all the trials, which increases the robustness of the fit even for low SNRs.

Our method is closely related to Bayesian modelling, and can be in fact seen as a Maximum a Posteriori (MAP) approach, but we are concentrating here on the nonlinear minimization aspect. Our model could be be extended in order to incorporate richer *a priori* information, or trial-to-trial variations in spatial patterns (i.e., topographies) of the signals.

The principles of the method and the mathematical framework are introduced first, followed by a description of the validation procedure and its results.

2 General Principles and Mathematical Framework

2.1 Decomposition into Realizations of Deformable Templates

We suppose that the signal contains classes of EEG or MEG activity that have a similar spatio-temporal structure. Such a structure will be approximated by a parametric template with parameters par. The signal $S(t,\theta)$, as a function of time t and spatial position θ, is modelled as the sum of a model signal $\hat{S}$ and a noise term:

$$S(t,\theta) = \hat{S}(t,\theta|par) + E(t,\theta) \ . \tag{1}$$

The model signal $\hat{S}$ is in turn composed of K repetitions (or trials) of N parametric templates

$$\hat{S}(t,\theta|par) = \sum_{n=1}^{N}\sum_{k=1}^{K} \beta_{n,k} T_n(t - t_{n,k}, \theta - \theta_{n,k}|par) \ . \tag{2}$$

In the above model, inter-trial variability is apparent in the form of a spatio-temporal shift by $(t_{n,k}, \theta_{n,k})$, and an amplitude modulation by $\beta_{n,k}$. Additional sources of inter-trial variability can be incorporated in the additional parameters par. The expected value of the noise $E(t,\theta)$ is assumed to be zero.

We further assume that a given template T_n, $n \in \{1...N\}$, can be decomposed as the product of a temporal pattern A_n and a spatial pattern (or topography) M_n (see Section 3.1 for more details).

$$T_n(t,\theta) = A_n(t)M_n(\theta) \ . \tag{3}$$

In the sequel, a simplified version of this model will be used, with $N = 1$, i.e. only one template, making the template index n no longer necessary. Moreover, the topography will be assumed stable across trials ($\theta_k = 0$), simplifying the model to

$$\hat{S}(t,\theta|par) = \sum_{k=1}^{K} \beta_k A(t - t_k|par)\, M(\theta) \ . \tag{4}$$

2.2 Time-Frequency Analysis

As we are interested in modelling signals across a wide range of frequencies (e.g., event-related potentials or induced oscillations), we propose to use time-frequency descriptors. With this in view, the Gabor atoms offer the best trade-off between time and frequency compactness. The temporal template is modeled as the linear combination of P Gabor atoms, in the real domain:

$$A(t) = \sum_{p=1}^{P} \beta_{k,p} e^{-\frac{1}{2\sigma_{k,p}^2}(t-d_{k,p})^2} cos(\omega_{k,p}(t - d_{k,p})). \tag{5}$$

The number of atoms P is fixed (see section 3.1); the template temporal shift $d_{k,p}$ is equal to the onset of the stimulation (i.e. the initial time for each trial). The trial-specific parameters to be estimated are, for each atom, its latency, amplitude, width and modulating frequency: $par = \{d_{k,p}, \beta_{k,p}, \sigma_{k,p}, \omega_{k,p}\}$.

The present study aims to model evoked potentials, hence the ratio between the width and the frequency is kept fixed (similar to Morlet wavelets). For bursts of oscillation, this constraint can be relaxed, in order to also adapt the number of oscillations to each trial.

2.3 Cost Function

The model defined by (1), (4) and (5) can be fitted to the data by the non-linear minimization of a cost function $C(par)$ composed of two parts. The first part $C_1(par)$ maximizes the fit to the data. The second part $C_2(par)$ minimizes the dispersion of the parameters around their mean and avoids over-fitting the noise. This can be formulated as:

$$C_1(par) = \sum_{t} \left[S(t) - \hat{S}(t|par)\right]^2, C_2(par) = \sum_{k,j,p} \left[\frac{par_{j,k}^p - \overline{par_j^p}}{std(par_j^p)}\right]^2, \tag{6}$$

with : t index of time samples, j index on parameters, p index on time-frequency atoms; $\overline{par_j^p}$ and $std(par_j^p)$ the sought values for the parameter mean and standard deviation across trials, respectively.

The complete cost function is

$$C(par) = C_1(par)/var(E) + \lambda\, C_2(par) \;, \tag{7}$$

where $var(E)$ is the variance of the background noise, and λ a regularization hyperparameter which balances the dispersion constraint.

The minimization is performed using the Levenberg-Marquardt algorithm, which is suited for minimizing cost functions consisting of sum of squares. We use the implementation provided in the immoptibox toolbox[1] [12]. In a first step, some quantities need to be estimated:

- the projection of the spatio-temporal data $S(t, \theta)$ into a single time-topography template,
- the initial values of the parameters $par^{init} = \{\beta_{k,p}, \sigma_{k,p}, d_{k,p}, \omega_{k,p}\}^{init}$,
- the hyperparameters $\lambda, var(E), \overline{par_j^p}$ and $std(par_j^p)$.

The next section presents strategies for estimating the time-topography signal projection, the hyperparameters and the initial values of the parameters.

3 Initialization of the Parameters

3.1 Time-Topography Decomposition

Many methods are available for decomposing spatio-temporal data (sensors × time) into fixed spatial topographies and corresponding time courses, as in (3). Examples of such methods include dipolar source localization with fixed dipoles, principal component analysis (PCA), independent component analysis (ICA), and PARAFAC (e.g. when including the frequency dimension). Such decompositions rely on the assumptions that (i) the spatial and temporal aspects of the activity of interest are independent of one another within a trial and (ii) that there is no spatial variability from one trial to the other. Albeit these are strong assumptions, they have however proven useful in a variety of situations. Moreover, they can be seen as a way of initializing spatially adaptive models such as (2).

The Singular Value Decomposition allows to project the data into a lower dimensional space that is tractable. In particular, if the data can be assumed to originate from a single source, the SVD allows to recover its spatial topography on the sensors. In a more realistic situation with several sources, the SVD can be performed as a dimension reduction preprocessing, prior to ICA. In order to select automatically the component that captures the temporal activity of the source, we assess the reproducibility of the component across trials. A score for each component is computed at each time point by dividing the mean energy by the standard deviation of the component; we select the component with highest score.

[1] Available at www2.imm.dtu.dk/ hbn/immoptibox/, in the Matlab (Mathworks, Natick, MA, USA) environment.

3.2 Initial Time-Frequency Atoms

The parameter initialization for the time-frequency atoms is performed via an iterative wavelet analysis. For this, Morlet wavelets are introduced, which are Gabor atoms with a fixed number of oscillations, defined in the frequency domain by:

$$\Psi_s^\xi(\omega) = \frac{\sqrt{s}}{(4\pi)^{\frac{1}{4}}} e^{-\frac{1}{2}(s\omega-\xi)^2} \tag{8}$$

The shifting frequency ξ determines the number of oscillations of the wavelet over its time-support. For a given shifting frequency ξ, the scale parameter s stretches or compresses the wavelet, controlling simultaneously the time-support (proportional to s) and the frequency (equal to $\xi/(2\pi s)$) at which the wavelet oscillates. The optimal number of oscillations depends on the type of activity under examination, smaller for evoked potentials/fields and larger for oscillations. Therefore a set of shifting frequencies is considered : $\xi \in \{1, 1.5, 3, 5, 9\}$.

An initial time-frequency decomposition $W_k^0(t, \omega)$ is obtained by projecting each trial $S_k(t)$ on a set of analyzing functions:

$$W_k^0(t, s, \xi) = \int S_k(t')\overline{\psi}_s^\xi(t - t')dt' \ . \tag{9}$$

In the above relation, the time index t belongs to a time window $[t_k, t_k + L]$ containing the kth trial (t_k defined in Section 2.2), and $\overline{\psi}$ denotes the complex conjugate of ψ. The energy for each ξ is then averaged across trials

$$TF^0(t, s, \xi) = \frac{1}{K}\sum_k |W_k^0(t - t_k, s, \xi)|^2. \tag{10}$$

The average energy $TF^0(t, s, \xi)$ could be normalized by the average power value in a baseline part of the window [1], [13]. One can also consider dividing by the standard deviation of the noise power estimated at the point of interest [6]. Such normalizations allow to be more robust to noise and to detect high-frequency activity that is hidden in the original signal due to the 1/f behavior of EEG and MEG.

The iterative parameter selection proceeds à la matching pursuit [14], iteratively subtracting from the single-trial data its projection on the atom $\psi_{s^0}^{\xi^0}$ whose parameters maximize the average energy:

$$(t^0, s^0, \xi^0) = argmax(TF^0(t, s, \xi))$$

This leads to a new set of trials $S_k^1(t)$ on which the above-described procedure can again be applied. The number of iterations P is determined by hand; however, one could consider using a quantitative criterion, based for example on the energy of the residuals after subtraction. The main difference with matching pursuit resides in the use of the data over a collection of trials, thereby taking advantage of the information arising from reproducibility across trials.

3.3 Constraint on Parameters Dispersion

The hyperparameters $\overline{par_j^p}$ and $std(par_j^p)$ help to reduce the parameter dispersion across trials, in order to increase robustness to noise. We choose to estimate these parameters from the data itself, in a first step that consists in minimizing only the first part $C_1(par)$ of the cost function (6) (i.e., without the control of the parameter dispersion). We make the assumption that the fit will be successful for a majority of trials, failing only in a small proportion of outliers due to the noise. The mean and standard deviation of each parameter are then estimated with a robust MM-estimator [15].

3.4 Regularization Hyperparameters

The hyperparameters $var(E)$ and λ appearing in (7) control the relative weights given on the one hand to the quality of the fit (6), and on the other hand to the constraint on dispersion $C2$ in (6).

The variance of the noise $var(E)$ is estimated on the residuals after the first fit (i.e., using only the first part of the cost function (6)), using robust estimators as in 3.3.

The regularization parameter λ is estimated with the L-curve method. The fit is performed using (7) for a series of λ ranging from 10^{-4} to 10^4, with a higher sampling around $\lambda = 1$. The minimization procedure results in optimal values C_1^{opt} and C_2^{opt}, for each λ. The L-curve method consists in finding the inflection point in the curve $C_2^{opt}(\lambda) = f(C_1^{opt}(\lambda))$. This point is estimated as the minimum of the cost function

$$c(\lambda) = \frac{C_1^{opt}(\lambda)}{std(C_1^{opt})} + \frac{C_2^{opt}(\lambda)}{std(C_2^{opt})} \tag{11}$$

with std standard deviation across values of λ.

4 Methodology of Evaluation

First of all, simulations were performed to evaluate the robustness of the method to different levels of noise, with a particular emphasis on the contribution of the regularization term C2 in (6). Secondly, the method was applied to real data originating from an oddball experiment [4].

4.1 Simulated Data

A series of 50 event-related potentials (ERPs) were computed, corresponding to a central radial source within a sphere, with 83 electrodes (10/10 system), at a sampling frequency of 1 kHz. The potentials consisted of a sum of Gaussian-shaped waves (N100-like and P300-like) and of high frequency oscillations (range 38-42 Hz) with a Gaussian envelope. The latency, amplitude, width and frequency parameters of the waves and oscillations were pseudo-random numbers with a

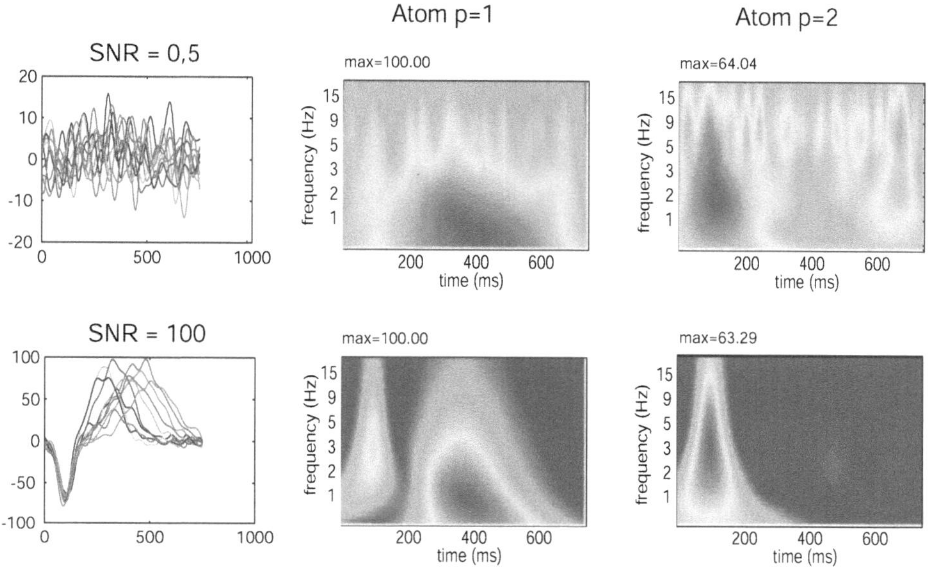

Fig. 1. Left column: Simulated data after spatial filtering, for a SNR of 0.5 (upper part) and 100 (lower part) (the SNR corresponds to the data before filtering). Middle and right column: time-frequency analysis used for the iterative definition of time-frequency atoms, for p=1 (first atom) and p=2 (second atom). The maximum value indicated is the maximum energy in the time-frequency plane with respect to the maximum energy of the first iteration (i.e, first atom).

truncated distribution, with values lying three standard deviations around the mean. The latency parameter was assigned a skewed distribution, similar to that of realistic reaction times. See figure 1 for an overview of the simulated signals.

Stationary background noise was simulated, with spatial and temporal correlations ressembling real EEG data. This noise was obtained by distributing dipoles uniformly within a sphere, with a random amplitude following a normal distribution [16]. Each channel was then filtered and scaled with an autoregressive filter, whose parameters had been fitted on real EEG data. The resulting correlated noise was added to the simulated ERPs, with a multiplicative factor corresponding to different values of the signal-to-noise ratio: SNR $\in \{0, 0.1, 0.5, 1, 3, 5, 10, 100, 10^6\}$. The SNR was computed as the ratio of the sums of squares across all channels. For the high frequency oscillations, the data and noise were first filtered with a 35-45 Hz bandpass filter before computing the scaling factor.

For each SNR, a singular value decomposition (SVD) was applied to the simulated data, and the time-course with the highest reproducibility across trials was retained. Reproducibility was assessed by computing the average energy across trials. The method was then applied on the time-course, across trials, as described in the previous sections.

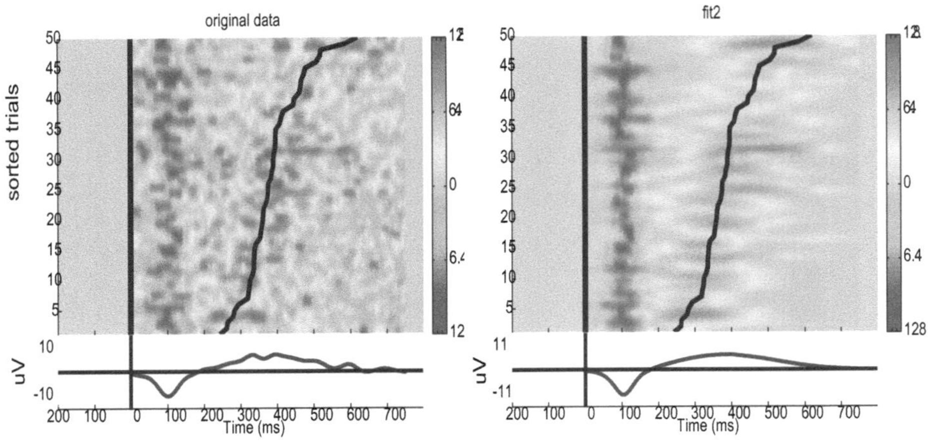

Fig. 2. Left: original data for a SNR of 1. For display purposes, the data is sorted with respect to the simulated latency of the second wave, an information that was not used during the fit. Right: fitted atoms, with constraint on parameter dispersion.

4.2 Real Data

We used an EEG dataset recorded within the MRI scanner, from an simultaneous EEG-fMRI oddball protocol presented in detail in [4]. In summary, the stimulation consisted in pure tones, with low frequency tones presented frequently, and high frequency tones presented rarely. The subject was asked to respond to the rare tones by a button press. This protocol is known to provoke a stereotyped positive response on the EEG around 300 ms, called P300.

5 Results

The data obtained after spatial filtering by SVD are presented in figure 1, along with the iterative time-frequency decomposition, for a SNR of 100 and a SNR of 0.5. This demonstrates that the iterative decomposition is robust even for low SNR. Figure 2 presents raster plots of the data across trials, for a SNR of 1, for the raw data (left plot) and for the estimated atoms (right plot). For display purposes, the data is sorted with respect to the simulated latency of the second wave, an information that was not used during the fit. The algorithm was able to recover the simulated waves. For each SNR, we have computed the correlation at each trial between the fitted data on a SNR of 10^6 and the fitted data at the SNR under consideration, with and without the constraint on parameter dispersion (figure 3). Without the constraint on the parameters, the quality of the fit deteriorates rapidly with decreasing SNR. The constraint allows the fit to maintain a good quality up to a SNR of 0.5.

The outcome of the fit on real data (auditory oddball in simultaneous EEG-fMRI) is presented in figure 4. The application of the proposed method results

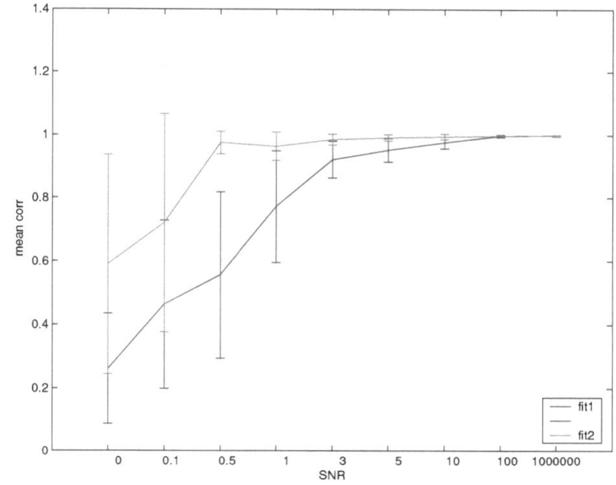

Fig. 3. Correlation between the fitted time-course at a given SNR and the fitted time-course for a SNR of 10^6, considered as the reference. The use of a constraint on parameter dispersion (fit2, in red, upper curve) improves the results compared to a fit without this constraint (fit1, in blue, lower curve).

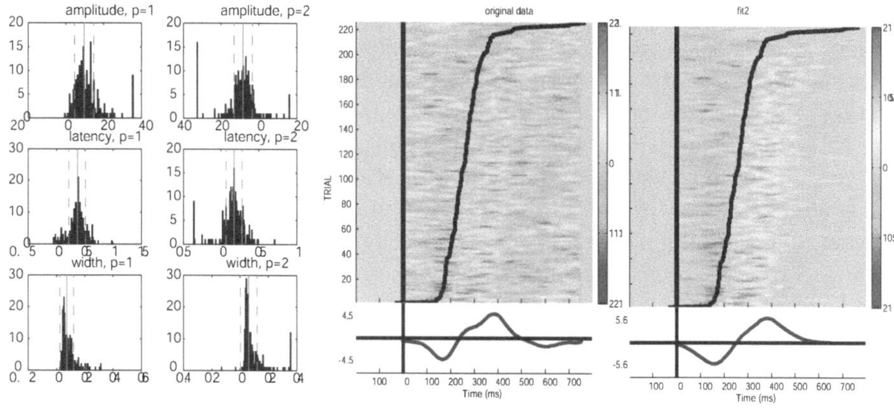

Fig. 4. Results for the oddball data. Left: histograms of parameters fitted in fit1 (no constraint on dispersion). The red (light grey) vertical bars show the mean and standard deviation of the parameters, which were not influenced by outliers (robust estimation). Middle: raster plot original data (y-axis: trials corresponding to rare events), sorted by reaction time (dark line). Right: result of the fitting procedure (fit2, with constraint on the parameters).

in a very significant denoising of this data, which had extremely low SNR due to the simultaneous fMRI scanning.

6 Discussion

A new method has been presented for estimating single-trial EEG or MEG activity, based on a non-linear fit. The method can be used for both transient (e.g., event-related potentials) and oscillatory (e.g., gamma bursts) activity, and for both evoked or induced activity.

The method aims to use all the structure present in the data. First, it takes advantage of the spatial structure via multivariate decomposition. Second, it uses the time-frequency structure via atomic decomposition. Third, reproducibility across trials is imposed via a constraint on parameter dispersion.

A novel method was introduced for estimating the initial time-frequency atoms used in the non-linear fit, which runs in an iterative manner. This method is similar to matching pursuit [14], with the originality of operating across trials. We use Gabor atoms, which have good time-frequency properties, but it could be interesting to learn the atom structure directly from the data. We also present a novel non-linear minimization framework, contrary to previous approaches using wavelet transforms [6], [7]. This leads to a more parcimonious (sparse) description of the data, in particular for large jitters in the parameters (for example latency jitters), which could result in higher robustness to noise.

The same data was used to estimate the hyper-parameters (mean and standard deviation of the parameters, used in the dispersion constraint) and the actual parameters of the time-frequency atoms. Such an approach must be performed with caution, since estimating (the hyper-parameters) and detecting (the parameters of the atoms) on the exact same dataset could lead to a bias of the results. However the risk of bias is low in our case, as the parameters for only *one* trial are being estimated, based on hyper-parameters estimated on *all* trials; i.e. the influence of the trial under investigation on the definition of the hyper-parameters is low. Moreover, the robust estimation of the hyper-parameters further lowers the influence of a given trial: if the parameters of a trial are outliers, they are not taken into account in the computation of the hyper-parameters, and therefore do not influence the estimation.

As shown by the tests on simulated and real data, the proposed method is robust to low signal-to-noise conditions. The introduction of a constraint on parameter dispersion, estimated from the data itself, significantly improves the quality of the fit. Future work will concentrate on the estimation of high-frequency (gamma) activity and on taking into account the structure of the noise.

Acknowledgment

The authors thank the team of the fMRI center of Marseille (Jean-Luc Anton, Bruno Nazarian and Muriel Roth) for the EEG-fMRI data.

References

1. Tallon-Baudry, C., Bertrand, O., Delpuech, C., Pernier, J.: Stimulus specificity of phase-locked and non-phase-locked 40 hz visual responses in human. J. Neurosci. 16(13), 4240–4249 (1996)
2. Jung, T., Makeig, S., Westerfield, M., Townsend, J., Courchesne, E., Sejnowski, T.: Analysis and visualization of single-trial event-related potentials. Human Brain Mapping 14, 166–185 (2001)
3. Canolty, R., Edwards, E., Dalal, S., Soltani, M., Nagarajan, S., Kirsch, H., Berger, M., Barbaro, N., Knight, R.: High gamma power is phase-locked to theta oscillations in human neocortex. Science 313(5793), 1626–1628 (2006)
4. Bénar, C., Schön, D., Grimault, S., Nazarian, B., Burle, B., Roth, M., Badier, J., Marquis, P., Liegeois-Chauvel, C., Anton, J.: Single-trial analysis of oddball event-related potentials in simultaneous EEG-fMRI. Human Brain Mapping (in press)
5. Quian Quiroga, R., Garcia, H.: Single-trial event-related potentials with wavelet denoising. Clin. Neurophysiol. 114(2), 376–390 (2003)
6. Benkherrat, M., Burle, B., Allain, S., Hasbroucq, T., Vidal, F.: Individual evoked potential extraction by multiresolution wavelets decomposition. In: Proceedings EUROCON2005 (2005)
7. Wang, Z., Maier, A., Leopold, D., Logothetis, N., Liang, H.: Single-trial evoked potential estimation using wavelets. Comput. Biol. Med. (in press)
8. Durka, P., Zygierewicz, J., Klekowicz, H., Ginter, J., Blinowska, K.: On the statistical significance of event-related eeg desynchronization and synchronization in the time-frequency plane. IEEE Trans. Biomed. Eng. 51(7), 1167–1175 (2004)
9. Kahana, M.: The cognitive correlates of human brain oscillations. J. Neurosci. 26(6), 1669–1672 (2006)
10. Fell, J., Fernandez, G., Klaver, P., Elger, C., Fries, P.: Is synchronized neuronal gamma activity relevant for selective attention? Brain Res. Rev. 42, 265–272 (2003)
11. Ranta-aho, P., Koistinen, A., Ollikainen, J., Kaipio, J., Partanen, J., Karjalainen, P.: Single-trial estimation of multichannel evoked-potential measurements. IEEE Trans. Biomed. Eng. 50(2), 189–196 (2003)
12. Madsen, K., Nielsen, H., Tingleff, O.: Methods for Non-Linear Least Squares Problems, 2nd edn. IMM DTU (2004)
13. Makeig, S.: Auditory event-related dynamics of the eeg spectrum and effects of exposure to tones. Electroencephalogr. Clin. Neurophys. 86(4), 283–293 (1993)
14. Mallat, S., Zhang, Z.: Matching pursuit with time-frequency dictionaries. IEEE Trans. Signal Processing 41(12), 3397–3415 (1993)
15. Croux, C., Dhaene, G., Hoorelbeke, D.: Robust standard errors for robust estimators. Research Report DTEW 0367, K.U.Leuven (2003)
16. de Munck, J., Vijn, P., da Silva, F.L.: A random dipole model for spontaneous brain activity. IEEE Trans. Biomed. Eng. 39(8), 791–804 (1992)

Imaging Brain Activation Streams from Optical Flow Computation on 2-Riemannian Manifolds

Julien Lefèvre[1], Guillaume Obozinski[2], and Sylvain Baillet[1]

[1] Cognitive Neuroscience and Brain Imaging Laboratory,
CNRS UPR640–LENA,
Université Pierre et Marie CURIE–Paris6, Paris, F-75013, France
{julien.lefevre,sylvain.baillet}@chups.jussieu.fr
[2] Department of Statistics, University of California,
Berkeley, CA 94720-3860, USA

Abstract. We report on mathematical methods for the exploration of spatiotemporal dynamics of Magneto- and Electro-Encephalography (MEG / EEG) surface data and/or of the corresponding brain activity at the cortical level, with high temporal resolution. In this regard, we describe how the framework and numerical computation of the optical flow — a classical tool for motion analysis in computer vision — can be extended to non-flat 2-dimensional surfaces such as the scalp and the cortical mantle. We prove the concept and mathematical well-posedness of such an extension through regularizing constraints on the estimated velocity field, and discuss the quantitative evaluation of the optical flow. The method is illustrated by simulations and analysis of brain image sequences from a ball-catching paradigm.

1 Introduction

Magnetoencephalography (MEG) and electroencephalography (EEG) respectively measure magnetic fields and electric potentials on the scalp surface, which provides investigation of neural processes with exquisite time resolution within the millisecond range. Estimation techniques of MEG/EEG generators have been considerably improving recently [5], thereby making electromagnetic brain mapping become a true functional imaging modality. However, most studies report on the classical brain mapping questions of 'Where?' and When?' specific brain processes have occurred, but rarely address 'How?' these latter might be embedded in space and time altogether.

The theory of *electrographic objects* [18] was the first computational approach with the objective of deciphering the 'Rosetta Stone' of brain language at the macroscopic scale. The concept of *spatiotemporal elements*, that were assumed to structurally sustain neural activity, was later reformulated by Lehmann in terms of *microstates* as 'building blocks of mentation' [14]. This concept emerged from empirical observations of the time-evolving topographies of scalp potential maps in EEG, which could be described as the succession of episodes of relatively-stable spatial configurations. Multiple techniques have been proposed to detect

N. Karssemeijer and B. Lelieveldt (Eds.): IPMI 2007, LNCS 4584, pp. 470–481, 2007.
© Springer-Verlag Berlin Heidelberg 2007

and characterize microstates and they have been applied in a great number of paradigms, from cognitive to clinical experimental neuroscience (e.g. [22]). However, they all refer to some static and geometrical analysis of EEG scalp patterns — through PCA analysis of time segments [17], dissimilarity measures on successive EEG topographies [24] — and have never been adapted to the analysis of brain image sequences so far.

Our contribution suggests a new framework to investigate the spatiotemporal dynamics of brain activations in terms of the estimation and analysis of their displacement field.

We first prove in Section 2 the concept and work at the theoretical aspects of the computation of optical flow on a 2-dimensional surface, through the generalization of existing variational formulations. In Section 3, we evaluate the consistency of the estimates and run realistic numerical simulations. Finally, the method is illustrated from experimental data in the context of a ball-catching experimental investigation with MEG.

2 Velocity Field of Neural Activity

In multiple applications, analysis of dynamical phenomena through the computation of a velocity vector field has contributed to the description and extraction of informational contents about the processes involved (see e.g. [7],[9]). Such approaches have barely been suggested for the analysis of structured patterns within brain signals and image sequences with high temporal resolution (e.g. using MEG/EEG or optical imaging). In [13], estimation of velocity fields was restricted to 2D images of narrow-band scalp EEG measures in the α range (i.e. typically within [7, 14] Hz), with limited quantitative analysis.

Our approach to the computation of the velocity vector field descends from optical flow techniques as introduced originally by Horn & Schunk [12]. These techniques have been demonstrating efficiency in the analysis of video sequences for about the last two decades (see e.g. [8, 15] which review a selection of computational methods associated with sound performance evaluation). The computation of vector flow is generally driven by basic assumptions which postulate conservation of brightness of moving objects. These restrictive hypotheses may not fit rigourously the exact nature of phenomena but have proven to yield commensurate estimations of vector fields provided they are valid locally in time and space [8]. The exquisite time-resolution of MEG/EEG images is generally compatible with these assumptions, as brain responses unfold to a large extent with substantial spatiotemporal smoothness.

In the context of brain imaging though, we are facing the issue of distributed intensity variations in 3D. Detection can be restricted to the cortical surface as a first approach, hence recent surface flattening tools could be applied [23] prior to using classical 2D flow estimators. However, such a transform entails multiple kinds of limitations: the required topological cuts in the closed surface of the brain induce linking problems at boundaries; moreover, local distortions of angles and distances are problematic when it comes to estimate the local orientation of the flow.

Here we introduce a formalism based on differential geometry to extend the computation of optical flow equations on non-flat surfaces (see [10] for an introduction), hence on the folded geometry of the brain.

2.1 Optical Flow on a Non-flat Domain

Let us define $\mathcal{M}$, a 2-Riemannian manifold representing the imaging support (i.e. the scalp or cortical surfaces), parameterized by the local coordinates system $\phi : p \in \mathcal{M} \mapsto (x_1, x_2) \in \mathbb{R}^2$. We introduce a scalar quantity defined in time on a 2-dimensional surface — e.g. brain activity from scalp MEG/EEG topographies or cortical activation maps — as a function $I(p,t) \in \mathcal{M}$, where $(p,t) \in \mathcal{M} \times \mathbb{R}$. We note $\mathbf{e}_\alpha = \partial_{x_\alpha} p := \partial_\alpha p$, the canonical basis of the tangent space $T_p\mathcal{M}$ at a point p of the manifold, and $T\mathcal{M} = \bigcup_p T_p\mathcal{M}$ the tangent bundle of $\mathcal{M}$.

$\mathcal{M}$ is equipped with a Riemannian metric, meaning that at each point p of manifold $\mathcal{M}$, there exists a positive-definite form:

$$g_p : T_p\mathcal{M} \times T_p\mathcal{M} \to \mathbb{R},$$

which is differentiable with respect to p. We later denote $(g_p)_{\alpha,\beta} = g_p\big(\mathbf{e}_\alpha, \mathbf{e}_\beta\big)$. A natural choice for g_p is the restriction of the Euclidian metric to $T_p\mathcal{M}$, which we have adopted for subsequent computations. For concision purposes, we will now only refer to g_p as g.

As in classical computation approaches to optical flow, we now assume that the activity of a point moving on a curve $c(t)$ in $\mathcal{M}$ is constant along time. The condition $\mathrm{d}I = 0$ yields :

$$\partial_t I + D_{c(t)} I(\dot{\mathbf{c}}) = 0, \tag{1}$$

where $D_{c(t)}I$ is the differential of I at point $c(t)$ applied to $\dot{\mathbf{c}} = \mathbf{V} = (V^1, V^2)$, the unknown vector field. We express the linear application $D_{c(t)}I$ as a scalar product and introduce $\nabla_{\mathcal{M}} I$, the gradient of I which is defined as the vector field satisfying at each point p :

$$\forall \mathbf{V} \in T_p\mathcal{M}, g(\nabla_{\mathcal{M}} I, \mathbf{V}) = D_p I\big(\mathbf{V}\big).$$

(1) can thereby be transformed into an optical-flow type of equation:

$$\partial_t I + g(\mathbf{V}, \nabla_{\mathcal{M}} I) = 0. \tag{2}$$

We note that (2) takes the same form as general conservation laws defined on manifolds in [19]. Here, only the component of the flow $\mathbf{V}$ in the direction of the gradient is accessible to estimation. This corresponds to the well-known *aperture problem* [12], which requires additional constraints on the flow to yield a unique solution. This approach classically reduces to minimizing an energy functional such as in [12]:

$$\mathcal{E}(\mathbf{V}) = \int_{\mathcal{M}} \left(\frac{\partial I}{\partial t} + g(\mathbf{V}, \nabla_{\mathcal{M}} I) \right)^2 \mathrm{d}\mu_{\mathcal{M}} + \lambda \int_{\mathcal{M}} \mathcal{C}(\mathbf{V}) \mathrm{d}\mu_{\mathcal{M}}, \tag{3}$$

where $d\mu_{\mathcal{M}}$ is a volume form on $\mathcal{M}$, for which we suggest $\sqrt{\det(g_{\alpha,\beta})}dx_1dx_2$ as a natural choice.

The first term is a measure of fit of the optical flow model to the data, while the second one acts as a spatial regularizer of the flow. The scalar parameter λ tunes the respective contribution of these two terms in the net energy cost $\mathcal{E}(\mathbf{V})$. Here we use the smoothness term from [12], which can be expressed as a Frobenius norm:

$$\mathcal{C}(\mathbf{V}) = \mathrm{Tr}({}^t\nabla\mathbf{V}.\nabla\mathbf{V}), \tag{4}$$

where

$$(\nabla\mathbf{V})_{\alpha}^{\beta} = \partial_{\alpha}V^{\beta} + \sum_{\gamma}\Gamma_{\alpha\gamma}^{\beta}V^{\gamma}$$

is the covariant derivative of $\mathbf{V}$, a generalization of vectorial gradient. $\partial_{\alpha}V^{\beta}$ is the classical Euclidian expression of the gradient, and $\sum_{\gamma}\Gamma_{\alpha\gamma}^{\beta}V^{\gamma}$ reflects local deformations of the tangent space basis since the Christoffel symbols $\Gamma_{\alpha\gamma}^{\beta}$ are the coordinates of $\partial_{\beta}\mathbf{e}_{\alpha}$ along $\mathbf{e}_{\gamma}$. This rather complex expression ensures the tensoriality property of $\mathbf{V}$, i.e. invariance with parametrization changes.

This constraint will tend to generate a regularized vector field with small spatial derivatives, that is a field with weak local variations. Such a regularization scheme may be problematic in situations where spatial discontinuities occur in the image sequences. For example, in the case of a moving object on a static background, the severe velocity discontinuities around the object contours are eventually blurred in the regularized flow field. In the case of brain activations revealed by MEG/EEG though, spatial patterns are naturally smooth thus we adopt the basic Horn & Schunk regularization scheme (see [25] for a taxonomy of other possible terms).

2.2 Variational Formulation

Variational formulation of 2D-optical flow equation has been first proposed by Schnörr in [20]. The advantage of such formulation is twofold. Theoretically, it ensures the problem is well-posed; that is there exists a unique solution in a specific and convenient function space e.g. a Sobolev spacen [20], or a space of functions with bounded variations [4]. Numerically, it allows to solve the problem on discrete irregular surfacic tessellations and to yield discrete solutions belonging to the chosen function space. We demonstrate these assertions in the case of Horn & Schunk isotropic smoothness priors, but the general framework remains the same for Nagel's anisotropic image-driven regularization approach [16].

Considering $\mathcal{M}$, we need to define a working space of vector fields $\Gamma^1(\mathcal{M})$ on which functional $\mathcal{E}(\mathbf{V})$ will be minimized. Let us first denote the Sobolev space $H^1(\mathcal{M})$ defined in [11] as the completion of $C^1(\mathcal{M})$ (the space of differentiable functions on the manifold) with respect to $\|\ .\ \|_{H^1}$ derived from the following scalar product :

$$< u, v >_{H^1} = \int_{\mathcal{M}} uv \ d\mu_{\mathcal{M}} + \int_{\mathcal{M}} g(\nabla u, \nabla v) \ d\mu_{\mathcal{M}}.$$

We chose a space of vector fields in which the coordinates of each element are located in a classical Sobolev space:

$$\Gamma^1(\mathcal{M}) = \left\{\mathbf{V} : \mathcal{M} \to T\mathcal{M} \ / \ \mathbf{V} = \textstyle\sum_{\alpha=1}^{2} V^\alpha \mathbf{e}_\alpha,\ V^\alpha \in H^1(\mathcal{M})\right\},$$

with the scalar product :

$$< \mathbf{U}, \mathbf{V} >_{\Gamma^1(\mathcal{M})} = \int_{\mathcal{M}} g(\mathbf{U}, \mathbf{V})\ \mathrm{d}\mu_{\mathcal{M}} + \int_{\mathcal{M}} \mathrm{Tr}({}^t\nabla\mathbf{U}\nabla\mathbf{V})\ \mathrm{d}\mu_{\mathcal{M}}.$$

$\mathcal{E}(\mathbf{V})$ can be simplified from (3) as a combination of the following constant, linear and bilinear forms :

$$\begin{aligned} K(t) &= \int_{\mathcal{M}} (\partial_t I)^2 \mathrm{d}\mu_{\mathcal{M}} , \\ f(\mathbf{U}) &= -\int_{\mathcal{M}} g(\mathbf{U}, \nabla_{\mathcal{M}} I)\partial_t I\ \mathrm{d}\mu_{\mathcal{M}}, \\ a(\mathbf{U}, \mathbf{V}) &= \underbrace{\int_{\mathcal{M}} g(\mathbf{U}, \nabla_{\mathcal{M}} I) g(\mathbf{V}, \nabla_{\mathcal{M}} I) \mathrm{d}\mu_{\mathcal{M}}}_{\textit{Fit to data}} + \lambda \underbrace{\int_{\mathcal{M}} \mathrm{Tr}({}^t\nabla\mathbf{U}\nabla\mathbf{V})\ \mathrm{d}\mu_{\mathcal{M}}}_{\textit{Regularizing term}} . \end{aligned}$$

Minimizing $\mathcal{E}(\mathbf{V})$ on $\Gamma^1(\mathcal{M})$ is then equivalent to the following problem :

$$\min_{\mathbf{V} \in \Gamma^1(\mathcal{M})} \big(a(\mathbf{V}, \mathbf{V}) - 2f(\mathbf{V}) + K(t)\big). \tag{5}$$

Lax-Milgram theorem ensures unicity of the solution with the following assumptions [3]:

1. a and f are continuous forms;
2. $\Gamma^1(\mathcal{M})$ is complete, the bilinear form $a(.,.)$ is symmetric and coercive (elliptic), that is, there exists a constant C such that :

$$\forall\ \mathbf{V} \in \Gamma^1(\mathcal{M}), a(\mathbf{V}, \mathbf{V}) \geq C \parallel \mathbf{V} \parallel^2_{\Gamma^1(\mathcal{M})} .$$

Moreover, the solution $\mathbf{V}$ to (5) satisfies:

$$a(\mathbf{V}, \mathbf{U}) = f(\mathbf{U}), \forall\ \mathbf{U} \in \Gamma^1(\mathcal{M}). \tag{6}$$

Continuity of f and a are straightforward. Completeness of $\Gamma^1(\mathcal{M})$ is ensured because any Cauchy sequence has components in $H^1(\mathcal{M})$ which are also Cauchy sequences since $\parallel . \parallel_{H^1}$ is bounded by $\parallel . \parallel_{\Gamma^1(\mathcal{M})}$.

Proof of coercivity can be adapted — analogously to flat domains [20] — thanks to isothermal coordinates. Indeed, the Korn–Lichtenstein theorem (1914) allows to find a system of coordinates for which the two basis vectors of tangent space are orthogonal. In this basis, calculus are similar to those in Euclidian case by introducing a multiplicative coefficient equal to the norm of the basis vectors.

The coercivity and therefore well-posedness requires only a similar assumption about linear independency of the two components of the gradient $\nabla_{\mathcal{M}} I$.

2.3 FEM Computation of the Optical Flow

Now that we have proven the well-posedness of the regularized optical flow problem on a manifold $\mathcal{M}$, we derive computational methods from the variational formulation, which are defined on a tessellation $\mathcal{M}_h$ which approximates the manifold.

Let us consider the vector space of continuous piecewise affine vector fields on $\mathcal{M}_h$ which belong to the tangent space at each node of the tessellation. A convenient basis is:

$$\mathbf{w}_{\alpha,i} = w(i)\mathbf{e}_\alpha(i) \text{ for } 1 \leq i \leq \mathrm{Card}(\mathcal{M}_h),\ \alpha \in \{1,2\},$$

where $w(i)$ stands for the continuous piecewise affine function which is 1 at node i and 0 at all other triangle nodes, and $\mathbf{e}_\alpha(i)$ is a basis of tangent space at node i.

The variational formulation in (6) yields a classical linear system:

$$\forall j\ \forall \beta \in \{1,2\},\ \sum_{i=1}^{\mathrm{Card}(\mathcal{M}_h)} \sum_{\alpha=1}^{2} a(\mathbf{w}_{\alpha,i}, \mathbf{w}_{\beta,j})\mathbf{V}_{\alpha,i} = f(\mathbf{w}_{\beta,j}), \tag{7}$$

where $\mathbf{V}_{\alpha,i}$ are the components of the velocity field $\mathbf{V}$ in the basis $\mathbf{w}_{\alpha,i}$. Note that $a(\mathbf{w}_{\alpha,i}, \mathbf{w}_{\beta,j})$ and $f(\mathbf{w}_{\beta,j})$ can be explicitly computed with first-order finite elements by estimating the integrals on each triangle T of the tessellation and summing the different contributions.

Practically, $\nabla_{\mathcal{M}} I$ is obtained on each triangle $T = [i,j,k]$ from the linear interpolation:

$$\nabla_{\mathcal{M}} I \sim I(i)\nabla_T w(i) + I(j)\nabla_T w(j) + I(k)\nabla_T w(k).,$$

with

$$\nabla_T w(i) = \frac{\mathbf{h_i}}{\| \mathbf{h_i} \|^2},$$

where $\mathbf{h_i}$ is the height of triangle T from vertex i.

Let us define $P_\mathbf{n}(i)$ as the projection operator onto the local tangent plane, which is obtained at node i by estimating the local normal $\mathbf{n}$ as the sum of normals of each triangle containing i. For each i, $\mathbf{e}_\alpha(i)$ is chosen as a basis of the kernel of $P_\mathbf{n}(i)$. The Christoffel symbols Γ^k_{ij} vanish in our discretization with first-order finite elements since the $\mathbf{e}_\alpha(i)$ have no variations on each triangle.

3 Simulations

We address the quantitative and qualitative evaluation of optical flow with simple and illustrative simulations on a selection of surfaces.

3.1 Angular Error Estimation Via Parallel Transport

Most of optical flow techniques are evaluated with quantitative comparison between the true velocity field $\mathbf{V}$ and the estimated optical flow $\hat{\mathbf{V}}$. This criterion can be reduced as the evaluation of an angular error (AE) between two vectors, taking into account their relative amplitude.

We introduce $||.|| = \sqrt{g(.,.)+1}$ and adapt the angular error estimate originally introduced in [6]:

$$AE(\mathbf{V}, \hat{\mathbf{V}}) = \arccos\left(\frac{g(\mathbf{V}, \hat{\mathbf{V}})+1}{||\mathbf{V}||.||\hat{\mathbf{V}}||}\right).$$

Nevertheless, there remains the nontrivial issue of defining a velocity field on a manifold. During the uniform translation of a uniformly-colored patch for instance, the velocity vectors of moving points are not parallel in the Euclidian sense anymore. Hence we extend the definition of parallelism via the notion of *parallel transport.*

Let us consider the centroid G of a translating illuminated patch with given velocity $\mathbf{V}_G$. In order to calculate the velocity at any point A of the patch, we transport $\mathbf{V}_G$ along γ, a geodesic curve joining G to A ($\gamma(0) = G, \gamma(1) = A$). Practically we have to solve the differential equation :

$$\nabla_{\dot{\gamma}(u)}\mathbf{Y}(u) = 0,$$

with

$$\nabla_{\dot{\gamma}(u)}\mathbf{Y}(u) = \sum_i \dot{\gamma}(t)^i (\nabla \mathbf{Y})_i^j \ , \ \mathbf{Y}(0) = \mathbf{V}_G.$$

The velocity at point A is obtained taking $\mathbf{Y}(1)$.

In the case of spherical geometry, the parallel transport along a geodesic reduces to a simple rotation whose axis is orthogonal to the plane containing the geodesic[1] (Fig. 1). The implementation of general parallel transport has not been addressed since it reaches far beyond the scope of this study.

The angular error provides a simple evaluation index as well as a quantitative criterion to adjust the regularizing parameter λ in (3), which was fixed to $\lambda = 0.1$ in the rest of the study.

3.2 Results on Synthetic Data

Two types of synthetic data were created. They approximate typical situations encountered when dealing with EEG or MEG images evolving on the surface of the head or on the cortical surface.

The first set of simulations illustrates the emergence and fading of activity within on a single region of the brain (see Fig. 2). Even if this situation infringes the hypothesis of intensity conservation across time 1, the radial structure of

[1] Note the parallel transport cannot be defined for diametrally-opposite points.

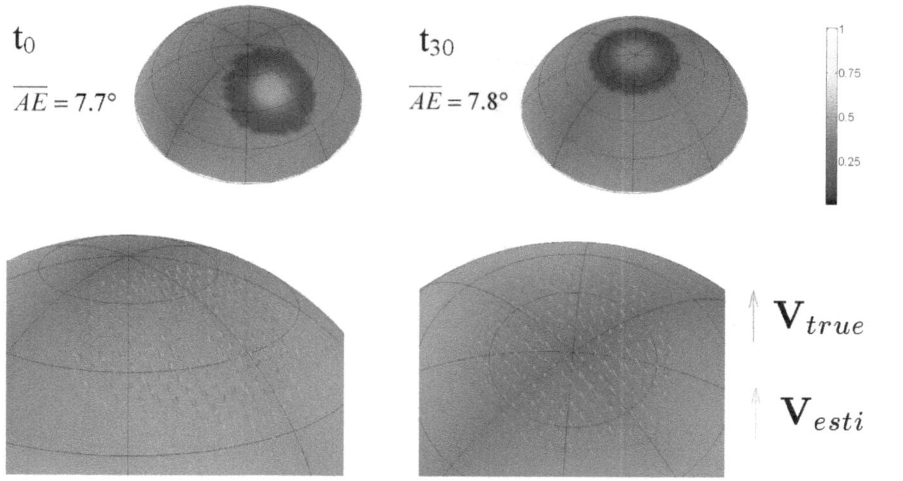

Fig. 1. Evaluation of computation of the vector flow: a patch with Gaussian distribution of intensity travels on a sphere. The outcome of the optical flow computation is shown in green and compared with the true velocity field in red at two time instants. Mean angular error AE is given in degrees.

optical flow gives an indication about how the system is evolving, spreading then collapsing.

The second kind of synthetic data simulates propagations of activity across distant brain regions. Fig. 1 shows the translation of a Gaussian patch of activity and compares the true displacement field with its optical-flow estimation. At each step of time, we indicate the mean angular error as defined in Section 3.1 for each point of the patch. A similar type of unfolding patterns of activation is shown Fig. 3 on real brain surface geometry. An approximation of a Gaussian patch propagates from a rather flat domain of the cortical manifold and travels down into a sulcal fold. We represent the velocity of the patch centroid and the mean optical flow projected on a plane containing the true displacement. We speculate the irregular angular error could be improved with the method exposed in Section 3.1.

4 Application to the Investigation of Spatiotemporal Dynamics of MEG Signals

4.1 The Electromagnetic Brain Imaging Problem

Magneto and electroencephalography stem from similar physical principles since they are directly related to the electromagnetical activity of neurons. Magnetic fields (and similarly electric potentials) are sampled on s sensors, $M_1, \ldots, M_s$, as a linear combination of p sources signals $S_1, \ldots, S_p$ which can be written as $M = AS$, where A is the gain matrix from the forward model.

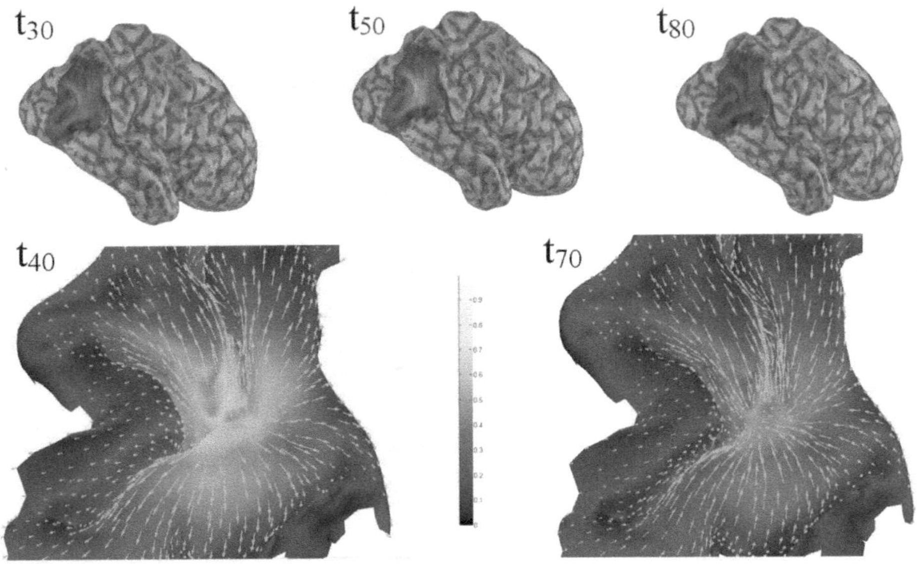

Fig. 2. Simulating local emergence and waning of brain activity with resulting flow. Top row illustrates the progressive emergence followed by fading of a 33 cm^2 region in the posterior medio-temporal brain area. The entire process unfolds within 100 time samples. Bottom row displays the corresponding distributions of vector flow; initially diverging from (left) then converging to (right) the center of the activation zone.

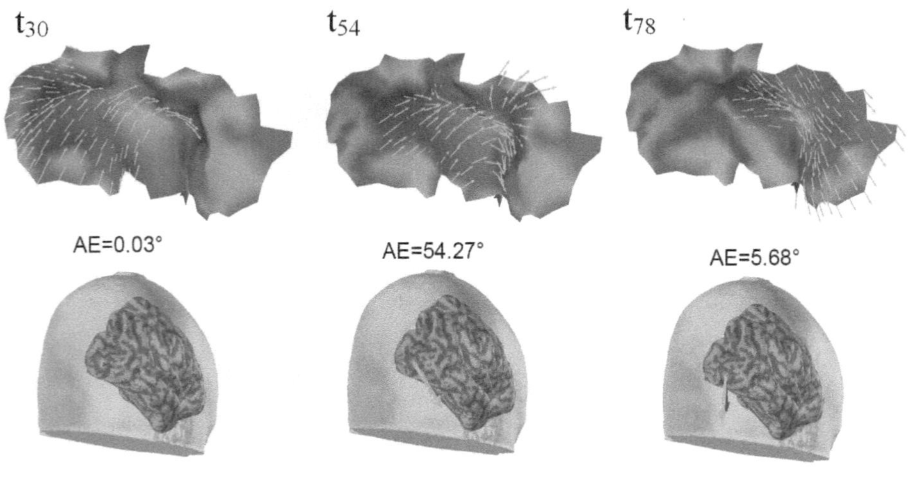

Fig. 3. Simulation of brain activation propagating at the surface of the cortex. Top row, from left to right: displacement field of an activation patch is translating along a predefined path during 100 steps of time. Bottom row: the mean vector field and true displacement are shown in green and blue, respectively, with indication of instantaneous angular error. For clarity purposes, only one brain hemisphere is shown within the scalp surface.

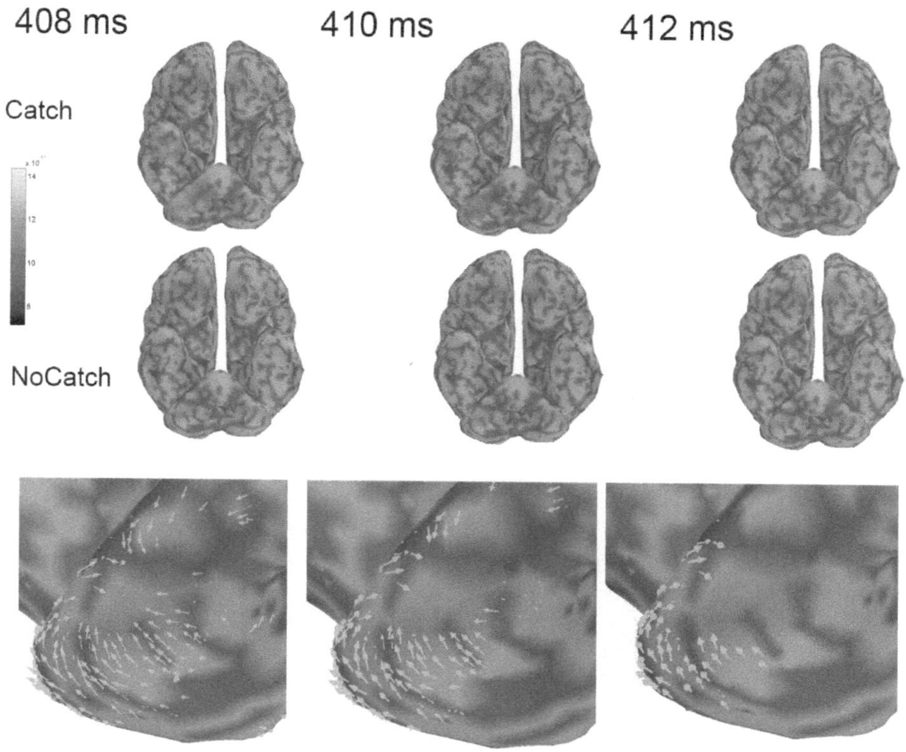

Fig. 4. MEG Activities in the *catch* (top) and *no-catch* (middle) experimental conditions. The corresponding velocity field in the catch condition is shown in green (bottom). The shrinking of activities specific to the *catch* condition is clearly elucidated by the convergent structure of the flow.

Electromagnetic brain mapping consists of the estimation of MEG/EEG sources S from scalp measures M. However, this inverse problem is underdetermined since there are far more possible cortical sources than sensors. s is typically on the order of a few hundreds while p amounts to about 10000 elemental sources constrained onto the surface of the cortical manifold, which was extracted from MRI image sequences [1]. Inverse modelling can therefore be approached as in many other image reconstruction applications, i.e. though the introduction of priors in addition to data. Here we used a weighted-minimum norm estimate (WMNE) of source amplitudes and its implementation in the BrainStorm software [2].

4.2 Evaluation on Experimental Data

We applied optical flow computation to magnetic evoked-fields in a ball-catching paradigm [21]. The subjects had to catch a free-falling tennis ball which fall was initiated at time $t = 0$ ms. The second experimental condition ('NoCatch') consisted for the subject in only looking at the ball falling without catching it.

Fig. 4 shows a rapid decrease of cerebellar activity around 40 ms after the ball hits the subject's hand (371 $\pm$ 7 ms). We can notice the convergent and radial structure of the flow. This phenomenon was not found in the NoCatch condition where no motor program was required at the time of ball-impact.

5 Conclusion

This article introduced an extension of computational approaches to optical flow on non-flat domains. The framework of Riemannian geometry allows to adapt a variational formulation for this ill-posed problem and to derive evaluation tools. We suggest new applications of the quantization of the displacement field to spatiotemporal data in MEG and EEG and to the question of neural information directionality. Results from simulations indicate the flow has satisfactory behavior in terms of spatial structure and angular errors for the application in question. Encouraging preliminary results have been presented from real experimental data. Ongoing developments consist in relating measures from this computational approach to their physiological origins. Particularly we intend to use these new indices for data mining and visualization, which could offer local and global descriptors of the brain dynamic.

Acknowledgements. This project is supported by the French Ministry of Research (ACI New Applications of Mathematics). Thanks to Patrice Senot (Laboratoire de Physiologie de la Perception et de l'Action, Collège de France & CNRS, Paris) for providing the data. Thanks to Stéphane Dellacherie (Commissariat à l'Énergie Atomique) for discussions about mathematical formulation.

References

[1] `http://brainvisa.info/`
[2] `http://neuroimage.usc.edu/brainstorm`
[3] Allaire, G.: Analyse numérique et optimisation. Editions de l'Ecole Polytechnique, first edn. (2005)
[4] Aubert, G., Deriche, R., Kornprobst, P.: Computing optical flow via variational techniques. SIAM Journal of Applied Mathematics 60(1), 156–182 (1999)
[5] Baillet, S., Mosher, J.C., Leahy R.M.: Electromagnetic brain mapping. IEEE Signal Processing Magazine (November 2001)
[6] Barron, J.L., Fleet, D.J., Beauchemin, S.S.: Performance of optical flow techniques. International Journal of Computer Vision 12, 43–77 (1994)
[7] Barron, J.L., Liptay, A.: Measuring 3-d plant growth using optical flow. Bioimaging 5, 82–86 (1997)
[8] Beauchemin, S.S., Barron, J.L.: The computation of optical flow. ACM Computing Surveys 27(3), 433–467 (1995)
[9] Corpetti, T., Heitz, D., Arroyo, G., Mémin, E., Santa-Cruz, A.: Fluid experimental flow estimation based on an optical-flow scheme. Experiments in fluids 40(1), 80–97 (2006)

[10] Do Carmo, M.P.: Riemannian Geometry. Birkhäuser (1993)
[11] Druet, O., Hebey, E., Robert, F.: Blow-up theory for elliptic PDEs in Riemannian geometry, chapter Background Material, pp. 1–12. Princeton University Press, Princeton, N.J (2004)
[12] Horn, B.K.P., Schunck, B.G.: Determining optical flow. Artificial Intelligence 17, 185–204 (1981)
[13] Inouye, T., Shinosaki, K., Toi, S., Matsumoto, Y., Hosaka, N.: Potential flow of alpha- activity in the human electroencephalogram. Neurosci Lett. 187, 29–32 (1995)
[14] Lehmann, D.: Quantitative and Topological EEG and MEG Analysis. In: Witte, H.H., Zwiener, U., Schack, B., Doering, A. (eds.) chapter From EEG waves to brain maps and to microstates of conscious mentation. Proceedings, Third Hans Berger Symposium, Jena 1996. Druckhaus Maier, Jena and Erlangen, Germany (1997), pp. 139–149 (1997)
[15] Liu, H., Hong, T., Herman, M., Camus, T., Chellapa, R.: Accuracy vs. efficiency trade-off in optical flow algorithms. Comput. Vision Image Understand 72, 271–286 (1998)
[16] Nagel, H.-H.: On the estimation of optical flow: relations between different approaches and some new results. Artificial Intelligence 33, 299–324 (1987)
[17] Pascual-Marqui, R.D., Michel, C.M., Lehmann, D.: Segmentation of brain electrical activity into microstates: Model estimation and validation. IEEE Trans. Biomed. Eng. 42, 658–665 (1995)
[18] Remond, A., Renault, B.: The theory of electrographic objects. Rev Electroencephalogr Neurophysiol Clin. 2(3), 241–256 (1972)
[19] Rossmanith, J.A., Bale, D.S., LeVeque, R.J.: A wave propagation algorithm for hyperbolic systems on curved manifolds. J. Comput. Phys. 199, 631–662 (2004)
[20] Schnörr, C.: Determining optical flow for irregular domains by minimizing quadratic functionals of a certain class. Int. J. Computer Vision 6(1), 25–38 (1991)
[21] Senot, P., Zago, M., Lacquaniti, F., McIntyre, J.: Anticipating the effects of gravity when intercepting moving objects: Differentiating up and down based on nonvisual cues. J Neurophysiol 94, 4471–4480 (2005)
[22] Strik, W.K., Chiaramonti, R., Muscas, G.C., Paganini, M., Mueller, T.J., Fallgatter, A.J., Versari, A., Zappoli, R.: Decreased eeg microstate duration and anteriorisation of the brain fields in mild and moderate dementia of the alzheimer type. Psychiatry Res., 75, 183–191 (1997)
[23] Van Essen, D.C., Drury, H.A., Joshi, S., Miller, M.I.: Functional and structural mapping of human cerebral cortex: Solutions are in the surfaces. Proc Natl. Acad. Sci. USA 95, 788–795 (1998)
[24] Wackermann, J., Lehmann, D., Michel, C.M., Strik, W.K.: Adaptive segmentation of spontaneous eeg map series into spatially defined microstates. Int J Psychophysiol., 14(3), 269–283 (1993)
[25] Weickert, J., Schnörr, C.: A theoretical framework for convex regularizers in pde-based computation of image motion. International Journal of Computer Vision 45(3), 245–264 (2001)

High Level Group Analysis of FMRI Data Based on Dirichlet Process Mixture Models

Bertrand Thirion[1], Alan Tucholka[2], Merlin Keller[1], Philippe Pinel[3], Alexis Roche[2], Jean-François Mangin[2], and Jean-Baptiste Poline[2]

[1] INRIA Futurs, Neurospin
bertrand.thirion@inria.fr
[2] CEA, DSV, I^{2}BM, Neurospin
[3] Unité INSERM 562 "Neuroimagerie Cognitive"
CEA Saclay, Bâtiment 145, 91191 Gif-sur-Yvette cedex, France

Abstract. Inferring the position of functionally active regions from a multi-subject fMRI dataset involves the comparison of the individual data and the inference of a common activity model. While voxel-based analyzes, e.g. Random Effect statistics, are widely used, they do not model each individual activation pattern. Here, we develop a new procedure that extracts structures individually and compares them at the group level. For inference about spatial locations of interest, a Dirichlet Process Mixture Model is used. Finally, inter-subject correspondences are computed with Bayesian Network models. We show the power of the technique on both simulated and real datasets and compare it with standard inference techniques.

1 Introduction

Functional neuroimaging aims at finding brain regions specifically involved in the performance of cognitive tasks. In particular, functional MRI (fMRI) is based on the detection of task-related Blood Oxygen-Level Dependent (BOLD) effect in the brain. Inference about putative regions of activity is generally based on several subjects (~10-15 subjects typically), and the current standard procedure consists in detecting voxels for which the average task-related BOLD signal increase is significant across subjects (Random/Mixed Effects analyzes, R/MFX)[2]. Such voxel-based inference schemes require the images to be warped to a common space, which is usually performed by coregistration of the anatomical, then functional data with a template image [1], generally the average T1 image provided by the Montreal Neurological Institute (MNI).

Traditional voxel-based inference suffers from several shortcomings. On the one hand, BOLD signal is not a quantitative measure of brain activity, i.e. the measured signals are uncalibrated, and it is unclear how signals acquired across subjects should be scaled. On the other hand, a given voxel does not necessarily represent the same anatomical and/or functional areas across subjects; mis-registrations remain after spatial normalization of the datasets. The magnitude of such local shifts is probably as far as 10 mm in many brain regions (this

N. Karssemeijer and B. Lelieveldt (Eds.): IPMI 2007, LNCS 4584, pp. 482–494, 2007.
© Springer-Verlag Berlin Heidelberg 2007

can be observed for regions like the the motor cortex or the visual areas [15,14] or the position of anatomical landmarks [3,6,8]). Inference is also hampered by the small number of subjects, and by unrealistic hypotheses used in some statistical models (e.g. modelling the data as a smooth random field [18]).

To deal with these issues, it has been proposed [4,5,15,17,7] to perform group analysis at a higher level than mere voxel-based BOLD signal. These structural approaches are motivated by several reasons: first, regional units might better represent functional brain modules than voxels ; second high-level models may be less sensitive to mis-registrations than voxel-based approaches ; third, one can assess the significance of a region by testing other features than the positivity of the average cross-subject signal. However, such approaches have to address a number of challenges:

- The first one is to find adequate descriptors of the individual data/structures of interest. Importantly, there is no consensus on this point. Scale-space blobs [4], large supra-threshold clusters [5,13], local maxima of the functional maps [16], anatomo-functional parcellations [15], watersheds [17] have been proposed. In this work we propose a perhaps more intuitive approach : we describe the maps through their blobs, i.e. the connected regions comprised between their critical points.
- Any description procedure will unavoidably yield false detections. In order to separate structures of interest from noise, it is essential to have some validity index about the selected structures. This point has certainly been neglected in previous contributions, and we address it more thoroughly in this work, where we associate the structurally defined ROIs with confidence levels.
- Structures of interest extracted at the subject-level should be compared across subjects. This is conceptually the most important part, since it consists in finding cross-subjects homologies at a high level of description. In this work, we improve the approach of [17] by using Bayesian Networks.
- Finally, one needs to have some ways to perform group inference, i.e. to make clear statements about brain regions involved in the task under consideration, with an explicit specificity control. This is not simple in high-level settings, since assessing the significance of a structure of interest across subjects is much more complex than testing the sign of an effect or the size of a region, using e.g. permutation techniques [5,9]. In this work, we rely on a Bayesian perspective : we assign to each region in each subject a posterior probability of being truly activated given its signal and position.

In the present work, we address the aforementioned issues in a sequential fashion, resulting in a pipeline of data processing. The different steps are described in Section 2, and some experiments on synthetic and real benchmark datasets in Section 3. In particular we illustrate the improvement in terms of sensitivity and reliability of fMRI group analyzes. Reliability is assessed by Jackknife subsampling in a population of 130 subjects, and we show that the results of the proposed method are less dependent on the particular subgroup of subjects under study than standard voxel-based tests. Technical issues and implications for neuroimaging studies are discussed in Section 4.

2 Materials and Methods

2.1 Notations

Let us assume that a group of S subjects take part in an fMRI acquisition protocol while they undergo a certain cognitive experiment. After some standard pre-processing (distortion correction, correction of differences in slice timing, motion correction, normalization), the dataset of each subject is analyzed in the General Linear Model (GLM) framework: Let c be a linear combination of the experimental conditions (termed a functional contrast) that is of particular interest. A certain statistic ϕ^s can be computed in each subject $s \in \{1, .., S\}$ to assess the presence of a positive effect in each voxel of the dataset. $(v \rightarrow \phi^s(v))$ is called a functional map, and is the basic input of our group analysis method, whose main steps are described in Fig. 1.

2.2 High-Level Descriptions of Individual Maps

The ϕ^s images are subject to a structural and a probabilistic analysis procedure.

Structural modelling. The structural model considers the critical points, i.e. the maxima, minima and saddle points of ϕ^s. ROIs are defined as blobs, i.e. sets of connected voxels that are comprised between two critical points. Let $(a_j^s)_{j=1..I(s)}$ be the corresponding regions for subject s. The smallest ROIs (less than e.g. 5 voxels) are merged into the region that includes them. This set of regions is naturally endowed with a tree structure, which describes the inclusion relationships between regions. The regions that correspond to maxima of the map are the leaves of the tree, while the saddle regions are branches. Each root of the tree corresponds to a connected supra-threshold region in the image. This graphical structure is used in order to define inter-subject correspondences (see Sec. 2.4). For each region a_j^s, let (t_j^s) be the spatial coordinates of the center of the areas in the subtree rooted in a_j^s. Only the regions above some threshold θ are considered. This is necessary, since low (close to 0) level sets of the maps are likely to represent noise only, thus having a non-informative structure. However, it is desirable to mitigate the impact of the hard threshold θ by endowing the regions with a significance value that represents the signal level in the ROI.

Probabilistic modelling. In order to obtain intra-subject estimates of the regions significance, the images ϕ^s are subject to mixture modeling (MM) with a Gamma-Gaussian MM, where the Gaussian mode represents the inactive mode, while the positive and negative Gamma modes represent positively and negatively activated voxels of the dataset. This model endows each voxel with a likelihood under the positive, null and negative hypotheses (which we denote H_1, H_0 and H_{-1}), $p(\phi^s(v)|H_i)$, for $i \in \{-1, 0, 1\}$, and with the corresponding posterior. The Gamma-Gaussian MM is estimated using an EM algorithm.

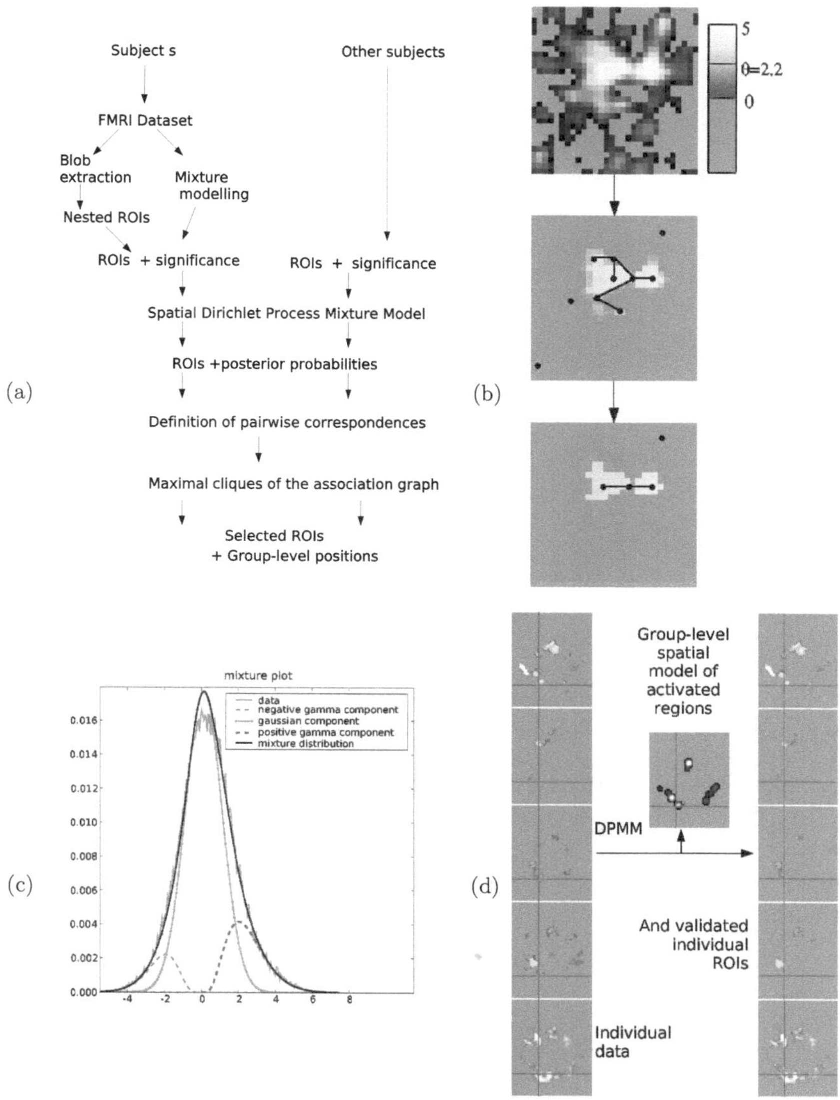

Fig. 1. Description of our method for structural analysis of group data. (a) Flowchart that represents the main steps of the method: intra-subject structural and statistical modeling, inter-subject spatial modeling, computation of correspondence probabilities and creation of region cliques. (b) The first step consists in a structural modeling, which finds the critical points of the functional image, and segments the blobs separated by the critical points. The smallest regions are merged into their parent regions. (c) In parallel, each dataset is subject to mixture modeling, in order to characterize the positively/negatively or non-activated regions of the dataset, given the values of each map ϕ_s. (d) The spatial model, a Dirichlet Process Mixture Model, defines the regions where the most reliable maxima are found across subjects, and validates the individual regions with high probability of being a true positive.

Putting things together. The voxel-based posterior probability of $(H_i), i \in \{0,1\}$[1] is pulled to the region level so that $p(H_1(a_j^s)|\phi^s) = min_{v \in a_j^s} p(H_1|\phi^s(v))$.

2.3 A Dirichlet Process Model for Spatial Data

The next step consists in validating the ROIs at the group level; the idea is to retain only spatially clustered regions, i.e. to improve the p-values $p(H_i(a_j^s)), i \in \{0,1\}$ based on spatial information. Formally, this analysis is performed in a Bayesian setting:

$$p(H_i(a_j^s)|t_j^s, \phi^s) = \frac{p(t_j^s|H_i(a_j^s), \phi^s)p(H_i(a_j^s)|\phi^s)}{p(t_j^s|\phi^s)} \tag{1}$$

where $p(t_j^s|\phi^s) = \sum_i p(t_j^s|H_i(a_j^s), \phi^s)p(H_i(a_j^s)|\phi^s)$. Moreover, we further assume the conditional independence of the positions of ROIs and of their significance given a certain hypothesis on these ROIs $p(t_j^s|H_i(a_j^s), \phi^s) = p(t_j^s|H_i(a_j^s))$. In order to estimate the spatial densities $p(t_j^s|H_i(a_j^s))$ we rely on two models:

- under H_0, the selected ROIs are distributed uniformly across the brain, so that $p(t_j^s|H_0(a_j^s)) = 1/|\Omega|$, where Ω is the brain volume.
- under H_1, the distribution $p(t_j^s|H_1(a_j^s))$ is also unknown, but is expected to be clustered in some regions of the brain. To model this density, we use a Gaussian Mixture Model with an unspecified number of components implemented through a Dirichlet Process Mixture Model (DPMM).

A Dirichlet Process $DP(\alpha, G)$ with a concentration parameter $\alpha > 0$ and a base measure G can be used as a nonparametric prior distribution on mixing proportion parameters in a mixture model when the number of components is unknown a priori [10,12]. The generative process for a mixture of Gaussian distributions with component means μ_k and DP prior $DP(\alpha, G)$ can be written

$$\begin{aligned} \pi|\alpha &\sim \text{Stick}(\alpha), \\ z_j|\pi &\sim \pi, \\ (\mu_k)_{k=1}^{\infty}|G &\sim G, \\ t_j^s|z_j^s, (\mu_k)_{k=1}^{\infty}, \sigma^2 &\sim \mathcal{N}(\mu_{z_j^s}, \sigma^2\mathbb{I}), \end{aligned} \tag{2}$$

where z_j^s is the variable that denotes the cluster with which a_j is associated. The base measure G is uniform over the brain volume, and the second-level densities are normal densities with fixed covariance, $\sigma^2\mathbb{I}$. The estimation of such models can be performed fairly easily using MCMC techniques. Gibbs sampling is carried out by integrating out all the random variables except z_j^s (collapsed Gibbs sampling). The algorithm iteratively samples z_j^s from

$$p(z_j^s = k|t_j^s, z_{-j}, \alpha) \propto p(t_j^s|t^{-s}, z_{-j}, z_j^s = k)p(z_j^s = k|z_{-j}, \alpha), \tag{3}$$

[1] Due to the thresholding above $\theta > 0$, the posterior probabilities $p(H_{-1}|\phi^s(v))$ of H_{-1} are systematically null.

where z_{-j} represents the values of z for the ROIs other than a_j^s and t^{-s} represents all the ROI positions in subjects other than s. The first term of Eq. (3) simply corresponds to a 3D Gaussian cluster model

$$p(t_j^s|t^{-s}, z_{-j}, z_j^s = k) = \mathcal{N}(t_j^s; \mu_k, \sigma^2\mathbb{I}) \tag{4}$$

or a constant if the component is empty. The second term comes from the partition structure of the Dirichlet process:

$$p(z_j^s = k|z_{-j}, \alpha) = \begin{cases} \frac{n_k^{-s}}{\alpha+N^{-s}} \text{ if } n_k^{-s} > 0, \\ \frac{\alpha}{\alpha+N^{-s}} \text{ otherwise,} \end{cases} \tag{5}$$

where n_k^{-s} is the number of instance of $z = k$ for all regions in subjects other than s and $N^{-s} = \sum_k n_k^{-s}$; $n_k^{-s} > 0$ amounts to considering that k is a previously seen component; k is unvisited otherwise. In our setting, we include an alternative case, in which the region a_j^s is false positive. The sampling scheme is thus

$$p(H_0(a_j^s)|t_j^s, \phi^s) = \frac{1}{c}\frac{1}{|\Omega|}p(H_0(a_j^s)|\phi^s), \tag{6}$$

$$p(H_1(a_j^s), z_j = k|t_j^s, z_{-j}, \alpha, \phi^s) = \frac{1}{c}\begin{cases} \frac{\alpha}{\alpha+N^{-s}}\frac{1}{|\Omega|}p(H_1(a_j^s)|\phi^s) \text{ if } n_k^{-s} = 0, \\ \frac{n_k^{-s}}{\alpha+N^{-s}}\mathcal{N}(t_j^s; \mu_k, \sigma^2\mathbb{I})p(H_1(a_j^s)|\phi^s) \end{cases} \tag{7}$$

otherwise,

where c is the normalizing constant. The parameters μ_k are updated naturally according to the current value of z_j. Once the Markov chain has run for long enough, the samples of the chain will be samples from the true posterior $p(H_i(a_j^s), z_j^s = k|t_j^s, z_{-j}, \alpha, \phi^s)$, and the approximate distribution of $p(H_i(a_j^s)|t_j^s, z_{-j}, \alpha, \phi^s)$ is given by averaging over the samples. Inference proceeds by selecting the regions a_j^s for which $p(H_1(a_j^s)|t_j^s, z_{-j}, \alpha, \phi^s)$ is above some threshold q. We found that 1000 iterations over all the ROIs of all subjects are sufficient to achieve a reliable estimate of the posterior.

In summary, the spatial model used here yields the posterior probabilities of the target regions being truly activated regions, given that truly activated regions should be clustered spatially across subjects. This procedure thus infers what are the true regions of activity among all the candidate regions, in each subject. In addition, the algorithm also yields the spatial likelihood of the position of activated regions $p(t|H_1)$, which is a second level of inference of the method. Next, we try to obtain a more explicit relationship between individual ROIs and to derive group-level clusters.

2.4 Finding Cross-Subject Correspondences in Structured Data

Although the DPMM yields a clustering of the individual regions through the z_j^s variables, the inter-subject correspondence implied by this model may not be very reliable, due to the relative simplicity of the Gaussian generative model.

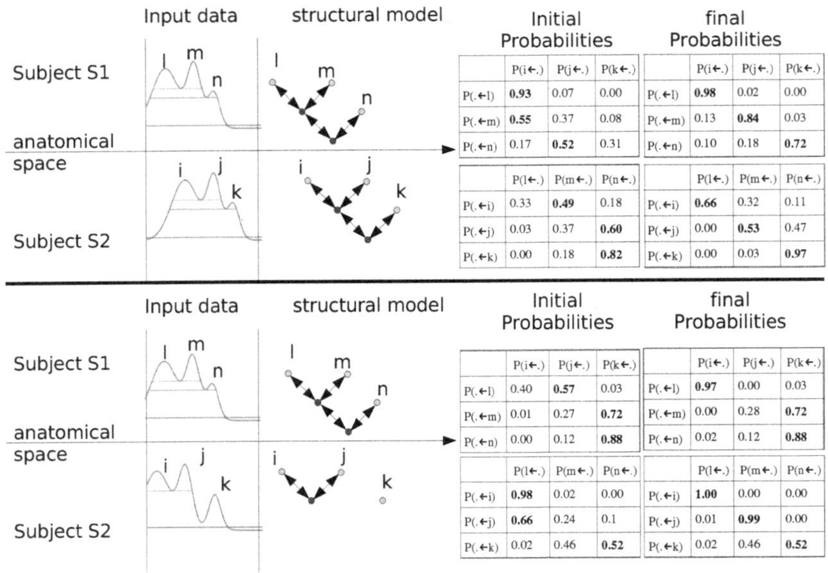

Fig. 2. Illustration of the probabilistic correspondence computation algorithm on a toy (1D) example: Recall that the input data corresponds to a synthetic model of the level sets of two activation maps of two subjects. The maps maxima are called (l, m, n) and (i, j, k) in the two subjects. (Top) the underlying structure is the same in the two subjects, but there is a translation, so that the trivial association scheme (see Eq. (9)) provides unreliable initial probabilities. After convergence of the probabilities through the BN model (see Eq. (8)), the probabilities are closer to the ground truth (diagonal terms get higher values). (Bottom) the underlying structure is different in the two subjects. Nevertheless, the algorithm considerably improves the correspondences.

In order to improve it, it is useful to take into account the topology of the individual patterns, which is coded in the graphical model of the nested level sets model defined in Sec. 2.2. Recall that these nested ROIs in each subjects are embedded in a *forest* (i.e. multiple trees) graphical model. Only the *leaves* of the forest will be included in the association model, since they represent maxima, i.e. putative foci of activity. Other (*saddle*, see section 2.2) regions are only used in order to code the large-scale structure of the functional activity pattern in the data. Probabilistic associations are searched for each pair of subjects. Given a reference subject s_1 and a target subject s_2, let $p(a_i^{s_2} \leftarrow a_j^{s_1})$ be the probability that region a_j in subject s_1 is associated with region a_i in subject s_2; let $a_{f(j)}^{s_1}$ be the *father* of $a_j^{s_1}$ in the graphical sense. The global association model is given by a Bayesian Network (BN) defined by the conditional probabilities:

$$p(a_k^{s_2} \leftarrow a_j^{s_1} | (a_l^{s_2} \leftarrow a_{f(j)}^{s_1})) \propto \delta_{father(a_k^{s_2})=a_l^{s_2}} \mathcal{K}_\sigma (t_j^{s_1} - t_k^{s_2} - (t_{f(j)}^{s_1} - t_l^{s_2})) \quad (8)$$

Here $\mathcal{K}_\sigma$ is a standard RBF kernel with parameter σ. The second term in Eq. (8) is crucial, since it implies that the children of two nodes in subjects s_1 and s_2 with a similar relative position will have a stronger probability of association, which is our core intuition. The associations are initialized at the leaf level as

$$p(a_i^{s_2} \leftarrow a_j^{s_1}) \propto \exp\left(-\frac{\|t_i^{s_2} - t_j^{s_1}\|^2}{2\sigma^2}\right) \tag{9}$$

The association probabilities are updated using a belief propagation (BP) algorithm [11]. This procedure is known to converge given that all the graphs involved in the model are trees. An interpretation and examples of this procedure are shown in Fig. 2.

2.5 Extracting Homologous Regions Across Subjects

Once all the probabilities of pairwise associations between individual ROIs are arranged in a common, asymmetric belief matrix B, it is possible to extract from it maximal cliques of strongly associated regions, using e.g. replicator dynamics. This point has been developed in [17], thus we do not detail it. The only difference is that we use only one pass of the clique extraction procedure.

Finally, all the cliques that contain maxima from at least ν subjects over S are retained. This method provides us with across subjects correspondences between activated regions. It does not require that all subjects are represented for a given activated region, and therefore is able to account for some inter-individual differences. In order to make group maps, we assume that the positions of the maxima t_j^s within each clique are normally distributed, and thus represent the cliques through their 95% confidence regions (CR) in the common (MNI) space.

The method requires few prior parameters:

- the initial threshold of activity maps θ is chosen to correspond to a p-value of 0.01 uncorrected for multiple comparisons. Note that this is a rather lenient choice. Importantly, the impact of this choice is mitigated by the fact that the ROIs are given a p-value which is related to their CNR (see section 2.2).
- $\alpha > 0$ is the parameter of the DPMM which controls the cluster creation process. $\alpha = 0.5$ is a standard choice (see [12] for a Bayesian choice of α).
- q controls the posterior significance of the regions. We choose $q = 0.5$.
- A spatial variability parameter σ is used in several parts of this work; we set systematically $\sigma = 10mm$ which is a reasonable estimation of inter-subject variability in fMRI group data analysis.
- ν is important since it explicitly controls the reproducibility of a region across subjects. For instance $\nu = \frac{S}{3}$ (our choice) yields regions that can be expected to be found in one third of the subjects.

Note that some of these parameters $(\theta, \alpha, \sigma, q)$ might be changed reasonably without creating inconsistencies, while ν has a more critical impact. The computation time of the method, implemented with a C/Python code based on nipy environment (http://projects.scipy.org/neuroimaging/ni/), is a couple of minutes minute for a dataset of 10 subjects on 3GHz Pentium IV PC running linux.

3 Simulations and Results

3.1 Cluster-Level ROC Curves Obtained on Synthetic Data

The algorithm was tested on synthetic datasets, which consisted in filtered noise, with activation added to the correlated noise. Ten distant regions are added with some signal in order to model spatially coherent activity in the group of subjects. The size of the activated regions varied from 20 to 50 voxels. According to the simulation, their mean position (center of mass) was jittered with isotropic normal shifts of 0, 1 or 2 voxels, which represents 0, 5.2 and 10.4mm standard deviation. The activation magnitudes were chosen to correspond to a mean CNR of either $-10dB$ or $-6dB$ in each dataset, which corresponds to a realistic CNR in fMRI datasets. In order to model inter-subject differences in the CNR, we let this value vary across subjects in the ranges [-18dB -6dB] and [-11 -3dB].

The CR maps, as well as the RFX maps computed on these datasets, are submitted to Receiver Operating Characteristic (ROC) Analysis. However, false or true positives are not computed at the voxel level, which does not really make sense, but at the cluster level (clusters comprise 10 voxels or more): each cluster whose centre falls less than 10mm apart from a simulated activity locus is counted as true, while the other clusters are counted as false positives. True and false positive clusters were computed while the q parameter (CR) or the threshold (RFX) is varied, resulting in a (sensitivity, specificity) plot (see Fig. 3(a)). Results were averaged over $n = 100$ repetitions of the simulation.

This shows that at different CNR and jitter levels, the specificity/sensitivity compromise is much more favorable with our method than with standard RFX analyzes techniques. We have also tested the robustness of the method with respect to mis-specification of first-level p-values, by resampling the values to make them have the histograms of unrelated datasets. This results in a mismatch between the empirical histogram and the true significance levels, hence biased first-level p-values. In that case, the performance of the proposed method decreases, but it remains similar to the RFX performance (see Fig. 3(b)).

3.2 Real fMRI Dataset

We used an event-related fMRI paradigm that comprised ten experimental conditions. This is described in more details in [17]. Among other tasks, the subjects had to perform subtractions, which resulted in maps of the computation activity, which we study here. 130 right-handed subjects participated in the study. Detailed acquisition parameters can be found in [17].

FMRI data pre-processing and statistical analysis were performed using the SPM2 software (www.fil.ucl.ac.uk, [2]). In particular, spatial normalization was performed using default parameters (non-rigid, low frequency deformation with 8*8*7 basis functions [1]); the normalized images were checked in all the subjects to prevent any gross mistake in the image coregistration.

For the sake of place, we limit ourself to a brief comparison of our method with a Mixed Effects analysis thresholded at the cluster level (CMFX, $p < 0.05$,

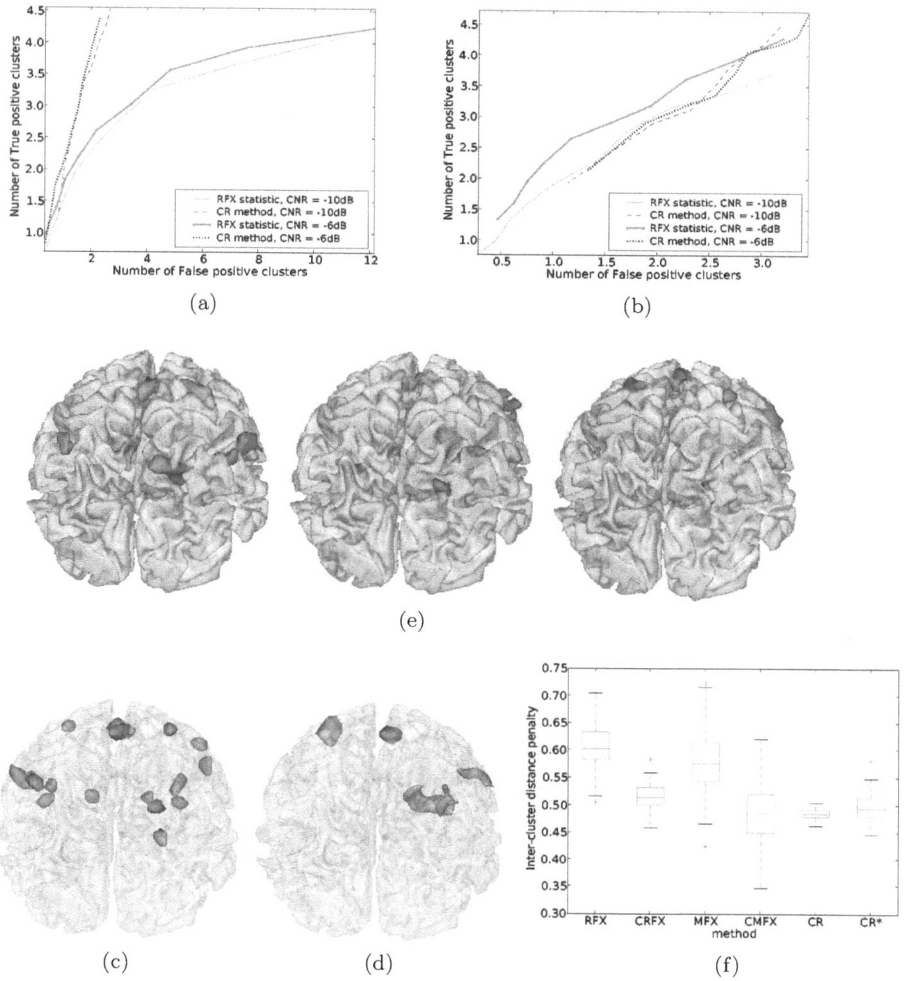

Fig. 3. (a) Cluster-level ROC curves for both RFX and our group analysis procedure. The number of detected regions (among 10 targets) is plotted against the number of false positive detections (at the cluster level) for our definition of the regions of activity at the group level, compared with traditional RFX inference. Simulated activated regions are jittered of 2 voxels in each direction. (b) The same, but based on the histogram of unrelated datasets (see main text). (c-e) Analysis of a particular group of 10 subjects: (c) confidence regions found with our method (17 regions) ; (d) regions found with a Mixed-Effects test, thresholded at the cluster level ($p < 0.05$ corrected, 5 regions) (e) Final significant regions of activity in three subjects of the datasets. (f) Inter-cluster distance penalty computed for 13 disjoint random samples of 10 subjects, and 6 different group analyzes techniques: Random Effects (RFX), cluster-level RFX (CRFX), Mixed Effects (MFX), cluster-level Mixed Effects (CMFX), our estimation of regions where activity occurs at the group level (CR), and the regions obtained with the method in [17] (CR*). CR, CR* and CMFX get the lowest penalty, which corresponds to an average inter-cluster distance of 6mm.

corrected) on a subset of 10 randomly chosen subjects. The results are given in Fig. 3(c,d) respectively. The proposed method extracts 17 regions of activity, while the CMFX extracts 5 supra-threshold clusters; the reason is that *i)* the CMFX merges several regions that are distinguished with our technique *ii)* some small activated clusters detected with our method are not significant for the CMFX test. Additionally, we present 3 individual maps in Fig. 3(e), in order to suggest that the results are not limited to group maps, but include individual patterns. Corresponding regions have the same color.

3.3 Assessment of the Reproducibility

Taking advantage of the large cohort, we controlled the reliability of the results obtained in small groups of subjects by assessing the reproducibility of the resulting regions across $R = 10$ disjoint groups of 13 subjects. We consider group-level binary maps obtained with different inference procedures, extract the clusters of size greater than $\eta = 10$ voxels and compute the following penalty, which measures how far supra-threshold clusters are from each other across groups:

$$\Psi = \frac{1}{R(R-1)} \sum_{r=1}^{R} \sum_{s \in \{1,..,R\}-\{r\}} \frac{1}{I(r)} \sum_{i=1}^{I(r)} min_{j \in \{1,..,I(s)\}} \psi(\|t_i^r - t_j^s\|), \qquad (10)$$

where (t_i^r) are the positions of the cluster centers, and $\psi(x) = 1 - \exp\left(-\frac{x^2}{2\sigma^2}\right)$. We do this for five statistics: voxel-based Random Effects, thresholded at $p < 0.001$, uncorrected (RFX), cluster-level RFX, where the map is thresholded at the $p < 0.01$,uncorrected level, then at the $p < 0.05$, corrected, cluster-level (CRFX), the same procedures and thresholds with Mixed-Effects models (MFX/CMFX), the group-level confidence regions obtained with our procedure and the procedure presented in [17] (CR/CR*). All the significance levels are obtained using permutation techniques, so that the tests can be considered as exact [9]. The results are given in Fig. 3(f). It turns out that the proposed method gets the lowest penalty in average, similar to CR* and CMFX, and moreover with less variability than the other methods. This proves its reliability for group studies. Note that the good results of CMFX are mitigated by the fact that this method only detects large clusters (see Fig. 3(d)).

4 Discussion

This paper presents three novelties in the field of group analysis of fMRI data: the first one consists in a conceptually simple, but useful framework for the structural description of individual maps, where the map is partitioned into a nested structure, which codes the topology of the activation patterns. The second one is the use of DPMM to model the positions of activated regions across subjects; the new features of this technique are that *i)* it does not require a pre-definition of the number or extent of putative regions of activity in the population *ii)* it can incorporate prior information on the significance of the regions, which was not available in previous contributions. Finally, we have introduced an improved correspondence estimation algorithm, which constrains the inter-subject pairings by the global organization of the activation patterns. These contributions improve previous work on structural modelling of group fMRI data [17], and allow a statistical assessment of the individual and group-level target regions.

The DPMM is used here in a quite basic setting, which certainly benefits the robustness of the method. Other use of the DPMM for fMRI data has been proposed in [7], with more complex hierarchical models, but in that case, the DPMM was used to model the signal itself, not a high-level representation of it. Our approach is thus computationally more efficient; moreover, low-level differences, such as those related to CNR, have less impact on the group model.

Our method is quite effective on synthetic datasets, especially when the activation position is jittered. Moreover, the method is quite robust to deviation from its underlying hypotheses (see Fig. 3(f)) ; it benefits the reliability of group analyses in terms of activation positions, with respect to the inter-group variability (see section 3.3). Although the present work was carried out using standard normalization procedures, thus MNI coordinates, it is worthwhile to note that these coordinates do not play any particular role, so that more adapted spatial coordinate systems (e.g. surface-based) are perfectly usable. This is an important matter for future developments. Lastly, our approach opens the way to intrinsic ROI-based group analysis, population comparison, which might be much more relevant than the current use of defining spheres in the MNI/Talairach space.

References

1. Ashburner, J., Friston, K.J.: Nonlinear Spatial Normalization Using Basis Functions. Hum. Brain Mapp. 7(4), 254–266 (1999)
2. Ashburner, J., Friston, K.J., Penny, W. (eds.): Human Brain Function, 2nd edn. Academic Press, San Diego (2004)
3. Collins, D.L., Le G., G., Evans, A.C.: Non-linear Cerebral Registration with Sulcal Constraints. In: Wells, W.M., Colchester, A.C.F., Delp, S.L. (eds.) MICCAI 1998. LNCS, vol. 1496, pp. 974–984. Springer, Heidelberg (1998)
4. Coulon, O., Mangin, J.-F., et al.: Structural Group Analysis of Functional Activation Maps. Neuroimage 11, 767–782 (2000)
5. Hayasaka, S., Nichols, T.E.: Validating Cluster Size Inference: Random Field and Permutation Methods. NeuroImage 20(4), 2343–2356 (2003)
6. Hellier, P., Barillot, C., et al.: Retrospective Evaluation of Intersubject Brain Registration. IEEE Trans. Med. Imag., 22(9), 1120–1130 (2003)
7. Kim, S., Smyth, P.: Hierarchical Dirichlet Processes with Random Effects. In: Advances in Neural Information Processing Systems, Vancouver (2006)
8. Mangin, J.-F., Rivière, D., et al.: Object-based Morphometry of the Cerebral Cortex. IEEE Trans. Med. Imag., 23(8), 968–982 (2004)
9. Mériaux, S., Roche, A., et al.: Combined Permutation Test and Mixed-effect Model for Group Average Analysis in fMRI. Hum. Brain Mapp., 27(5), 402–410 (2006)
10. Neal, R.M.: Markov Chain Sampling Methods for Dirichlet Process Mixture Models. Journal of Computational and Graphical Statistics 9(2), 249–265 (2000)

11. Pearl, J.: Probabilistic Reasoning in Intelligent Systems: Networks of Plausible Inference, 2nd edn. Morgan Kaufmann Publishers, Inc, San Francisco (1988)
12. Rasmussen, C.E.: The Infinite Gaussian Mixture Model. In. Advances in Neural Information Processing Systems 12, 554–560 (2000)
13. Simon, O., Kherif, F., et al.: Automatized Clustering of Human Parietofrontal Networks. NeuroImage 11, 1192–1202 (2004)
14. Stiers, P., Peeters, R., et al.: Mapping Multiple Visual Areas in the Human Brain with a Short fMRI Sequence. NeuroImage 29(1), 74–89 (2006)
15. Thirion, B., Flandin, G., et al.: Dealing with the Shortcomings of Spatial Normalization. Hum. Brain Mapp., 27(8), 678–693 (2006)
16. Thirion, B., Pinel, P., et al.: Finding landmarks in the Functional Brain: Detection and Use for Group Characterization. In: Duncan, J.S., Gerig, G. (eds.) MICCAI 2005. LNCS, vol. 3750, pp. 476–483. Springer, Heidelberg (2005)
17. Thirion, B., Roche, A., et al.: Improving Sensitivity and Reliability of fMRI Group Studies through high level Combination of Individual Subjects Results. In: Proc. MMBIA 2006, New York, USA, June17-18, 2006 (2006)
18. Worsley, K.J.: An Improved Theoretical P value for SPMs Based on Discrete Local Maxima. NeuroImage 28(4), 1056–1062 (2005)

Insight into Efficient Image Registration Techniques and the Demons Algorithm

Tom Vercauteren[1,2], Xavier Pennec[1], Ezio Malis[3], Aymeric Perchant[2], and Nicholas Ayache[1]

[1] Asclepios Research Group, INRIA Sophia-Antipolis, France
[2] Mauna Kea Technologies, 9 rue d'Enghien Paris, France
[3] Icare Research Group, INRIA Sophia-Antipolis, France

Abstract. As image registration becomes more and more central to many biomedical imaging applications, the efficiency of the algorithms becomes a key issue. Image registration is classically performed by optimizing a similarity criterion over a given spatial transformation space. Even if this problem is considered as almost solved for linear registration, we show in this paper that some tools that have recently been developed in the field of vision-based robot control can outperform classical solutions. The adequacy of these tools for linear image registration leads us to revisit non-linear registration and allows us to provide interesting theoretical roots to the different variants of Thirion's demons algorithm. This analysis predicts a theoretical advantage to the symmetric forces variant of the demons algorithm. We show that, on controlled experiments, this advantage is confirmed, and yields a faster convergence.

1 Introduction

As the integration of information from multiple images finds more and more applications in the fields of biomedical research and clinical applications, the efficiency of the image registration procedures becomes a crucial point for the end-users. Correspondingly there is a growing interest from the scientific community to better understand and optimize the registration procedures.

In this paper, we present an efficient approach to image registration that encompass both linear and non-linear registration with a focus on mono-modal image registration. In this setting, registration is classically performed by optimizing a similarity criterion such as the mean squared error. Literature on image registration and optimization theory already provide a wealth of algorithms that can be used to solve this problem. However they do not always use all the specificity of mono-modal image registration. *Our first contribution* is to shed a new light on this problem by showing that the tools that have recently been developed by Malis [1] in the field of vision-based robot control can be used for biomedical image registration and that they outperform the well-known optimizers. The efficient second-order minimization (ESM) technique [1] takes advantage of the specificity of mono-modal image registration to boost its convergence rate. It is

N. Karssemeijer and B. Lelieveldt (Eds.): IPMI 2007, LNCS 4584, pp. 495–506, 2007.
© Springer-Verlag Berlin Heidelberg 2007

not tailored to a particular class of spatial transformations and can thus be used for a broad class of problems.

Looking at non-linear image registration, one of the most efficient methods is the demons algorithm proposed by Thirion [2]. Several variants of the algorithm have been proposed depending on how the *forces* are computed. In [3,4] an *ad hoc* symmetrization of the demons force similar to the one proposed by Thirion was shown to improve the results of the original demons algorithm. In [5] the authors showed that the demons algorithm had connection with gradient descent schemes. However, to the best of our knowledge, the different variants of the demons have not been given a strong unified theoretical justification. *Our second and main contribution* is to show that the image registration framework we use in this work provides strong theoretical roots to the demons algorithm and that the different variants are related to the use of different optimizers. One of the main results of our theoretical analysis is to show that the symmetric forces variant is related to the ESM scheme. This study thus explains why, from a theoretical point of view, the symmetric forces demons algorithm seems to be more efficient in practice. *Our third contribution* is to provide evidence that, in practice, using symmetric forces indeed leads to a higher convergence rate.

The paper is organized as follows. In Section 2, we develop a unified framework for mono-modal image registration and show how the classical optimizer fit in the framework. Section 3 focuses on the efficient second-order minimization (ESM) with an emphasis on sound mathematical treatment. A practical example is worked out to compare the performance of the different approaches. In Section 4 we show how to extend the framework for the study of the demons algorithm. Finally Section 5 concludes the paper.

2 Registration Using Newton Methods on Lie Groups

2.1 Image Registration Model

Given a *fixed image* $F(.)$ and a *moving image* $M(.)$ in a D-dimensional space, intensity-based image registration is treated as an optimization problem that aims at finding the spatial mapping that will align the fixed and moving images. The transformation $s(.)$, $\mathbb{R}^D \to \mathbb{R}^D$, $p \mapsto s(p)$, models the spatial mapping of points from the fixed image space to the moving image space. The similarity criterion $Sim(F, M \circ s)$ measures the quality of a given transformation. In this paper we will only consider the mean squared error similarity measure which forms the basis of the intensity-based image registration algorithms:

$$Sim(F, M \circ s) = \frac{1}{2} \|F - M \circ s\|^2 = \frac{1}{2\,|\Omega_P|} \sum_{p \in \Omega_P} |F(p) - M(s(p))|^2, \quad (1)$$

where Ω_P is the region of overlap between F and $M \circ s$.

In order to register the fixed and moving images, we need to optimize (1) over a given space of spatial transformations. This can often be done by parameterizing the transformations. However most of the spatial transformations we use do not form vector spaces but only Lie groups (e.g. rigid body, affine, projective, diffeomorphisms...), meaning that we can invert or compose these transformations and obtain a spatial transformation of the same type. We thus need to perform an optimization procedure on a Lie group such as in [1,6,7].

2.2 Newton Methods for Lie Groups

Optimization problems on Lie groups can often be related to constrained optimization by embedding the Lie group in an Euclidean space. The classical way of dealing with the structure of the group is to use Lagrange multipliers or when the constraints are simple to have an *ad hoc* procedure to preserve the constraints (e.g. renormalize a quaternion to have a unit quaternion). In this work we use an alternative strategy known as geometric optimization which uses local canonical coordinates [6]. This strategy intrinsically takes care of the geometric structure of the group and allows the use of unconstrained optimization routines.

Let $\mathcal{G}$ be a Lie group for the composition $\circ$. We refer the reader to the standard textbooks for a detailed treatment of Lie groups. To any Lie group can be associated a Lie algebra $\mathfrak{g}$, whose underlying vector space is the tangent space of $\mathcal{G}$ at the neutral element Id. This Lie algebra captures the local structure of $\mathcal{G}$. The Lie group and the Lie algebra are related through the group exponential which is a diffeomorphism from a neighborhood of 0 in $\mathfrak{g}$ to a neighborhood of Id in $\mathcal{G}$. Let $\boldsymbol{e}_1, \dots, \boldsymbol{e}_n$ be a basis of the Id-tangent space $T_{\mathrm{Id}}(\mathcal{G})$ corresponding to a basis of $\mathfrak{g}$. Canonical coordinates provide local coordinate charts so that for any $x \in \mathcal{G}$ in some neighborhood of s, there exists a vector $\boldsymbol{u} = \sum_i u_i \boldsymbol{e}_i \in T_{\mathrm{Id}}(\mathcal{G})$ such that $x = s \circ \exp(\boldsymbol{u}) = s \circ \exp(\sum_i u_i \boldsymbol{e}_i)$. They can be used to get the Taylor expansion of a smooth function φ on $\mathcal{G}$:

$$\varphi\left(s \circ \exp(\boldsymbol{u})\right) = \varphi(s) + J_s^{\varphi}.\boldsymbol{u} + \frac{1}{2}\boldsymbol{u}^T.H_s^{\varphi}.\boldsymbol{u} + O(\|\boldsymbol{u}\|^3), \tag{2}$$

where $[J_s^{\varphi}]_i = \frac{\partial}{\partial u_i}\varphi(s \circ \exp(\boldsymbol{u}))\big|_{\boldsymbol{u}=0}$ and $[H_s^{\varphi}]_{ij} = \frac{\partial^2}{\partial u_i \partial u_j}\varphi(s \circ \exp(\boldsymbol{u}))\big|_{\boldsymbol{u}=0}$. It is shown in [6], that this expansion allows us to adapt the classical Newton-Raphson method by using an intrinsic update step,

$$s \leftarrow s \circ \exp(\boldsymbol{u}) \tag{3}$$

where $\boldsymbol{u}$ solves $H_s^{\varphi}.\boldsymbol{u} = -J_s^{\varphi T}.\varphi(s)$. As in the vector space case, this algorithm has a local quadratic convergence, and is independent of the chosen basis of $\mathfrak{g}$.

In many cases, using the Newton-Raphson method is not advocated or simply not possible. The Hessian matrix is indeed often difficult or impossible to compute, is not numerically well-behaved and convergence problem may arise when it is not definite positive. To address these problems in the context of non-linear least squares optimization, most of the available efficient methods (e.g. Levenberg-Marquardt) are related to the Gauss-Newton method [8].

Let $\phi(.) = \frac{1}{2}\|\boldsymbol{\varphi}(.)\|^2 = \frac{1}{2}\sum_p \varphi_p(.)^2$ be a sum of squared smooth functions. The Gauss-Newton method is based on a linear approximation of $\boldsymbol{\varphi}$ in a neighborhood of the current estimate. From (2), we have $\varphi(s \circ \exp(\boldsymbol{u})) = \varphi(s) + J_s^{\varphi}.\boldsymbol{u} + O(\|\boldsymbol{u}\|^2)$. By keeping only the linear part we obtain a quadratic approximation that we use to derive the Gauss-Newton method on a Lie group:

$$\phi(s \circ \exp(\boldsymbol{u})) = \frac{1}{2}\left\|\varphi(s \circ \exp(\boldsymbol{u}))\right\|^2 \approx \frac{1}{2}\left\|\varphi(s) + J_s^{\varphi}.\boldsymbol{u}\right\|^2. \quad (4)$$

It is well known that if J_s^{φ} has full rank, this equation admits a unique minimizer which is the solution of the so-called normal equations: $\left(J_s^{\varphi T}.J_s^{\varphi}\right).\boldsymbol{u} = -J_s^{\varphi T}.\varphi(s)$. By using this solution in the intrinsic update step, $s \leftarrow s \circ \exp(\boldsymbol{u})$, we get the Gauss-Newton method for Lie Groups. In a vector space, the local convergence of the Gauss-Newton (and Levenberg-Marquardt) method is in general not quadratic. In the Lie group setting, we also see that (4) is a first-order approximation. We must therefore also expect only local linear convergence.

2.3 Gauss-Newton for Image Registration

For the registration problem (1), the Gauss-Newton algorithm can be used with the following function involved in the nonlinear least squares problem:

$$\varphi_p(s \circ \exp(\boldsymbol{u})) = F(p) - M \circ s \circ \exp(\boldsymbol{u})(p). \quad (5)$$

We now need to know how to compute the Jacobian $J_s^{\varphi_p}$ of this function.

In practice, we need a computational representation. By Whitney's theorem, we know that there exists an embedding Θ, $\mathcal{G} \to \mathbb{R}^N$, $s \mapsto \Theta(s)$ of the Lie group in an Euclidean space. This embedding also allows us to represent the Lie algebra. An example is the matrix representation of the common spatial transformations (e.g. rigid body, affine, projective) in homogeneous coordinates. In practice, this Euclidean representation is used to compute the spatial transformation (using e.g. matrix multiplication in homogeneous coordinates). Let us denote $w(\Theta(s), p)$ the expression, in the Euclidean embedding space $\mathbb{R}^N$, of the transformation of a point $p \in \mathbb{R}^D$ through the mapping $s \in \mathcal{G}$. Using this Euclidean representation, the chain rule and the fact that the differential map of the exponential at Id is the identity, the Jacobian of (5) can be decomposed as (cf. appendix):

$$J_s^{\varphi_p} = \frac{\partial}{\partial \boldsymbol{u}^T}\varphi_p(s \circ \exp(\boldsymbol{u}))\bigg|_{\boldsymbol{u}=0} = -\nabla_p^T(M \circ s).J^{w_p}.\boldsymbol{e}_\Theta, \quad (6)$$

where $\nabla_p(M \circ s)$ is the gradient of the warped moving image ($D \times 1$ vector), $J^{w_p} = \frac{\partial w(X,p)}{\partial X^T}\big|_{X=\Theta(\mathrm{Id})}$ is the derivative of the mapping action expressed the Euclidean embedding space ($D \times N$ matrix) and $\boldsymbol{e}_\Theta = [\Theta(\boldsymbol{e}_1), \dots, \Theta(\boldsymbol{e}_n)]$ stacks the basis vectors of $\mathfrak{g}$ expressed in the Euclidean embedding space ($N \times n$ matrix). A practical case for 2D rigid-body registration is given in Section 2.3.

3 Efficient Second-Order Minimization (ESM)

Image registration (especially mono-modal) is not any generic optimization problem, the algorithms can take advantage of the specificity of the problem to develop more efficient schemes. We focus on the efficient second-order minimization

(ESM) procedure of [1] that uses the following fact: when the images are aligned with the optimal spatial transformation s^{opt}, the fixed image and the warped image as well as their gradient should be very close to each other.

The main idea behind the ESM is that we can use this information to improve the search direction of the Newton methods. The Newton-Raphson uses the value of φ_p, its first and second derivatives around 0 to build a second-order polynomial approximation of φ_p. The Gauss-Newton case discards the second derivative and can thus only build a first-order polynomial. What we do with the ESM is to use the value of φ_p, its first derivative around 0 as well as its first derivative around s^{opt} to build a second-order polynomial without the need of second derivative information. The ESM is thus a second-order minimization method that does not need the computation of the Hessian matrix.

3.1 A Second-Order Linearization

With the ESM, the information about the Hessian that is discarded with the Gauss-Newton iteration is recovered with a Taylor expansion of a Jacobian calculated at the optimal transformation. Such an information can only be used in the image registration settings because we should have $\nabla_p M \circ s^{\text{opt}} \approx \nabla_p F$ up to a noise term. In order to use this very special property, let us define a generalization of the Jacobian used in Section 2.2:

$$J_s^{\varphi}(\boldsymbol{u}) = \frac{\partial}{\partial \boldsymbol{v}^T} \varphi(s \circ \exp(\boldsymbol{v}))\Big|_{\boldsymbol{v}=\boldsymbol{u}}. \tag{7}$$

Note that $J_s^{\varphi}(0) = J_s^{\varphi}$. By using a first-order Taylor expansion around 0 we get:

$$J_s^{\varphi}(\boldsymbol{u}) = J_s^{\varphi}(0) + \boldsymbol{u}^T.H_s^{\varphi} + O(\|\boldsymbol{u}\|^2),$$

that can be rewritten as $\boldsymbol{u}^T.H_s^{\varphi} = J_s^{\varphi}(\boldsymbol{u}) - J_s^{\varphi}(0) + O(\|\boldsymbol{u}\|^2)$. By incorporating this expression into (2), this provides us with a true second-order approximation:

$$\begin{aligned} \varphi\left(s \circ \exp(\boldsymbol{u})\right) &= \varphi(s) + J_s^{\varphi}(0).\boldsymbol{u} + \frac{1}{2}\left(J_s^{\varphi}(\boldsymbol{u}) - J_s^{\varphi}(0)\right).\boldsymbol{u} + O(\|\boldsymbol{u}\|^3) \\ &= \varphi(s) + \frac{1}{2}\left(J_s^{\varphi}(\boldsymbol{u}) + J_s^{\varphi}\right).\boldsymbol{u} + O(\|\boldsymbol{u}\|^3) \end{aligned} \tag{8}$$

The non-linear least squares problem of Section 2.2 can thus be revisited to get a second-order approximation of (4):

$$\phi(s \circ \exp(\boldsymbol{u})) = \frac{1}{2}\|\varphi(s) + \frac{1}{2}\left(J_s^{\varphi}(\boldsymbol{u}) + J_s^{\varphi}\right).\boldsymbol{u}\|^2. + O(\|\boldsymbol{u}\|^3) \tag{9}$$

The computation of $J_s^{\varphi}(\boldsymbol{u})$ is a difficult problem in the general setting. Even if we get a closed-form expression of it, a minimization problem that involves this term might not be easy to solve in practice. In order to be able to use (9), we need to use the special properties of our optimization problem.

From the current transformation s, the optimum step $\boldsymbol{u}_s^{\text{opt}}$ that an optimizer can make is such that $s^{\text{opt}} = s \circ \exp(\boldsymbol{u}_s^{\text{opt}})$. From a computational point of view, the main result of the ESM procedure is that, for this optimal step, the product $J_s^{\varphi}(\boldsymbol{u}_s^{\text{opt}}).\boldsymbol{u}_s^{\text{opt}}$ is linear in $\boldsymbol{u}_s^{\text{opt}}$. This allows for a simple minimization of (9).

The idea is to replace the gradient of the optimally warped image $M \circ s^{\text{opt}} = M \circ s \circ \exp(\boldsymbol{u}_s^{\text{opt}})$ by its *equivalent*, the gradient of the fixed image F. We then get a simple linear approximation: $J_s^{\varphi}(\boldsymbol{u}_s^{\text{opt}}).\boldsymbol{u}_s^{\text{opt}} \approx \nabla_p^T F.J^{w_p}.\boldsymbol{e}_\Theta.\boldsymbol{u}_s^{\text{opt}}$ as shown in the appendix. This can be used with (8) to get:

$$\boldsymbol{\varphi}\left(s \circ \exp(\boldsymbol{u}_s^{\text{opt}})\right) = \boldsymbol{\varphi}(s) + J_s^{\text{ESM}}.\boldsymbol{u}_s^{\text{opt}} + O(\|\boldsymbol{u}_s^{\text{opt}}\|^3) \tag{10}$$

$$J_s^{\text{ESM}_p} \triangleq -\frac{1}{2}\left(\nabla_p^T F + \nabla_p^T (M \circ s)\right).J^{w_p}.\boldsymbol{e}_\Theta \tag{11}$$

where we omit the image noise and where J^{w_p} and $\boldsymbol{e}_\Theta$ are given in Section 2.3. This efficient procedure can thus be summarized by the following algorithm:

Algorithm 1 (ESM and Gauss-Newton for Image Registration)

- *Choose a starting spatial transformation* s
- *Iterate until convergence:*
  - *Given* s, *let*
    - $J^p = -\frac{1}{2}\left(\nabla_p^T F + \nabla_p^T (M \circ s)\right).J^{w_p}.\boldsymbol{e}_\Theta$ *for ESM*
    - $J^p = -\nabla_p^T (M \circ s).J^{w_p}.\boldsymbol{e}_\Theta$ *for Gauss-Newton*
  - *Compute the update* $\boldsymbol{u}$ *by solving the linear system* $(J^T.J).\boldsymbol{u} = -J^T.\boldsymbol{\varphi}(s)$ *using e.g. a QR factorization of* J
  - *Let* $s \leftarrow s \circ \exp(\lambda \boldsymbol{u})$, *with* $\lambda = 1$ *or is given by a line search*

Note that the two options have the same computational complexity since $\nabla_p F$ needs only be computed once during initialization.

3.2 A Practical Example: 2D Rigid Body Transformations

Let us now focus on the optimization of (1) for the Lie group $SE(2)$ of 2D rigid body transformations. In order to use the optimization method presented in Algorithm 1, we need to know what the corresponding Lie algebra $\mathfrak{se}(2)$ is and to be able to compute the exponential map and the necessary Jacobian.

A 2D rigid body transformation r is composed of a rotation of angle α followed by a translation $\tau = (\tau^x, \tau^y)$. This Lie group $SE(2)$ can be represented using homogeneous coordinates by a 3×3 matrix group of the form $\Theta(r) = \left[\begin{smallmatrix} R_\alpha & \tau \\ 0 & 1 \end{smallmatrix}\right]$, where R_α is a rotation matrix. Since we have a matrix Lie group, the exponential map coincides with the matrix exponential. In this special case, we even have a closed-form expression of the matrix exponential. Thanks to this matrix representation (which is the Euclidean embedding space used in Section 2.3), we see that the Lie Algebra can be represented by the vector space of matrices of the form $\left[\begin{smallmatrix} dR_\alpha & d\tau \\ 0 & 0 \end{smallmatrix}\right]$, where dR_α is any skew-symmetric matrix and $d\tau$ is any vector. We thus see that a convenient basis of $\mathfrak{se}(2)$ is given (in matrix form) by $\Theta(\boldsymbol{e}_1) = \left[\begin{smallmatrix} 0 & -1 & 0 \\ 1 & 0 & 0 \\ 0 & 0 & 0 \end{smallmatrix}\right]$, $\Theta(\boldsymbol{e}_2) = \left[\begin{smallmatrix} 0 & 0 & 1 \\ 0 & 0 & 0 \\ 0 & 0 & 0 \end{smallmatrix}\right]$ and $\Theta(\boldsymbol{e}_3) = \left[\begin{smallmatrix} 0 & 0 & 0 \\ 0 & 0 & 1 \\ 0 & 0 & 0 \end{smallmatrix}\right]$. In order to use Algorithm 1, the only expression we still need to compute is J^{w_p}. The spatial

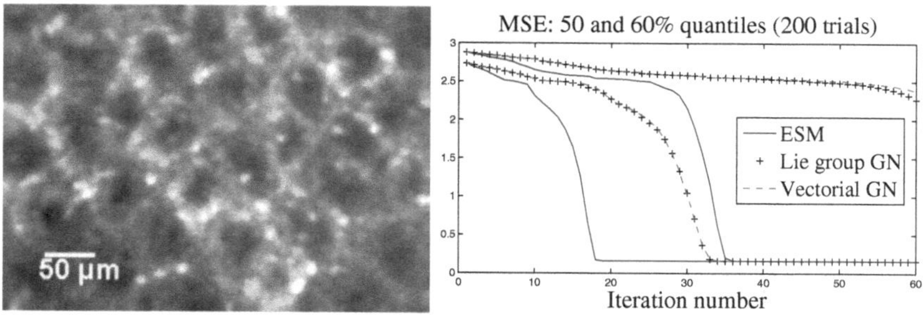

Fig. 1. Simple convergence experiment using two consecutive live mouse colon images of a dynamic fibered confocal microscopy (FCM) sequence (left, image courtesy of D. Vignjevic, S. Robine, D. Louvard, Institut Curie, Paris). We initialize the different optimizers with a random rigid body transformations to compare them. The random generator is Gaussian centered around the optimal transformation (validated by an expert), uses $\sigma_\alpha = 0.3$ rad for the rotation part and $\sigma_\mathcal{T} = 10$ pixels for the translation parts so as to get a sufficient number of divergent optimizations. The ESM is both faster to converge with 50% of the trials converging in less than 19 iterations vs. 34 for the Gauss-Newton and more robust as 60% converge in less than 36 iterations with ESM but we never reach 60% of convergence with the Gauss-Newton.

transformation $r(p)$ of a point p through a 2D rigid body transformation r is a simple matrix multiplication and this leads to $J^{w_p} = \begin{bmatrix} p_x & 0 & 0 & p_y & 0 & 0 & 1 & 0 & 0 \\ 0 & p_x & 0 & 0 & p_y & 0 & 0 & 1 & 0 \end{bmatrix}$. After some basic simplifications we obtain a simple expression: $J^{w_p}.e_\Theta = \begin{bmatrix} -p_y & 1 & 0 \\ p_x & 0 & 1 \end{bmatrix}$.

Registration results: In the context of tracking for vision-based robot control, a detailled comparison of the optimization schemes showed that, for the space of homographies, the ESM outperformed classical solutions [9]. In this section, we compare the performance of the ESM optimizer with respect to the Gauss-Newton optimizer on a real-life biomedical image registration problem. A $2D+t$ dynamic sequence is acquired with a fibered confocal microscope (FCM) and we need to perform a rigid body registration between the consecutive frames. In order to get a statistically meaningful example, we chose two representative frames and compared the optimizers with random starting points. Since the emphasis is on the comparison of the various schemes and not on the final performance, no multi-resolution scheme was used. Our results in Fig. 1 show that the analysis of [9] can be extended to the problem of biomedical image registration. We indeed see that for rigid body registration the ESM has a faster convergence rate and is more robust than the Gauss-Newton optimizer.

4 An Insight into the Demons Algorithm

In [2], the author proposed to consider non-linear registration as a diffusion process. He introduced *demons* that push according to local characteristics of the images in a similar way Maxwell did for solving the Gibbs paradox. The forces are inspired from the optical flow equations and the method alternates between computation of the forces and their regularization by a simple Gaussian smoothing. This results into a computationally efficient algorithm. Several teams [5,10,11] have worked towards providing theoretical roots to the demon's in order to understand the underlying assumptions and potentially modify them.

The goal of this section is twofold. We first go one step further in providing theoretical explanations of the demons and show that the different variants of of this algorithm can all be cast into the image registration framework derived above. One of the main results of this analysis is to show that the symmetric forces demons can be cast to the ESM optimization method of [1]. This variant should therefore be the most efficient one. Our second goal is thus to verify if the theoretical advantage of the symmetric variant are noticeable in practice.

4.1 An Alternate Optimization Framework

In order to end-up with the global minimization of a well posed criterion, it was proposed in [11] to introduce a hidden variable in the registration process: correspondences. The idea is to consider the regularization criterion as a prior on the smoothness of the transformation s. Instead of requiring that point correspondences between image pixels (a vector field c) be exact realizations of the transformation, one allows some error at each image point. Considering a Gaussian noise on displacements, we end-up with the global energy:

$$E(c, s) = \|\frac{1}{\sigma_i}(F - M \circ c)\|^2 + \frac{1}{\sigma_x^2} \operatorname{dist}(s, c)^2 + \frac{1}{\sigma_T^2} \operatorname{Reg}(s) \qquad (12)$$

where σ_i accounts for the noise on the image intensity, σ_x accounts for a spatial uncertainty on the correspondences and σ_T controls the amount of regularization we need. We classically have $\operatorname{dist}(s, c) = \|c - s\|$ and $\operatorname{Reg}(s) = \|\nabla s\|$ but the regularization can also be modified to handle fluid-like constraints [11].

The interest of this auxiliary variable is that an alternate optimization over c and s decouples the complex minimization into simple and very efficient steps:

Algorithm 2 (Demons Algorithm as an Alternate Optimization)

- *Choose a starting spatial transformation (a vector field) s*
- *Iterate until convergence:*
  - *Given s, compute a correspondence update field $\boldsymbol{u}$ by minimizing $E_s^{\text{corr}}(\boldsymbol{u}) = \|F - M \circ (s + \boldsymbol{u})\|^2 + \frac{\sigma_i^2}{\sigma_x^2} \|\boldsymbol{u}\|^2$ with respect to $\boldsymbol{u}$*
  - *If a fluid-like regularization is used, let $\boldsymbol{u} \leftarrow K_{\text{fluid}} \star \boldsymbol{u}$. The convolution kernel will typically be a Gaussian kernel.*
  - *Let $c \leftarrow s + \boldsymbol{u}$*
  - *If a diffusion-like regularization is used, let $s \leftarrow K_{\text{diff}} \star c$ (else let $s \leftarrow c$). The convolution kernel will also typically be a Gaussian kernel.*

We focus on the first step of this alternate minimization and refer the reader to [11] for a detailed coverage of the regularization questions.

4.2 The Symmetric Forces Demons as an ESM Optimization

As one can see in Algorithm 2, the minimization of $E_s^{\text{corr}}(\boldsymbol{u})$ is very close to the mean squared error image registration problem (1) we have been focusing on. The space of free-form deformations used within the demons algorithm is a simple vector space. It is therefore a trivial Lie group where the group composition is the addition of free-form deformation fields, and the group exponential simply maps a free-form deformation field onto itself. This implies that the optimization step $s \circ \exp(\boldsymbol{u})$ we have been using so far is simply expressed by an addition $s + \boldsymbol{u}$. The only remaining difference lies in the term $\|\boldsymbol{u}\|^2$. We now show that the same framework allows us to take care of this additional term.

The efficient image registration tools we showed in the previous sections can easily be applied to get the following approximations:

$$F(p) - M \circ (s + \boldsymbol{u})(p) \approx F(p) - M \circ s(p) + J^p.\boldsymbol{u}(p)$$

where $J^p = -\nabla_p^T(M \circ s)$ with Gauss-Newton, $J^p = -\frac{1}{2}\left(\nabla_p^T F + \nabla_p^T(M \circ s)\right)$ with ESM and $J^p = -\nabla_p^T F$ with Thirion's rule. As shown previously, the approximation order depends on this choice of J^p. These approximations can be used to rewrite the correspondence energy used in the demons algorithm:

$$E_s^{\text{corr}}(\boldsymbol{u}) \approx \frac{1}{2\,|\Omega_P|} \sum_{p \in \Omega_P} \left\| \begin{bmatrix} F(p) - M \circ s(p) \\ 0 \end{bmatrix} + \begin{bmatrix} J^p \\ \frac{\sigma_i(p)}{\sigma_x} I \end{bmatrix} .\boldsymbol{u}(p) \right\|^2,$$

where we recall that Ω_P is the overlap between F and $M \circ s$.

As opposed to the global transformation case (e.g. 2D rigid body transformations) we see that here, the approximations given for each pixel are independent from each other. This greatly simplifies the minimization of E_s^{corr} by splitting it into very simple systems for each pixel. We indeed only need to solve, at each

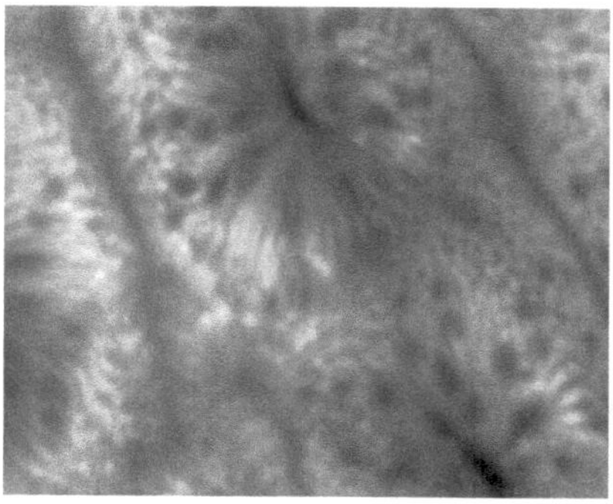

(a) Original image

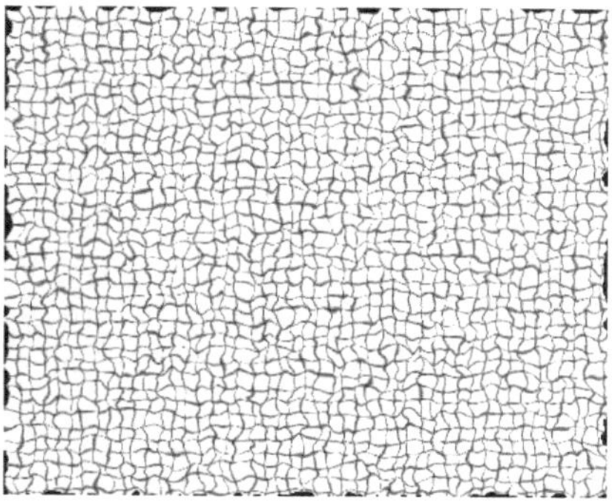

(b) Random warped grid

Fig. 2. Experiment using a random warp on a normal human colonic mucosa image (FCM). Image Courtesy of PD. Dr. A. Meining, Klinikum rechts der Isar, Munich.

pixel p, the following normal equations:

$$\left[J^{pT} \; \frac{\sigma_i(p)}{\sigma_x} I\right] \cdot \begin{bmatrix} J^p \\ \frac{\sigma_i(p)}{\sigma_x} I \end{bmatrix} .\boldsymbol{u}(p) = -\left[J^{pT} \; \frac{\sigma_i(p)}{\sigma_x} I\right] \cdot \begin{bmatrix} F(p) - M \circ s(p) \\ 0 \end{bmatrix}$$

$$\left(J^{pT}.J^p + \frac{\sigma_i^2(p)}{\sigma_x^2} I\right).\boldsymbol{u}(p) = -(F(p) - M \circ s(p)).J^{pT}$$

From the Sherman-Morrison formula (matrix inversion lemma) we finally have:

$$\boldsymbol{u}(p) = -\frac{F(p) - M \circ s(p)}{\|J^p\|^2 + \frac{\sigma_i^2(p)}{\sigma_x^2}} J^{pT} \tag{13}$$

We see that if we use the local estimation $\sigma_i(p) = |F(p) - M \circ c(p)|$ of the image noise, and the ESM approximation of J^p we end up with the exact expression of the symmetric forces demons algorithm. Note that σ_x then controls the maximum step length: $\|\boldsymbol{u}(p)\| \leq \sigma_x/2$.

4.3 Demons Results

To compare the performance of the different variants of the demons algorithm, we present some results using synthetic data. We use a fibered confocal microscopy image as our original image. For each random experiment, we generate a random (MRF) smooth deformation field and warp the original image. We add some random noise both to the original and the warped image. We then run the different demons algorithm starting with an identity spatial transformation.

We used the same set of parameters for all the experiments: a maximum step length of 2 pixels, a Gaussian *fluid-like* regularization with $\sigma_{\text{fluid}} = 1$ and a Gaussian *diffusion-like* regularization with $\sigma_{\text{diff}} = 1$. As previously, no multi-resolution scheme was used because the emphasis is on the comparison of the various schemes and not the final performance. We can see on Fig. 3 that the

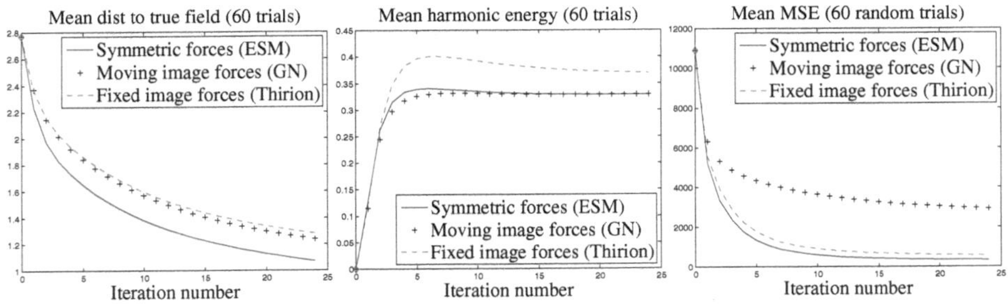

Fig. 3. Registration on 100 random experiments such as the one presented in Fig. 2. Note the faster convergence of the symmetric forces demons in terms of images intensities agreement (MSE), smoothness of the non-linear spatial transformation (harmonic energy) and more importantly in terms of distance to the actual spatial transformation.

symmetric forces variants converges faster in terms of MSE, smoothness and more importantly in terms of distance to the actual field.

5 Conclusion

We showed in this paper that some tools that have recently been developed in the field of vision-based robot control can outperform classical image registration algorithms by exploiting the special nature of the image registration problem. We have focused on mono-modal registration but the ESM scheme can also be extended to handle more complex intensity relationships. Robust estimation techniques can be used to account for outliers in the cost function and we plan to investigate on iterative intensity matching for the optimization of other simple similarity metrics such as the correlation coefficient and the correlation ratio.

The adequacy of the ESM for linear image registration led us to revisit non-linear registration and especially the demons algorithm. By using the ESM, the matrix inversion lemma and the local estimation of the image noise, we improved our understanding of the demons algorithm. This analysis predicted a theoretical advantage to the symmetric forces variant of the demons algorithm which we confirmed on the practical side.

If the confluence of the ESM theory and the alternate minimization framework of the demons algorithm indeed leads to a unified theoretical explanation of the demons, it could still be argued that all the aspects of the Lie group structure used in the ESM theory are not fully exploited there. We believe contrastingly that this Lie group point of view makes this theory much more powerfull. The final goal of understanding an algorithm is indeed to improve it. One of the main limitations of the demons algorithm is that it doesn't provide diffeomorphic transformations contrarily to the algorithms developed in [12,13]. Our next goal will be to show how the ESM theory can be used in combination with the Lie group structure of diffeomorphic transformations to adapt the demons algorithm to this Lie group.

References

1. Malis, E.: Improving vision-based control using efficient second-order minimization techniques. In: Proc. IEEE ICRA'04 Apr 2004 (2004)
2. Thirion, J.-P.: Image matching as a diffusion process: An analogy with Maxwell's demons. Medical Image Analysis 2(3), 243–260 (1998)
3. Wang, H., Dong, L., O'Daniel, J., Mohan, R., Garden, A.S., Ang, K.K., Kuban, D.A., Bonnen, M., Chang, J.Y., Cheung, R.: Validation of an accelerated 'demons' algorithm for deformable image registration in radiation therapy. Physics in Medicine and Biology 50(12) (2005)
4. Rogelj, P., Kovačič, S.: Symmetric image registration. Medical Image Analysis 10(3), 484–493 (2006)
5. Pennec, X., Cachier, P., Ayache, N.: Understanding the Demon's Algorithm: 3D non-rigid registration by gradient descent. In: Taylor, C., Colchester, A. (eds.) Medical Image Computing and Computer-Assisted Intervention – MICCAI'99. LNCS, vol. 1679, Springer, Heidelberg (1999)

6. Mahony, R., Manton, J.H.: The geometry of the Newton method on non-compact Lie-groups. J. Global Optim. 23(3), 309–327 (2002)
7. Lee, P.Y., Moore, J.B.: Gauss-Newton-on-manifold for pose estimation. J. Indus. Management Optim. 1(4), 565–587 (2005)
8. Madsen, K., Nielsen, H.B., Tingleff, O.: Methods for non-linear least squares problems. Lecture Notes, Informatics and Mathematical Modelling, Technical University of Denmark, DTU (1999)
9. Benhimane, S., Malis, E.: Homography-based 2d visual tracking and servoing. Joint Issue of IJCV and IJRR on Vision and Robotics (2007) (to appear)
10. Modersitzki, J.: Numerical Methods for Image Registration. Oxford University Press, Oxford, UK (2004)
11. Cachier, P., Bardinet, E., Dormont, D., Pennec, X., Ayache, N.: Iconic feature based nonrigid registration: The PASHA algorithm. CVIU — Special Issue on Nonrigid Registration 89(2-3), 272–298 (2003)
12. Marsland, S., Twining, C.: Constructing diffeomorphic representations for the groupwise analysis of non-rigid registrations of medical images. IEEE Trans. Med. Imag. 23(8), 1006–1020 (2004)
13. Beg, M.F., Miller, M.I., Trouvé, A., Younes, L.: Computing large deformation metric mappings via geodesic flows of diffeomorphisms. Int'l J. Comp. Vision 61(2) (2005)

Appendix

Derivation of (6)**:** We apply the chain rule to $J_s^{\varphi_p} = -\frac{\partial M \circ s \circ e^{\boldsymbol{u}}}{\partial \boldsymbol{u}^T}\big|_{\boldsymbol{u}=0}$ and get (using the Euclidean embedding space),

$$[J_s^{\varphi_p}]_i = -\frac{\partial M \circ s(q)}{\partial q^T}\bigg|_{q=p} . \frac{\partial w(X,p)}{\partial X^T}\bigg|_{X=\Theta(\mathrm{Id})} . \frac{\partial \Theta(\exp(u_i \boldsymbol{e}_i))}{\partial u_i}\bigg|_{u_i=0}$$
$$= -\nabla_p^T (M \circ s). \frac{\partial w(X,p)}{\partial X^T}\bigg|_{x=\Theta(\mathrm{Id})} .\Theta(\boldsymbol{e}_i),$$

where we used that the differential map of the exponential at Id is the identity.

Derivation of (10)**:** We start by incorporating $\boldsymbol{u}_s^{\mathrm{opt}}$ into $M \circ s \circ e^{\boldsymbol{v}}$ by writing it as $M \circ s \circ e^{\boldsymbol{u}_s^{\mathrm{opt}}} \circ e^{-\boldsymbol{u}_s^{\mathrm{opt}}} \circ e^{\boldsymbol{v}}$. By using the chain rule we find that $J_s^{\varphi_p}(\boldsymbol{u}_s^{\mathrm{opt}})$ can be decomposed into a product of three terms. The first one is given by:

$$\frac{\partial}{\partial q^T} M \circ s \circ e^{\boldsymbol{u}_s^{\mathrm{opt}}}(q)\bigg|_{q=e^{-\boldsymbol{u}_s^{\mathrm{opt}}} \circ e^{\boldsymbol{u}_s^{\mathrm{opt}}}(p)} = \nabla_p^T (M \circ s^{\mathrm{opt}}) = \nabla_p^T F + \varepsilon,$$

where ε is a noise term. The second term is the same as the one appearing in (6): $\frac{\partial w(X,p)}{\partial X^T}\big|_{X=\Theta(e^{-\boldsymbol{u}_s^{\mathrm{opt}}} \circ e^{\boldsymbol{u}_s^{\mathrm{opt}}})} = J^{w_p}$. And finally, the last term is given by $\frac{\partial \Theta(e^{-\boldsymbol{u}_s^{\mathrm{opt}}} \circ e^{\boldsymbol{u}})}{\partial \boldsymbol{u}^T}\big|_{\boldsymbol{u}=\boldsymbol{u}_s^{\mathrm{opt}}}$. This last term is in general very difficult to compute but in fact we only need to compute its product with $\boldsymbol{u}_s^{\mathrm{opt}}$. This appears to be a directional derivative. We can thus also write it as a rate of change to get:

$$\frac{\partial \Theta(e^{-\boldsymbol{u}_s^{\mathrm{opt}}} \circ e^{\boldsymbol{u}_s^{\mathrm{opt}} + t\boldsymbol{u}_s^{\mathrm{opt}}})}{\partial t}\bigg|_{t=0} = \frac{\partial \Theta(e^{t\boldsymbol{u}_s^{\mathrm{opt}}})}{\partial t}\bigg|_{t=0} = \boldsymbol{e}_{\Theta}.\boldsymbol{u}_s^{\mathrm{opt}}.$$

Divergence-Based Framework for Diffusion Tensor Clustering, Interpolation, and Regularization

Torsten Rohlfing[1], Edith V. Sullivan[2], and Adolf Pfefferbaum[1,2]

[1] Neuroscience Program, SRI International, Menlo Park, CA, USA
torsten@synapse.sri.com, dolf@synapse.sri.com
[2] Department of Psychiatry and Behavioral Sciences, Stanford University, Stanford CA, USA
edie@stanford.edu

Abstract. This paper introduces a novel framework for diffusion tensor combination, which can be used for tensor averaging, clustering, interpolation, and regularization. The framework is based on the physical interpretation of the tensors as the covariance matrices of Gaussian probability distributions. The symmetric Kullback-Leibler divergence provides a natural distance measure on these distributions, which leads to a closed-form expression for the distance between any two diffusion tensors, as well as for the weighted average of an arbitrary number of tensors. We illustrate the application of our technique in four different scenarios: (a) to combine tensor data from multiple subjects and generate population atlases from ten young and ten older subjects, (b) to perform k-means clustering and generate a compact Gaussian mixture of multiple tensors, (c) to interpolate between tensors, and (d) to regularize (i.e., smooth) noisy tensor data. For boundary-preserving regularization, we also propose a non-linear two-stage smoothing algorithm that can be considered remotely similar to a median filter.

1 Introduction

Diffusion tensor magnetic resonance imaging (DT-MRI) is an increasingly popular method for non-invasive mapping of *in vivo* brain connectivity [1]. The most common applications of DT-MRI currently are voxel-based comparisons [2] and fiber tracking [3]. In voxel-based studies, statistics are performed on scalar fields derived from the tensor data, e.g., fractional anisotropy (FA) maps. Fiber tracking, on the other hand, uses the complete tensor information to extract geometrical models that represent the course of white matter fiber tracts through the brain. Methods are also being developed that perform statistics on tensors directly (e.g., Xu *et al.* [4]).

To apply many common image processing tasks (e.g., smoothing, interpolation, averaging) to tensor images, multiple tensors must be combined in a meaningful way. For averaging, these tensors originate from corresponding positions in multiple images, whereas for interpolation and smoothing they originate from a local neighborhood of a given location in a single image. It is possible simply to add the tensor matrices element by element [5], but this ignores the fact that the manifold of diffusion tensors does not define a Euclidean vector space. More appropriate tensor combination schemes have therefore been proposed, such as the geodesic approach by Fletcher & Joshi [6] or the algebraic framework by Batchelor *et al.* [7]. Both are motivated by the *abstract mathematical properties* of the diffusion tensors, e.g., their positive definiteness.

N. Karssemeijer and B. Lelieveldt (Eds.): IPMI 2007, LNCS 4584, pp. 507–518, 2007.
© Springer-Verlag Berlin Heidelberg 2007

We introduce herein a new framework for the combination of multiple diffusion tensors that is motivated by the *physical interpretation* of the tensors. These are the covariance matrices of Gaussian probability distributions of local Brownian motion of hydrogen atoms [1]. Unlike [6] and [7], our combination method also has the advantage of providing a *closed-form* (i.e., non-iterative) solution for the weighted average of an arbitrary number of diffusion tensors. It also provides a closed-form expression for a distance measure between any two tensors. Compared with our method, the frameworks put forth by Fletcher & Joshi [6] and Batchelor *et al.* [7] require iterative procedures.

As a proof of concept, this paper presents initial results of applying our new framework to four different scenarios. First, we use it to construct inter-subject population atlases by averaging several diffusion tensor images (DTI). Such atlases are potentially useful, for example, in cross-sectional studies of disease effects and longitudinal studies of aging and brain disease. Second, we use tensor average and distance to construct a k-means clustering algorithm [8] and generate Gaussian mixture representations of multiple tensor fields. Third, we illustrate the application of our framework for regularization (i.e., smoothing) of noisy tensor fields. Fourth, we illustrate the interpolation between different tensors that is useful for tensor image reformatting.

2 Methods

In the original (and still most commonly used) diffusion imaging method [1], the diffusion tensor represents the covariance matrix of a zero-mean multivariate Gaussian probability distribution. For general Gaussian distributions, Myrvoll [9] developed a divergence-based clustering framework. We describe below the application of this framework to Gaussian diffusion distributions. The mathematical details are substantially simplified compared with [9], because *a priori* all distributions must have zero means. Thus, Myrvoll's iterative joint estimation of centroid mean and covariance matrix is reduced to a closed-form expression for the covariance matrix.

Divergence-based Tensor Distance. For two arbitrary probability distributions f and g over a domain Ω (here: $\Omega = \mathbb{R}^3$), the symmetric Kullback-Leibler (SKL) divergence is a distance measure (but not a metric) that is defined as

$$d(f,g) = \int_\Omega f \log \frac{f}{g} + \int_\Omega g \log \frac{g}{f}. \tag{1}$$

When f and g are zero-mean multivariate Gaussians with covariance matrices $\mathbf{\Sigma}_f$ and $\mathbf{\Sigma}_g$, then Eq. (1) can be evaluated in closed form as

$$d(f,g) = \frac{1}{2} \operatorname{trace} \left(\mathbf{\Sigma}_f \mathbf{\Sigma}_g^{-1} + \mathbf{\Sigma}_f^{-1} \mathbf{\Sigma}_g - 2\mathbf{I} \right). \tag{2}$$

Simple Tensor Average. For M zero-mean Gaussians with covariance matrices $\mathbf{\Sigma}_m$, $m = 1, \dots, M$, their "centroid" is the zero-mean Gaussian that minimizes the total distance (2) from all M input Gaussians. This centroid, therefore, follows the common definition of the mean (or average) of the input Gaussians. Its covariance matrix $\mathbf{\Sigma}_c$ can be computed as the solution of the simplified matrix Ricatti equation

$$\sum_{m=1}^{M} \mathbf{\Sigma}_m - \mathbf{\Sigma}_c \left(\sum_{m=1}^{M} \mathbf{\Sigma}_m^{-1} \right) \mathbf{\Sigma}_c = \mathbf{0}. \tag{3}$$

We determine $\mathbf{\Sigma}_c$ by computing the eigensystem of the 6×6 block matrix

$$\mathbf{M} = \left(\begin{array}{c|c} \mathbf{0} & \sum_{m=1}^{M} \mathbf{\Sigma}_m \\ \hline \sum_{m=1}^{M} \mathbf{\Sigma}_m^{-1} & \mathbf{0} \end{array} \right). \tag{4}$$

To determine the solution of Eq. (3) from the block matrix $\mathbf{M}$, let $\vec{v}_1$ through $\vec{v}_3$ be those three of its eigenvectors for which the real part of the corresponding complex eigenvalue is positive. Furthermore, for $i = 1, 2, 3$ let $\vec{u}_i$ denote the upper halves (first three elements) of $\vec{v}_i$ and $\vec{w}_i$ the lower halves of $\vec{v}_i$. Then the 3×3 matrix product

$$\mathbf{\Sigma}_c = \left(\vec{u}_1 \,\vdots\, \vec{u}_2 \,\vdots\, \vec{u}_3 \right) \left(\vec{w}_1 \,\vdots\, \vec{w}_2 \,\vdots\, \vec{w}_3 \right)^{-1} \tag{5}$$

is a positive semi-definite solution of Eq. (3). Details of the derivation and the relevant proofs of existence are provided by Myrvoll [9] and the references therein. A shorter summary is also given in [10].

k-Means Clustering. Tensor average and distance as introduced above are sufficient to implement a k-means clustering algorithm [8] for diffusion tensors. The topic of clustering is an active field of research in its own right and is well beyond the scope of this paper. For now, we use an *ad hoc* implementation of a simple iterative clustering algorithm. All input tensors are first combined to form an initial centroid. They are then grouped by their distances to that centroid, where the number of groups is the user-defined number of output clusters. This initial clustering is then iteratively refined by alternatingly updating cluster centroids and tensor-to-cluster assignments.

Weighted Tensor Average and Regularization. Using a real-valued vector $\vec{w} \in \mathbb{R}^M$ of weights, where $\sum_{m=1}^{M} w_m = 1$, the weighted average $\mathbf{\Sigma}_c^{(\vec{w})} = w_1 \mathbf{\Sigma}_1 \oplus \cdots \oplus w_m \mathbf{\Sigma}_m$ can be computed by analogously solving the eigensystem equation of the modified matrix

$$\mathbf{M}_{\vec{w}} = \left(\begin{array}{c|c} \mathbf{0} & \sum_{m=1}^{M} w_m \mathbf{\Sigma}_m \\ \hline \sum_{m=1}^{M} w_m \mathbf{\Sigma}_m^{-1} & \mathbf{0} \end{array} \right). \tag{6}$$

The weighted tensor average allows for the divergence-based regularization of tensor images by using weights of a filter kernel (e.g., Gaussian) in the weighted average.

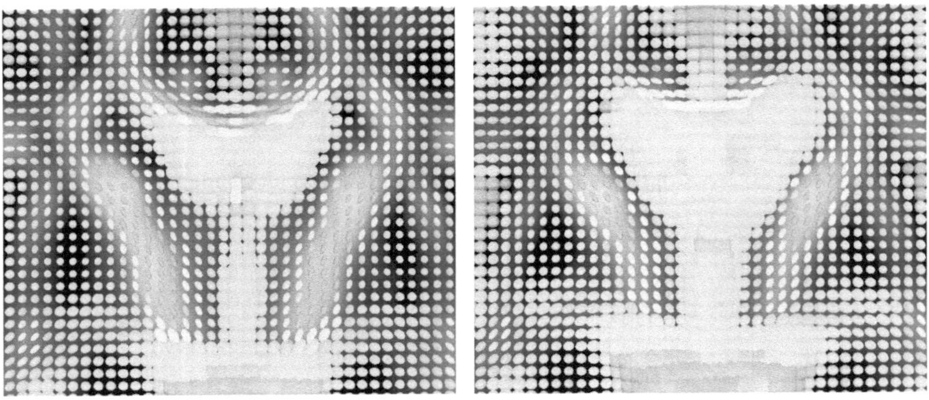

(a) (b)

Fig. 1. Ellipsoid glyph visualization of average tensor fields (coronal slice through lateral ventricles, corpus callosum, and basal ganglia). The FA map of each tensor field is shown in the image background. (a) Average of 10 young subjects. (b) Average of 10 older subjects.

The appropriateness of the definition in Eq. (6) follows from the following three observations: (a) Eq. (5) is invariant under multiplication of $\mathbf{M}$ with a positive real number. (b) Rational weights $w_m \in \mathbb{Q}^+$ can be replaced with integers by multiplying each of them with the product of all denominators; the resulting matrix then represents an inflated set of input tensors, which are replicated in exact proportion to their relative weights. (c) The generalization to irrational weights $w_m \in \mathbb{R}^+ \setminus \mathbb{Q}$ follows from continuity of mapping $\mathbf{M} \mapsto \mathbf{\Sigma}_c$ (the eigenvalues of a matrix are the roots of a polynomial, i.e., a function in $\mathcal{C}^\infty$).

Tensor Interpolation. Interpolation between two tensors, $\mathbf{\Sigma}_1$ and $\mathbf{\Sigma}_2$, can also be expressed as a special case of the weighted tensor average: the linear interpolation between two tensors is computed as the weighted average $\mathbf{\Sigma}_{12}(w) = (w-1)\mathbf{\Sigma}_1 \oplus w\mathbf{\Sigma}_2$ for $w \in [0,1]$. Higher-order interpolation kernels can be applied accordingly.

3 Results

In this section, we demonstrate the application of our framework for tensor averaging, clustering, regularization, and interpolation. First, tensor averaging is applied to tensor data from young and elderly healthy individuals. Second, we illustrate the potential benefits of k-means clustering for diffusion tensors on a set of synthetic tensor fields. Third, tensor regularization is illustrated using synthetic noisy tensor data. Finally, tensor interpolation is illustrated between multiple synthetic tensors.

3.1 Tensor Averaging

DTI data were acquired on a 3 T GE scanner with the following parameters: FOV = 24 cm; 2.5 mm isotropic voxel size; T_R = 11,000 ms; T_E = 97.6 ms; slice thickness

= 2.5 mm; inter-slice gap = 0 mm; slices = 62; six non-collinear gradient orientations +x +y, +y +z, +x +z, -x +y, -y +z, +x -z (each repeated with opposite gradient polarity); 1.5 Gauss/cm with 32 ms duration and 34 ms separation, resulting in a b-value of 860 s/mm².

We acquired data on two groups of healthy subjects: ten young subjects (mean = 28.6, range = 22–37 years, 17.2 years of education; five men, five women) and ten older subjects (mean = 72.2, range = 65–79 years, 16.3 years of education; five men, five women). The older subjects were part of an ongoing study on aging [11]. One subject from the young group (23.8 year old woman) was randomly picked as the reference subject. From the $b = 0$ image of this subject, nonrigid coordinate transformations were computed to the $b = 0$ image of each of the remaining subjects. In a multi-resolution strategy, the nonrigid transformation had an initial control point spacing of 40 mm, which was refined three times to a final resolution of 5 mm. The benefits of higher spatial resolutions of the deformation appear marginal, based on the limited resolution and geometric fidelity of the diffusion-weighted images (DWI). Through the respective transformations, all seven images ($b = 0$, and b_1 through b_6) from each subject were warped into the coordinate system of the reference subject. The method used for tensor reconstruction is described in detail in Appendix A.1, and for image registration in Appendix A.2.

The divergence-based averages of the tensor images from all ten young and all ten older subjects are shown using ellipsoid glyphs (Fig. 1(a,b)). The average of the older subjects shows greater diffusivity (i.e., increased tensor volume) and decreased anisotropy (i.e., more spherical tensors) than the young group. This is consistent with published studies on the effects of aging on FA [12].

3.2 k-Means Clustering

A synthetic example of k-means clustering and Gaussian superposition of tensor fields is shown in Fig. 2. Ten synthetic noisy input tensor fields were generated, five with a horizontal simulated "fiber," and the other five with a vertical fiber. The clustering algorithm was set to generate two output clusters and was generally successful at distinguishing between the horizontal and vertical tensors (Fig. 2(c),(d)). The superposition of the centroids of both clusters (Fig. 2(e)) thus represents a mixture in which both fiber directions are preserved. This is a substantial improvement over the simple tensor average (Fig. 2(f)), in which tensors degenerate to isotropic distributions. The assignment which cluster represents which centroid is essentially arbitrary, so the horizontal, vertical, and spherical tensors are split somewhat randomly between the two clusters. The single spherical tensor in the crossing region in Fig. 2(e) illustrates a weakness of the k-means clustering algorithm (but *not* the divergence-based tensor combination framework), especially for even numbers of inputs. It is simply not always possible for the clustering algorithm to determine how many modes there truly are in the input data, independent of the type of input data and distance measure used.

3.3 Tensor Field Regularization

In Fig. 3, a synthetic noisy tensor field is regularized using our framework. The noise-free tensor field (Fig. 3(a)) was generated by tensor reconstruction from simulated DWI

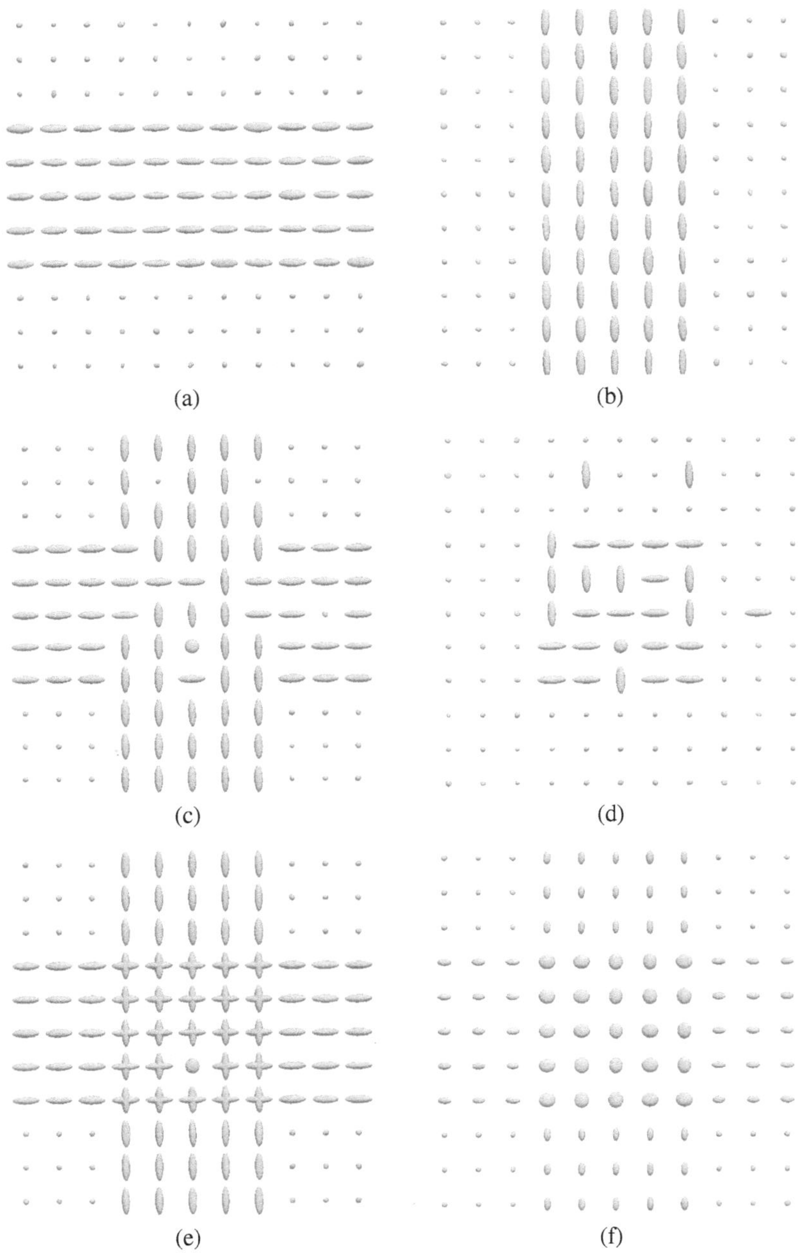

Fig. 2. Synthetic example for k-means clustering with ten inputs and two output clusters. (a) One out of five input tensors fields with a horizontal "fiber." (b) One out of five input fields with a vertical "fiber." (c) Tensor field showing centroids of cluster #1. (d) Tensor field showing centroids of cluster #2. (e) Superposition of cluster centroid tensor fields (c) and (d). (f) Simple tensor average of the input images.

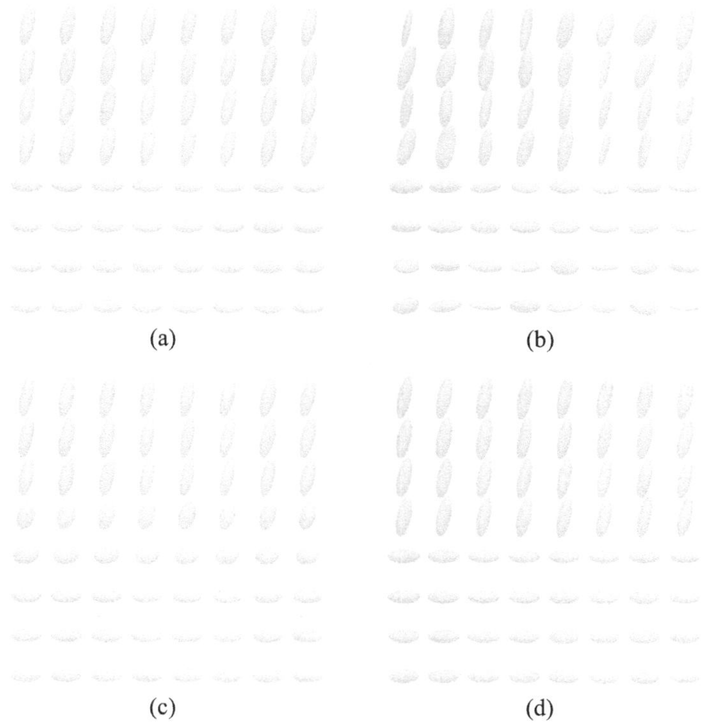

Fig. 3. Divergence-based tensor field regularization (synthetic example). (a) Noise-free tensor field. (b) Noisy tensor field. (c) Noisy tensor field after smoothing. (d) Noisy tensor field after two-stage smoothing with distance percentile threshold. All four images show the same central 8×8 pixels from a three-dimensional 20×20×10 volume.

(6 gradient directions). The upper half of the field contains tensors oriented mostly along the y direction, the lower half contains tensors oriented along the x direction. The total size of the simulated tensor field was 20×20×10 pixels, which provided sufficient field of view for the smoothing kernel, but only the central 8×8 pixels are shown here. The noisy tensor data (Fig. 3(b)) was generated by tensor reconstruction from the same images after adding Gaussian noise to each of them.

The visualization in Fig. 3(c) shows the noisy tensor field after regularization with a Gaussian kernel (2 pixels full width at half maximum). The noise was substantially reduced, but tensors along the boundary between the two homogeneous regions (upper and lower half) are mixed and combined into less anisotropic tensors.

The visualization in Fig. 3(d) shows the noisy tensor field after regularization with a two-stage algorithm for thresholded smoothing. In the first pass, the tensors in a local neighborhood are combined using the same kernel used in Fig. 3(c). Then, for each of the combined tensors, its distance to the combined tensor is computed according to Eq. (2). The 50% of tensors that are closest to the first-pass combined tensor are then combined again with their previous kernel weights, and the result is the final

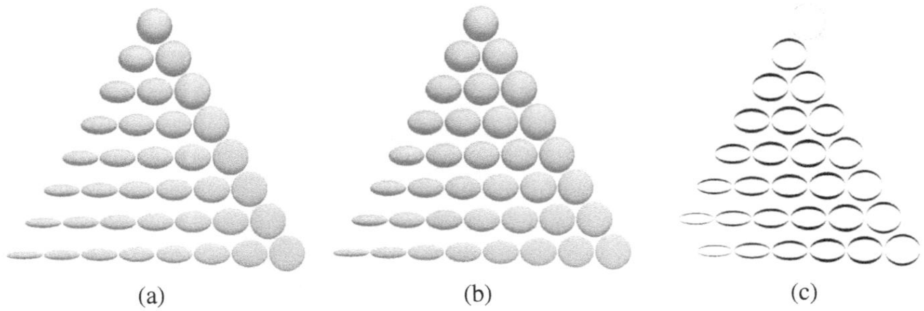

Fig. 4. Barycentric interpolation between anisotropic (bottom left), oblate (bottom right), and isotropic tensors (top). (a) Divergence-based interpolation. (b) Arithmetic interpolation. (c) Differences between the tensor contours in (a) and (b).

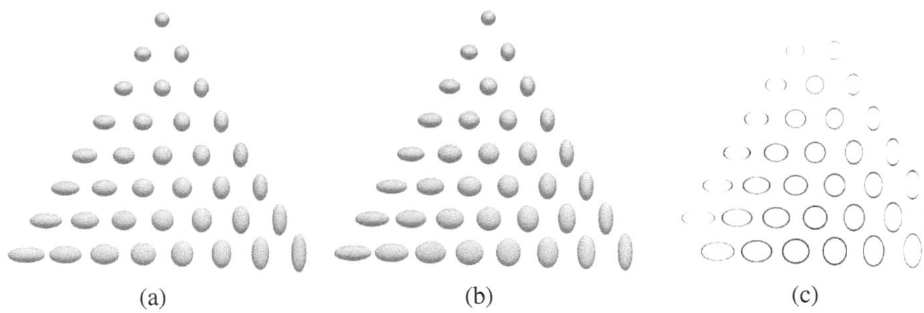

Fig. 5. Barycentric interpolation between anisotropic tensors oriented along the x (bottom left), y (bottom right), and z direction (top). (a) Divergence-based interpolation. (b) Arithmetic interpolation. (c) Differences between the tensor contours in (a) and (b).

regularized output tensor. This procedure resembles a median filter in that both improve the boundary preservation while performing effective regularization. The 50% distance threshold can be adjusted to trade between better regularization (higher threshold) or better boundary preservation (lower threshold). The optimum value may depend on the relative size of filter kernel and image structures.

3.4 Tensor Interpolation

Interpolation between tensors is illustrated in two examples. In Fig. 4, we interpolate between three anisotropic tensors, each of which is oriented along a different coordinate axis (x, y, and z). In Fig. 5, we interpolate between an anisotropic (bottom left), an oblate (bottom right), and a spherical tensor (top). Each interpolation example is represented over an equilateral triangle. The three sides of each triangle represent linear interpolation between the two tensors on the adjacent corners. Tensors inside the triangles are the barycentric combination of the tensors at all three corners.

In each example, we compare the interpolation using our framework with arithmetic interpolation, i.e., the element-wise interpolation between the tensor matrices. Visual

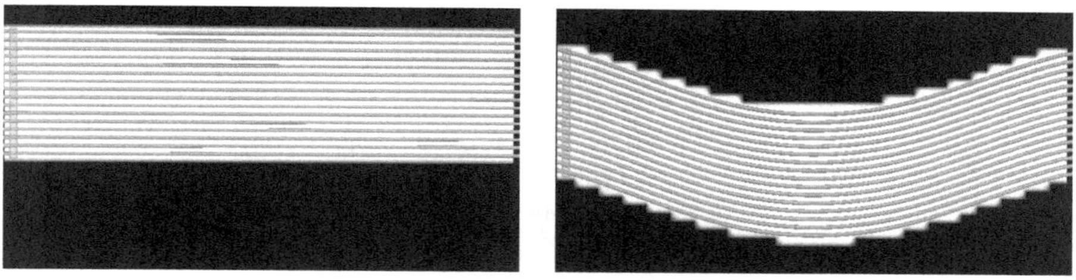

(a) (b)

Fig. 6. Reoriented tensor reconstruction illustrated using a numerical phantom. (a) Tracked fibers along straight tracts originating from 16×16 region on the left, shown in red. Fiber count = 256. (b) Tracked fibers along deformed tract originating from 16×16 region on the left, shown in red. Fiber count = 254. Fibers were tracked using the DTI module of Slicer [17].

inspection of the difference images of the tensor outlines (Figs. 4(c) and 5(c)) indicates that our framework is biased in favor of more anisotropic tensors. Because anisotropic tensors are more direction specific than isotropic ones, the former can be considered to carry more useful information.

4 Discussion

This paper has introduced a novel combination framework for diffusion tensors based on a divergence distance measure between Gaussian distributions. We have demonstrated its application to tensor averaging, interpolation, regularization, and clustering. To the best of our knowledge, this paper is also the first to propose retrospective k-means clustering of multiple diffusion tensor images and to demonstrate this technique as an effective means of producing a compact, information-preserving representation of tensor superpositions.

The basic tensor combination approach proposed herein competes with other methods, such as the geodesic approach [6], or the algebraic framework [7]. Compared with these methods, ours has the advantage of providing closed-form solutions for the distance between any two tensors and for the weighted average of an arbitrary number of diffusion tensors, at least to the extent that solving Eq. (3), which involves computing the eigensystem of a non-symmetric 6×6 matrix, is considered a closed-form operation.

We note that our derivation a combination framework for diffusion tensors is based entirely on selecting an appropriate distance measure between two tensors, in our case the symmetric Kullback-Leibler divergence, Eq. (1). This is analogous to both Fletcher & Joshi and to Batchelor *et al.*, albeit with a different distance measure as the foundation of our framework.

It is not clear, which published tensor combination method performs better, and the answer probably depends on the application. However, our distribution-based model is physically well motivated and possesses convenient computational properties. It is also conceptionally more consistent than other methods with representing complex combinations of tensors as probabilistic superpositions, e.g., by means of Gaussian mixtures.

Such mixtures have used as inputs to a Monte-Carlo fiber tracking algorithm [13]. Herein, we have generated such a mixture in a synthetic example in Section 3.2.

Our next goal is to apply the k-means methodology used herein to obtain compact probabilistic population representations of actual multi-subject DTI data. This could be considered a generalization and extension of a method by Parker & Alexander [14], who represented crossings of two fibers in a *single* subject. Compared with simply averaging tensors across subjects, the k-means clustering almost entirely preserves their directional specificity, thus minimizing degeneration of tensors in the combined tensor images. As recently shown by Behrens *et al.* [15], probabilistic fiber tracking in such Gaussian mixture fields has the potential of improving the detection of minor tracts in areas of fiber crossings. Our next step will be to generate the Gaussian superpositions from multiple subjects rather than a single one.

Acknowledgments

This work was supported by the National Institute on Alcohol Abuse and Alcoholism, Grants AA05965 and AA12388, and the National Institute on Aging, Grant AG17919.

References

1. Basser, P.J., Mattiello, J., LeBihan, D.: MR diffusion tensor spectroscopy and imaging. Biophys. J. 66(1), 259–267 (1994)
2. Shimony, J.S., McKinstry, R.C., Akbudak, E., et al.: Quantitative diffusion-tensor anisotropy brain MR imaging: Normative human data and anatomic analysis. Radiology 212(3), 770–784 (1999)
3. Mori, S., Crain, B.J., Chacko, V.P., et al.: Three-dimensional tracking of axonal projections in the brain by magnetic resonance imaging. Ann.Neurol. 45(2), 265–269 (1999)
4. Xu, D., Mori, S., Shen, D., et al.: Spatial normalization of diffusion tensor fields. Magn. Reson. Med. 50(1), 175–182 (2003)
5. Jones, D.K., Griffin, L.D., Alexander, D.C., et al.: Spatial normalization and averaging of diffusion tensor MRI data sets. NeuroImage 17(2), 592–617 (2002)
6. Fletcher, P.T., Joshi, S.: Principal geodesic analysis on symmetric spaces: Statistics of diffusion tensors. In: Sonka, M., Kakadiaris, I.A., Kybic, J. (eds.) Computer Vision and Mathematical Methods in Medical and Biomedical Image Analysis. LNCS, vol. 3117, pp. 87–98. Springer, Heidelberg (2004)
7. Batchelor, P.G., Moakher, M., Atkinson, D., et al.: A rigorous framework for diffusion tensor calculus. Magn. Reson. Med. 53(1), 221–225 (2005)
8. MacQueen, J.: Some methods for classification and analysis of multivariate observations. In: Proceedings, Fifth Berkeley Symposium on Mathematical Statistics and Probability vol. 1., University of California Press, pp. 281–296 (1967)
9. Myrvoll, T.A.: Adaptation of Hidden Markov Models using Maximum a Posteriori Linear Regression with Hierarchical Priors. PhD thesis, Norwegian University of Science and Technology, Trondheim (2002)
10. Myrvoll, T.A., Soong, F.K.: Optimal clustering of multivariate normal distributions using divergence and its application to HMM adaptation. In: Proceedings (ICASSP '03). 2003 IEEE International Conference on Acoustics, Speech, and Signal Processing, 2003, vol. I, pp. 552–555. IEEE Press, New York (2003)

11. Sullivan, E.V., Adalsteinsson, E., Pfefferbaum, A.: Selective age-related degradation of anterior callosal fiber bundles quantified in vivo with fiber tracking. Cereb. Cortex 16(7), 1030–1039 (2005)
12. Salat, D., Tuch, D., Greve, D., et al.: Age-related alterations in white matter microstructure measured by diffusion tensor imaging. Neurobiol. Aging 26(8), 1215–1227 (2005)
13. Behrens, T.E.J., Woolrich, M.W., Jenkinson, M., et al.: Characterization and propagation of uncertainty in diffusion-weighted MR imaging. Magn. Reson. Med. 50(5), 1077–1088 (2003)
14. Parker, G.J., Alexander, D.C.: Probabilistic Monte Carlo based mapping of cerebral connections utilising whole-brain crossing fibre information. In: Taylor, C.J., Noble, J.A. (eds.) IPMI 2003. LNCS, vol. 2732, pp. 684–695. Springer, Heidelberg (2003)
15. Behrens, T., Johansen Berg, H., Jbabdi, S., et al.: Probabilistic diffusion tractography with multiple fibre orientations: What can we gain? NeuroImage 34(1), 144–155 (2007)
16. Alexander, D.C., Pierpaoli, C., Basser, P.J., et al.: Spatial transformations of diffusion tensor magnetic resonance images. IEEE Trans. Med. Imag. 20(11), 1131–1139 (2001)
17. 3D Slicer, available online: `http://www.slicer.org`.
18. Rueckert, D., Sonoda, L.I., Hayes, et al.: Nonrigid registration using free-form deformations: Application to breast MR images. IEEE Trans. Med. Imag. 18(8), 712–721 (1999)
19. Studholme, C., Hill, D.L.G., Hawkes, D.J.: An overlap invariant entropy measure of 3D medical image alignment. Pattern Recognit. 32(1), 71–86 (1999)
20. Rohlfing, T., Maurer, J.C.R., Bluemke, D.A., et al.: Volume-preserving nonrigid registration of MR breast images using free-form deformation with an incompressibility constraint. IEEE Trans. Med. Imag. 22(6), 730–741 (2003)

A Appendix

A.1 Nonridigly Reoriented Tensor Reconstruction

Let $\mathbf{T} : \mathbb{R}^3 \to \mathbb{R}^3$ be the coordinate transformations from the reference subject image to the image from one of the other subjects. If $\vec{g}_1$ through $\vec{g}_K$ are the gradient directions used for acquisition of the DWI for the other subject, then at each pixel $\vec{x}$ in the reference image the diffusion tensor is of the reformatted image is reconstructed based on the directions

$$\mathbf{J}_{\mathbf{T}}^{-1}(\vec{x})\vec{g}_1, \ldots, \mathbf{J}_{\mathbf{T}}^{-1}(\vec{x})\vec{g}_K, \tag{7}$$

where $\mathbf{J}_{\mathbf{T}}^{-1}$ is the inverse of the Jacobian matrix of $\mathbf{T}$ at pixel $\vec{x}$. If $\mathbf{T}$ is a rigid transformation, this results in a rotation of the gradient directions according to the global rotation between reference and subject anatomy. For nonrigid transformations, this rotation is locally different for each pixel, and there may be shear. By enforcing a positive Jacobian determinant throughout image space, it is guaranteed that the Jacobian matrix is non-singular, which in turn guarantees that the gradient directions remain non-collinear.

This method does not require eliminating shear components of the transformation [16]. Nonetheless, we found that penalizing shear during the registration and applying only the orthogonal part of the Jacobian helped avoid numerical problems associated with angular resolution of the directional sampling when using the minimal number of six gradient directions. Unlike approaches that re-orient the tensors, our method is directly applicable to non-Gaussian models of diffusion. It may also be better suited for high-angular-resolution data, because it does not approximate shear by a rotation.

The effectiveness of the tensor reconstruction method with locally reoriented gradients was tested using a numerical phantom (Fig. 6). DWIs were simulated as they would result from imaging a horizontal fiber tract with a square 16×16 pixel cross-section using 6 simulated diffusion gradients. Tensors were reconstructed from these DWI and fibers were tracked from one end of the tract. The DWI were then deformed using a B-spline deformation [18], with the center of the tract displaced by approximately 8 pixels (the control points in the plane cutting the tract in half were all move by 10 pixels). Tensors were reconstructed using locally reoriented gradients, and fibers were tracked from one end of the tract. As Fig. 6 clearly demonstrates, the tracked fibers follow the deformed tract perfectly and appear to remain parallel. Out of 256 original fibers in the undeformed tract, only two were lost in the deformed tract due to interpolation effects on the tract boundary.

A.2 Shear-Constrained Nonrigid Inter-subject Image Registration

To register images from different subjects, we applied the B-spline algorithm by Rueckert *et al.* [18] to register the $b = 0$ images. The image similarity measure was normalized mutual information, E_{NMI}, as defined by Studholme *et al.* [19]. To prevent folding of the deformation field, we added a folding prevention term. To minimize shear components of the nonrigid transformations, which could impact the angular sampling of the reoriented diffusion gradient directions (see next section), we also incorporated a local shear penalty constraint. The total registration cost function thus is

$$E_{\text{total}} = E_{\text{NMI}} + w_{\text{folding}} E_{\text{folding}} + w_{\text{shear}} E_{\text{shear}} \tag{8}$$

The folding constraint E_{folding} is a weakly weighted version of the volume preservation constraint introduced by Rohlfing *et al.* [20], which enforces a positive Jacobian determinant at each pixel in the image. The local shear constraint E_{shear} is computed via a QR decomposition of the local Jacobian $\mathbf{J}$,

$$\mathbf{J} = \begin{pmatrix} q_{xx} & q_{xy} & q_{xz} \\ q_{yx} & q_{yy} & q_{yz} \\ q_{zx} & q_{zy} & q_{zz} \end{pmatrix} \begin{pmatrix} r_{xx} & r_{xy} & r_{xz} \\ 0 & r_{yy} & r_{yz} \\ 0 & 0 & r_{zz} \end{pmatrix}, \tag{9}$$

where the first matrix of the decomposition is orthogonal, and the second contains scales and shears. The shearing constraint term is then defined using the coefficients of the second matrix as

$$E_{\text{shear}} = \sum_{\vec{x} \in \Omega} w_{\text{shear}}(\vec{x}) (r_{xy}^2 + r_{xz}^2 + r_{yz}^2), \tag{10}$$

where $w(\vec{x})$ is a local rigidity constraint weight. We used here the FA map of the reference subject's tensor image, multiplied by 10^{-2}, i.e.,

$$w_{\text{shear}}(\vec{x}) = 10^{-2}\,\text{FA}_{\text{ref}}(\vec{x}). \tag{11}$$

Anisotropic areas (e.g., white matter) are thus warped with relatively little shear, while the more lenient shear constraint in regions with isotropic diffusion keeps the warping flexible enough to recover the complex inter-subject coordinate correspondences.

Localized Components Analysis

Dan Alcantara[1,a], Owen Carmichael[1,a,b], Eric Delson[2,3], Will Harcourt-Smith[2,3], Kirsten Sterner[3], Stephen Frost[4], Rebecca Dutton[5], Paul Thompson[5], Howard Aizenstein[6,a], Oscar Lopez[6,b], James Becker[6,a,b,c], and Nina Amenta[1,a]

[1] [a]Computer Science and [b]Neurology Departments, University of California, Davis
[2] Lehman College of the City University of New York
[3] NYCEP, American Museum of Natural History
[4] Anthropology Department, University of Oregon
[5] Neurology Department and Laboratory of Neuro Imaging, University of California, Los Angeles
[6] [a]Psychiatry, [b]Neurology, and [c]Psychology Departments, University of Pittsburgh

Abstract. We introduce **Localized Components Analysis** (LoCA) for describing surface shape variation in an ensemble of biomedical objects using a linear subspace of *spatially localized* shape components. In contrast to earlier methods, LoCA optimizes explicitly for localized components and allows a flexible trade-off between localized and concise representations. Experiments comparing LoCA to a variety of competing shape representation methods on 2D and 3D shape ensembles establish the superior ability of LoCA to modulate the locality-conciseness trade-off and generate shape components corresponding to intuitive modes of shape variation. Our formulation of locality in terms of compatibility between pairs of surface points is shown to be flexible enough to enable spatially-localized shape descriptions with attractive higher-order properties such as spatial symmetry.

1 Introduction

The parameterization of an ensemble of biomedical shapes is a key step in a broad array of scientific and medical applications that require quantification of the shape properties of physical objects. In this paper, shape parameterization refers to the problem of converting a representation of the delineating boundary of an object in 2D or 3D into a concise vector of numbers that captures its salient shape characteristics. Converting the potentially complex boundary of a biological object such as an organ or bone into a small set of *shape parameters* facilitates a variety of statistical analyses, including the characterization of shape variability across an ensemble; comparison of object shape between groups; and the tracking of shape change over time. It is important to present the results of these analyses in an intuitive way to encourage the connection of the shape analysis to domain-specific physical or biological processes. For instance, the interpretability of statistical tests of brain region shape differences between healthy and diseased subjects would be enhanced if differences could

N. Karssemeijer and B. Lelieveldt (Eds.): IPMI 2007, LNCS 4584, pp. 519–531, 2007.
© Springer-Verlag Berlin Heidelberg 2007

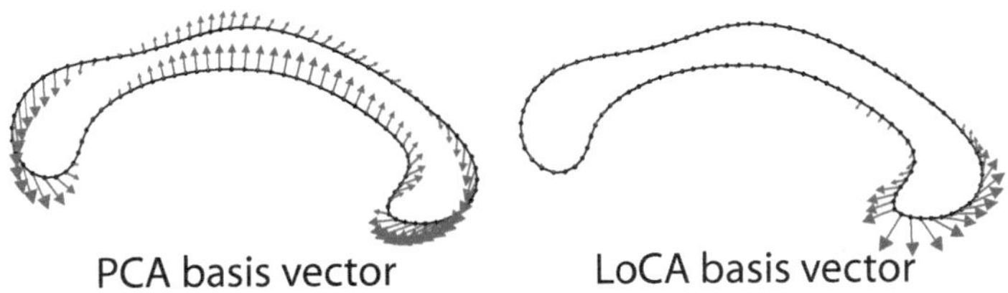

Fig. 1. Shape characteristics of corpora callosa captured by basis vectors generated with PCA and LoCA. Arrows start at points tracing the average corpus callosum; their magnitudes indicate the degree that points move when the corresponding shape parameter is varied.The PCA vector represents a complex, global pattern of shape characteristics while the LoCA vector focuses on the genu.

be presented in terms of a small number of parameters, each of which represents an easily-grasped aspect of region shape. This could promote interpretations of the shape difference in terms of disease causes or effects.

Our goal is to encourage interpretability of results by generating shape parameterizations that are both *concise*– capturing salient shape characteristics in a small number of parameters– and *spatially localized*– accounting for the shape of a spatially restricted sub-region in each parameter. The hypothesis underlying this paper is that spatially-localized and concise shape parameterizations are more intuitive for end users because they allow them to conceptualize object shape in terms a small number of object parts, which are often affected differentially by physical phenomena. In the above example, shape change due to disease processes is known to occur in spatially-localized brain sub-regions in a variety of disorders [1]. In addition, concise parameterizations are attractive because the statistical power of tests on those parameters is reduced as little as possible by corrections for multiple comparisons [2].

We follow the *linear subspace* paradigm of expressing each shape as a linear combination of prototypical, or *basis* shapes. That is, if each shape is represented as a vector $\mathbf{v}_j$ of the $2m$ or $3m$ coordinates of m points sampled from its boundary (*i.e.*, $\mathbf{v}_j = [\mathbf{v}_{j,1}, \mathbf{v}_{j,2}, \cdots \mathbf{v}_{j,m}], \mathbf{v}_{j,k} = [x_k, y_k]$ for 2D shapes), $\mathbf{v}_j$ is approximated as a linear combination of k basis vectors $\{\mathbf{e}_1, \mathbf{e}_2, \cdots \mathbf{e}_k\}$:

$$\mathbf{v}_j^k = \sum_{i=1}^{k} \alpha_{j,i} * \mathbf{e}_i$$

The shape parameters are the coefficients $\alpha_{j,i}$. Linear subspace methods are attractive because their linearity in $\mathbf{e}_i$ allows them to be manipulated using standard tools from linear algebra.

However, linear subspace methods do not inherently encourage locality. Figure 1 (left) depicts a typical $\mathbf{e}_i$ generated by the classical linear subspace method, principal components analysis (PCA), applied to tracings of the *corpus callosum* (CC), a human brain region. The basis shape summarizes a complex pattern of shape characteristics across the entirety of the CC. Therefore, if the corresponding α_i differs between groups, the explanation of the group difference in physical terms is complex. Figure 1 (right), by contrast, shows a typical $\mathbf{e}_i$ generated by the method presented below; differences in the corresponding α_i between groups gives rise to a simple physical explanation in terms of the *genu*, the CC subregion whose shape is captured by the $\mathbf{e}_i$.

We present Localized Components Analysis (LoCA), a method that optimizes the $\mathbf{e}_i$ for spatial locality and conciseness simultaneously. It improves on previous linear subspace methods by explicitly optimizing for localized shape parameters and by allowing the user to modulate the tradeoff between locality and conciseness with greater flexibility than previous methods. The resulting shape components could provide succinct summaries of spatially-localized changes to biomedical structures due to a variety of physical phenomena; for example, LoCA could provide a concise summary of the spatially-localized CC shape changes that are thought to accompany diseases such as HIV / AIDS [3]. In primate evolution, LoCA could summarize the shape similarities between the skulls of genetically related species using a few intuitive parameters.

We summarize related techniques in Section 2, and present LoCA in Section 3. A thorough set of experiments in Section 4 shows the intuitiveness and flexibility gained by LoCA over established linear subspace methods when applied to human CC, colobine monkey skulls, and primate *humeri* (upper arm) bones.

2 Related Work

PCA has been used to find concise bases for shape spaces in medical image analysis [4], morphometrics [5], computer graphics [6], and many other contexts. In PCA, $\mathbf{e}_i$ is the ith eigenvector of the covariance matrix of the example $\mathbf{v}_j$ vectors; therefore, the $\mathbf{e}_i$ are orthogonal and $\mathbf{v}_j^k$ is the best k-th order approximation of $\mathbf{v}_j$ under the L_2 norm. Two algorithms independently named Sparse PCA (S-PCA) encourage as many entries in $\mathbf{e}_i$ to be zero as possible, either by iteratively adjusting the PCA basis [7] or by iteratively constructing sparse orthogonal vectors [8] [9][1]. Empirically the $\mathbf{e}_i$ often represent shape in a small number of spatially-localized subregions [9] [11]. Similarly, while independent components analysis (ICA) and principal factor analysis (PFA) do not directly optimize a locality-related objective function when estimating $\mathbf{e}_i$, they appear to generate spatially-localized components anyway [12] [13]. Alternatively, pre-defined spatially located regions of interest can be integrated into PCA [14]. Our approach is inspired by S-PCA and follows a similar strategy of adjusting the $\mathbf{e}_i$ provided by PCA; but we explicitly optimize for spatially-localized, rather than sparse, $\mathbf{e}_i$. Unlike [14] we allow the decomposition into local regions to emerge from the data.

Networks of localized medial geometric primitives have the potential to capture local shape in a concise set of parameters [15]. We feel that medial and surface-based representations could capture complementary shape information. We note, however, that networks of medial primitives can be challenging to construct in an automated way and may therefore be more labor-intensive than the approach we present.

[1] A third, unrelated Sparse PCA sparsifies the $\mathbf{v}_j$ before applying standard PCA [10].

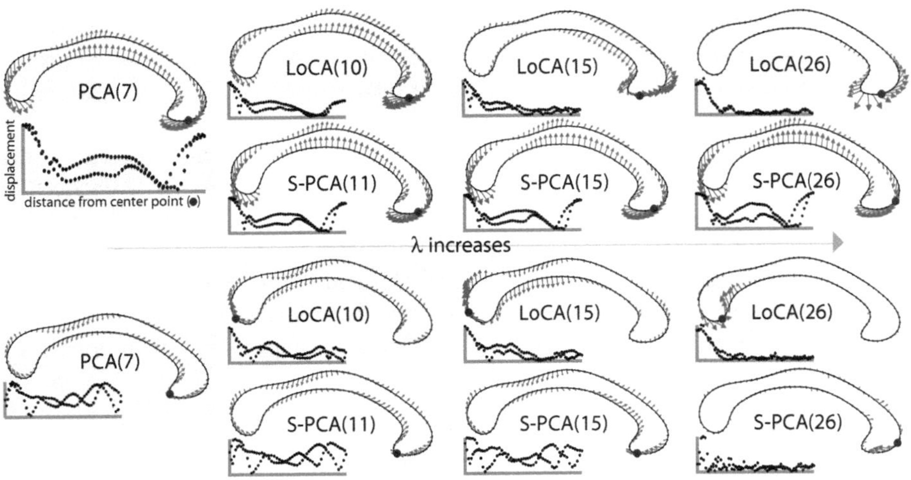

Fig. 2. Effect of λ on the first (top) and third (bottom) basis vectors, where vectors are ordered by the amount of shape variation captured. As λ increases, the number of vectors required to capture 90% of the variation (in parentheses) increases. For small values of λ, vectors capturing substantial variation represent a global deformation of the entire shape. As λ is increased, more of the LoCA vectors become local deformations, until the entire basis consists of local vectors. S-PCA becomes sparse more slowly, so that the first vector is still a global deformation on the right. The third vector is sparse, but there is some perturbation across the entire shape. Each vector is accompanied by a graph showing its locality, where every point in the graph represents a point on the outline. The *center point* is defined as the point minimizing E_{loc}, as described in Section 3.

An alternative approach for determining spatially-localized differences between shape ensembles is to perform statistical tests that compare corresponding $\mathbf{v}_{j,k}$ between groups; spatial maps then color-code each $\mathbf{v}_{j,k}$ by the effect size or p value of the test. Visual inspection of the renderings has revealed spatially-localized shape differences in a variety of medical conditions (see, *e.g.*, [1]); however, m is generally so large that the significance threshold of the statistical tests must be reduced dramatically to guard against detection of spurious group differences [2]. This reduces the sensitivity of spatial mapping techniques to detect subtle shape differences. LoCA uses a linear subspace to reduce the number of variables required for localized shape comparisons, and therefore boost the power of statistical tests.

3 Methods

PCA produces the most concise basis possible under the L_2 norm; that is, for each k, $\sum_{j=1}^{n} ||\mathbf{v}_j - \mathbf{v}_j^k||_{L_2}$ is minimized when $\mathbf{e}_1 \cdots \mathbf{e}_k$ are the first k eigenvectors of the covariance matrix of the $\mathbf{v}_j$. We use a formulation of PCA as the minimization of an energy function E_{var}, and modify it by minimizing $E_{var} + \lambda E_{loc}$, where E_{loc} is a new energy term that summarizes the spatial locality of the $\mathbf{e}_i$. The λ balances the tradeoff between the competing interests of conciseness and locality (Figure 2).

Energy Function. Each successive PCA component accounts for as much of the shape variation as possible; that is, the distribution of shape variation over the PCA basis vectors is as concentrated as possible on the leading $\mathbf{e}_i$. More formally, one can define the relative variance β_i of each basis vector $\mathbf{e}_i$ as

$$\beta_i = \frac{\sum_{j=1}^{n} \langle (\mathbf{v}_j - \mu), e_i \rangle^2}{\sum_{j=1}^{n} ||\mathbf{v}_j - \mu||^2}$$

where μ represents the mean of the data vectors $\mathbf{v}_j$. The entropy of the distribution $-\sum_{i=1}^{k} \beta_i \log \beta_i$ is minimized, over all orthogonal bases, by the PCA basis, so we define this to be E_{var}, as in [7]. The S-PCA construction in that paper balances E_{var} against another energy function that rewards sparse $\mathbf{e}_i$– that is, as many entries as possible in each $\mathbf{e}_i$ are encouraged to have zero magnitude. We instead optimize for locality, defining E_{loc} as follows.

We encourage each $\mathbf{e}_i$ to have simultaneous nonzero entries corresponding to points p_i and p_j if and only if p_i and p_j are close to each other. To do so, we introduce a *pairwise compatibility matrix* $\mathbf{B}$ whose entries $\mathbf{B}[i,j]$ tend toward 1 when p_i and p_j are near each other, and tend towards 0 when they are distant; we define $\mathbf{B}$ below. The $\mathbf{B}$ matrix defines a cost function C:

$$C(\mathbf{e}_i, p_c) = \sum_{j=1}^{m} (\mathbf{B}[c,j] - ||\mathbf{e}_{i,j}||_{L_2})^{\kappa}$$

The $\mathbf{e}_i$ have unit length, so both $\mathbf{B}[c,j]$ and $||\mathbf{e}_{i,j}||$ vary between 0 and 1. Intuitively, points p_c and p_j contribute significantly to C if: 1. p_c and p_j are incompatible, but $\mathbf{e}_{i,j}$ has high magnitude; or 2. p_c and p_j are compatible, but $||\mathbf{e}_{i,j}||$ is close to 0. The exponent κ can take on any value between 1 and 2 to deal with outlier effects. For our experiments, κ was 1.5.

For each basis vector $\mathbf{e}_i$, each p_c yields a different C. We define the locality of $\mathbf{e}_i$ using the best possible p_c, that is, the one that minimizes this cost function C. Each p_c differs in the distribution of its distances to all other p_j– for example, points at one end of a humerus bone in Figure 5 are extremely distant from many points at the opposite end of the bone, while points in the middle are not. So we normalize C as follows:

$$E_{loc} = \sum_{i} \min_{p_c} \frac{C(\mathbf{e}_i, p_c)}{\max_{\mathbf{e}_{bad}} C(\mathbf{e}_{bad}, p_c)}$$

The denominator for a given p_c is simply $\sum_j max(|B[c,j]-1|, |B[c,j]-0|)^{\kappa}$. It needs to be computed only once.

The compatibility $\mathbf{B}[i,j]$ can be computed in whatever way is appropriate for the data set; here, $\mathbf{B}[i,j]$ is based on the distance $D(p_i, p_j)$ between p_i and p_j. For the CC data set considered below, D is the geodesic distance computed from dense surface meshes. For the 3D humeri and skull data sets, D is computed from an adjacency graph constructed between the landmarks. The compatibility is $\mathbf{B}[i,j] = f(D(p_i, p_j))$, where f is a function that modulates D to adjust its range to [0, 1]. We chose a sinusoidal f that is non-zero over a half-period: $f(x) = 0.5(\cos(\pi \frac{x}{\rho}) + 1)$. Larger ρ select for groups of points which co-vary over larger spatial extents. It was set to 0.25 in all of the experiments below.

Optimization. Our optimization procedure is similar to that used in [7]. PCA provides an initial orthonormal basis $\mathbf{e}$, and every possible pair $\mathbf{e}_i, \mathbf{e}_j$ are rotated together in the two-dimensional plane they span. Because the rotating pair is kept orthogonal to each other and stay in their 2D plane, the basis remains orthonormal throughout optimization. Each pair is rotated by the angle θ that minimizes $E_{var} + \lambda E_{loc}$. The optimal θ is found numerically using Brent's method [16]. Notice that since E_{var} and E_{loc} are both summations of terms that each depend solely on an individual $\mathbf{e}_i$, only the terms corresponding to the current $\mathbf{e}_i, \mathbf{e}_j$ pair need to be updated during optimization.

The pairs are rotated in decreasing order of shape variation accounted for. The set of all $\mathbf{e}_i, \mathbf{e}_j$ pairs are adjusted repeatedly, and optimization ceases when adjusting them changes the objective function less than a fixed threshold. Between 50 and 150 iterations were required for each experiment below.

Data Preparation. We assume that we are given an ensemble of n objects, each represented by m points on its boundary, and the compatibility matrix $\mathbf{B}$. Overall differences in object scale, rotation and translation over the ensemble are removed through generalized Procrustes alignment [5]. The resulting scaled and aligned data sets are used as input to the above optimization.

4 Results

Below, we compare LoCA to PCA, ICA, and S-PCA on three data sets: CCs, colobine monkey skulls, and humeri from various primates[2]. For each basis, locality is evaluated visually using renderings of the entries in each basis vector, and through locality graphs (see Figure 2). Conciseness of each basis is assessed quantitatively by charting $\sum_{j=1}^{n} ||\mathbf{v}_j - \mathbf{v}_j^k||_{L_2}$ over all k, and more specifically by recording the number of $\mathbf{e}_i$ required to capture 90% of shape variation, *i.e.* reduce this reconstruction error to 10%.

LoCA behavior depends strongly on λ, the parameter that modulates the tradeoff between conciseness and locality. For $\lambda = 0$, LoCA reduces to PCA. For small λ, LoCA basis vectors accounting for the highest amounts of shape variation resemble PCA basis vectors, while the rest of the basis is clearly localized (Figure 2). For larger λ, all LoCA basis vectors are local, and the bases require more basis vectors to account for shape variation in the data. In Figures 3, 5, and 6, LoCA and S-PCA basis vectors are depicted for the smallest value of λ for which the bases lacked global basis vectors. S-PCA performs similarly to LoCA for small values of λ, in agreement with earlier S-PCA results [7]. However, S-PCA required a much larger basis– more basis vectors for 10% reconstruction error– before the global basis vectors disappeared; this is likely due to the very

[2] Movies and larger images are at: http://idav.ucdavis.edu/~dfalcant/loca.html

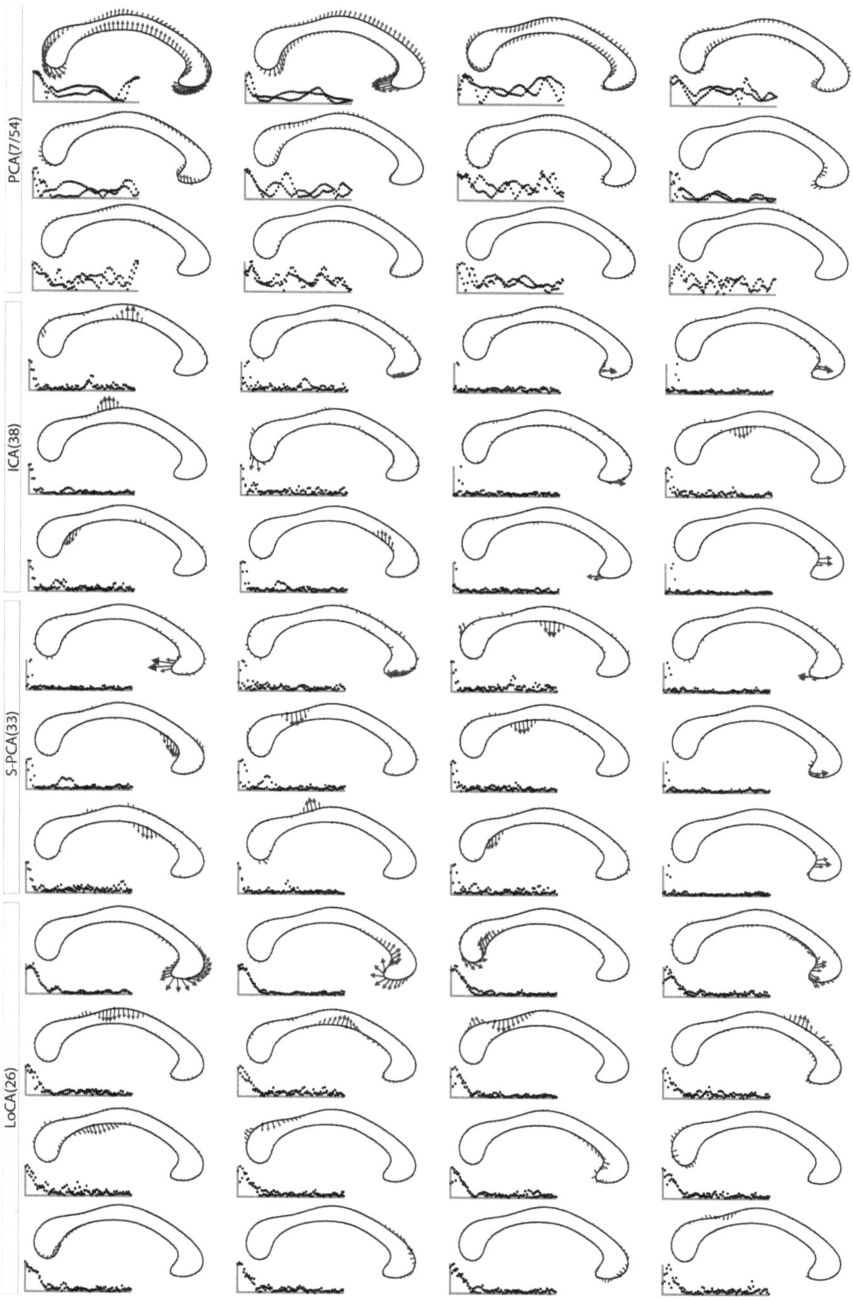

Fig. 3. Corpora callosa basis comparison. Out of 54 basis vectors, the first few are shown. LoCA successfully captures the major shape deformations of the genu and splenium in the first four vectors, while both ICA and S-PCA spread this variation over several vectors.

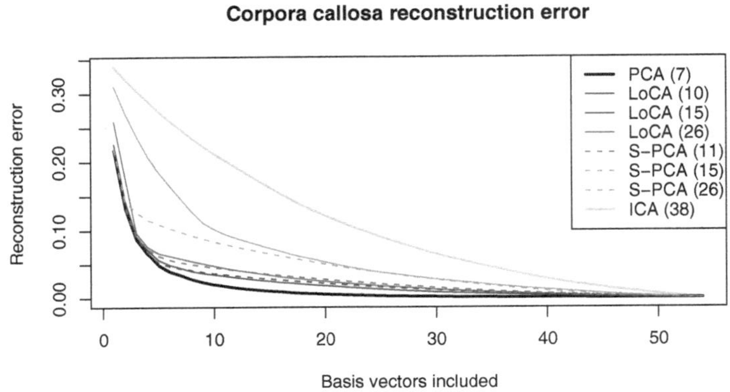

Fig. 4. Reconstruction error when using only the first k vectors of the basis. The numbers in parentheses denote the number of vectors required to capture 90% of variation in the data set. LoCA bases are compared with S-PCA bases which have essentially the same reconstruction error for 10, 15, or 26 vectors respectively. These choices correspond to the different λ settings used in Figure 2. Using fewer vectors, S-PCA has lower reconstruction error because the first few S-PCA vectors represent global deformations (as seen in Figure 2).

high spatial locality of S-PCA basis vectors. Also, more of them were required to describe the deformation of any extended surface region.

Corpora Callosa. 55 healthy subjects and HIV/AIDS patients received high-resolution magnetic resonance brain scans as part of a previously-described study [3]. The CC was manually traced on all scans using a reliable, repeatable protocol, and sparse landmarks were placed on all traces using the Witelson criteria [17]. 103 point correspondences were established between all CC traces based on the Witelson landmarks using a sparse-to-dense correspondence algorithm [18].

Figure 3 compares the basis vectors from each method that captured the most shape variation. PCA required 7 basis vectors for 90% of shape variation, while ICA required the most at 38. Note the global effects of PCA vectors, the extreme locality of ICA and S-PCA, and the spatially broader effects of LoCA. Major deformations of meaningful CC sub-regions, the genu and splenium, are represented by the first four LoCA vectors, while the next six represent deformations of the corpus callosum's long central body.

Reconstruction error for all methods is graphed in Figure 4. ICA requires a large number of components for accurate shape reconstruction, and PCA requires the fewest; S-PCA and LoCA require more basis vectors for bases that are more local or sparse (*i.e.*, higher λ). Note, however, that for comparable reconstruction error curves, S-PCA bases tend to contain global shape components while LoCA does not; for example, compare LoCA(26) and S-PCA(26) in Figures 4 and 2.

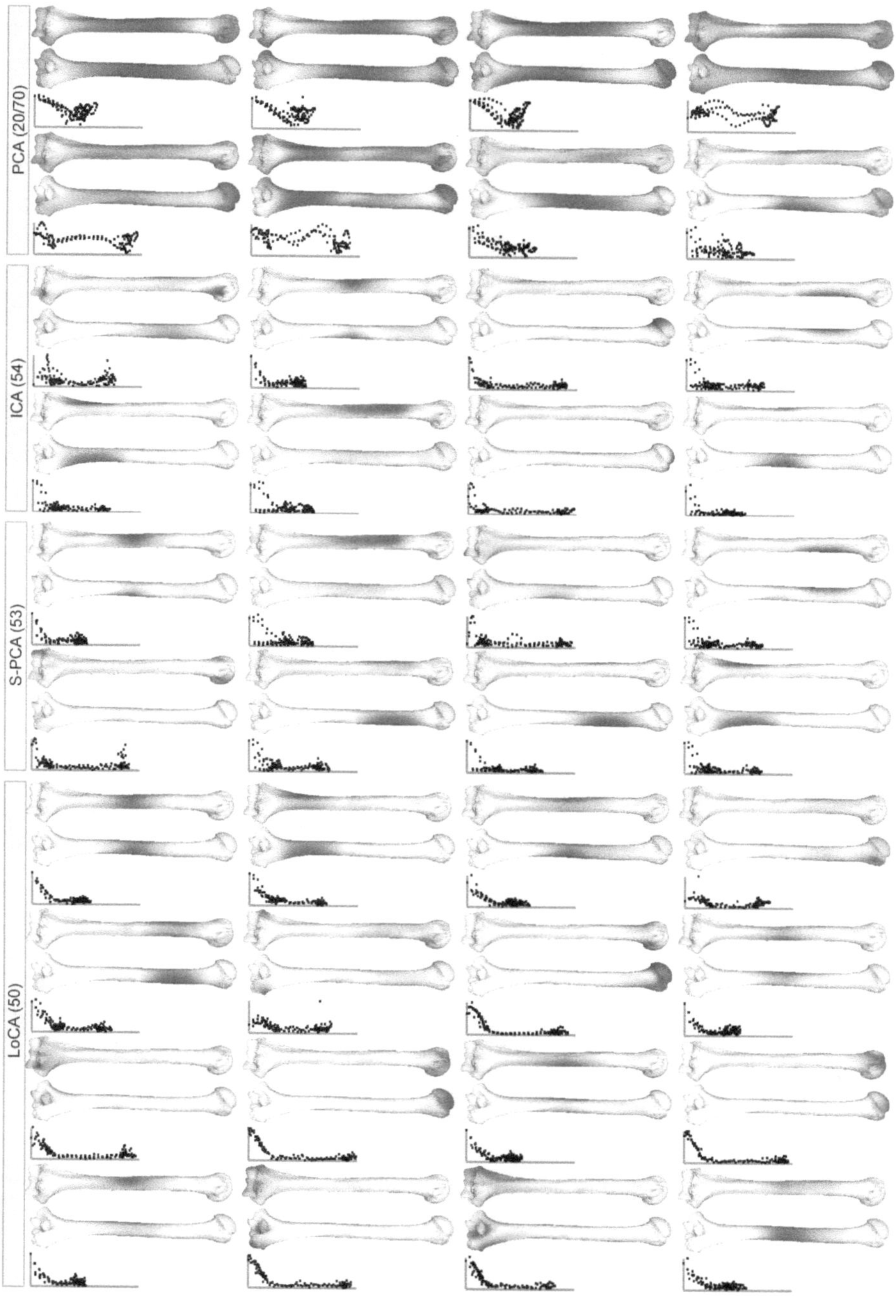

Fig. 5. Front and back views of displacements on primate humeri. Displacements of the landmark points are computed using different methods, and then interpolated onto the mesh using a thin-plate-spline. Darker locations indicate greater displacement magnitudes. LoCA components describe the articular surfaces at the two extremities as well as deformations of the shaft.

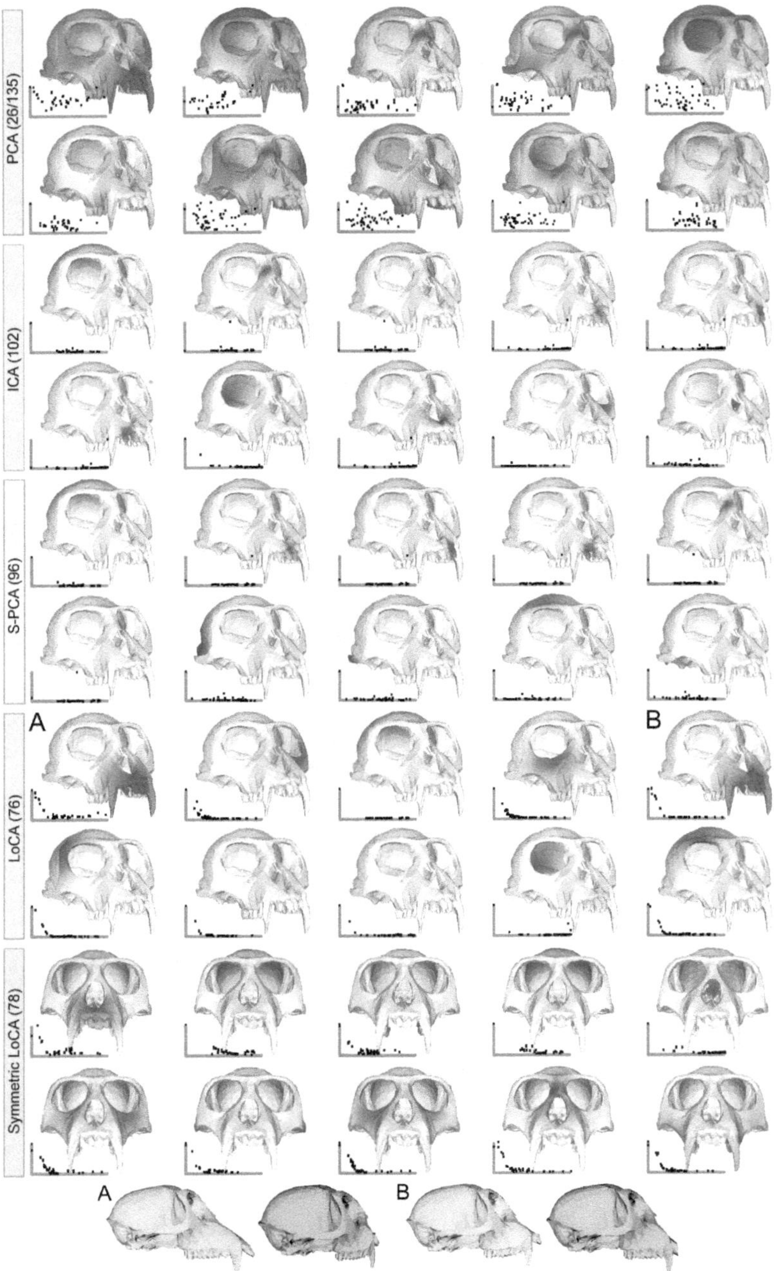

Fig. 6. Cranial basis comparison, colored by displacement magnitude. Both S-PCA and ICA produce vectors that move single teeth, while LoCA has vectors that move the entire jaw at once. The side views of vectors A and B differentiate their effects: A represents prognathism (snout elongation), while B represents facial kyphosis (teeth straightening). Note that since the crania are shown from a single angle, vectors representing motion on the bottom of the cranium appear completely white.

Humeri. 3D surface models of human, gorilla, and chimpanzee humerus bones were obtained by scanning the bones using a laser range scanner as part of a long-term project on of primate evolutionary morphology. The 3D models were annotated by a single human operator (D.A.) in a graphical interface by placing curves at anatomical landmarks on the shaft and proximal and distal extremities of the bone. A curve on the proximal extremity followed the length of the articular neck. Three curves were traced longitudinally along ridges that spanned the length of the shaft. On the distal extremity, curves followed the ridge of the olecranon fossa, the ridge along the medial limit of the trochlea, the ridge along the lateral limit of the capitulum, and the ridge between the trochlea and capitulum. Surface points sampled from these curves were the input to the shape parameterization methods.

The first few basis vectors of the results are shown in Figure 5. LoCA identified basis vectors that intuitively describe deformations of the two joint surfaces at the extremities, as well as deformations of sub-regions of the long body.

Colobine Monkey Crania. The shape space was built from a set of 235 crania from colobine monkeys (Subfamily *Colobinae*, Family *Cercopithecidae*), from six Asian species. Each cranium was marked with 45 corresponding landmark points. Various comparative primate morphologists manually marked each cranium with 45 landmark points using a Microscribe 3D digitizer [19], as part of data collection for a long-term project on Old World monkey cranial evolution. Results are shown in figure 6. The landmarks are shown on a *Colobus guereza* cranium, which is colored as in 5.

The usefulness of the compatibility matrix $\mathbf{B}$ for creating localized bases with higher-order characteristics is also illustrated in Figure 6. To encourage spatially symmetric components, landmark points were reflected across the midsagittal plane; *i.e.* points were transformed across the symmetry plane from the right to left side of the skull. Compatibility $\mathbf{B}[i, j]$ was computed between the reflected points, so that two points at corresponding locations across the midsagittal plane (*e.g.*, right and left cheek) were highly compatible. The resulting "Symmetric LoCA" basis intuitively captures shape variability in corresponding right and left skull features in each component.

5 Discussion

LoCA provided a superior trade-off of conciseness and locality than ICA or S-PCA for a broad range of data sets, at a cost of greater computation time. Future work will focus on designing compatibility matrices for a wide range of shape applications, using non-geodesic distance metrics and user-defined object regions of interest. We will also generate localized bases whose vectors vary significantly in their spatial suppport; currently, the range of possible spatial supports is limited to a degree by the distance modulating function f.

References

1. Carmichael, O.T., Thompson, P.M., Dutton, R.A., Lu, A., Lee, S.E., Lee, J.Y., Kuller, L.H., Lopez, O.L., Aizenstein, H.J., Meltzer, C.C., Liu, Y., Toga, A.W., Becker, J.T.: Mapping ventricular changes related to dementia and mild cognitive impairment in a large community-based cohort. In: IEEE International Symposium on Biomedical Imaging (ISBI) (2006)
2. Curran-Everett, D.: Multiple comparisons: philosophies and illustrations. Am. J Physiol Regul Integr Comp. Physiol 279(1), R1–R8 (2000)
3. Thompson, P., Dutton, R., Hayashi, K., Lu, A., Lee, S., Lee, J., Lopez, O., Aizenstein, H., Toga, A., Becker, J.: 3d mapping of ventricular and corpus callosum abnormalities in hiv/aids. NeuroImage 31(1), 12–23 (2006)
4. Cootes, T.F., Hill, A., Taylor, C.J., Haslam, J.: The use of active shape models for locating structures in medical images. Image and Vision Computing 12(6), 355–366 (1994)
5. Bookstein, F.L.: Morphometric tools for landmark data: Geometry and Biology. Cambridge Univ. Press, New York (1991)
6. Allen, B., Curless, B., Popovic, Z.: The space of human body shapes: reconstruction and parameterization from range scans. In: Proceedings of ACM SIGGRAPH, pp. 587–594 (2003)
7. Chennubhotla, C., Jepson, A.: Sparse PCA: Extracting multi-scale structure from data. Proc. ICCV, Vancouver, pp. 641–647. IEEE, Washington, DC, USA (2001)
8. Zou, H., Hastie, T., Tibshirani, R.: Sparse principal component analysis. Journal of Computational and Graphical Statistics 15(2), 265–286 (2006)
9. Sjöstrand, K., Stegmann, M.B., Larsen, R.: Sparse principal component analysis in medical shape modeling. In: Reinhardt, J.M., Pluim, J.P.W. (eds.): In:Proc. SPIE Medical Imaging: Image Processing. vol. 6144 (2006)
10. Johnstone, I.M., Lu, A.Y.: Sparse principal components analysis. In: Proceedings, IMS Mini-Meeting on Functional Data Analysis, (2003)`http://www.stat.ufl.edu/symposium/2003/fundat/Archive/`
11. Stegmann, M.B., Sjöstrand, K., Larsen, R.: Sparse modeling of landmark and texture variability using the orthomax criterion. In: Reinhardt, J.M., Pluim, J.P.W., eds.: Proc. SPIE Medical Imaging: Image Processing. vol. 6144 (2006)
12. Üzümcü, M., Frangi, A., Sonka, M., Reiber, J., Lelieveldt, B.: ICA vs. In: Ellis, R.E., Peters, T.M. (eds.) MICCAI 2003. LNCS, vol. 2878, pp. 451–458. Springer, Heidelberg (2003)
13. Ballester, M.A.G., Linguraru, M.G., Aguirre, M.R., Ayache, N.: On the adequacy of principal factor analysis for the study of shape variability. In: Fitzpatrick, J.M., Reinhardt, J.M., eds.: In: Proc. SPIE Medical Imaging: Image Processing. vol. 5747 (2005)
14. Vermaak, J., Perez, P.: Constrained subspace modeling. In: Conf. Computer Vision and Pattern Recog, CVPR'03, Madison, Wisconsin (June 2003)
15. Pizer, S., Fritsch, D., Yushkevich, P., Johnson, V., Chaney, E., Gerig, G.: Segmentation, registration, and measurement of shape variation via image object shape. IEEE Trans. Med. Imaging 18(10), 851–865 (1999)
16. Press, W., Teukolsky, S., Vetterling, F.B.: Numerical Recipes In C, 2nd edn. Cambridge University Press, Cambridge (1992)
17. Witelson, S.: Hand and sex differences in the isthmus and body of the corpus callosum: a postmortem morphological study. Brain 112, 799–835 (1989)

18. Ghosh, D., Amenta, N.: Landmark transfer using deformable models. Technical Report CSE-2007-6, Department of Computer Science, University of California, Davis (2007)
19. Frost, S.R., Marcus, L.F., Bookstein, F.L., Reddy, D.P., Delson, E.: Cranial allometry, phylogeography, and systematics of large-bodied papionins (primates: Cercopitihecinae) inferred from geometric morphometric analysis of landmark data. The Antatomical Record Part A 275A, pp. 1048–1072 (2003)

Regional Appearance in Deformable Model Segmentation

Joshua V. Stough, Robert E. Broadhurst,
Stephen M. Pizer, and Edward L. Chaney

Medical Image Display & Analysis Group (MIDAG)
University of North Carolina, Chapel Hill NC 27599, USA
stough@cs.unc.edu

Abstract. Automated medical image segmentation is a challenging task that benefits from the use of effective image appearance models. In this paper, we compare appearance models at three regional scales for statistically characterizing image intensity near object boundaries in the context of segmentation via deformable models. The three models capture appearance in the form of regional intensity quantile functions. These distribution-based regional image descriptors are amenable to Euclidean methods such as principal component analysis, which we use to build the statistical appearance models.

The first model uses two regions, the interior and exterior of the organ of interest. The second model accounts for exterior inhomogeneity by clustering on object-relative local intensity quantile functions to determine tissue-consistent regions relative to the organ boundary. The third model analyzes these image descriptors per geometrically defined local region.

To evaluate the three models, we present segmentation results on bladders and prostates in CT in the context of day-to-day adaptive radiotherapy for the treatment of prostate cancer. Results show improved segmentations with more local regions, probably because smaller regions better represent local inhomogeneity in the intensity distribution near the organ boundary.

1 Introduction

Automated segmentation of objects in medical images is a challenging task that benefits from the use of effective image appearance models. Some models that have shown success are those that analyze intensity patterns with respect to larger-than-voxel-scale regions of the image in the vicinity of and including the organ of interest. Such methods are compatible with the idea that the appearance of an organ in an image is in part a function of the position and intensities of neighboring organs and volumes and their tissue mixtures. In this paper we compare appearance models at three regional scales that statistically characterize image intensity near object boundaries for use in deformable model segmentation.

In Bayesian deformable model segmentation, a geometric model for an object of interest is deformed via its shape parameters to fit the image data. The

N. Karssemeijer and B. Lelieveldt (Eds.): IPMI 2007, LNCS 4584, pp. 532–543, 2007.
© Springer-Verlag Berlin Heidelberg 2007

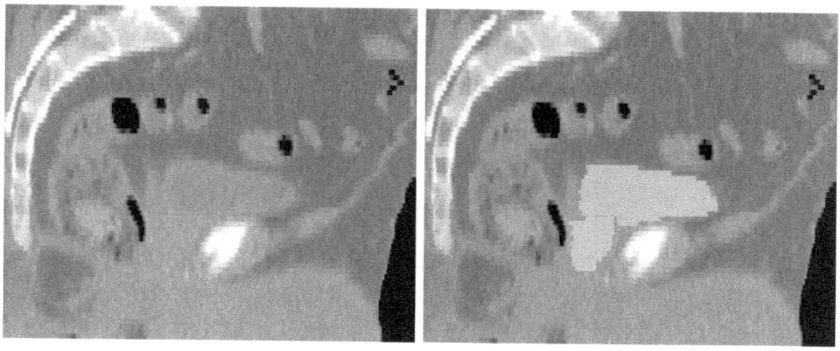

Fig. 1. Example sagittal CT slice of the male pelvis (left), with the bladder and prostate highlighted (right). Note the lack of contrast around the organs of interest.

optimization proceeds according to an objective function that includes a term measuring geometry-to-image match, or "image match" for short, which is the result of the image appearance model. Some previous image matches depend on a voxel-scale dense correspondence across training cases. Such image matches include those based on intensity profiles that are either associated with individual image points [1] or averaged over similar image points [2], and those based on tuples that are formed from intensity-derived features at an ordered collection of these points [3]. These schemes are effective in situations where objects have a consistent voxel-scale structural relationship with one another. However, in segmenting organs in the male pelvis for example, one cannot expect the same tissue-mixture at a voxel-scale correspondence (see Fig. 1).

Region-based methods address this concern by modeling intensity distributions in object-relative regions. These approaches typically sample image intensities within the object interior or separately the interior and exterior. Some of the resulting intensity models use foreground/background intensity ranges [4], or use summary statistics such as mean and variance [5] [6]. Such simplifications of regional intensity distributions limit the information captured by the appearance model. Recently developed methods use an appropriate parameterization of the full intensity distribution for a region and either compute an image match with respect to a single reference distribution [7] [8], or directly model the variability in the intensity distribution as seen in training [9].

In [9] the authors sample from the interior and exterior regions and convert the resulting distributions to regional intensity quantile functions (RIQFs), which are amenable to linear statistical methods such as principal component analysis (PCA). Their appearance model is then based on probabilities of the regional distributions. As with previous approaches, the method has a significant drawback: the use of a single global exterior. Any such model oversimplifies the appearance by failing to account for the inhomogeneity in the local intensity distributions exterior to the object. While it may be reasonable to model intensities in the interior of an organ as samples from a single distribution, the exterior may consist of neighboring organs, bones, and fat and connective tissue, the intensities of which should not be considered samples from a single source. While using a single exterior has the advantage of a more stable approximation of appearance, this must be balanced against the lack of positional sensitivity that more local regions provide.

In this paper we explore this balance by experimentally comparing the efficacy in segmentation of image models at three scales. The three models use RIQFs to capture intensity distribution variability. As a baseline for comparison, the first model, "global", uses two regions, the interior and exterior of the organ of interest, as in [9]. The second model, "local-clustered", attempts to reflect the inhomogeneity in the intensity distribution around the exterior by determining local distribution-consistent region types relative to the object boundary. The region types are formed by clustering on local RIQFs. We then partition the object boundary according to region type and apply PCA on the cluster populations. For the third model, "local-geometric", we separately train the intensity distribution and its variability at each object-relative local region.

Section 2 reviews the intensity quantile methodology and describes the three image appearance models. Section 3 describes the segmentation framework and presents results on bladders and prostates in CT in the context of adaptive radiotherapy for prostate cancer. In section 4, we conclude and posit future directions.

2 Quantile Functions and Image Match

We begin with a description of RIQFs, followed by details of the three appearance models. For each regional scale we will construct the image match function.

2.1 Regional Intensity Quantile Functions

[9] describes an approach to image match that probabilistically represents the appearance of an object in an image. The basic unit of appearance is the regional intensity quantile function (RIQF), derived from the intensity histogram within an object-relative region, such as the interior near the object boundary. Quantile functions are a useful parameterization of one-dimensional distributions. For example, RIQFs have the advantage that certain common changes in a distribution, such as mean shift and variance scaling, are represented as linear changes in the RIQF feature space. Given the RIQFs from a region corresponding across image cases, PCA can therefore be used to characterize the variability in that region's intensity distribution.

We briefly review the construction of the RIQF in the context of the distance metric that provides linearity. Let q and r be the continuous, one-dimensional intensity distributions in two regions between which we wish to measure the similarity. The Mallows distance [10] between q and r, with cumulative distribution functions Q and R, respectively, is defined as

$$M_p(q,r) = \left(\int_0^1 |Q^{-1}(t) - R^{-1}(t)|^p dt \right)^{1/p} . \tag{1}$$

An n-dimensional RIQF is then the discretized inverse cumulative distribution function on intensities in a region, i.e., $Q^{-1}(t)$ or $R^{-1}(t)$ in the above equation. Let these discretized quantile functions be denoted $\mathbf{q}$ or $\mathbf{r}$. Coordinate j of $\mathbf{q}$ or $\mathbf{r}$ stores the average of the $[\frac{j-1}{n}, \frac{j}{n}]$ quantile of the intensity distribution for that region, i.e, $\mathbf{q}_j = \int_{(j-1)/n}^{j/n} Q^{-1}(t)dt$. After discretization, the Mallows distance above corresponds (up to a scale factor) to the L_p vector norm between $\mathbf{q}$ and $\mathbf{r}$,

$$M_p(q,r) \approx \left(\frac{1}{n} \sum_{j=1}^{n} ||\mathbf{q}_j - \mathbf{r}_j||^p \right)^{(1/p)} . \tag{2}$$

Through quantile functions, regional intensity distributions are understood as points in an n-dimensional Euclidean space in which distance corresponds to the M_2 metric, and mean and variance changes in intensities are linear.

2.2 Global Regions

In the following sections we describe the construction of the RIQF training populations and the image match used in segmentation, for each of the global, local-clustered, and local-geometric appearance models. The image match itself in each case is a sum over regions of log probabilities in the context of Bayesian deformable model segmentation (sec. 3.1). Our data consist of CT images of the male pelvic region and corresponding manual segmentations of bladders and prostates used for training both the shape and appearance models (sec. 3). Each object is trained separately.

With the global regions model we analyze the intensity patterns near the organ boundary, interior and exterior to it. For each training image I_p, we construct the RIQFs $\mathbf{q}^{in,p}$ and $\mathbf{q}^{out,p}$ through sampling relative to the manual segmentation. The contribution of a voxel is Gaussian weighted by its distance to the surface. The σ for this voxel weighting is a parameter of the training: ours is such that the contribution is negligible farther than 1 cm. We then apply PCA separately to the two RIQF sets,$\{\mathbf{q}^{in,p}, \forall p\}$ and $\{\mathbf{q}^{out,p}, \forall p\}$, to obtain Gaussian models of the intensity variation inside and outside the organ. For segmenting a target case then, the image is similarly sampled relative to a prospective model. We treat the two regions as though they were independent, so the match computed is the sum of the log probabilities of the interior and exterior target RIQFs.

2.3 Local-Clustered Regions

The impetus for the local-clustered appearance model [11] is that more local regions will better specify the exterior than the common single homogeneous region approach. The question is what constitutes a region. For our purposes, consider that an organ or other volume whose local intensity distributions are distinguishable from those of neighboring volumes constitutes such a region. Examples of such volumes are neighboring organs and fat deposits. These regions

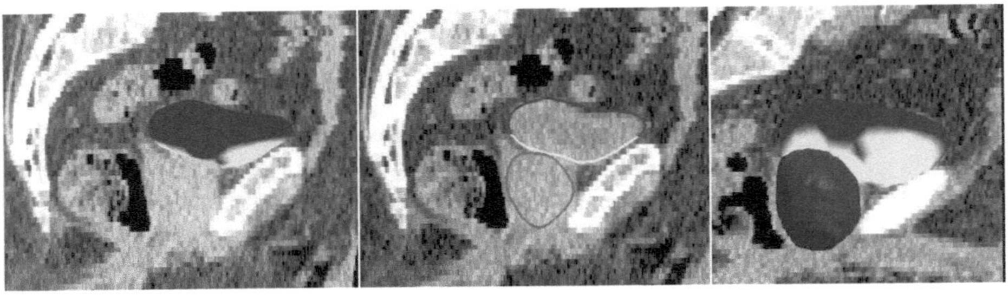

Fig. 2. Sagittal views of a male pelvis in CT, with bladder boundary colored by region type. Left: a 3D view. Middle: the in-plane contour also colored by region type, with the prostate shown for reference. Right: an off-sagittal 3D view of the same bladder, now with the prostate also in 3D and in the foreground.

are a cause of intensity inhomogeneity in the organ exterior. We avoid modeling the 3D shapes of these regions and for our appearance model consider them only as they affect the local distributions near the boundary of the object of interest. We determine region types, corresponding to these different organs and volumes, through clustering on the RIQFs of smaller regions.

Over all training images I_p, we compute RIQFs $\mathbf{q}^{i,p}$ for many local exterior regions anchored to individual geometrically defined points on the object boundary indexed by i. The interior of the object is treated as one region. As in the global case, the contribution of a voxel to $\mathbf{q}^{i,p}$ is weighted by its distance to the surface but further is equal to zero if its closest point on the surface is not close enough to point i–ensuring locality. Computing these weights involves minimal additional computation through our sampling scheme (see sec. 3.1). Parameters for this model are the density of points on the surface and the "close enough" distance, in addition to the Gaussian distance weight of the global region model.

We then cluster the pooled set of RIQFs for all boundary points and images, $\{\mathbf{q}^{i,p}, \forall i, p\}$, using Fuzzy C-means Clustering [12]. The Euclidean feature space distances inherent in this method hold for RIQFs (see sec. 2.1). We specify

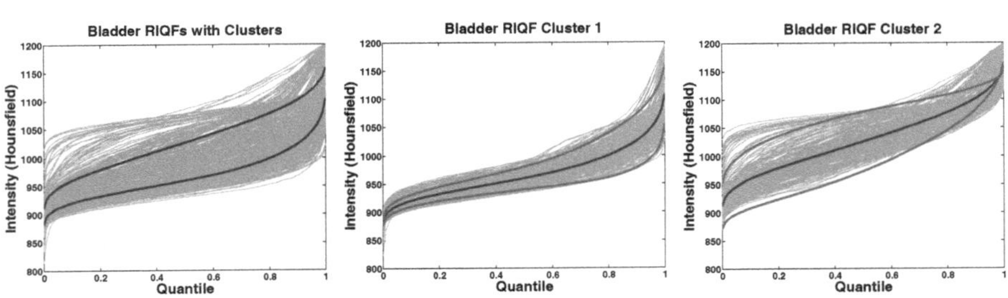

Fig. 3. Clustering on local RIQFs for the bladder exterior. Left shows the pooled data with cluster centers overlaid (two clusters). The middle and right images show the two cluster populations with mean and ± 2 standard deviations overlaid. The reasonable separation into lighter and darker distributions is evidenced in Fig. 2.

the number of clusters. The results are the set of RIQF cluster centers $\{\mu_k\}$ and cluster membership scores $\{u_k^{i,p}, \forall i, p\}$ over all positions and images that minimize the sum of score-weighted distance in the M_2 metric used:

$$\{\mu_k\} = \min_{\{\tilde{\mu}_1, \ldots, \tilde{\mu}_K \in \Re^n\}} \sum_{\forall i,p} \sum_{k=1}^{K} u_k^{i,p} * ||\mathbf{q}^{i,p} - \tilde{\mu}_k||^2, \tag{3}$$

with $u_k^{i,p} \in [0,1]$ and $\sum_k u_k^{i,p} = 1$ for given i and p.

The last two steps for training the local-clustered model are to partition the object boundary according to representative region type and to separately characterize the variability in the cluster populations. To partition the object model boundary, we use the explicit correspondence across training cases required of our shape model (see sec. 3.1). Each point i is assigned the region type/cluster center k that maximizes $\sum_p u_k^{i,p}$, the sum of cluster membership scores for that point over all images. Finally, we perform PCA on the individual cluster populations, resulting in Gaussian models of the RIQF variability per region type. Each point i is then assigned the PCA model of its cluster.

During target segmentation, the image is sampled relative to a prospective model to populate the set of RIQFs $\{\mathbf{q}^i, \forall i\}$. For each point i, we compute the probability of $\mathbf{q}^i$ with respect to the principal modes and variances of that point's region type. The image match is then the sum of the log probabilities over all points, weighted by the points' comparative importance (related to how many voxels contributed to each local RIQF).

Confirming evidence for this approach is found in the spatial distribution of region-type on the boundary that we observe in training. When we look for two clusters on the bladder data (Fig. 3), the resultant boundary partition corresponds to lighter and darker local distribution areas (Fig. 2). This is anatomically justified because the bladder is surrounded mostly by lower intensity bowel and fat, with much brighter tissue from the pubic bone area and prostate inferior to it. There is similar evidence for the prostate, which has brighter tissue exterior to it in the pubic bones areas and bladder, with darker tissue elsewhere.

2.4 Local-Geometric Regions

A problem with the global model is that through considering only a single exterior region it sacrifices all positional sensitivity. The appearance model is not specific enough, in that there could be many large-scale regions with the same aggregate tissue mixture. The local-clustered model attempts to capture the exterior inhomogeneity and replaces a single Gaussian model of intensity with a number of local region-type Gaussian models, thus leading to a better specified appearance. However, when we analyze the RIQF data we see that these region-types still over-generalize the local intensity distribution at many particular points on the object boundary. Figure 4 shows a point's regional data relative to the cluster populations. Neither cluster population is representative

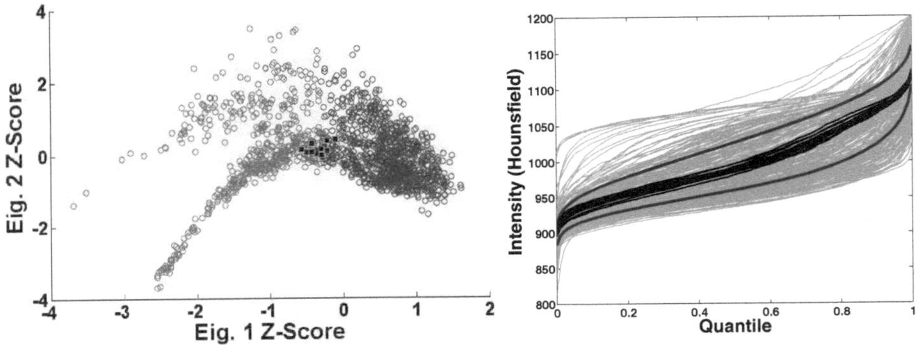

Fig. 4. Plots showing the over-generalization of the local-clustered scheme, for bladder data. Left shows the data projected onto the first two eigen directions of the pooled PCA space, colored according to cluster type (two clusters). Right shows the pooled curve plots, with cluster centers. The highlighted data are the local RIQFs for a particular geometrically corresponding point across training. Note that either cluster population poorly represents that point's variability.

of that point's variability; yet the RIQFs themselves are tightly grouped (at least in that projection). So we must use an even more specific model.

The local-geometric appearance model addresses the weaknesses of both previous models. In training, the local RIQFs are sampled as in the local-clustered model. However in this scheme, we analyze the variability at each point on its own, applying PCA to the set $\{\mathbf{q}^{i,p}, \forall p\}$, for each point i, thereby constructing a more specific Gaussian model for each local region. At target time then, we treat the local regions as though they were independent. We compute a probability for each point i with respect to the principal modes and variances of that point's PCA model. The image match is then the weighted sum of log probabilities, as in the previous models.

3 Experimental Results

We compare the efficacy of the three appearance models in the context of deformable model segmentation of bladders and prostates. These organs present a very challenging segmentation problem due to the lack of contrast between the bladder and prostate and the large variability of the bladder across days (Fig. 1). We run the same experiment three times, with the only difference being the image match model. Our data consists of five patient image sets, each of approximately 16 daily CT scans of the male pelvic area taken during radiotherapy courses. The images have an in-plane resolution of 512 × 512 with voxel dimensions of 0.98 mm × 0.98 mm and an inter-slice distance of 3 mm. We also are provided expert manual segmentations of the bladder and prostate in every image. We consider the patients separately, segmenting the images from one patient in a leave-one-day-out study, where training is based on all days for the patient except the target day. In section 3.1 we discuss our segmentation framework. In section 3.2 we present segmentation results.

3.1 The Segmentation Framework

In this section we discuss our shape model, its use in segmentation, and the particular parameters of our experiment. We use discrete medial representations, or "m-rep", models to describe the shape of prostates and bladders [13]. An m-rep is a discretely sampled grid of medial atoms, where each atom consists of a hub and two equal-length spokes. The boundary of the object model passes orthogonally through the spoke ends. Properties, such as spoke length and orientation, are interpolated between atoms in the grid. The model defines a coordinate system which provides an explicit correspondence between deformations of the same m-rep model (e.g., those m-reps making up a training set) and the 3D volume in the object boundary region. This leads to a constructive approach to sampling an image relative to an object, stepping along profiles normal to the surface that are provided by the m-rep.

To extract m-reps from images, we perform Bayesian deformable model segmentation, with a semi-automatic initialization [13]. To start, a mean bladder or prostate model is positioned in a target image using a similarity transform computed from two prostate landmarks. After initialization, we optimize the posterior $p(m|I)$ of the geometric parameters given the image data. This is equivalent to optimizing the sum of the log prior $p(m)$ and the log likelihood $p(I|m)$, which measure geometric typicality and image match, respectively. Geometric typicality and the initial mean models are based on the statistics of m-rep deformation over the training set [14].

There are several parameters that specify the appearance models we use. The choice of region depth has already been discussed. For the clustered and geometric local models, we use a boundary point density that places 306 points on the bladder model surface and 290 on the prostate at fixed object relative coordinates. We set the number of clusters to be two for both object exteriors (see sec. 2.3). Our experiments show that while small changes in these parameters do affect specific results, they do not change the overall conclusions.

3.2 Segmentation Results

We consider the relative segmentation accuracy of the three appearance models by comparing automatically generated results against the expert manual segmentations. As our measures, we use average surface distance (ASD) and volume overlap given by the Dice Similarity Coefficient (DSC) [15], which is intersection over average. We will describe the results of the global model, then the local-clustered model relative to the first, and finally the local-geometric appearance model relative to the first two. Tables 1 and 2 show bladder and prostate results for each patient and appearance model, while Fig. 5 contains trend graphs over the pooled patient data.

Table 1. Bladder median overlap and surface distance per patient. See sec. 3.2 for meaning of the abbreviations.

Patient	GlobDSC	ClustDSC	LocalDSC	GlobASD	ClustASD	LocalASD
1	91.0%	92.0	93.1	1.43mm	1.50	1.16
2	93.5	93.6	94.0	1.23	1.15	1.09
3	90.9	91.3	92.8	1.58	1.48	1.21
4	93.7	93.9	95.1	1.16	1.14	0.92
5	89.7	89.9	90.9	2.13	1.98	1.80

Table 2. Prostate median overlap and surface distance per patient

Patient	GlobDSC	ClustDSC	LocalDSC	GlobASD	ClustASD	LocalASD
1	90.2%	91.8	90.7	0.98mm	0.82	0.93
2	92.0	92.3	94.2	1.34	1.26	0.97
3	92.3	92.0	93.0	0.95	0.94	0.83
4	93.9	94.2	94.2	0.97	0.93	0.90
5	91.3	90.0	91.9	1.59	1.78	1.44

The global interior/exterior appearance model results in a median volume overlap of 91.2% for bladders and 92.1% for prostates, with an overlap greater than 90% in about 50 of 80 total target bladders and 60 of 80 prostates. In terms of average surface distance, global regions results in a median ASD of 1.40mm for bladders and 1.03mm for prostates with 50 of 80 bladders and 65 of 80 prostates having ASD less than 1.5mm. These results are good in the context of the male pelvis in CT, exceeding the agreement we observe between experts.

Segmentations using the local-clustered regions appearance scheme improve upon the global results in 57.5% (46 of 80) of bladders and 53.8% (43 of 80) of prostates over all patients. Considered separately (as they are trained and segmented), this appearance model improves bladder and prostate segmentations in a majority of three of the five patient image sets. In the successful patients, bladders are improved in 68.1% (30 of 44) of images while prostates are improved in 67.3% (33 of 49). These results are encouraging considering that even in the patient sets that are not improved in a majority of the images, the results are not significantly worse (see Tables 1 and 2).

The local-geometric model notably improves results over the first two methods, as evidenced in Fig. 5. In every cumulative measure, this method provides better fits overall. As well, the tables show that in terms of both volume overlap and average surface distance measures, local-geometric is the best method in 4 of 5 patient prostate sets and all 5 patient bladder sets. The improvements are more pronounced in the bladder because there is more room for improvement. The prostate's mostly rigid day-to-day change is well captured by the initial transform in the segmentation algorithm (sec. 3.1).

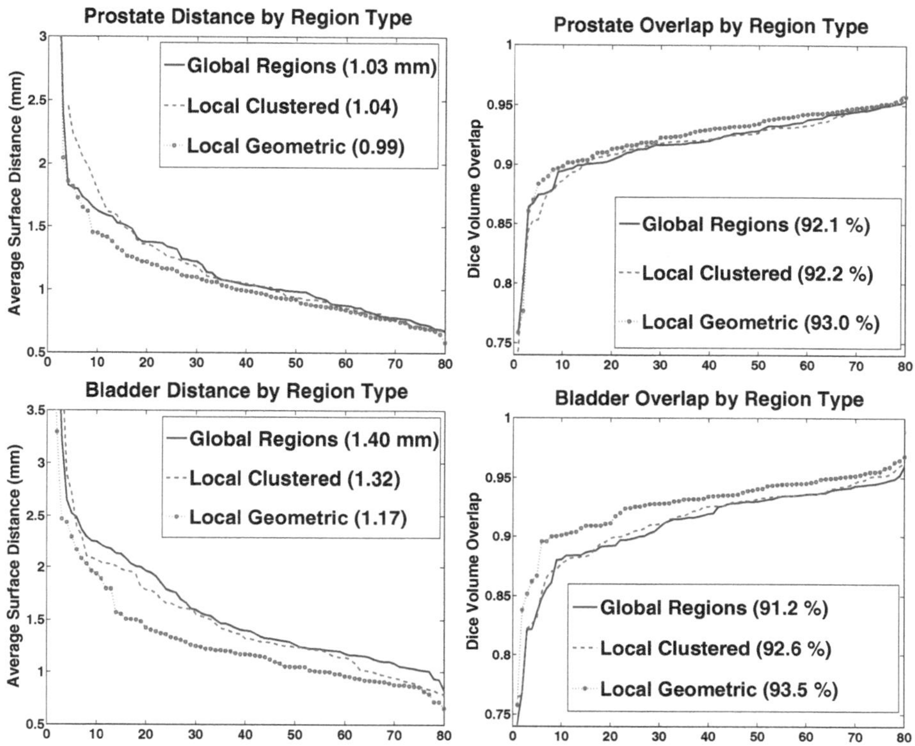

Fig. 5. Comparisons of the three appearance models by organ (prostate and bladder by row), average surface distance (left column) and volume overlap (right column). The comparisons are with respect to expert manual segmentations. The data for each model is sorted independently over all patients to show trends, so the abscissa is image number and does not correspond across models. The numbers in parentheses are median values. While the local-clustered model just outperforms the global, the local-geometric appearance model is clearly superior.

4 Conclusions

In this paper, we compared the efficacy of three statistical appearance models based on RIQFs, where the difference in the models is in regional scale. The first model, the common global interior/exterior regions approach, provides good results and is computationally inexpensive. However, it is not a realistic model, in that it assumes the exterior of an organ has no distinguishing features which can be useful to segmentation. The second model, local-clustered, gives a boundary partition consistent with anatomy and leads to somewhat improved results over the global method. However, this model imposes an inaccurate appearance on many particular local regions. The final appearance model, which analyzes the RIQFs per local region, provides the most specific local appearance at every point and results in the best segmentations overall.

Our analysis asserts several directions for continuing research. One area of future research is to control the kind of distribution variability we are attempting to capture in the RIQF framework. PCA and Euclidean clustering on quantile functions is appropriate only to the extent that the variability in the observed distributions is captured by operations that are linear in the RIQF feature space. Some variability, such as changes in the mixture of multiple sources, is non-linear in this space, so it should be accounted for prior to PCA. At the moment when we train with the local-geometric appearance model, we do not explicitly ensure mixture-consistent regions. In the local-clustered model we may get some mixture-consistency in the cluster in that there is distance between observed distributions that differ in mixture.

A key to improving the performance of the local regional methods is correspondence. The geometric correspondence the methods rely on is a baseline for finding what local image intensity distributions to expect, but the *image* correspondence comes from how the neighboring objects are configured with respect to the object of interest. The image correspondence is in general too strongly tied to the geometric correspondence. For example, the region representing the bladder may change position relative to the prostate surface across days, while the geometric correspondence of the prostates will not. The result is a false association of bladder type and non-bladder type distributions based upon geometric correspondence that is a source of confusion in the appearance model. We will address this problem through an extended local-clustered approach, where we model the changes in the region type partition on the object surface.

Other ongoing research involves both the joint modeling of the local RIQFs, which would obviate the assumption of independence in our image match, and a multiscale segmentation scheme that takes advantage of the positional sensitivity the local regions provide. Finally, we look to improve the local-clustered method through better clustering in the space of local RIQFs, such as that proposed by [16]. We would like a clustering that captures the disparate shapes and relative counts of the ideal cluster populations–bone, bowel, fat, etc., rather than only light versus dark RIQFs.

Acknowledgements

We are grateful for algorithmic and code contributions from Gregg Tracton and Graham Gash. We thank Joshua Levy for authoring the software pipeline allowing for fast processing of our data set. Finally, we thank the reviewers for their thoughtful comments. This work was funded under NIBIB P01 EB02779.

References

1. Cootes, T.F., Cooper, D., Taylor, C.J., Graham, J.: Active shape models - their training and application. Computer Vision and Image Understanding 61(1), 38–59 (1995)
2. Stough, J., Pizer, S.M., Chaney, E.L., Rao, M.: Clustering on image boundary regions for deformable model segmentation. In: IEEE International Symposium on Biomedical Imaging (ISBI) (2004)

3. Scott, I.M., Cootes, T.F., Taylor, C.J.: Improving appearance model matching using local image structure. In: Taylor, C.J., Noble, J.A. (eds.) IPMI 2003. LNCS, vol. 2732, pp. 258–269. Springer, Heidelberg (2003)
4. Zhu, S.C., Yuille, A.L.: Region competition: Unifying snakes, region growing, and bayes/MDL for multiband image segmentation. IEEE Transactions on Pattern Analysis and Machine Intelligence 18(9), 884–900 (1996)
5. Tsai, A., Anthony Yezzi, J., Wells, W., Tempany, C., Tucker, D., Fan, A., Grimson, W.E., Willsky, A.: A shape-based approach to the segmentation of medical imagery using level sets. IEEE Transactions on Medical Imaging 22(2), 137–154 (2003)
6. Chan, T.F., Vese, L.A.: Active contours without edges. IEEE Transactions on Image Processing 10(2), 266–277 (2001)
7. Freedman, D., Radke, R.J., Zhang, T., Jeong, Y., Lovelock, D.M., Chen, G.T.Y.: Model-based segmentation of medical imagery by matching distributions. IEEE Transactions on Medical Imaging 24(3), 281–292 (2005)
8. Rubner, Y., Puzicha, J., Tomasi, C., Buhmann, J.M.: Empirical evaluation of dissimilarity measures for color and texture. Computer Vision and Image Understanding 84, 25–43 (2001)
9. Broadhurst, R.E., Stough, J., Pizer, S.M., Chaney, E.L.: A statistical appearance model based on intensity quantile histograms. In: IEEE International Symposium on Biomedical Imaging (ISBI) (2006)
10. Levina, E.: Statistical Issues in Texture Analysis. PhD thesis, University of California at Berkley (2002)
11. Stough, J.V., Broadhurst, R.E., Pizer, S.M., Chaney, E.L.: Clustering on local appearance for deformable model segmentation. In: IEEE International Symposium on Biomedical Imaging (ISBI) (2007)
12. Bezdec, J.C.: Pattern Recognition with Fuzzy Objective Function Algorithms. Plenum Press, New York (1981)
13. Pizer, S.M., Fletcher, T., Fridman, Y., Fritsch, D.S., Gash, A.G., Glotzer, J.M., Joshi, S., Thall, A., Tracton, G., Yushkevich, P., Chaney, E.L.: Deformable m-reps for 3d medical image segmentation. International Journal of Computer Vision - Special UNC-MIDAG issue 55(2), 85–106 (2003)
14. Fletcher, P.T., Lu, C., Pizer, S.M., Joshi, S.: Principal geodesic analysis for the study of nonlinear statistics of shape. IEEE Transactions on Medical Imaging 23(8), 995–1005 (2004)
15. Dice, L.R.: Measures of the amount of ecologic association between species. Ecology 26, 297–302 (1945)
16. Gath, I., Geva, A.: Unsupervised optimal fuzzy clustering. IEEE Transactions on Pattern Analysis and Machine Intelligence 11(7), 773–780 (1989)

Fully Automated Registration of First-Pass Myocardial Perfusion MRI Using Independent Component Analysis

J. Milles[1], R.J. van der Geest[1], M. Jerosch-Herold[2], J.H.C. Reiber[1], and B.P.F. Lelieveldt[1]

[1] Division of Image Processing, Department of Radiology, Leiden University Medical Center, Leiden, The Netherlands
J.R.Milles@lumc.nl
[2] Advanced Imaging Research Center, Oregon Health & Science University, Portland, USA

Abstract. This paper presents a novel method for registration of cardiac perfusion MRI. The presented method successfully corrects for breathing motion without any manual interaction using Independent Component Analysis to extract physiologically relevant features together with their time-intensity behavior. A time-varying reference image mimicking intensity changes in the data of interest is computed based on the results of ICA, and used to compute the displacement caused by breathing for each frame. Qualitative and quantitative validation of the method is carried out using 46 clinical quality, short-axis, perfusion MR datasets comprising 100 images each. Validation experiments showed a reduction of the average LV motion from 1.26±0.87 to 0.64±0.46 pixels. Time-intensity curves are also improved after registration with an average error reduced from 2.65±7.89% to 0.87±3.88% between registered data and manual gold standard. We conclude that this fully automatic ICA-based method shows an excellent accuracy, robustness and computation speed, adequate for use in a clinical environment.

1 Introduction

The use of first-pass, gadolinium-enhanced, myocardial perfusion magnetic resonance imaging (MRI) for early ischemia detection has been proposed in the early years of that imaging modality [1]. This acquisition technique has now been clinically validated and offers a valid non-invasive alternative to SPECT and PET for the assessment of myocardial perfusion [2, 3, 4]. However, requirement of perfusion MRI is to image every slice every heartbeat. As a result little time is available for image acquisition, leading to poor image quality.

First-pass myocardial perfusion MR image sequences can be roughly decomposed in 4 main phases shown in Figure 1. Those phases present different contrast according to the circulation of the contrast agent. The first frames, before contrast agent reaches the heart ventricles, mainly show the surrounding organs and the heart inner anatomy is barely visible. Then contrast agent enters the myocardium

N. Karssemeijer and B. Lelieveldt (Eds.): IPMI 2007, LNCS 4584, pp. 544–555, 2007.
© Springer-Verlag Berlin Heidelberg 2007

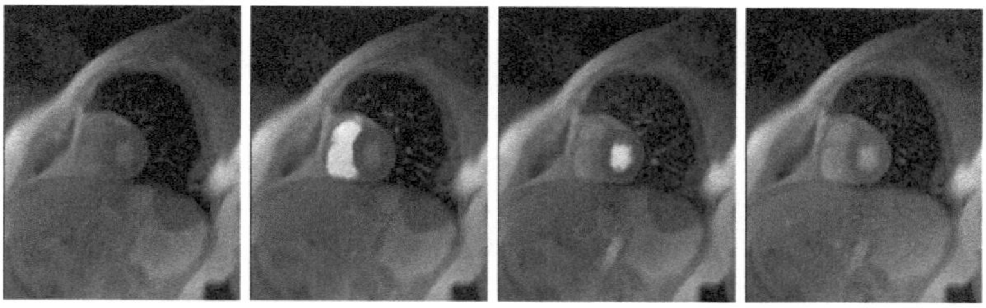

Fig. 1. Example of four time points taken from a first-pass perfusion MRI acquisition. From left to right: before the bolus reaches the heart, bolus in the right ventricle, bolus in the left ventricle and diffusion in the myocardial wall.

via the right ventricle, highlighting its geometry. The bolus subsequently appears in the left ventricle and finally diffuses in the left ventricular wall. Total acquisition time for a typical full dataset is between 45 seconds and one minute with 40 to 50 frames being typically acquired. This is too long to perform the whole acquisition in one breath hold. Therefore, protocols combining breath hold followed by a series of shallow breathing phases are commonly used. Such a succession of breathing phases can lead to the acquisition of images with a varying diaphragm position and thus a varying heart position within the image.

Post-processing usually consists of a registration step followed by manual segmentation of the myocardium. A characteristic feature for perfusion MRI is the dramatic contrast variation with time that has to be taken into account for a proper registration. This contrast variation awareness can be implemented implicitly, by choosing a similarity measure emphasizing non-linear intensity variation between reference and original image, or explicitly by using a time-varying reference image. Typically a fixed reference image is obtained by selecting a frame where contrast agent has reached both LV and RV cavities. A minimization scheme is then used to register each image of the sequence with the reference frame using rigid [5,6,7] or non-rigid [8,9,10] registration schemes. The two main types of time-varying reference images are the "cascading" scheme [11,12], where subsequent images are registered, and modeling of the intensity variations within the different features of interest [13,14,15]. This variety of methods shows that, as yet, there is no clear consensus on which technique is optimal for first-pass perfusion MRI registration.

This paper presents a novel approach for registration of perfusion data. As shown in Figure 1, the representation of the heart varies dramatically during the whole acquired sequence. As a result, the sequence can be roughly considered as the superimposition of different sources with distinct spatial location and dynamic behavior. Our approach aims at separating those different sources using Independent Component Analysis (ICA) in order to enable automated image interpretation and post-processing. In this paper, we demonstrate this concept by focusing on the issue of registration of in-plane motion throughout time.

The contributions of this work are twofold:

- We develop a novel method to automatically identify and locate perfusion events in time and space.
- Based on this, we present a fully automatic algorithm for registration of perfusion data using a spatially static reference image with dynamic contrast variation corresponding to the original, unregistered, data for each time point.

2 Methods

2.1 Overview

Our method is composed of a semantic analysis step followed by a multi-resolution registration step. The semantic analysis step, described in Section 2.2, aims at fully automatically extracting the relevant information regarding perfusion, both in time and space. The registration steps, described in Section 2.3, is actually build around a common registration module that performs ICA computation, time-varying reference computation and motion estimation. This gives a flexible framework that can be quickly and efficiently adapted to other types of perfusion data.

2.2 Semantic Analysis of the Perfusion Sequence

Independent Component Analysis. ICA is a blind source separation method that has already been successfully applied to various problems arising in signal and image processing [16] including medical image analysis [17,18]. ICA decomposes measured mixed signals X into a set of statistically independent sources S and their corresponding weights A.

Let $\mathbf{x}_t = [I_t(x_1, y_1), I_t(x_1, y_2), \ldots, I_t(x_m, y_n)]$ be the vectorized representation of a $m \times n$ image I_t acquired at time t. Using that notation, a set of images acquired at subsequent p time points can be written $\mathbf{X} = [\mathbf{x}_{t1}^T \mathbf{x}_{t2}^T \ldots \mathbf{x}_{tp}^T]^T$. The ICA model is for such a dataset formulated as follows

$$\mathbf{X} \approx \bar{\mathbf{X}} + \mathbf{AS} \tag{1}$$

The matrix $\mathbf{S} \in \mathbb{R}^{k \times mn}$, where k is the number of retained components, defines the independent components (ICs) and $\mathbf{A} \in \mathbb{R}^{p \times k}$ the weight coefficient matrix. $\bar{\mathbf{X}}$ is defined by

$$\bar{\mathbf{X}} = [\bar{\mathbf{x}}_{t1}^T \bar{\mathbf{x}}_{t2}^T \ldots \bar{\mathbf{x}}_{tp}^T]^T \tag{2}$$

where $\bar{\mathbf{x}}_t$ is the average image intensity for image I_t.

From dimensional analysis, $\mathbf{A}$ is expected to represent the time-intensity evolution of the k feature images contained in $\mathbf{S}$. The result of applying ICA on a slice level of a perfusion time sequence is shown in Figure 2.

ICA determines independent components up to a, possibly negative, scaling. In our application, we use the computed components for pattern recognition

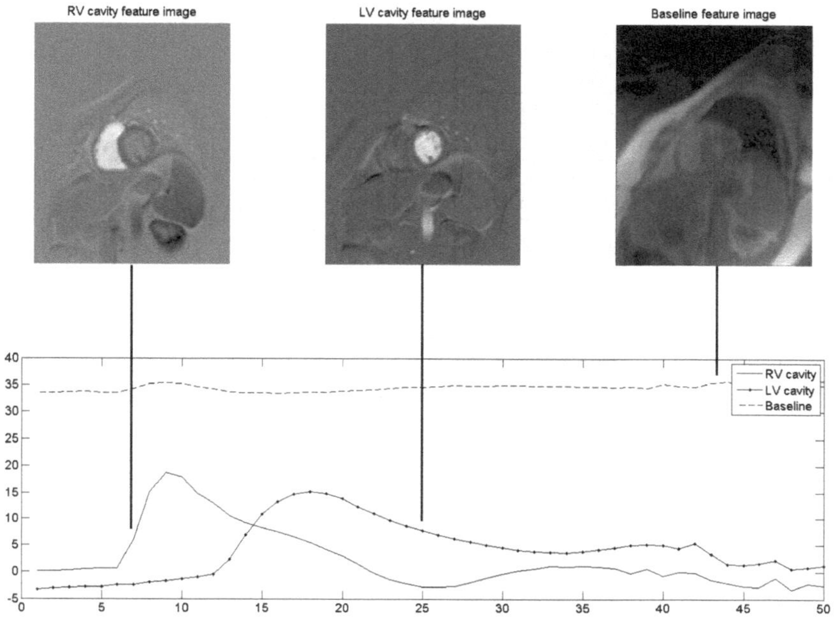

Fig. 2. Example of feature images (top row) and weighting factors obtained using ICA. The feature images depict events separated in time whereas the weighting curves show a similar shape to the one expected for time-intensity curves for corresponding regions of interest.

purpose. As a result, the absolute value of the scaling factor is not critical. However, in order to simplify the labeling step, we correct for the sign before semantic labeling. This is performed by computing the mean values of the weighting coefficients for each IC. A negative mean value indicates that the corresponding IC needs to be inverted.

Automatic Semantic Labeling of the Independent Components. For our purpose we chose to focus on the three first events of a perfusion sequence, that is the baseline, before the contrast agent is visible, and the bolus passage through the right and left ventricles. ICA initialization being random, pairs of computed independent components and weighting coefficients are unsorted. For further post-processing the proper semantic label is assigned to each component. This is realized by integrating knowledge about the time-intensity behavior of those features as the circulation of the contrast agent is governed by physiology and thus is patient-independent.

Contrast in the baseline IC does not depend on bolus passage. As a result, weights related to the baseline IC should be approximately constant throughout the whole acquisition. Bolus passage in the RV and LV cavity present the shape of a gamma-variate function [19] with RV cavity peaking before LV cavity.

Table 1. Criteria used for automated labeling and corresponding IC ranking, 1 being most probable and 3 least probable

Sorting Criterion	Ordering	1	2	3
Mean weight value	Descending	Baseline	RV	LV
Maximum weight value	Descending	Baseline	RV	LV
Time point of maximum	Ascending	Baseline	RV	LV

Identifying the corresponding ICs thus consists in recognizing two weighting vectors presenting a significant contributions, i.e. a high mean value, and a clear maximum. Contrast agent systematically entering the RV cavity before the LV cavity, position of their respective maximum provides relevant information for labeling.

Automated labeling of ICs is performed by combining this knowledge into a majority voting system. Each computed IC is ranked according to several criteria, as described by Table 1. The obtained matrix is then processed to label each component with its most likely meaning. Compared to manual labeling, this automated step achieves 98% correct identification for the baseline feature image and 88% for both LV and RV feature images.

LV mask generation. The ROI in which registration has to be performed can be roughly described as the rectangle centered on the left ventricle that fully comprises it. Based on the labeled components obtained from the previous two steps, a coarse LV blood pool segmentation can be obtained by thresholding the LV component image thanks to its high contrast w.r.t. the background, as shown in Figure 2. Its center of gravity $C_{\text{LV}} = (x_{\text{LV}}, y_{\text{LV}})$ gives a good estimate of the location for the LV center. To fully comprise the left ventricle, we make the assumption that the LV radial extent r_{LV} is the same in every azimuth. The distance $d_{\text{LV-RV}}$ between LV and RV blood pool centers of gravity then provide a good over-estimation of the LV radial extent. The LV mask can then be defined as $ROI = (|x - x_{\text{LV}}| < d_{\text{LV-RV}}) \cap (|y - y_{\text{LV}}| < d_{\text{LV-RV}})$.

2.3 ICA-Based Registration

The registration module. For each frame, a reference image is computed based on the computed ICA. This reference is a linear combination of the 3 feature images weighted by their respective weighting coefficients for that frame. Its characteristic features present the same intensity values as the original image to be matched against up to a multiplicative factor. It is computed over the ROI obtained via the semantic analysis step, as described in Section 2.2. This ROI is displaced over a displacement range in both x and y directions to obtain a cost matrix $M(\delta x, \delta y)$. The maximum value of this cost matrix provides the optimal displacement $(\delta x_{\text{optimal}}, \delta y_{\text{optimal}})$, which is used to correct the input dataset.

Multi-resolution scheme. Exploration of the data showed that 15 pixels, corresponding to roughly a 2cm displacement, was a reasonable over-estimation of the maximum displacement in one given dimension. Instead of exploring a 15×15 search space, we chose to use a coarse-to-fine multi-resolution scheme where two successive 5×5 search spaces are explored, one after sub-sampling by a factor 2 in each spatial dimensions and the other at full resolution. The gain in our case is a reduction of the search space dimension by more than 75%.

Further reduction of the search space was achieved by using the semantic labeling described previously, which allows for fully automatically selecting the relevant time intervals based on the weighting coefficient values. In our case, we chose to focus on the time interval between the peaking of the RV bolus and the end of the acquisition. This allows to only consider frames where contrast agent is present and to reduce the number of frames to process by 20% on average.

This multi-resolution scheme allows for processing a slice level composed of 50 frames in around 1 minute using Matlab on a standard laptop PC. This computation time is suitable for use in clinical routine.

3 Experimental Set-Up

3.1 Perfusion CMR Data

The proposed algorithm was validated using 46 datasets obtained from 35 participants of the Multi-Ethnic Study of Atherosclerosis (MESA) [20]. Images were T1-weighted, acquired using a fast gradient echo pulse sequence (TR 225 ms, TE 1 ms, flip angle 18°). Three slices in a short-axis orientation were obtained (in-plane resolution: 1.37×1.37 mm^2, slice thickness: 8 mm, slice gap: 8 mm). Participants were asked to hold their breath for 12 to 18 seconds. A Gadolinium-DTPA (Gd-DTPA) bolus (Magnevist, Berlex, Wayne, New Jersey) of 0.04 mmol per kg of body weight was injected, starting at the third or fourth heartbeat, followed by a saline flush of 10 ml. The first pass of the injected contrast agent bolus through the right and left ventricles and its first recirculation were captured in 50 heartbeats. 46 datasets, composed of 2 slice levels and 50 images per slice level, were selected randomly, allowing for testing for robustness with regard to the acquisition protocol.

The datasets used for this validation were subsequently manually processed by medical experts. Endocardial and epicardial contours were traced on a reference frame and adjusted to each frame constituting the sequence. The myocardium region of interest (ROI) was divided into sectors to the obtain time-intensity curves used for independent studies [21].

3.2 Validation Procedure

LV center motion. Reference LV motion is assessed using the manual LV endocardial contour centroid position $C(t) = (x_C(t), y_C(t))$ variation in time. For each dataset, the parameters $C_{\text{before}}(t)$ and $C_{\text{after}}(t)$ are computed respectively before and after registration. They contain the position of LV endocardial contour centroid for each time point $C = \{C(t), t = 1 \ldots N_{\text{frames}}\}$. Variations of C_{before} and C_{after} around their respective average values $\bar{C}_{\text{before}}$ and $\bar{C}_{\text{after}}$ gives a clear indication of the amplitude of the motion affecting a given dataset. Standard deviation, minimum and maximum values of the distance between C and $\bar{C}$ computed before and after registration are thus relevant parameters to evaluate the improvement, if any, provided by a registration algorithm. Moreover, studying those parameters across the whole population of evaluation datasets gives clear indications regarding the overall robustness of the method.

Global myocardial perfusion curve. The primary goal of perfusion CMR is the extraction of perfusion-related parameters from time-intensity curves. Computation of such curves is currently done by manually drawing endo- and epicardial contours for each acquired frame, yielding our gold standard. To evaluate the efficiency of our method, we assume that the obtained dataset is not affected by motion anymore, allowing to only select one endocardial and one epicardial manual contours for the whole slice level. We chose to select those contours from the already existing set of contours mentioned in the previous section. To automate the selection of the optimal set of contours, we make the assumption that myocardium presents a low standard deviation w.r.t. intensity levels on a MIP image. As a result, the two optimal contours are obtained by selecting the pair of endo- and epicardial contours that minimize standard deviation within the myocardial ROI for a MIP image obtained from the registered slice. Improvement is studied by using the same set of contours on the original data.

We investigated the accuracy of the time-intensity curves obtained after registration by computing the Normalized Mean Squared Error (NMSE) and the squared Pearson correlation coefficient R^2 between the normalized perfusion curve obtained from manual contours and the normalized perfusion curve obtained from unregistered or registered data using only one set of contours.

Finally, we studied the possible incursion of either the LV or RV blood pool within the ROI by computing the standard deviation $\sigma_{\boldsymbol{x}}(t) = SD(I(\boldsymbol{x}, t), \boldsymbol{x} \in ROI)$ of intensity values inside the ROI for each frame. The standard deviation over time $\sigma_{\boldsymbol{x},t} = SD(\sigma_{\boldsymbol{x}}(t), t \in [1 \ldots n_{\text{frames}}])$ for such a parameter gives an indication of possible misaligned ROI as the asymptotic lowest value is obtained when no motion is corrupting the dataset. Standard deviation is then only affected by perfusion defects and acquisition artefacts such as noise and intensity non-uniformity. If one of the contrast agent-filled cavity enters the ROI, standard deviation for that particular frame will increase. As a result, the standard deviation over time for the whole slice level will increase.

4 Results

4.1 LV Center Motion

Results for LV center motion are illustrated in Figures 3 and 4 and summarized in Table 2. Figure 3 shows that myocardium is much more homogeneous after

Table 2. Quantitative results obtained for LV center motion criterion, $SD(C - \bar{C})$, in pixels

	Mean	SD	Median	Min	Max
Original	1.26	0.87	1.15	0	5.36
Registered	0.64	0.46	0.49	0	2.36

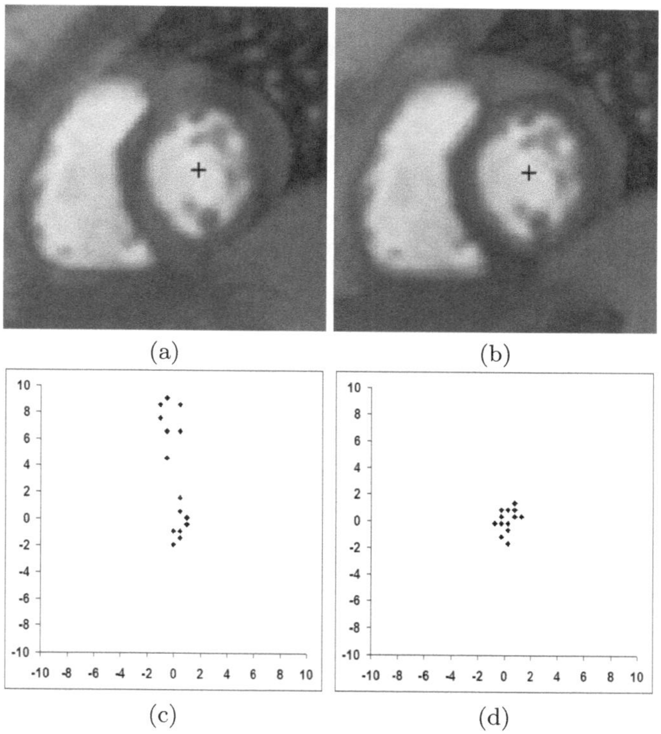

Fig. 3. Example of MIP images before registration (a) and after registration (b). The myocardium in (b) appears darker than in (a), showing that motion of the LV cavity is limited by the registration step. The scatter plots shown in (c) and (d) depict the corresponding position of the LV center w.r.t. its average position throughout the whole perfusion sequence. They clearly demonstrate the reduction in motion amplitude.

registration, as hyper-intensities due to post-LV bolus motion are compensated for. This is confirmed by the curves displayed in Fig. 4. Those curves show that there is a significant reduction in motion after using the proposed method. The area under the curve is increased by 17% after registration and 88% of the datasets show a standard deviation of the distance to the average position lower or equal to 1 pixel. In the original dataset, such a limited range of motion is obtained in only 31.5% of the cases.

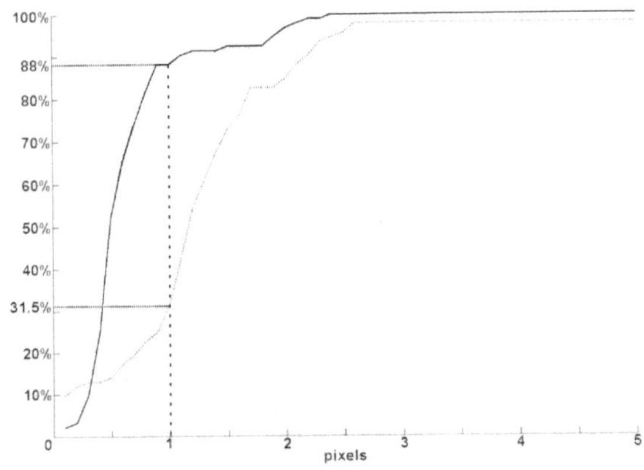

Fig. 4. Curves depicting motion range over the population before (dotted line) and after (solid line) registration. For example, 88% of the registered datasets show an overall motion inferior to 1 pixel, which was the case for only 31.5% of the original datasets.

Average LV center motion, characteristic of intra-slice variability, is reduced on average by almost 49.2% to 0.64 pixel after registration. Standard deviation of LV center motion, depicting inter-data variability, is reduced by 47.1% and is below 0.5 pixel. Median value is also reduced, by 57.4%. Minimum value is left unchanged, that being a good sign as the original minimal LV center displacement was 0. Finally, the averaged maximum LV center displacement is also reduced, from 5.36 pixels to 2.36 pixels, hence a 56% decrease, showing that the proposed method is robust even for large displacements.

4.2 Time-Intensity Curves

Registration increases the accuracy of computed perfusion parameters not only by correcting for a punctual error in time-intensity curves due to a misaligned frame, but also by making sure that the plotted dynamics are correct. Numerical results can be found in table 3.

First, accuracy in terms of dynamics has been improved as shown by the squared Pearson correlation coefficient (R^2) values. The average value across the datasets is increased, with a significantly reduced standard deviation. This means that time-intensity curves after registration present a good matching with the manual gold standard in terms of dynamics.

Second, NMSE is, on average, significantly reduced, average estimated error being now below 1%. Standard deviation of NMSE is reduced by 50% across the whole set of data, proving the robustness of our method in terms of perfusion curves. However, a punctual error can be observed as the maximum value for NMSE, which is lower after registration than before, is still high.

Table 3. Quantitative results obtained for Time-intensity curves. Average NMSE is in percent, average and standard deviation of $\sigma_{x,t}$ within the myocardial ROI in A.U.

		Mean	SD	Median	Min	Max
R^2	Original	0.88	0.16	0.97	0.19	1
	Registered	0.92	0.10	0.98	0.50	1
Average	Original	2.65	7.89	0.05	0	48.58
NMSE	Registered	0.87	3.88	0.03	0	34.05
$\sigma_{x,t}$	Original	2.33	2.30	1.52	0.28	12.42
	Registered	1.31	1.14	1.04	0.30	7.80

Finally, values for $\sigma_{x,t}$ show a significant decrease, meaning that there is far less unwanted incursion of the ventricles within the ROI after registration.

5 Discussion

We presented a fully automated registration algorithm designed for first-pass myocardial perfusion MR image sequence. Validation described in Section 4 shows that this method compares favorably in terms of accuracy and robustness with manual segmentation, which is the current gold-standard. A strong point for our method is the fact that only a few parameters are used, namely the number of independent components and the size of the registration window, thanks to the higher level reasoning allowed by the use of ICA. Moreover, computation speed, often a major drawback for registration method, is suitable for use in a clinical environment. This trade-off between accuracy, robustness and speed has been achieved via a careful choice of assumptions that are discussed here.

One point of debate is the ideal similarity measure to be used with perfusion data. Sum of Squared Differences (SSD) is a classic similarity measure used for intra-modality registration but sensitive to contrast variations. Our method overcomes that problem as the reference image mimics the intensity variation observable during the acquisition. Another popular choice for a similarity measure is the Mutual Information (MI) or its normalized version (NMI). Both are derived from inter-modality registration techniques. They are optimal in the sense that they can cope with varying contrast. However, such measures are computationally more expensive than either SSD or cross-correlation, a crucial point when the measure is included in an iterative scheme like registration. In the current setting, computation time for a 50 frames slice level is lower than 1 minute, which is fast enough to be used for off-line analysis of perfusion data.

Finally, a comparison of sector-wise perfusion curves before and after registration with the manual gold standard may have been a possibility for time-intensity curves-wise evaluation. However, sector definition is extremely sensitive to local contour variation and reference point selection. Moreover, the number of sectors and their positioning are still up to debate. Using global myocardial perfusion curves allows to overcome those problems, not to forget the reduction in noise due to taking into account a region with a larger extent. Computing standard deviation of intensities within the ROI allows for detecting any contrast agent-filled cavity incursion. Its lower boundary is indeed set in the ideal case of a perfectly centered ROI where only noise and natural intensity variations caused by possible perfusion defect are possible causes for intensity variations.

6 Conclusion

We presented a fully automated method for registration of first-pass perfusion MRI data. This method uses ICA to extract relevant features about the perfusion sequence, which both describe the anatomy and the perfusion timeline. Anatomically relevant features allow for the computation of a reference image optimized for each acquired frame, subsequently reducing the computational burden by using a faster and more robust similarity criterion. Timeline description is also used to reduce the computational load as only the time interval where contrast agent is present is taken into account. Obtained results, both in terms of accuracy, robustness and computation speed, are very good compared to existing methods and are good enough to envision use in a clinical environment. Future work will be directed toward the use of obtained feature images to automatically segment the myocardial wall, leading to a fully integrated and automated pipeline for perfusion data processing.

Acknowledgements

Financial support by the European Commission under the Marie Curie Programme (grant # HPMI-2002-00175) is gratefully acknowledged. This research was also supported by R01-HL-65580-01 and contracts N01-HC-95159, N01-HC-95163. The authors thank the other investigators, the staff and the participants of the MESA study for their valuable contributions. A full list of participating MESA investigators and institutions can be found at http://www.mesa-nhlbi.org.

References

1. McNamara, M.T., Higgins, C.B., Ehman, R.L., Revel, D., Sievers, R., Brasch, R.C.: Acute myocardial ischemia: Magnetic resonance contrast enhancement with Gadolinium-DTPA. Radiology 153, 157–163 (1984)
2. Wilke, N.M., Jerosch-Herold, M., Zenovich, A., Stillman, A.E.: Magnetic resonance first-pass myocardial perfusion imaging: Clinical validation and future applications. Journal of Magnetic Resonance Imaging 10, 676–685 (1999)
3. Schwitter, J., Nanz, D., Kneifel, S., Bertschinger, K., Buchi, M., Knusel, P.R., Marincek, B., Luscher, T.F., von Schulthess, G.K.: Assessment of myocardial perfusion in coronary artery disease by magnetic resonance: A comparison with positron emission tomography and coronary angiography. Circulation 103, 2230–2235 (2001)
4. Panting, J.R., Gatehouse, P.D., Yang, G.Z., Jerosch-Herold, M., Wilke, N., Firmin, D.N., Pennell, D.J.: Echo-planar magnetic resonance myocardial perfusion imaging: Parametric map analysis and comparison with Thallium SPECT. Journal of Magnetic Resonance Imaging 13, 192–200 (2001)

5. Bidaut, L.M., Vallee, J.P.: Automated registration of dynamic MR images for the quantification of myocardial perfusion. Journal of Magnetic Resonance Imaging 13, 648–655 (2001)
6. Bansal, R., Funka-Lea, G.: Integrated image registration for cardiac MR perfusion data. In: MICCAI (2002), pp. 659–666 (2002)
7. Dornier, C., Ivancevic, M.K., Thevenaz, P., Vallee, J.P.: Improvement in the quantification of myocardial perfusion using an automatic spline-based registration algorithm. Journal of Magnetic Resonance Imaging 18, 160–168 (2003)
8. Gallippi, C.M., Gregg, E.T.: Automatic image registration for MR and ultrasound cardiac images. In: Insana, M.F., Leahy, R.M. (eds.) IPMI 2001. LNCS, vol. 2082, pp. 148–154. Springer, Heidelberg (2001)
9. Gao, J., Ablitt, N., Elkington, A., Yang, G.Z.: Deformation modeling based on PLSR for cardiac magnetic resonance perfusion imaging. In: Dohi, T., Kikinis, R. (eds.) MICCAI 2002. LNCS, vol. 2488, pp. 612–619. Springer, Heidelberg (2002)
10. Olafsdottir, H., Stegmann, M.B., Ersboll, B.K., Larsson, H.B.W.: A comparison of FFD-based nonrigid registration and AAMs applied to myocardial perfusion MRI. In: SPIE Medical Imaging (2006)
11. Breeuwer, M., Spreeuwers, L., Quist, M.: Automatic quantitative analysis of cardiac MR perfusion images. In: Proceedings of SPIE Medical Imaging, pp. 733–742 (2001)
12. Gupta, S.N., Solaiyappan, M., Beache, G.M., Arai, A.E., Foo, T.K.F.: Fast method for correcting image misregistration due to organ motion in time-series MRI data. Magnetic Resonance in Medicine 49, 506–514 (2003)
13. Delzescaux, T., Frouin, F., De Cesare, A., Philipp-Foliguet, S., Zeboudj, R., Janier, M., Todd-Pokropek, A., Herment, A.: Adaptive and self-evaluating registration method for myocardial perfusion assessment. Magnetic Resonance Materials in Physics, Biology and Medicine 13, 28–39 (2001)
14. Delzescaux, T., Frouin, F., De Cesare, A., Philipp-Foliguet, S., Todd-Pokropek, A., Herment, A., Janier, M.: Using an adaptive semiautomated self-evaluated registration technique to analyze MRI data for myocardial perfusion assessment. Journal of Magnetic Resonance Imaging 18, 681–690 (2003)
15. Stegmann, M., Olafsdottir, H., Larsson, H.: Unsupervised motion-compensation of multi-slice cardiac perfusion MRI. Medical Image Analysis 9, 394–410 (2005)
16. Hyvarinen, A., Oja, E.: Independent component analysis: Algorithms and applications. Neural Networks 13, 411–430 (2000)
17. Carroll, T.J., Haughton, V.M., Rowley, H.A., Cordes, D.: Confounding effect of large vessels on MR perfusion images analyzed with independent component analysis. American Journal of Neuroradiology 23, 1007–1012 (2002)
18. Quigley, M.A., Haughton, V.M., Carew, J., Cordes, D., Moritz, C.H., Meyerand, M.E.: Comparison of independent component analysis and conventional hypothesis-driven analysis for clinical functional MR image processing. American Journal of Neuroradiology 23, 49–58 (2002)
19. Jerosch-Herold, M., Teja Seethamraju, R., Swingen, C.M., Wilke, N.M., Stillman, A.E.: Analysis of myocardial perfusion MRI. Journal of Magnetic Resonance Imaging 19, 758–770 (2004)
20. Bild, D.E., Bluemke, D.A., Burke, G.L., Detrano, R., Diez Roux, A.V., Folsom, A.R., Greenland, P., Jacob, J.D.R., Kronmal, R., Liu, K., Nelson, J.C., O'Leary, D., Saad, M.F., Shea, S., Szklo, M., Tracy, R.P.: Multi-ethnic study of atherosclerosis: Objectives and design. American Journal of Epidemiology 156, 871–881 (2002)
21. Wang, L., Jerosch-Herold, M., Jacobs, D.R., Shahar, E., Folsom, A.R.: Coronary risk factors and myocardial perfusion in asymptomatic adults: The Multi-Ethnic Study of Atherosclerosis. Journal of American College of Cardiology 47, 565–572 (2006)

Octree Grid Topology Preserving Geometric Deformable Model for Three-Dimensional Medical Image Segmentation

Ying Bai[1], Xiao Han[2], and Jerry L. Prince[1]

[1] Johns Hopkins University, Baltimore MD 21218
[2] CMS, Inc., St. Louis, MO 63132

Abstract. Topology-preserving geometric deformable models (TGDMs) are used to segment objects that have a known topology. Their accuracy is inherently limited, however, by the resolution of the underlying computational grid. Although this can be overcome by using fine-resolution grids, both the computational cost and the size of the resulting surface increase dramatically. In order to maintain computational efficiency and to keep the surface mesh size manageable, we have developed a new framework, termed OTGDMs, for topology-preserving geometric deformable models on balanced octree grids (BOGs). In order to do this, definitions and concepts from digital topology on regular grids were extended to BOGs so that characterization of simple points could be made. Other issues critical to the implementation of OTGDMs are also addressed. We demonstrate the performance of the proposed method using both mathematical phantoms and real medical images.

1 Introduction

Front propagation using level set methods [1] and their application in deformable models – geometric deformable models (GDMs) [2,3,4]are well established and extensively used in medical image segmentation. Topology preserving geometric deformable models (TGDMs) [5,6,7] were recently introduced in order to provide the ability to maintain topology of segmented objects while preserving the other benefits of GDMs. For example, in medical imaging many organs to be segmented have boundary topologies equivalent to that of a sphere. While many applications such as visualization and quantification may not require topologically correct segmentations, there are some applications — e.g., surface mapping and flattening and shape atlas generation — that cannot be achieved without correct topology of the segmented objects.

GDMs represent the evolving surface implicitly as a level set of a higher dimensional function. The resolution of the implicit surface is therefore restricted by the resolution of the sampling grid that defines the level set function, as demonstrated in Figs. 1(a)–(c). Accurate solution and representation of shapes with fine anatomical details (e.g., the folded sulci and gyri on the cortex) requires the use of a fine resolution grid. This dramatically increases the computation time of GDMs and produces surface meshes with prohibitive size, however, especially

N. Karssemeijer and B. Lelieveldt (Eds.): IPMI 2007, LNCS 4584, pp. 556–568, 2007.
© Springer-Verlag Berlin Heidelberg 2007

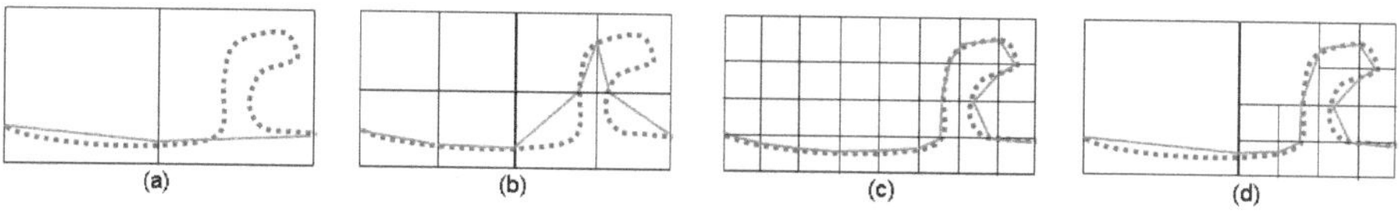

Fig. 1. Implicit surface resolution: the dotted contour is the truth contour; the solid contour is the implicit contour embedded in each sampling grid. (a) A coarse resolution grid cannot resolve contour details. (b) A refined grid represents the truth contour better. (c) A more refined grid provides a more accurate representation. (d) An adaptive grid with local refinement provides an accurate and efficient multiresolution shape representation.

on highly resolved 3D medical images. Adaptive grid techniques [8,9,10,11,12,13] address the resolution problem of GDMs by locally refining the sampling grid in order to resolve details and concentrate computational efforts where more accuracy is needed (as shown in Fig. 1(d)).

Although numerical schemes to implement level set methods on adaptive grids are well developed, there is little literature on the issue of defining digital connectivity rules for adaptive grids. Without such rules, it is difficult to guarantee homeomorphisms between the implicit surfaces and the corresponding boundaries of segmented objects on an adaptive grid. Digital connectivity rules for adaptive grids are also necessary in order to design a topology preserving level set method on adaptive grids. The method introduced by Han et al. [5] for regular grids maintains the topology of the implicit surface by controlling the topology of the corresponding binary object segmentation. This is achieved by applying the *simple point* criterion [14] from the theory of digital topology [15], preventing the level set function from changing sign at non-simple points. Until now, this topology preservation mechanism could not be used on adaptive grids because there was no characterization of "simple points" on adaptive grids.

In this paper, we propose a new topology-preserving level set method based on the balanced octree grids (BOGs) (i.e., octree grids for which the maximum cell edge length ratio between adjacent grid cells is 2). We first briefly review the digital topology framework for the adaptive grid that we recently proposed [16]. We then present a topology preserving geometric deformable model for adaptive octree grids (OTGDM), which is based on our new characterization of simple points on BOGs that extends the original characterization on the uniform grid in [14]. Several experiments are used to demonstrate the performance of OTGDM on both computational phantoms and real medical images.

2 Digital Topology Framework on BOGs

In [16], we extended basic digital topology concepts to BOGs, providing a unique and topologically consistent digital embedding scheme for implicit surfaces defined on BOGs. In the following, we summarize the concepts of "neighbor points"

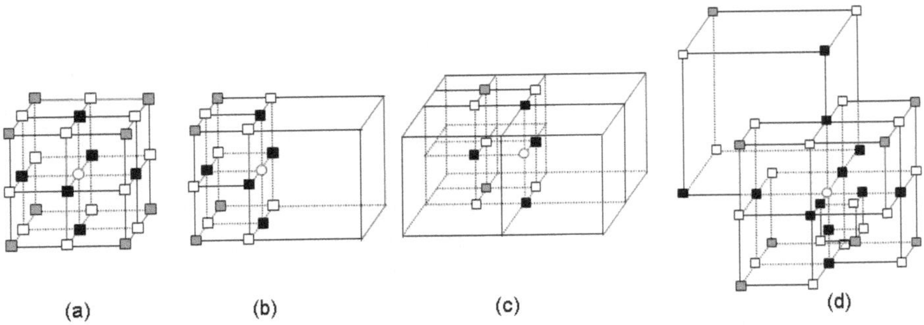

Fig. 2. 3D neighborhoods on balanced octree grids

and "invalid cases", which will be used in the characterization of "simple points" on BOGs presented later.

The concept of *neighbor points* is fundamental in classical digital topology theory [15]. In [16], grid points on an octree grid are defined to be *edge(E)-neighbors*, *square(S)-neighbors*, or *cube(C)-neighbors* if they share an edge, a face, or a cube, respectively, of leaf cells of the octree. (*Leaf cells* are cells that have no child cells.) Fig. 2 shows an example of neighborhoods on a BOG. Fig. 2(a) shows a uniform neighborhood and Figs. 2(b)–(d) show examples of non-uniform neighborhoods. The white circle in each figure indicates the root point of the neighborhoods; black squares are the E-neighbors; white squares are the points that are added to the E-neighbors to yield the S-neighbors; and gray squares are the points that are added to S-neighbors to yield the C-neighbors. Analogous definitions of *neighborhood*, *adjacency*, *path*, and *connectivity* can be found in [16].

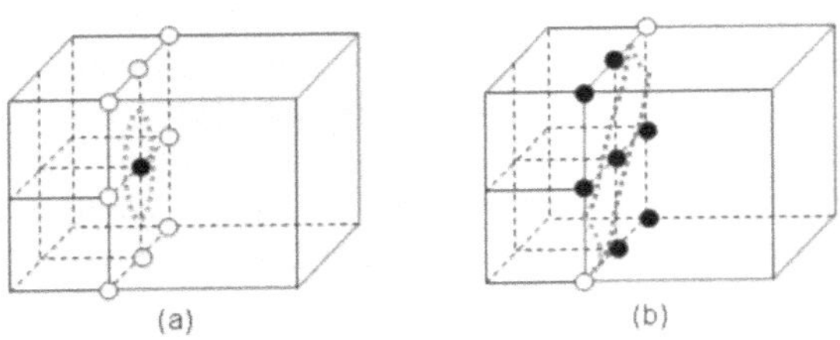

Fig. 3. Examples of invalid cases on interface of resolution transition

Using the above neighborhood and connectivity definitions, inconsistencies can still occur at the interface(s) between grid cells of different resolution (referred as *transition face*) as illustrated in Fig. 3. Assume E-connectivity for the black foreground points, and S-connectivity for the white background points. In Fig. 3(a), the black point is shared only by the fine resolution grid cells and forms a single connected component on the transition face. This foreground component does not exist, however, if we look at the coarse side of the transition face. Similarly, in Fig. 3(b), the two white background points are disconnected and form two connected components at the fine resolution side of the transition face, whereas they are connected as one connected component by the coarse cell. As a result, the embedded isosurface will have a discontinuity at the transition face. To eliminate these inconsistencies and thus guarantee unique and valid surface embedding on BOGs, we define such cases as *invalid case* [16] where the numbers of connected components (for both foreground and background) formed by the grid points on two sides of a transition face are not equal. Invalid cases are explicitly checked and prevented to happen in the OTGDM algorithm, as will be described later.

3 A Topology-Preserving Level Set Method on BOGs

In this section, we present a new topology-preserving level set method on BOGs. The overall algorithm is first summarized and the details about each step are then discussed.

We adopt the narrowband framework [17] in the following implementation and we assume a general GDM model as can be summarized by the following equation:

$$\frac{\partial \Phi(\boldsymbol{x},t)}{\partial t} = [F_{\text{prop}}(\boldsymbol{x},t) + F_{\text{curv}}(\boldsymbol{x},t)]|\nabla\Phi(\boldsymbol{x},t)| + \boldsymbol{F}_{\text{adv}}(\boldsymbol{x},t)\cdot\nabla\Phi(\boldsymbol{x},t) \quad (1)$$

where F_{prop}, F_{curv}, and $\boldsymbol{F}_{\text{adv}}$ denote user-designed force (or speed) terms that control the model deformation. In particular, F_{curv}, the curvature force, controls the regularity (smoothness) of the implicit surface. F_{prop} and $\boldsymbol{F}_{\text{adv}}$ are two forms of image forces (scalar and vector respectively) that drive the surface to the desired object boundary.

Octree-based TGDM algorithm

1. Initialize the adaptive grid according to the initial surface topology and adaptation metric (cf. Section 3.1). Initialize the level set function to be the signed distance function of the initial surface.
2. Build the narrow band by finding all grid points within a distance threshold of the implicit surface (zero level set of the current level set function).
3. Update the level set function at each point in the narrow band iteratively as follows:
   (a) Compute the new value of $\Phi(\boldsymbol{x},t)$ using Eq. (1).
   (b) If there is no sign change, accept the new value and move on to the next point. Otherwise, go to Step 3(c).
   (c) Test whether the sign change at this point yields a valid configuration (cf. Section 2). If yes, go to Step 3(d). Otherwise, move on to the next point.
   (d) Test whether the current point is a simple point by computing two topological numbers (cf. Section 3.2)). If the point is simple accept the new value. Otherwise, set the level set function to be a small number with the same sign as its original value.

4. If the zero level set is near the boundary of the current narrow band, reinitialize the level set function to be a signed distance function and go to Step 2.
5. Test whether the zero level set has stopped moving (i.e., no sign change happens at any point inside the narrow band in two or three consecutive iterations). If yes, stop; otherwise, go to the next iteration. ■
6. Extract the zero-value isosurface using an adaptive connectivity-consistent marching cells algorithm (cf. Section 3.3).

A few comments about OTGDM. First, the reinitialization step is a straightforward extension of the fast marching method to the non-uniform cartesian grid. Different grid sizes are handled by the modified finite difference operator [17]. Second, the simple point check can be omitted, and the algorithm becomes a standard geometric deformable model on an adaptive octree grid (OSGDM).

3.1 Adaptive Grid Generation

We generate a BOG following two criteria: first, the BOG should embed the initial implicit surface with correct topology; second, the BOG should adapt its resolution according to the geometrical shape of the final surface. We discuss these two considerations below.

Initial surface topology
To guarantee that the final surface has the correct topology, we must start with an initial surface that has the correct topology. Assume that we are given an initial implicit surface defined on the uniformly sampled grid; by definition, it has the correct topology, which can be arbitrary and unknown. To initialize an implicit surface on a BOG while preserving topology, we apply the bottom-up cell merging algorithm that we presented in [16]. The algorithm starts from the original uniform grid and treats it as an octree grid that is at its finest possible resolution. The leaf cells of this octree grid are then traversed level-by-level from bottom to up. At each level, the leaf cells are evaluated one-by-one to see if they can be merged without changing the topology of the underlying isosurface and without generating invalid cases. Details of this algorithm can be found in [16]. After applying the cell-merging algorithm and balancing the grid, we obtain a BOG that embeds the initial surface with the correct topology.

Image-based adaptivity metric
We now refine the initial BOG so that it has finer cells where image details predict the need for a higher resolution surface representation. The concept of an *adaptivity metric*, which is derived from the image volume, is used. This metric estimates the local geometrical properties of the final surface boundary — if it should come to rest at the given image location — and the BOG is adapted accordingly. A classical adaptivity metric is the magnitude of the image gradient (cf. [8]), wherein computational grid is refined at high gradient regions and coarsened elsewhere. This metric cannot help to reduce the size of the final surface mesh on the adaptive octree grid, however, since the grid will be uniformly refined along the entire object boundary. In this work, we have used

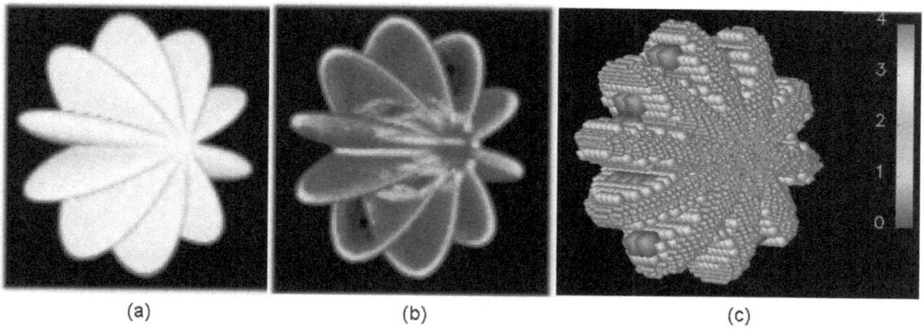

Fig. 4. Illustration of grid adaptation for a harmonic sphere phantom image

the max-curvature — i.e., the larger absolute value of the two principal curvatures — estimated from the volumetric gray-level image using the method in [18]. To achieve more robust estimation (in noise, for example), we apply an anisotropic smoothing to the image before using curvature estimation (cf. [19]). Once curvature $\kappa(\mathbf{x})$ is estimated, we define a refinement rule to be:

$$l(\mathbf{x}) = \mathbf{i}, \quad \text{if } \mathbf{t_{i-1}} < \frac{\kappa(\mathbf{x})}{\kappa_{\mathbf{max}}} \leq \mathbf{t_i}$$

where $\mathbf{x}$ denotes a octree grid node, and $l(\mathbf{x})$ denotes the minimum level of the leaf cells sharing node $\mathbf{x}$. If the highest level of the octree is l_{max}, then $i = 1, \ldots, l_{max}$. κ_{max} is the maximum of $\kappa(\mathbf{x})$. The t_i's are user-selectable thresholds to flexibly tune the grid resolution for different images.

Fig. 4 shows one example of grid generation for a mathematical phantom that has a modulated spherical shape as shown in Fig. 4(a). We estimated the max-curvature from the image volume, and Fig. 4(b) shows that the larger values (indicated by bright colors) occur on the ridges and valleys. We then generated an adaptive grid using the above refinement rule. Fig. 4(c) shows all the leaf cells on the adaptive grid that the final reconstructed surface cut through. The color map shows the resolution scale of the grid cells. It is observed that the grid resolution is finer in the high-curvature ridge and valley regions, and is coarser in the flat regions.

3.2 Simple Point Characterization on BOGs

An efficient algorithm to determine a simple point on a *uniform grid* was presented in [14]. The method requires the definition of a geodesic neighborhood and topological numbers. We follow the spirit of [14] to characterize a simple point on BOGs, using the digital topology framework summarized in Section 2. Let us denote the domain of digital images on a BOG to be Ω, and the n-neighborhood of a point x on a BOG by $N_n(x)$, and the set comprising the neighborhood of x with x removed by $N_n^*(x)$, where $n \in \{E, S, C\}$. We define *geodesic neighborhood* and *topological numbers* on BOGs as follows:

DEFINITION 3.1 ***(Geodesic Neighborhood).*** *Let $X \subset \Omega$ and $x \in \Omega$. The geodesic neighborhood of x with respect to X of order k is the set $N_n^k(x, X)$ defined recursively by: $N_n^1(x, X) = N_n^*(x) \cap X$ and $N_n^k(x, X) = \cup\{N_n(y) \cap N_M^*(x) \cap X, y \in N_n^{k-1}(x, X)\}$, where $M = C$ in the balanced octree grid.*

DEFINITION 3.2 ***(Topological Numbers).*** *Let $X \subset \Omega$ and $x \in \Omega$. The topological numbers of the point x relative to the set X are: $T_E(x, X) = \#C_E (N_E^2(x, X))$, $T_{E^+}(x, X) = \#C_E(N_E^3(x, X)), T_S(x, X) = \#C_S(N_S^2(x, X)), T_C(x, X) = \#C_C(N_C^1(x, X))$ in the balanced octree grid, where $\#$ denotes the cardinality of a set.*

Note that in defining topological numbers, the notation "E^+" means the E-connectivity whose dual connectivity is S-connectivity. Once the topological numbers are known, the following proposition gives a characterization of simple point on BOGs.

PROPOSITION 3.1 *A point x on a balanced octree grid is simple if and only if $T_n(x, X) = 1$ and $T_{\bar{n}}(x, \bar{X}) = 1$, where $(n, \bar{n})$ is a pair of compatible connectivities (cf. [16]) on the balanced octree grid.*

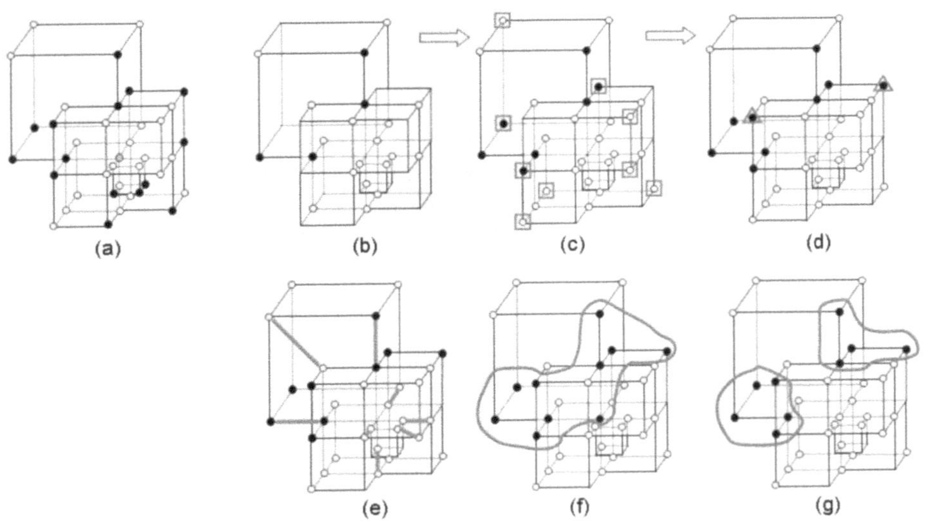

Fig. 5. An example of constructing geodesic neighborhood on a BOG

Fig. 5 illustrates the computation of topological numbers for a particular example. The root point is the gray point in the center of Fig. 5(a). All points in its neighborhood are marked as either black or white circles representing foreground and background respectively. Assume black circles have E-connectivity and white circles have S-connectivity. The highlighted black and white points in Fig. 5(b) are the first-order E-neighbors in the foreground (black) and the first-order S-neighbors in the background (white), respectively. In Fig. 5(c), the points in squares are the second order neighbors added to the geodesic neighborhood. In Fig. 5(d), the points in triangles are the third order neighbors added to the geodesic neighborhood. All the points in Fig. 5(d) consist of the complete geodesic neighborhood for the root point. A straightforward computation of the topological numbers requires counting the number of connected components within geodesic neighborhoods, which can be navigated by leaf cell edges on the adaptive grid. For example, when computing the foreground topological number in this case, we start from the root point and search in the E-connected directions for the first-order neighbors in the foreground. When we search in the left direction, we find the paired black points (as they are both one leaf cell edge away from the root point). This pair of points is automatically counted as belonging to the same connected component. Next, the neighbors of these two points in the foreground inside the geodesic neighborhood are also counted into the same connected component, and so on. All the paired points connected by solid lines in Fig. 5(e) are counted in this manner. In this example, $T_{E^+}(x, X) = 2$ and $T_S(x, \bar{X}) = 1$. Therefore the considered root point is not simple. Fig. 5(f) and Fig. 5(g) show how the topology of the implicit surface changes if the root point is changed from foreground to background.

It is important to note that the above characterization of simple points is only valid on a BOG that has no invalid configurations. Therefore, if a level set function is about to change sign at a given node, we must first check to see whether the sign change would create an invalid configuration; if not, then it is appropriate to check the simple point property.

3.3 Connectivity Consistent Isosurface Extraction on BOGs

The final surface mesh must be extracted using an adaptive connectivity-consistent marching cells (ACCMC) algorithm (cf. [5,16]). The ACCMC algorithm prevents "cracks" that can happen on the interface of resolution transition by re-tessellating the coarse resolution cell so that it agrees with the fine resolution cells on the transition face. The triangulation scheme is carefully designed to prevent self-intersection of surface patches inside a coarse cell that has transition face(s).

4 Experiments

4.1 Harmonic Sphere Phantom

In the first experiment, we used the harmonic sphere image phantom shown in Fig. 4(a) and performed a quantitative analysis of the efficiency and accuracy of the proposed method. The original image has a size of 128 × 128 × 128, and the true surface is known. Since topology is not an issue here, we applied a GDM on uniform grids of different sizes and an OSGDM on a BOG (with finest resolution equivalent to that of the finest uniform grid). We then measured the errors of these results by computing the distance from each vertices of the truth surface to the other surfaces. All the models were initialized with a small sphere inside the

Table 1. Harmonic sphere experiment results

Grid Size	Mean Error (voxel)	Max Error (voxel)	Triangle Number	Time (min)
64 × 64 × 64 SGDM	0.43	3.39	34000	2
128 × 128 × 128 SGDM	0.14	1.42	137660	16
256 × 256 × 256 SGDM	0.09	0.94	548992	130
OSGDM	0.12	1.23	108990	9

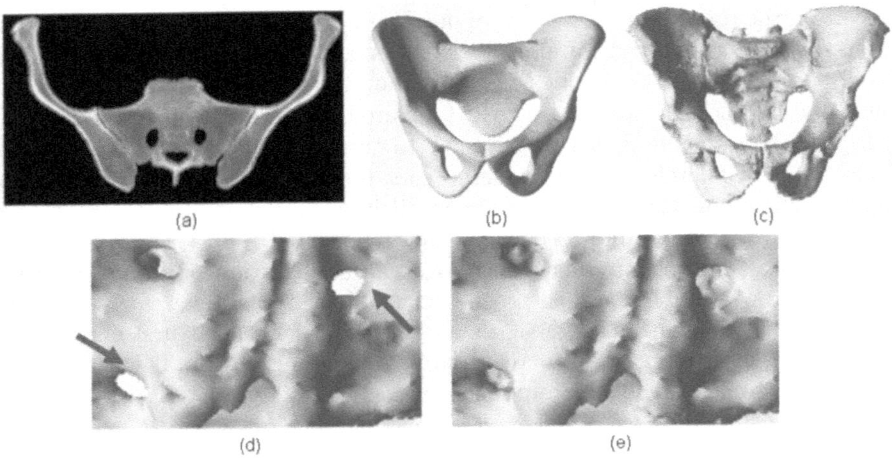

Fig. 6. Pelvic bone experiment (see text for details)

object. The results are summarized in Table 1. The 256^3 uniform grid result has the best accuracy but it takes the most computation time and has the largest mesh size. Compared with the 128^3 uniform grid result, the OSGDM result has better accuracy with smaller mesh size and less computation time.

4.2 CT Pelvic Bone

In the second experiment, we tested OTGDM on a CT image of a pelvic bone which has size 512 × 512 × 280. Fig. 6(a) shows a 2D slice of this 3D image. The topology of a pelvic bone surface is assumed to be genus 3 (Euler Number = −4) [20], i.e., the surface should only have 3 handles.

We started from an initial shape template that has the correct topology (shown in Fig. 6(b)), and then applied an OTGDM with finest resolution equivalent to that of the original image grid to reconstruct a topologically correct pelvic bone surface (shown in Fig. 6(c)). The topology of the reconstructed surface is verified to be correct (i.e., Euler number is computed to be −4). Due to noise and other artifacts, applying OSGDM on this image yielded a segmentation with incorrect topology (Euler number is −60). Fig. 6(d)–(e) show a close up view of

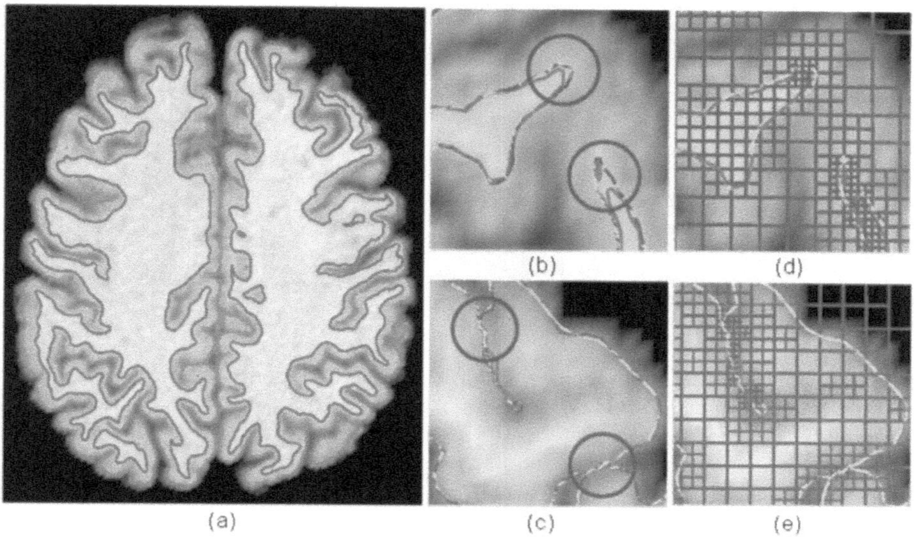

Fig. 7. Cortical surfaces (cross-section views): (a) OTGDM results overlaid on MR brain image (blue–inner surface, red–outer surface); (b)-(c) close-up views of inner and outer surfaces reconstructed by three types of grid: red–coarse uniform grid TGDM result, blue–fine uniform grid TGDM result, yellow–OTGDM result); (d)-(e) close-up views of BOGs used by OTGDM (shown in blue)

the OSGDM result and the OTGDM result. We see that the OSGDM result has undesirable small handles (indicated by arrows), whereas in the OTGDM result those handles are all eliminated.

4.3 MR Human Brain

In the last experiment, we applied the proposed method to extract the inner and the outer cortical surfaces for two MR brain images. The original images both have a size of $256 \times 256 \times 198$. The overall reconstruction methodology that we used is called "CRUISE," as described in [6]. We ran the CRUISE procedure on the original image until the deformable surface reconstruction step. We then started from a topologically correct estimate of the GM/WM interface, and applied TGDM on three different computational grids to extract the inner and outer cortical surfaces. The first one used a fine uniform computational grid (double size of the original image). The second one used a coarse uniform computational grid (of the original image size). The third one applied the proposed OTGDM, whose finest grid resolution is same as the fine uniform grid. The image derived forces are computed initially on the coarse uniform grid, and interpolated to the fine uniform grid for the first implementation. The topology of the OTGDM results are all verified to be correct (i.e., the Euler number of all extracted surface meshes is 2). The results and their close-up views are shown in Fig. 7. The improvement of accuracy by using a fine resolution grid appears

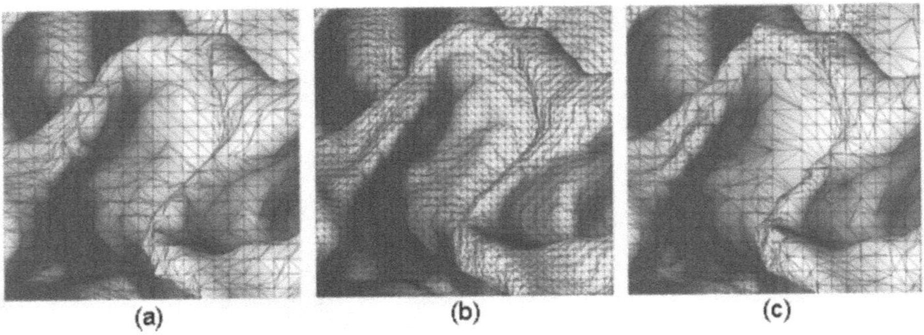

Fig. 8. triangle meshes: left – coarse uniform grid TGDM result; center – fine uniform grid TGDM result; right – OTGDM result

subtle in most places; however, we can still observe that the fine grid TGDM result and the OTGDM result capture anatomical details (such as the deeply folded sulci and gyri indicated by circles) better than the coarse grid TGDM result. Fig. 8 shows a close-up 3D view of the three inner surface meshes. As we can see, the OTGDM surface mesh is a multi-resolution representation and has large triangles in regions that are relatively flat and small triangles in regions with high curvature. The average mesh sizes and computation time for all the surface results are: fine uniform grid TGDM result – 2,771,000 triangles (40 mins); coarse uniform grid TGDM result – 659,000 triangles (5 mins); OTGDM – 968,000 triangles (12 mins).

We also conducted a landmark-based study of accuracy for these surface results of the two subjects. The landmark picking procedure is described in [6]. A total of 420 landmark points are used for each brain subject, corresponding to 14 fundi, 14 banks, and 14 gyri crowns near major sulci. The landmark errors for the results on three computational grids are shown in Table 2. It can be seen that a fine uniform grid provides the best accuracy, that is, the smallest landmark error. The computation time and the surface mesh size is consider-

Table 2. Landmark Errors for Inner and Outer Cortical Surfaces (in mm)

		Subject 1					Subject 2				
Region	Grid	mean SD	std SD	mean AD	std AD	max AD	mean SD	std SD	mean AD	std AD	max AD
Overall Inner	OG	-0.05	0.62	0.45	0.43	2.28	-0.16	0.61	0.49	0.39	2.15
	DG	-0.08	0.53	0.39	0.36	1.73	-0.17	0.56	0.45	0.37	1.83
	AG	-0.08	0.53	0.39	0.36	1.67	-0.15	0.57	0.46	0.36	1.84
Overall Outer	OG	-0.50	0.44	0.54	0.40	1.91	0.12	0.61	0.46	0.41	2.49
	DG	-0.31	0.38	0.39	0.30	1.71	0.13	0.54	0.40	0.35	2.17
	AG	-0.35	0.39	0.40	0.32	1.74	0.12	0.55	0.40	0.36	2.10

SD: signed distance in mm, AD: absolute distance in mm
OG: original size grid, DG: double size grid, AG: adaptive octree grid.

ably increased, however. The coarse uniform grid is the fastest and produces the smallest triangle mesh, at the cost of having a larger error. OTGDM produces comparable landmark error as the fine uniform grid TGDM and the resulting surface mesh size and the computation cost are slightly larger than that of the coarse uniform grid TGDM result.

5 Discussion and Conclusion

We have proposed a topology-preserving geometric deformable model for the adaptive octree grid (OTGDM); it is based on new digital topology concepts that we have developed for adaptive octree grids. Experiments show that the proposed method correctly preserves the digital topology of the implicit surface(s) embedded on the adaptive grid, saves computation time, and yields fewer triangles in the final surface(s).

We have additional comments on two issues. The first issue is about the introduction of "invalid cases". It appears that the grid configurations defined to be invalid can possibly be allowed by introducing several new types of connectivities on BOGs. Such a strategy will considerably increase the complexity of the connectivity-consistent isosurface algorithm. A further concern is that having these many connectivities makes the characterization of simple point an almost intractable problem in 3D. The introduction of "invalid cases" greatly reduces the extra complexity in the study of connectivity on BOGs. The second issue is about the generation of BOGs. Currently we generate BOGs only once before running OTGDM algorithm, which proves to be efficient for segmentation purpose since only the final solution is of concern. Dynamic grid refinement may be desirable for some applications and designing a topology-preserving dynamic refinement scheme is part of our future work.

References

1. Osher, S., Sethian, J.A.: Fronts propagating with curvature-dependent speed: Algorithms based on Hamilton-Jacobi formulations. J. Comput. Phys. 79, 12–49 (1988)
2. Caselles, V., Kimmel, R., Sapiro, G.: Geodesic active contours. International Journal of Computer Vision 22, 61–79 (1997)
3. Malladi, R., Sethian, J.A., Vemuri, B.C.: Shape modeling with front propagation: A level set approach. IEEE Trans. PAMI 17, 158–175 (1995)
4. Yezzi, A., Kichenassamy, S., Olver, P., Tannenbaum, A.: A geometric snake models for segmentation of medical imagery. IEEE Trans. Med. Imag. 16, 199–209 (1997)
5. Han, X., Xu, C., Prince, J.L.: A topology preserving level set method for geometric deformable models. IEEE Trans. Patt. Anal. Machine Intell. 25, 755–768 (2003)
6. Han, X., Pham, D.L., Tosun, D., Rettmann, M.E., Xu, C., Prince, J.L.: Cortical reconstruction using implicit surface evolution. NeuroImage 23, 997–1012 (2004)
7. Sundaramoorthi, G., Yezzi, A.J.: More-than-topology-preserving flows for active contours and polygons. In: ICCV pp. 1276–1283 (2005)
8. Terzopoulos, D., Vasilescu, M.: Sampling and reconstruction with adaptive meshes. In: Proc. CVPR'91, Lahaina, HI, pp. 70–75 (1991)
9. Milne, R.B.: Adaptive Level Sets Methods Interfaces. PhD thesis, Dept. Math., UC Berkely (1995)

10. Sussman, M., Almgren, A.S., Bell, J.B., Colella, P., Howell, L.H., Welcome, M.L.: An adaptive level set approach for incompressible two-phase flow. J. Comput. Phys. 148, 81–124 (1999)
11. Xu, M., Thompson, P.M., Toga, A.W.: An adaptive level set segmentation on a triangulated mesh. IEEE Trans. Medical Imaging 23(2), 191–201 (2004)
12. Droske, M., Meyer, B., Schaller, C., Rumpf, M.: An adaptive level set method for medical image segmentation. In: Insana, M.F., Leahy, R.M. (eds.) IPMI 2001. LNCS, vol. 2082, Springer, Heidelberg (2001)
13. Sochnikov, V., Efrima, S.: Level set calculations of the evolution of boundaries on a dynamically adaptive grid. Int. J. Numer. Meth. Engng 56, 1913–1929 (2003)
14. Bertrand, G.: Simple points, topological numbers and geodesic neighborhoods in cubic grids. Pattern Recognition Letters 15, 1003–1011 (1994)
15. Kong, T.Y., Rosenfeld, A.: Digital topology: Introduction and survey. CVGIP: Image Understanding 48, 357–393 (1989)
16. Bai, Y., Han, X., Prince, J.L.: Octree-based topology-preserving isosurface simplification. In: IEEE Workshop on Mathematical Methods in Biomedical Image Analysis (MMBIA 2006), New York (2006)
17. Sethian, J.A.: Level Set Methods and Fast Marching Methods. Cambridge University Press, Cambridge, UK (1999)
18. Thirion, J.-P., Gourdon, A.: Computing the differental characteristics of isointensity surfaces. CVIU 61, 190–202 (1995)
19. Malladi, R., Sethian, J.A.: Image processing via level set curvature flow. In: Proc. Natl. Acad. Sci. U.S.A, pp. 7046–7050 (1995)
20. Lamecker, H., Seebass, M., Hege, H., Deuflhard, P.: A 3d statistical shape model of the pelvic bone for segmentation. In: SPIE, pp. 1341–1351 (2004)

High-Dimensional Entropy Estimation for Finite Accuracy Data: *R*-NN Entropy Estimator

Jan Kybic

Center for Machine Perception, Czech Technical University, Prague, Czech Republic
kybic@fel.cvut.cz,
http://cmp.felk.cvut.cz/~kybic

Abstract. We address the problem of entropy estimation for high-dimensional finite-accuracy data. Our main application is evaluating high-order mutual information image similarity criteria for multimodal image registration. The basis of our method is an estimator based on k-th nearest neighbor (NN) distances, modified so that only distances greater than some constant R are evaluated. This modification requires a correction which is found numerically in a preprocessing step using quadratic programming. We compare experimentally our new method with k-NN and histogram estimators on synthetic data as well as for evaluation of mutual information for image similarity.

1 Introduction

Nonparametric entropy and mutual information estimation from finite number of samples is an important tool in diverse domains such as statistics [1], computational chemistry [2], or measuring information contents of signals such as neural spike trains [3]. For multimodal image registration, mutual information is the image similarity measure of choice [4,5,6]. Instead of measuring mutual information of scalar image intensities, in some cases it is advantageous to use more complex multidimensional features, such as color, output of spatial filters, texture descriptors, or intensities of neighborhood pixels [7,8,9,10]. However, due to the lack of good estimators, most approaches are limited to low dimensions or have to use strong assumptions such as normality. Histogram and kernel estimators do not work well in high dimensions ($d \gtrapprox 5$) [11,12,13,3] when the bins are simultaneously too large and almost empty. Nearest neighbor (NN) distance estimators [14,15,3,16] look promising, if their two principal problems can be circumvented — the computational complexity of the nearest neighbor search [17] and the artifacts and singularities when applied to finite accuracy (quantized) data. Here we attempt to solve the second problem by using a new estimator called R-NN, combining k-NN and kernel estimator approaches.

1.1 Entropy Estimation

Let us have N samples $X = \{\mathbf{x}_1, \ldots, \mathbf{x}_N\}$, from an unknown probability density $f(\mathbf{x})$ in a d-dimensional space, $\mathbb{R}^d$. The task is to estimate the Shannon information entropy $H_{\text{true}}(f) = -\int f(\mathbf{x}) \log \mathbf{x} \, \mathrm{d}\mathbf{x}$. We consider estimators of the form

N. Karssemeijer and B. Lelieveldt (Eds.): IPMI 2007, LNCS 4584, pp. 569–580, 2007.
© Springer-Verlag Berlin Heidelberg 2007

$$H(X) = \frac{1}{N} \sum_{i=1}^{N} h(\mathbf{x}_i; X) \qquad \text{with} \qquad h(\mathbf{x}_i; X) \approx -\log f(\mathbf{x}_i) \tag{1}$$

If $h(\mathbf{x}_i; X)$ is an unbiased estimator of $-\log f(\mathbf{x}_i)$, then $H(X)$ is an unbiased estimator of $H_{\text{true}}(f)$ [15].

1.2 Kernel Estimator

For $H(X)$ to be a non-parametric estimator, $h(\mathbf{x}_i; X)$ must depend only on the neighborhood of $\mathbf{x}_i$ [13]. We describe the neighborhood compactly by the dependency of the number of points $q(r)$ on the neighborhood size[1] r.

$$q_i(r) = \left| \{ \|\mathbf{x} - \mathbf{x}_i\|_\infty \leq r; \mathbf{x} \in X \} \right| \tag{2}$$

Fixing the neighborhood radius R, we obtain an estimator for $-\log f(\mathbf{x}_i)$

$$h_{\text{ker}}(\mathbf{x}_i; X) = -\log \frac{q_i(R)}{V_d(R) N} \tag{3}$$

where $V_d(R) = (2R)^d$ is the volume of the neighborhood. This is a plug-in kernel estimator for a constant kernel, equivalent to an averaged shifted histogram (ASH) [13].

1.3 Nearest-Neighbor Estimator

The distance to the k-th nearest neighbor is

$$\varrho_i(k) = \min_{r \geq 0} \{ r; q_i(r) > k \} \tag{4}$$

An estimator based on the distance $\varrho_i(1)$ to the nearest-neighbor (NN) of $\mathbf{x}_i$ is due to [14] and was later extended to k-th nearest-neighbor (k-NN) [15,16]. Its formulation for the ℓ_∞ norm [17] is

$$h_{\text{NN}}(\mathbf{x}_i; X) = h_0(r, k) = -\psi(k) + \psi(N) + d \log 2r \qquad \text{for} \qquad r = \varrho_i(k) \tag{5}$$

where ψ is the digamma function[2]. The estimator (5) is asymptotically unbiased [14,3]. Its variance can be reduced by choosing higher k [16]. The k-NN estimator works reasonably well even in high dimensions (we have tested it for $d = 25 \sim 50$) and for small sample sizes. The computational bottleneck is the nearest neighbor search (all-NN search) but acceleration techniques exist, based on space partitioning and approximative search [17,18,19,20,21,22]. Graph-based estimators for Rényi entropy [23,24] behave similarly to the k-NN estimators.

[1] We are using the ℓ_∞ (maximum) norm for better compatibility with rectangular bins. The ℓ_2 (Euclidean) norm can also be used with minimal changes.

[2] $\psi(k) = -\gamma + \sum_{i=1}^{k-1} 1/i$, where where $\gamma \approx 0.577$ is the Euler constant.

Real data is often quantized or known only with limited accuracy. Due to the presence of the $\log r$ factor in (5), the results will fluctuate highly if small values of $\varrho_i(k)$ are inaccurate; if some $\varrho_i(k)$ are zero, the estimator diverges. A possible solution is to add low-amplitude perturbation to the data [15] or to switch to a histogram-like estimator for $r < R$, for some fixed R [17]. Singh [16] advocates the use of $k > 1$. However, the first approach increases variance, the second performs poorly in the transition region, and the third does not guarantee to eliminate the problem.

1.4 Proposed Approach

Consider the case of finite accuracy data where no distances smaller than a given R can be reliably measured. The k-NN estimator h_{NN} (5) works well for low densities f, when the distance between neighboring points is much larger than the measurement accuracy. Conversely, the kernel estimator h_{ker} (3) works best for high densities f, when the distance between points is smaller than the kernel size. Hence, we propose to construct a new estimator, called R-NN, combining the advantages of the two approaches with a smooth transition between [25]. A numerically calculated correction is used to preserve unbiasedness.

2 Method

For a fixed R, we take the k-NN estimator h_{NN} (5), varying the k for each $\mathbf{x}_i$ so that $\varrho_i(k) > R$. This gives us a naive R-NN estimator $h_{\mathrm{naive}}(\mathbf{x}_i; X) = h_0(r,k)$ where (from now on we will drop the subscript i for brevity)

$$h_0(r,k) = -\psi(k) + \psi(N) + d \log 2r \quad \text{with} \quad k = q(R), \quad r = \varrho(k) \tag{6}$$

The expected value of $h_0(r,k) = h_{\mathrm{naive}}(\mathbf{x}_i; X)$ for a fixed $\mathbf{x}_i$ is

$$\mathrm{E}\big[h_0\big]_{X\setminus\{\mathbf{x}_i\}} = \sum_{k=1}^{N-1} \int_{r>R} h_0(k,r)\, p(k,r)\, \mathrm{d}r \tag{7}$$

where $p(k,r)$ is the probability density of observing k points (including $\mathbf{x}_i$) in the neighborhood R and the $(k+1)$-th point (the k-th NN) at distance $r > R$. It can be obtained using the trinomial formula [15]

$$p(k,r) = \frac{(N-1)!}{(k-1)!(N-k-1)!}(2^d R^d f)^{k-1}(1-2^d R^d f)^{N-k-1} 2^d d\, r^{d-1} f \tag{8}$$

where we assume that $f = f(\mathbf{x}_i)$ is constant in a sufficiently large neighborhood of $\mathbf{x}_i$. The restriction $r > R$ makes the naive estimator (6) biased. The expected value $\mathrm{E}\big[h_0\big]$ can be calculated numerically (see Appendix A). A typical dependency of the bias B_0 on the density f

$$B_0(f) = \log f + \mathrm{E}\big[h_0\big] \tag{9}$$

is shown in Figure 1. The bias goes to zero for $f \to 0$ as the h_0 estimator approaches h_{NN}, and also as $f \to \infty$ as h_0 approaches[3] h_{ker}. The numerical

[3] Using the fact that $\psi(N) \approx \log N$ for large N.

calculation of $B_0(f)$ becomes inaccurate for high f. A deeper problem is that the assumption of a locally constant f in a neighborhood r is contradictory for high f, since the probability $V_d(r)f$ must not exceed 1. We therefore constrain $f < f_{\max}$ for a suitable $f_{\max}$.

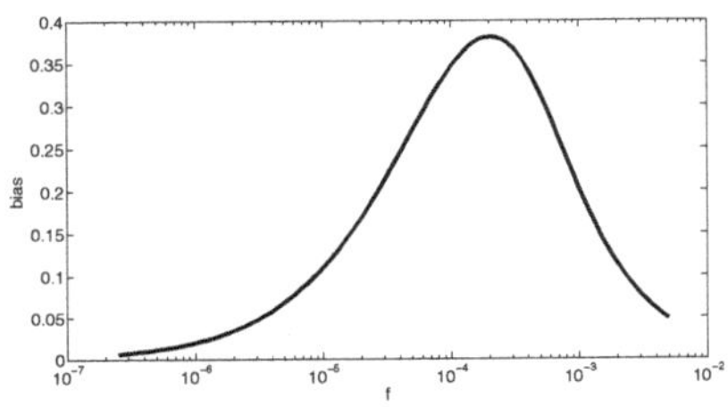

Fig. 1. Bias $B_0(f)$ of the naive estimator h_0 for $N = 1000$, $d = 2$ and $R = 1$

2.1 Corrected *R*-NN Estimator

Let us add a correction $\tilde{h}$ to the naive estimator h_0

$$h(r,k) = h_0(r,k) + \tilde{h}(r,k) \quad \text{with} \quad k = q(R), \quad r = \varrho(k) \tag{10}$$

so that the corrected estimator h is unbiased

$$\mathrm{E}\big[h\big] = -\log f \qquad \text{for} \quad f < f_{\max} \tag{11}$$

Note that we can assume without loss of generality that $R = 1$. The correction for general R' is then obtained as $\tilde{h}'(r,k) = \tilde{h}(r/R',k)$ for $f' < (R')^{-d} f_{\max}$. To see it, consider estimating entropy $H(R'X)$ and $f' = (R')^{-d} f$.

As finding $\tilde{h}$ analytically seems to be difficult, we attempt a numerical solution. We require (11) to hold for $f_1 = f_{\min}, f_2, \dots, f_F = f_{\max}$ for sufficiently small $f_{\min}$ and distributing $\log f_i$ uniformly. The correction $\tilde{h}$ is represented as a linear combination

$$\tilde{h}(r,k) = [k \leq K] \sum_{i=1}^{M} a_{ik} \varphi_i(r) \tag{12}$$

where the basis functions φ_i are piecewise linear on each interval $[r_i, r_{i+1}]$ and satisfying $\varphi_i(r_j) = \delta_{ij}$. We choose $r_1 = R$, sufficiently large r_M and K, and uniformly distributed $\log r_i$.

2.2 Quadratic Programming Formulation

The expected value of the estimator h (10) with correction $\tilde{h}$ (12) is

$$\mathrm{E}\big[h\big] = \mathrm{E}\big[h_0\big] + \mathrm{E}\big[\tilde{h}\big] = \mathrm{E}\big[h_0\big] + \sum_{k=1}^{K} \sum_{i=1}^{M} a_{ik} P_{ik} \tag{13}$$

$$\text{where} \quad P_{ik}(f) = \int_{r>R} \varphi_i(r)\, p(k,r)\, \mathrm{d}r \tag{14}$$

See Appendix B for details on calculating P_{ik}. For numerical reasons, we shall require the bias of h to be bounded by some small constant γ for all $f \in \{f_1, \ldots, f_F\}$. Using (9,10,13) leads to a system of $2F$ linear inequalities

$$-\gamma \leq B_0(f) + \sum_{k=1}^{K} \sum_{i=1}^{M} a_{ik} P_{ik}(f) \leq \gamma \qquad \text{for} \quad f \in f_1, \ldots, f_F \tag{15}$$

In addition we shall require $a_{Mk} = 0$ for all $k \leq K$ to prevent the discontinuity of $h(r,k)$ at $r = r_M$. Then (15) can be written in a matrix form as

$$\mathsf{A}\mathbf{a} \leq \mathbf{c} \tag{16}$$

where $\mathbf{a} = (a_{11}, \ldots, a_{M-1,K})$ is a linearized vector of unknowns.

To prevent indeterminacy of (16), we use a quadratic programming formulation: minimize a quadratic criterion $Q(\mathbf{a})$ under the conditions (16) with

$$Q(\mathbf{a}) = \frac{1}{2}\mathbf{a}^T \mathsf{H} \mathbf{a} + \mathbf{u}^T \mathbf{a} \tag{17}$$

A natural choice for Q would be the variance $\mathrm{Var}[h](f)$. Unfortunately, this choice requires numerical integration and is both time-consuming and inaccurate, leading to an ill-posed or infeasible minimization problem. We have therefore decided to minimize the following simple finite-difference-based criterion instead, taking advantage of the fact that Q serves primarily as a regularization, the final solution is determined mainly by the constraints (16).

$$Q(\mathbf{a}) = \sum_{k=1}^{K} \sum_{i=1}^{M-1} (a_{i+1,k} - a_{i,k})^2 + \sum_{k=1}^{K-1} \sum_{i=1}^{M-1} (a_{i,k+1} - a_{i,k})^2 \tag{18}$$

The criterion (18) expresses our preference for 'smooth' $\tilde{h}$, motivated by the well-known formula $\mathrm{Var}[g(x)] \approx g'(\mathrm{E}[x])^2 \mathrm{Var}[x]$. The corresponding Hessian H is very sparse, positive definite, and easy to calculate. The quadratic programming problem (17),(16) is solved by the MINQ algorithm [26].

It remains to determine a good value of γ in (15). We proceed iteratively, starting with $\gamma = \max_f |B_0(f)|$ and halving γ in each step. We stop if the solution cannot be found, or if the criterion increase is suspiciously large compared to the previous one, which signals overfitting.

3 Experiments

A typical shape of the correction $\tilde{h}(k,r)$ is shown in Figure 2 together with the shape of the uncorrected and corrected estimators h_0 and h. The width and position of the peak in $\tilde{h}$ depends on N and d. The parameter M influences the smoothness and F the accuracy. We found that $M = 100$ and $F = 1000$ give good results, with calculation of the estimator parameters taking several minutes. Higher values of M and F require more time and the calculation is often numerically unstable. The estimation itself is as fast as the k-NN estimator, with typical image similarity criterion taking between several seconds and one minute to evaluate, if acceleration techniques for the neighborhood search are used [17].

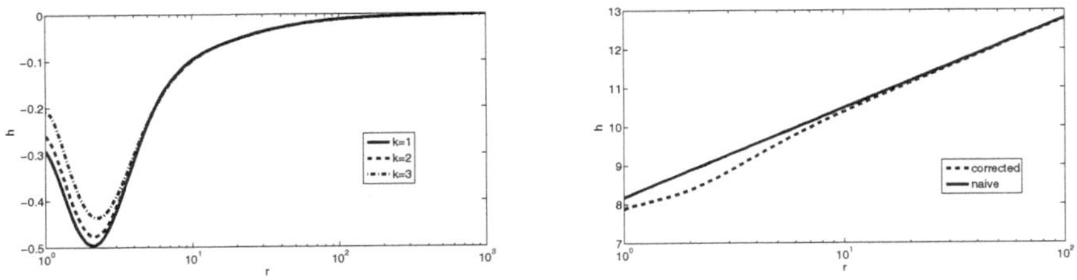

Fig. 2. The correction $\tilde{h}(r,k)$ for $N = 1000$, $d = 1$, shown as a function of r for $k = 1, 2, 3$ (left). The naive and corrected estimators (h_0 resp. h) for $k = 1$ (right).

Table 1. Estimating entropy of unit covariance normal data using k-NN, R-NN and histogram estimators, $d = 2$, $N = 1000$. Best values in each column are set in bold.

estimator	bias	variance	MSE
k-NN, $k = 1$	0.0099	0.0660	0.0045
k-NN, $k = 2$	0.0101	0.0519	0.0028
k-NN, $k = 5$	0.0197	0.0423	0.0022
k-NN, $k = 10$	0.0300	0.0405	0.0025
histogram	0.0349	0.0386	0.0027
R-NN, $R = 10^{-4}$	0.0099	0.0660	0.0045
R-NN, $R = 10^{-3}$	0.0100	0.0661	0.0045
R-NN, $R = 10^{-2}$	0.0102	0.0628	0.0040
R-NN, $R = 10^{-1}$	**0.0080**	0.0433	**0.0019**
R-NN, $R = 1$	0.0437	**0.0358**	0.0032

3.1 Entropy Estimation of Normal Data

Table 1 shows the bias, variance and mean squared error (MSE) for the k-NN, R-NN and histogram estimators (with optimal bin-width [13]) for estimation of entropy of normal data with unit covariance matrix in two dimensions ($d = 2$) from $N = 1000$ sample points. The experiment was repeated 100 times. For very small R the R-NN estimator is equivalent to the k-NN estimator; for higher R the variance decreases while bias remains essentially constant until R becomes comparable to the standard deviation of the data. Histogram estimator has a slightly lower variance but much higher bias.

3.2 Entropy Estimation for Quantized Normal Data

In Figure 3 we compare the k-NN, histogram (bin size 1), and R-NN estimators on 2D isotropic normal data quantized with step 1 as a function of the standard deviation σ. For σ comparable with the quantization step, histogram has the lowest bias and the lowest MSE. For σ much larger than the quantization step, the k-NN estimators perform best in terms of bias and MSE. It appears indeed that $k = 4$ is a good choice [16]. The R-NN estimators are a good compromise — they are almost as good as k-NN estimators for large σ (the difference is negligible for $\sigma = 10^3 \sim 10^4$) while offering significant improvement for small σ. In the high dimensional case ($d = 10$, MSE shown in Figure 3, bottom right), R-NN estimators outperform k-NN for small σ. Note that high R values may not be used in this case, since often no points fall outside the R neighborhood. Conversely, the k-NN estimator performs badly due to high bias for $k \geq 3$.

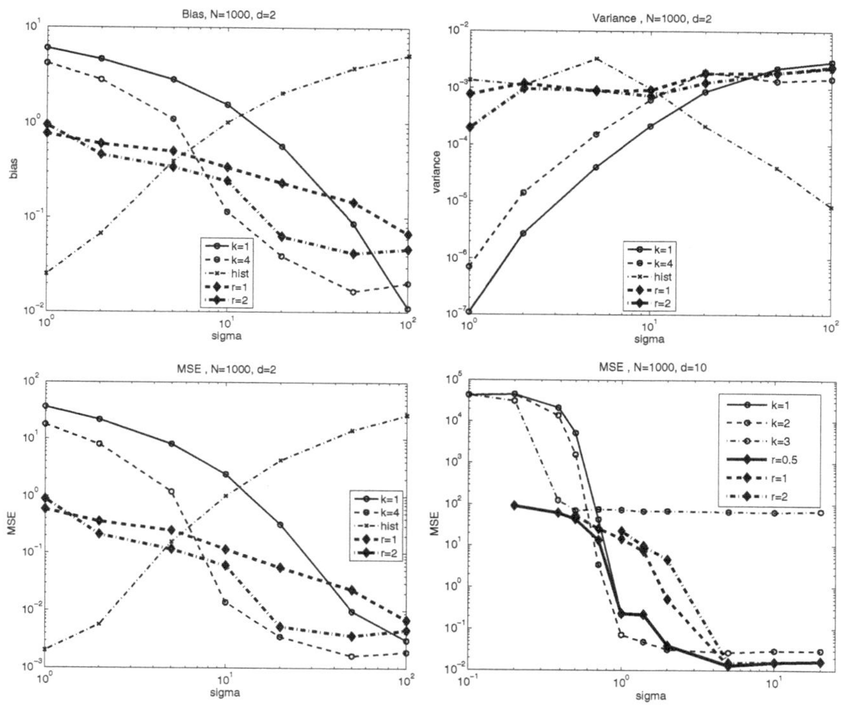

Fig. 3. The bias (top left), variance (top right), and MSE (bottom left) for several entropy estimators — k-NN with $k = 1$, $k = 4$, histogram estimator, and R-NN with $r = 1, r = 2$ — as a function of the standard deviation. The input are $N = 1000$ samples of a 2D ($d = 2$) Gaussian random variable with covariance matrix $\sigma^2 I$, rounded to the nearest integer. Bottom right image is the MSE for $d = 10$, $N = 1000$ for k-NN estimator with $k = 1, 2, 3$ and R-NN with $r = 0.5, r = 1.0, r = 2.0$.

3.3 Mutual Information as an Image Similarity Criterion

We have evaluated mutual information $I(X,Y) = H(X) + H(Y) - H(X,Y)$ between two scalar images (as it is done in image registration) as a function of their horizontal shift. The difficulty of this particular case lies in suppressing quantization artifacts (peaks) for integer shifts and obtaining a smooth dependence on the shift for easy optimization. We use 100×100 pixel centered regions from approximately registered T1 and T2 magnetic resonance images (Figure 4) of the same brain slice [27]. For the histogram estimator (Figure 5, top left), bin size is critical; bins too small lead to quantization artifacts, while bins too large

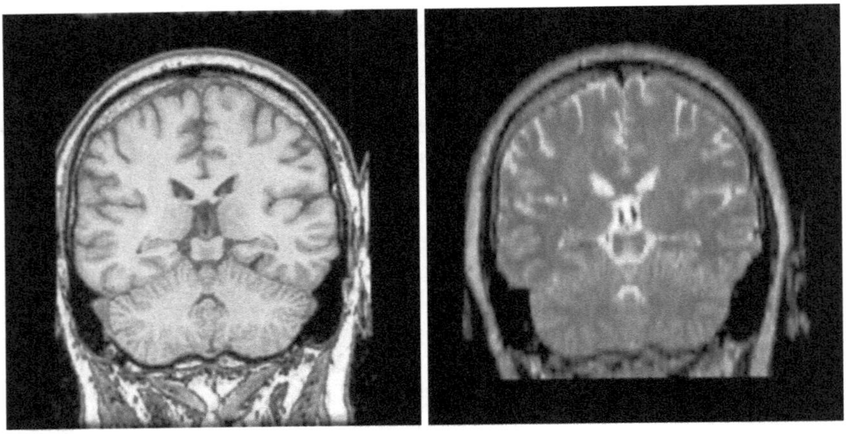

Fig. 4. 2D MRI images used for testing, T1 (left) and T2 (right)

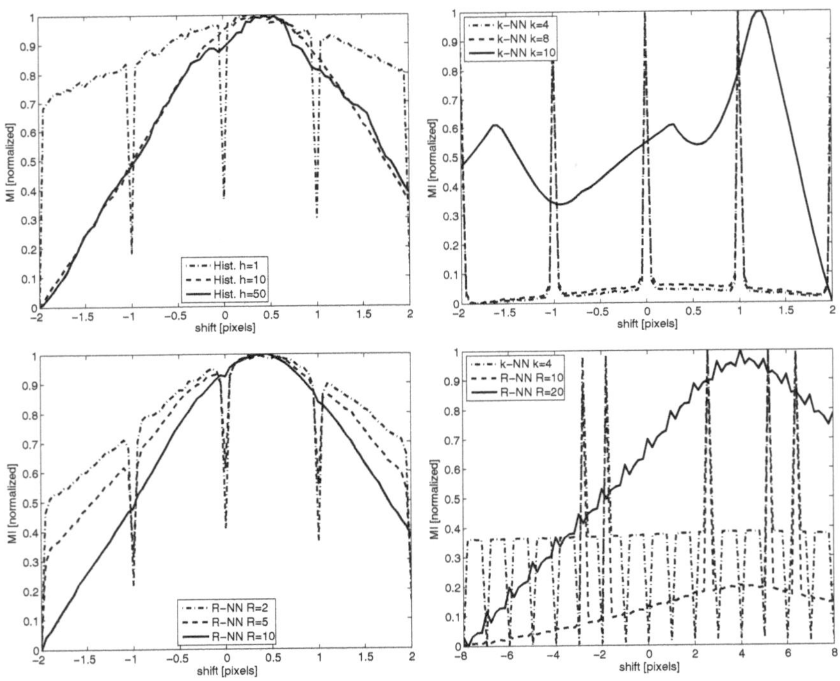

Fig. 5. Scalar mutual information criterion as a function of the horizontal shift, evaluated by histogram estimator (top left), k-NN estimator (top right), and R-NN estimator (bottom left). All values were normalized to $[0, 1]$ for easy visualization. The optimum shift is around 0.5 pixels. The bottom right graph shows the color MI criterion as a function of shift for two color colposcopy images for k-NN and R-NN estimators.

distort the curve shape. k-NN estimator performs poorly in this case, for $k \leq 8$ there are strong peaks on integers, for $k > 8$ the dependency is lost. The result of the R-NN estimator, for $R \geq 10$, is as good as the histogram.

Finally, we show also the color MI criterion as a function of shift for color colposcopy images [28]. While the k-NN estimator has artifacts for all k tested, the R-NN estimation is quite usable for $R = 20$, albeit noisy.

4 Conclusions

We have presented a new entropy estimator based on two quantities, the number of points k in a neighborhood of size R and the distance to the closest point r farther than R. The estimator behaves like an averaged histogram for high densities and like an NN estimator for low densities, smoothly varying between the two, combining their particular strengths. Finding the estimator is formulated as a constrained optimization problem (quadratic programming). The limited accuracy of this numerical procedure especially for high values of N, d, and f is currently the biggest setback of the new method. Nevertheless, our experiments show that the new method outperforms its ancestors in a number of situations, it deals successfully with the limited accuracy effects and is usable in a practical setting.

Acknowledgements

This work was sponsored by the Czech Ministry of Education, Project MSM6840770012.

References

1. Beirlant, J., Dudewicz, E.J.L.G., van der Meulen, E.C.: Nonparametric entropy estimation: an overview. International J. Math. Stat. Sci. (6), 17–39 (1997)
2. Harner, E.J., Singh, H., Li, S., Tan, J.: Computational challenges in computing nearest neighbor estimates of entropy for large molecules. Computing Science and Statistics, 35 (2003)
3. Victor, J.D.: Binless strategies for estimation of information from neural data. Physical Review E,66(5), 051903(15) (2002)
4. Viola, P., Wells III, W.M.: Alignment by maximization of mutual information. International Journal of Computer Vision (2), 137–154 (1997)
5. Pluim, J.P.W., Maintz, J.B.A., Viergever, M.A.: Mutual-information-based registration of medical images: A survey. IEEE Transactions on Medical Imaging 22(8), 986–1004 (2003)
6. Maes, F., Collignon, A., Vandermeulen, D., Marchal, G., Suetens, P.: Multimodality image registration by maximization of mutual information. IEEE Transactions on Medical Imaging 16(2), 187–198 (1997)
7. Pluim, J.P.W., Maintz, J.B.A., Viergever, M.A.: Image registration by maximization of combined mutual information and gradient information. IEEE Transactions Med. Imag. 19(8) (August 2000)
8. Rueckert, D., Clarkson, M.J., Hill, D.L.G., Hawkes, D.J.: Non-rigid registration using higher-order mutual information. In: Proceedings of SPIE Medical Imaging,: Image Processing 2000, pp. 438–447 (2000)

9. Russakoff, D.B., Tomasi, C., Rohlfing, T., Maurer, Jr,C.R.: Image similarity using mutual information of regions. In: Pajdla, T., Matas, J. (eds.) ECCV 2004. LNCS, vol. 3023, pp. 596–607. Springer, Heidelberg (2004)
10. Sabuncu, M.R., Ramadge, P.J.: Spatial information in entropy-based image registration. In: Gee, J.C., Maintz, J.B.A., Vannier, M.W. (eds.) WBIR 2003. LNCS, vol. 2717, pp. 132–141. Springer, Heidelberg (2003)
11. Darbellay, G.A., Vajda, I.: Estimation of the information by an adaptive partitioning of the observation space. IEEE Transactions on Information Theory 45(4), 1315–1321 (1999)
12. Miller, E.G.: A new class of entropy estimators for multi-dimensional densities. In: Proceedings of ICASSP2003 (2003)
13. Scott, D.W. (ed.): Multivariate Density Estimation : Theory, Practice, and Visualization. In: Wiley Series in Probability and Mathematical Statistics, John Wiley & Sons, New York (1992)
14. Kozachenko, L.F., Leonenko, N.N.: On statistical estimation of entropy of random vector. Probl. Inf. Trans. (in Russian) 23(9) (1987)
15. Kraskov, A., Stögbauer, H., Grassberger, P.: Estimating mutual information. Physical Review E, (69 066138) (2004)
16. Singh, H., Misra, N., Hnizdo, V., Fedorowicz, A., Demchuk, E.: Nearest neighbor estimates of entropy. American journal of mathematical and management sciences 23(3–4), 301–321 (2003)
17. Kybic, J.: Incremental updating of nearest neighbor-based high-dimensional entropy estimation. In: Duhamel, P., Vandendorpe, L. eds.: ICASSP2006, Toulouse, France, IEEE, III–804 DVD proceedings (2006)
18. Callahan, P.B., Kosaraju, S.R.: A decomposition of multi-dimensional point-sets with applications to k-nearest-neighbors and n-body potential fields. In: Proceedings 24th Annual AMC Symposium on the Theory of Computing 1992. pp. 546–556 (1992)
19. Smid, M.: Closest-point problems in computational geometry. In: Sack, J.-R.(ed.) Handbook on Computational Geometry, North Holland, Amsterdam (To appear) (1997)
20. Beis, J.S., Lowe, D.G.: Shape indexing using approximate nearest-neighbour search in high-dimensional spaces. In: Proceedings of Conference on Computer Vision and Pattern Recognition, June 1997, pp. 1000–1006 (1997)
21. Preparata, F.P., Shamos, M.I.: Computational geometry: An introduction. Texts and Monographs in Computer Science. Springer, Heidelberg (1985)
22. Sedgewick, R.: Algorithms. Addison-Wesley, Reading (1989)
23. Hero, A.O., Ma, B., Michel, O., Gorman, J.: Applications of entropic spanning graphs. IEEE Signal Proc. Magazine 19(5), 85–95 (2002)
24. Neemuchwala, H., Hero, A., Carson, P.: Image matching using alpha-entropy measures and entropic graphs. Signal Process. 85(2), 277–296 (2005)
25. Šára, R.: A modification of Kozachenko-Leonenko entropy estimator for quantized data. (Unpublished notes 2006)
26. Neumaier, A.: MINQ — general definite and bound constrained indefinite quadratic programming. (1998) `http://www.mat.univie.ac.at/neum/software/minq/`.
27. Johnson, K.A., Becker, J.A.: (The whole brain atlas) `http://www.med.harvard.edu/AANLIB/`
28. García-Arteaga, J.D., Kybic, J., Li, W.: Elastic image registration for movement compensation in digital colposcopy. In Jan, J., Kozumplík, J., Provazník, I., (eds.): Buiosignal: Analysis of Biomedical Signals and Images, Brno, Czech Republic June 2006, Eurasip, pp. 236–238 Vutium Press (2006)

A Expected Value of the Naive Estimator

We rewrite expression (7) by taking terms independent of r out of the integral and by substituting $\xi = 2^d r^d f$:

$$\mathrm{E}\big[h_0\big] = \sum_{k=1}^{N-1} \frac{(N-1)!}{(k-1)!(N-k-1)!} (2^d R^d f)^{k-1} I_1(N,k,f,R)$$

$$\text{with} \quad I_1(N,k,f,R) = \int_{\alpha}^{1} \big(\log\xi - \log f + \psi(N) - \psi(k)\big)(1-\xi)^{N-k-1}\,\mathrm{d}\xi$$

where $\alpha = 2^d R^d f$ and the upper integration limit comes from the fact that ξ is a probability. The integral I_1 is broken into two:

$$I_1 = \big(-\log f + \psi(N) - \psi(k)\big) \int_{\alpha}^{1} (1-\xi)^{N-k-1}\,\mathrm{d}\xi + \underbrace{\int_{\alpha}^{1} \log\xi (1-\xi)^{N-k-1}\,\mathrm{d}\xi}_{I_2}$$

The first integral is standard, the second one can be integrated by parts

$$I_2 = \frac{1}{N-k} \log\alpha\,(1-\alpha)^{N-k} + \frac{1}{N-k} \underbrace{\int_{\alpha}^{1} \frac{(1-\xi)^{N-k}}{\xi}\,\mathrm{d}\xi}_{I_3}$$

After substitution $z = 1-\xi$, we obtain:

$$I_3 = \int_{0}^{1-\alpha} \frac{z^{N-k}}{1-z}\,\mathrm{d}z = -\int_{0}^{1-\alpha} \sum_{i=0}^{N-k-1} z^i\,\mathrm{d}z + \int_{0}^{1-\alpha} \frac{1}{1-z}\,\mathrm{d}z = -\sum_{i=1}^{N-k} \frac{(1-\alpha)^i}{i} - \log\alpha$$

The last expression is delicate to calculate, since $\sum_{i=1}^{\infty} \frac{(1-\alpha)^i}{i} = -\log\alpha$.

B Calculating the Coefficients *P*

The integral (14) can be written as follows

$$P_{ik} = \frac{(N-1)!}{(k-1)!(N-k-1)!} (2^d R^d f)^{k-1} (I^- + I^+)$$

$$\text{with} \quad I^- = \int_{r_{i-1}}^{r_i} (1-2^d r^d f)^{N-k-1} \frac{r-r_{i-1}}{r_i - r_{i-1}}\, 2^d r^{d-1} d\,\mathrm{d}r$$

$$I^+ = \int_{r_i}^{r_{i+1}} (1-2^d r^d f)^{N-k-1} \frac{r_{i+1}-r}{r_{i+1} - r_i}\, 2^d r^{d-1} d\,\mathrm{d}r$$

Substituting $\xi = 2^d r^d f$ and $\xi_i = 2^d r^d f_i$ we get

$$I^+ = \frac{1}{r_{i+1} - r_i} \left(r_{i+1} \int_{\xi_i}^{\xi_{i+1}} (1-\xi)^{N-k-1} \mathrm{d}\xi - \frac{1}{2 f^{1/d}} \int_{\xi_i}^{\xi_{i+1}} \xi^{1/d} (1-\xi)^{N-k-1} \, \mathrm{d}\xi \right)$$

and similarly for I^-. The first integral is standard, the second one is related to the non-regularized incomplete beta function:

$$\int_0^{\xi_i} \xi^{1/d} (1-\xi)^{N-k-1} \, \mathrm{d}\xi = B(\xi_i; \frac{1}{d} + 1, N - l)$$

Kernel-Based Manifold Learning for Statistical Analysis of Diffusion Tensor Images

Parmeshwar Khurd, Ragini Verma, and Christos Davatzikos

Section of Biomedical Image Analysis, Dept. of Radiology,
University of Pennsylvania, Philadelphia, USA
khurdp@uphs.upenn.edu

Abstract. Diffusion tensor imaging (DTI) is an important modality to study white matter structure in brain images and voxel-based group-wise statistical analysis of DTI is an integral component in most biomedical applications of DTI. Voxel-based DTI analysis should ideally satisfy two desiderata: (1) it should obtain a good characterization of the statistical distribution of the tensors under consideration at a given voxel, which typically lie on a non-linear submanifold of $\Re^6$, and (2) it should find an optimal way to identify statistical differences between two groups of tensor measurements, e.g., as in comparative studies between normal and diseased populations. In this paper, extending previous work on the application of manifold learning techniques to DTI, we shall present a kernel-based approach to voxel-wise statistical analysis of DTI data that satisfies both these desiderata. Using both simulated and real data, we shall show that kernel principal component analysis (kPCA) can effectively learn the probability density of the tensors under consideration and that kernel Fisher discriminant analysis (kFDA) can find good features that can optimally discriminate between groups. We shall also present results from an application of kFDA to a DTI dataset obtained as part of a clinical study of schizophrenia.

1 Introduction

Diffusion tensor imaging (DTI) has become an important modality for studying white matter structure in brain imaging and other biomedical applications [1]. Several such applications require a group-wise statistical analysis of DT images which can identify regional differences between two groups of DT images. However, statistical analysis of DTI is complicated by the fact that we now have a 3×3 positive-definite symmetric matrix or diffusion tensor at each voxel instead of a single value as in the case of scalar images.

In conventional methods of performing such an analysis, scalar or vector images are first computed from the DTI dataset and then spatially normalized to a common template. A statistical p-value map is then computed from these scalar or vector images with the application of standard tests for statistical inference. Commonly used scalar images for such analyses include the fractional anisotropy (FA) and the apparent diffusion coefficient (ADC) [1]. Non-scalar features [2] such as the principal eigendirections of the tensors have also been used

N. Karssemeijer and B. Lelieveldt (Eds.): IPMI 2007, LNCS 4584, pp. 581–593, 2007.
© Springer-Verlag Berlin Heidelberg 2007

in some analyses. However, a main disadvantage of these methods is that they do not use the complete information available in the DTI dataset, but rather make the *a priori* assumption that group differences will affect specific quantities to be extracted from the diffusion tensor, such as FA. Moreover, differences in these scalar maps may be mutually difficult to interpret.

A voxel-based statistical analysis should ideally try to learn the density and the manifold structure pertinent to the specific tensors under consideration and determine the degree of separation between two groups of tensors. Methods for statistical analysis of tensors have been recently developed that utilize the full tensor information by trying to learn the underlying structure of the data. These methods fall into two categories: methods based upon Riemannian symmetric spaces [3,4] and methods based upon manifold learning [5]. Methods based upon Riemannian symmetric spaces [3,4] rely upon the assumption that the tensors around a given voxel from various subjects belong to a principal geodesic (sub)-manifold and that these tensors obey a normal distribution on that sub-manifold. The basic principle of these methods is sound, namely that statistical analysis of tensors must be restricted to the appropriate manifold of positive definite symmetric tensors, which is known to be a cone embedded in $\Re^6$. However, there is no guarantee that the representations of the tensors on this sub-manifold will have normal distributions, and most importantly, restricting the analysis on the manifold of positive definite symmetric tensors is of little help in hypothesis testing studies, since the tensors measured at a given voxel or neighborhood from a particular set of brains typically lie on a much more restricted submanifold. Our main goal is to determine the statistical distribution of tensors on this submanifold. In the approaches based upon manifold learning [5], the focus was on learning embeddings (or features) parameterizing the underlying manifold structure of the tensors. The learned features belonged to a low-dimensional linear manifold parameterizing the higher-dimensional tensor manifold and were subsequently used for group-wise statistical analysis. The main problem with manifold learning approaches [6] is that although they estimate the embedding of the manifold that represents the tensor measurements fairly well, they fail to estimate the probability distribution (non-Gaussian) on the (flattened) manifold itself. From experiments with simulated data, we have found that such an approach does not completely parameterize the probability density of the tensors under consideration and that the learned features do not always identify the differences between the two groups.

We shall present an integrated kernel-based approach to voxel-based analysis that accurately estimates the underlying distribution of the tensor data, obtains a highly informative linear representation for the tensors and uses this representation to determine statistically optimal ways of separating the tensor data. We shall build upon related approaches in [5]. We present our methods in Sec. 2 and the results from various experiments on simulated and real data in Sec. 3.1 and Sec. 3.2. We shall establish that higher-dimensional kernel principal component analysis (kPCA) features are very effective in learning the required probability density of the tensors from a voxel and that kernel Fisher discriminant analysis (kFDA) can optimally discriminate between groups of tensors. We shall also apply our methods to a clinical DTI dataset of healthy controls and schizophrenic patients in Sec. 3.3. We conclude with Sec. 4.

2 Methods

2.1 Kernel-Based Approach to Group-Wise Voxel-Based DTI Statistical Analysis

A DT image consists of a 3×3 positive-definite symmetric matrix or tensor T at each voxel in the image. We may represent this tensor as $T = \sum_{i=1}^{3} \lambda_i \mathbf{v}_i \mathbf{v}_i^T$, where $\lambda_i > 0$ and $\mathbf{v}_i$ represent the eigenvalues and eigenvectors of the tensor, respectively. Pathology can bring about subtle changes in eigen values or angular changes in the eigen vectors, that can be partially seen in measures of anisotropy and diffusivity computed from the tensor, such as FA and ADC, although eigen vector changes can only be seen in full tensor color maps. Group-wise voxel-based statistical analysis of DTI data involves normalizing all DT images to a common DTI template using a suitable technique [7,8,9] and then using an appropriate statistical test to infer regional differences between groups based upon the tensors at (or around) a voxel. We form a voxel-based dataset by collecting tensors from each location as samples. Such samples should ideally be formed using the tensors at a voxel from all subjects, in conjunction with the deformation field used to normalize the tensors. In this paper, we focus on the former term, however our approach readily extends to the latter, as well as to neighborhood information from tensors around a voxel under consideration, albeit at the cost of increasing the dimensionality of the measurements and the embedding space. The samples in our voxel-based dataset will have unknown statistical distributions on complex unknown non-linear manifolds. Therefore, it is particularly important to analyze the underlying structure in our dataset and to use this structure to estimate features that can identify group differences.

We have found that kernel-based techniques (kPCA and kFDA) are ideally suited for performing such an analysis. The common idea behind kernel-based techniques is to transform the samples into a higher-dimensional reproducible kernel Hilbert space (RKHS). Using the "kernel trick", any algorithm that can be written in terms of inner products in the RKHS, can be readily formulated in the original space in terms of the kernel. Moreover, hyperplanes in the RKHS, such as the ones spanned by principal eigenvectors or the ones separating two sets of samples, become nonlinear hyper-surfaces in the original space, thereby allowing us to nonlinearly span or separate groups of samples for the purposes of density estimation or classification, respectively. We can hence easily perform various calculations such as computing projections onto directions in the RKHS, although we cannot visualize this space itself. Figure 1 illustrates the idea behind obtaining such projections.

From our voxel-based samples, we can obtain highly informative projections using the kPCA technique, as described later in Sec. 2.2. Although we could extract useful features from this higher-dimensional kPCA representation to aid

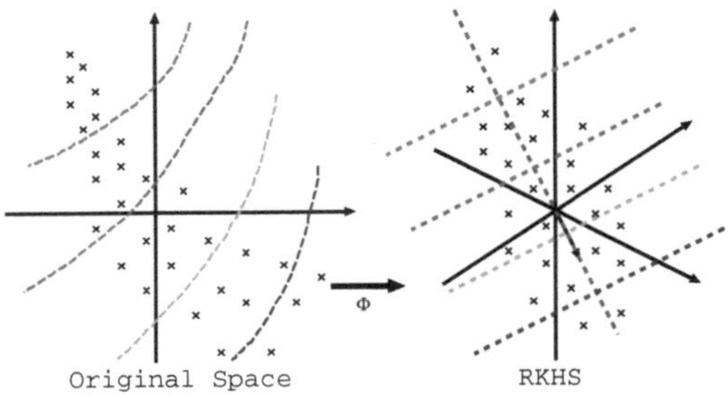

The mapping $\boldsymbol{\Phi}$ takes points (marked with crosses) from the original space to the RKHS. Hyperplanes having constant projections onto a vector in the RKHS become curved lines in the original space. Such curved lines can give us important insight into how the corresponding RKHS projection parameterizes the original points.

Fig. 1. Kernel-based projections

us in inferring differences between groups, it would be better to perform this inference step in an automated and optimal manner. For this purpose, we shall use the kFDA technique described in Sec. 2.3, which finds scalar projections onto a single RKHS direction that can optimally discriminate between groups. Having obtained our kernel-based features, we can then apply standard statistical tests such as the Hotelling T^2 test in the case of kPCA or the t-test in the case of the kFDA to obtain a voxel-wise p-value map. We note that the projections found by kPCA and kFDA lie along directions in the linear RKHS and hence linear tests for statistical inference can be reliably applied to these projections in order to identify separation between groups. Regions with low p-values indicate the regions with significant differences between the two groups.

Before we present the kPCA and kFDA techniques in detail, here is a brief note on our mathematical conventions: We denote vectors by bold-faced lower case letters, e.g. $\mathbf{x}$, and matrices by upper-case letters, e.g. A. We use $\mathbf{e}$ to denote the vector of all 1's and I to denote the identity matrix. We occasionally use $\mathbf{e}_m$ to denote a vector of all 1's in m-dimensional space. We use the superscripts ^{T} and $^{-1}$ to denote the matrix transpose and the matrix inverse respectively. We denote the sample mean of a set of vectors $\{\mathbf{x}_i, i = 1, \cdots, K\}$ by $\bar{\mathbf{x}}$. We denote the inner product of two vectors $\mathbf{x}_i, \mathbf{x}_j$ by $< \mathbf{x}_i, \mathbf{x}_j >$. We shall assume that our group-wise study involves a statistical analysis of the DT images of N subjects, with N_+ subjects in one class (the positive class) and the remaining N_- subjects in a second class (the negative class).

2.2 Kernel Principal Component Analysis (kPCA)

We now describe the kPCA technique [10] which can find a rich linear representation of our voxel-based samples as well as provide an accurate estimate of the probability density underlying these samples. In conventional PCA, we find out principal directions in the vector space of the samples that maximize the variance of the projections of the samples along those directions and which also minimize the least-squares representation error for the samples. In kPCA, we find similar principal eigendirections in the higher-dimensional RKHS. Let us denote the nonlinear mapping of point $\mathbf{x}$ into the Hilbert space by $\boldsymbol{\Phi}(\mathbf{x})$, and let us denote the underlying kernel by $k(.,.)$, where $< \boldsymbol{\Phi}(\mathbf{x}_i), \boldsymbol{\Phi}(\mathbf{x}_j) >= k(\mathbf{x}_i, \mathbf{x}_j)$.

Since a principal eigenvector $\mathbf{v}$ in the higher-dimensional Hilbert space lies in the span of the vectors $\mathbf{\Phi}(\mathbf{x}_i) - \bar{\mathbf{\Phi}}, i = 1, \cdots, N$, it can be conveniently represented as $\mathbf{v} = \sum_i \alpha_i(\mathbf{\Phi}(\mathbf{x}_i) - \bar{\mathbf{\Phi}})$, where $\boldsymbol{\alpha}$ is an N-dimensional vector. Projections of any sample along the eigenvector $\mathbf{v}$ can now be conveniently computed using this new representation in the kernel basis.

The entire kPCA procedure is summarized below [6]:

1. Form the kernel matrix K, where $K_{ij} = k(\mathbf{x}_i, \mathbf{x}_j), i = 1, \cdots, N, j = 1, \cdots, N$.
2. Center the kernel matrix to obtain $K_c = (I - \frac{1}{N}\mathbf{e}\mathbf{e}^T)K(I - \frac{1}{N}\mathbf{e}\mathbf{e}^T)$.
3. Eigen-decompose K_c to obtain its eigenvectors $\boldsymbol{\alpha}^{(i)}$ and eigenvalues $\lambda_i, i = 1, \cdots, N$.
4. Normalize the eigenvectors $\boldsymbol{\alpha}^{(i)}$ to have length $\frac{1}{\sqrt{\lambda_i}}$ so that the eigenvectors $\mathbf{v}^{(i)}$ in the RKHS have unit length.
5. The ith kPCA component for training sample $\mathbf{x}_k$ is given by: $< \mathbf{\Phi}(\mathbf{x}_k) - \bar{\mathbf{\Phi}}, \mathbf{v}^{(i)} >= \lambda_i \alpha_k^{(i)}$
6. For a general test point $\mathbf{x}$, the ith kPCA component is: $< \mathbf{\Phi}(\mathbf{x}) - \bar{\mathbf{\Phi}}, \mathbf{v}^{(i)} >= \sum_m \alpha_m^{(i)} k(\mathbf{x}, \mathbf{x}_m) - \frac{1}{N} \sum_{m,n} \alpha_m^{(i)} k(\mathbf{x}, \mathbf{x}_n)$

In addition to finding the orthogonal directions of maximal variance in the higher-dimensional RKHS, kPCA also provides an estimate of the probability density underlying the samples. It has been pointed out in [11] that kPCA with a Gaussian radial basis function kernel amounts to orthogonal series density estimation using Hermite polynomials. In Sec. 3.1, we shall present a simulated example (see Fig. 2) where kPCA obtained a very good parameterization of the density underlying the dataset. We also note that the kPCA components constitute a linear representation of the dataset in the RKHS, which considerably simplifies any further analysis such as the application of tests for statistical inference.

2.3 Kernel Fisher Discriminant Analysis (kFDA)

As described earlier, often the goal is not only to nonlinearly approximate the probability density from a number of samples, as in Sec. 2.2, but also to nonlinearly separate two groups of samples belonging to separate classes. We now examine this problem using kernel-based discriminants. We describe the kFDA technique [10,12], which focuses on finding nonlinear projections of the tensorial data which can optimally discriminate between the two groups. Kernel FDA finds a direction $\mathbf{w}$ in the higher-dimensional RKHS so that a projection along this direction maximizes a separability measure known as the Rayleigh coefficient (or the Fisher discriminant ratio). Let $\bar{\mathbf{\Phi}}^+$ denote the Hilbert-space mean for the samples in the positive class, corresponding to the N_+ DT images from the first group, and let $\bar{\mathbf{\Phi}}^-$ denote the mean for the negative class, corresponding to the N_- DT images from the second group. Let Σ^+ and Σ^- denote the sample covariance matrices for the positive and negative classes respectively. The Rayleigh coefficient is then given by:

$$J(\mathbf{w}) = \frac{(\mathbf{w}^T(\bar{\mathbf{\Phi}}^+ - \bar{\mathbf{\Phi}}^-))^2}{\mathbf{w}^T(\Sigma^+ + \Sigma^- + cI)\mathbf{w}},$$

where the scalar c is used to introduce regularization. As in kPCA, the optimal solution $\mathbf{w}^*$ maximizing $J(\mathbf{w})$ can again be conveniently represented using the samples, i.e. $\mathbf{w}^* = \sum_n \alpha_n^* \mathbf{\Phi}(\mathbf{x}_n)$, and projections along this direction can be easily obtained. A convenient analytical solution for $\boldsymbol{\alpha}^*$ is provided in [12]:

$$\boldsymbol{\alpha}^* = \frac{1}{c}\big[I - J(cI + JKJ)^{-1}JK\big]\mathbf{a},$$

$$\text{where } \mathbf{a} = \mathbf{a}^+ - \mathbf{a}^-,\ \mathbf{a}^+ = \begin{bmatrix} \frac{1}{N_+}\mathbf{e}_{N_+} \\ 0 \end{bmatrix},\ \mathbf{a}^- = \begin{bmatrix} 0 \\ \frac{1}{N_-}\mathbf{e}_{N_-} \end{bmatrix},\ J = \begin{bmatrix} J^+ & 0 \\ 0 & J^- \end{bmatrix},$$

$$J^+ = \frac{1}{\sqrt{N_+}}\Big(I - \frac{1}{N_+}\mathbf{e}_{N_+}\mathbf{e}_{N_+}^T\Big),\ J^- = \frac{1}{\sqrt{N_-}}\Big(I - \frac{1}{N_-}\mathbf{e}_{N_-}\mathbf{e}_{N_-}^T\Big),$$

and where K represents the un-centered kernel matrix. An alternative quadratic programming approach to obtaining the solution $\boldsymbol{\alpha}^*$ is provided in [10].

To summarize, we have presented the kPCA technique which can estimate the probability density and yield a rich linear representation for any voxel-based tensor dataset and the kFDA technique which uses this representation to extract features that can identify group differences in a statistically optimal manner.

3 Results and Discussion

We have applied the kernelized framework to the group analysis of real and simulated DTI data with the aim of demonstrating that kPCA is able to capture the statistical distribution underlying such datasets and that application of kFDA facilitates optimal group-based separation.

3.1 Statistical Analysis of Simulated Tensors

We shall first apply our kernelized framework to group analysis of simulated (non-imaging) tensor datasets where we know the ground-truth underlying structure in the dataset and can therefore easily validate our results. We consider tensor datasets with changes in the principal eigenvalue as well as in one of the angles describing the principal eigendirection. Such subtle changes emulate pathology-induced changes that affect the eigenvalue and eigenvector and an analysis of subtle changes of this nature may be of particular importance in studying complex brain disorders such as schizophrenia which result in non-focal regional changes. We have found that kPCA is well-suited for parameterizing the density for such datasets and that kFDA can effectively highlight the differences that discriminate between groups. For ease of visualization, we present representative results on a dataset with variation in the radial and angular directions instead of on a tensorial dataset with changes in the principal eigenvalue and eigendirection.

kPCA representation: Our dataset consisted of points forming a semi-circular band (see Fig. 2(a)) and was generated using 36 angles (in the $0 - 144$ degrees range) and 6 radial values (in the range $1.3 - 1.8$) resulting in a total of 216 points.

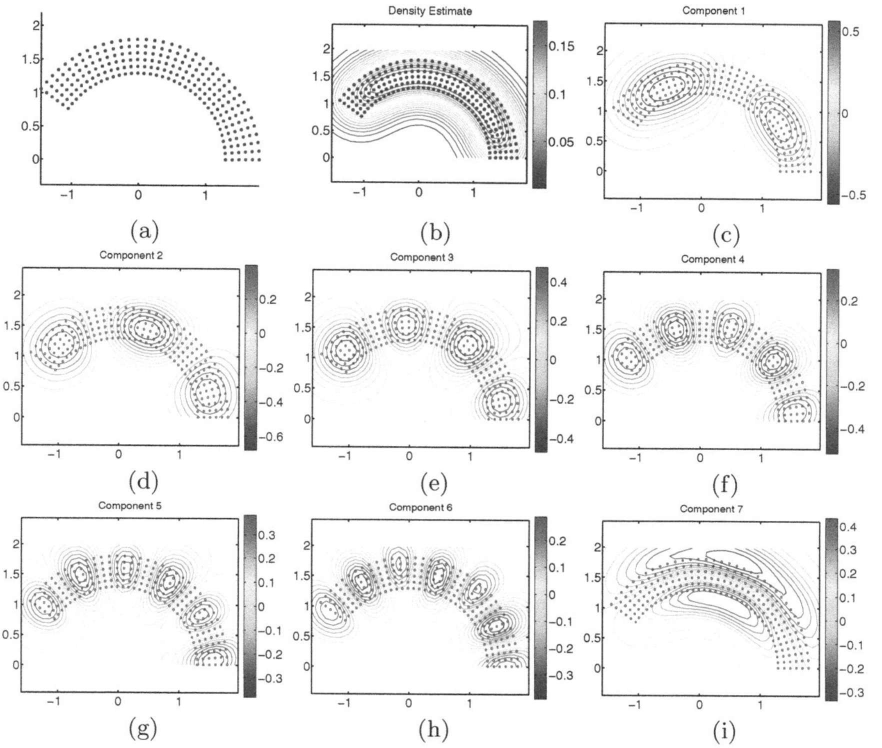

Fig. 2. (a) Dataset, (b) Contour plot for kernel probability density estimate, (c) Contour plot for 1st kPCA component, (d) Contour plot for 2nd kPCA component, (e) Contour plot for 3rd kPCA component, (f) Contour plot for 4th kPCA component, (g) Contour plot for 5th kPCA component, (h) Contour plot for 6th kPCA component, and (i) Contour plot for 7th kPCA component (Please see text for explanation)

We applied kPCA to this dataset using a Gaussian radial basis function (RBF) as our kernel with the kernel width σ^2 set to 0.1. The kernel width parameter was chosen to be a suitable function of the average distance between nearest neighbors $\mathbf{x}_i$ and $\mathbf{x}_j$, i.e. $||\mathbf{x}_i - \mathbf{x}_j||$ and the number of samples, and our choice was motivated by the desire to obtain meaningful representations for the different kPCA components as well as a reasonably good probably density estimate for the entire dataset. The iso-contours for our kernel probability density estimate (using all kPCA components), shown in Fig. 2(b), indicate that the estimated density is roughly constant in the central regions where data points are uniformly present and that the density estimate smoothly fades to zero as we approach the data points lying along the borders. The iso-contour plots for 7 principal kPCA components, shown in Fig. 2(c)-(i), represent the hyperplanes having constant projections onto the corresponding 7 RKHS eigen-vectors, as explained earlier in Fig. 1. It can be seen that the first 6 components (Fig. 2(c)-(h)) represent the angular changes in the data using varying scales, e.g., the third kPCA component (Fig. 2(e)) divides the angular variation in the data into four

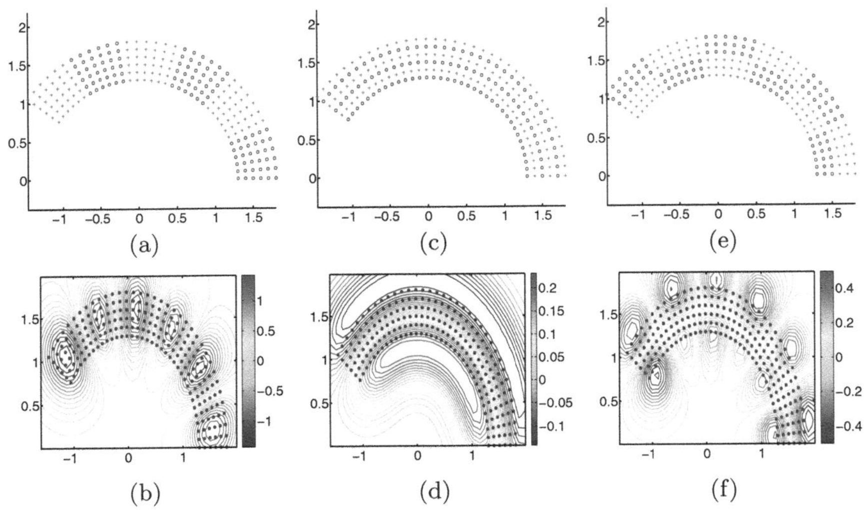

Fig. 3. (a) Samples with angle-based labels. (b) Contour plot for kFDA projection corresponding to (a). (c) Samples with radius-based labels. (d) Contour plot for kFDA projection corresponding to (c). (e) Samples with labels determined by both angle and radius. (f) Contour plot for kFDA projection corresponding to (e). (Blue labels marked 'o' indicate one class and red labels marked '+' indicate the other class in (a), (c) and (e). Colors refer to the online version of the paper.)

regions and alternately assumes positive and negative values as we move along the angular direction across these four regions. We may also observe that the seventh kPCA component (Fig. 2(i)) individually captures the radial change in the data and that it smoothly increases from negative to positive values as we step along the data in the radial direction.

kFDA projections: The previous synthesized dataset addressed the issue of estimating the probability density of these samples. We now reformulate this experiment as one requiring classification, i.e., as an experiment aiming to find the optimal separator between two groups of samples, as depicted by red and blue labels in Fig. 3(a), (c) and (e). We assigned labels in the angular direction to this dataset as shown in Fig. 3(a) and applied kFDA, which successfully discriminated between the two groups, as shown Fig. 3(b). (The kFDA projection in Fig. 3(b) roughly corresponds to the 5th kPCA component in Fig. 2(g).) We also assigned labels in the radial direction to this dataset as shown in Fig. 3(c) and applied kFDA, which again discriminated very well between the two groups, as seen in Fig. 3(d). (The kFDA projection in Fig. 3(d) roughly corresponds to the 7th kPCA component in Fig. 2(i).) We also conducted experiments where the labels were assigned to indicate changes in both the radial and angular directions and we have found that the kFDA projection (which did not correspond to any kPCA component) still separated the groups in an optimal manner (please see Fig. 3(e) and Fig. 3(f)).

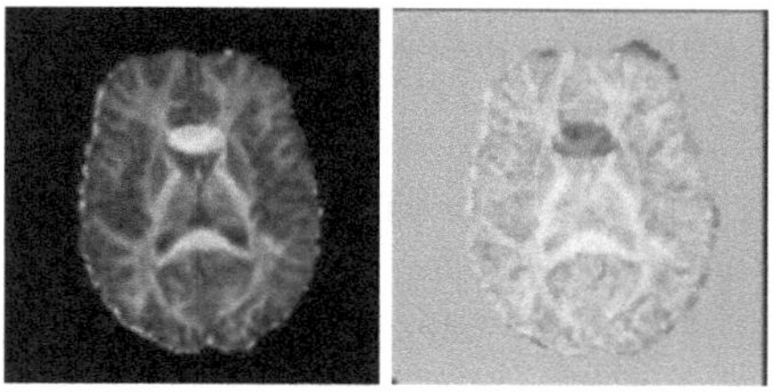

(a) (b)

Fig. 4. (a) ROI with changes (highlighted) overlaid on the template FA map. (b) kFDA voxel-wise p-map (with significant low p-values highlighted) overlaid on the same FA map. Low p-value regions in (b) match the true ROI in (a).

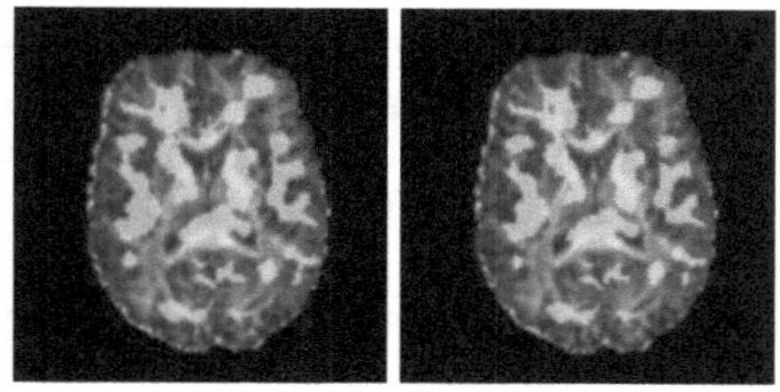

(a) (b)

Fig. 5. (a) Schizophrenia kFDA p-map thresholded at 0.02 and overlaid on the template FA map. (b) Schizophrenia kFDA p-map thresholded using a false discovery rate of 0.18 and overlaid on the template FA map. Significant p-values after thresholding are highlighted in (a), (b).

Comparison to manifold learning: Manifold learning techniques such as ISOMAP (isometric mapping) [5] have also been proposed for DTI statistical analysis. We performed such an analysis using two approaches, ISOMAP [6], on the lines of [5], and MVU (maximum variance unfolding) [13], both of which correctly identify the underlying manifold of dimension 2 when applied to the dataset in Fig. 2(a), with MVU doing better than ISOMAP in separating the angular and radial changes in the data into its two components. An application of the Hotelling T^2 test on the MVU or ISOMAP embeddings, when group labels were assigned as in Figs. 3(a) or 3(c), yielded higher p-values, indicating less significant differences, than those found by applying a t-test on the kFDA projections or on the appropriate kPCA components, indicating that both MVU and ISOMAP were unable to identify the statistical distribution on the manifold like kPCA or determine projections like kFDA that separate the groups.

Having successfully validated our methods on a simulated non-imaging dataset with radial and angular variation, we shall now validate them on real DTI data with simulated changes in both the tensor eigenvalues and eigenvectors that emulate this joint radial and angular variation.

3.2 Statistical Analysis of DTI Datasets with Simulated Changes

Dataset Description: Our DTI dataset consisted of scans of 36 healthy volunteers (17 male and 19 female), acquired at dimensions $128 \times 128 \times 40$ and a voxel size of $1.72 \times 1.72 \times 3.0$ mm. These DT images were warped to a template, which was chosen as the scan of an additional healthy subject. We then identified an ROI on the template in the corpus callosum, as shown in Fig. 4(a), and introduced random changes in the principal eigenvalue and the azimuthal angle for the principal eigenvector of each tensor into the appropriate ROI for all unwarped subject DT images. The random changes were designed to slightly increase the principal eigenvalue and the principal azimuthal angle, on average, but were subtle enough so that these changes could not be visibly easily discerned on an FA map or a colormap for the principal direction. The DT images with the introduced random changes were then warped back to the template resulting in 36 DT images belonging to the abnormal class.

The simplest approach to forming the voxel-based sample vector is to use the 6-independent components of the tensor at a voxel. However, we can potentially obtain more significant regional differences by incorporating neighborhood information around a voxel into our samples, in two different ways. In one approach, which we call the "long-vector" approach, we form a local spherical neighborhood around each voxel and combine the 6-independent components from each tensor in the local neighborhood into a long vector, which we use as our sample. In an alternative approach, we first smooth the DTI [14] data and then use the 6-independent tensor components at a voxel as our sample. We shall now present results obtained by applying kPCA and kFDA to these different sample types.

Results Using kPCA, kFDA and Other Techniques: We have shown the central axial slice of the 3-D p-value map found from an application of kFDA and the t-test in Figure 4(b). We may observe that significant regions identified in Figure 4(b) match the true ROI very well. In Table 1, we have presented a detailed quantitative performance comparison of different approaches to discovering the true ROI. Our performance measure was the percentage overlap of voxels in the detected ROI (p-value map thresholded at a cut-off of 0.1) with the voxels in the true ROI. We have applied the different approaches to the original DTI dataset as well as to a smoothed version of the DT images, smoothed in the Log-Euclidean domain [14] using an isotropic truncated Gaussian filter with the filter σ set to 4 mm . This choice for smoothing yielded good results for the technique in [5]. For the long-vector results, we used a spherical neighborhood of 4 mm radius that contained 39 voxels. The Gaussian RBF kernel width parameter σ^2 was set to $4e-4$ in all kernel-based results not using the long-vector and this value was multiplied by the number of neighborhood voxels when the long-vector approach was used.

Rows 1 and 2 in Table 1 present results from conventional ADC and FA analyses and row 3 presents results using the ISOMAP technique from [5]. Since the ADC and FA concentrate on eigenvalue differences, they are not particularly sensitive in detecting the ROI. The ISOMAP technique (row 3) performs better than these two approaches, but it is hampered by the fact it does not use knowledge of the statistical distribution underlying the tensors. Knowledge of this statistical distribution led to enhanced results using the kPCA technique, as can be seen in rows 4-8. Rows 4 and 5 present results using the 6 independent tensor components as the sample vector, whereas rows 6-8 use the long-vector approach. We may observe that kPCA, when used appropriately, is very sensitive in detecting the ROI. While the long-vector kPCA approach yielded poor results on the original DT data, it yielded good results on the smoothed DTI. From these kPCA results, we may also observe a general difficulty with using this method and the ISOMAP-based method, which stems from the fact that

Table 1. Percentage overlap of detected ROI (p-value map thresholded at a cut-off of 0.1) with the true ROI (Please see text for explanation)

	Analysis Method	Original DTI	Smooth DTI
1.	ADC	14.92	21.71
2.	FA	39.14	42.39
3.	ISOMAP- 3 components	35.60	44.46
4.	kPCA- 3 components	60.41	72.53
5.	kPCA- 8 components	54.95	62.48
6.	kPCA-long-vector 3 components	13.44	53.32
7.	kPCA-long-vector 8 components	44.46	75.18
8.	kPCA-long-vector 12 components	51.70	81.83
9.	kFDA	57.90	71.64
10.	**kFDA-long-vector**	**79.17**	**83.31**
11.	kFDA-long-vector-cross-validated	56.72	51.55

we do not know the discriminatory component(s) in these representations, making it hard to select the component(s) on which the subsequent statistical tests must be applied. The kFDA approach (rows 9-11), on the other hand, does not suffer from this problem. **As seen from row 10, kFDA employing the long-vector approach on smooth DT images yields the best performance among all methods compared.**

We note that kFDA is the only technique in Table 1 that uses the class labels while computing its features and hence it requires a special form of cross-validation. We divided our data equally into training and testing samples. We then learned discriminatory directions on the training samples, used these directions to obtain projections for the testing samples and then applied the t-test on these test sample projections. Such a naive cross-validation approach would reduce performance considerably because the training is performed on half the number of samples and also partly because the p-values are computed from a fewer number of testing samples. However, row 11 in Table 1 indicates that the kFDA performance remains significantly better than several other approaches.

3.3 Statistical Analysis of Schizophrenia DTI Dataset

In addition to the 36 healthy volunteers used in Sec. 3.2, our dataset now additionally included scans of 34 schizophrenic patients (21 male and 13 female), again warped to the template. We first smoothed this dataset and applied kFDA with the 6 tensor components and the t-test voxel-wise (using the same smoothing and kernel parameters as in Sec. 3.2) to obtain a p-value map showing regional differences. The resulting significant regions, after thresholding the p-value map at a cut-off of 0.02 and removing small spurious clusters, are shown in Fig. 5(a). Kernel FDA has found a number of white matter regions such as the corpus callosum and the internal capsule and gray matter regions such as some regions in the fronto-temporal cortex that have been implicated in other studies of schizophrenia. We plan to investigate the clinical significance of our findings in future work. (We note that we found similar significant regions when the p-value maps were alternatively thresholded using a false discovery rate [15] of 0.18, as shown in Fig. 5(b).)

4 Conclusion

Using both simulated and real data, we have established that kernel-based methods pave the way to resolving major issues in group-wise DTI statistical analysis, namely, the density estimation of voxel-based tensors (in the presence of non-linearity), the appropriate representation of these tensors on a manifold and the subsequent use of this representation in the identification of features that can optimally identify region-based group differences. In particular, we have shown that kFDA can form the basis of a highly sensitive method for group-wise DTI statistical analysis. Such a method can open up numerous avenues of research in various DTI applications requiring large scale group analysis such as studies of various brain disorders involving prognosis, diagnosis or progression of disease. Future work will involve optimal kernel selection in kFDA [12] and more sophisticated cross-validation of our kFDA results using permutation tests on the DTI dataset with simulated changes as well as on the schizophrenia DTI dataset.

Acknowledgements

This work was supported by the National Institute of Health via grants R01MH070365, R01MH079938 and R01MH060722.

References

1. LeBihan, D., Mangin, J.F., et al.: Diffusion tensor imaging: Concepts and applications. J. of Magnetic Resonance Imaging 13, 534–546 (2001)
2. Wu, Y.C., Field, A.S., et al.: Quantitative analysis of diffusion tensor orientation: Theoretical framework. Magnetic Resonance in Medicine 52, 1146–1155 (2004)
3. Lenglet, C., Rousson, M., Deriche, R., Faugeras, O.: Statistics on the manifold of multivariate normal distributions: Theory and application to diffusion tensor MRI processing. Journal of Math. Imaging and Vision 25(3), 423–444 (2006)
4. Fletcher, P.T., Joshi, S.: Principal geodesic analysis on symmetric spaces: Statistics of diffusion tensors. In: Sonka, M., Kakadiaris, I.A., Kybic, J. (eds.) Computer Vision and Mathematical Methods in Medical and Biomedical Image Analysis. LNCS, vol. 3117, pp. 87–98. Springer, Heidelberg (2004)
5. Verma, R., Davatzikos, C.: Manifold based analysis of diffusion tensor images using isomaps. In: IEEE Int. Symp. on Biomed, Imaging, pp. 790–793. IEEE, Washington, DC, USA (2006)
6. Burges, C.: Geometric Methods for Feature Extraction and Dimensional Reduction. In: Data Mining and Knowledge Discovery Handbook, Kluwer Academic Publishers, Dordrecht (2005)

7. Zhang, H., Yushkevich, P., et al.: Deformable registration of diffusion tensor MR images with explicit orientation optimization. Medical Image Analysis 10(5), 764–785 (2006)
8. Cao, Y., Miller, M., Mori, S., Winslow, R., Younes, L.: Diffeomorphic matching of diffusion tensor images. In: CVPR-MMBIA, 67 (2006)
9. Xu, D., Mori, S., Shen, D., van Zijl, P., Davatzikos, C.: Spatial normalization of diffusion tensor fields. Magnetic Resonance in Medicine 50(1), 175–182 (2003)
10. Scholkopf, B., Smola, A.: Learning with Kernels. The MIT Press, Cambridge, MA (2002)
11. Girolami, M.: Orthogonal series density estimation and the kernel eigenvalue problem. Neural Computation 14(3), 669–688 (2002)
12. Kim, S.J., Magnani, A., Boyd, S.: Optimal kernel selection in kernel Fisher discriminant analysis. In: ACM Int. Conf. on Machine Learning 2006 (2006)
13. Saul, L.K., Weinberger, K.Q., Ham, J.H., Sha, F., Lee, D.D.: Spectral methods for dimensionality reduction. In: Semisupervised Learning, MIT Press, Cambridge, MA (2006)
14. Arsigny, V., Fillard, P., et al.: Medical Image Computing and Computer-Assisted Intervention. In: Duncan, J.S., Gerig, G. (eds.) MICCAI 2005. LNCS, vol. 3749, pp. 115–122. Springer, Heidelberg (2005)
15. Genovese, C., Lazar, N., Nichols, T.: Thresholding of statistical maps in functional neuroimaging using the false discovery rate. NeuroImage 15, 870–878 (2002)

An Anatomical Equivalence Class Based Joint Transformation-Residual Descriptor for Morphological Analysis

Sajjad Baloch, Ragini Verma, and Christos Davatzikos

University of Pennsylvania, Philadelphia, PA

Abstract. Existing approaches to computational anatomy assume that a perfectly conforming diffeomorphism applied to an anatomy of interest captures its morphological characteristics relative to a template. However, biological variability renders this task extremely difficult, if possible at all in many cases. Consequently, the information not reflected by the transformation, is lost permanently from subsequent analysis. We establish that this residual information is highly significant for characterizing subtle morphological variations and is complementary to the transformation. The amount of residual, in turn, depends on transformation parameters, such as its degree of regularization as well as on the template. We, therefore, present a methodology that measures morphological characteristics via a lossless morphological descriptor, based on both the residual and the transformation. Since there are infinitely many [transformation, residual] pairs that reconstruct a given anatomy, which collectively form a nonlinear manifold embedded in a high-dimensional space, we treat them as members of an *Anatomical Equivalence Class* (AEC). A unique and optimal representation, according to a certain criterion, of each individual anatomy is then selected from the corresponding AEC, by solving an optimization problem. This process effectively determines the optimal template and transformation parameters for each individual anatomy, and removes respective confounding variation in the data. Based on statistical tests on synthetic 2D images and real 3D brain scans with simulated atrophy, we show that this approach provides significant improvement over descriptors based solely on a transformation, in addition to being nearly independent of the choice of the template.

1 Introduction

The problem of quantitatively characterizing normal and pathologic anatomy is usually addressed in computational anatomy through high dimensional diffeomorphic shape transformations [1,2,3,4,5] that warp individuals to a common template and vice-versa. Various descriptors are then derived from these transformations for quantifying morphological characteristics, leading to a wide range of approaches such as *deformation based morphometry* (DBM) [6,7,8], *voxel based morphometry* (VBM) [9,10,11], and *tensor based morphometry* (TBM) [12,13]. Accuracy of these methods, however, depends on the ability to establish perfect correspondences between subjects and a template, which may, in general, not be

N. Karssemeijer and B. Lelieveldt (Eds.): IPMI 2007, LNCS 4584, pp. 594–606, 2007.
© Springer-Verlag Berlin Heidelberg 2007

possible due to anatomical variability across individuals. For instance, a biologically meaningful diffeomorphism that warps a single-folded sulcus to a bifolded sulcus may not exist. As a result, a shape transformation would likely fail to capture the shape of the sulcus, resulting in the loss of residual information. In this paper, we establish that the residual may carry more important information than the transformation itself, and, therefore, consider a *complete morphological descriptor*[1] (CMD) of the form [Transformation, Residual].

CMD requires additional consideration due to its dependence on transformation parameters such as the degree of conformity achieved by the transformation, which is determined by some regularization parameter(s), as well as on the selection of a template. Since the selection of these parameters is an open question in computational anatomy, a complete representation does not lead to a unique descriptor. By varying these parameters, one may, in fact, generate an entire class of infinitely many anatomically equivalent descriptors, all representing the same anatomy via different transformations and respective residuals. This class, the *Anatomical Equivalence Class* (AEC), is generally a nonlinear manifold embedded in a high dimensional space. In this paper, we address the problem of non-uniqueness of this anatomical descriptor by representing each anatomy with an "optimal" descriptor, referred to as *Optimal Morphological Signature* (OMS), which is estimated by minimizing the variance of an ensemble, while allowing each CMD to slide along its respective AEC. The hypothesis is that by minimizing the variance due to confounding factors, one may overcome arbitrariness in selecting these parameters, thereby enhancing the ability to detect morphological abnormalities. Our results indicate that this morphological representation provides generally better and more robust detection of group morphological differences than the transformation alone. Moreover, it is nearly invariant to template selection, and the amount of flexibility in the transformation, thus avoiding their arbitrary selection.

2 Morphological Descriptor Framework

2.1 Motivation

Computational anatomy typically involves characterizing anatomical differences between a subject S and a template T by mapping the template space Ω_T to the subject space Ω_S through a diffeomorphism $h \in \mathcal{H}_S : \Omega_T \rightarrow \Omega_S, \mathbf{x} \mapsto h(\mathbf{x})$, where $\mathcal{H}_S$ is the set of all diffeomorphic transformations that maximize some similarity criterion between T and normalized subject S_T. Resulting transformation h then carries information about morphological differences between a subject and a template [6,2,7,14,9,12,10,8,11,13]. This, however, requires a diffeomorphism that perfectly warps a subject to the template, i.e., $T(\mathbf{x}) - S(h(\mathbf{x})) = 0, \forall \mathbf{x} \in \Omega_T$. Moreover, h must define anatomical correspondences, instead of simply matching

[1] The term "complete" is used, since this morphological descriptor does not discard any image information.

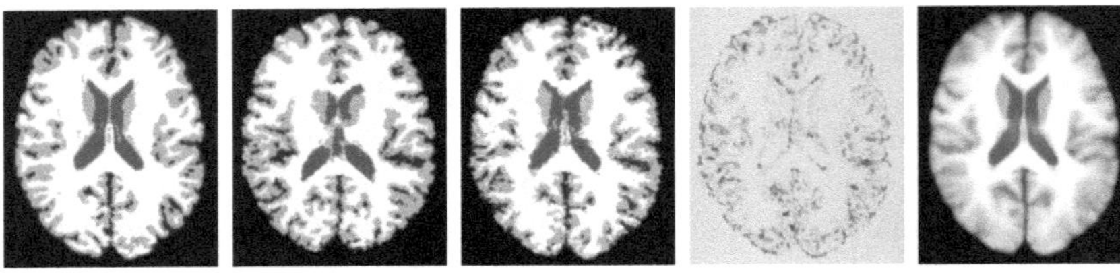

(a) (b) (c) (d) (e)

Fig. 1. (a) Template; (b) A representative subject; (c) Spatial normalization of (b); (d) Corresponding residual; (e) Crispness of the mean of 31 spatially normalized subjects indicates relatively good anatomical correspondence

images. Achieving both of these goals is usually not possible, thereby resulting in a residual error:

$$R_h(\mathbf{x}) := T(\mathbf{x}) - S(h(\mathbf{x})), \mathbf{x} \in \Omega_T \qquad (1)$$

This is shown with an illustrative example in Fig. 1, based on the spatial normalization of 31 subjects using a deformable registration method [5]. While the accuracy of the registration is demonstrated by the clarity of the average brain given in Fig. 1(e), spatial normalization of a typical subject (Fig. 1(b)) to the template (Fig. 1(a)) still produces significant residual shown in Fig. 1(d). A study based solely on a warping transformation irreversibly loses this residual information. Although one may argue that a more flexible and aggressive registration may further minimize the residual, this is often impossible to achieve using biologically consistent transformations. Our approach herein is to use a template warping algorithm that is flexible enough, yet respecting anatomical correspondences and then capture the resulting residual in an $\mathcal{M}_h := (h, R_h)$ descriptor, referred to as CMD.

2.2 Anatomical Equivalence Class Framework

CMD, $\mathcal{M}_h$, defined in the previous section not only depends on the underlying anatomy but also on transformation parameters, resulting in a non-unique representation of the anatomy. An entire family of anatomically equivalent CMDs may be generated by varying $h \in \mathcal{H}_S$. This unwanted variation usually confounds subsequent analyses, and, therefore, must be eliminated. We approach this problem by first approximating the range of variation in $\mathcal{M}_h$. Since it is not possible to sample all possible transformations and to evaluate their respective residuals for all possible templates, we examine a restricted family of transformations $h_{\lambda,\tau} \in \mathcal{I}_S \subset \mathcal{H}_S$, by perturbing $h_{\lambda,\tau}$ through two parameters, namely $\lambda \in \mathbb{R}_+$ and $\tau \in \mathcal{T}^m$, where $\mathcal{T}$ represents the set of all possible templates. The first parameter λ represents the level of regularity (smoothness) in $h_{\lambda,\tau}$, as determined by viscosity in viscous fluid registration, for instance, or Young's modulus in elastic registration. For notational consistency, we reparameterize the regularization parameter such that small λs correspond to aggressive transformations, and, hence,

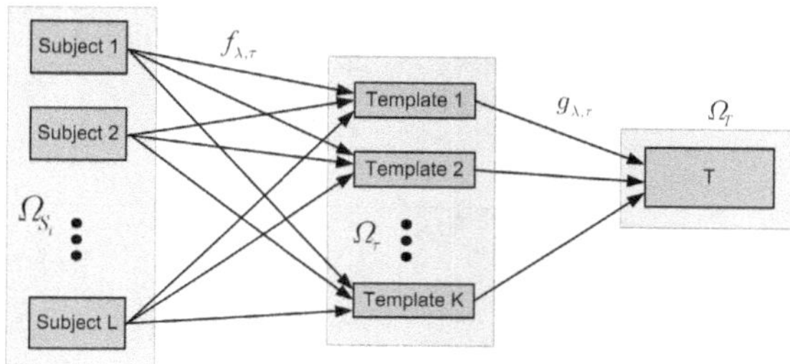

Fig. 2. Constructing AECs: Each subjects is normalized to Ω_T via intermediate templates at different smoothness levels of the warping transformations

small residuals. The second parameter, τ, denotes a sequence of m intermediate templates, $\tau := \tau_1 \rightarrow \ldots \rightarrow \tau_m$, between S and T. For a given smoothness, λ, individual anatomies are first normalized to intermediate templates τ through $f_{\lambda,\tau} \in \mathcal{F}_S$ as shown in Fig. 2. Intermediate results are then warped to T through $g_{\lambda,\tau} \in \mathcal{G}_S$, since we ultimately need to go to a single reference space, Ω_T. $\mathcal{F}_S$ and $\mathcal{G}_S$ respectively denote sets of all $\tau - S \circ f_{\lambda,\tau}$ and $T - (S \circ f_{\lambda,\tau}) \circ g_{\lambda,\tau}$ minimizing diffeomorphisms. As a result $h_{\lambda,\tau} := f_{\lambda,\tau} \circ g_{\lambda,\tau}$ takes S to the template T, with τ perturbing the path taken by $h_{\lambda,\tau}$ from an individual to the template by providing a sequence of milestones that may facilitate registration. A poor choice of intermediate templates increases the amount of the residual, whereas appropriately selected intermediate templates may find paths for the transformation $h_{\lambda,\tau}$ that result in minimal residuals. In many instances, a different choice of T may result in different registration results, as shown in Fig. 3(d) and (e). This inconsistency will be eliminated in subsequent formulation by viewing how registration responds to different intermediate templates. In short, introduction of τ and λ provides variability in $(h_{\lambda,\tau}, R_{h_{\lambda,\tau}})$ necessary to account for template and parameter bias, which allows us to consider the restriction of $\mathcal{H}_S$:

$$\mathcal{I}_S := \{h_{\lambda,\tau} = f_{\lambda,\tau} \circ g_{\lambda,\tau} \in \mathcal{H}_S : g_{\lambda,\tau} \in \mathcal{G}_S, f_{\lambda,\tau} \in \mathcal{F}_S, \lambda \in \mathbb{R}_+, \tau \in \mathcal{T}^m\},$$

for subsequent analysis. The anatomies, which are otherwise not well represented by the template T, may be captured effectively through $\mathcal{I}_S$ (Fig. 4). By introducing this variability in $(h_{\lambda,\tau}, R_{h_{\lambda,\tau}})$ carefully restricted to λ and τ, we generate a class of equivalent anatomical representations, $\mathcal{A}(S) = \{\{\mathcal{M}_h(\mathbf{x}) : S(h(\mathbf{x})) = T(\mathbf{x}) - R_h(\mathbf{x}), \forall \mathbf{x} \in \Omega_T\}, \forall h \in \mathcal{I}_S\}$, referred to as AEC. For notational simplicity, we combine the two parameters, τ and λ, in $\boldsymbol{\theta}$ to represent AEC as:

$$\mathcal{A}(S) = \{\{(\mathcal{M}_{h_{\boldsymbol{\theta}}}(\mathbf{x})) : S(h_{\boldsymbol{\theta}}(\mathbf{x})) = T(\mathbf{x}) - R_{h_{\boldsymbol{\theta}}}(\mathbf{x}), \forall \mathbf{x} \in \Omega_T\}, \forall \boldsymbol{\theta} \in \boldsymbol{\Theta}\}, \quad (2)$$

where $\mathcal{M}_{h_{\boldsymbol{\theta}}}(\mathbf{x})$ denotes CMD $(h_{\boldsymbol{\theta}}(\mathbf{x}), R_{h_{\boldsymbol{\theta}}}(\mathbf{x}))$. An AEC maps each anatomy to a (generally nonlinear) manifold in an n-dimensional space as shown schematically in Fig. 5(a), where n is the dimensionality of CMD. Although the resulting AEC is rich with an entire range of variability in $R_{h_{\boldsymbol{\theta}}}$, one may not arbitrarily select $\boldsymbol{\theta}$

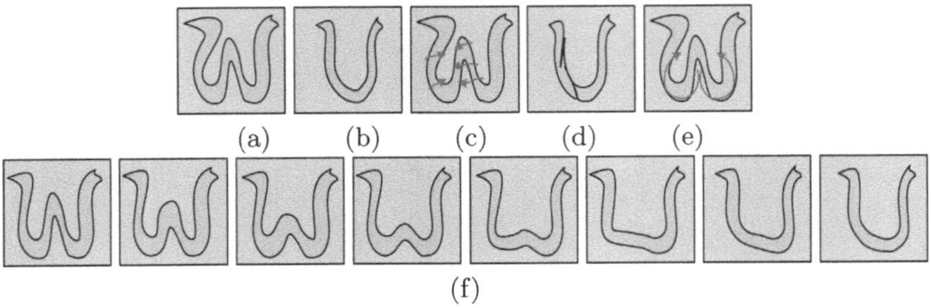

Fig. 3. (a) Template; (b) Subject; (c) Deformation field for direct warping – middle of W is mapped to a limb of V; (d) Warped subject; (e) Sequence of transformations obtained through intermediate templates of (f) may open up a W-fold to a V-fold by guiding registration; (f) Intermediate templates for (e)

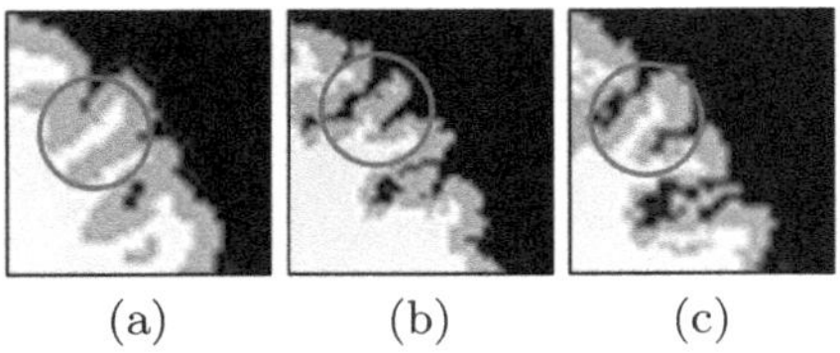

Fig. 4. Intermediate templates aid registration: (a) Template; (b) Direct warping of Fig. 1(c); (c) Warping via an intermediate template

for analysis. It should be noted that a small residual does not necessarily correspond to the best CMD. For instance, the residual may be reduced by selecting small λs, but it may lead to an overly aggressive registration, which introduces noise and erroneous correspondence as shown in Fig. 3(d), where viscous fluid based registration was employed [1]. It is, therefore, important to find the optimal parameter selection, which requires a metric for carrying out intersubject comparisons based on AEC manifolds. One may define distance between two anatomies as infimum separation between their anatomical manifolds as shown in Fig. 5(b), i.e., $\text{Dist}(S_A, S_B) := \inf(\{d(\mathcal{M}^A_{h_A}, \mathcal{M}^B_{h_B}) : \forall h_A \in \mathcal{F}_{S_A}, \forall h_B \in \mathcal{F}_{S_B}\})$, where d represents Euclidean distance defined on the space of CMDs. While this works for two subjects, comparing three or more anatomies becomes problematic as illustrated in the figure, where $\text{Dist}(S_A, S_C) \nleq \text{Dist}(S_A, S_B) + \text{Dist}(S_B, S_C)$, which is no longer a metric. We circumvent this problem by representing each AEC through OMS, which allows directly employing a Euclidean metric for groupwise comparisons.

Since we are mainly interested in volumetric variations among subjects representing tissue growth or death, in subsequent discussion, we utilize Jacobian determinant (JD), J_{h_θ}, of $h_{\boldsymbol{\theta}}$ to construct the proposed AEC through $\mathcal{M}_{h_\theta} = (J_{h_\theta}, R_{h_\theta})$ descriptors. Moreover, we consider a single milestone ($m = 1$) between S and T, with τ representing a single intermediate template in $\mathcal{T}$.

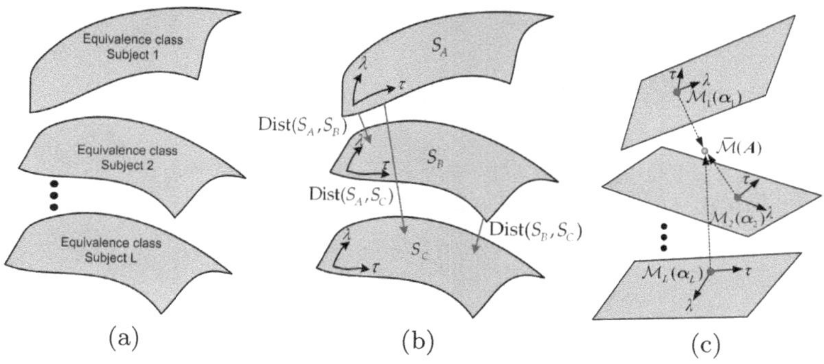

Fig. 5. (a) Nonlinear manifold structure of AEC; (b) Problem with Euclidean distance based comparisons; (c) Approximation with hyperplanes

The idea of AEC was first proposed in [15], where *tissue density maps* [10] were employed with λ as the sole confounding factor. Its major limitation was the assumption that all AECs were collinear and could be approximated by a single hyperplane. We extend this idea by providing a robust way to eliminate non-uniqueness of CMDs and present a general framework that incorporates all confounding factors in $\boldsymbol{\theta}$.

2.3 Optimal Morphological Signature

Optimal choice of $\boldsymbol{\theta}$ for one subject may be different from that for the others, which intuitively follows from the fact that different anatomies are affected differently by it. For instance, a subject with bifolded sulci will prefer similar structures in the template. It is, therefore, imperative to find an appropriate τ and λ for each subject that is optimized for the underlying anatomy, leading to optimal parameters $\boldsymbol{\Theta} = (\boldsymbol{\theta}_1, \ldots, \boldsymbol{\theta}_L)$ for L subjects.

In order to define our criterion for optimality of Θ, we first consider two anatomies. If we were to slide along the respective AECs, we would find two representations that have minimum distance. We consider these two representations as the ones that best highlight differences between the two anatomies, since together they eliminate confounding effects of λ and τ. More generally, for L anatomies, we allow their representations to slide along respective AECs in order to minimize the cumulative of pairwise distances of all individuals:

$$\boldsymbol{\Theta}^* = \arg \min_{\substack{\boldsymbol{\Theta}=(\boldsymbol{\theta}_1,\ldots,\boldsymbol{\theta}_L) \\ \mathcal{M}_k(\boldsymbol{\theta}_k)\in\mathcal{A}(S_k),k=1,\ldots,L}} \sum_{i=1}^{L}\sum_{\substack{j=1 \\ j\neq i}}^{L} d^2(\mathcal{M}_i(\boldsymbol{\theta}_i), \mathcal{M}_j(\boldsymbol{\theta}_j)), \tag{3}$$

where d denotes the Euclidean distance, and $\mathcal{M}_i(\boldsymbol{\theta}_i) = (J_{h_{\boldsymbol{\theta}_i}}, R_{h_{\boldsymbol{\theta}_i}})$ is the CMD of subject i at the correspondence $\boldsymbol{\Theta} = (\boldsymbol{\theta}_1, \ldots, \boldsymbol{\theta}_L)$. It can be shown that the criterion of Eq. (3) minimizes the variance of morphological descriptors over entire ensemble w.r.t. confounding factors, leading to:

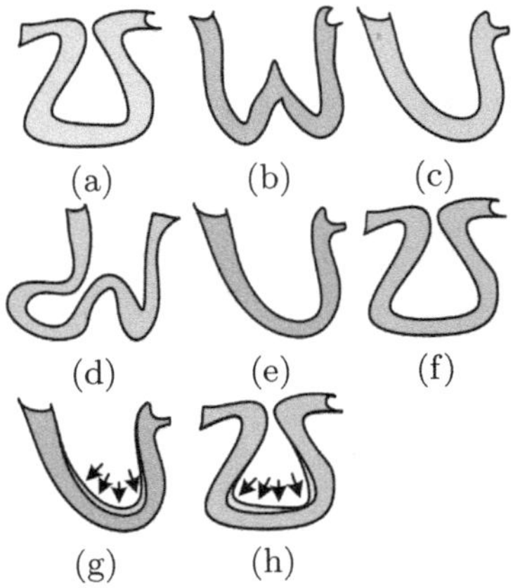

Fig. 6. (a)-(d) Normalizing templates $T_1, \ldots, T_4$; (e)-(f) Subjects S_1 and S_2; (g)-(h) Deformation fields for S_1 and S_2.

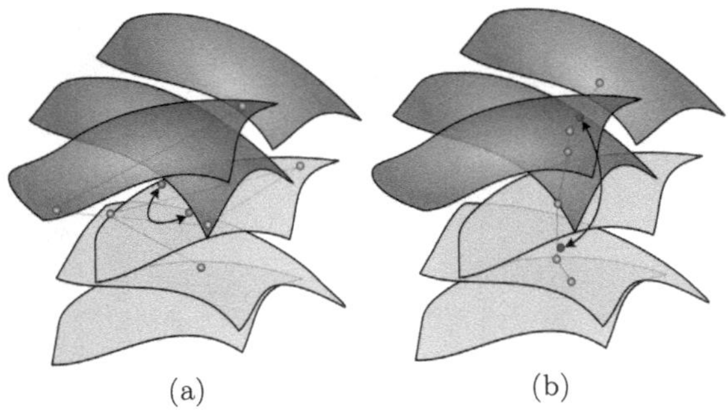

Fig. 7. OMS versus CMD: (a) Randomly selecting CMDs (random parameter selection) from AECs reduces the inter-group separation. Dots marked with arrows represent group means; (b) OMS results in optimal separation between the two groups.

$$\boldsymbol{\Theta}^* = \arg \min_{\substack{\boldsymbol{\Theta}=(\boldsymbol{\theta}_1,\ldots,\boldsymbol{\theta}_L) \\ \mathcal{M}_k(\boldsymbol{\theta}_k)\in\mathcal{A}(S_k),k=1,\ldots,L}} \sum_{i=1}^{L} d^2\left(\mathcal{M}_i(\boldsymbol{\theta}_i), \bar{\mathcal{M}}(\boldsymbol{\Theta})\right), \tag{4}$$

where $\bar{\mathcal{M}}(\boldsymbol{\Theta}) = \frac{1}{L}\sum_{i=1}^{L}\mathcal{M}_i(\boldsymbol{\theta}_i)$ represents the mean descriptor. The resulting OMS, $\mathcal{M}_i(\boldsymbol{\theta}_i^*)$, corresponding to optimal parameters, $\boldsymbol{\theta}_i^*$, for each individual, effectively allows us to select optimal intermediate template and transformation individually for each anatomy. This is a very important aspect of our approach, which is better explained with a schematic example given in Fig. 6. Suppose S_1 and S_2 are two anatomies under study, and $T_1, \ldots, T_4$ are the normalizing templates. Eq. (4) finds for each individual corresponding templates such that the resulting (JD, residual) are as similar as possible. Resultantly, T_3 and T_1 will be selected for S_1 and S_2 respectively, since they yield very similar transformations and residuals. Selecting a different template, on the other hand, results in dissimilar transformations, and possibly dissimilar residuals (depending on the smoothness level). When generalized to L subjects and $\mathcal{T}$, Eq. (4) yields optimal transformation parameters for each subject as shown Fig. 7. An analysis based on random CMD selection results in poor inter-group separation (Fig. 7(a)). Eq. (4), on the other hand, helps in removing this randomness of CMDs to provide an optimal separation between the two groups (Fig. 7(b)). Additionally, by constraining each OMS to its respective AEC, it preserves inter-subject and inter-group anatomical differences.

In order to solve the optimization problem of Eq. (4), we need to define the structure of AEC manifolds shown in Fig. 5(a). For simplicity we approximate the AECs with hyperplanes as shown in Fig. 5(c). If $\{\mathbf{V}_j^{(i)}, j = 1, \ldots, n\}$ are the principal directions of the AEC of ith subject, and $\hat{\mathcal{M}}_i$ is the corresponding mean, then the linear hyperplane approximating the corresponding AEC manifold is given by:

$$\mathcal{M}_i(\boldsymbol{\theta}) = \hat{\mathcal{M}}_i + \sum_{j=1}^{n} \alpha_{ij} \mathbf{V}_j^{(i)}, \tag{5}$$

where $\alpha_{ij}, j = 1, \ldots, n$ capture transformation dependent parameters, $\boldsymbol{\theta}_i$. The objective function of Eq. (4), therefore, becomes:

$$\boldsymbol{A}^* = \arg \min_{\boldsymbol{A}:=(\boldsymbol{\alpha}^1,\ldots,\boldsymbol{\alpha}^L)} \sum_{i=1}^{L} d^2 \left(\hat{\mathcal{M}}_i + \sum_{j=1}^{n} \alpha_{ij} \mathbf{V}_j^{(i)}, \bar{\mathcal{M}}(\boldsymbol{A}) \right), \tag{6}$$

where:

$$\bar{\mathcal{M}}(\boldsymbol{A}) = \frac{1}{L} \sum_{i=1}^{L} \left(\hat{\mathcal{M}}_i + \sum_{j=1}^{n} \alpha_{ij} \mathbf{V}_j^{(i)} \right), \tag{7}$$

is the mean descriptor of all subjects, and $\boldsymbol{\alpha}^i = (\alpha_{i1}, \ldots, \alpha_{in})$. In order to stay on individual manifolds, the optimization is constrained to $\boldsymbol{\alpha}_i^{\min} \leq \boldsymbol{\alpha}_i \leq \boldsymbol{\alpha}_i^{\max}$, where $\boldsymbol{\alpha}_i^{\min}$ and $\boldsymbol{\alpha}_i^{\max}$ depend on the corresponding principal modes.

Solution to this constrained problem is an algorithm that allows moving along individual hyperplanes, in order to minimize the objective function. At each optimization iteration, an update of $\mathcal{M}_i(\boldsymbol{\alpha}_i)$ (Fig. 5(c)) is computed, which yields the current floating mean $\bar{\mathcal{M}}(\boldsymbol{A})$ given by Eq. (7). The procedure is repeated until the minimum of Eq. (6) is attained. Analytically it leads to the following solution subject to constraints given above:

$$\boldsymbol{\alpha}_i^* = \mathbf{V}^{(i)^T} \left[\frac{1}{L-1} \sum_{k \neq i} \left(\hat{\mathcal{M}}_k + \mathbf{V}^{(k)} \boldsymbol{\alpha}_k \right) - \hat{\mathcal{M}}_i \right] \quad i = 1, \ldots, L. \tag{8}$$

When combined with Eq. (5), optimal correspondence of Eq. (8) yields OMS, $\mathcal{M}_i^*$, which is then used for subsequent analysis. The first term within braces represents the mean across a smaller subset of subjects excluding ith subject. $\boldsymbol{\alpha}_i^*$ is, therefore, the projection to the principal axes of the difference between the mean across other users and the subject mean. Eq. (8), hence, presents a direct way of estimating the optimal signatures.

OMS, $\mathcal{M}_i^*$, provides the optimal combination of JD and the corresponding residual in addition to optimal selection of transformation parameters, λ and τ, which, herein, makes subsequent analysis invariant to transformation parameters.

3 Experiments

In this section, we provide experimental results to support our hypothesis that residual carries significant amount of information for identifying group differences and that OMS yields superior performance by maintaining group separation between normal and pathologic anatomies. We considered two datasets:

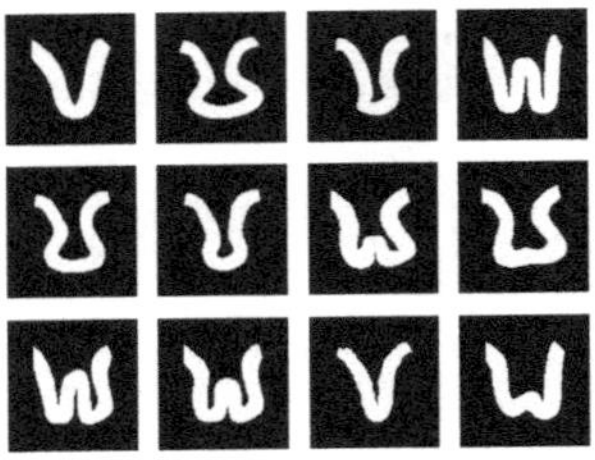

Fig. 8. Templates $T_1, \ldots, T_{12}$ simulating gray matter folds

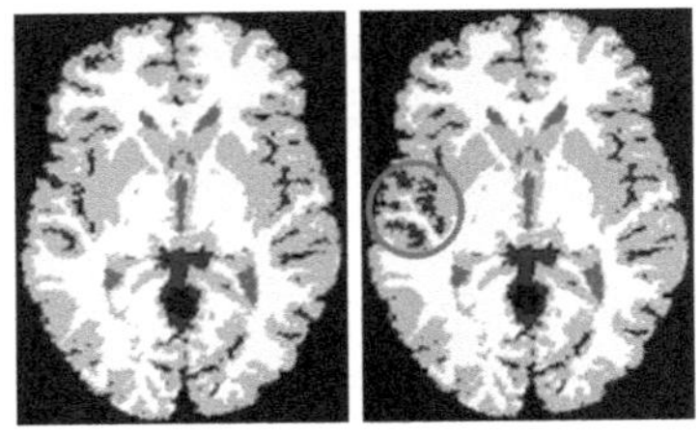

Fig. 9. (a) A subject without atrophy; (b) With 10% simulated atrophy

1. A 2D dataset of 60 subjects was generated by introducing random variability in 12 manually created templates given in Fig. 8. This variability across subjects is close to anatomical differences encountered in real gray matter folds. 5% atrophy was introduced in center one-third of the fold of 30 subjects to simulate patient data. All subjects were spatially normalized to T_{12} via $T_1, \ldots, T_{11}$, for smoothness levels of $\lambda = 0, \ldots, 42$ to construct individual AECs.
2. The second dataset consisted of real MRI scans of 31 subjects. To simulate patient data, 10% atrophy was introduced in 15 randomly selected subjects in a spherical region as shown in Fig. 9 using the simulator of [16]. Five intermediate templates were selected for spatial normalization to generate AECs for all subjects with smoothing levels of $\lambda = 0, \ldots, 7$.

3.1 Results and Discussion

For both datasets, we performed two types of tests on CMDs and OMSs: (1) t-tests on individual $\log J_{h_{\lambda,\tau}}$ and $R_{h_{\lambda,\tau}}$ components, and (2) T^2 test on ($\log J_{h_{\lambda,\tau}}$, $R_{h_{\lambda,\tau}}$) descriptor, for finding significance of differences between healthy and pathologic anatomies. For CMDs, we randomly selected intermediate templates for each subject before conducting tests for all smoothness levels λ. Note that residual was smoothed with a Gaussian filter with various selections of smoothness parameter σ prior to statistical tests mainly due to two reasons. First, it ensures the Gaussianity of the smoothed residual. Second, since the residuals appear only on tissue boundaries, even if tissue atrophy is in the interior of the structure, smoothing produces a more spatially uniform residual. JD, on the other hand, was not smoothed for the T^2 test due to its inherent smoothness.

Based on statistical tests, p-value maps were computed for all values of σ (and λ for tests on CMDs). Since the minimum of a p-value map provides the best performance for group differences, we computed minimum of each p-value map for both datasets. Minimum $\log_{10} p$ plots as a function of σ are given in Figs. 10 and 11 for 2D and 3D datasets respectively. It may be observed from results based on CMDs for both datasets that residual achieves considerably lower p values as compared with JD, which indicates the significance of residual for capturing group differences. The significance of both log JD and the residual increases with

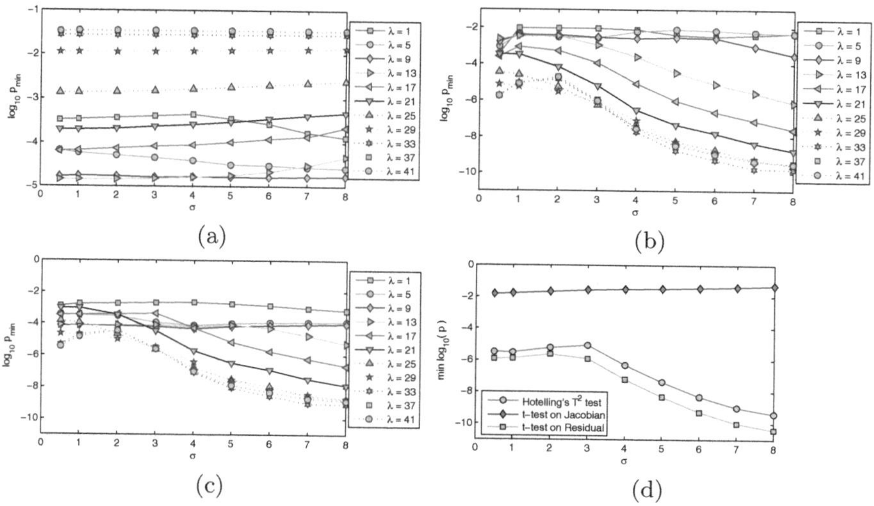

Fig. 10. Minimum p-value plots for synthetic dataset: (a) t-test on AEC based log JD; (b) t-test on AEC based Residual; (c) T^2-test on AEC based $(\log J_{h_{\lambda,\tau}}, R_{h_{\lambda,\tau}})$; (d) Statistical tests on OMS

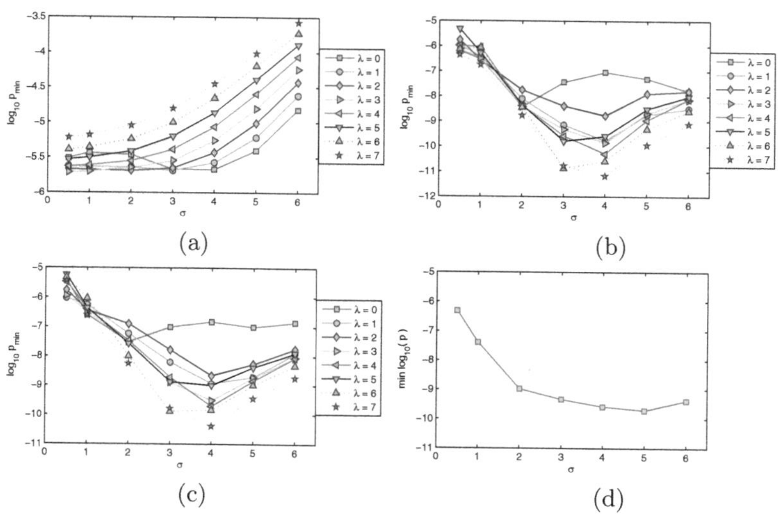

Fig. 11. Minimum p-value plots for real 3D dataset: (a) t-test on AEC based $\log J_{h_{\lambda,\tau}}$; (b) t-test on AEC based $R_{h_{\lambda,\tau}}$; (c) T^2-test on AEC based $(\log J_{h_{\lambda,\tau}}, R_{h_{\lambda,\tau}})$; (d) T^2-test on OMS

σ and λ up to a point after which it starts degrading. Similarly, T^2 test also shows best performance for intermediate values of λ ($\lambda = 33$ for 2D and $\lambda = 7$ for 3D), which means that an overly aggressive transformation is not required

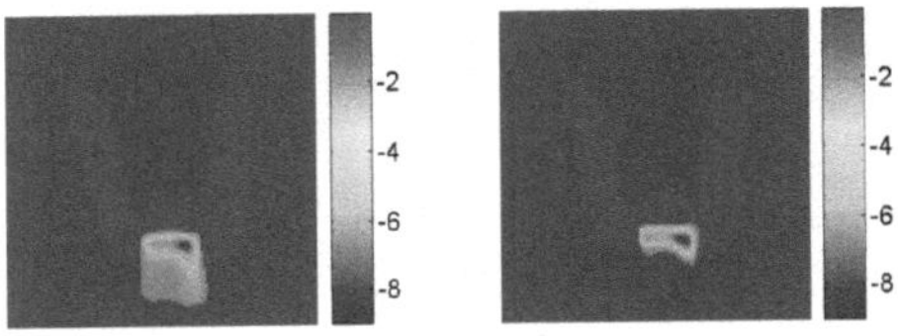

(a) (b)

Fig. 12. T^2-test based $\log_{10} p$-value maps for 2D simulated data at $\sigma = 8$ thresholded to $p \leq 10^{-2}$: (a) CMD $\lambda = 33$; (b) OMS

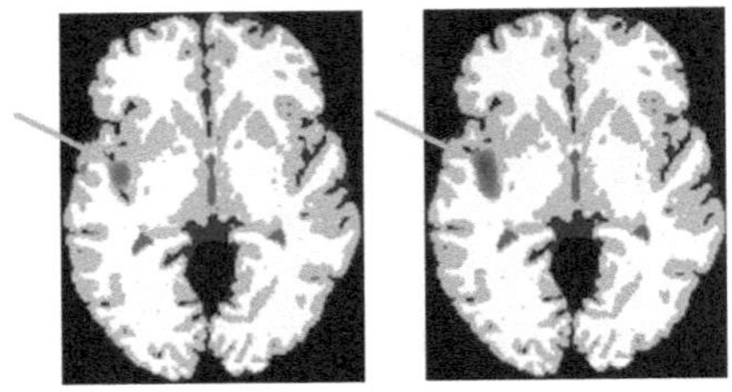

(a) (b)

Fig. 13. T^2 test based p-value maps for 3D dataset corresponding to best results for each descriptor thresholded to $p \leq 10^{-5}$: (a) CMD $\lambda = 7, \sigma = 4$; (b) OMS with $\sigma = 5$; (c) OMS with $\sigma = 5$ thresholded to $p \leq 10^{-3}$

for capturing anatomical differences. These observations are in accordance with our hypothesis that residual carries important anatomical information that is complementary to the transformation. An analysis based solely on JD loses this information, thereby degrading the performance of subsequent diagnostic tests. The dependence of $(J_{h_{\lambda,\tau}}, R_{h_{\lambda,\tau}})$ on λ is eliminated through optimization as indicated by OMSs for 2D, which shows an improved performance versus CMDs ($p = 10^{-9.5}$ at $\sigma = 8$ for OMS vs $p = 10^{-8.5}$ at $\sigma = 8$, $\lambda = 33$ for CMDs). For 3D dataset, the optimal signatures provide a performance similar to the CMDs, with the latter performing slightly better ($p = 10^{-9.75}$ against $p = 10^{-10.5}$). On the other hand, OMS appears to be relatively insensitive to σ with a better dynamic range. For instance, the variation in p-values for OMS in the range $\sigma = 2$–6 is $10^{-0.75}$, whereas that for CMDs is $10^{3.5}$, which makes CMDs much more sensitive to σ. Small variations in σ, therefore, may considerably degrade CMD-based analysis. OMS is, hence, not only more robust but also maintains the separation between the two groups as indicated by very low p-values.

Another advantage of OMS may be observed from appropriately thresholded p-value maps for 2D and 3D datasets given in Figs. 12 and 13 respectively. Clearly, OMS helps in precisely localizing atrophy, which is in accordance with the objective function of Eq. (6). On the other hand, CMDs fail to localize atrophy, and occasionally result in false positives.

4 Conclusions

In this paper, we have presented a morphological descriptor for computational anatomy with two major contributions. First, the transformation was combined with the residual for a complete (lossless) description of the anatomy. Second, each anatomy was represented with a rich class of descriptors, that incorporates smoothness of the transformation and the choice of intermediate templates. Independence to these parameters was established through OMS, which was estimated using a manifold sliding algorithm. Since each OMS was forced to stay on the corresponding AEC manifold, it maintains inter-group differences, which was validated through statistical tests on synthetic 2D as well as real 3D data.

Tests confirmed our hypothesis that residual provides remarkably better group separation than the JD. Results clearly indicated that residual contains not only important, but critical morphological information, and should, therefore, be an integral part of any morphological descriptor, if not the most important part. Marginal gain was achieved by using the OMS, when compared to the absolutely best result that can be obtained from individual pairs of (transformation, residual). Although this may indicate that the optimization along AEC manifolds could well be omitted, it is argued that the robustness and independence of the results from template and transformation parameters are important reasons to perform this optimization, even if it does not significantly improve detection power at the absolutely optimal set of parameter values. Moreover, future work on estimating the nonlinear structure of these manifolds, instead of approximating them linearly, may further increase the significance of the optimization procedure.

Acknowledgements. This work was supported by the NIH-funded Grant R01-AG14971. The authors extend special thanks to Professor Dinggang Shen for interesting and stimulating discussions.

References

1. Christensen, G., Rabbit, R., Miller, M.: A deformable neuroanatomy textbook based on viscous fluid mechanics. In: Proc. CISS'93 1993, pp. 211–216 (1993)
2. Miller, M., Banerjee, A., et al.: Statistical methods in computational anatomy. Statistical Methods in Medical Research 6, 267–299 1, 2 (1997)
3. Miller, M., Younes, L.: Group actions, homeomorphisms, and matching: a general framework. International Journal of Computer Vision 41(1), 61–84, 1 (2001)
4. Ashburner, J., Friston, K.: Nonlinear spatial normalization using basis functions. Human Brain Mapping 7(4), 254–266, 1 (1999)
5. Shen, D., Davatzikos, C.: HAMMER: Hierarchical attribute matching mechanism for elastic registration. IEEE TMI 21(11), 1421–1439 1,3 (2002)
6. Davatzikos, C., et al.: A computerized approach for morphological analysis of the corpus callosum. Journal of Comp. Assisted Tomography 20(1), 88–97 1, 2 (1996)
7. Ashburner, J., et al.: Identifying global anatomical differences: deformation-based morphometry. Human Brain Mapping 6(6), 348–357 1, 2 (1998)
8. Chung, M., Worsley, K., et al.: A unified statistical approach to deformation-based morphometry. NeuroImage 14(3), 595–600 1, 2 (2001)
9. Ashburner, J., Friston, K.J.: Voxel-based morphometry – the methods. NeuroImage 11(6), 805–821 1, 2 (2000)
10. Davatzikos, C., Genc, A., Xu, D., Resnick, S.: Voxel-based morphometry using RAVENS maps: methods and validation using simulated longitudinal atrophy. Neuroimage 14, 1361–1369 1,2,5 (2001)

11. Chetelat, G., et al.: Mapping gray matter loss with voxel-based morphometry in mild cognitive impairment. Neuroreport 13(15), 1939–1943 1, 2 (2002)
12. Thompson, P., et al.: Growth patterns in the developing human brain detected using continuum-mechanical tensor mapping. Nature 404(6774), 190–193 1,2 (2000)
13. Leow, A., Klunder, A., et al.: Longitudinal stability of mri for mapping brain change using tensor-based morphometry. Neuroimage 31(2), 627–640 1,2 (2006)
14. Joshi, S.: Large deformation diffeomorphisms and Gaussian random fields for statistical characterization of brain sub-manifolds. PhD thesis, Washington University, St. Louis 2 (1998)
15. Makrogiannis, S., et al.: Anatomical equivalence class: A computational anatomy framework using a lossless shape descriptor. IEEE TMI (Accepted) 5
16. Karaçhali, B., Davatzikos, C.: Simulation of tissue atrophy using a topology preserving transformation model. IEEE TMI 25(5), 649–652 9 (2006)

Incorporation of Regional Information in Optimal 3-D Graph Search with Application for Intraretinal Layer Segmentation of Optical Coherence Tomography Images

Mona Haeker[1,2], Xiaodong Wu[1], Michael Abràmoff[1,3], Randy Kardon[3], and Milan Sonka[1,3]

[1]Departments of Electrical & Computer Engineering, [2]Biomedical Engineering, and [3]Ophthalmology & Visual Sciences, The University of Iowa, Iowa City, IA 52242, USA
{mona-haeker, milan-sonka}@uiowa.edu

Abstract. We present a method for the incorporation of regional image information in a 3-D graph-theoretic approach for optimal multiple surface segmentation. By transforming the multiple surface segmentation task into finding a minimum-cost closed set in a vertex-weighted graph, the optimal set of feasible surfaces with respect to an objective function can be found. In the past, this family of graph search applications only used objective functions which incorporated "on-surface" costs. Here, novel "in-region" costs are incorporated. Our new approach is applied to the segmentation of seven intraretinal layer surfaces of 24 3-D macular optical coherence tomography images from 12 subjects. Compared to an expert-defined independent standard, unsigned border positioning errors are comparable to the inter-observer variability (7.8 ± 5.0 μm and 8.1 ± 3.6 μm, respectively).

1 Introduction

Even though medical images commonly exist in three or more dimensions, the ability to efficiently and accurately segment images in 3-D or 4-D remains a challenging problem. For example, in order to make many 3-D segmentation approaches practical, optimality of the resulting segmentation is often not guaranteed because of the computational demands in searching a large solution space [1,2].

Nevertheless, Li *et al.* [3] recently presented a low-polynomial time graph-based approach for the *optimal* multi-surface segmentation of 3-D or higher dimensional data. This was an extension of the approach for the optimal detection of single surfaces presented by Wu and Chen [4] to the multiple surface case. In these approaches [3,4], the surface segmentation problem is transformed into that of finding a minimum-cost closed set in a constructed vertex-weighted geometric graph. The edges of the graph are defined so that each closed set in the graph corresponds to a feasible surface (or set of feasible surfaces). Furthermore, the vertex costs are assigned so that the cost of each closed set directly

N. Karssemeijer and B. Lelieveldt (Eds.): IPMI 2007, LNCS 4584, pp. 607–618, 2007.
© Springer-Verlag Berlin Heidelberg 2007

corresponds to the cost of the set of surfaces. The closed set with the minimum cost (corresponding to the optimal set of surfaces) is then determined by finding a minimum s-t cut in a closely-related graph. Note that even though the surfaces are ultimately found by finding a minimum-cost s-t cut in a constructed graph, these approaches [3,4] are fundamentally different than the "graph cut" methods of Boykov *et al.* (e.g., [5]).

While the edges of the graph are important in determining what it means for a surface to be feasible, it is the cost function that determines what set of surfaces is optimal. As originally presented in [3, 4] and used by all of the applications to date (e.g., [6, 7]), the cost of a set of surfaces is defined as a summation of cost values associated with voxels on the surfaces (i.e., the cost of a voxel with respect to a particular surface reflects the unlikeliness that the voxel would be part of the surface). While such "on-surface" costs can incorporate both image edge and regional information [7], the incorporation of regional information is often limited to a region immediately surrounding the voxel for which the cost is defined (especially in cases of multiple surface detection). In some applications, better cost functions could likely be defined if "true" regional information could be incorporated. This involves extending the definition of the cost of a set of surfaces to also include the summation of in-region cost values in addition to the on-surface cost values. The in-region cost value for a voxel associated with a particular region would reflect the unlikeliness of that voxel belonging to the region. Using the segmentation of the intraretinal layers of optical coherence tomography (OCT) images as an example application, this paper presents how true regional information can be incorporated into the 3-D graph search.

2 OCT Imaging Background

With its first introduction in 1991 [8], OCT is a relatively new imaging modality. One of its most common uses is within the ophthalmology community, where the high-resolution cross-sectional images resulting from OCT scanners are used for the diagnosis and management of a variety of ocular diseases such as glaucoma, diabetic macular edema, and optic neuropathy. The macula and region surrounding the optic nerve are two locations commonly scanned. For the images used in this work, a macular scanning protocol was used that involved the acquisition of six linear radial scans in a spoke pattern centered at the fovea (Fig. 1(a–c)). An example image series using this protocol is shown in Fig. 1(d).

Even though intraretinal layers are visible on these macular scans, current commercial systems (e.g., Stratus OCT-3, Carl Zeiss Meditec, Inc., Dublin, CA, USA) only segment and provide thickness measurements for the total retina. As each layer may be affected differently in the presence of ocular disease, an intraretinal layer segmentation approach is needed in order to correlate the individual layer properties with disease state. We have previously reported a method for the division of the retina into five intralayers (corresponding to six surfaces) using only on-surface costs in the graph search [7]. However, even though the graph search theoretically allowed for the simultaneous detection of many surfaces,

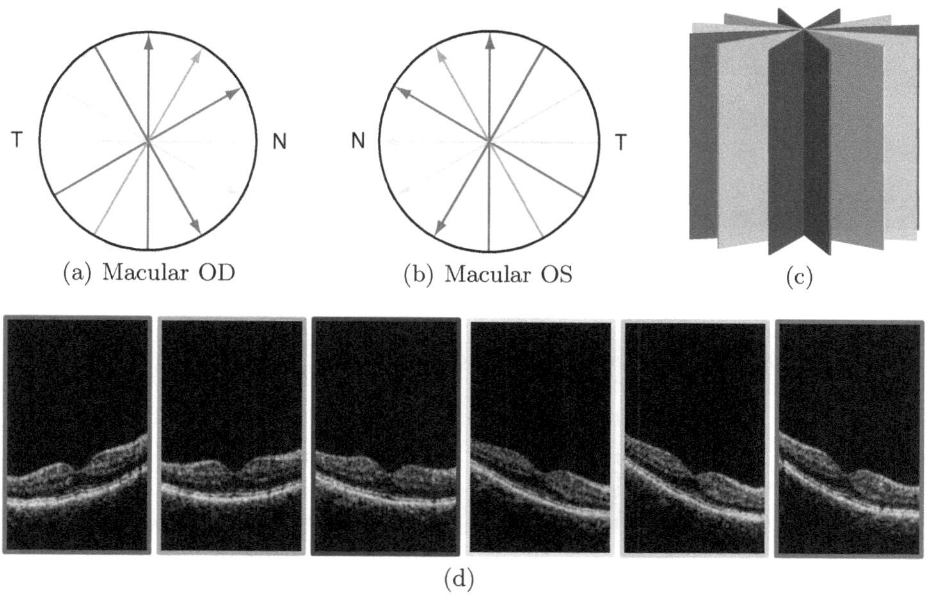

Fig. 1. Macular scanning protocol. (a) OD = right eye. (b) OS = left eye. (c) Schematic view of 3-D image in which each color reflects one 2-D scan. (d) Six example scans in one macular series.

we found the three interior surfaces in a sequential fashion because of the limitations of incorporating regional information into on-surface costs. The method reported in this work for incorporating in-region costs allowed us to instead find four interior surfaces simultaneously. The surfaces we desired to find are shown in Fig. 2, with Fig. 2(c) providing an example 3-D view of three of the surfaces.

3 The Multiple Surface Segmentation Problem

In very general terms, the multiple surface segmentation problem can be thought of as an optimization problem with the goal being to find the set of surfaces with the minimum cost – such cost being edge and/or region based – so that the found surface set is feasible. In this section, we define what is meant by a feasible surface set and the cost of a set of surfaces.

3.1 Feasible Surface Set

Consider a volumetric image $I(x, y, z)$ of size $X \times Y \times Z$. We focus on the case in which each surface of interest can be defined with a function $f(x, y)$ mapping (x, y) pairs to z-values; however, note that the graph search can be extended to work with closed surfaces as well [9]. Associated with each (x, y) pair is a column of voxels in which only one of the voxels – the voxel at $(x, y, f(x, y))$ – intersects the surface. Each column also has a set of neighbors. For example, a

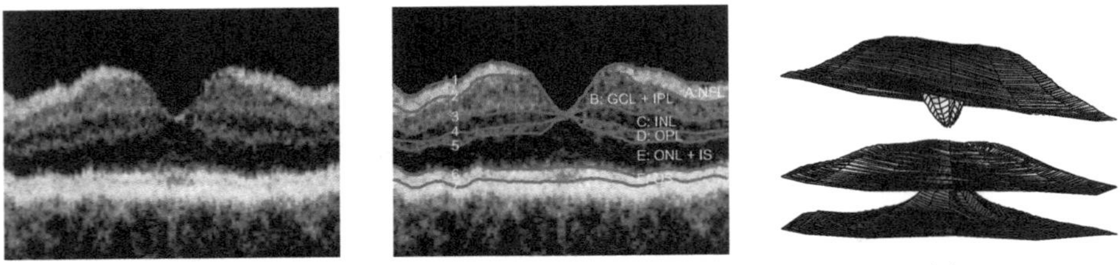

(a) (b) (c)

Fig. 2. Intraretinal surfaces and layers of macular OCT images. (a) One 2-D image. (b) Seven surfaces (labeled 1-7) and six corresponding intralayers (labeled A through F). (c) Example 3-D visualization of surface 1, 3, and 5.

typical set of neighbors for the column associated with (x, y) are the columns associated with $(x+1, y)$, $(x-1, y)$, $(x, y+1)$, and $(x, y-1)$. Other neighborhood relationships are also possible. One common example is to add a "circularity" neighbor relationship for images that were unwrapped from a cylindrical coordinate system. An example of this would be if the column associated with $(0, y_0)$ was considered to be a neighbor to the column associated with $(X-1, y_0)$. A single surface is considered feasible if it satisfies certain smoothness constraints. In particular, if (x_1, y_1, z_1) and (x_2, y_2, z_2) are voxels on the surface from neighboring columns in the x-direction, then $|z_1 - z_2| \leq \Delta_x$, where Δ_x is a specified smoothness parameter. A similar constraint exists for neighboring columns in the y-direction ($|z_1 - z_2| \leq \Delta_y$).

For a set of surfaces, additional constraints are added to model the desired relationships between the surfaces. For example, it may be known that one surface is always above another surface and that the distance between the surfaces is at least δ^l voxels, but no more than δ^u voxels. More specifically, for each pair of surfaces $f_i(x, y)$ and $f_j(x, y)$, a constraint may be added to require that $\delta^l \leq f_i(x, y) - f_j(x, y) \leq \delta^u$ for all (x, y), where δ^l and δ^u are specified surface interaction parameters associated with the pair of surfaces. While in general a pair of surfaces may be allowed to cross, having crossing surfaces does not make sense when defining regional costs, and thus we will also assume that δ^l and δ^u have the same sign.

In summary, a set of surfaces are considered feasible if each individual surface in the set satisfies the given smoothness constraints for the surface and if each pair of surfaces satisfies the surface interaction constraints.

3.2 Cost of a Feasible Surface Set

Given a set of n non-intersecting surfaces $\{f_1(x, y), f_2(x, y), \ldots, f_n(x, y)\}$, the surfaces naturally divide the volume into $n+1$ regions (Fig. 3). Assuming the surfaces are labeled in "increasing" order, the regions can be labeled $R_0, \ldots, R_n$, where R_i reflects the region that lies between surface i and surface $i+1$ (with region boundary cases R_0 and R_n being defined as the region with lower z-values

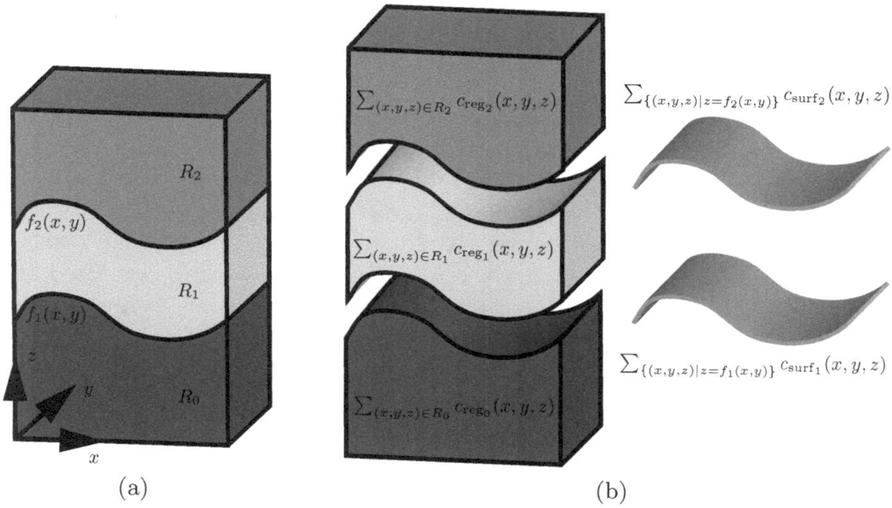

Fig. 3. Example schematic cost of two surfaces for the multiple surface segmentation problem. The two surfaces divide the volume into three regions.

than surface 1 and the region with higher z-values than surface n, respectively). Each voxel could thus have $2n + 1$ real-valued costs associated with it: n on-surface costs corresponding to the unlikeliness of belonging to each surface and $n+1$ in-region costs associated with the unlikeliness of belonging to each region. Let $c_{\text{surf}_i}(x, y, z)$ represent the on-surface cost function associated with surface i and $c_{\text{reg}_i}(x, y, z)$ represent the in-region cost function associated with region i. Then, the cost $C_{\{f_1(x,y),f_2(x,y),\ldots,f_n(x,y)\}}$ associated with the set of surfaces can be defined as

$$C_{\{f_1(x,y),f_2(x,y),\ldots,f_n(x,y)\}} = \sum_{i=1}^{n} C_{f_i(x,y)} + \sum_{i=0}^{n} C_{R_i} \; , \tag{1}$$

where

$$C_{f_i(x,y)} = \sum_{\{(x,y,z)|z=f_i(x,y)\}} c_{\text{surf}_i}(x, y, z) \; , \tag{2}$$

and

$$C_{R_i} = \sum_{(x,y,z)\in R_i} c_{\text{reg}_i}(x, y, z) \; . \tag{3}$$

Note that $C_{f_i(x,y)}$ reflects the cost associated with voxels on surface i and C_{R_i} reflects the cost associated with voxels belonging to region i.

Thus, the multisurface segmentation problem becomes to find the surface set $\{f_1(x, y),\ f_2(x, y),\ \ldots,\ f_n(x, y)\}$ that minimizes Equation (1) such that each surface individually satisfies the smoothness constraints and each pair of surfaces satisfies the given surface interaction constraints.

4 Transforming the Multiple Surface Segmentation Problem into the Minimum-Cost Closed Set Problem

As was described in [3], a directed graph $G = (V, E)$ can be defined such that each feasible surface set corresponds to a closed set in the graph. A closed set is subset V_{CS} of the vertices V such that no edges leave the closed set. The cost of a closed set is the summation of the costs of all the vertices. Because of the direct correspondence between the vertices in the graph and voxels in the image, it is easiest to visualize the graph vertices as being organized as n volumes of vertices, one for each surface to be found. First, edges are added to each volume of vertices such that each closed set within this volume corresponds to a surface satisfying the given surface smoothness constraints. Essentially, the corresponding closed set includes all the vertices corresponding to the surface voxels plus all the "lower" vertices. This is done by adding two types of edges: intracolumn edges and intercolumn edges. The intracolumn edges ensure that all vertices below a given vertex (within one column) are also included in the closed set. The intercolumn edges ensure that the smoothness constraints are satisfied. Next, intersurface edges are added between the volumes of vertices to enforce the surface interaction constraints. This makes each non-empty closed set in the entire graph correspond to a feasible set of surfaces.

As an example, we will consider the added edges for one vertex associated with a voxel towards the center of the image (i.e., a vertex not involved in boundary conditions). It will be associated with two intracolumn directed edges: one directed towards the vertex below it in the column and one from the vertex above it. Two intercolumn edges will also exist for each neighboring column in the x-direction (y-direction): one directed to the vertex in the neighboring column that has a z-value that is Δ_x (Δ_y) smaller and one from the vertex in the neighboring column that has a z-value that is Δ_x (Δ_y) greater. Finally, for each corresponding column in the volume associated with a surface interaction constraint, two intersurface edges are associated with the vertex: one to the vertex in the corresponding column with a z-value that is δ^u smaller and one from the vertex in the corresponding column with a z-value that is δ^l smaller. Slightly different edges must be used in the "boundary cases" in which any of those vertices do not exist [3].

The cost of each vertex in the graph is set such that the cost of each closed set corresponds to the cost (within a constant) of the set of surfaces. The weight $w_i(x, y, z)$ of each vertex ($i = 1, 2, \ldots, n$) can be defined as the summation of a term related to the on-surface costs ($w_{\text{on-surf}_i}(x, y, z)$) and a term related to the in-region costs ($w_{\text{in-reg}_i}(x, y, z)$):

$$w_i(x, y, z) = w_{\text{on-surf}_i}(x, y, z) + w_{\text{in-reg}_i}(x, y, z) . \qquad (4)$$

For on-surfaces costs, the basic idea is to assign the cost of each vertex the on-surface cost of the corresponding voxel minus the on-surface cost of the voxel

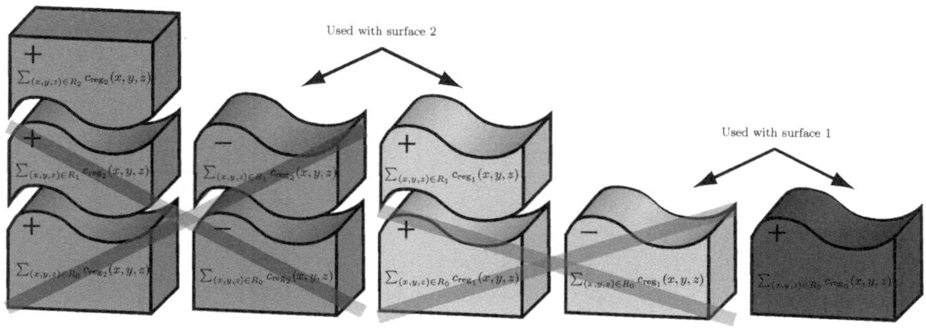

Fig. 4. Schematic showing how the assignment of in-region costs to vertices produces the desired overall cost

below it [4,3]:

$$w_{\text{on-surf}_i}(x,y,z) = \begin{cases} c_{\text{surf}_i}(x,y,z) & \text{if} \quad z=0 \\ c_{\text{surf}_i}(x,y,z) - c_{\text{surf}_i}(x,y,z-1) & \text{otherwise} \end{cases} . \quad (5)$$

For in-region costs, the cost of each vertex is assigned the in-region cost of the region below the surface associated with the vertex minus the in-region cost of the region above the surface associated with the vertex:

$$w_{\text{in-reg}_i}(x,y,z) = c_{\text{reg}_{i-1}}(x,y,z) - c_{\text{reg}_i}(x,y,z) . \quad (6)$$

Because the use of in-region costs is new and perhaps less intuitive, Fig. 4 illustrates why such a transformation works. The cost of the closed set $C(V_{CS_i})$ associated with surface i using the in-region costs becomes

$$C(V_{CS_i}) = \sum_{(x,y,z)\in R_0 \bigcup \cdots \bigcup R_{i-1}} c_{\text{reg}_{i-1}}(x,y,z) - \sum_{(x,y,z)\in R_0 \bigcup \cdots \bigcup R_{i-1}} c_{\text{reg}_i}(x,y,z) . \quad (7)$$

Recognizing that many of costs associated with each individual region cancel when added together and the fact that $\sum_{(x,y,z)\in R_0 \bigcup \cdots \bigcup R_n} c_{\text{reg}_n}(x,y,z)$ is a constant K, the cost for the closed set associated with the entire set of surfaces $C(V_{CS})$ reduces to

$$C(V_{CS}) = -K + \sum_{i=0}^{n} \sum_{(x,y,z)\in R_i} c_{\text{reg}_i}(x,y,z) , \quad (8)$$

which, within a constant, is equivalent to the desired in-region component of the cost of the set of surfaces.

5 Application to OCT Intraretinal Layer Segmentation

5.1 Overall Segmentation Approach

To increase the signal to noise ratio on the macular OCT images, up to six raw macular series were first aligned and registered together using the methods

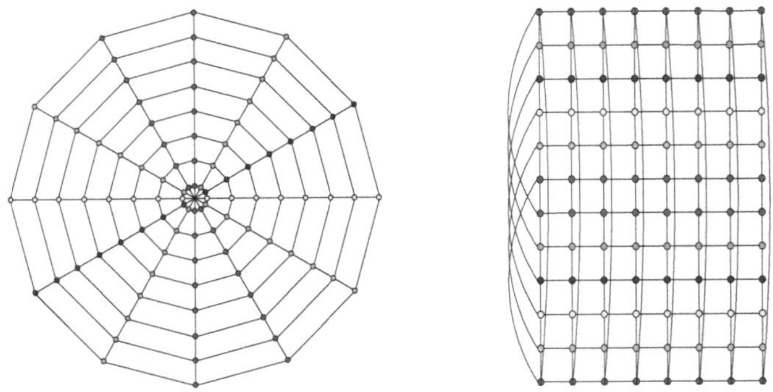

(a) (b)

Fig. 5. Base graph showing neighborhood relationship. The edges indicate neighborhood connectivity of one column of z-values at a (r, θ) pair to another. For each edge shown, smoothness constraints existed between the corresponding columns. (a) Base graph using cylindrical coordinates. (b) Base graph using unwrapped coordinate system (as was stored in the computer).

described in [7]. This left one composite 3-D image for each eye. As a preprocessing step, a speckle-reducing anisotropic diffusion method was applied [10]. Boundaries 1, 6, and 7 were simultaneously found first using the graph search with only on-surface costs. The remaining boundaries were then simultaneously found using only in-region costs.

5.2 Surface Set Feasibility for Macular OCT Images

The acquisition setup of the macular scans (Fig. 1) made it natural to use a discrete cylindrical coordinate system when working with each 3-D image (the z-axis coincided with the intersection of the six 2-D composite scans). The coordinates of each voxel could thus be described with the triple (r, θ, z), where r reflected the distance of the voxel from the z-axis, θ reflected the angular location of the voxel (12 values in 30 degree increments), and z reflected the row of the voxel in the corresponding 2-D image. Note that with this coordinate system, voxels in the left half of each 2-D image had a different θ value than those in the right half (for example, for the vertical 2-D scan shown in red in Fig. 1, voxels in the right half of the image had a θ value of 90 while those in the left half had a θ value of 270). Each surface could be defined with a function $f(r, \theta)$, mapping (r, θ) pairs to z-values. The base graph in Fig. 5 schematically shows the neighborhood relationship for the columns and the corresponding smoothness constraints.

In addition, surface interaction constraints were added between each pair of surfaces $f_i(r, \theta)$ and $f_{i+1}(r, \theta)$. Because of the different nature of the surfaces near the fovea (layers often become much thinner), the surface interaction constraints towards the center of the image (r values less than 15) were correspondingly defined to allow for smaller distances between surfaces.

5.3 Surface Set Costs for Macular OCT Images

The on-surface cost functions for surfaces 1, 6, and 7 were the same as those used in our prior work [7] (each involved the combination of an edge term and a localized region-based term) and thus we will focus on the use of in-region cost terms for the simultaneous detection of the remaining four interior surfaces (surfaces 2, 3, 4, and 5).

Motivated by the observation that the intensity of each of the five interior regions could be described as being dark, medium, or bright (region A was bright, region B was medium, region C was dark, region D was medium, region E was dark), the in-region cost values were set based on fuzzy membership functions. Based on Gaussians, each membership function mapped a normalized image intensity value to a value between 0 and 1, with higher values reflecting a greater likelihood of belonging to the particular intensity group. The corresponding cost value was then defined as 1 minus the membership value. Fig. 6 shows an example plot of these membership functions and their corresponding cost values. More specifically, the dark membership function, $\mathrm{dark}_{\mathrm{mem}}(x)$, was defined as

$$\mathrm{dark}_{\mathrm{mem}}(x) = \begin{cases} 1 & \text{for } x \leq \Delta d \\ e^{-(x-\Delta d)^2/2\sigma^2} & \text{for } x > \Delta d \end{cases}, \tag{9}$$

the medium membership function, $\mathrm{med}_{\mathrm{mem}}(x)$, was defined as

$$\mathrm{med}_{\mathrm{mem}}(x) = \begin{cases} e^{-(x-(c_m-\Delta m))^2/2\sigma^2} & \text{for } x < c_m - \Delta m \\ 1 & \text{for } c_m - \Delta m \leq x \leq c_m + \Delta m \\ e^{-(x-(c_m+\Delta m))^2/2\sigma^2} & \text{for } x > c_m + \Delta m \end{cases}, \tag{10}$$

and the bright membership function, $\mathrm{bright}_{\mathrm{mem}}(x)$, was defined as

$$\mathrm{bright}_{\mathrm{mem}}(x) = \begin{cases} e^{-(x-(1-\Delta b))^2/2\sigma^2} & \text{for } x < 1 - \Delta b \\ 1 & \text{for } x \geq 1 - \Delta b \end{cases}. \tag{11}$$

Note that the precise membership functions used could be described by the five parameters Δd, Δm, and Δb, c_m, and σ. To allow for varying membership functions for each image, Δd, c_m, and Δb were estimated from the image data by computing the mean intensity value of regions that were assumed to have a dark, medium, or bright intensity. The assumed dark region was taken as 50–70 μm above surface 7, the assumed medium region was taken as a 40–60 μm below surface 1 (not including the middle voxels closest to the fovea), and the assumed bright region was taken as 0–24 μm below surface 7. These estimates could be taken because surfaces 1, 6, and 7 had already been determined.

6 Experimental Methods for OCT Intraretinal Segmentation

The intraretinal layer segmentation algorithm was applied to fast macular scans from 12 subjects with unilateral chronic anterior ischemic optic neuropathy. Note

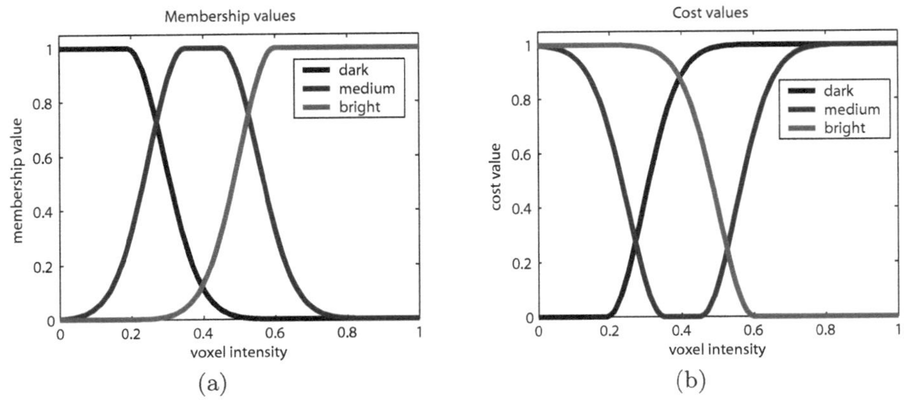

Fig. 6. Example dark, medium, and bright membership functions and corresponding cost values

that the unilateral nature of the disease meant that we had data for 24 eyes, 12 of which were affected by optic neuropathy, 12 of which were not. In almost all cases (21/24 eyes), six repeated series ($6 \times 6 = 36$ raw scans) were used to create the 3-D composite image for each eye. (Each of the remaining three eyes used fewer than six repeated series to create the 3-D composite image.) The resulting 24 3-D composite images were each comprised of 6 composite 2-D scans (144 total composite 2-D scans) of size 128×1024 pixels. The physical width and height of the 2-D raw scans (and thus also the composite scans) was 6 mm $\times$ 2 mm, resulting in a pixel size of approximately 50 μm (horizontally) $\times$ 2 μm (vertically).

One raw scan from each eye was independently traced by two human experts with the average of the two tracings being used as the reference standard. The experts did not attempt to trace borders that were not considered visible. The algorithmic result on the corresponding composite 2-D scan was converted into the coordinate system of the raw scan (inversely transforming the alignment/registration) and the mean and the maximum unsigned border positioning errors for each border were computed (the middle 30 pixels were not included to exclude the fovea). The unsigned border positioning errors were also computed using one observer as a reference standard for the other. For each border, a paired t-test was used to test for significant differences in the computed mean border positioning errors (p-values < 0.05 were considered significant).

7 OCT Intraretinal Segmentation Results

The computed unsigned and maximal border position errors are summarized in Table 1. Except for the unsigned border positioning errors for surface 2 and surface 4 (which both were significantly greater, $p < 0.001$ and $p = 0.04$, respectively), the computed mean errors for all the surfaces were significantly lower or not significantly different from that between the human observers ($p < 0.001$ for

Table 1. Summary of unsigned border positioning errors† for 24 scans

	Algorithm vs. Avg. Observer		Observer 1 vs. Observer 2	
Border	Mean	Maximum	Mean	Maximum
1	4.0 ± 1.2	16.9 ± 9.0	5.9 ± 1.3	16.4 ± 5.0
2*	11.2 ± 5.2	37.1 ± 11.9	5.8 ± 1.2	21.5 ± 8.6
3*	10.0 ± 4.7	29.0 ± 9.3	8.4 ± 3.3	26.0 ± 11.8
4*	10.4 ± 5.1	31.4 ± 14.3	7.7 ± 2.1	22.7 ± 6.6
5	9.1 ± 6.5	27.1 ± 13.2	9.4 ± 4.4	28.5 ± 12.5
6	3.5 ± 2.0	13.1 ± 7.5	7.8 ± 2.8	19.3 ± 5.6
7	7.8 ± 2.5	22.5 ± 7.2	11.5 ± 4.6	24.8 ± 5.8

† Mean ± SD in μm. For each boundary, differences were not computed for the middle 30 pixels (out of 128) to exclude the fovea.
* Errors were not computed for those scans in which boundary was determined to not be visible by at least one expert.

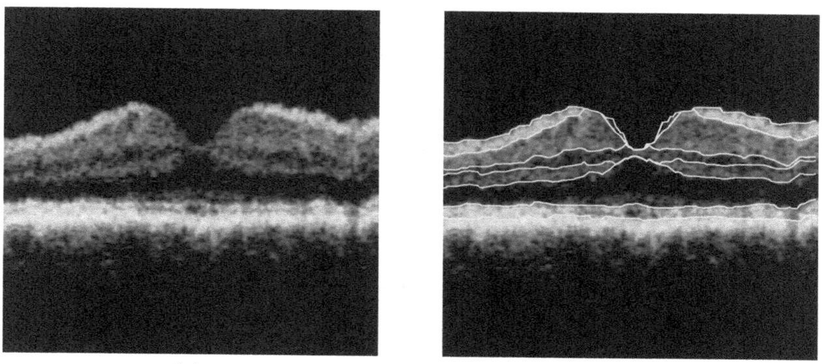

(a) (b)

Fig. 7. Example result shown on a 2-D scan from one of the 3-D images

surface 1; $p = 0.11$ for surface 3; $p = 0.80$ for surface 5; $p < 0.001$ for surface 6; $p = 0.004$ for surface 7). The overall mean (all borders combined) unsigned border positioning error for the algorithm was 7.8 ± 5.0 μm with an overall maximum unsigned border positioning error of 24.7 ± 12.9 μm. This was comparable to the overall mean and maximum border positioning errors computed between the observers which were 8.1 ± 3.6 μm and 22.8 ± 9.2 μm, respectively, and compared well with the true 9–10 μm resolution of the OCT imaging system reported in the literature [11]. An example result is shown in Fig. 7.

8 Discussion and Conclusion

We have presented how in-region cost terms may be added to the optimal 3-D graph search approach and demonstrated its applicability to the intraretinal layer segmentation of macular OCT images. In fact, we chose to only use in-region cost terms for the interior surfaces to help to show how surfaces may be found using only in-region cost terms. With the resulting segmentation errors being similar to that found between two observers, our results were very good overall. Nevertheless, we anticipate that incorporating both on-surface and in-region cost terms will help to provide a better segmentation than that from using either type of cost alone.

References

1. McInerney, T., Terzoppoulos, D.: Deformable models in medical image analysis: A survey. Medical Image Analysis 1(2), 91–108 (1996)
2. Suri, J.S., Liu, K., Singh, S., Laxinarayan, S.N., Zeng, X., Reden, L.: Shape recovery algorithms using level sets in 2-D/3-D medical imagery: A state-of-the-art review. IEEE Trans. Inform. Technol. Biomed. 6(1), 8–28 (2002)
3. Li, K., Wu, X., Chen, D.Z., Sonka, M.: Optimal surface segmentation in volumetric images – a graph-theoretic approach. IEEE Trans. Pattern Anal. Machine Intell. 28(1), 119–134 (2006)
4. Wu, X., Chen, D.Z.: Optimal net surface problems wih applications. In: Widmayer, P., Triguero, F., Morales, R., Hennessy, M., Eidenbenz, S., Conejo, R. (eds.) ICALP 2002. LNCS, vol. 2380, pp. 1029–1042. Springer, Heidelberg (2002)
5. Boykov, Y.Y., Jolly, M.P.: Interactive graph cuts for optimal and region segmentation of objects in N-D images. In: Proc. of the Eighth IEEE International Conference on Computer Vision (ICCV), vol. 1, pp. 105–112. IEEE Computer Society, Washington, DC, USA (2001)
6. Zhao, F., Zhang, H., Wahle, A., Scholz, T.D., Sonka, M.: Automated 4D segmentation of aortic magnetic resonance images. In: British Machine Vision Conference (BMVA). vol. 1, pp. 247–256 (2006)
7. Haeker, M., Sonka, M., Kardon, R., Shah, V.A., Wu, X., Abràmoff, M.D.: Automated segmentation of intraretinal layers from macular optical coherence tomography images. In: Proceedings of SPIE Medical Imaging 2007: Image Processing. vol. 6512., SPIE (2007)
8. Huang, D., Swanson, E.A., Lin, C.P., Schuman, J.S., Stinson, W.G., Chang, W., Hee, M.R., Flotte, T., Gregory, K., Puliafito, C.A.: Optical coherence tomography. Science 254(5035), 1178–1181 (1991)
9. Li, K., Millington, S., Wu, X., Chen, D.Z., Sonka, M.: Simultaneous segmentation of multiple closed surfaces using optimal graph searching. In: Christensen, G.E., Sonka, M. (eds.) IPMI 2005. LNCS, vol. 3565, pp. 406–417. Springer, Heidelberg (2005)
10. Yu, Y., Acton, S.T.: Speckle reducing anisotropic diffusion. IEEE Trans. Image Processing 11(11), 1260–1270 (2002)
11. Costa, R.A., Skaf, M., Melo, L.A.S., Calucci, D., Cardillo, J.A., Castro, J.C., Huang, D., Wojtkowski, M.: Retinal assessment using optical coherence tomography. Prog. Retin. Eye Res. 25(3), 325–353 (2006)

Localized Maximum Entropy Shape Modelling

Marco Loog

Department of Computer Science, Nordic Bioscience A/S
University of Copenhagen, Herlev
Copenhagen, Denmark
loog@diku.dk

Abstract. A core part of many medical image segmentation techniques is the point distribution model, i.e., the landmark-based statistical shape model which describes the type of shapes under consideration. To build a proper model, that is flexible and generalizes well, one typically needs a large amount of landmarked training data, which can be hard to obtain. This problem becomes worse with increasing shape complexity and dimensionality.

This work presents a novel methodology applicable to principal component-based shape model building and similar techniques. The main idea of the method is to make regular PCA shape modelling more flexible by using merely covariances between neighboring landmarks. The remaining unknown second order moments are determined using the maximum entropy principle based on which the full covariance matrix—as employed in the PCA—is determined using matrix completion.

The method presented can be applied in a variety of situations and in conjunction with other technique facilitating model building. The experiments on point distributions demonstrate that improved shape models can be obtained using this localized maximum entropy modelling.

1 Introduction

In the past decade, the approach to segmentation, using statistical shape models and the like, has received a lot of attention and a considerable amount of literature in the field has been devoted to this subject.

A core issue in statistical shape modelling is to build the prior shape model. Typically, the model building is based on examples shapes, which are obtained through the manual delineation by an expert of the shapes of interest in medical images. A reoccurring difficulty in the process is to collect enough data in order to be able to build a shape model that both has an adequate generalization ability and a high specificity. On the one hand, the model should capture enough of the variations in the class of shapes under consideration to ensure that everything that has to be modelled can actually be modelled. On the other, the model should avoid modelling more than necessary.

In this paper, we shall take the small amount of training instances as a given fact and focus on the problem of building a shape model under such circumstances. More specifically, we considers statistical shape model building based

N. Karssemeijer and B. Lelieveldt (Eds.): IPMI 2007, LNCS 4584, pp. 619–629, 2007.
© Springer-Verlag Berlin Heidelberg 2007

on the principal components of the shape covariance matrix, which is the approach pursued in well-known active shape modelling [1]. We should, however, stress that the general principle is more broadly applicable.

When there is not enough training data, a PCA model will be overly constrained and not generalize well to new shapes of the same class. In PCA, one typically employs the full sample covariance matrix, which describes second order covariations between *all* landmarks in the model. Arguably, this is too restrictive in the small sample case, and we propose to relax this constraint by merely modelling local covariations between landmark points which are all within a same neighborhood. Still, to actually perform PCA, one does need a full covariance matrix and we suggest to fill in the unspecified covariances by "assuming the least" and cast the problem into a maximum entropy formulation [2,3]. As a results of the maximization of the entropy, typically a *full rank* covariance matrix is obtained from which a larger number of sensible modes can be extracted than from the original sample covariance matrix.

1.1 Related Work

Many of the other techniques employed to make statistical shape models more flexible do this by adding a second (covariance) matrix to the sample covariance [4,5,6,7]. The actual form of this second matrix is, for example, obtained through finite element methods or based on regularization or smoothing principles, which can also be modelled through certain assumptions about the prior probability. Similar to these methods is the adaptive focus method [8] and its variations (see [9]), in which individual shapes are explicitly manipulated so to increase their influence on the final PCA and partly overcome the small sample problem. The shape manipulation can be seen as a different way of providing prior information to the model. Another class is concerned with expanding the representation basis to model the shapes with, typically in an hierarchical way, e.g. using wavelets, [10,11,12,13]. Subsequently, explicitly or implicitly assuming certain independencies between representations at different levels, these levels can be modelled separately and a more flexible overall model is obtained.

Our approach is in some sense complementary to the previously mentioned. The way we use prior knowledge in shape modelling here is by explicitly *not* modelling those interactions between landmarks which seem too restrictive, too uncertain, or simply improper. The unmodelled part is then taken care of by the maximum entropy principle. Such an approach can be integrated into most, if not all, of the methods previously mentioned, both where it involves determining a covariance matrix and when the goal is the estimation of some other parameters.

2 Local Covariations and Maximum Entropy

The methodology is presented within the context of point distribution models [1] in which shapes are represented by the coordinates of a set of n landmark points placed alongside the object boundary. The landmarks are taken to correspond between different shape instances. Subsequently, employing Procrustes analysis, the correspondence is used to align all shapes into a common coordinate frame, removing translation, rotation, and scaling variations.

Following the alignment, all d-dimensional shapes are represented in an Euclidean nd-dimensional space, in which the shape variability is analyzed using principal component analysis (PCA), i.e., an eigenvalue decomposition of the covariance matrix is carried out which yields eigenvectors that can be interpreted as the primary shape variations w.r.t. the mean shape, i.e., the so-called modes of shape variation, describing a joint displacement of landmarks. By a linear combination of the mean shape and these modes of variation, it should be possible to approximate each relevant shape. Usually only a small number of modes is needed to capture most of the variation in the training set. One of the main questions, however, is how this shape model behaves on unseen data.

Given N ($N < dn$) shapes, the standard method only allows for the extraction of $N-1$ non-degenerate modes of variation, which, especially in the small sample case, is most often too restrictive to describe the shape class properly. One too restrictive assumptions the PCA model makes is that the interactions, or covariations, between all landmark points are explicitly modelled. This means that every single landmark influences every other landmark in the shape, no matter how far they are located from each other. As few examples do not allow for an accurate estimation of the full covariance matrix from the data, it would be beneficial to reduce the number of covariances estimated directly from the data.

2.1 Local Entries of the Covariance Matrix

Arguably, from the position of one landmark, another landmark's position can be more accurately predicted the closer both points are to each other. Being well enough able to predict shape variations locally, the prediction of a global shape would also be roughly possible. This leads us to avoiding the estimation of covariances for the data of landmarks that are spatially remote: For every landmark, the k nearest neighbors are determined and merely their (co)variances are estimated.

As we need a full covariance matrix to perform PCA, all unspecified entries have to be filled out such that the matrix becomes a proper covariance matrix. This is a so-called matrix completion problem, which is generally nontrivial to solve [14,15]. E.g., in order to make the model maximally flexible, one would like to assume independence between landmarks not in the same local neighborhood, which would imply the associated covariance to be zero. However, generally, setting all non-neighborhood matrix entries to zero does *not* result in a positive semidefinite matrix.

We can be certain that a positive semidefinite solution exists (e.g. take the sample covariance matrix), however if there are more solutions—which should be the case for our approach to work, we need a criterion that picks out a unique one. We suggest to use a maximum entropy approach for this [2,3]. Assuming that the covariance matrix specifies a Gaussian model, the (differential) entropy

h_C equals

$$h_C = \frac{1}{2}\ln((2\pi)^{nd}\det C))\,, \tag{1}$$

where C is the covariance matrix, and the maximum entropy solution can be obtained by matrix completion under the constraint that the determinant of the matrix is maximized [2], because

$$h_C \propto \det(C)\,. \tag{2}$$

This optimization problem can be readily solved through semidefinite programming [16], however we used a more heuristic approach [17] which turns out to work more efficient for our purpose. The latter approach finds the global maximum by cycling iteratively through all of the unspecified matrix entries and solving, explicitly, the associated one-variable problem that maximizes the determinant. For a description of the optimization strategy and related pseudo-code, we refer to [17].

2.2 Rationale of Maximum Entropy

The rationale of maximum entropy is that one obtains the distribution which assumes the least about the unknown parameters [3]. Or rather, in a way it avoids modelling dependencies and interactions that are spurious. In the current case, this means that it tries to fill in the unspecified entries in such a way that the landmarks are taken *as independent as possible*. This behavior can also be seen from the trace and the determinant of the covariance matrices. All positive semidefinite solutions to the matrix completion problem, have the same trace, as the diagonal is fully specified (because a landmark is always its own first nearest neighbor). This means that the total variance that is being modelled is the same for all solutions. However, the maximum entropy solution attains this total variance and at the same time maximizes the determinant. This means that it tries to distribute the eigenvalues of the matrix as evenly as possible; the more uniformly distributed the eigenvalues are, the higher the determinant is[1], i.e., the more spherical the Gaussian distribution becomes.

Note, by the way, that a maximum entropy completed covariance matrix will generally have a positive determinant, i.e., the matrix is full rank, implying that all eigenvectors have a positive eigenvalue associated to them and there are no degenerate, eigenvalue zero, shape modes in the model.

3 Illustrative Experiments

To illustrate the effect of using the localized maximum entropy covariance matrix, the lung field segmentations in standard chest radiographs, as described in [18], are used. This data set was chosen because of the amount of segmentations available, which allows us to refrain from leave-one-out experiments or

[1] All of this is rather reminiscent of the arithmetic-geometric inequality.

other cross-validation techniques and simply use a separate train and test set. In addition, the visualization of the effect is easier because it concerns 2D data. Last, but not least, the data is already landmarked and all is made publicly available[2].

3.1 Data and Experimental Settings

Lung segmentations are provided for 247 images with a total of 94 landmarks to represent both lung fields. 64 images were used for testing and the remaining 183 images were used in the test phase. Experiments were conducted using 4, 8, 16, and 32 shapes in the training set and the number of neighbors k, based on which the local modelling was performed, was taken to be 3, 7, or 15. The percentage of initially *unspecified* entries in the 188×188-covariance matrix for these choices of k is considerable—about 97%, 92%, and 81%, respectively.

The performance is measured using often employed measures for generalization and specificity (see e.g. [19] or [20]). Compactness could have been used as well, however the models obtained by means of maximum entropy will, by construction, have better compactness compared to the regular PCA model. The eigenvalues become more and more similar to each other as the entropy increases, while the trace remains fixed, implying that the leading eigenvalues become smaller. For this reason, the focus is on model generalization ability and model specificity.

3.2 Results

Figure 1 displays, for a training set containing four shapes, examples of the first four and modes of variation obtained be regular PCA. The corresponding first four modes for the approach proposed using local modelling based on 3 neighbors are displayed in Figure 2. Mode variations are shown using the notorious ± 3 standard deviations from the mean shape. Figure 3 shows four additional modes obtainable using local maximum entropy modelling. Clearly, for regular PCA the last modes (the light gray shapes in the bottom righthand corner of Figure 1) provides no additional shape variability as its standard deviation equals zero. The maximum entropy modes provides more than $N-1$ plausible shape variations. In addition, in Figure 3, note that higher order modes seem to have the tendency to model more and more localized shape variability, e.g. all of them model either something in the right or in the left, but not in both lungs.

Plots for the specificity and the generalization ability against the number of modes are shown in Figure 4. The curves on the left give the generalization ability of the four models (i.e., regular PCA and localized maximum entropy with $k = 3$, 7, and 15 neighbors). Those on the right provide the specificity. Top graph shows the results for 4 training instances, the second for 8, the third one for 16, and bottom one for 32 training shapes. In general, the lower the curve is situated, the better the model performs.

[2] `www.isi.uu.nl/Research/Databases/`

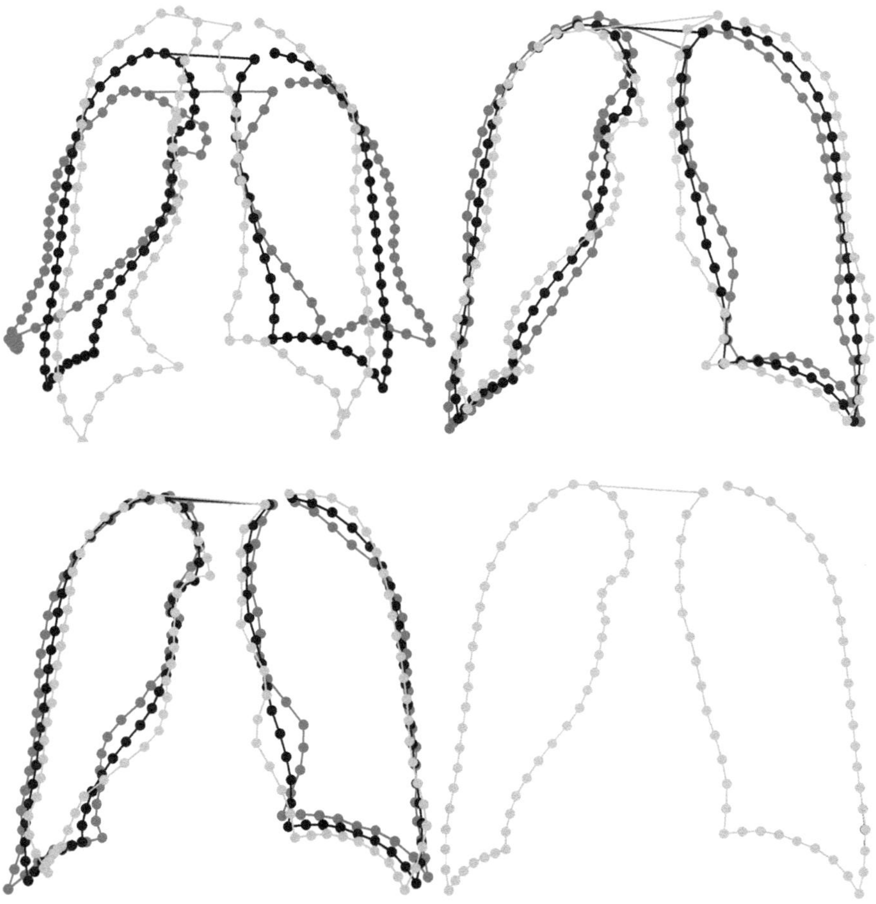

Fig. 1. Left to right, top to bottom: Modes of variation for $N = 4$ training samples using regular PCA. The mean shape is in black, while the light and dark gray shapes give the variations with ± 3 standard deviations.

From the graphs, we see that the localized maximum entropy models tend to provide better generalization ability than a regular PCA model. On the other hand, the specificity often increases w.r.t. the PCA model. The gain in generalization ability is often considerably larger than the loss w.r.t. specificity when using maximum entropy. The actual tradeoff between these two entities should decide whether or not a maximum entropy model should be employed.

Note that in the top graph only the very unconstrained $k = 3$ model improves upon regular PCA. The other choices of neighborhood size, are apparently still too restricted to gain anything over normal PCA. As the number of training examples increases the situation gradually changes. The improvement in generalization ability for 8 (and partly also for 16) training instances is very convincing. In the bottom graph, where 32 training instances are used, the very flexible

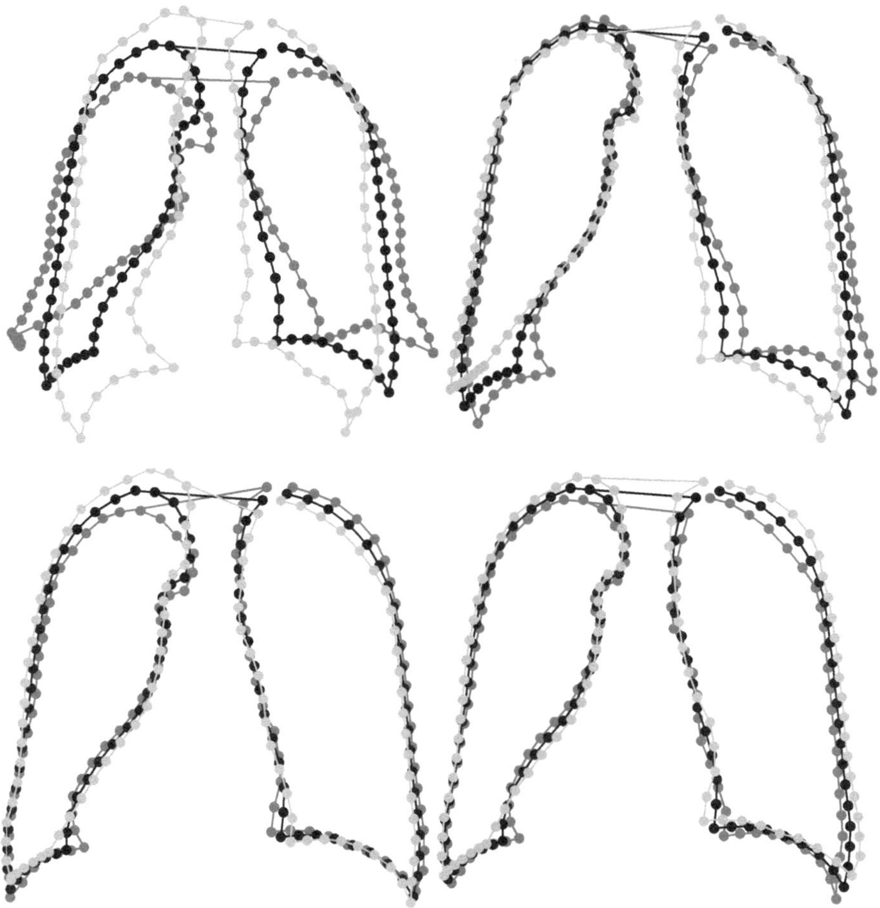

Fig. 2. Left to right, top to bottom: Modes of variation for $N = 4$ training samples obtained by localized maximum entropy model, in which the neighborhood consists of the $k = 3$ nearest neighbors. The mean shape is in black, while the light and dark gray shapes give the variations with ± 3 standard deviations.

model does not seem to be better than regular PCA anymore, however now the two other shape models seem to provide some improvements.

4 Discussion and Conclusion

In this work, the original PCA-based point distribution model was made more flexible by restricting the data-driven modelling of interactions merely to local interactions between neighboring landmark points. This results in a covariance matrix with a considerable amount of unspecified covariance entries, which we proposed to specify based on a maximum entropy approach, i.e., the entries are chosen such that the matrix becomes positive definite (a full rank covariance

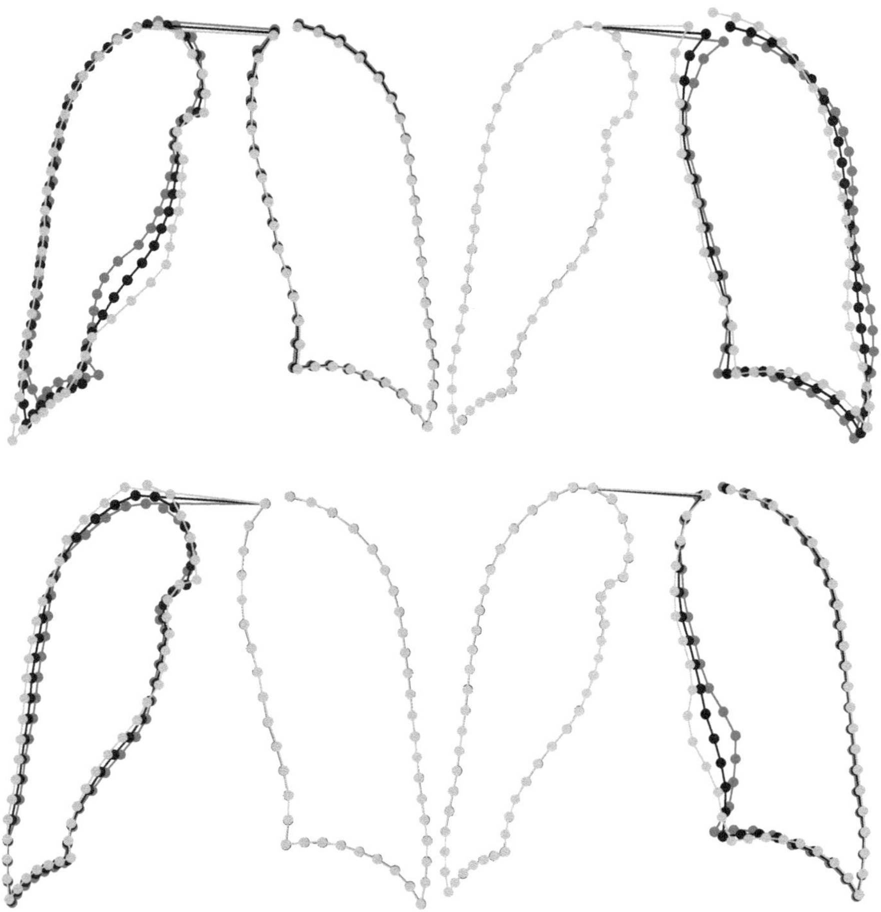

Fig. 3. Left to right, top to bottom: Four additional $k = 3$ local maximum entropy modes for $N = 4$ training samples. (See also Figure 2.) The mean shape is in black and the light and dark gray shape show the variations with ± 3 standard deviations.

matrix) and at the same time maximizes the determinant of the resulting matrix. In this way, a model is obtained that keeps the localized interactions as independent as possible and as such increases the model's ability to generalize on previously unseen shapes.

In the experiments, when using our maximum entropy approach, it turned out that an accurate enough shape model could be built using only 16 training shapes. Even training on 8 instances would be acceptable, as in this an average absolute landmark error of only 1 millimeter can be obtained. In addition, the method also slightly improved the standard PCA approach when 32 training samples were used, and seems therefore also beneficial to use when dealing with moderate sample sizes.

Future research aims at applying the method to 3D data. In such situations the ability of regular PCA to capture the essential shape variations becomes even

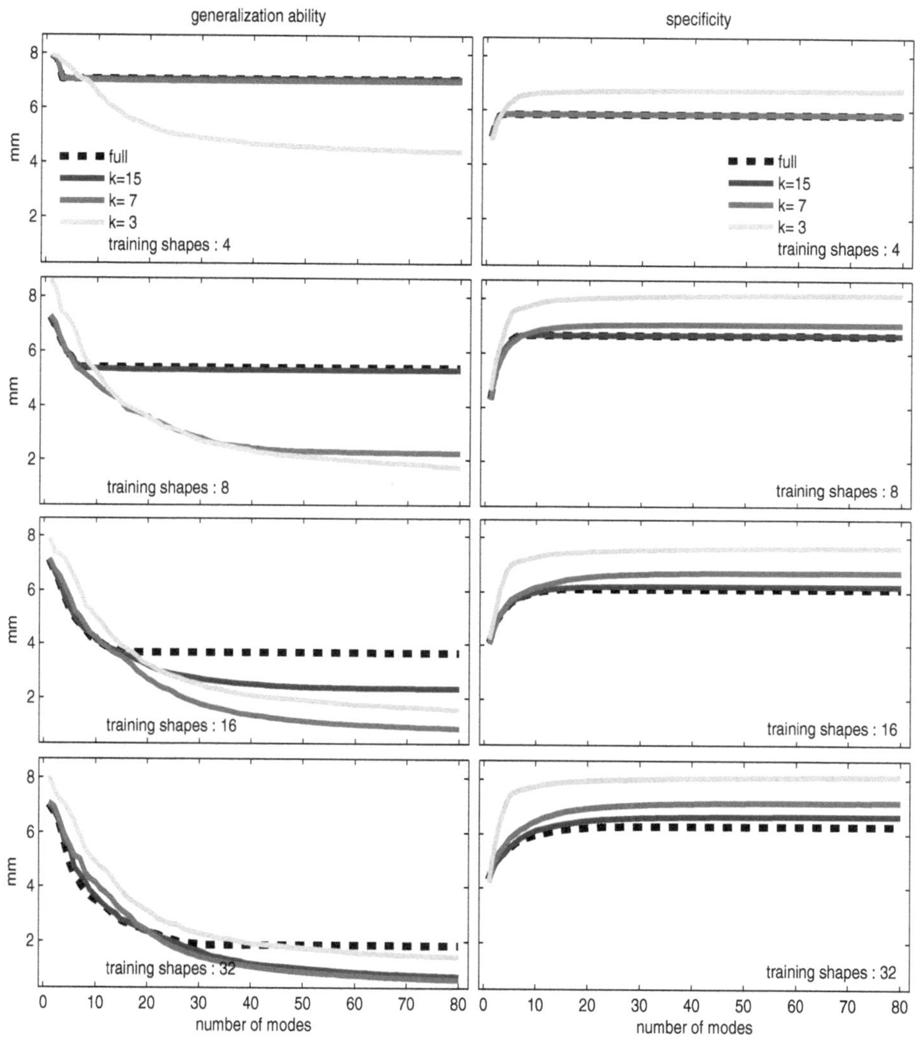

Fig. 4. Left : plots of the reconstruction error, indicating the generalization ability of the models. Right : the 'nearest neighbor' error [19,20], indicating the specificity of the models. The performance of the sample covariance PCA model is given by the black dashed graphs. Errors are measured on the test set. The mean absolute landmark deviation in millimeters is reported.

less and the need for local modelling increases. The results presented indicate that the method should work good in this situation as well.

As remarked in the introduction, the suggested modelling approach can be considered complementary to many already existing methods to improve small sample-based shape modelling. In addition, our method also makes it possible to improve nonlinear shape models [21,22] in the same way as presented here.

Nonlinear modelling calls for relatively more data, as the model becomes more complex. Localized maximum entropy modelling can aid in dealing with such models.

Finally, we are very interested in a possible link with work like presented in [23]. It would be interesting to see in what way our explicit local modelling does actually result in localized, and possible better interpretable, modes of variation.

Acknowledgment

Dr. M. De Bruijne is kindly acknowledged for making several point distribution modelling tools available to me.

References

1. Cootes, T.F., Taylor, C.J., Cooper, D., Graham, J.: Active shape models—their training and application. Computer Vision and Image Understanding 61, 38–59 (1995)
2. Cover, T.M., Thomas, J.A.: Elements of Information Theory. Wiley Interscience, New York (1991)
3. Jaynes, E.T.: On the rationale of maximum-entropy methods. In: Proceedings of the IEEE, vol. 70, pp. 939–952 (1982)
4. Cootes, T.F., Taylor, C.J.: Combining point distribution models with shape models based on finite-element analysis. Image and Vision Computing 13, 403–409 (1995)
5. de Bruijne, M., van Ginneken, B., Viergever, M., Niessen, W.: Adapting active shape models for 3D segmentation of tubular structures in medical images. In: Taylor, C.J., Noble, J.A. (eds.) IPMI 2003. LNCS, vol. 2732, pp. 136–147. Springer, Heidelberg (2003)
6. Wang, Y., Staib, L.H.: Elastic model based non-rigid registration incorporating statistical shape information. In: Wells, W.M., Colchester, A.C.F., Delp, S.L. (eds.) MICCAI 1998. LNCS, vol. 1496, pp. 1162–1173. Springer, Heidelberg (1998)
7. Wang, Y., Staib, L.H.: Boundary finding with prior shape and smoothness models. IEEE Transactions on Pattern Analysis and Machine Intelligence 22, 738–743 (2000)
8. Shen, D., Davatzikos, C.: An adaptive-focus statistical shape model for segmentation and shape modeling of 3-D brain structures. IEEE Transactions on Medical Imaging 20, 257–270 (2001)
9. Lötjönen, J., Antila, K., Lamminmäki, E., Koikkalainen, J., Lilja, M., Cootes, T.: Artificial enlargement of a training set for statistical shape models: Application to cardiac images. In: Frangi, A.F., Radeva, P.I., Santos, A., Hernandez, M. (eds.) FIMH 2005. LNCS, vol. 3504, pp. 92–101. Springer, Heidelberg (2005)
10. Davatzikos, C., Tao, X., Shen, D.: Hierarchical active shape models using the wavelet transform. IEEE Transactions on Medical Imaging 22, 414–423 (2003)
11. Mohamed, A., Davatzikosh, C.: Shape representation via best orthogonal basis selection. In: Barillot, C., Haynor, D.R., Hellier, P. (eds.) MICCAI 2004. LNCS, vol. 3216, pp. 225–233. Springer, Heidelberg (2004)
12. Nain, D., Haker, S., Bobick, A., Tannenbaum, A.R.: Multiscale 3D shape analysis using spherical wavelets. In: Duncan, J.S., Gerig, G. (eds.) MICCAI 2005. LNCS, vol. 3750, pp. 459–467. Springer, Heidelberg (2005)

13. Zhao, Z., Aylward, S.R., Teoh, E.K.: A novel 3D partitioned active shape model for segmentation of brain MR images. In: Duncan, J.S., Gerig, G. (eds.) MICCAI 2005. LNCS, vol. 3749, pp. 221–228. Springer, Heidelberg (2005)
14. Johnson, C.R.: Matrix completion problems: A survey. In: Proceedings of Symposia in Applied Mathematics. Providence, Rhode Island, American Mathematical Society 1990, vol. 40, pp. 171–198 (1990)
15. Laurent, M.: In: Matrix completion problems. (Interior–M) of The Encyclopedia of Optimization, vol.III, pp. 221–229. Kluwer Academic Publishers, Dordrecht (2001)
16. Boyd, S., Vandenberghe, L.: Convex Optimization. Cambridge University Press, Cambridge (2004)
17. Glunt, W., Hayden, T.L., Johnson, C.R., Tarazaga, P.: Positive definite completions and determinant maximization. Linear Algebra and its Applications 288, 1–10 (1999)
18. van Ginneken, B., Stegmann, M., Loog, M.: Segmentation of anatomical structures in chest radiographs using supervised methods: a comparative study on a public database. Medical Image Analysis 10, 19–40 (2006)
19. Davies, R.H.: Learning Shape: Optimal Models for Analysing Natural Variability. Ph.D. Thesis, Division of Imaging Science and Biomedical Engineering, University of Manchester, UK (2002)
20. Styner, M.A., Rajamani, K.T., Nolte, L.P., Zsemlye, G., Székely, G., Taylor, C.J., Davies, R.H.: Evaluation of 3D correspondence methods for model building. In: Taylor, C.J., Noble, J.A. (eds.) IPMI 2003. LNCS, vol. 2732, pp. 63–75. Springer, Heidelberg (2003)
21. Romdhani, S., Gong, S., Psarrou, A.: A multi-view non-linear active shape model using kernel PCA. In: Proceedings of the 10th British Machine Vison Conference, Nottingham, UK, vol. 2, pp. 483–492. BMVA Press (1999)
22. Sozou, P., Cootes, T.F., Taylor, C.J., Mauro, E.D.: A non-linear generalisation of point distribution models using polynomial regression. Image and Vision Computing 13, 451–457 (1995)
23. Larsen, R., Eiriksson, H., Stegmann, M.B.: Q-MAF shape decomposition. In: Niessen, W.J., Viergever, M.A. (eds.) MICCAI 2001. LNCS, vol. 2208, pp. 837–844. Springer, Heidelberg (2001)

Computer Aided Detection of Pulmonary Embolism with Tobogganing and Mutiple Instance Classification in CT Pulmonary Angiography

Jianming Liang and Jinbo Bi

Computer Aided Diagnosis and Therapy
Siemens Medical Solutuions USA, Inc., Malvern, PA 19355

Abstract. Pulmonary embolism (PE) is a very serious condition causing sudden death in about one-third of the cases. Treatment with anti-clotting medications is highly effective but not without complications, while diagnosis has been missed in about 70% of the cases. A major clinical challenge, particularly in an Emergency Room, is to quickly and correctly diagnose patients with PE and then send them on to therapy. Computed tomographic pulmonary angiography (CTPA) has recently emerged as an accurate diagnostic tool for PE, but each CTPA study contains hundreds of CT slices. The accuracy and efficiency of interpreting such a large image data set is complicated by various PE look-alikes and also limited by human factors, such as attention span and eye fatigue. In response to this challenge, in this paper, we present a fast yet effective approach for computer aided detection of pulmonary embolism in CTPA. Our proposed approach is capable of detecting both acute and chronic pulmonary emboli with a distinguished feature of incrementally reporting any detection immediately once becoming available during searching, offering real-time support and achieving 80% sensitivity at 4 false positives. This superior performance is contributed to our novel algorithms (concentration oriented tobogganing and multiple instance classification) introduced in this paper for candidate detection and false positive reduction.

1 Introduction

Pulmonary embolism (PE) is the third most common cause of death in the US with at least 650,000 cases occurring annually. PE is a sudden blockage in a pulmonary artery, and is caused by an *embolus* that is usually formed in the legs and travels in the bloodstream through the heart before reaching the lungs. PE is a very serious condition that can cause sudden death in about one-third of the cases. Most of those who die do so within 30 to 60 minutes after symptoms start. Anti-clotting medications are highly effective in treating PEs, but sometimes can lead to subsequent hemorrhage and bleeding. Therefore, they should be only given to those who really need. A major clinical challenge, particularly in an ER (Emergency Room) scenario, is to quickly and correctly diagnose patients with PE and then send them on to treatment – a prompt and accurate diagnosis is the key to survival.

However, PE is among the most difficult conditions to diagnose because its primary symptoms are vague, non-specific, and may have a variety of other causes, making it hard to separate out the critically ill patients suffering from PE. The diagnosis of PE

N. Karssemeijer and B. Lelieveldt (Eds.): IPMI 2007, LNCS 4584, pp. 630–641, 2007.
© Springer-Verlag Berlin Heidelberg 2007

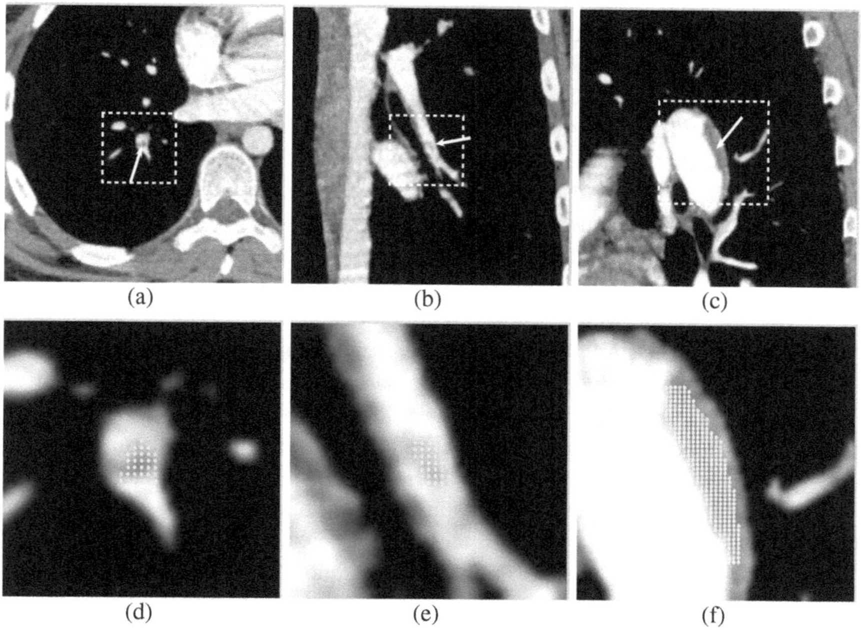

Fig. 1. The emboli appears as dark regions residing in bright vessel lumen. Our toboggan-based approach is capable to detect both acute (a, b) and chronic (c) pulmonary emboli, offering simultaneous detection and segmentation (d, e, f). The clot in (b) was actually missed by our radiologists, but correctly detected by our system, and confirmed by the radiologists.

is missed more than 400,000 times in the US each year, and approximately 100,000 patients die who would have survived with the proper diagnosis and treatment.

Computed tomographic (CT) pulmonary angiography (CTPA) has become first-line diagnosis technique for PE. Significant PEs are detectable given the high spatial resolution of modern CT scanners. A CT image is a large 3D volumetric image, which consists of hundreds of images, each representing one slice of the lung. Clinically, manual reading of these slices is laborious, time consuming and complicated by various PE look-alikes (false positives) including respiratory motion artifacts, flow-related artifacts, streak artifacts, partial volume artifacts, stair step artifacts, lymph nodes, and vascular bifurcation, among many others. The accuracy and efficiency of interpreting such a large image data set is also limited by human factors, such as attention span and eye fatigue. Consequently, it is highly desirable to have a computer aided detection (CAD) system to assist radiologists in detecting and characterizing emboli in an accurate, efficient and reproducible way. Such a CAD system has to achieve an extremely high detection sensitivity with as few as false positives to acquire clinical acceptance. It also needs to satisfy stringent real-time requirement due to the emergency nature of PE cases.

A number of computer aided diagnosis methods have been developed [1–4]. These existing methods are all based on sophisticated vessel segmentation, namely, first segmenting the pulmonary vessel structure and then searching for PEs within the segmented vessels, because PEs only exist in pulmonary arteries. However, vessel segmentation is computationally time-consuming and has been problematic in small vasculature where subsegmental PEs often occur [1]. Furthermore, the normal regions of pulmonary vessels are enhanced with contrast material. There is no need to search for PE in the enhanced normal regions. Therefore, even if the pulmonary vascular structure is correctly segmented, large part of it would be excluded anyway. In this paper, we present a fast yet effective toboggan-based approach for automated PE detection in CTPA without vessel segmentation. Another distinguished feature of our approach is its highly interactiveness and real-time response. For clinical use, all the detections reported by a CAD systems must be reviewed and approved by radiologists. The existing PE CAD systems adopts a pipe-line architecture and only report the final detection at the end of execution, implying that the radiologist has to wait until the end of the system run in order to review and approve any detections. However, in an ER (Emergency Room) scenario, radiologists only have a small time window (2-3 minutes) to read a case and make the diagnosis. They cannot wait till the end of run to examine all the CAD detection. To meet this requirement, our approach is capable to report any PE detection once available in real time for radiologist to review and approve, while it continues searching for additional PEs. These capabilities are founded on our two novel algorithms introduced in this paper: concentration oriented tobogganing algorithm for candidate detection and mutiple instance classification algorithm for false positive reduction.

2 Basic Tobogganing

Pulmonary embolism may be acute or chronic. They are only existing in pulmonary arteries and generally attached to the vessel wall (see Fig. 1). Due to the nature of their formation, CTPA reveals emboli, whether acute or chronic, as dark regions with Hounsfield Units (HU) between -50 HU and 100 HU, residing in contrast enhanced bright vessel lumen. However, due to partial volume effects, the pixels around the vessel boundaries are also in the same HU range. Therefore, a major challenge for automatic PE detection is to effectively separate the emboli from the vessel wall and to quickly remove partial volume effects around the vessel boundaries while correctly preserving the PE pixels. In response to this challenge, we have come up with an idea: sliding all the voxels with Hounsfield Units (HU) between -50 HU and 100 HU to its neighbor with minimal HU value and collecting all voxels that don't slide into regions with Hounsfield Unit below -50 HU. This idea is illustrated in Fig. 2 and explained in the following.

This algorithm is called tobogganing [5], which takes its name from the processing analogy of sliding down a steep hill and will be referred as "basic tobogganing" in this paper to be differentiated from a new tobogganing algorithm, called concentration oriented tobogganing, to be presented in Section 3. A basic operation in tobogganing is "sliding". A pixel v with intensity $P(v)$ and neighbors $N(v)$ slides down to pixel g:

$$g = \underset{\mathrm{t} \in \mathrm{N(v)} \cup \{\mathrm{v}\}}{\arg\min} \; P(t). \tag{1}$$

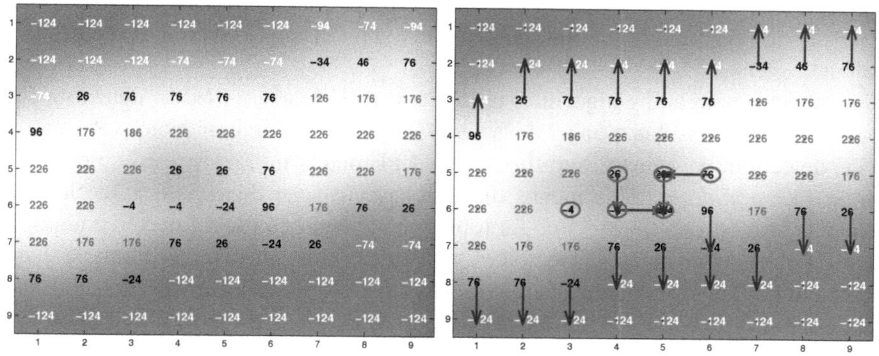

Fig. 2. An illustration of our idea for PE detection with basic tobogganing algorithm. In this small PE image, CT values below -50 HU are printed in "white", CT values above 100 HU in "gray" and all others in "dark". Naturally, all the CT values for PE pixels are in "dark". However, due to partial volume effects, the CT values for those pixels around the artery boundaries are also in "dark". Our idea can effectively detect the PE (circled) and remove the partial volume effects.

In cases where a pixel is surrounded by more than one pixel with the same minimal intensity value, the first pixel found with this value can be chosen or other more sophisticated strategies may be used in selecting a neighbor. A pixel that cannot slide to any of its neighbors is called a *concentration*. All the pixels that slide down to the same concentration form a toboggan *cluster* with a unique *label*.

The basic tobogganing algorithm operates as follows: Each unlabeled pixel slides till reaching a labeled pixel or a unlabeled new concentration. If it reaches a labeled pixel, the label is propagated back to all the pixels along the sliding path, otherwise, a new label is generated and then propagated back along the path. All the sliding directions may be recorded during the process. Referring to the simple PE image in Fig. 2, for detecting PE, we scan the image in row by row, but only selectively slide those pixels with CT values between -50 HU and 100 HU. For illustration, we use 2D four-connected neighborhood. The arrows indicate the sliding directions. During the tobogganing, the first pixel with CT value between -50 HU and 100 HU is pixel (7,2), which slides towards to pixel (7,1). Since the CT value of pixel (7,1) is -74 HU, and is pre-labeled as "air", label "air" is propagated back to pixel (7,2). During the tobogganing process, the first pixel collected as PE pixel is pixel (4,5), because it slides down to pixel (4,6) and then concentrates at pixel (5,6) with CT value above -50 HU. Consequently, a PE label is generated and assigned to pixel (5,6) and propagated back to pixels (4,6) and (4,5). When it is done for all the pixels in the image, the "dark" pixels around the arteries have all merged into darker regions with CT values below -50 HU and all the PE pixels stand out (circled in red). In this example, two toboggan clusters are formed for the detected PE pixels: The pixel (3,6) constitutes a single-pixel toboggan cluster, while all other pixels forms one cluster with concentration at pixel (5,6). To achieve the goal of PE detection, the adjacent toboggan clusters (with detected

PE pixels) must be merged into a connected component, called a PE *candidate*, so that a detection position (3D point) can be derived by ultimate erosion to represent the candidate.

This basic tobogganing algorithm is intuitive and clearly useful in detecting PEs. However, a problem is that it only labels the PE voxels, providing suspicious PE regions. For PE detection, we must group the detected PE pixels into connected components, forming PE *candidates*. This means that we have to scan the whole 3D volumetric image data at least two times – one for tobogganing and one for connected component analysis, before reporting any detected PEs. In other words, the user (radiologist) has to wait the completion of two scans before reviewing and approving any PE detections. To overcome this drawback, we introduce concentration oriented tobogganing in the next section.

3 Concentration Oriented Tobogganing

3.1 The Algorithm

During the PE search process, our goal is, once a PE pixel is encountered, to extract a whole PE candidate from the pixel immediately and send it to the user (radiologist) for review and approval. A PE candidate consists of multiple toboggan clusters. Naturally, in order to achieve the goal, we must first have an algorithm which can extract a toboggan cluster from any given pixel and provide the external boundary pixels of the cluster. The process of extracting a toboggan cluster from a given pixel is referred as concentration oriented tobogganning and formulated as an algorithm in Appendix which is iteratively invoked for detecting PEs. The idea is illustrated in Fig. 3 and detailed as follows.

Basically, the concentration oriented tobogganing algorithm has two steps. It first searches for concentration c from the given pixel s and then expands from the found concentration c to extract the whole toboggan cluster C. The expansion includes a base step and an iterative step. In the base step, it includes the concentration c as the first pixel in the cluster and pushes all its neighbors with CT values between -50 HU and 100 HU into an active list A. In the iterative step, it selects pixel q with the minimal CT value from the active list A, if the selected pixel toboggans to an already clustered pixel, then conditionally pushes its neighbors to the active list A to ensure the uniqueness of the pixels in the active list, otherwise, the selected pixel belongs to the cluster's external boundary B. The iterative step is repeated till the active list A is empty. This concentration oriented tobogganing algorithm is repeatedly applied on all those external boundary pixels, until a whole PE candidate has been extracted.

Referring to Fig. 3, when our example image is scanned in row by row, the first PE pixel encountered is (4,5), because it does not merge into regions with CT value below -50 HU. Therefore, we wish to extract the whole PE from the pixel at (4,5). Fig. 3.(a) illustrates Step A of the algorithm: finding the concentration. It regards the starting location as the current location, slides it to its neighbor with minimal CT value, then selects the neighbor as the current location and slides it until reaching a concentration. Once the concentration is found, if its CT value is between -50 HU and 100 HU, Step B is initiated to expand from the concentration to cover a whole toboggan cluster and

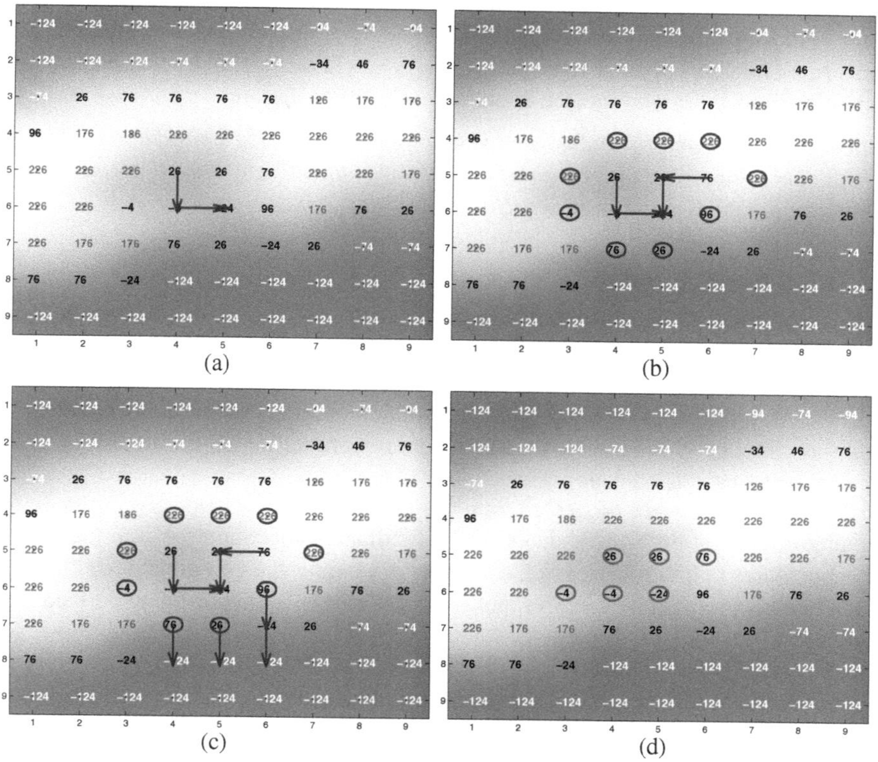

Fig. 3. Using the concentration oriented toboggan algorithm for PE detection. (a) Step A of the algorithm: Finding the concentration. (b) Step B: Expanding from the concentration to cover a whole toboggan cluster and providing all the external boundary pixels (circled). (c) Repeatedly apply the algorithm on all those external boundary pixels with CT value between -50 HU and 100 HU to form a PE candidate, leading to an identical result (d) as in Fig. 2.(b).

provide all the external boundary pixels (circled) as shown in Fig. 3.(b). In this example, the concentration (5,6) is included into the cluster and then all its neighbors with CT values in the PE HU range are pushed into an active list. A pixel with the minimal CT value is selected from the active list. In this case, it is pixel (4,6). Since it slides towards pixel (5,6), which has been included into the cluster, its neighbors are conditionally pushed into the active list. The condition is that the neighbor must have CT value in the PE HU range, is not included in the cluster and is not in the active list. A new pixel with the minimal CT value is selected from the active list. For this time, it is pixel (3,6), but it does not slides towards any pixels within the cluster, therefore, it is a pixel on the external boundary of the cluster, and no processing is performed on its neighbors. Repeatedly select a new pixel from the active lust and process it in the same way till the active list is empty. Once done, we obtain all the pixels within the cluster, namely, (4,5), (4,6), (5,5), (5,6) and (6,5), as well as the pixels along the external boundary of the cluster (circled in Fig. 3.(b)). The concentration oriented tobogganing algorithm is then iteratively applied on each of the external boundary pixels with CT value in the PE HU range. Any additional extracted toboggan cluster is merged into the previously extracted toboggan clusters, and any additional external boundary pixels are also merged. Once no external boundary pixel is left, all the toboggan clusters are extracted and merged, automatically forming a connected component – a PE candidate.

Proposition 3.1. *Concentration oriented tobogganing provides identical PE detections as basic tobogganing, but it has an advantage of reporting any detection immediately once becoming available during searching.*

3.2 Detection Performance

We have collected 177 cases with 872 clots marked by expert chest radiologists at four different institutions (two North American sites and two European sites). They are divided into two sets: training (45 cases with 156 clots) and testing (132 cases with 716 clots). The training cases were used in the development process for algorithm developing, improving and testing, while the testing cases were only used for algorithm testing and were never used for development.

All the 177 cases were processed with our concentration oriented algorithm, which generated a total of 8806 candidates: 2431 candidates appear in the training set and 6375 candidates in the test set. Each candidate is a connected component – a cluster of voxels, and represented by a representative point with a 3-D coordinate derived from the cluster of voxels.

Each candidate was then labeled as a PE or not based on 3-D landmark ground truth provided by the experts. In order to automatically label each candidate, each PE pointed out by an expert landmark is semi-automatically extracted and segmented. Therefore, the ground truth for each PE is also a cluster of voxels (*i.e.*, the segmented PE). Any candidate that was found to be intersected with any of the segmented PEs in the ground truth was labeled as a PE. Multiple candidates may intersect with the same segmented PE, that is, multiple candidates may correspond to a single PE. Each PE is assigned with a unique identifier, therefore, multiple candidates may be labeled with the same PE identifier.

Our algorithms successfully detected 90.38% (141/156) of the PE in the training cases and 90.1%(645/716) of the PE in the testing cases. On average, the total computation time for each case is about 2 minutes on a 2.4GHz P4 PC and the first detection if any in a case is reported within 27 seconds. However, the concentration oriented algorithm also produces candidates that do not intersect with any PEs. These candidates are regarded as *false positives*. On average, 47.5 and 40.3 false positives for each case are generated for the training set and the test set, respectively. However, a system that "cries wolf" too often will be rejected out of hand by radiologists. Thus, the goal is to detect as many true PEs as possible, subject to a constraint on false positives, usually within 4 false positives per case. Therefore, we design a novel classification framework based on mathematical programming to reduce false positives in the next section.

4 False Positive Reduction

For clinical acceptability, it is critical to control false positive rates and detect as many true PEs as possible. A PE can be large, or have an elongated shape along the vessel, or split at the vessel bifurcation. Multiple candidate clusters may exist to intersect with a single PE. As long as one of the candidates is identified and visualized to physicians, the entire PE can be easily traced out. Consequently, it is sufficient to detect one candidate for each PE. Correct classification of every candidate instance is not as important as the ability to detect at least one candidate that points to a specific PE. Based on this concept, a novel multiple instance classification algorithm is devised to reduce false positives.

4.1 Feature Computation

A set of 116 descriptive properties, called *features*, are computed for each candidate. These features were all image-based features and were normalized to a unit range. The features can be categorized into several groups: those indicative of voxel intensity distributions within the candidate, those summarizing distributions in neighborhood of the candidate, and those that describe the 3-D shape of the candidate and enclosing structures. These features, in conjunction with each other, capture candidate properties that can disambiguate true emboli from typical false positives, such as dark areas that result from poor mixing of bright contrast agents with blood in veins, and dark connective tissues between vessels. These features are not necessarily independent, and may be correlated with each other, especially within the same group.

4.2 Mutiple Instance Classification

Assume that totally ℓ candidates are extracted, each represented by a feature vector $\mathbf{x}_i$ associated with a label y_i. The label $y_i = 1$ if the candidate overlays on a PE, or otherwise $y_i = -1$. Let I^+ and I^- be two index sets containing indices of candidates that intersect with PEs and do not intersect with PEs, respectively. Let m be the total number of PEs marked by expert radiologists for the n images. Denote I_j as the index set of the candidates that intersect with the j-th PE, $j = 1, \cdots, m$. Notice that $\cup_{j=1,\cdots,m} I_j = I^+$ but any two index sets I_j's are not necessarily disjoint since there may exist a candidate cluster that intersects with more than one segmented PEs.

Support vector machine (SVM) [6–8] has been a successful methodology for classification and regression. It constructs linear classification functions of the form $\mathbf{w}^T\mathbf{x}+b$ by minimizing the hinge error defined as $\xi = \max\{0, 1 - y(\mathbf{w}^T\mathbf{x} - b)\}$ for all candidates. We derive a more effective classification approach by exploring the key observation that once a candidate in I_j is classified as a positive, then the j-th PE is considered being identified. This consideration suggests the classifier to focus on different PEs instead of multiple candidates within a single PE. Especially it facilitates the reduction of false positives by possibly ignoring extremely noisy candidates that intersect with some PEs where, for the same PE, other associated candidates can be easily classified correctly. A geometric interpretation is illustrated in a 2-D feature space as in Fig.4 where standard SVMs focus on separating all candidates to correct sides whereas our learning algorithm classifies at least one true PE candidate into one side and others on the other side, thus successfully removing all false detections.

Mathematically, distinguishing at least one candidate for each PE from the negative class is equivalent to the statement that as long as the minimum of the errors (ξ) that are occurred on the candidates associated with a PE is 0, then that PE is detected. For

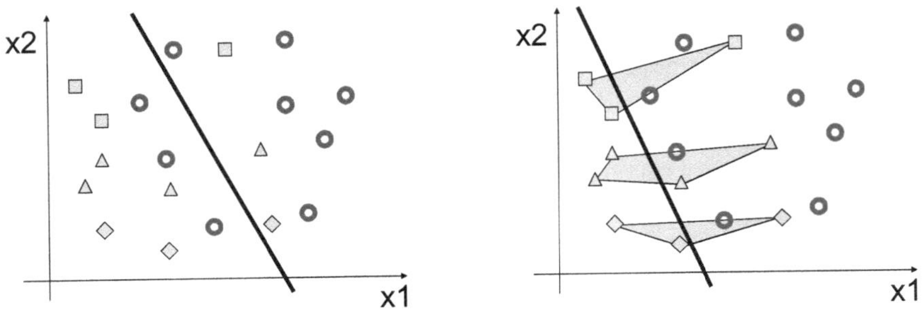

Fig. 4. Illustration of the classification. (Left) the linear separation boundary by standard SVM where circles represent false detections, and the symbols (diamond, box and triangle) each represent one PE with multiple candidates. (Right) the linear separation boundary by our multiple instance classification algorithm with more significant false positive reduction.

example, if a PE is associated with 3 candidates, and a classifier generates $\xi_1 = 0$ for the first candidate, $\xi_2 = 5,\ \xi_3 = 100$ for the other two candidates, the classifier detects the PE. Correspondingly, this implies to construct the classifier by solving the following optimization problem:

$$\begin{array}{ll} \min_{\mathbf{w},\xi} & \gamma||\mathbf{w}||_1 + \sum_{j=1}^{m} \min\{\xi_i,\ i \in I_j\} + \sum_{i \in I^-} \xi_i \\ \text{s.t.} & \mathbf{w}^T x_i + b \geq 1 - \xi_i,\ i \in I^+, \\ & \mathbf{w}^T x_i + b \leq -1 + \xi_i,\ i \in I^-, \\ & \xi_i \geq 0,\ i = 1, \cdots, \ell. \end{array} \tag{2}$$

However, this optimization problem is computationally difficult to solve, because it involves a minimization of the to-be-determined variables ξ in the evaluation of the objective function, and it is neither differentiable nor convex. Hence, it is necessary to devise a tractable optimization problem that is equivalent. To this end, we prove that problem (2) is equivalent to the quadratic program (3), as characterized by the following theorem:

$$\begin{array}{ll} \min_{\mathbf{w},\xi,\boldsymbol{\lambda}} & \gamma||\mathbf{w}||_1 + \sum_{j=1}^{m} (\sum_{i \in I_j} \lambda_i \xi_i) + \sum_{i \in I^-} \xi_i \\ \text{s.t.} & \mathbf{w}^T x_i + b \geq 1 - \xi_i,\ i \in I^+, \\ & \mathbf{w}^T x_i + b \leq -1 + \xi_i,\ i \in I^-, \\ & \xi_i \geq 0,\ i = 1, \cdots, \ell, \\ & \sum_{i \in I_j} \lambda_i = 1, \lambda_i \geq 0,\ i \in I_j,\ j = 1, \cdots, m. \end{array} \tag{3}$$

Theorem 4.1. *An optimal solution $\hat{\mathbf{w}}$ of Problem (2) is also optimal to Problem (3) with properly chosen λ, and vice versa.*

Proof. First of all, we prove that an optimal solution of Problem (3) has nonzero λ's only on the candidates for which the classifier achieves $\min\{\xi_i,\ i \in I_j\},\ \forall\, j$.

Let $(\hat{\mathbf{w}}, \hat{\boldsymbol{\xi}}, \hat{\boldsymbol{\lambda}})$ be the optimal solution of Problem (3). For notational convenience, denote the objective of Problem (3) as $\mathcal{J}(\mathbf{w}, \boldsymbol{\xi}, \boldsymbol{\lambda}) = \gamma||\mathbf{w}||_1 + \sum_{j=1}^{m} (\sum_{i \in I_j} \lambda_i \xi_i) + \sum_{i \in I^-} \xi_i$. Then let $\hat{\mathcal{J}}$ be the objective value attained at the optimal solution. Notice

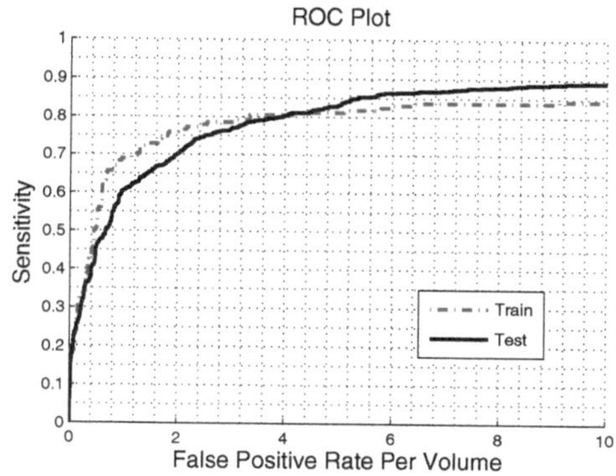

Fig. 5. The ROC plot of the final system

that the hinge loss $\hat{\boldsymbol{\xi}}$ is uniquely determined by $\hat{\mathbf{w}}$ as $\hat{\xi}_i = \max\{0, 1 - y_i(\mathbf{w}^T\mathbf{x}_i + b)\}$ for each candidate $\mathbf{x}_i$.

If $\exists\, j \in \{1, \cdots, m\}$, and $\exists i_0 \in I_j$, such that $\lambda_{i_0} > 0$ but $\hat{\xi}_{i_0} \neq \min\{\xi_i, i \in I_j\}$. Then let $\xi_{I_j} = \min\{\xi_i, i \in I_j\} < \hat{\xi}_{i_0}$. Then $\tilde{\mathcal{J}} = \hat{\mathcal{J}} - \lambda_{i_0}\xi_{i_0} + \lambda_{i_0}\xi_{I_j} < \hat{\mathcal{J}}$. This contradicts to the optimality of $(\hat{\mathbf{w}}, \hat{\boldsymbol{\xi}}, \hat{\boldsymbol{\lambda}})$.

By this contradiction, $\forall i, j$, such as $\lambda_i > 0$, the corresponding ξ_i has to be the minimum loss that the classifier achieves on the j-th PE. This implies that at the optimality of Problem (3), $\mathcal{J} = \gamma||\mathbf{w}||_1 + \sum_{j=1}^{m} \min\{\xi_i,\ i \in I_j\} + \sum_{i\in I^-} \xi_i$ which is the same as the objective of Problem (2).

4.3 System Performance

Our classification algorithm has dramatically reduced the false positive rate down to 4 false positives per patient while maintaining the high detection sensitivity. Fig.5 depicts the Receiver Operating Characteristics (ROC) plot of our final system that combines the candidate detection, feature computation, and classification. As shown in Fig.5, the final system detects 80% of the PEs, respectively, for the training study set and the test set at 4 false positive per patient.

5 Discussions and Conclusions

We view our method as toboggan-based because the idea is originally inspired by the work of Fairfield [5] and of Mortensen and Barrett [9]. The basic tobogganing algorithm presented in Section 2 is a modified version of the algorithm in [5, 10]. Nevertheless, each of the research groups has different aims in mind. Fairfield aimed to enhance the contrast of images by tobogganing, while Mortensen and Barrett used tobogganing with the aim to group the pixels to reduce the underlying graph in livewire for efficient interactive image segmentation. Clearly, our aim is to separate objects (PEs in this case) from adjacent (connected) objects (vessel walls in this case) and remove partial volume effects. Given the general nature of the idea, the algorithm has been successfully applied to other applications, for instance, detecting colonic polyps in CT images.

We also would like to contrast our concentration oriented tobogganing algorithm with a few of existing related algorithms in the literature including: watershed, hierarchical tobogganing, intelligent paint, and intelligent scissor" (*i.e.*, "live-wire"). There is a rich set of algorithms in the watershed literature. The most related ones are rainfalling simulation [11] and the watershed technique based on hill climbing reported in [12]. The basic toboggan algorithm first reported by Fairfield largely went unnoticed in the watershed community. Rainfalling simulation can be regarded as an extension of Fairfield's algorithm for handling "plateau". The watershed technique based on hill climbing reported in [12] requires that *all* the minima be found in advance and marked with distinct labels followed by "hill climbing". This implies that we would not be able to obtain a watershed region till the whole image has been scanned and processed. "Hierarchical tobogganing" is to repeatedly apply the basic toboggan algorithm, forming toboggan hierarchy. "Intelligent paint" is built on top of hierarchical tobogganing to allow the user to interactively "select" the pre-formed toboggan regions at a user pre-specified toboggan hierarchical level, based on cost-ordered region collection. "Intelligent scissor" or interactive "live-wire" aims to compute an optimal path from a selected seed point to *every* other point in the image based on unrestricted graph search, so that the user can move the mouse freely in the image plane and interactively "select" a desired path among all the optimal paths based on the current cursor position. The underlying algorithm is Dijkstra's algorithm, which computed a shortest path from a given point to every other point in the image. However, for large images, the underlying graph created in live-wire for search become large, the interactiveness of livewire would be comprised due to the fundamental limitation of Dijkstra's algorithm. Therefore, Mortensen and Barrett [9] proposed toboggan-based livewire, in which the basic toboggan algorithm is applied to reduce the underlying graph in livewire to achieve highly efficient interaction in image segmentation. In short, all the discussed algorithms cannot meet our requirement to extract a toboggan cluster from an initial site without processing any pixels beyond its external boundary.

In conclusion, we have developed a novel approach for computer aided detection of pulmonary embolism. Our approach has a set of distinguished features, requiring no vessel segmentation, reporting any detection incrementally in real time, and detecting both acute and chronic pulmonary emboli, achieving 80% sensitivity at 4 false positives.

References

1. Masutani, Y., MacMahon, H., Doi, K.: Computerized detection of pulmonary embolism in spiral CT angiography based on volumetric image analysis. IEEE Transactions on Medical Imaging 21(12), 1517–1523 (2002)
2. Quist, M., Bouma, H., van Kuijk, C., van Delden, O., Gerritsen, F.: Computer aided detection of pulmonary embolism on multi-detector CT. In: RSNA, Chicago, USA, November 2004, (Conference Poster) (2004)
3. Zhou, C., Hadjiiski, L.M., Patel, S., Chan, H.-P., Chan, B.: Computerized detection of pulmonary embolism in 3D computed tomographic (CT) images. In: RSNA, Chicago, USA, November 2004, (abstract) (2004)
4. Park, S., Bajaj, C., Gladish, G., Cody, D.: Automatic pulmonary embolos detection and visualization, (2004) poster at `http://www.ices.utexas.edu/~smpark`

5. Fairfield, J.: Toboggan contrast enhancement for contrast segmentation. In: IEEE Proceedings of 10th International Conference on Pattern Recognition, vol. 1, Atlantic City, June 1990, pp. 712–716 (1990)
6. Vapnik, V.: The Nature of Statistical Learning Theory. Springer, New York (1995)
7. Boser, B.E., Guyon, I.M., Vapnik, V.N.: A training algorithm for optimal margin classifiers. In: Haussler, D. (ed.): Proceedings of the 5th Annual ACM Workshop on Computational Learning Theory 1992, pp. 144–152 (1992)
8. Zhu, J., Rosset, S., Hastie, T., Tibshirani, R.: 1-norm support vector machines. In: Thrun, S., Saul, L., Schölkopf, B. (eds.): Advances in Neural Information Processing Systems, vol. 16, MIT Press, Cambridge, MA (2004)
9. Mortensen, E.N., Barrett, W.A.: Toboggan-based intelligent scissors with a four parameter edge model. In: Proceedings of IEEE Conference on Computer Vision and Pattern Recognition, Fort Collins, CO, June 1999, pp. 452–458 (1999)
10. Mortensen, E.N.: Simultaneous multi-frame subpixel boundary definition using toboggan-based intelligent scissors for image and movie editing. Ph.D. dissertation, Department of Computer Science, Brigham Young University, Provo, UT 2000 (2000)
11. stoevi, S.: Rafsi- A fast watershed algorithm based on rainfalling simulation (2000) [Online]. Available: `citeseer.ist.psu.edu/stoev00rafsi.html`
12. Roerdink, J., Meijster, A.: The watershed transform: Definitions, algorithms and parallelization techniques (1999) [Online]. Available: `citeseer.ist.psu.edu/roerdink01watershed.html`

Appendix: A Concentration Oriented Tobogganing Algorithm

Input:
- s {initial site}
- p = P(v) {toboggan potential p of voxel v}
- lt {the low threshold}
- ht {the high threshold}

Output:
- C {toboggan cluster containing initial site s; initially empty}
- B {external boundary pixels of cluster C; initially empty}

Data Structures:
- A {Active list of voxels; initially empty}

Functions:
- E = N(v) {get neighbors E of voxel v}
- g = tob(v) {$g = \arg\min_{t \in N(v) \cup \{v\}} P(t)$ }
- A = update(A,v) {$\forall$ r $\in$ N(v), A $\leftarrow$ r, if (r $\notin$ A) and (r $\notin$ C) and (P(r) $\in$ [lt, ht]) }
- q = pop(A) {$q = \arg\min_{a \in A} P(a)$ }

Steps:

```
{Step A: Find concentration c of initial site s}
   c = s;
   repeat
      q = c; c = tob(q);
   until (q = c)
{Step B: Expand from concentration c}
   if (P(c) ∈ [lt, ht]) begin
      {Step B.1: Base step}
         C ← c; A = update(A, c);
      {Step B.2: Iterative step}
         repeat
            q = pop(A); r = tob(q);
            if r ∈ C begin {include q into cluster C and update A}
               C ← q; A = update(A,q);
            end else begin {include q into external boundary B}
               B ← q;
            end
         until A is empty
   end
```

Measures for Pathway Analysis in Brain White Matter Using Diffusion Tensor Images*

Laura Astola, Luc Florack, and Bart ter Haar Romeny

Eindhoven University of Technology, PO Box 513, NL-5600 MB Eindhoven, The Netherlands

Abstract. In this paper we discuss new measures for connectivity analysis of brain white matter, using MR diffusion tensor imaging. Our approach is based on Riemannian geometry, the viability of which has been demonstrated by various researchers in foregoing work. In the Riemannian framework bundles of axons are represented by geodesics on the manifold. Here we do not discuss methods to compute these geodesics, nor do we rely on the availability of geodesics. Instead we propose local measures which are directly computable from the local DTI data, and which enable us to preselect viable or exclude uninteresting seed points for the potentially time consuming extraction of geodesics. If geodesics are available, our measures can be readily applied to these as well.

We consider two types of geodesic measures. One pertains to the connectivity saliency of a geodesic, the second to its stability with respect to local spatial perturbations. For the first type of measure we consider both differential as well as integral measures for characterizing a geodesic's saliency either locally or globally. (In the latter case one needs to be in possession of the geodesic curve, in the former case a single tangent vector suffices.) The second type of measure is intrinsically local, and turns out to be related to a well known tensor in Riemannian geometry.

Keywords: DTI, geodesics, brain white matter connectivity, geodesic deviation, Riemann tensor, Ricci tensor.

1 Introduction

The traditional MR-DTI data matrix gives a Gaussian probabilistic model for the diffusion of water molecules in six different directions in each volume element of a 3D image. If diffusivity is large in a certain direction, then the time a water molecule travels a given distance in this direction is short. Thus the positive definite data matrix can be interpreted as reciprocally proportional to a Riemannian metric tensor as is pointed out by O'Donnell et al. [1] and Lenglet et al. [2]. Having a metric tensor attached to each point (on a compact manifold), we can solve for the shortest path, i.e. a minimal geodesic between a given

* The Netherlands Organisation for Scientific Research (NWO) is gratefully acknowledged for financial support.

N. Karssemeijer and B. Lelieveldt (Eds.): IPMI 2007, LNCS 4584, pp. 642–649, 2007.
© Springer-Verlag Berlin Heidelberg 2007

pair of points. For this purpose, there are various numerical methods ranging from techniques similar to Dijkstra's algorithm [3,4,5], level set methods [2,6], to solving the discretized Hamilton-Jacobi equation of propagating wavefronts [7].

Whatever the method for computing geodesics, one has to appreciate that although a coherent bundle of axons with resolvable thickness is likely to produce geodesics in (uncorrupted) DTI data, an arbitrarily chosen geodesic is unlikely to correspond to a bundle of axons. (Geodesics "run all over the place", so to speak.) Therefore, we propose a set of measures for the connection strength of a geodesic, both locally as well as globally (Section 2), and for its sensitivity to small spatial perturbations of the initial seed point (Section 3). A large connection strength implies that a candidate geodesic is more likely to correspond to an actual axon bundle (or other physical water channel). The stability measure, on the other hand, quantifies the amount of deviation from nearby geodesics, akin to the relative acceleration of freely falling particles in an inhomogeneous gravitational field (metric). One expects this deviation to be small in fibrous tissue in which the fibres are well aligned, and large in chaotic regions.

In short, we answer the question whether and to which extent a geodesic can be seen as a representative member of an articulated, coherent bundle of neighbouring geodesics, and which points are (un)likely to be part of such a structure.

2 Geodesics Versus DTI Fibres

In white matter microstructures inhibit the free Brownian motion of water molecules. the myelinated neurons in brain white matter favor diffusion along and impede diffusion across their tangent directions. Therefore, along a meaningful bundle of axons, the diffusivity is relatively large.

In the following we use Einstein summation convention: $a_i b^i \equiv \sum_{i=1}^{n} a_i b^i$. On a compact simply connected manifold, every pair of points can be connected by a geodesic, i.e. a curve of extremal energy (with affine parameter t)

$$E(\gamma) = \frac{1}{2} \int_0^T g_{ij}(\gamma(t)) \dot{\gamma}^i(t) \dot{\gamma}^j(t) dt, \tag{1}$$

or equivalently, of the (parametrization independent) length functional

$$L(\gamma) = \int_0^T \sqrt{g_{ij}(\gamma(t)) \dot{\gamma}^i(t) \dot{\gamma}^j(t)} dt \ . \tag{2}$$

Here we want to measure the quality of a geodesic as a carrier of diffusion, i.e. how likely it is for the geodesic to actually be generated by a bundle of fibres (or other physical water channel). As a measure of the relative diffusivity along a geodesic we take the ratio of lengths or energies given by the Euclidean and diffusion induced Riemannian metric tensors, respectively. Let $g = D^{-1}$, where D is the DTI matrix field, with components g_{ij} relative to a coordinate basis: $g(x) = g_{ij}(x) dx^i \otimes dx^j$, and let $\gamma(t)$ be a parameterized geodesic for the metric

g, starting at point $p = \gamma(0)$, with tangent $\dot{\gamma}(t)$. The proposed measures are then given by

$$m_E(\gamma) = \frac{\int_0^T \delta_{ij}\dot{\gamma}^i(t)\dot{\gamma}^j(t)dt}{\int_0^T g_{kl}(\gamma(t))\dot{\gamma}^k(t)\dot{\gamma}^l(t)dt} \quad \text{resp.} \quad m_L(\gamma) = \frac{\int_0^T \sqrt{\delta_{ij}\dot{\gamma}^i(t)\dot{\gamma}^j(t)}dt}{\int_0^T \sqrt{g_{kl}(\gamma(t))\dot{\gamma}^k(t)\dot{\gamma}^l(t)}dt} \ . \tag{3}$$

It should be stressed that neither equals the so-called validity index, cf. [7].

In the neighbourhood of point p on γ, the limit of each ratio in Eq. (3) for $T \to 0$ gives us a local measure of the connection strength:

$$m_E(V) = \frac{\delta_{ij}V^iV^j}{g_{kl}(p)V^kV^l} \quad \text{resp.} \quad m_L(V) = \frac{\sqrt{\delta_{ij}V^iV^j}}{\sqrt{g_{kl}(p)V^kV^l}}, \tag{4}$$

where $V = \dot{\gamma}(0)$.

If we denote by $V^+ \equiv \text{argmax}\,(m(V))$ the principal eigenvector of $D = g^{-1}$ with eigenvalue λ_+, say, then

$$m_E(V^+) = \lambda_+ \quad \text{resp.} \quad m_L(V^+) = \sqrt{\lambda_+} \tag{5}$$

are indeed (up to monotonic transformations) the most reasonable a priori *local* measures.

Thus locally, in anisotropic voxels, our measure gives maxima in the direction of the eigenvector that corresponds to the largest eigenvalue of the DTI-tensor, and coincides with traditional largest eigenvalue fibre tracking. However, by splitting up the integrals in (3) over a partitioning of the curve γ into subcurves γ_α, we may apply the integral measures to any curve segment γ_α, and measure possible variations in diffusivity along the curve to any desired level of discretization. In this way we obtain a set of integral connectivity measures for an arbitrary partitioning of a given (not necessarily geodesic) curve. If $\gamma = \cup_{\alpha=1}^N \gamma_\alpha$ is a partitioning of a curve $\gamma : [0, T] \to \mathbb{R}^3$ into any number N of curve segments $\gamma_\alpha : [t_{\alpha-1}, t_\alpha] \to \mathbb{R}^3$ (with $t_0 = 0$, $t_N = T$), then from Eq. (3) we obtain an arbitrarily large set of submeasures,

$$m_E^{(\alpha)} = m_E(\gamma_\alpha) \quad \text{resp.} \quad m_L^{(\alpha)} = m_L(\gamma_\alpha) \ . \tag{6}$$

If a curve (segment) γ corresponds to an actual fibre bundle, then both $m_E(\gamma)$ and $m_L(\gamma)$ will be large, since the denominator will be small. Note also that the magnitudes of $m_{L,E}(\gamma)$ are not biased w.r.t. the length of the curve (unlike numerator and denominator separately, which do scale with curve length, cf. the similar but non-invariant measure proposed by Prados [8]). This motivates our choice for Eq. (3).

3 Geodesic Deviation

The concept of geodesic deviation pertains to the relative acceleration by which two hypothetical test particles in “free fall” along two neighbouring geodesics

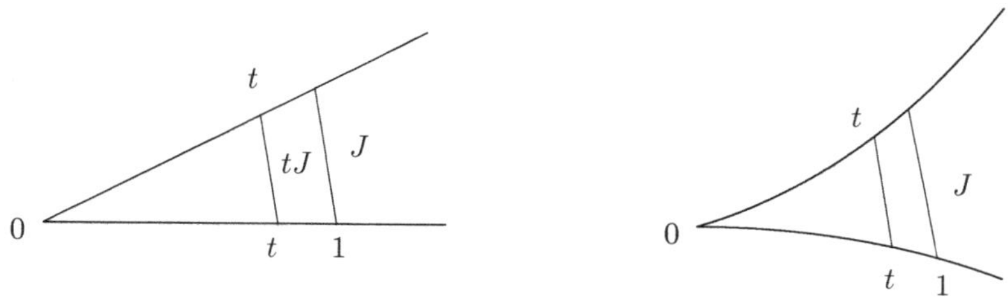

Fig. 1. Left: $\ddot{J} = 0$ (no geodesic deviation). Right: $\ddot{J} > 0$ as a result of curvature.

separate. That is, if one moves along two geodesics that start out from the same seed point at $t = 0$, say, with initial velocity vectors of equal magnitude, differing only in relative directions, one naturally observes that their mutual distance increases. This geodesic separation as such is trivial. In a flat space it is linear in t, so that the relative acceleration between the two points vanishes identically. However, in a curved space this is different (just think of the great circles of a sphere, which are geodesics if one is confined to its curved surface, cf. Fig. 1). In general there is a deviation from the lowest order linear behaviour, which will (initially) cause either an acceleration or deceleration in the mutual separation of the points. One can show that, if $J(t)$ denotes the separation vector[1] connecting any point $\gamma(t)$ on a fiducial geodesic at time t to a corresponding one on a neighbouring geodesic indicated by the relative separation vector $J(t)$, then

$$\frac{D^2 J(t)}{dt^2} + R(\gamma'(t), J(t))\gamma'(t) = 0\,. \tag{7}$$

The symbol D denotes covariant derivative, and R is the so-called Riemann curvature. One can show that the magnitude of the relative separation vector $J(t)$ initially evolves as

$$|J(t)| = t - \frac{1}{6}\langle R(V,W)V,W\rangle t^3 + \mathcal{O}(t^4)\,, \tag{8}$$

in which $V = \gamma'(0)$ and $W = J'(0)$. Thus the interesting quantity is the coefficient of the $\mathcal{O}(t^3)$ term, which contains all relevant curvature information responsible for geodesic deviation.

In a local coordinate system Eq. (7) becomes

$$\frac{D^2 J^i(t)}{dt^2} + R^i_{jkl}(\gamma(t))\frac{d\gamma^j(t)}{dt}\, J^k(t)\, \frac{d\gamma^l(t)}{dt} = 0\,. \tag{9}$$

[1] Formally $J(t)$ is defined in terms of the exponential map, $J(t) = (d\exp_p)_{tV} tW$, in which p is the base point of interest, V is a tangent to a fiducial geodesic, and W a second tangent which "selects" a neighbouring geodesic. We refer to the literature for details.

Following do Carmo's index convention [9], the Riemann curvature tensor—second term in Eq. (7)—is defined as

$$R(X,Y)Z = R^l_{ijk} X^i Y^j Z^k \frac{\partial}{\partial x_l}, \tag{10}$$

in terms of its components, which are given by the functions (spatial arguments $x \in \mathbb{R}^3$ are implicit)

$$R^m_{ijk} = \Gamma^l_{ik}\Gamma^m_{jl} - \Gamma^l_{jk}\Gamma^m_{il} + \frac{\partial}{\partial x_j}\Gamma^m_{ik} - \frac{\partial}{\partial x_i}\Gamma^m_{jk}, \tag{11}$$

in which the Christoffel symbols are defined as

$$\Gamma^k_{ij} = \frac{1}{2} g^{kl} \left\{ \frac{\partial g_{jl}}{\partial x^i} + \frac{\partial g_{li}}{\partial x^j} - \frac{\partial g_{ij}}{\partial x^l} \right\}. \tag{12}$$

(Recall that $g^{ij}(x)$ are just the entries of the DTI matrix at point x, and $g_{ij}(x)$ the entries of its inverse.)

Although a detailed explanation of this geometric analysis is far beyond the scope of this paper, it suffices to appreciate the heuristics of our approach. The interested reader is referred to do Carmo [9] or any other suitable text book on Riemannian geometry for further details and proofs.

In this section, our next goal is to obtain a measure for geodesic deviation that (i) is a purely local entity, and (ii) involves only the geodesic direction (i.e. $V = \gamma'(0)$) and does not prefer any extrinsically chosen plane through V, in other words, does not contain the vector $W = J'(0)$. To this end we may average the relevant coefficient of Eq. (8) over all independent vectors W_a, $a = 1, \ldots, n-1$, perpendicular to $V = \gamma'(0)$. In this way one obtains the so-called Ricci curvature:

$$\mathrm{Ric}_p(V) = \frac{1}{n-1} \sum_{a=1}^{n-1} \langle R(V, W_a)V, W_a \rangle . \tag{13}$$

In particular, in the 3-dimensional case at hand, we have two mutually orthonormal vectors $W_1, W_2 \perp V$, and we may obtain the average as:

$$\mathrm{Ric}_p(V) = \frac{1}{2\pi} \int_0^{2\pi} \langle R(V, \cos\theta W_1 + \sin\theta W_2)V, \cos\theta W_1 + \sin\theta W_2 \rangle d\theta \tag{14}$$

$$= \frac{1}{2} \sum_{a=1}^{2} \langle R(V, W_a)V, W_a \rangle , \tag{15}$$

which indeed agrees with the general definition, Eq. (13). Although the r.h.s. still contains the basis $\{W_a\}_{a=1}^{n-1}$ that spans the plane orthogonal to V, the result must be independent of its actual choice. To see that this is indeed the case, substitute the coordinate expressions of all geometric quantities involved into Eq. (13), using $V = V^i \frac{\partial}{\partial x_i}$, $W_a = W_a^i \frac{\partial}{\partial x_i}$, and Eq. (10). We obtain

$$
\begin{aligned}
\mathrm{Ric}_p(V) &= \frac{1}{n-1} \sum_{a=1}^{n-1} \langle R^l_{ijk} V^i W_a^j V^k \frac{\partial}{\partial x_l}, W_a^m \frac{\partial}{\partial x_m} \rangle \\
&= \frac{1}{n-1} \sum_{a=1}^{n-1} R^l_{ijk} V^i V^k W_a^m W_a^j g_{lm} \\
&= \frac{1}{n-1} \sum_{a=1}^{n-1} R_{ijkm} V^i V^k W_a^m W_a^j ,
\end{aligned}
\tag{16}
$$

in which we have defined $R_{ijkm} = g_{lm} R^l_{ijk}$. In n dimensions $\{W_1, W_2, \ldots, W_{n-1}, V\}$ constitutes an orthonormal basis, as a result of which we have

$$
\sum_{a=1}^{n-1} W_a^j W_a^m = g^{jm} - V^j V^m . \tag{17}
$$

Substitution into Eq. (16) yields, abbreviating $R_{ik} = g^{mj} R_{ijkm}$,

$$
\begin{aligned}
\mathrm{Ric}_p(V) &= \frac{1}{n-1} R_{ijkm} V^i V^k (g^{jm} - V^j V^m) \\
&= \frac{1}{n-1} R_{ik} V^i V^k - \frac{1}{n-1} \sum_{h=1}^{n-1} R_{ijkm} V^i V^k V^j V^m
\end{aligned}
$$

By virtue of the symmetries of the Riemann tensor the last summand vanishes, and so we end up with

$$
\mathrm{Ric}_p(V) = \frac{1}{n-1} R_{ij} V^i V^j . \tag{18}
$$

Eq. (18) is our main result with respect to geodesic deviation. (In our case, $n=3$, but the proportionality factor is immaterial.) Note that it satisfies our previous requirements, i.e. it depends only on differential DTI properties, and only involves a directional argument. Thus one does not need to know the geodesics in order to compute geodesic deviation. This greatly facilitates the computation. In fact, given a unit tangent vector V, Eq. (18) can be obtained by a somewhat lengthy but completely straightforward algebraic combination of partial derivatives of the DTI image of orders $0, 1, 2$. The algorithm is as follows:

1. Compute the metric g_{ij} by pointwise inversion of the DTI matrix g^{ij}.
2. Compute the Christoffel symbols Γ^k_{ij}, Eq. (12).
3. Compute the components of the Riemann tensor R^l_{ijk}, Eq. (11).
4. Obtain the Ricci tensor by contraction: $R_{ij} = R^k_{ijk}$.
5. Specify the components of a unit tangent V^i, and contract onto the Ricci tensor so as to obtain the proposed measure for geodesic deviation: $R_{ij} V^i V^j$.

The second and third steps require the computation of derivatives up to second order. This can e.g. be done in the usual way within the framework of scale space theory, taking into account a scale parameter that admits a sufficiently accurate extraction of second order derivatives (a Gaussian scale slightly larger than one voxel may already yield acceptable results depending on noise level, cf. [10,11]). The algorithm may be augmented with a scale selection procedure for optimal performance, since the "right" scale for pathway analysis is not known a priori. This highly interesting but nontrivial option is not further pursued here.

4 Conclusions

We have proposed two different types of differential geometric measures for DTI pathway analysis, and operational schemes to compute them. The first one, the connection strength, is a zeroth order differential property that gives information about the relative diffusivity along a given curve. Curves with large connection strengths are more likely to correspond to actual elongated structures of axons or other physical water channels. Our connectivity measure can be applied to any not necessarily geodesic curve, to an arbitrary segment and, in the limit, even to any point of such a curve. For the preselection of viable seed points for geodesics, it is, apart from quantifying their connectivity, likewise useful to compute their geodesic deviation as a measure for local stability and coherence. We have argued that the Ricci curvature in the direction of largest diffusion is an appropriate measure for this. A positive Ricci curvature, which depends on second order derivatives of the DTI image, indicates the presence of bundles of geodesics that are well aligned. Combination of the two types of measures can be used to single out suitable seed points for, and to judge the saliency of, a fiducial geodesic.

References

1. O'Donnell, L., Haker, S., Westin, C.F.: New approaches to estimation of white matter connectivity in diffusion tensor mri: Elliptic PDEs and geodesics in a tensor-warped space. In: Dohi, T., Kikinis, R. (eds.) MICCAI 2002. LNCS, vol. 2488, pp. 459–466. Springer, Heidelberg (2002)
2. Lenglet, C., Deriche, R., Faugeras, O.: Inferring white matter geometry from diffusion tensor MRI: Application to connectivity mapping. In: Pajdla, T., Matas, J. (eds.) ECCV 2004. LNCS, vol. 3024, pp. 127–140. Springer, Heidelberg (2004)
3. Dijkstra, E.W.: A note on two problems in connexion with graphs. Numerische Mathematik 1(1), 267–271 (1959)
4. Kimmel, R., Sethian, J.A.: Computing geodesic paths on manifolds. In: Proceedings of the National Academy of Sciences, vol. 95, pp. 8431–8435 (1998)
5. Tsitsiklis, J.N.: Efficient algorithms for globally optimal trajectories. IEEE Transactions on Automatic Control 40(9), 1528–1538 (1995)
6. Osher, S., Sethian, J.A.: Fronts propagating with curvature-dependent speed: Algorithms based on Hamilton-Jacobi formulations. Journal of Computational Physics 79, 12–49 (1988)

7. Jackowski, M., Kao, C.Y., Qiu, M., Costable, R.T., Staib, L.H.: White matter tractography by anisotropic wavefront evolution and diffusion tensor imaging. Medical Image Analysis 9, 427–440 (2005)
8. Prados, E., Soatto, S., Lenglet, C., Pons, J.P., Wotawa, N., Deriche, R., Faugeras, O.: Control theory and fast marching techniques for brain connectivity mapping. In: Proceedings of the IEEE Computer Society Conference on Computer Vision and Pattern Recognition, New York, USA, June 2006, vol. 1, pp. 1076–1083. IEEE Computer Society Press, New York, USA (2006)
9. Carmo, M.P.d.: Riemannian Geometry. Second edn. Mathematics: Theory & Applications. Birkhäuser, Boston (1993)
10. Blom, J., Haar Romeny, B.M.t., Bel, A., Koenderink, J.J.: Spatial derivatives and the propagation of noise in Gaussian scale-space. Journal of Visual Communication and Image Representation 4(1), 1–13 (1993)
11. Florack, L.M.J., Duits, R.: Regularity classes for locally orderless images. In: Griffin, L.D, Lillholm, M. (eds.) Scale Space Methods in Computer Vision. LNCS, vol. 2695, pp. 255–265. Springer, Heidelberg (2003)

Estimating the Mesorectal Fascia in MRI

Sarah Bond, Niranjan Joshi, Styliani Petroudi, and Mike Brady

Wolfson Medical Vision Laboratory, Department of Engineering Science,
University of Oxford, Oxford, OX1 3PJ, UK

Abstract. Apart from chemoradiotherapy, surgery by total mesorectal resection is currently the only curative therapy for colorectal cancer. However, this often has a poor outcome, especially if there are affected lymph nodes too close to the resection boundary. The circumferential resection margin (CRM) is defined as the shortest distance from an affected region to the mesorectal fascia (MF), and should be at least 1mm. However, this 3D distance is normally estimated in 2D (from image slices) and takes no account of uncertainty of the position of the MF. We describe a system able to estimate the location of the MF with a measure at each point along it of the uncertainty in location, and which then estimates the CRM in three dimensions. The MF localisation algorithm combines anatomical knowledge with a level set method based on: a non-parametric representation of the distribution of intensities, and the use of the monogenic signal to detect portions of the boundary.

1 Introduction

Colorectal cancer is primarily a disease of the developed world. Approximately 500,000 new cases are reported annually. The survival rate at 5 years is just 50%, primarily because of metastatic spread to the liver and pelvis. The primary imaging modality used for the detection, diagnosis and for staging colorectal cancer is MRI. Specifically, a widely used clinical protocol comprises axial small field of view T2 weighted MR images (TE = 90ms, TR = 3500-5000ms, α = 90deg, slice thickness = 3mm) acquired using a 1.5T MRI machine. Our datasets are 3-D, each comprising 512 x 512 x 25 voxels of size 1mm x 1mm x 3mm. The datasets acquired at our site exhibited a substantial bias field, with a particularly bright artefact near the coccyx and extending over several MR slices. There is a diversity of tissue classes in colorectal MR images, and several of them have substantial texture. Since it is relatively insensitive to the tissue class definitions, and since the bias field varies substantially across the image, we applied the Parametric Bias Field Correction (PABIC) method [1] which models the bias field explicitly using Legendre polynomials. We have found that second order Legendre polynomials suffice for a good approximation to the bias field. The bias field varies minimally between slices, so is easily be approximated across the whole 3-D dataset.

Conventionally, a tumour is staged using the TNM method: T refers to whether or not the tumour has invaded: the submucosa (T1); circular or longitudinal muscle layers (T2); or through the muscularis propria subserosa and/or into non-peritonealised perirectal tissues (T3) or other structures (T4); N refers to whether there is no regional lymph node metastasis (N0); there are metastases in up to three lymph nodes (N1); or

N. Karssemeijer and B. Lelieveldt (Eds.): IPMI 2007, LNCS 4584, pp. 650–661, 2007.
© Springer-Verlag Berlin Heidelberg 2007

more than 3 (N2); and whether there are not (M0) or are (M1) distant metastases. The relevant sentinel lymph nodes are located in the mesorectum, the region of fat surrounding the rectum. Based on our previous work [2], [3], in the remainder of this paper, we assume that: the lymph nodes have been detected, that they have been delimited accurately, and that their status (affected or not) has been determined.

Currently, apart from chemoradiotherapy (used in 65% of cases), surgery is considered to be the only curative therapy. Since local excision surgery continues to gain acceptance slowly, surgery is predominantly by "total" resection of the mesorectum (TMR). This is often quite traumatic surgery, frequently necessitating use of a stoma post-surgery. Clinicians consider very carefully the likely success of surgery before proceeding. One of the major reasons for poor outcome following a TRM is the presence of affected lymph nodes too close to the resection margin, nominally the mesorectal fascia. The circumferential resection margin (CRM) is "defined" as the shortest distance from an affected lymph node to the mesorectal fascia. It has been proposed [4] that the TRM be planned so that the CRM is at least 1mm, or, if this is not possible, that the surgical option be dismissed. To this end, [4] proposed that "thin section" MRI should be used to estimate the CRM.

This assumes that all affected lymph nodes have been detected and their often small sizes estimated accurately (incorporating partial volume estimation); as noted above, in this paper we assume that this has been done. It also requires the bounding surface of the mesorectum (the MF) to be located completely and accurately; and the CRM estimation to take due account of the MRI spatial sampling and the relative orientation of MRI slices to the local axial direction of the colorectum/mesorectum. The first of these two problems is surprisingly difficult, not least for clinicians planning surgery, and is the main focus of this paper. In Section 2, we combine anatomical knowledge with a level set method based on: a non-parametric representation of the distribution of intensities inside the putative MF and an estimate of MF feature locations using monogenic signal analysis. As a result of this process, a measure of the uncertainty in the position of the MF is estimated at each boundary location. Finally, in Section 3 we propose a method for estimating the CRM which incorporated the uncertainty in the position of the MF.

2 Determining the Mesorectal Fascia

Accurate localisation of the MF is a difficult segmentation problem because: (a) there is negligible contrast at several points along the MF, at least for the imaging protocol used clinically; (b) there are substantially different kinds of contrast change (texture step changes near the coccyx, thin line changes near the bladder wall, etc.) at different points along the MF; (c) the intensities inside the MF show substantial variation between individuals, and this impacts on the detection of the lymph nodes, blood vessels, the colorectum, and a variety of folds; and (d) there is a substantial range of tissue types, with varying amounts of musculature and fat forming the band flanking the MF, so it is difficult to constrain the intensity distribution in this band. Even the clinicians find it hard to segment the MF, as is seen in two annotations of consecutive slices in Fig. 1, where the location of the MF clearly changes far too much.

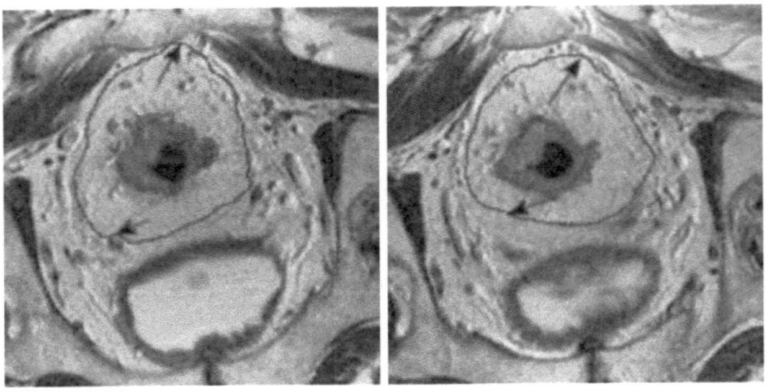

Fig. 1. Two consecutive slices in a dataset, with annotations of the tumour and MF by an experienced radiologist, showing the huge unpredictability in radiology labelling

To determine the MF, we proceed in two stages. First, we initialise the mesorectum (hence its boundary) by mobilising contextual anatomical knowledge [2], [3]. This is a completely automatic process which has given a satisfactory initialisation in every case we have tried. The algorithm begins by locating the hip bones (straightforward), and from these the centre of the colorectum and coccyx. We find that the colorectum can be accurately delineated across the slices of the dataset using a Kalman snake. The inscribed circle formed by the centres of the approximately spherical hip bones and the coccyx forms the initial approximation to the MF. We experimented with further refining this circular approximation using spherical harmonics [3]; but we found that, in practice, the result is often not much changed from the initial circular approximation. While this initialisation forms a satisfactory basis for staging (lymphs) and assessing the effect of chemoradiotherapy [2], it is insufficiently accurate for CRM estimation and for surgical planning. Nevertheless, the inscribed circle is a good initialisation for the following level set step. We have implemented many of the published level set schemes (in ITK) and have found the Chan-Vese framework most suitable for our purpose. However, the Chan-Vese framework relies crucially upon: (a) estimating the intensity (or other) probability density function (pdf) inside the evolving level set; and (b) a model of features to which the level set should be attracted. Regarding (a), we have applied a novel PDF estimation scheme; regarding (b) we have applied monogenic signal analysis.

2.1 NPMM-ICLS Level Set Formulation

For simplicity, consider the case of 2-dimensional (2D) images. Let Y_1 denotes intensity variable (all variables will be denoted by upper case letters in this subsection and their particular values will be denoted by lower case letters). Continuous random variables X_1 and X_2 denote positional variables in 2D. We divide the image into several piecewise sections. The intensity variable Y_1 is deterministically related with the positional variables over these piecewise sections. Typically this relationship is polynomial. Our objective is to determine the PDF of the intensity values, given the nature of randomness in the positional variables and the deterministic relationship. In this paper it is assumed that Y_1 is related with the positional variables through the bilinear interpolation over a piecewise section joining centres of four mutually neighbouring pixels. This case was originally proposed in [5]. Next it is assumed that the positional variables are uniformly distributed over this piecewise bilinear region i.e. $f_{X_1,X_2}(x_1,x_2) = 1$ for $0 \leq x_1, x_2 \leq 1$, where $f(.)$ denotes a PDF. It is straightforward to derive the following equations:

$$y_1(x_1,x_2) = ax_1x_2 + bx_1 + cx_2 + d, \;\; y_2(x_1,x_2) = x_1 \tag{1}$$

$$x_2(y_1,y_2) = \frac{y_1 - by_2 - d}{ay_2 + c}, \;\; x_1(y_1,y_2) = y_2 \tag{2}$$

where Y_2 is a dummy variable. The joint PDF f_{Y_1,Y_2} can then be calculated using the transformation formula for functions of random variables [6]. In the present case,

$$f_{Y_1,Y_2}(y_1,y_2) = f_{X_1,X_2}(y_2, \frac{y_1 - by_2 - d}{ay_2 + c})|J| \tag{3}$$

where, $|J|$ is the Jacobian and is equal to $|1/(ay_2 + c)|$ in this case. Therefore,

$$f_{Y_1,Y_2}(y_1,y_2) = \frac{1}{ay_2 + c} \tag{4}$$

subject to,

$$0 \leq y_2 \leq 1 \quad \text{and} \quad 0 \leq \frac{y_1 - by_2 - d}{ay_2 + c} \leq 1 \tag{5}$$

The marginal PDF f_{Y_1} is obtained by integrating out the dummy variable Y_2 over the ranges given in Equation (5).

Note that the specific geometry of a configuration is determined by values of the coefficients in Equation (1). In their original proposition [5], the authors point out that there are 24 such configurations, corresponding to 4! ways of arranging the values of the four corner pixels of the piecewise bilinear section. We have proved that we can reduce the number of configurations, which makes our implementation both less complex and considerably faster than the original one. However, for reasons of space we omit the implementation details. The PDF obtained over each piecewise bilinear section is added and normalised to get the PDF of the given image region.

We then move on to model the image histogram as a non-parametric mixture model (NPMM) of the PDFs [7]. Note that we also take into account the partial volume effect (PVE). The observed image is assumed to be obtained from an idealised high resolution image through a downsampling process. We assume that each pixel in the high resolution image belongs only to a pure class. On the other hand, a pixel in the observed image may either belong to a pure class or to a partial class. A partial class is identified with the fraction of each pure class present in that pixel. We refer to the PDFs of pure and partial tissue as *basis PDFs*. The basis PDFs are directly estimated from image regions using the method described in the previous subsection. The weights associated with the basis PDFs in the mixture model are the prior probabilities of the occurrence of the tissue classes. We now note that,

$$P(Y) = \sum P(Y|X)P(X) \tag{6}$$

where, $P(Y)$ is the overall intensity distribution, $P(Y|X)$ are the basis PDFs corresponding to each pure and partial class, and $P(X)$ is the prior PDF of all the classes. $P(Y)$ and $P(Y|X)$ are estimated using the NP-windows method described previously. To estimate $P(X)$, we arrange the system of linear equations given in eqn.(6) in vector form: $\mathbf{p_y} = \mathbf{P_{y,x}}\,\mathbf{p_x}$ where, $\mathbf{p_y}$ and $\mathbf{p_x}$ are vectors, and $\mathbf{P_{y,x}}$ is a matrix whose columns represent the basis PDFs. In order to estimate $\mathbf{p_x}$, we seek a least squares solution to this equation. However, we note that since $\mathbf{p_x}$ represents a PDF; its elements must follow the positivity and summability constraints of a PDF. Hence we formulate the problem as follows:

$$\begin{aligned} \hat{\mathbf{p}}_\mathbf{x} &= arg\min_{\mathbf{p_x}} \quad \frac{1}{2}(\mathbf{P_{y,x}}\,\mathbf{p_x} - \mathbf{p_y})^T\,(\mathbf{P_{y,x}}\,\mathbf{p_x} - \mathbf{p_y}) \\ &\text{subject to,} \qquad \mathbf{I}\,\mathbf{p_x} \geq \mathbf{0} \qquad \text{and} \qquad \mathbf{u}^T\,\mathbf{p_x} = 1 \end{aligned} \tag{7}$$

where, $\mathbf{I}$ is the identity matrix, $\mathbf{u}$ is a vector with all its elements equal to 1, and $\hat{\mathbf{p}}_\mathbf{x}$ is the inequality constrained least squares (ICLS) estimate of prior PDF of tissue classes. The basis PDFs and the mixture weights then can be used in a *maximum a posteriori* (MAP) framework to find optimal labelling of the image pixels. Fig. 2 illustrates various PDFs involved in the segmentation of MF.

In order to introduce spatial regularisation in the above segmentation solution, we incorporate the NPMM method outlined above into a level set framework. Suppose we have $x_1, x_2, \ldots, x_n$ pure classes. We consider n separate level sets functions $\phi_1, \phi_2, \ldots, \phi_n$, one per pure class. For small n, it makes sense to use separate level sets functions for each class. We evolve each level set function separately. For each evolution equation we consider the following region based force.

$$F_{1n} = \log\left[\frac{P(Y|x_n)P(x_n)}{\sum_{i,i\neq n} P(Y|x_i)P(x_i)}\right] \tag{8}$$

The likelihood probabilities $P(Y|x_i)$ are the basis functions of the NPMM, and are estimated using the NP windows method. The mixture weights or the *a priori* probabilities are calculated using the NPMM-ICLS algorithm described in previously. To

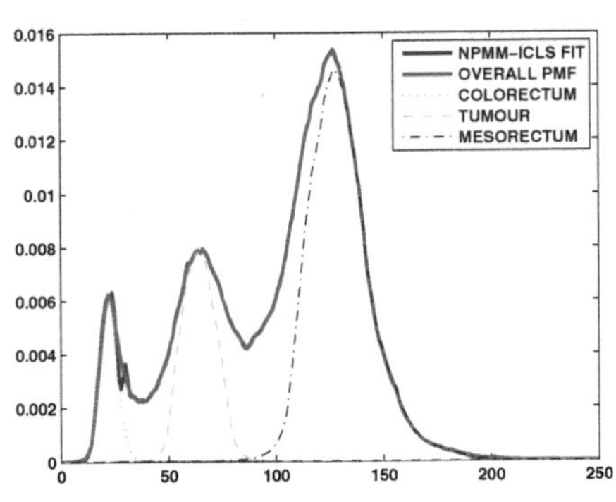

Fig. 2. Various probability distributions for a single slice of a colorectal MR dataset

address the PVE, we formulate a second regional force term which discourages the level sets from entering into a region which NPMM deems as a partial volume region. Let $f_{x_1}, f_{x_2}, \ldots, f_{x_n}$ be the fractions of pure classes present in a pixel. The inhibition force term is:

$$F_{2n} = \sum_{i,i \neq n} f_{x_i}, \tag{9}$$

and so the overall evolution equation of the nth level set function is:

$$\frac{\partial \phi_n}{\partial t} = [\kappa + \alpha F_{1n} - \beta F_{2n}]|\nabla \phi_n| + \gamma \mathbf{A} \cdot \nabla \phi_n, \tag{10}$$

where κ is the curvature term and $\mathbf{A}$ represents a vector field, referred to as the advection term in the level sets literature. The advection term takes into account the boundary information. We have used magnitude of intensity gradients to represent the boundary but also explore alternatively the use of monogenic signals.

2.2 Monogenic Signals

We noted earlier that the *type* of intensity change marking the boundary of the MF changes substantially along its length. Typically, we find texture step changes near the coccyx, thin line changes near the bladder wall, and step changes at other locations. The exact types and placement of these intensity changes varies from person to person. This implies that any feature detector that is specific to a particular kind of feature (eg step edge) will tend to miss whole portions of the MF boundary, even where it is (at least to a clinician) "obvious". The net result is that the boundary of the MF, as detected by the level set algorithm, is under-constrained at such segments. Fortunately, in the late 1980s, Owens and Morrone proposed an alternative approach, based on the observation that the components a Fourier series expansion of "pure" examples of features (step, roof, spike, ...) are all in phase, and that this is true only at such features. This leads to an alternative definition of a feature as a signal/image location at which local phase measurements are all in close agreement: they called this *phase congruency*. Note that a high value of phase congruency corresponds to the detection of a feature point; the associated (shared) phase value and the local energy further characterise the feature point. As such, phase congruency detects all the features around the MF, not just the clear step edges.

Note that the definition requires that the *local phase* be computed at each point in a signal. The computation of local phase requires the application to the signal of quadrature pairs of filters (a typical, though not optimal, example consists of even and odd Gabor filters). Quadrature is most conveniently defined via the Hilbert Transform, which produces for a given filter $f(t)$ its quadrature partner $f^H(t)$. Kovesi [8] proposed an implementation of phase congruency based on a specific set of quadrature filters, namely log-Gabor filters and showed some very encouraging results on a wide range of signal changes. Unfortunately, the Hilbert Transform is only defined for signals $s(t)$, and so Kovesi's implementation of Phase Congruency for images $I(x, y)$ interpolated a set of 1D signals $s_i(t|x, y)$ centred on each image location (x, y). The resulting directional phase congruency measures were then combined to form a single measure in order to detect and assign types to feature points. This is both inefficient and the rules for combining directional phase congruency measures tend to be rather heuristic.

Fortunately, Felsberg and Sommer [9] have shown how to use the Riesz transform to extend the Hilbert transform to 2D, 3D and arbitrarily higher dimensional images. The transfer functions of the Riesz transform is

$$H_1(\omega_1, \omega_2) = i\frac{\omega_1}{\sqrt{\omega_1^2 + \omega_2^2}}, H_2(\omega_2, \omega_2) = i\frac{\omega_1}{\sqrt{\omega_1^2 + \omega_2^2}}. \tag{11}$$

In the space domain, the Riesz transform is given by

$$h_1(x_1, x_2) = -\frac{x_1}{2\pi(x_1^2 + x_2^2)^{\frac{3}{2}}}, h_2(x_1, x_2) = -\frac{x_2}{2\pi(x_1^2 + x_2^2)^{\frac{3}{2}}} \tag{12}$$

The *monogenic signal* is then defined as the 3D vector formed by the image and its Riesz transform:

$$f_M(x_1, x_2) = (f(x_1, x_2), (h_1 \otimes f)(x_1, x_2), (h_2 \otimes f)(x_1, x_2)), \tag{13}$$

where $\otimes$ denotes the convolution. The image and the monogenic signal can be shown to have the following properties:

$$\begin{aligned} A_f(x_1, x_2) &= \sqrt{f^2(x_1, x_2) + (h_1 \otimes f)^2(x_1, x_2) + (h_2 \otimes f)^2(x_1, x_2)} \\ f(x_1, x_2) &= A_f(x_1, x_2)\cos(\phi) \\ (h_1 \otimes f) &= A_f \sin(\phi)\cos(\theta) \\ (h_2 \otimes f) &= A_f \sin(\phi)\sin(\theta), \end{aligned} \tag{14}$$

where $A_f(x_1, x_2)$ is the local energy of the image f(x1, x2) at the location (x_1, x_2), $\phi \in [0, \pi)$ is the local phase, and $\theta \in [-\pi, \pi)$ is the local orientation of the feature:

$$\theta = \arctan 2(\frac{h_2 \otimes f}{h_1 \otimes f}), \phi = \arccos(\frac{f}{A_f}). \tag{15}$$

In practice, the image $f(x_1, x_2)$ is often made bandpass by filtering with a rotationally symmetric filter, say $g(x_1, x_2) \otimes f(x_1, x_2)$, for example with a difference of Gaussians. This is by no means the only choice of bandpass filter; but we do not discuss this issue further in this paper. In the case of band pass filtering, the monogenic signal becomes:

$$f_M(x_1, x_2) = ((g \otimes f)(x_1, x_2), (h_1 \otimes g \otimes f)(x_1, x_2), (h_2 \otimes g \otimes f)(x_1, x_2)) \tag{16}$$

The Riesz Tranform then generates two odd filters $h_i(x_1, x_2) \otimes g(x_1, x_2)$ which are oriented at 90 degrees to each other, one oriented in the ω_1 direction in the Fourier domain, the other in the ω_2 direction. This enables a fast implementation. Let $F(\omega_1, \omega_2)$

be the Fourier Transform of $f(x_1, x_2)$, and F^{-1}denote the inverse Fourier Transform, each term of the monogenic signal can be obtained as following:

$$\begin{aligned} (g \otimes f)(x_1, x_2) &= real(\mathrm{F}^{-1}(G(\omega_1, \omega_2) \cdot F(\omega_1, \omega_2))) \\ (g \otimes h_1 \otimes f)(x_1, x_2) &= \mathrm{F}^{-1}(G(\omega_1, \omega_2) \cdot H_1(\omega_1, \omega_2) \cdot F(\omega_1, \omega_2)) \\ (g \otimes h_2 \otimes f)(x_1, x_2) &= \mathrm{F}^{-1}(G(\omega_1, \omega_2) \cdot H_2(\omega_1, \omega_2) \cdot F(\omega_1, \omega_2)) \end{aligned} \quad (17)$$

The monogenic signal has previously been applied to non-rigid registration [10]. Having had some encouraging results in these diverse cases, and having noted the varying type of boundary feature type, we have incorporated the monogenic signal (as phase congruency) into the advection term of level set framework (Eqn. 10), in order to attract the level set to a range of feature types, by using it instead of the gradient field used previously.

3 Results

3.1 Segmentation of the MF

Our NPMM level set method was tested on 5 axial MRI datasets, taken using the standard clinical protocol at our site. These datasets cover a range of patients, with tumours of varying sizes. A typical slice of the 3D segmentation using intensity information only can be seen in Fig. 3, and the corresponding 3D representation is shown in Fig. 3. The results are compared to manual segmentations of the MF drawn on the datasets by an expert clinician, Table 1. It can be seen that the automated segmentation is very close to the manual segmentation, but the relatively large standard deviation is probably due to the inconsistency in the radiologist segmentations as shown previously in Fig. 1.

To take into account boundary information we used magnitude of the evolution forces. To appreciate the effectiveness of these, we colour coded force information at

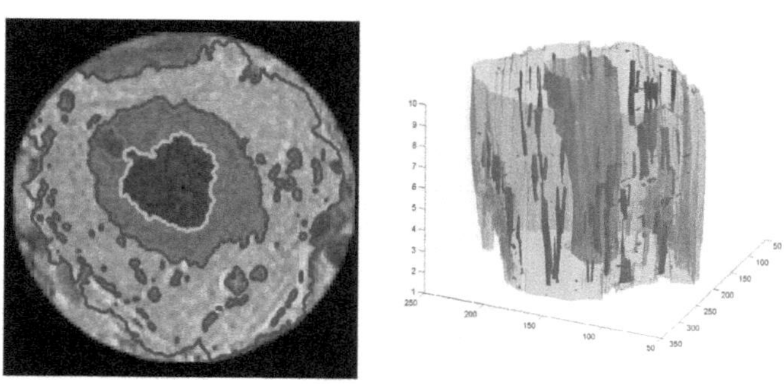

Fig. 3. Left: Level sets segmentation of a colorectal MR image slice using NPMM-ICLS algorithm, with colour code of green - colorectum, red - tumour, blue - mesorectum. Right: Segmentation of the Mesorectal Fascia in 3D, showing also the colorectum and tumour, blood vessels and lymph nodes within the mesorectum

Table 1. Comparison of Automatic Segmentation using Level Sets with Manual Clinical Segmentation

Patient	Mean difference (mm)	Standard deviation (mm)
1	3.4	2.4
2	2.6	1.9
3	2.2	1.8
4	2.0	1.6
5	2.3	2.0

each pixel lying in a narrow band around the boundary and overlaid them. A typical example is shown in Figure 4. We observe that the evolving surface is stopped effectively at the "yellow" bands where the gradient information dominates. As noted above, discontinuities in the yellow bands are for two reasons. First, any individual patient's MF is not easily completely delineated in the T2 weighted MR image. Second, there is a variety of signal changes around the MF. This is the problem that is addressed using the monogenic signal.

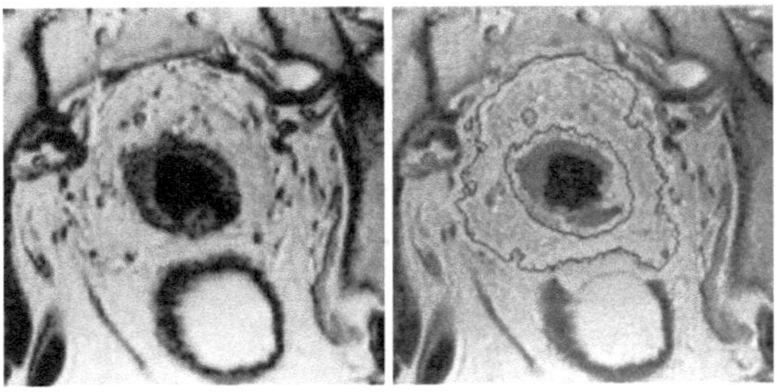

Fig. 4. A colorectal MR image slice overlayed with the force information used for the evolution of level set surface representing the mesorectal fascia. The surface expands in blue region and contracts in yellow region. The black contour represents the current position of the surface.

Based on the level set method described in the previous section, we suppose that the MF has been detected as a surface $\mathbf{r}(u,v)$ in some global coordinate frame. Suppose that the surface normal at each coordinate (u,v) is $\mathbf{n}(u,v)$ and denote the allowed uncertainty in the location of the MF as a measure $\epsilon(u,v)$.

The method outlined in the previous section can provide, for each location (u,v) a possible measurement of $\epsilon(u,v)$. This is done using the force $F(u,v)$ from the level set which is visualised inside and outside the zero level set in Fig. 4. The differences between the forces inside and outside the zero level set $\Delta F(u,v) = |F_{inside}(u,v) - F_{outside}(u,v)|$ are compared with the errors at each point on a test dataset. A function was found empirically (using examples of clinical intra-observer variability) to model the maximum and minimum errors and this is given by $\epsilon(u,v) = \alpha e^{\pm\beta\Delta F(u,v)}$, where $\alpha = 3$ and $\beta = 85$.

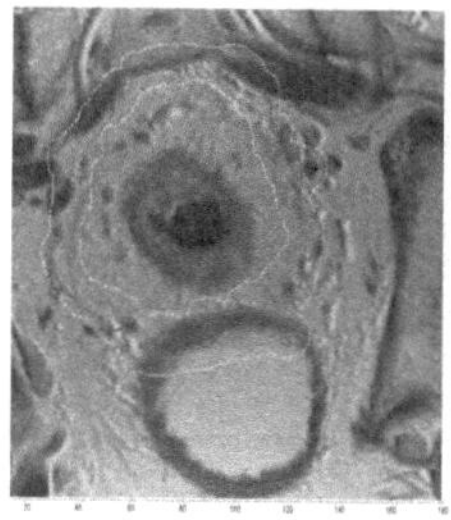

Fig. 5. Segmentation of the Mesorectal Fascia, showing the minimum and maximum bounding area

Table 2. Comparison of Minimum and Maximum Values of Automatic Segmentation using Level Sets with Manual Clinical Segmentation

Patient	Mean difference between Min ± Standard Deviation (mm)	Mean difference between Max ± Standard Deviation (mm)
1	2.6 ± 2.1	4.2 ± 2.3
2	2.1 ± 1.6	3.8 ± 2.2
3	1.9 ± 1.4	3.9 ± 2.2
4	1.8 ± 1.4	2.7 ± 1.9
5	2.2 ± 1.4	3.5 ± 2.5

Using this method the maximum and minimum bounding areas of the mesorectal fascia can be found and these are shown in Fig. 5. This was done in 3D for all our datasets and the manual clinical segmentations all lied within this bounding region. The distances between the manual segmentation and the minimum and maximum boundaries are shown in Table 2. Again the mean error is low but with a relatively high standard deviation.

Finally we found a segmentation of the MF by incorporating the phase congruency from the monogenic signal. It can be seen in Fig. 6 that the level set is stopped at finer ridges that are the MF boundary, instead of being attracted to the stronger intensity edges of different anatomies.

3.2 Estimating the CRM

Now consider a cancerous region at a position $\mathbf{x}$, and suppose that $\mathbf{r}(u, v)$ is the nearest point on the MF. Evidently, $\mathbf{r}(u, v) - \mathbf{x}$ is parallel to $\mathbf{n}(u, v)$. If the maximum extent of the lymph node in the direction $\mathbf{n}(u, v)$ towards the MF is estimated (subject to PVE) as being at the location $\mathbf{y_n}$, then the clinical CRM criterion is based on $||\mathbf{y_n} - \mathbf{r}(u, v) - \epsilon(u, v)|| < 1\text{mm}$.

We calculated the CRM at each point on the MF using this minimum distance between the MF, and the tumour, using the intensity level set segmentations. We did this for the initial estimated MF and also the worst case, minimum MF. This was repeated

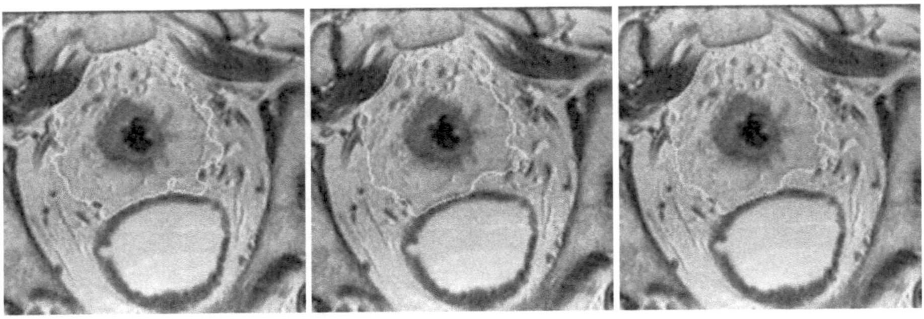

Fig. 6. A comparison of the MF segmentation using just intensity information on the left, incorporating edge information from the phase congruency map in the middle, and the segmentations overlaid on the right

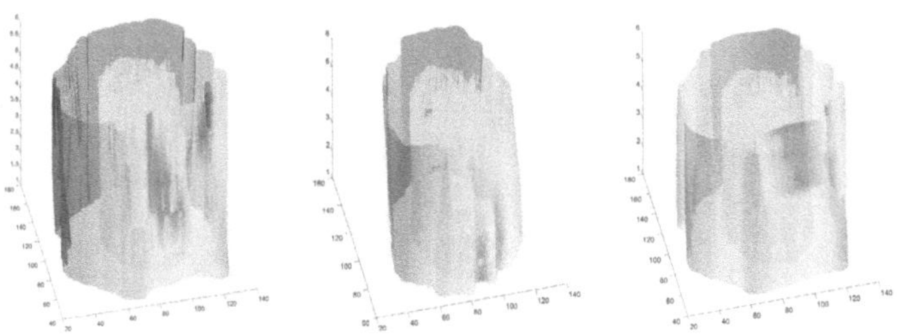

Fig. 7. An example segmentation of the Mesorectal Fascia, showing the magnitude of the CRM, showing our normal estimate (left), a worst case estimate (centre), and a best case estimate (right)

with the same 5 datasets used previously and results for Patient 1 are displayed in 3D in Fig. 7. The regions where the CRM is low are coloured in red, and those regions with a larger margin are coloured in blue. This was considered very useful by our collaborating clinicians.

We also compare our values of the CRM with those of the clinician. We do not expect these values to be the same since the clinician will always estimate the values using the 2D axial MRI slices. The results in Petroudi 2006 [11] highlight how the CRM, traditionally accurately accessible post-surgically from histopathology, cannot be measured accurately in MRI, unless the whole 3D dataset is considered. This is because there is usually an offset angle between the normal to the imaging plane, and the principal axis of the anatomical volume, defined by the direction of the colorectum.

The results of comparing our estimates of the minimum CRM with that of the clinician are shown in Table 3. The substantial differences highlight the potential errors in the clinical CRM estimates using current manual techniques, and re-enforce the need for accurate of evaluation of such measures, which have a great impact in the evaluation

Table 3. Comparison of CRM from Automatic Segmentation using Level Sets with Manual Clinical Estimation

Patient	Minimum clinical CRM (mm)	Automatic estimation of CRM at clinical minimum (Normal/Worst case) (mm)	Automatic estimation of overall minimum CRM (Normal/Worst Case) (mm)
1	1.0	5.4/0.8	3.8/0.0
2	11.8	7.7/7.2	6.9/0.0
3	5.6	4.9/3.3	2.8/0.0
4	12.8	12.8/11.4	6.6/3.3
5	12.6	12.2/12.0	5.8/3.7

of treatment. A further validation of our work could be carried out using the results from post-surgery histopathology, and this is the subject of our future work.

References

1. Styner, M., Brechbuhler, C., Szckely, G., Gerig, G.: Parametric estimate of intensity inhomogeneities applied to MRI. IEEE TMI 19, 153–165 (2000)
2. Bond, S.:DPhil thesis: Image analysis for patient management in colorectal cancer (2006)
3. Bond, S., Brady, M.: Image analysis for patient management in colorectal cancer. CARS (2005)
4. Brown, G., Richards, C., Newcombe, J., Dallimore, N., Radcliffe, A., Carey, D., Bourne, M., Williams, G.: Rectal carcinoma: Thin-section mr imaging for staging in 28 patients. Radiology 211, 215–222 (1999)
5. Kadir, T., Brady, M.: Non-parametric estimation of probability distributions from sampled signals. Technical report, OUEL No: 2283/05 (2005) available at `http://www.robots.ox.ac.uk/~timork/PDFEstimation/TR-2283-05.pdf`
6. Papoulis, A., Pillai, S.U.: Probability, random variables and stochastic processes. McGraw-Hill, New York (2002)
7. Joshi, N., Brady, M.: A non-parametric model for partial volume segmentation of MR images. BMVC (2005)
8. Kovesi, P.: Image features from phase congruency. Videre: Journal of computer vision research, 1 (1999)
9. Felsberg, M., Sommer, G.: The monogenic signal. IEEE TSP 49, 3136–3144 (2001)
10. Mellor, M., Brady, M.: Non-rigid multimodal image registration using local phase. MIA 4, 330–343 (2005)
11. Petroudi, S., Brown, G., Bond, S., Brady, M.: Circumferential resection margin assessment on MRI of rectal cancer. EMBC (2006)

A Marginalized MAP Approach and EM Optimization for Pair-Wise Registration

Lilla Zöllei[1], Mark Jenkinson[2], Samson Timoner[3], and William Wells[4]

[1] A. A. Martinos Center, MGH, USA
lzollei@nmr.mgh.harvard.edu
[2] FMRIB Centre, University of Oxford, UK
mark@fmrib.ox.ac.uk
[3] Scalable Display Technologies, USA
samson@ai.mit.edu
[4] Radiology Department, BWH, USA
sw@bwh.harvard.edu

Abstract. We formalize the pair-wise registration problem in a *maximum a posteriori* (MAP) framework that employs a multinomial model of joint intensities with parameters for which we only have a prior distribution. To obtain an MAP estimate of the aligning transformation alone, we treat the multinomial parameters as nuisance parameters, and marginalize them out. If the prior on those is uninformative, the marginalization leads to registration by minimization of joint entropy. With an informative prior, the marginalization leads to minimization of the entropy of the data pooled with pseudo observations from the prior. In addition, we show that the marginalized objective function can be optimized by the Expectation-Maximization (EM) algorithm, which yields a simple and effective iteration for solving entropy-based registration problems. Experimentally, we demonstrate the effectiveness of the resulting EM iteration for rapidly solving a challenging intra-operative registration problem.

1 Introduction

The field of medical image registration has been very active in the past two decades. Although numerous alignment methods have been introduced, only limited attention has been devoted to study the relationship among the available methods and the justification for their preference, implicit and explicit hypothesis and their performance[1,2]. Currently, a significant number of methods build upon the maximum likelihood framework because of its intuitive nature and ease of implementation. According to this approach, correct alignment is obtained if we find the transformation that makes the the current observations most probable. Recently, with the abundance of available data sets, using prior information to guide registration has received significant attention. Such techniques allow for more robustness and a larger capture range in the implementation, and with respect to the transformation domain, they facilitate the introduction of smoothness constraints on the deformation models.

N. Karssemeijer and B. Lelieveldt (Eds.): IPMI 2007, LNCS 4584, pp. 662–674, 2007.

© Springer-Verlag Berlin Heidelberg 2007

When relying on prior models, however, it is challenging to find the appropriate balance between previous and current observations. For example, it is not obvious how the level of confidence in the model can be automatically encoded and / or changed over time. Preliminary efforts using both model- and data-related terms have introduced both sequential and unified algorithms with arbitrary weighing terms [3,4]. In this work, we focus on the establishment of a *maximum a posteriori* (MAP) framework that allows for making use of prior information about both the transformation and the joint statistics of the observed intensity distributions. By treating the former as nuisance parameters, we can marginalize them out and define our registration goal as a posterior on the transformation components. Depending on how informative the prior is on the joint statistics, we demonstrate implicit relationships with currently used methods. We also introduce an attractive optimization framework over our marginalized formulation – the Expectation-Maximization (EM) algorithm allows us to compute the registration update in a simple and elegant way.

2 Problem Formulation

2.1 Marginalized MAP Formulation of Registration

Given multi-modal input data sets, u and v, our goal is to find transformation T that that brings those into correct alignment. In addition to the unknown transformation parameters, we introduce another set of parameters, Θ, that encode a discrete joint probability distribution. This model is used in such a way that, if the intensities in the two images are discretized to take values in $\{I_1, I_2, ..., I_K\}$ then the probability of corresponding voxels (at location j) having discrete intensity values of $T(u)_j = I_a$ and $v_j = I_b$ is $p(u, v|T) = p(T(u)_j = I_a, v_j = I_b) = \Theta(a, b)$. If we use a simplified, one-dimensional indexing for the parameters of the discrete joint probability model, $\Theta = \{\theta_1, ..., \theta_g\}$ encodes information about intensity joint value occurrences as parameters of an unknown multinomial model, where $\forall i \;\; \theta_i \geq 0$ and $\sum_{i=1}^{g} \theta_i = 1$. This model can also incorporate any additive noise.

The posterior parameter distribution of the transformation variable T and the joint statistics model Θ with respect to the image observations is $p(T, \Theta|u, v)$. In order to align the data sets, this quantity is to be maximized. For our registration purposes though, it is more attractive to compute the posterior on just the transformation parameters. This is manageable given a prior model on the joint statistics parameters that can be marginalized out. Assuming independence between the transformation and the joint distribution models, the posterior distribution of the transformation variable T with respect to solely the image observations is:

$$p(T|u, v) \propto \int P(u, v|T, \Theta)P(T)P(\Theta)d\theta \quad . \tag{1}$$

In Eq.(1), the $P(u, v|T, \Theta)$ term indicates the likelihood function of the transformation and the model parameters given the input observations, and the right-most two terms are prior distributions over the T and Θ parameters respectively. Optimizing over such a quantity provides a convenient formulation of the registration objective, if we assume that we have prior knowledge about both the transformation and the joint statistics. The most optimal set of transformation parameters $\hat{T}$ are then the ones that optimize the following objective function:

$$\hat{T} = \arg\max_{T} \log p(T|u,v) \quad . \tag{2}$$

2.2 The Likelihood Term

Using the multinomial model for ordered data, the likelihood of the image observations given the offsetting transformation and an unknown joint probability model is

$$p(u,v|T,\Theta) \propto \prod_{j} \theta_j^{n_j(T)} \quad , \tag{3}$$

where $n_j(T)$ is the number of voxel pairs that map to the intensity bin associated with θ_j (i.e. $T(u)_j = I_a$ and $v_j = I_b$) and $\sum_{i=1}^{g} n(T)_i = N$ is the total number of observations. Note that the values of n_j depend on the transformation T, and this dependency is made explicit in this notation.

2.3 Prior on the Joint Statistics Model

For the registration problem, the multinomial distribution is a convenient choice of representation as the θ_i parameters naturally correspond to the widely used histogram encoding of the joint statistics of images given g number of components. Additionally, prior information about such parameters can be expressed by using the Dirichlet distribution, the conjugate prior to a multinomial distribution. We choose the following encoding

$$\text{Dirichlet}(\Theta; w) = \frac{1}{Z(w)} \prod_{i=1}^{g} \theta_i^{(w_i-1)} = \Gamma(w_0) \prod_{j} \frac{\theta_j^{(w_j-1)}}{\Gamma(w_j)} \quad , \tag{4}$$

where $\forall i, w_i > 0$ and $\sum_{i=1}^{g} w_i = w_0$. We may interpret w_0 as the total number of pseudo measurements observed to obtain information about the model and w_i as the individual frequency counts for the joint distribution parameters. The higher the former number is, the greater our confidence becomes in the values of the prior observations.

2.4 The Proposed Objective Function

Using Eq.(3) and Eq.(4), we write the posterior probability on T from Eq.(1) as

$$p(T|u,v,w) \propto P(T) \int \left(\prod_{i} \theta_i^{n_i(T)} \right) \Gamma(w_0) \left(\prod_{j} \frac{\theta_j^{(w_j-1)}}{\Gamma(w_j)} \right) d\theta \tag{5}$$

$$\propto P(T)\frac{\Gamma(w_0)}{\Gamma(N+w_0)}\left(\prod_j \frac{\Gamma(n_j(T)+w_j)}{\Gamma(w_j)}\right) \quad , \tag{6}$$

where we derived Eq.(6) by identifying a Dirichlet distribution with parameters $n_j(T)+w_j$ and using the fact that the integral of the distribution over its domain is equal to one. Therefore, the objective function of our proposed marginalized MAP registration method becomes

$$\hat{T} = \arg\max_T \log\left[P(T)\frac{\Gamma(w_0)}{\Gamma(N+w_0)}\left(\prod_{j=1}^{g} \frac{\Gamma\left(n_j(T)+w_j\right)}{\Gamma(w_j)}\right)\right] \tag{7}$$

$$= \arg\max_T \left[\log P(T) + \sum_{j=1}^{g} \log \Gamma\left(n_j(T)+w_j\right) + C\right] \quad . \tag{8}$$

2.5 Special Cases: Strength of Priors

In the following, we demonstrate how our objective function changes with respect to the nature of the prior, and we also examine the equivalence of our novel objective function of Eq.(8) with some widely used methods. These relationships help us better explain why these registration techniques are expected to converge to the correct alignment configuration.

Uninformative Prior: First we choose an uninformative prior. This means that the prior does not favor any solutions *a priori* and the current observations are going to be solely responsible for the solution to be computed. As an uninformative prior (whose use achieves an equivalence with the maximum likelihood (ML) solution of the problem), we choose to use Jeffreys' prior [5]. These are not affected by any transformations applied to the variables. Accordingly, we set, $w_0 = 1$ and $\forall i, w_i = \frac{1}{g}$, or in words, we assume to have only one prior observation, and it is distributed over all the existing bins (where g represents the total number of bins used in the multinomial model). Consequently,

$$\log p(T|u,v,w) \rightarrow \log P(T) + \sum_j \log \Gamma\left(n_j(T)+\frac{1}{g}\right) + \mathrm{C} \quad . \tag{9}$$

The information theoretic joint entropy [6], measuring uncertainty related to the joint occurrence of the input random variables, is defined by :

$$\mathrm{H}\left(\frac{\mathrm{n}}{\mathrm{N}}\right) \equiv -\sum_{\mathrm{j}} \frac{\mathrm{n_j}}{\mathrm{N}} \log \frac{\mathrm{n_j}}{\mathrm{N}} = -\frac{1}{\mathrm{N}}\sum_{\mathrm{j}} \mathrm{n_j}\log \mathrm{n_j} + \log \mathrm{N} \quad , \tag{10}$$

where $\sum_j n_j = N$. For the most part, the differences between expressions $\left(\sum_j n_j \log(n_j)\right)$ and $\left(\sum_j \log \Gamma(n_j)\right)$ are small ("first order" version of the Stirling approximation). Therefore, we may re-write the registration objective function using an uninformative prior as

$$\hat{T} = \arg\max_T \log p(T|u, v, w) \approx \arg\min_T \left[c\mathrm{H}\left(\frac{\mathrm{n(T)} + \frac{1}{\mathrm{g}}}{\mathrm{N}+1} \right) - \log \mathrm{P(T)} \right] \quad . \tag{11}$$

This approximation, ignoring the transformation prior, is equivalent to the widely used minimization of joint entropy method [7]. Although widely used, the justification of using that metric in registration has long been debated. Formally, joint entropy is maximum likelihood method. While others have discussed a similar equivalence between ML and joint entropy [8], the present marginalization approach provides a rigorous demonstration of its validity.

Informative Prior: When the priors are informative, or in words, when we have access to a sufficient number of pseudo observations (w_j) from, for example, training data sets, they allow for a more certain belief in their information content. In such a case, the objective function can be approximated by

$$\hat{T} = \arg\max_T \log p(T|u, v, w) \approx \arg\min_T \left[\mathrm{H}\left(\frac{\mathrm{n(T)} + \mathrm{w}}{\mathrm{N} + \mathrm{w_0}} \right) - \log \mathrm{P(T)} \right] \quad . \tag{12}$$

According to Eq.(12), prior information is introduced into the framework by *pooling* together corresponding samples from the previously aligned (prior distribution model) and from the current, to-be-aligned cases. Throughout the optimization, the model observations remain fixed and act as anchor points to bring the other samples into a more likely configuration. Interestingly, this formulation is closely related to another type of entropy-based registration algorithm. Sabuncu et al. introduced a registration technique based on minimizing Renyi entropy, where the entropy measure is computed via a non-plug-in entropy estimator on pooled data [9]. This estimator is based upon constructing the EMST (Euclidean Minimum Spanning Tree) and using the edge length in that tree to approximate the entropy. The reason that such an arrangement would provide a favorable solution has not been previously theoretically justified.

Strong Prior: Lastly, we briefly mention the scenario, where the prior information is very strong.

$$\log p(T|u, v, w) \approx \log P(T) + \sum_j \left(\log \Gamma(w_j) + n_j(T) \frac{\Gamma'(w_j)}{\Gamma(w_j)} \right) + \mathrm{C} \tag{13}$$

$$\approx \log P(T) + \sum_j \left(w_j \log(w_j) + n_j(T) \log(w_j) \right) + \mathrm{C} \quad . \tag{14}$$

In Eq.(13) a first order approximation of $\log \Gamma(n_j(T)+w_j)$ around w_j was written out, with Γ' indicating the derivative of the Gamma function. In Eq.(14), the approximation for $\sum_j \log \Gamma(w_j)$ from Eq.(11) and $\frac{\Gamma'(n)}{\Gamma(n)} \approx \log(n)$ are used, where the latter is valid for a large range of n. The only term that depends on $n_j(T)$ is $\sum_j n_j(T)\log(w_j)$, thus

$$\hat{T} = \arg\max_T \log p(T|u,v,w) \approx \arg\max_T \left[\log P(T) + \sum_j (n_j(T)\log(w_j))\right] \quad . \tag{15}$$

If we re-express the sum in Eq.(15) as a sum over data points, we can see that this formulation is equivalent to an approximate maximum likelihood approach, where the current samples are, indeed, evaluated under the previously constructed model distribution [10]. Chung et al. experimentally showed that the performance of this similarity measure is not always sufficiently accurate[11]. That finding is now explained by the fact that this objective function considers the model with such a high level of confidence that might not be justified by the number of previous observations.

3 EM Optimization for the Marginalized MAP Registration Problem

The above described objective functions could be optimized in several ways. In general, we can differentiate between gradient- and non-gradient-based techniques. Using gradient-based information in the optimization procedure often results in significant computational advantages, however, they might also require challenging approximation of some terms. For example, when using the multinomial model, update terms need to be estimated from a discrete distribution and also it is required to calculate the partial derivative of *changing* (non-fixed) joint statistics parameters with respect to the to-be-optimized transformation components. Although close approximations exist, one might worry about their accuracy. To escape such computational difficulties, we might optimize both of the above marginalized formulations by using the Expectation-Maximization (EM) algorithm [12]. This framework, from the statistical computing literature, is known to have good properties as an optimizer and the resulting iteration is attractive from a practical standpoint. If we consider the input images as observations and the Θ parameters as hidden information, the EM algorithm defines the solution to $\hat{T} = \arg\max_T \log p(T|u,v)$ as iteratively obtaining the best current solution ($\hat{T}_{\text{next}}$) based upon:

$$\hat{T}_{\text{next}} = \arg\max_T \mathrm{E}_{\Theta|u,v,\hat{T}_{\text{old}}}\left[\log P(T,\Theta|u,v)\right] \tag{16}$$

$$= \arg\max_T \mathrm{E}_{\Theta|u,v,\hat{T}_{\text{old}}}\left[\log P(T|u,v,\Theta) + \log P(\Theta)\right] \tag{17}$$

$$= \arg\max_T \mathrm{E}_{\Theta|u,v,\hat{T}_{\text{old}}}\left[\log(P(u,v|T,\Theta)P(T)) + \sum_{j=1}^{g}(w_j-1)\log\theta_j\right] \tag{18}$$

where Bayes rule was applied in order to express the conditional probability term on the registering transformation. Continuing with the manipulation

$$\hat{T}_{\text{next}} = \arg\max_T \mathrm{E}_{\Theta|u,v,\hat{T}_{\text{old}}} \left[\log \prod_j \theta_j^{n_j(T)} + \log P(T) + \sum_{j=1}^{g} (w_j - 1) \log \theta_j \right] \quad (19)$$

$$= \arg\max_T \left[\log P(T) + \mathrm{E}_{\Theta|u,v,\hat{T}_{\text{old}}} \left[\sum_{j=1}^{g} (n(T)_j + w_j - 1) \log \theta_j \right] \right] \quad (20)$$

$$= \arg\max_T \left[\log P(T) + \sum_{j=1}^{g} (n(T)_j + w_j - 1) \, \mathrm{E}_{\Theta|u,v,\hat{T}_{\text{old}}} [\log \theta_j] \right] \quad (21)$$

If we define $l_j \equiv \log \theta_j$, then we can define the two steps of the EM algorithm: maximization (M) and expectation (E) as follows:

$$\mathbf{M-step}: \quad \hat{T}_{\text{next}} = \arg\max_T \left[\log P(T) + \sum_{j=1}^{g} (n(T)_j + w_j - 1) \, l_{j_{\text{old}}} \right] \quad (22)$$

$$\mathbf{E-step}: \quad l_{j_{\text{next}}} = \mathrm{E}_{\Theta|u,v,\hat{T}_{\text{old}}} [l_j] , \quad (23)$$

In words, the M-step searches for transformation T that optimizes the sum of expectation over the log model parameters and a transformation prior; and the E-step calculates the expectation of these log parameters given the current best estimate of the transformation parameters. Note that in this framework, we need to pay special attention to the scenario where the θ_j parameters tend to zero and we also have to enforce the property that the parameters add to one. More details on these special cases are discussed below.

3.1 Evaluating the E-Step

In order to evaluate the expression in the E-step, we may use the following form for the posterior on Θ given the input images and the transform:

$$P(\Theta|u,v,T) = \frac{P(u,v|\Theta,T)P(\Theta)}{\int_\Theta P(u,v|\Theta,T)P(\Theta)d\theta} \quad . \quad (24)$$

Computing the expectation term thus becomes:

$$\mathrm{E}_{\Theta|u,v,\hat{T}} [\log \theta_l] = \int_\Theta \log \theta_l P(\Theta|u,v,\hat{T}) d\theta = \int_\Theta \log \theta_l \frac{P(u,v|\Theta,\hat{T})P(\Theta)}{\int_\Theta P(u,v|\Theta,\hat{T})P(\Theta)d\theta} d\theta. \quad (25)$$

Using our multinomial model and the Dirichlet distribution as its prior, the numerator in Eq.(25) has the form of another unnormalized Dirichlet distribution.

Therefore, if we define a new Dirichlet distribution with parameters β, where $\beta_i = (n(\hat{T})_i + w_i)$, we may write

$$\mathrm{E}_{\Theta|u,v,\hat{T}}\left[\log\theta_l\right] = \int_{\Theta} \log\theta_l \; \frac{\prod_{j=1}^{g} \theta_j^{n(\hat{T})_j} \frac{1}{Z(w_0)} \prod_{k=1}^{g} \theta_k^{(w_k-1)}}{\int_{\Theta} \prod_{j=1}^{g} \theta_j^{n(\hat{T})_j} \frac{1}{Z(w_0)} \prod_{k=1}^{g} \theta_k^{(w_k-1)} d\theta} d\theta \quad (26)$$

$$= \mathrm{E}_{\mathrm{Dir}(\Theta;\beta)}\left[\log\theta_l\right] \quad . \quad (27)$$

The expression in Eq.(27) is the expected value of the $(\log\theta_l)$ parameters given a Dirichlet distribution parameterized by β. As the Dirichlet distribution belongs to the family of exponential functions, the expectation over its sufficient statistics can be computed as the derivative of the logarithm of the normalization factor with respect to its natural parameters[13]. Writing the Dirichlet distribution in its exponential form results in

$$\mathrm{Dir}(\Theta; w) = \exp\left(\sum_{i=1}^{g}(w_i - 1)\log\theta_i + \log\Gamma(w_0) - \sum_{i=1}^{g}\log\Gamma(w_i)\right) \quad . \quad (28)$$

Given this form, we see that the sufficient statistics are indeed the $(\log\theta_l)$ parameters. Therefore, the expectation term we are concerned with can be expressed by using the Digamma (or Psi) function which is the first derivative of the log Gamma functions [14].

$$\mathrm{E}_{\mathrm{Dir}(\Theta;\beta)}\left[\log\theta_l\right] = \Psi(\beta_l) - \Psi(\beta_0) = \Psi(n(\hat{T})_l + w_l) - \Psi(N + w_0) \quad . \quad (29)$$

In the following, we approximate the Digamma expressions in Eq.(29) by using $\Psi(x) \approx \log(x - .5)$ [15]. This approximation is very accurate in the positive real domain, except for values in the range of $[0, 1]$. A value in that particular range would correspond to the extreme scenario of an "empty bucket", where there are neither current nor prior observations associated with a particular model parameter. In order to make the approximation hold even in such a scenario, we differentiate between two cases: uninformative and informative priors. In the case of uninformative priors, we propose to use Laplace priors [5] instead of zero counts for the Dirichlet parameters. Consequently, when no prior / pseudo information is available for the model, we initialize all parameters uniformly as one. The case of informative priors requires more attention. Although the total sum of pseudo information in this case is significant, we cannot directly assume that it holds for all individual Dirichlet parameters. Thus in that case we explicitly require that each pseudo count should hold at least one count. With such specifications we can ensure that our approximation holds regardless of the nature of the prior information and that the argument of the log function, in the case of the parameter update, does not approach zero (which could be a concern as mentioned while defining the EM framework). Thus the E-step of the EM algorithm is expressed as

$$(\bar{l}_l)_{\mathrm{next}} = \Psi\left(n(\hat{T}_{\mathrm{old}})_l + w_l\right) - \Psi(N + w_0) \quad (30)$$

$$\approx \log\left(n(\hat{T}_{\text{old}})_l + w_l - .5\right) - \log(N + w_0 - .5) \tag{31}$$

$$= \log\left(\frac{n(\hat{T}_{\text{old}})_l + w_l - .5}{N + w_0 - .5}\right) \quad . \tag{32}$$

This rule assigns the logarithm of normalized sum of the pseudo and observed counts minus a constant to the most current $\log(\theta)$ parameters. This pooling of current and pseudo counts for describing joint intensity statistics has been already discussed in Sec.2.5. We point out that, in order to enforce the relationship $\sum_{i=1}^{g} \theta_i = 1$, we compute the E-step for all $1 \le j \le (g-1)$ and we assign the last remaining parameter as $(\bar{l}_g)_{\text{next}} = \log\left[1 - \sum_{i=1}^{g-1} \exp((\bar{l}_i)_{\text{next}})\right]$.

3.2 Evaluating the M-Step

Using the results from the E-step, we may now express the M-step (the most current estimate of the registration parameter), which indeed results in a simple formulation of the problem:

$$\hat{T}_{\text{next}} = \arg\max_T \mathrm{E}_{\Theta|u,v,\hat{T}_{\text{old}}} \left[\log P(u, v, \Theta|T)\right] \tag{33}$$

$$= \arg\max_T \left[logP(T) + \sum_{j=1}^{g} (n(T)_j + w_j - 1)\, \mathrm{E}_{\Theta|u,v,\hat{T}_{\text{old}}} [l_j] \right] \tag{34}$$

$$= \arg\max_T \left[\log P(T) + \sum_{j=1}^{g} (n(T)_j + w_j - 1) \log\left(\frac{n(\hat{T}_{\text{old}})_j + w_j - .5}{N + w_0 - .5}\right)\right] \tag{35}$$

$$= \arg\max_T \left[\log P(T) + \sum_{j=1}^{g} n(T)_j \log\left(n(\hat{T}_{\text{old}})_j + w_j - .5\right)\right] \tag{36}$$

Therefore, ignoring the prior on transformation T, our objective function in the M-step is the maximization of a log likelihood term. When solving the optimization problem with a non-informative set of priors, the solution approaches an *iterated* ML framework. This result underlies the fact that an MAP framework with a non-informative prior produces results that are equivalent to the ML solution. The best transformation parameters therefore are calculated by using old, currently the best, model estimates. In the scenario where we have significant amount of prior information with respect to the model, again, the pseudo and the current observations are pooled together.

We note that the expression in Eq.(36) can be further simplified to result in an information theoretic framework that comprises of a data- and model-related term. The former measures the KL-divergence between two categorical distributions over the parameters describing the current joint statistics and that including *pseudo* observations from the prior model and the latter computes the entropy of the estimated joint statistics of the observations.

$$\hat{T}_{\text{next}} \approx \arg\max_T \left[\log P(T) - \mathrm{D_{KL}}\left(n(T) \parallel n(\hat{T}_{\text{old}}) + w_j - .5\right) - \mathrm{H}\left(\mathrm{n(T)}\right)\right] \quad (37)$$

$$\approx \arg\min_T \left[\mathrm{D_{KL}}\left(p_T \parallel p_{\hat{T}_{\text{old}},w}\right) + \mathrm{H}\left(\mathrm{p_T}\right) - \log \mathrm{P(T)}\right] \quad (38)$$

In summary, the utilization of the EM framework provides an iterative method for the transformation parameter estimation where the model parameter updates are computed in an efficient and principled manner.

4 Experimental Results

In this section, we present our experimental results from an iterated registration algorithm that uses uninformative priors. The resulting EM solution to the ML (in θ) formulation is demonstrated on a complex intra-operative non-rigid brain registration problem. We introduced a prior on the deformation field that approximates a fluid flow model. The algorithm also facilitates (on the EM iterations) a quadratic approximation to the search problem that may be quickly solved. That would not be justified if the multinomial model were not constant within the iterations. Preliminary experimental results for the scenario where we do have access to informative prior information was presented in [16]. At each iteration, our non-rigid registration algorithm defines the prior probability on configurations phenomenologically, using linear elastic deformation energy and Boltzmann's Equation, as $P(T) \propto \exp(-E/\tau)$. Configurations of the deforming anatomy are parameterized by the coordinates of the vertices of an adaptive tetrahedral mesh. Using standard methodology of the Finite Element Method (FEM) [17], the stress-strain integral is linearized about the current configuration, yielding a quadratic approximation for the energy in terms of displacements from the current configuration, $E \approx \Delta_T^T K \Delta_T$,where K is a banded elasticity matrix. At each iteration, the log likelihood, $\log P(n(T)_{\text{old}}|\Delta_T)$, is approximated by a second order Taylor expansion. This is centered on a nearby local maximum of the likelihood function that we locate using a greedy method. The resulting quadratic expression is combined with the quadratic prior term, and the resulting approximation to the posterior probability is easily solved as a linear system. This iterative method resets the elastic energy to zero at each iteration. Papademetris et al. [18] call this "history free" approach the *incremental approach*, and point out that, in a limiting case, it is equivalent to the fluid model [19].

Figures 1 (a) and (b) show two MRI images of the same brain taken during brain surgery. The images contain 256x256x124 voxels with 0.9375x0.9375x1.5 mm spacing. According to visual comparison, deformation between the two images mostly occurs near the incision. The result of the non-rigid registration algorithm is shown in Fig. 1 (c). The warped image is very similar to the target image. In particular, the small displacement of the left and right ventricles was captured and the boundaries near the incision appear to be in appropriate

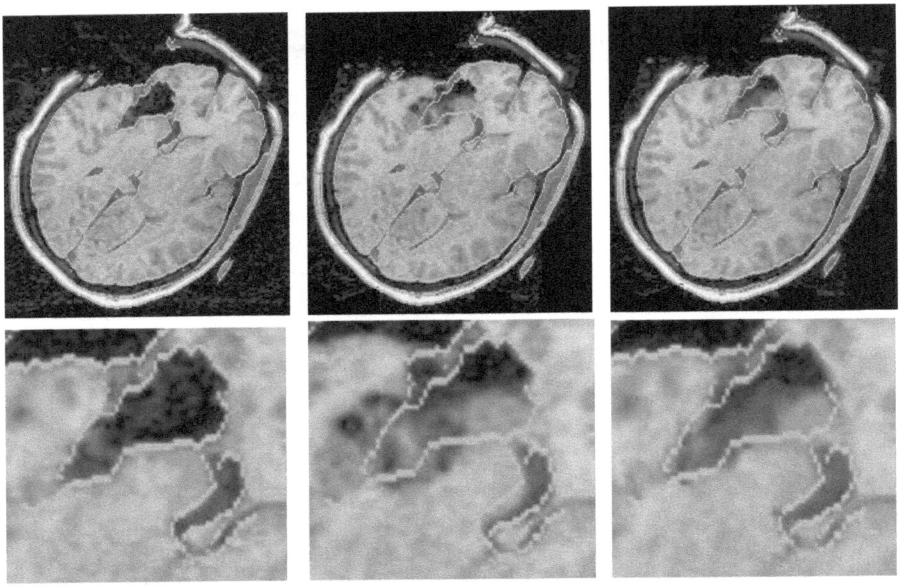

(a) Intra-operative slice at t_1 (b) Intra-operative slice at t_2 (c) Deformed acquisition

Fig. 1. MRI acquisition of the brain: (a) taken during surgery with edges highlighted; (b) taken later in the surgery, with the edges from (a) overlaid; (c) deformed the former image onto the latter, with the edges of (a) overlaid

places as well. The final match used 8500 mesh nodes, and the entire matching process was finished in less than 6 minutes on a 2 Ghz desktop computer. To validate our registration results, we compared manually located landmarks in the initial and the deformed images. The majority of the motion was captured by our non-rigid registration algorithm, with disagreements typically not more than the voxel size. More details on the experimental setup and the validation results is described in dissertation work [20].

5 Conclusion

We introduced an MAP framework for the pair-wise registration problem that allowed us to include prior information about not only the transformation parameter space but also the joint intensity statistics of the inputs. Treating the latter as nuisance parameters and marginalizing them out allowed us to establish a close relationship between our method and certain entropy-based objective functions. We also demonstrated that using an EM-based optimization framework the aligning transformations can be computed in a principled and computationally attractive manner.

Acknowledgements

This work was supported by grants NIH U41-RR019703, NCRR NAC P41-RR13218, NSF CISST/ERC EEC9731748, NCRR P41-RR14075, NCRR R01 RR16594-01A1, NINDS R01 NS052585-01 and by the UK BBSRC.

References

1. Zöllei, L., Fisher, J., Wells, W.: A unified statistical and information theoretic framework for multi-modal image registration. In: Taylor, C.J., Noble, J.A. (eds.) IPMI 2003. LNCS, vol. 2732, pp. 366–377. Springer, Heidelberg (2003)
2. Roche, A., Malandain, G., Ayache, N.: Unifying maximum likelihood approaches in medical image registration. International Journal of Imaging Systems and Technology 11(7180), 71–80 (2000)
3. Chung, A., Gan, R., Wells, W.: Robust multi-modal image registration based on prior joint intensity distributions and minimization of kullback-leibler distance. Technical Report HKUST-CS07-01, HKUST (2007)
4. Gütter, C., Xu, C., Sauer, F., Hornegger, J.: Learning based non-rigid multi-modal image registration using kullback-leibler divergence. In: Gerig, G., Duncan, J. (eds.) MICCAI. LNCS, vol. 2, pp. 255–263. Springer, Heidelberg (1973)
5. Gelman, A., Carlin, J., Stern, H., Rubin, D.: Bayesian Data Analysis. CRC Press LLC, Boca Raton, FL (2003)
6. Cover, T., Thomas, J.: Elements of Information Theory. John Wiley & Sons, Inc, New York (1991)
7. Studholme, C., Hill, D., Hawkes, D.: An overlap invariant entropy measure of 3d medical image alignment. Pattern Recognition 32(1), 71–86 (1999)
8. Zhu, Y., Cochoff, S.: Likelihood maximization approach to image registration. IEEE Transactions on Image Processing 11(12), 1417–1426 (2002)
9. Sabuncu, M., Ramadge, P.: Graph theoretic image registration using prior examples. In: Proceedings of European Signal Processing Conference (Sept 2005)
10. Leventon, M., Grimson, W.: Multi-modal Volume Registration Using Joint Intensity Distributions. In: Wells, W.M., Colchester, A.C.F., Delp, S.L. (eds.) MICCAI 1998. LNCS, vol. 1496, pp. 1057–1066. Springer, Heidelberg (1998)
11. Chung, A., Wells, I.W., Norbash, A., Grimson, W.: Multi-modal Image Registration by Minimizing Kullback-Leibler Distance. In: Dohi, T., Kikinis, R. (eds.) MICCAI 2002. LNCS, vol. 2489, pp. 525–532. Springer, Heidelberg (2002)
12. Dempster, A.P., Laird, N.M., Rubin, D.: Maximum likelihood from incomplete data via the em algorithm. Journal of the Royal Statistical Society 39(1), 1–38 (1977)
13. Blei, D., Ng, A., Jordan, M.: Latent dirichlet allocation. Journal of Machine Learning Research 3, 993–1022 (2003)
14. Minka, T.: Estimating a dirichlet distribution. Notes (2003)
15. Abramowitz, M., Stegun, I.A.: Handbook of Mathematical Functions. Dover, New York (1964)
16. Zöllei, L., Wells, W.: Multi-modal image registration using dirichlet-encoded prior information. In: Pluim, J.P.W., Likar, B., Gerritsen, F.A. (eds.) WBIR 2006. LNCS, vol. 4057, pp. 34–42. Springer, Heidelberg (2006)
17. Zenkiewicz, O., Taylor, R.: The Finite Element Method, 4th edn. McGraw-Hill, Berkshire, England (1989)

18. Papademetris, X., Onat, E.T., Sinusas, A.J., Dione, D.P., Constable, R.T., Duncan, J.S.: Specification and Compositional Verification of Real-Time Systems. LNCS, vol. 0558, pp. 36–49. Springer, Heidelberg (2001)
19. Christensen, G., Rabbit, R., Miller, M.: Deformable templates using large deformation kinematics. IEEE Transactions on Image Processing 5(10), 1435–1447 (1996)
20. Timoner, S.: Compact Representations for Fast Nonrigid Registration of Medical Images. PhD thesis, Massachusetts Institute of Technology (July 2003)

Geometry Driven Volumetric Registration

Gheorghe Postelnicu, Lilla Zollei, Rahul Desikan, and Bruce Fischl

MGH/MIT/HMS Athinoula A. Martinos Center for Biomedical Imaging, Charlestown, MA
{postelni,lzollei,rahul,fischl}@nmr.mgh.harvard.edu

Abstract. In this paper, we propose a novel method for the registration of volumetric images of the brain that attempts to maximize the overlap of cortical folds. In order to achieve this, relevant geometrical information is extracted from a surface-based morph and is diffused throughout the volume using the Navier operator of elasticity. The result is a volumetric warp that aligns the folding patterns.

1 Introduction

Pairwise brain registration is one of the active areas of research in the medical imaging community. Different algorithms have tackled the generic problem of registering information from two brain scans in various ways. Volumetric registration (see [1] for a survey) seeks a 3D deformation field which is driven by either raw intensity information or features derived from image intensities. A different approach is to extract geometric features from surface models of structures such as the neocortex, and to reformulate the complex correspondence problem in a *surface matching* framework.

Each of these approaches has advantages and weaknesses. Surface-based methods [2,3,4] have been shown to accurately align the highly complex folding pattern of the human cerebral cortex, and to result in increased statistical power presumably due to their alignment of functionally homologous regsions accross subjects. This accuracy stems from the direct use of geometric information that is generally unavailable to volumetric methods and the relatively close relationship between folding patterns and functional properties of the neocortex. Conversely, volumetric methods [5,6,7,8], while frequently failing to align corresponding cortical folds, provide a correspondence field in the whole brain, and align subcortical and ventricular structures as well as the cortex (regions that are outside of the domain of classical surface-based registrations).

In this paper, we propose a method which combines the two approaches. This is done by integrating surface-based information into a volumetric registration procedure. The result is a 3D deformation field which aligns the folding patterns of the the two scans. While the idea of using surface registration to drive volumetric deformation fields is not new [9,10,11], this is the first paper to explicitly concentrate on the accurate registration of the cortical sheet in 3D space.

The current work can be seen as growing out of the non-linear registration literature that aims at integrating prescribed displacements into a volumetric

N. Karssemeijer and B. Lelieveldt (Eds.): IPMI 2007, LNCS 4584, pp. 675–686, 2007.
© Springer-Verlag Berlin Heidelberg 2007

morph: [9] proposes a linear and incremental method for performing volumetric deformations, and [10,11,12] use various types of surfaces and matching algorithms that are then interpolated in the rest of the image to yield a dense deformation field, while [13] uses explicitly extracted sulcal traces together with feature vectors. Perhaps the closest related work to this article is by Liu et al. [14], where the geometrical information carried by the brain surfaces is explicitely used in the registration process. However, it should be mentioned that the surface similarity is maximized after the volumetric warping, which we believe makes it susceptible to local minima.

2 Methods

We present the process of registering two structural brain scans, *fixed* and *moving*. Each of the scans is independently processed to obtain an accurate topologically correct reconstruction of the cortical surfaces (see [15,16,17,18,19] for details). Then, we perform a surface-based registration, independently for each of the surfaces (4/brain - left and right pial and gray/white respectively). This registration takes place in spherical coordinates and aims at maximizing the similarity of the folding patterns, while remaining topologically correct and controlling the amount of allowed metric distortions.

The result of the surface registration algorithm provides the input to the volumetric registration we present in this paper. Using a regularizer from the theory of elasticity, we build a displacement field which is driven by the surface registration. The resulting morph yields surfaces that are as close as possible to the target surfaces, while being topologically correct and respecting the anatomical variability between individuals.

2.1 Surface Registration

The surface-based registration of our choice is briefly described below [3]. The first step is to transform the cortical surface into a spherical representation with moderate metric distortions [20]. The algorithm aims at iteratively minimizing the following energy in the spherical space:

$$J = J_p + \lambda_A J_A + \lambda_d J_d \tag{1}$$

where J_p measures the alignment, based on the cortical depth and the curvature information, while the other two terms act as regularizers. J_A is a topology-preservation term, while J_d controls the amount of metric distortion allowed:

$$J_A = \frac{1}{2T}\sum_{i=1}^{T}\left(A_i^n - A_i^0\right)^2 \qquad J_d = \frac{1}{4V}\sum_{i=1}^{V}\sum_{n\in N(i)}\left(d_{in}^n - d_{in}^0\right)^2 \qquad d_{in} = \|x_i - x_n\|$$

Here, superscripts denote time with 0 being the starting point, T and V are the number of triangles and vertices in the tesselation, x_i^n is the position of vertex i at iteration n, $N(i)$ is the set of neighbors of the ith vertex and A_i denotes the *oriented* area of triangle i. The result of the surface registration is a 1-to-1 mapping that transports each surface of the fixed scan to its counterpart surface in the moving image $F_{reg} : \mathcal{S}_{fixed} \rightarrow \mathcal{S}_{moving}$, where S can be any of the left/right pial/white surfaces of the brain.

2.2 Volumetric Warping

When the surface registration is completed, we obtain a displacement vector field which provides a 1-to-1 mapping between the hemisphere surfaces of the fixed and moving brain scans in the Euclidean space. We now show how to diffuse this vector field from the cortical surfaces to the rest of the volume.

Let Ω be the source image domain. We define an arbitrary transformation $\phi : \Omega \rightarrow \mathbb{R}^3$ of the source image as: $\phi(x) = x+u(x)$ where $u : \Omega \rightarrow \mathbb{R}^3$ denotes the displacement field. The goal here is to find a function ϕ such that $\phi\left(x_{surf}^{fixed}\right) = F_{reg}\left(x_{surf}^{fixed}\right)$, for any $x_{surf}^{fixed} \in \mathcal{S}$, where $\mathcal{S}$ is one of the surfaces of the fixed brain scan. Since the surfaces represent a space of co-dimension 1, in order for this problem to be well-posed, we impose an additional regularity constraint. We require that the displacement field we are searching to be an *elastic deformation*, i.e. a smooth, orientation-preserving deformation which satisfies the equations of static equilibrium in elastic materials. This means that we (additionally) require u to satisfy

$$\mathcal{L}(u) = 0 \tag{2}$$

where $\mathcal{L}$ is an operator we define below.

The choice of the operator $\mathcal{L}$ and the discretization method to numerically extrapolate the displacement field has numerous solutions that have been proposed in the registration litterature. Some of the better known are the thin plate splines, proposed by Bookstein [21], or the free-form deformations proposed by Rueckert et al [22]. We have chosen to use the Navier operator from the linearized elasticity theory together with the finite element method. This choice was motivated by the high level of flexibility needed in order to satisfy the constraints imposed by the displacement fields obtained on the 4 surfaces of the brain image.

2.3 Elasticity Operator

In order to solve the problem stated above, we use the equilibrium equation for elastic materials. This states that at equilibrium, the elastic energy equals the external forces applied to the body $\mathcal{L}(u) = f$ [23].

$$\mathcal{L}(u) = -\operatorname{div}\left[(I + \nabla u)\,\hat{S}\right] \tag{3}$$

where the second Piola-Kirchoff stress tensor $\hat{S} : \bar{\Omega} \rightarrow \mathcal{M}^3$ is defined as

$$\hat{S} = \lambda\,\mathrm{tr}(\hat{E})I + 2\mu\,\hat{E} \quad \text{and} \quad \hat{E} = \frac{1}{2}\left(\nabla u^T + \nabla u + \nabla u^T\,\nabla u\right)$$

is the Green-St. Venant strain tensor. Here λ and μ are the *Lamé* elastic constants that characterize the elastic properties of an isotropic material. The linear approximation to the above operator uses the Fréchet derivative of $\mathcal{L}$

$$\mathcal{L}(u) = \mathcal{L}(0) + \mathcal{L}'(0)u + o(u) \Rightarrow f = \mathcal{L}(u) \approx \mathcal{L}'(0)u$$

since no deformation occurs in the absence of external forces. Finally, $\mathcal{L}'(0)u$ is computed by dropping the non-linear terms in $\mathcal{L}(u)$, which results in $\mathcal{L}'(0)u = -\operatorname{div} S$ with $S = \lambda \operatorname{tr}(E)I + 2\mu E$ the linearized stress tensor and $E = \frac{1}{2}\left(\nabla u + \nabla u^T\right)$ the linearized strain tensor. Hence, the linear approximation of (2) can be written as

$$\mathcal{L}'(u) = -\operatorname{div} S = f \tag{4}$$

The main drawback of (4) is that it is only valid for small-magnitude deformations. To overcome this, we implement an extension of the linear model, as presented in [9]. Namely, given external forces that describe large displacements, one can iteratively solve for small linear increments using the linearized Navier equation (4): $\mathcal{L}\left(u^{n+1}\right) = \mathcal{L}'\left(u^n\right)\left(u^{n+1} - u^n\right) + o\left(u^{n+1} - u^n\right)$ or, by neglecting the last term,

$$f^{n+1} - f^n = \mathcal{L}\left(u^{n+1}\right) - \mathcal{L}\left(u^n\right) \approx \mathcal{L}'\left(u^n\right)\left(u^{n+1} - u^n\right) \tag{5}$$

Using this iterative process, the solution of (5) converges to the solution of (2) (see [23] for the proof).

The Lamé constants λ and μ are specified as functions of *Young's modulus of elasticity* $\mathcal{E}$ and the *Poisson ratio* ν: $\lambda = \frac{\mathcal{E}\nu}{(1+\nu)(1-2\nu)}$ and $\mu = \frac{\mathcal{E}}{2(1+\nu)}$. In all our experiments we used $\mathcal{E} \equiv 1$ and $\nu = 0.3$.

2.4 Finite Element Method

Using the notation introduced in the previous subsection, equation (4) can be re-written as a minimization problem by considering the potential energy of an elastic body submitted to externally applied forces

$$\mathbb{E} = \frac{1}{2}\int_\Omega \left[\lambda \left\|\nabla \cdot u\right\|^2 + 2\mu \sum_{i,j=1}^{3} e_{ij}^2(u)\right] \mathrm{d}x + \int_\Omega f \cdot u \,\mathrm{d}x \tag{6}$$

with $e_{ij}(u) = \frac{1}{2}\left(\partial_i u_j + \partial_j u_i\right)$.

One common way to tackle a minimization problem for (6) is to use the Finite Element Method. This consists in dividing the domain Ω using an assemblage of discrete finite elements interconnected at nodal points at the element boundaries (tetrahedra in our case). The continuous field u within each element can be approximated as a linear function of the displacements at the nodal points - the computation is detailed in [24]. The first term in (6) results in a sparse symmetric matrix K, also called the stiffness matrix, whereas the external forces result in a vector F. By using the linear approximations mentioned, (6) can be re-written

$$\mathbb{E}_{mesh} = U^T K U + U^T F \tag{7}$$

hence by minimizing (6) wrt. the nodal displacements $\frac{d\mathbb{E}_{mesh}(U)}{dU_i} = 0$, equation (4) can be written as

$$KU = F \tag{8}$$

2.5 Specifying the External Forces

All that remains to be specified for equation (8) is the vector of external forces F. As mentioned previously, the input to our problem is actually a set of prescribed displacements.

One way of implementing prescribed displacements as external forces when solving a FEM problem is described in [9]. It consists of modifying the matrix K and the vector F so that the value of the variable U_i we want to prescribe is forced. This is implemented by setting $K_{ij} = \delta_{ij}$ and $K_{ji} = \delta_{ji}\, \forall j$ and subtracting the appropriate quantity on the right hand side. However, numerical experiments showed that this way of constraining the stiffness matrix is too strong and it can cause topology problems (i.e. noninvertible regions). Indeed, in the current problem domain, where anatomical differences between the two brains are to be expected (such as a split fold), such hard constraints are undesirable, as they result in overfitting the warp field.

We have instead opted for an implementation of prescribed displacements using penalty weighting. This means that we use the displacements given by the surface registration F_{reg} to modify equation (4). Indeed, without external constraints, the elasticity problem simply reads $KU = 0$, with a trivial solution.

Suppose we want to impose a constraint $u(x) = v$. We start by determining the tetrahedron T_i such that $x \in T_i$ and we know that we must have $\sum_{j=1}^{4} N_j^{T_i}(x) U_j^{T_i} = v$, where N_j are the barycentric coordinates of x in T_i. Then we impose the condition by modifying (7) so that the energy becomes

$$E_{mesh}^{mod} = U^T K U + \alpha U^T (A_i U - B_i) \tag{9}$$

where A_i are the barycentric coordinates of $x \in T_i$ and $B_i = v$ (which are immersed in the global array U using the correspondence table of the nodes of tetrahedron T_i). In (9), α is the weight placed on the constraints. In all of our experiments we used a constant weight for all displacement vectors, although this could change in the future. For instance, a surface similarity measure could be used to better condition the morph.

2.6 Handling Topology Problems

After each iteration of the elastic solver, we check for potential topology problems, i.e. tetrahedra with negative Jacobian. Indeed, in spite of using the incremental model and solving the elasticity equation in more iterations, topology problems do appear. There are two general techniques used for performing mesh untangling: smoothing or, more generally, solving an optimization problem aiming at locally fixing tangles (see [25] for an algorithm that combines the two).

In our case, the goal pursued was to solve the tangles from the deformed mesh (i.e. inverted tetrahedra in the deformed configuration) while modifying the displacement field as little as possible. This task is facilitated by the fact that in the absence of displacements, the initial mesh is guaranteed to be topologically correct. Thus, we opt for a local smoothing-based algorithm, which we formulate as the solution of a local linear elastic problem.

We segment the regions with topological defects into local connected components. We then solve a linear elastic equation within each local cluster, the external forces being the displacements on the boundary of the cluster. Finally, we discard the initial displacements inside the cluster and replace them with the solution of the system.

We repeat the above clustering procedure until there are no more tetrahedra with topology problems. Although there is no formal proof of it, the above procedure has solved all the topological problems we were experiencing in the tests we ran thus far.

2.7 Implementation

To resume, the execution of the pipeline described in this section results in the following:

1. compute surfaces for each of the brain images (2 surfaces per hemisphere - pial and gray/white);
2. perform surface registration for each of the surfaces independently in spherical coordinates;
3. recover sparse displacement fields $x_i^{fixed} \to y_i^{moving}$;
4. regress out affine transform from the displacement field A; this results in the updated sparse displacement field $x_i^{fixed} \to A^{-1}\left(y_i^{moving}\right) = z_i$;
5. apply linear incremental model in n steps; i.e. loop $j = 1 \ldots n$
   (a) get current morphed positions $\phi_j \circ \phi_{j-1} \circ \ldots \phi_1(x_i) = x_i^j$ and create sparse displacement field $v_i^j = \frac{1}{n-j+1}(z_i - x_i^j)$
   (b) create tetrahedral mesh based on current surface positions and initialize the stiffness matrix and the external forces;
   (c) solve the linear system;
   (d) handle potential topology problems.

We use TetGen [26,27] to build a Delaunay tetrahedral mesh which is adapted to the input surfaces and PETSc [28,29] to solve the linear system at each step. Generally, we place a constraint on the volume of the tetrahedra that are near the surfaces (so that they have a lower volume), since it is expected that the morph will require greater flexibility in those areas.

It should also be noticed that prior to the elastic registration we apply an affine registration. This is motivated by the fact that the linearized version of the elastic operator does not satisfy the axiom of material frame-indifference [23,30]. This means that the linearized elastic energy increases when the object is rotated. This occurs because the linearized operator drops the quadratic terms. Even though the linear incremental model approximates the Navier operator as the number of steps $n \to \infty$, applying the affine transform prior to performing the elastic registration allows to decrease n, which results in a significant computational time gain.

3 Results

We illustrate the utility of the method through two experiments. First, we show how the elastic warping can succesfully recover the nonlinear deformation caused in the brain due to autopsy and fixation. Subsequently, we present a more ambitious experiment, where we use the pairwise surface correspondence to obtain a warp between brain images of different subjects. As will be seen, this is a more challenging problem, being inherently ill-posed.

3.1 Registration of ex-vivo Scans with the Corresponding in-vivo Scan

In this case, the imaging protocol for the ex-vivo tissue is different due to the reduced T1 contrast observed post-mortem, so a Multi Echo Flash protocol is used. This makes the pre-processing required to obtain the surfaces for the ex-vivo images a little more challenging, but does not affect the registration algorithm proposed here.

We present in figure 1 the result of the volumetric warp applied to the ex-vivo image so that it matches the in-vivo one. The resulting correspondence is almost perfect, since the underlying anatomy is the same and the deformation is a truly mechanical one. However, we remind the reader that the correspondence is not perfect near the lateral ventricles, because none of the cortical surfaces we have used crosses that area.

Also, it should be noted that in this case only the surfaces from one hemisphere were used in the process, as we only had one hemisphere available for the ex-vivo imaging. Nevertheless, the resulting match is excellent, and highlights the insensitivity of the procedure to the underlying image contrast, as the geometric features are of course invariant to the contrast properties.

3.2 Inter-subject Registration

In this section, we show results from a comparison of our morphing method with the morph produced by the publicly available version of HAMMER [31][1] . We selected eleven subjects for which we had labels that had been manually drawn on the surface [33] and we morphed each of them on a randomly chosen subject

[1] We would like to mention that the HAMMER version we have uses the gray/white matter segmentation produced by FAST [32] exclusively to produce the attribute vectors. As such, it is possible that results improve with different inputs to the attribute vector.

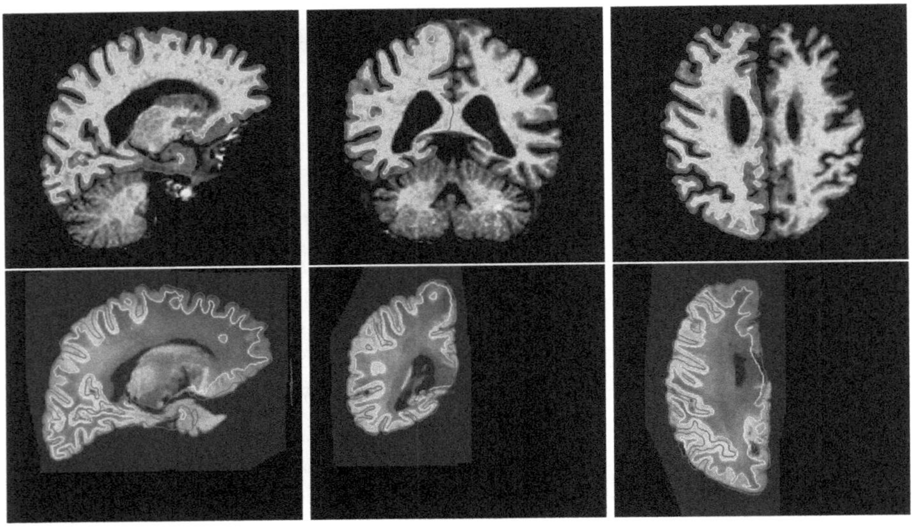

Fig. 1. Results of the surface-driven morph between an ex-vivo hemisphere and an in-vivo scan of the same subject. Surfaces are from the in-vivo data (pial surface in red and gray/white surface in yellow).

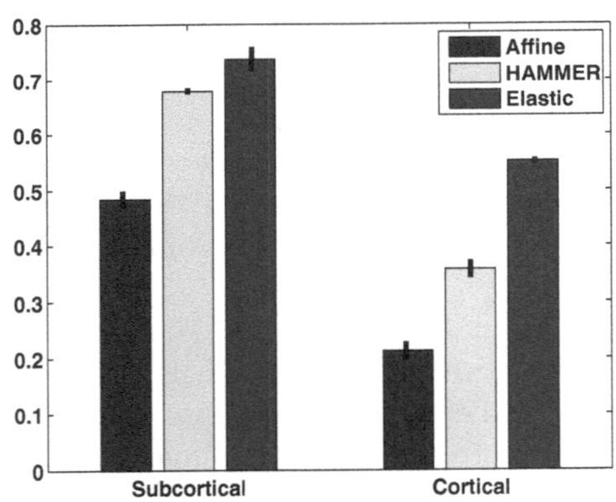

Fig. 2. Average DICE measures with standard error for cortical and subcortical areas over 10 brains. As expected, the measure for cortical areas shows the surface-based morph out-performs HAMMER by 20%. Surprisingly, HAMMER is also out-performed for sub-cortical areas, although our morph does not use any information from these regions.

which played the role of template. We then performed a DICE measure separately for the cortical and subcortical areas and compared the results produced by FLIRT [34] (i.e. 12 DOFs) and HAMMER.

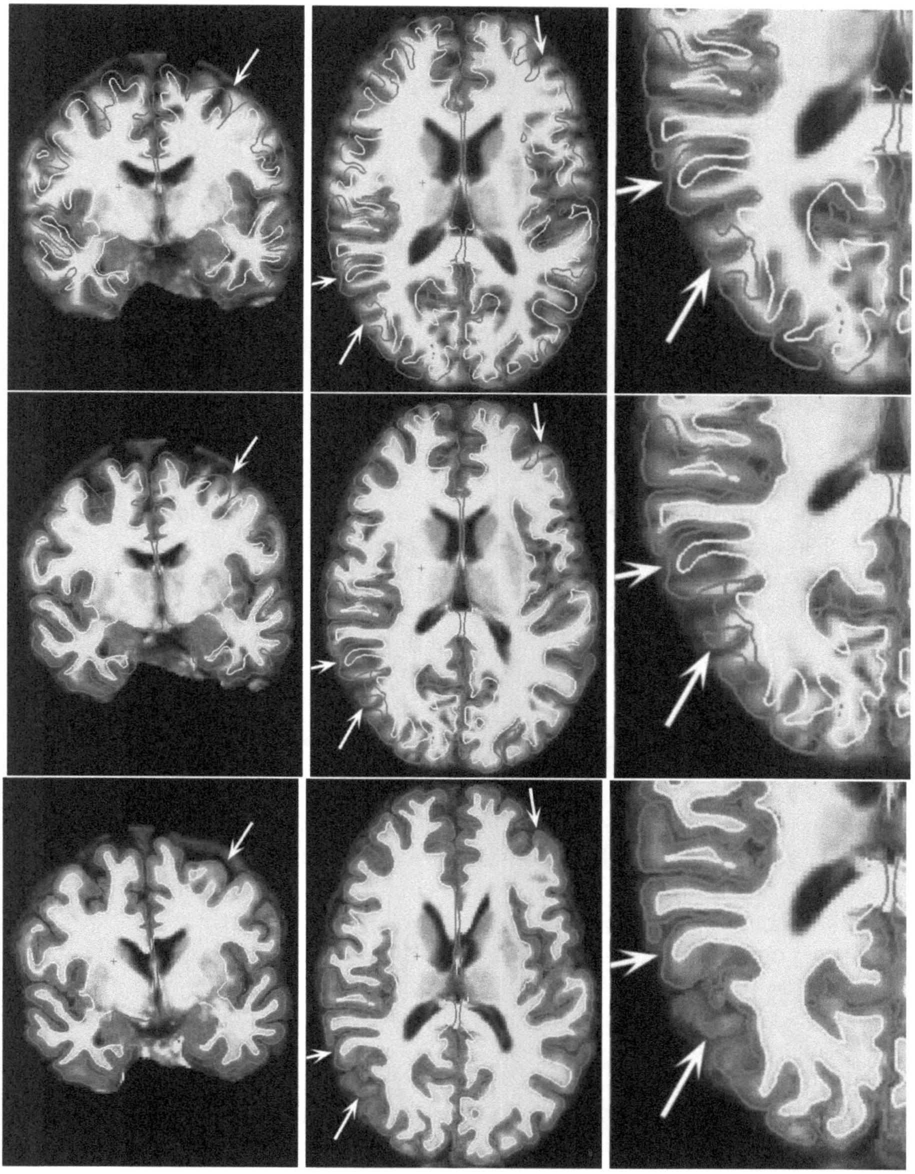

Fig. 3. Visual Comparison of inter-subject registration. Surfaces are from the atlas (pial surfaces in red and gray/white surfaces in yellow). Upper row - FLIRT. Middle row - HAMMER. Bottom row - result of the surface-based morph. It is apparent the HAMMER result is trapped in local minima in certain regions, which does not happen for the surface-based morph. Gyri where large differences occur emphasized with an arrow. It seems reasonable to believe local mis-registrations occur due to a poor initialization.

The validation measures we used were DICE measures on two sets of labels. Using [35], we created a label volume independently for each brain image with each of the major subcortical structures. In addition, we filled the cortical ribbon with manual surface-based labels from [33] for each of the subjects to generate volumetric labels for surface folding patterns. The DICE results were divided into two sets to illustrate the differences in these structures: the sparse displacement fields were explicitly generated to align cortical folds. The degree to which the volumetric morph generated from the surface registration also aligns subcortical regions thus reflects how well predicted the position and shape of subcortical structures are from the folding patterns, with potential implications for neurodevelopment.

To be more specific, the measure we used to compare the degree of overlap between two volumes V_1 and V_2 for a set of labels $S = \{s_i, i = 1 \dots n\}$ is given by

$$\mathrm{DICE}_S\left(V_1, V_2\right) = \frac{\sum_{i=1}^{n} \left|\left[V_1 = s_i\right] \cap \left[V_2 = s_i\right]\right|}{\sum_{i=1}^{n} \left|\left[V_1 = s_i\right] \cup \left[V_2 = s_i\right]\right|} \tag{10}$$

The morph was executed with $n = 13$ iterations for the linear incremental model and the results are summarized in figure 2. An example of the alignment achieved is shown in figure 3. As was to be expected, the cortical measure is higher by 20% for the surface driven morph than HAMMER (as can be seen in figure 3, HAMMER can get caught in local minima, resulting in over-deformed gyri). Surprisingly, the results also show we outperform HAMMER for subcortical regions, despite the lack of any specific information from these regions in the morph.

4 Conclusion and Future Work

We presented a technique for computing a dense volumetric registration field that was shown to align cortical folding patterns as well as deep brain structures. This was achieved by using a surface-driven morph, together with a regularizer taken from the theory of elasticity to compute a volumetric registration.

Another finding from the present study that has potentially interesting neuroscientific applications is that the alignment of cortical folds also appears to align subcortical structures, indicating that the folds are good predictors of the position/shape of deep brain regions.

In future work, we will use this volumetric field to initialize a volumetric registration algorithm to further align non-cortical structures. We anticipate that this technique will resolve one of the main difficulties with volumetric registration: they do not in general align cortical folding patterns.

Acknowledgments

Support for this research was provided in part by the National Center for Research Resources (P41-RR14075, R01 RR16594-01A1 and the NCRR BIRN Morphometric Project BIRN002, U24 RR021382), the National Institute for Biomedical Imaging and Bioengineering (R01 EB001550), the National Institute for

Neurological Disorders and Stroke (R01 NS052585-01) as well as the Mental Illness and Neuroscience Discovery (MIND) Institute, and is part of the National Alliance for Medical Image Computing (NAMIC), funded by the National Institutes of Health through the NIH Roadmap for Medical Research, Grant U54 EB005149. Information on the National Centers for Biomedical Computing can be obtained from http://nihroadmap.nih.gov/bioinformatics.

References

1. Maintz, J., Viergever, M.: A survey of medical image registration. Medical Image Analysis 2(1), 1–36 (1998)
2. Thompson, P., Hayashi, K., et al.: Detecting dynamic and genetic effects on brain structure using high-dimensional cortical pattern matching. In: Proc. International Symposium on Biomedical Imaging 2002 (2002)
3. Fischl, B., Sereno, M.I., Tootell, R., Dale, A.M.: High-resolution inter-subject averaging and a coordinate system for the cortical surface. Human Brain Mapping (8), 272–284 (1999)
4. Davatzikos, C., Bryan, N.: Using a deformable surface model to obtain a shape representation of the cortex. IEEE Trans. Med. Imag. 15(6), 785–795 (1996)
5. Bajcsy, R., Kovacic, S.: Multi-resolution elastic matching. Computer Vision, Graphics, and Image Processing 46, 1–21 (1989)
6. Davatzikos, C.: Spatial transformation and registration of brain images using elastically deformable models. Computer Vision and Image Understanding 66(2), 207–222 (1997)
7. Christensen, G., Joshi, S., Miller, M.: Volumetric transformation of brain anatomy. IEEE Trans. Med. Imaging 16(6), 864–877 (1997)
8. Fischl, B., Salat, D.H., van der Kouwe, A.J., Segonne, F., Dale, A.M.: Sequence-independent segmentation of magnetic resonance images. NeuroImage 23(1), 69–84 (2004)
9. Peckar, W., Schnorr, C., Rohr, K., Stiehl, H.S.: Parameter-free elastic deformation approach for 2d and 3d registration using prescribed displacements. J. Math. Imaging Vis. 10(2), 143–162 (1999)
10. Ferrant, M., Nabavi, A., Macq, B.M., Jolesz, F.A., Kikinis, R., Warfield, S.K.: Registration of 3d intraoperative mr images of the brain using a finite element biomechanical model. IEEE Trans. Med. Imaging 20(12), 1384–1397 (2001)
11. Toga, P.M., Toga, A.W.: A surface-based technique for warping three-dimensional images of the brain. IEEE Trans. Med. Imaging 15(4), 402–417 (1996)
12. Peckar, W., Schnorr, C., Rohr, K., Stiehl, H.S.: Two-step parameter-free elastic image registration with prescribed point displacements. In: ICIAP (1), pp. 527–534 (1997)
13. Collins, D., LeGoualher, G., Caramanos, Z., Evans, A., Barillot, C.: Cortical constraints for non-linear cortical registration. In: Proceedings of the International Conference on Visualization in Biomedical Computing, pp. 307–316 (1996)
14. Liu, T., Shen, D., Davatzikos, C.: Deformable registration of cortical surfaces via hybrid volumetric and surface warping. NeuroImage 22, 1790–1801 (2004)
15. Segonne, F., Dale, A.M., et al.: A hybrid approach to the skull-stripping problem in mri. NeuroImage 22, 1160–1175 (2004)
16. Dale, A.M., Fischl, B., Sereno, M.I.: Cortical surface-based analysis i: Segmentation and surface reconstruction. NeuroImage 9(2), 179–194 (1999)

17. Fischl, B., Sereno, M.I., Dale, A.M.: Cortical surface-based analysis ii: Inflation, flattening, and a surface-based coordinate system. NeuroImage 9(2), 195–207 (1999)
18. Fischl, B., Liu, A., Dale, A.M.: Automated manifold surgery: Constructing geometrically accurate and topologically correct models of the human cerebral cortex. IEEE Trans. Med. Imaging 20(1), 70–80 (2001)
19. Segonne, F., Grimson, E., Fischl, B.: Genetic algorithm for the topology correction of cortical surfaces. In: Christensen, G.E., Sonka, M. (eds.) IPMI 2005. LNCS, vol. 3565, pp. 393–405. Springer, Heidelberg (2005)
20. Fischl, B., Dale, A.M., Sereno, M.I., Tootell, R., Rosen, B.: A coordinate system for the cortical surface. NeuroImage, (7) (1998)
21. Bookstein, F.: Principal warps: Thin-plate splines and the decomposition of deformations. IEEE Transactions on Pattern Analysis and Machine Intelligence 11(6), 567–585 (1989)
22. Rueckert, D., Sonoda, L., Hayes, C., Hill, D., Leach, M., Hawkes, D.: Non-rigid registration using free-form deformations: Applications to breast mr images. IEEE Trans. Med. Imag. 18(8), 712–721 (1999)
23. Ciarlet, P.: Mathematical Elasticity. Three-Dimensional Elasticity. vol. I, North-Holland, Amsterdam (1988)
24. Zienkewickz, O., Taylor, R.: The Finite Element Method. McGraw Hill Book Co. New York (1987)
25. Freitag, L., Plassman, P.: Local optimization-based untangling algorithms for quadrilateral meshes (2001)
26. Si, H., Gaertner, K.: Meshing piecewise linear complexes by constrained delaunay tetrahedralizations. In: Proceedings of the 14th International Meshing Roundtable 2005, pp. 147–163 (2005)
27. Si, H.: On refinement of constrained delaunay tetrahedralizations. In: Proceedings of the 15th International Meshing Roundtable (2006)
28. Balay, S., Buschelman, K., Eijkhout, V., Gropp, W.D., Kaushik, D., Knepley, M.G., McInnes, L.C., Smith, B.F., Zhang, H.: PETSc users manual. Technical Report ANL-95/11 - Revision 2.1.5, Argonne National Laboratory (2004)
29. Balay, S., Gropp, W.D., McInnes, L.C., Smith, B.F.: Efficient management of parallelism in object oriented numerical software libraries. In: Arge, E., Bruaset, A.M., Langtangen, H.P. (eds.) Modern Software Tools in Scientific Computing, pp. 163–202. Birkhäuser Press (1997)
30. Picinbono, G., Delingette, H., Ayache, N.: Non-linear and anisotropic elastic soft tissue models for medical simulation. In: ICRA2001: IEEE International Conference Robotics and Automation, Seoul Korea (2001) Best conference paper award.
31. Shen, D., Davatzikos, C.: Hammer: Hierarchical attribute matching mechanism for elastic registration. IEEE Trans. Med. Imaging 21(11), 1421–1439 (2002)
32. Zhang, Y., Brady, M., Smith, S.: Segmentation of brain mr images through a hidden markov random field model and the expectation maximization algorithm. IEEE Trans. Med. Imag. 20(1), 45–57 (2001)
33. Desikan, R., Segonne, F., Fischl, B., et al.: An automated labeling system for subdividing the human cerebral cortex on mri scans into gyral based regions of interest. NeuroImage 31(3), 968–980 (2006)
34. Jenkinson, M., Bannister, P., Brady, J., Smith, S.: Improved optimisation for the robust and accurate linear registration and motion correction of brain images. NeuroImage 17(2), 825–841 (2002)
35. Fischl, B.: Automatically parcellating the human cerebral cortex. Cerebral Cortex 14, 11–22 (2004)

A Recursive Anisotropic Fast Marching Approach to Reaction Diffusion Equation: Application to Tumor Growth Modeling

Ender Konukoglu*, Maxime Sermesant, Olivier Clatz, Jean-Marc Peyrat, Hervé Delingette, and Nicholas Ayache

Asclepios Research Project, INRIA Sophia Antipolis, France
ender.konukoglu@sophia.inria.fr

Abstract. Bridging the gap between clinical applications and mathematical models is one of the new challenges of medical image analysis. In this paper, we propose an efficient and accurate algorithm to solve anisotropic Eikonal equations, in order to link biological models using reaction-diffusion equations to clinical observations, such as medical images. The example application we use to demonstrate our methodology is tumor growth modeling. We simulate the motion of the tumor front visible in images and give preliminary results by solving the derived anisotropic Eikonal equation with the recursive fast marching algorithm.

1 Introduction

One of the main gaps between mathematical models explaining biological phenomena and medical applications is due to the inconsistency between the number of observations available clinically and needed mathematically. While building more realistic models is very important to improve our insight on the general phenomena, creating reduced models is essential in using mathematical models in specific clinical situations.

Reaction-diffusion equations like:

$$u_t = \nabla \cdot (D\nabla u) + f(u) \tag{1}$$

arise in many different biological models, where one describes the change of a density u in time with an anisotropic diffusion characterized by the tensor D and a reaction term $f(u)$. We can give examples to such situations like tumor growth, electrophysiology and wound healing. However, available observations are often sparse and incomplete and these models are often computationally costly. Thus, making the adjustment of complete models to a specific case is difficult. This is why reduced models are of great interest. In the case of Equation 1, one can

* This work has been partly supported by the European Health-e-Child project (IST-2004-027749) and by the CompuTumor project (http://www-sop.inria.fr/asclepios/projects/boston/).

N. Karssemeijer and B. Lelieveldt (Eds.): IPMI 2007, LNCS 4584, pp. 687–699, 2007.
© Springer-Verlag Berlin Heidelberg 2007

approximate the motion of a single iso-contour of u in terms of its arrival times T using the anisotropic Eikonal equation

$$F\sqrt{\nabla T^t D \nabla T} = 1 \tag{2}$$

based on the fact that reaction-diffusion equations admit traveling wave solutions in certain cases [1,2]. This form is preferable because it does not require the whole distribution of u to compute the motion of a single iso-contour, it can reduce the number of unknown parameters based on the form of F and it can be solved faster. Aiming at clinical applications, it is essential to solve this *front tracking approximation* given in Equation 2 efficiently and accurately.

In this paper, we propose a new fast algorithm to solve the anisotropic Eikonal equation and improve the current front tracking approximation by taking into account the convergence properties of the reaction-diffusion equations. For demonstration, we apply these methods to tumor growth modeling, more specifically, to modeling glial based ones. These tumors account for approximately 40-45% of all primary intracranial tumors, forming the largest class in this pathology, [3]. Characteristics of this type of tumors vary a lot within the group, and when faced with one, understanding its aggressiveness and correct grading is very crucial in therapy planning and might improve prognosis. Although medical imaging is not the sole source of information used for this, it plays an important role in understanding the pattern and speed of invasion of healthy tissue by cancerous cells. One of the most important hints that can be obtained from images is the progression of the visible tumor front. Therefore mathematically describing and simulating the motion of this front would help the grading process and therapy planning.

2 Recursive Anisotropic Fast Marching

Anisotropic Eikonal equations, given as Equation 2, poses extra difficulties for fast numerical schemes compared to its isotropic counterpart, $F|\nabla T| = 1$. There have been different ways proposed to solve such equations or in general convex, static Hamilton-Jacobi equations using single-pass methods [4], or iterative methods [5,6]. Single-pass methods start from points where time (T) values are already known and follow the characteristic direction of the PDE to compute T at other points. This approach is based on the fact that in equations such as Eqn. 2, the value of T at a point is only determined by a subset of its neighboring points, which lie along the characteristic direction [7]. In isotropic case these methods are very efficient because they follow gradient direction, which coincides the characteristic direction [8]. In other words, they only use immediate neighbors of a point with lower values of T to compute the new arrival time at that point using an upwind scheme. In the anisotropic case, characteristic direction does not necessarily coincide with gradient direction and the same idea used for isotropic case yields false results, see Fig. 1. In order to deal with this, Sethian and Vladimirsky enlarged the neighborhood around a point used to compute

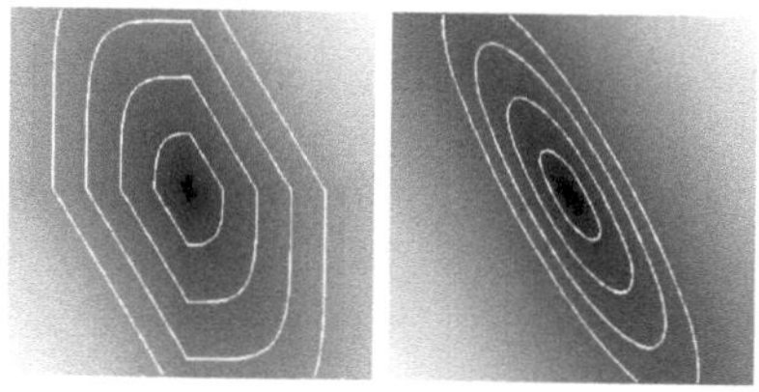

Fig. 1. $F\sqrt{\nabla T^t D \nabla T}$ with a constant anisotropic D solved using isotropic Fast Marching Method (left) and the solution solved by anisotropic methods (right)

the new arrival time such that characteristic direction remains within the neighborhood [4]. But size of the enlarged neighborhood increases with increasing anisotropy of D. This would result in large number of points used to calculate new values and a high computational load in case of high anisotropies. Iterative methods start from an initial distribution of T, use an upwind, monotone and consistent discretization of the equation and iterate over the domain until convergence [5]. However, depending on the spatial variation of D these methods might need high number of iterations to converge and they need an ordering of the mesh to sweep the domain, which might not be trivial to obtain for general meshes.

2.1 Algorithm

Recursive anisotropic fast marching, proposed here, is based on the single-pass idea and it uses immediate neighborhood to compute arrival times. As a novel step, it includes a recursive correction scheme taking into account the fact that due to anisotropy the immediate neighborhood used for computation may not always contain the characteristic direction. This algorithm works efficiently under general meshes, very high anisotropies and highly varying D fields. Moreover, it can be applied to more general forms of static, convex Hamilton-Jacobi equations, which is beyond the scope of this article.

Algorithm 1. Anisotropic Fast Marching: Initialization

for all $X \in KNOWN$ **do**
  for all $Y_i \in \mathcal{N}(X)$ and $Y_i \in FAR$ **do**
    compute $T(Y_i) \leftarrow \text{UPDATE}(Y_i, X)$
    remove Y_i from FAR and add Y_i to $TRIAL$
  end for
end for

The overall algorithm is similar to the original fast marching method proposed for the isotropic Eikonal equation. The main differences are the recursive correction scheme and the computation of T values. The initialization steps are the same: we go over points whose value are already known (kept in the $KNOWN$ list), compute their unknown neighbors' values using only known points (kept in the FAR list) trial T values and add these neighbors to the $TRIAL$ list while removing them from the FAR list, see Algorithm 1. By neighborhood $\mathcal{N}(X)$ we mean all points directly connected to the point X in some preferred connectivity sense (e.g. 4-8 in 2D and 6-18-26 in 3D cartesian grid). The isotropic fast marching algorithm follows same operations throughout its main loop. The $TRIAL$ point with the minimum value of T, Y, is removed from the $TRIAL$ list, added to the $KNOWN$ list, trial values of unknown neighbors of Y are computed, if they are in the FAR list they are added to the $TRIAL$ list and removed from the FAR one, and if they are already in the $TRIAL$ list their values are updated.

In order to take into account the anisotropy, we insert the recursive correction in the main loop. Before trial values of unknown neighbors of Y are computed, we recompute its known neighbors' values. The reason for this is that when values of these points were computed Y was not used since it was not known. Hence, in their computation the characteristic direction may not have been contained in their known neighborhood, which was used to compute their T value. If we obtain a lower value of T during the recomputation we update the value and add the point to the $CHANGED$ list, which holds known points whose values have been changed. This correction is based on the fact that the lowest T value for a point is obtained when the characteristic direction is contained in the neighborhood used for the computation [6]. Every time the main loop restarts it checks if the $CHANGED$ list is empty, if this is not the case then instead of taking a point from the $TRIAL$ list it takes from the $CHANGED$ list. In other words the main loop tries to empty the $CHANGED$ list first. The pseudo code for the algorithm gives a clear summary in Algorithm 2.

2.2 Local Solver

Up to now we have not detailed the computation of $T(X)$ value using $\mathcal{N}(X)$. We have defined $\mathcal{N}(X)$ as the set of immediate neighbors of X and naturally there exists a set of elements corresponding to this neighborhood, set of triangles ($\triangle_X$) in 2D or set of tetrahedras (TET_X) in 3D. $T(X)$ is calculated inside every element using linear interpolation between nodes and solving a minimization problem, $T(X) = f_{1D}(X,Y)$ for 1D, $T(X) = f_{2D}(X,Y,Z)$ for 2D and $T(X) = f_{3D}(X,Y,Z,W)$ for 3D, using nodes of the element neighboring X.

$$f_{1D}(X,Y) = T(Y) + \frac{[\mathbf{v}_{1D}^t D^{-1}\mathbf{v}_{1D}]^{1/2}}{F} \tag{3}$$

$$f_{2D}(X,Y,Z) = \min_{p\in[0,1]}\{T(Y)p + T(Z)(1-p) + \frac{[\mathbf{v}_{2D}(p)^t D^{-1}\mathbf{v}_{2D}(p)]^{1/2}}{F}\} \tag{4}$$

$$f_{3D}(X,Y,Z,W) = \min_{p,q\in[0,1]\times[0,1]}\{[T(Y)p + T(Z)(1-p)]q + T(W)(1-q) + \frac{[\mathbf{v}_{3D}(p,q)^t D^{-1}\mathbf{v}_{3D}(p,q)]^{1/2}}{F}\} \tag{5}$$

Algorithm 2. Anisotropic Fast Marching: Main Loop with Recursive Correction

```
while TRIAL or CHANGED lists are not empty do
  if CHANGED list is not empty then
    X ← argmin_{X∈CHANGED} CHANGED
    remove X from CHANGED
  else
    X ← argmin_{X∈TRIAL} TRIAL
    remove X from TRIAL and add X to KNOWN
  end if
  for all X_i ∈ N(X) and X_i ∈ KNOWN do
    compute T̄(X_i) ← UPDATE(X_i, X)
    if T̄(X_i) < T(X_i) then
      T(X_i) ← T̄(X_i)
      add X_i to CHANGED list
    end if
  end for
  for all Y_i ∈ N(X) and Y_i ∈ TRIAL ∪ FAR do
    compute T̄(Y_i) ← UPDATE(Y_i, X)
    if Y_i ∈ TRIAL and T̄(Y_i) < T(Y_i) then
      T(Y_i) ← T̄(Y_i)
    else if Y_i ∈ FAR then
      T(Y_i) ← T̄(Y_i)
      remove Y_i from FAR and add Y_i to TRIAL
    end if
  end for
end while
```

where $\mathbf{v}_{1D} = \overrightarrow{YX}$, $\mathbf{v}_{2D}(p) = \overrightarrow{YX}p + \overrightarrow{ZX}(1-p)$ and $\mathbf{v}_{3D}(p,q) = [\overrightarrow{YX}p + \overrightarrow{ZX}(1-p)]q + \overrightarrow{WX}(1-q)$. The common term $[\mathbf{v}^t D^{-1} \mathbf{v}]^{1/2}/F$ visible in all these equations is the time difference between a point connected to X with vector $\mathbf{v}$ and $T(X)$ under the effect of the diffusion tensor D. It is derived from the group velocity idea for which the details can be found in [9].

As in the original fast marching algorithm we only use known points in $\mathcal{N}(X)$ to compute the value at X. In other words when in the case of a tetrahedral element we use Equation 5 when all nodes are known, Equation 4 when 2 nodes are known and Equation 3 when only 1 node is known, see Algorithm 3. The minimization of Equation 4 has an analytical solution however, the one in Equation 5 is not trivial. Instead of solving it with a minimization algorithm, which would increase the computational load, we use the quadratic equation in $T(X)$ obtained by discretizing equation $F\sqrt{\nabla T^t D \nabla T} = 1$ on the nodes of the tetrahedral element. We check if this computed value of $T(X)$ satisfies the causality condition, which is that the characteristic direction should lie inside the element used. Practically this is just computing ∇T using the new computed $T(X)$ on the element and checking if $D\nabla T$ vector resides within the tetrahedra. If this is

Algorithm 3. Computation of $\overline{T}(X_i) = UPDATE(X_i, X)$

```
IN 2D
T̄(X_i) ← ∞
for all △(XX_iY) ∈ △^X_{X_i} = {△(XX_iY)|Y ∈ N(X_i)} do
  if Y ∈ KNOWN then
    T̄(X_i) ← min(T̄(X_i), f_2D(X, X_i, Y))
  else
    T̄(X_i) ← min(T̄(X_i), f_1D(X, X_i))
  end if
end for
IN 3D
T̄(X_i) ← ∞
for all TET(XX_iYZ) ∈ TET^X_{X_i} = {TET(XX_iYZ)|Y, Z ∈ N(X_i)} do
  if Y, Z ∈ KNOWN then
    T̄(X_i) ← min(T̄(X_i), f_3D(X, X_i, Y, Z))
  else if Y ∈ KNOWN then
    T̄(X_i) ← min(T̄(X_i), f_2D(X, X_i, Y))
  else if Z ∈ KNOWN then
    T̄(X_i) ← min(T̄(X_i), f_2D(X, X_i, Z))
  else
    T̄(X_i) ← min(T̄(X_i), f_1D(X, X_i))
  end if
end for
```

the case, the minimum lies inside the tetrahedra and it is approximated with the computed $T(X)$. If this is not the case we search the minimum on the triangular sides of the tetrahedra using f_{2D}. This method was proposed by Qian *et al.* [6] and it speeds up the overall algorithm greatly.

We have tested the proposed algorithm by solving $F\sqrt{\nabla T^t D \nabla T} = 1$ in 2D, 3D cartesian grid and on surfaces using triangulation. These results are shown in Fig. 2. Computation times for these results can be found in Table 1, where we also compare our algorithm with the sweeping algorithm proposed in [6], for which we used our own implementation done in the best way possible. Comparison is only done for cases in 2D cartesian grid based on the examples provided in the mentioned reference. The sweeping method has been iterated until convergence, where the maximum number of iterations was 12 in the variable D case. In the recursive anisotropic fast marching algorithm the size of the $CHANGED$ list did not exceed 3 for these cases. The following computational times were obtained with Matlab7.1 for 2D cases and C++ for 3D cases on a 2.4GHz Intel Pentium machine with 1Gb of RAM. Cases given in Table 1 correspond to images shown in Fig. 2. The proposed algorithm is fast and visually accurate even in the case of very high and variable anisotropy. Moreover, applying the explained method to general meshes bears no difficulty. In our experiments with triangular meshes on 2D and on surfaces, the algorithm was appearently much faster.

Table 1. Computational times

Case (D is anisotropic in all cases)	Sweeping Method [6] (seconds)	Fast Marching (seconds)
2D: constant D, 64×64 grid	24.43	16.15
2D: constant D, 128×128 grid: Fig. 2(a)	91.06	63.39
2D: spirally varying D, 64×64 grid: Fig. 2(c)	80.6076	13.56
2D: spirally varying D, 128×128 grid	319.34	49.48
3D: constant D, $64 \times 64 \times 18$ grid: Fig. 2(g)		26
3D: helix D, $64 \times 64 \times 64$ grid: Fig. 2(h)		65
3D: constant D, 13000 node mesh: Fig. 2(e)		2

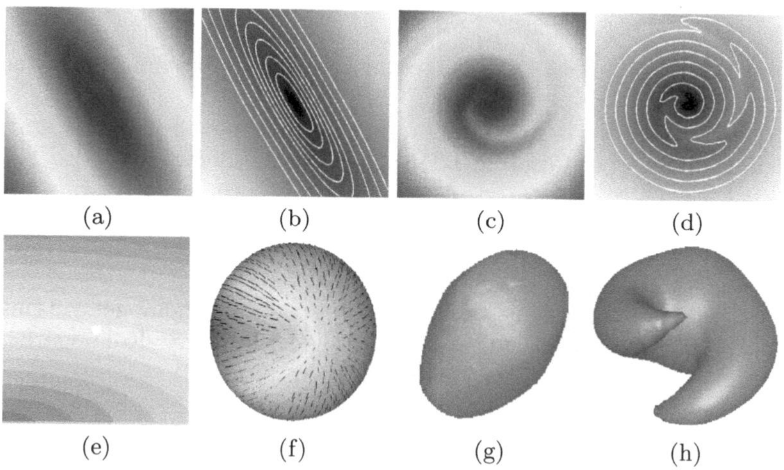

Fig. 2. a) 2D cartesian grid, high anisotropy in 120° increasing distance from blue to red, b) iso-contours of a, c) 2D cartesian grid, D is highly anisotropic inside a spiral following it, isotropic in other regions, d) iso-contours of c, e) 2D triangular mesh with 13000 nodes anisotropy in x direction, colors represent iso-contours, f) 2D triangular mesh on a surface D is anisotropic and principle eigenvector is shown in black lines, colors represent iso-contours, g) 3D cartesian grid, anisotropic D h) 3D cartesian grid, D is highly anisotropic inside a helix following it, isotropic in other regions.

3 Approximating the Front Motion: Time Varying Speed

Reaction-diffusion models explain the change of the distribution of densities by combination of diffusion and reaction processes. Usually, one is interested in the motion of an iso-contour (front) of such distributions, which can be attained by an anisotropic Eikonal equation $F\sqrt{\nabla T^t D \nabla T} = 1$. In this approximation, the speed term $F = F(x)$ is normally set to a function constant in time [10]. But the convergence properties of the reaction-diffusion system is then neglected, which can lead to important errors. Taking this into account, we propose to use

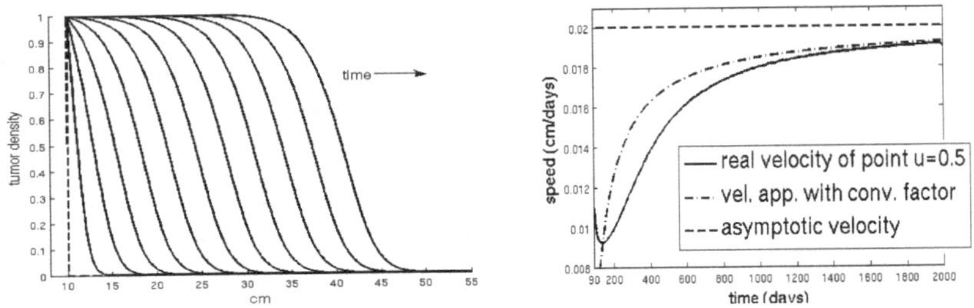

Fig. 3. Left: Front evolution starting from a step function under Equation 6. Right: Speed of the point $u = 0.5$ on the front is plotted along with the asymptotic speed and the speed approximation including convergence term.

a time varying function $F = F(x, T)$ to have a better approximation of the front motion.

In order to obtain the approximation for the motion of the front we start from the reaction-diffusion equation in 1-D with constant coefficients:

$$u_t = du_{xx} + \rho f(u) \qquad (6)$$
$$u(x, 0) = U$$

where $f(u)$ has a homogeneous stable state at $u = 1$ and a homogeneous unstable state at $u = 0$. Equation 6, which is also called the Fisher-Kolmogorov equation, admits traveling wave solutions in the form of $u(x, t) = u(x - vt) = u(\xi)$, where v is the asymptotic speed of the wavefront, [11,12]. In other words, initial conditions evolve in time to uniformly translating front shapes, see Fig. 3. This allows us to formulate the motion of a single point on the wavefront $u = u_0$ by simply describing the arrival time of the point $u = u_0$ as $T_x = 1/v$, where T is the arrival time function. The value of the asymptotic speed depends on the initial condition U. All initial conditions that are steep enough, meaning $\lim_{x\to\infty} u(x, 0) = 0$, converge to the travelling wave moving with an asymptotic speed: $2\sqrt{df'(0)}$, where $f'(0)$ denotes the derivative at $u = 0$ [1]. This suggests that for all practical modeling problems we can use this asymptotic value in the arrival time formulation to approximate the motion of the front. However, it was shown that convergence of the front speed to the asymptotic one is

$$v(t) = 2\sqrt{df'(0)} - \frac{3}{2t}\sqrt{\frac{d}{f'(0)}} \qquad (7)$$

independent of the initial condition and the u_0 value being tracked, [13,2]. This convergence rate is algebraic and rather slow. Thus, using a time varying $v(t)$ as given in Equation 7 is a better approximation of the actual speed than using the asymptotic one, see Fig. 3. The convergence to a traveling wave behavior of the Equation 6 applies to higher dimensions when coefficients are constant and the initial condition has non-curved iso-contours. In this case the initial condition converges to a traveling plane having a cross section looking as a 1D wavefront with the time varying velocity given as $v(t) = 2\sqrt{f'(0)\mathbf{n}^t D\mathbf{n}} - 3/(2t)\sqrt{\mathbf{n}^t D\mathbf{n}/f'(0)}$, where $\mathbf{n}$ is the normal of the moving plane.

Convergence properties of the reaction-diffusion equation is only valid when the front is not curved and parameters of the equation are constants. Models using Equation 1 does not necessarily have constant parameters and the front they describe can be curved. In order to formulate the motion of the general front using the construction explained above, we make the assumption that **within a voxel** front is planar and parameters of the reaction-diffusion equation are constants, which are taken as values at that voxel. Under these assumptions, we derive the arrival time formulation for the front in 3D as:

$$|\nabla T| = 1/v(t) = \left[2\sqrt{f'(0)\mathbf{n}^t D\mathbf{n}} - \frac{3}{2T}\sqrt{\frac{\mathbf{n}^t D\mathbf{n}}{f'(0)}} \right]^{-1} \tag{8}$$

where $\mathbf{n}$ can be replaced by $\nabla T/|\nabla T|$. This simply leads to the anisotropic Eikonal equation given as:

$$\sqrt{\nabla T^t D \nabla T} = \frac{2\sqrt{f'(0)}T}{4f'(0)T - 3} \tag{9}$$

4 Application: Predicting the Motion of Tumor Front

There has been a large amount of mathematical models proposed to describe the growth dynamics of glial tumors, e.g. [14,15]. Those trying to explain growth and invasion dynamics based on observations from medical images, describe these processes using cell densities and average behavior [15], consisting of fewer equations and parameters. Such models are based on reaction-diffusion formalism introduced in [11], which uses reaction-diffusion type equations. Although these models are successful in explaining underlying dynamics of the tumor growth, they encounter some problems in adapting to patient data. Given images, in order to compute the growth they require tumor cell density values at every point. What is available in conventional modalities like MR and CT is not cell densities, but an enhanced homogeneous looking region and its boundary with the brain tissue, the tumor front, as seen in Fig. 4(a). Moreover, numerical load of such simulations, depending on the mesh size used, can be very heavy.

In this paper for demonstration, we use the front approximation given in Section 3 to describe the motion of the tumor front and use the recursive anisotropic fast marching algorithm to simulate its motion. The specific reaction-diffusion model we base our approximation on is proposed by Clatz *et al.* [16]. Their model for tumor growth can be given by the following reaction-diffusion equation:

$$\frac{\partial u}{\partial t} = \nabla \cdot (D(\mathbf{x})\nabla u) + \rho u(1-u) \tag{10}$$

$$D(\mathbf{x})\nabla u \cdot \vec{n}_{\Sigma} = 0 \tag{11}$$

where u is the tumor cell density, $D(\mathbf{x})$ is the diffusion tensors, ρ is the proliferation rate of tumor cells and $\vec{n}_\Sigma$ is the normal direction at the boundaries, which in the case of the brain are skull and ventricles. The first term in Equation 10, $\nabla \cdot (D(\mathbf{x})\nabla u)$, defines invasion of brain tissue by tumor cells using a diffusion process. The second term in the same equation, $\rho u(1-u)$ describes proliferation of tumor cells using logistic growth. Based on the experiments done by Giese *et al.* [17], which shows that tumor cells move faster on myelin sheath, $D(\mathbf{x})$ is set as a spatially varying tensor, becoming isotropic on grey matter and anisotropic on white matter following fiber tracts as defined in Equation 12.

$$D(\mathbf{x}) = \begin{cases} d_g\mathbf{I} & \text{if } \mathbf{x} \text{ is in grey matter} \\ \mathbf{V}(Diag(d_w\lambda_1, 0, 0) + d_g\mathbf{I})\mathbf{V}^t & \text{if } \mathbf{x} \text{ is in white matter} \end{cases} \quad (12)$$

where d_g and d_w are speed of diffusion in grey matter and white matter respectively, $\mathbf{I}$ is the 3x3 identity matrix, λ_1 is the principal eigenvalue and $\mathbf{V}$ is the eigenvector matrix of the water diffusion tensor obtained from DT-MRI. By construction d_w/d_g can have a large value resulting in a high anisotropy.

The front approximation for this model can be given as:

$$\sqrt{\nabla T^t D \nabla T} = \frac{2\sqrt{\rho T}}{4\rho T - 3} \quad (13)$$

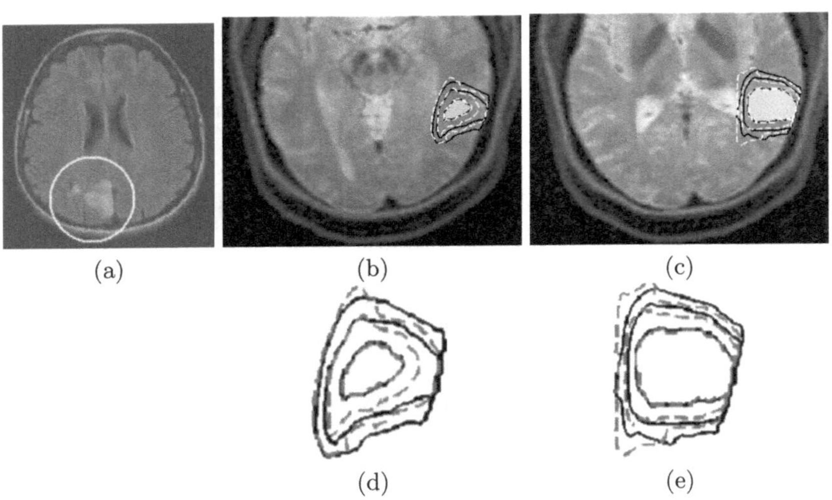

Fig. 4. a) A low grade glioma (inside the white circle) showing a single contour around a homogeneous prolongation of Flair MRI. b,c) Different axial slices of an artificially grown tumor. Grey region shows the visible part of the tumor at day 90. Black contours shows the location of $u = 0.1$ front of the artificial tumor at days 180 and 240. White contours show same locations computed by the front approximation. d,e) Same contours as shown in b,c. Black solid is the actual location and red dashed are approximated locations. Discrepancies between contours is a result of curvature and boundary effects, which were not taken into account in the current state of the front approximation.

In order to have a realistic simulation and to compare the results of the front approximation and the reaction-diffusion model, we have grown an artificial tumor using real boundary conditions, white-grey matter segmentation and diffusion tensor images (DTI) taken from a healthy subject. We set the diffusion coefficients as $d_g = 0.001$ and $d_w = 0.1$ and the proliferation rate as an average rate of $\rho = 0.012$ [15]. The artificial tumor is grown for 240 days using the formulation given in Equation 10 and 11. We took the time of diagnosis as day 90, where we obtain the first image as in Fig. 4(b) and observe the tumor front, taken as $\gamma = \{\mathbf{x}|u(\mathbf{x}, 90) = 0.1\}$. We set this contour as the boundary condition of Equation 13 ($T(\gamma) = 90$) and we solved it using the recursive anisotropic fast marching algorithm. Fig. 4(c) and (d) compare the motion of the front computed by the reaction-diffusion model (solid blue curves) and computed by the front approximation (dashed red curves). Observe that the speed of invasion is well captured by the front approximation formulation given in Equation 13. The pattern of invasion on the other hand shows some differences visible in Fig. 4. There are two reasons for these differences: (1) the front approximation is based on un-curved tumor fronts, however, curvature plays a role in smoothing and slowing down the front, (2) the Neumann boundary conditions are not captured by the approximation which creates differences near the boundary. The computation time for reaction-diffusion model to grow the tumor for 240 days was 4500 seconds while fast marching algorithm computed the motion of the γ front throughout the whole brain in 250 seconds, which corresponds to a growth simulation of 2500 days. This yields a speed up of nearly 180 folds. Implementations were done in C++ using GMM library on a 2.4GHz Intel Pentium processor with a 1Gb memory.

5 Discussions

In this paper, we proposed the recursive anisotropic fast marching algorithm and to use the time varying speed term in front approximation formulation for reaction-diffusion models in order to create the link between mathematical models and clinical observations. The fast marching algorithm is successful in handling high anisotropies, which are often encountered in biological modeling, on general meshes. We demonstrated the usage of proposed tools by simulating the motion of the tumor front, visible in medical images.

Formulating the motion of the tumor front sets a link between observations in images and the mathematical models explaining the growth dynamics. Fast and efficient algorithms like the recursive fast marching method explained here gives us an easy tool to adapt growth models to specific patient cases and do simulations. It can also help us quantify the speed of growth and invasion by solving an inverse problem to estimate the parameters like diffusion coefficients. We have seen that the formulation is successful in capturing the speed of invasion, however, the patterns have differences. In the future, we would like to explore new ways to integrate the effect of curvature and boundaries in the formulation to get better approximation.

Although we have concentrated on tumor growth modeling in this paper, front approximations for reaction-diffusion equations and the proposed algorithm can be useful in other modeling problems as well. Such an example is the electrophysiological model of the heart, where one is interested in computing the excitation times throughout the organ. This problem is similar to tumor growth, in the sense that it requires following the motion of a front. Moreover, this application requires fast computations, which is possible with the method presented in this work.

The recursive fast marching method explained here is a general tool and can be used for lots of different applications than simulating the motion of a wavefront, such as fiber tracking or geophysics. Moreover, the algorithm can also be used for solving general static, convex Hamilton-Jacobi equations encountered in computer vision and material science. The future work consists in characterizing convergence properties of the recursive fast marching algorithm.

References

1. Aronson, D., Weinberger, H.: Multidimensional nonlinear diffusion arising in population genetics. Advances in Mathematics 30 (1978)
2. Ebert, U.: W.S.: Front propagation into unstable states: universal algebraic convergence towards uniformly translating pulled fronts. Physica D: Nonlinear Phenomena 146 (2000)
3. Tovi, M.: Mr imaging in cerebral gliomas analysis of tumour tissue components. Acta Radiol. Suppl. (1993)
4. Sethian, J., Vladimirsky, A.: Ordered upwind methods for static hamilton-jacobi equations: theory and algorithms. SIAM J. Numer. Anal. 41 (2003)
5. Kao, C., Osher, S., Tsai, Y.: Fast sweeping methods for static hamilton-jacobi equations. SIAM J. Numer. Anal. 42 (2005)
6. Qian, J., Zhang, Y., Zhao, H.: A fast sweeping method for static convex hamilton-jacobi equations. UCLA Comp. and App. Math. Reports, 06-37 (2006)
7. Kevorkian, J.: Partial differential equations: Analytical solution techniques. Springer, Heidelberg (2000)
8. Sethian, J.: Level set methods and fast marching methods: Evolving interfaces in computational geometry, fluid mechanics, computer vision, and materials science. Cambridge University Press, Cambridge (1999)
9. Qian, J., Symes, W.: Paraxial eikonal solvers for anisotropic quasi-p travel times. J. Comp. Physics, 173 (2001)
10. Keener, J., Sneyd, J.: Mathematical physiology. Springer, Heidelberg (1998)
11. Murray, J.: Mathematical Biology. Springer, Heidelberg (2002)
12. Maini, P., McElwain, D., Leavesley, D.: Traveling wave model to interpret a wound-healing cell migration assay for human peritoneal mesothelial cells. Tissue Eng. 10 (2004)
13. Bramson, M.: Convergence of solutions of the kolmogoroff equations to traveling waves. Mem. Am. Math. Soc (1983)
14. Cristini, V., Lowengrub, J., Nie, Q.: Nonlinear simulation of tumor growth. Journal of Math. Biol. 46 (2003)
15. Swanson, K., Alvord, E., Murray, J.: Virtual brain tumours (gliomas) enhance the reality of medical imaging and highlight inadequacies of current therapy. British Journal of Cancer, 86 (2002)

16. Clatz, O., Sermesant, M., Bondiau, P., Delingette, H., Warfield, S., Malandain, G., Ayache, N.: Realistic simulation of the 3d growth of brain tumors in mr images coupling diffusion with biomechanical deformation. IEEE T.M.I. 24(10) (2005)
17. Giese, A., Kluwe, L., Laube, B., Meissner, H., Berens, M., Westphal, M.: Migration of human glioma cells on myelin. Neurosurgery, 38(4) (1996)

Population-Based Fitting of Medial Shape Models with Correspondence Optimization

Timothy B. Terriberry[1], James N. Damon[2], Stephen M. Pizer[1], Sarang C. Joshi[4], and Guido Gerig[1,3]

[1] Dept. of Computer Science, Univ. of North Carolina, Chapel Hill, NC 27599, USA
[2] Dept. of Mathematics, Univ. of North Carolina, Chapel Hill, NC 27599, USA
[3] Dept. of Psychiatry, Univ. of North Carolina, Chapel Hill, NC 27599, USA
[4] Dept. of Biomedical Engineering, Univ. of Utah, Salt Lake City, UT 84112, USA
{tterribe,pizer,gerig}@cs.unc.edu, jndamon@math.unc.edu, sjoshi@sci.utah.edu

Abstract. A crucial problem in statistical shape analysis is establishing the *correspondence* of shape features across a population. While many solutions are easy to express using boundary representations, this has been a considerable challenge for medial representations. This paper uses a new 3-D medial model that allows continuous interpolation of the medial manifold and provides a map back and forth between it and the boundary. A measure defined on the medial surface then allows one to write integrals over the boundary and the object interior in medial coordinates, enabling the expression of important object properties in an object-relative coordinate system. We use these integrals to optimize correspondence during model construction, reducing variability due to the model parameterization that could potentially mask true shape change effects. Discrimination and hypothesis testing of populations of shapes are expected to benefit, potentially resulting in improved significance of shape differences between populations even with a smaller sample size.

1 Introduction

In questions of statistical shape analysis, the foremost is how such shapes should be represented. The number of parameters required for a given accuracy and the types of deformation they can express directly influence the quality and type of statistical inferences one can make. Most methods of establishing correspondence in a population use features on the boundary [1,2,3,4], since in many imaging modalities the interior of objects have a uniform appearance with poorly localized features. However our research uses a medial model parametrization, which represents a solid object using a skeleton of a lower dimension and naturally expresses intuitive changes such as "bending", "twisting", and "thickening", but where establishing correspondence is more difficult. As a descriptor of *shape*, the medial axis can be used to provide a detailed quantitative and qualitative analysis that simpler object descriptors, such as volume, surface area, pose, etc., cannot. Pizer et al. give an overview and comparison of definitions and numerous methods for computing of a medial axis [5]. Yet the reversal of the original

N. Karssemeijer and B. Lelieveldt (Eds.): IPMI 2007, LNCS 4584, pp. 700–712, 2007.
© Springer-Verlag Berlin Heidelberg 2007

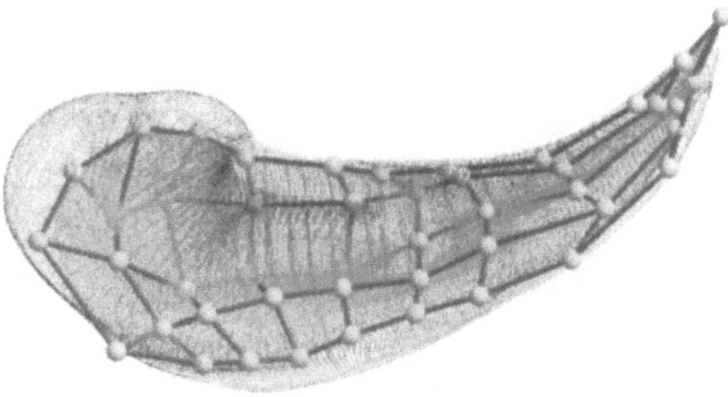

Fig. 1. A dense sampling of a medial model of a left caudate defined continuously using subdivision surfaces, with volume overlap $V_{\text{Dice}} = 93.46\%$

relationship, from an object describing a medial axis to a medial axis describing an object, is the critical idea that makes medial representations effective image analysis tools. It replaces an inherently unstable and ill-defined problem—computing the medial axis of an object from its boundary—with a well-defined and stable one: computing the boundary of an object from its medial axis. An object is then modeled by deforming a template medial axis until the associated boundary matches that of the target object.

Näf et al. use the medial axis to measure local bone thickness and to describe the sulco-gyral foldings of the human brain [6]. Zhang et al. use the medial axis for articulated shape matching [7]. They use Siddiqi et al.'s shock detection algorithm to construct the medial axis and classify the voxels according to Giblin and Kimia's taxonomy directly via [8]. Golland et al. use "fixed-topology skeletons" for 2D shape classification [9,10]. Similar to Golland's fixed-topology skeletons, Pizer et al. introduce a sampled medial representation called (discrete) *m-reps* used for segmentation [11,12]. Bouix et al. apply the medial axis to estimate the local width of the hippocampus [13]. They propose two different approaches to solving the problem of identifying corresponding points between different subjects: projecting the axis onto a plane and rigidly aligning it or using nonlinear deformations to warp the axis to a common template shape. Styner et al. [14] use sampled medial descriptions for shape modeling and analysis in clinical studies of hippocampi and lateral ventricles. They use boundary correspondence established via spherical harmonics (SPHARMs) when initializing the medial model fitting process, but do not enforce it during the individual optimization for each subject, allowing features to wander independently.

Statistical analysis of populations requires appropriate solutions for *robust parameterizations* of shape models and *establishing correspondence* across a class of objects that is meaningful given the specific task and application domain. An inherent problem in any shape representation, one must ensure that the parameters of the representation in some sense control the "same" features of the resulting shape. Otherwise, noise in the parameterization can overwhelm the size of any shape change effect, reducing or eliminating the power of the tests.

The method presented here does *not* provide yet another means for determining the correspondence between shapes. Instead, it takes the stance that correspondence is inherently specific to the problem domain. Without some input governing the process whereby the representation is constructed results are unpredictable. Our modeling scheme can use any existing correspondence on the boundary, defined via prior or learned knowledge of the target population, to establish correspondence on the medial representation. This in turn requires a unique link between locations on the boundary and on the medial parametrization. In principle, the medial geometry provides an intrinsic link between the boundary and the medial axis that allows one to use the appropriate representation for the desired analysis task. Every (non-singular) point on the medial axis lies at the center of ball which is tangent to the boundary in two places, and the field of vectors from the points on the axis to their associated points of tangency, called *spokes*, provides this link. This relationship was explored in [15], and [16,17] provide an analysis of the differential geometry in arbitrary dimension. However with the discrete version of m-rep models [11], the connection with the boundary is given only at a coarse set of discrete points and the interpolation given by [18] to recover a dense sampling does not respect the intrinsic medial geometry. Correspondence is established only approximately using a regularizing term in the model fit optimization, which requires determining an appropriate weight and trades off homology for goodness of fit. More recent work on interpolation does respect the intrinsic medial geometry [19], but it sacrifices the uniqueness of the representation, requires expensive numeric integration, and only approximately interpolates the original model.

An alternative approach to discrete skeletons, *cm-reps*, considers the dual problems of designing a discrete computer representation and computing a continuous mathematical representation from it as a coupled system [20,21,22,23]. A continuous representation inherently provides the necessary connection between the medial axis and the boundary and thus is chosen for this paper.

2 Group-Wise Model Fitting with Explicit Correspondence Optimization

This paper addresses the problem of producing a collection of models that represent a set of shapes to be used in statistical tests. The basic approach is to start with a template object, described medially with a fixed branching topology, to align a copy of that template to each target shape, and then to deform it to match. This work only considers fitting a model to an existing, segmented shape, such as a binary image or a triangulated surface.

The following sections begin by describing a method for sampling a continuous medial axis and then show how this sampling can be used to approximate medial integrals. The complete process for fitting a single model to a single target

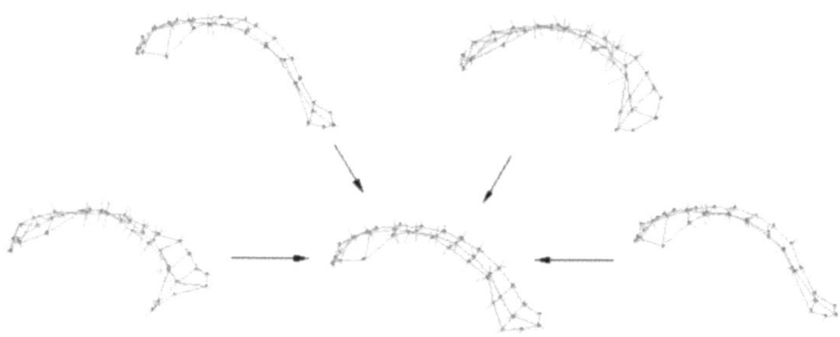

Fig. 2. The entire population of objects is mapped to a common coordinate system to optimize correspondence

shape follows. This involves aligning a template to the target shape and deforming it using a multi-scale constrained optimization. Finally, the process for a single shape is extended to a technique for producing a population of models with a common correspondence. This is integrated directly into the deformation stage by constructing deformations approximately transverse to the fitting process. The models are mapped to a common coordinate system and the control points are adjusted to achieve a parameterization that matches an explicit correspondence given on the boundary, as illustrated in Figure 2. This is done by taking advantage of the inherent link between the boundary and the medial axis given by a continuous medial model, moving the problem of formulating correspondence to the boundary, where most of the information lies.

The specific discretized representation for the target shapes used here are binary images, $I(x) : \mathbb{R}^3 \to \{0,1\}$, defined to be 1 when x is in the shape's interior, and 0 elsewhere. Other representations like triangle meshes could be used as well, as described in [24].

2.1 Approximating Medial Integrals

The main mathematical tool used in this paper is the medial integral, which we approximate via numeric integration. This section describes the procedure.

Sampling the Medial Axis. The first step is to define a sampling of the medial axis. We use the subdivision surface approach presented in [23] for our 3D continuous medial axis representation, illustrated in Fig. 1. This divides the medial axis into a fixed number of patches which can be evaluated analytically at arbitrary points using B-splines or other fast evaluation methods [25]. Each patch gives a continuous function m, the position of a point on the axis, and r, the radius of the maximally inscribed sphere, defined over a square domain $(u, v) \in [0,1]^2$. The exact expressions for m and r and their derivatives can be found in [24] and are omitted for space reasons. The unit spoke vectors $U^{\pm}$ pointing towards the two points of tangency on the boundary and the two boundary points themselves are computed directly from derivatives of m and r by

$$U^{\pm} = -\nabla r \pm \sqrt{1 - \|\nabla r\|^2} \cdot \mathcal{N} , \qquad \mathcal{B}^{\pm} = m + rU^{\pm} , \tag{1}$$

where ∇r is the Riemannian gradient and $\mathcal{N}$ is the unit normal vector to the medial surface. A single sample is then placed at the center of each patch with extent $(\Delta u, \Delta v) = (1, 1)$ and recursively subdivided until

$$\|\mathcal{B}_u^{\pm} \Delta u \times \mathcal{B}_v^{\pm} \Delta v\| < \tau^2 \tag{2}$$

for some threshold τ, which ensures the sample area of the boundary is sufficiently small on both sides of the medial axis. A sample set $\mathbb{S}$ is then constructed from these samples, containing the tuple (m, r, U) and all its derivatives, where U is one of the two spoke vectors $U^{\pm}$. Each point on the medial axis contributes two sample values, one for each spoke vector, in order to integrate over both sides of the medial axis.

Numeric Integration in Medial Coordinates. Damon showed how to rewrite volume and surface integrals of a medially defined region in terms of medial integrals [26]. We begin with a motivational example: some simple volume integrals over the object interior Ω for moments up through second order, which we will use to align a template to the target shape. Given a Borel measurable and Lebesgue integrable function $g : \Omega \to \mathbb{R}$,

$$\tilde{g}(m, r, U) \triangleq \int_0^1 g(m + t \cdot rU) \cdot \det\left(\mathbf{I} - t \cdot rS_{\text{rad}}\right) dt , \tag{3}$$

$$\int_{\Omega} g \, dV = \int_{\tilde{M}} \tilde{g} \, dM = \int_{\tilde{M}} \tilde{g} \cdot (U \cdot \mathcal{N}) \, dA . \tag{4}$$

Here $\tilde{M}$ is the *double* of the medial axis M, indicating that integration is performed over both sides, with $\mathcal{N}$ chosen to point towards the same side as U. The term $dM \triangleq (U \cdot \mathcal{N}) dA$ is the *medial measure* defined by Damon [26], which accounts for the failure of U to be orthogonal to M. $\mathbf{I}$ is the identity matrix and S_{rad} is Damon's *radial shape operator*, which measures the rate of change of U along M. In three dimensions S_{rad} can be expressed as a 2×2 matrix computed from derivatives of m and r as described in [24]. Then for simple functions g we can write analytic expressions for $\tilde{g}$ using the *mean radial curvature*, $H_{\text{rad}} \triangleq \frac{1}{2}\text{trace}(S_{\text{rad}})$, and the *Gaussian radial curvature*, $K_{\text{rad}} \triangleq \det\left(S_{\text{rad}}\right)$:

$$\text{For } g(x) = 1,\ \tilde{g} = r - r^2 H_{\text{rad}} + \frac{1}{3} r^3 K_{\text{rad}} \ . \tag{5}$$

$$\begin{aligned}\text{For } g(x) = x,\ \tilde{g} = m \cdot & \left(r - r^2 H_{\text{rad}} + \frac{1}{3} r^3 K_{\text{rad}} \right) \\ & + U \cdot \left(\frac{1}{2} r^2 - \frac{2}{3} r^3 H_{\text{rad}} + \frac{1}{4} r^4 K_{\text{rad}} \right) \ .\end{aligned} \tag{6}$$

$$\begin{aligned}\text{For } g(x) = xx^T,\ \tilde{g} = mm^T & \cdot (r - r^2 H_{\text{rad}} + \frac{1}{3} r^3 K_{\text{rad}}) \\ & + (mU^T + Um^T) \cdot \left(\frac{1}{2} r^2 - \frac{2}{3} r^3 H_{\text{rad}} + \frac{1}{4} r^4 K_{\text{rad}} \right) \\ & + UU^T \cdot \left(\frac{1}{3} r^3 - \frac{1}{2} r^4 H_{\text{rad}} + \frac{1}{5} r^5 K_{\text{rad}} \right) \ .\end{aligned} \tag{7}$$

The complete volume integrals may now be approximated for any choice of $\tilde{g}$ by

$$\int_{\Omega} g \, dV \approx \sum_{(m,r,U) \in \mathbb{S}} \tilde{g} \cdot \Delta M \ , \qquad \Delta M \triangleq |U \cdot (m_u \times m_v)| \Delta u \Delta v \ . \tag{8}$$

These integrals allow the computation of the volume, center of mass, and second order moment tensor of a medially-defined object. Surface integrals over the boundary are even easier. For a Borel measurable function $h : \mathcal{B} \to \mathbb{R}$,

$$\int_{\mathcal{B}} h \, d\mathcal{B} = \int_{\tilde{M}} \tilde{h} \cdot \det (\mathbf{I} - r S_{\text{rad}}) \ dM \ , \tag{9}$$

$$\approx \sum_{(m,r,U) \in \mathbb{S}} \tilde{h} \cdot (1 - 2r H_{\text{rad}} + r^2 K_{\text{rad}}) \Delta M \ , \tag{10}$$

where $\tilde{h}(m, r, U) \triangleq h(m + rU)$.

2.2 Single-Subject Model Fitting

Before describing the correspondence optimization, this section outlines the fitting process for a single target shape. First, a similarity transform is applied to the template to align it to the target using its center of mass, volume, and the eigenvectors of the second order moment tensor to define the translation, scale, and rotation, respectively. More robust alignment methods are possible, but this was sufficient for the objects considered in this paper.

We then convert the binary image to a multiscale level-set representation I_σ by convolving it with a Gaussian for various choices of σ and choosing a level ℓ_0 for each scale that maximizes the volume overlap with the original image. We deform the template to match the level set at the coarsest scale, and then successively refine it to match each finer scale. Our objective function is given by the squared error integrated over the surface using (10):

$$F_I^\sigma = \sum_{(m,r,U) \in \mathbb{S}} (I_\sigma(m + rU) - \ell_0)^2 \cdot w_i \ , \quad w_i = |\det (\mathbf{I} - r S_{\text{rad}}) \, \Delta M| \tag{11}$$

We use nonlinear conjugate gradient (CG) optimization, with a quadratic penalty function to ensure the model is valid—that is, to ensure that the square root in (1) is real and that no spokes cross inside the object. At points outside the feasible region, the weight w_i is taken to be zero if (1) cannot be evaluated, and the absolute value in w_i handles the case of overfolding. The nonlinear CG method periodically restarts when the next step fails certain orthogonality constraints. We call all the steps between two restarts a *macro step* and hold $\mathbb{S}$ and w_i fixed for its duration. This avoids the need to compute their derivatives and avoids descent towards the trivial global minimum of a zero-volume Ω.

2.3 Correspondence Optimization

In order to optimize the correspondence of a group of medially-defined objects $\mathcal{M}^{(j)}$, we borrow an idea from recent work on computing unbiased, symmetric atlases [27,28] and represent the known correspondence via a series of maps ϕ_j that project each shape into a common coordinate system. In the absence of any other prior information, this coordinate system is constructed by Procrustes aligning the target shapes and mapping each point to the linear average of all corresponding points. The map is extended to medially defined points (m, r, U) by projecting $m+rU$ onto the target shape along the U direction, which is normal to the model boundary. This leads to an objective function for correspondence:

$$F_C^j = \sum_{(m,r,U)\in\mathbb{S}} (\phi_j(m,r,U) - \mu_i)^2 \cdot w_i \ . \tag{12}$$

Here μ_i is the average of the *medially* corresponding points after projection by ϕ_j, that is, those from the same patch, with the same (u, v) coordinates, in multiple models. We use the same sampling $\mathbb{S}$ for each model to ensure this is well-defined, continuing to subdivide in all the models so long as any one violates the threshold in (2). Like w_i, we fix μ_i for the duration of a CG macro step.

In order to avoid interfering with the model fitting process, the deformations allowed in the correspondence optimization are constructed to be approximately transverse to it. That is, we define a *base model* $\mathcal{M}_0^{(j)}$—taken to be the latest result of the model fitting optimization—and restrict the motion of control points so that their corresponding limit points "slide" along it. For small deformations, within the approximation accuracy of the interpolation, this does not change the shape of the model. The neighborhood of each limit point on $\mathcal{M}_0^{(j)}$ is parameterized using the bilinear map Φ given in [29], which is G^2 and has simple analytic derivatives. Then the control point values that give the desired limit points are recovered by solving a linear system. This system is fixed for a given subdivision surface topology and admits a sparse *LU* decomposition, whose size is linear in the number of control points [30], making this extremely efficient.

Optimization then proceeds by trading back and forth between model fitting and correspondence optimization. This ensures the approximate transversality holds as the the process nears convergence, since this approximation is not very accurate for the initial, large step sizes. First a macro step optimizing F_I^σ is taken for each model, then μ_i is updated and a macro step optimizing F_C^j is taken for each subject j. The two processes do not compete with each other, and so no weight parameter is needed to trade off between the two. The problem is well over-constrained for any modest level of subdivision, so an exact match with the input boundary correspondence will not, in general, be obtained. However, the result conforms to growth or deformation consistent with the medial model, even if the input correspondence does not.

3 Results

We applied our method to a population of synthetic ellipsoids and to a collection of 3D brain objects provided by an ongoing clinical neuroimaging study.

3.1 Ellipsoid Data

A simple test population was created from an ellipsoid deformed by a set of 20 diffeomorphisms of the form [31]

$$\Psi_{\alpha,\beta,\gamma}(x,y,z) \triangleq \begin{bmatrix} x \\ e^{\gamma x}(y\cos(\beta x) - z\sin(\beta x)) \\ e^{\gamma x}(y\sin(\beta x) + z\cos(\beta x)) + \alpha x^2 \end{bmatrix} , \tag{13}$$

where the α, β, and γ parameters control bending, twisting, and tapering, respectively. These parameters were drawn from normal distributions with standard deviations 1.5, 1.05, and 2.12, respectively, and the resulting deformation was applied to a standard ellipsoid with axis lengths of $(1/2, 1/3, 1/4)$ centered around the origin. The result was converted to a $128 \times 128 \times 128$ binary image.

For this data set, ground-truth correspondence is known. Therefore ϕ_j is set to $\Psi^{-1}_{\alpha_j,\beta_j,\gamma_j}$. Although this map does describe the deformation applied to obtain the target object, it may not be physically realistic, since one would not, for example, expect two points on the top and bottom of an ellipsoid with the same x coordinate to still have the same x coordinate after bending it. We constructed a template by averaging models fit without correspondence optimization, and fit it to the population using 10 scale levels for σ with an iteration limit of $K_{\max} = 200$ macro steps. At each level, the subdivision threshold τ was set to $\frac{1}{2}\sigma$. Each iteration comprised one macro step optimizing the binary image match, F_I^{σ}, followed by one macro step optimizing the correspondence match for each subject, F_C^j. The optimization only stopped when one of the stopping criteria for CG was encountered for every model, which in this case meant it proceeded to the iteration limit at every scale. The average Dice coefficient of the volume overlap (also computed with a medial integral) was $V_{\text{Dice}} = 96.88\%$, which was actually slightly higher than the 96.72% obtained without correspondence optimization. The continuing evolution of the correspondence optimization even after the image match optimization has converged for a particular subject likely gives it the chance to escape a local minimum and accounts for this small improvement.

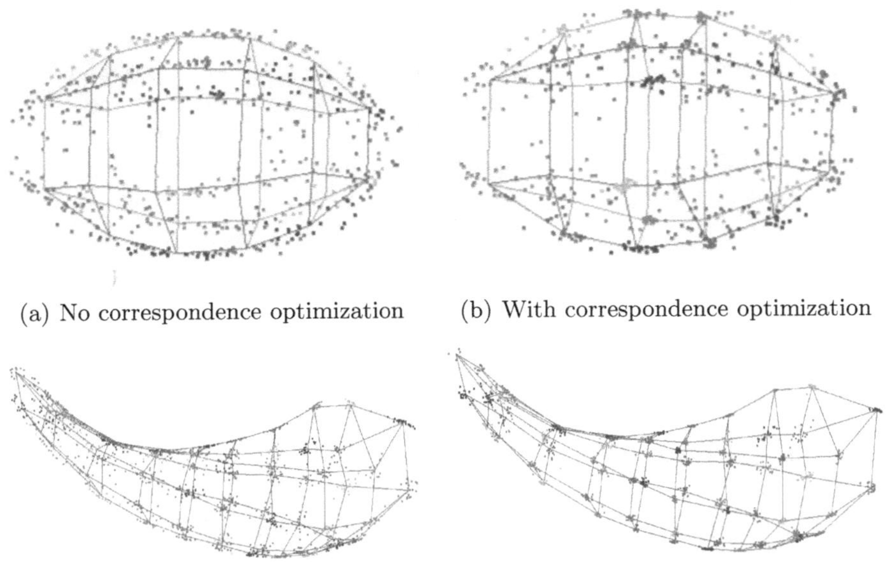

(a) No correspondence optimization (b) With correspondence optimization

(c) No correspondence optimization (d) With correspondence optimization

Fig. 3. Clusters of corresponding points in the reference coordinate system, both with and without correspondence optimization enabled. Deformed ellipsoids (top) and left caudate structures (bottom) are shown. Points with the same color belong to the same cluster. The wireframe model connects the cluster centers. Enabling correspondence optimization gives much tighter clusters, especially near the center of the ellipsoid, where the parameterization is most ambiguous. Significant improvement is also shown in the tail region of the caudate.

In order to visually evaluate how well the surface correspondence was maintained by the medial model, the top row of Fig. 3 shows the endpoints of the spokes associated with each control point mapped into the reference coordinate system via ϕ_j for the models fit both with and without correspondence optimization enabled. When correspondence optimization is enabled, these points form much tighter clusters, especially towards the center of the ellipsoid, where the radius changes more slowly. This is precisely the place where the parameterization is most ambiguous, allowing the correspondence match to produce tight clusters without sacrificing fit quality. The clusters on the ends are not as tight, but for the most part they are still well-separated, unlike their counterparts obtained by fitting models individually.

3.2 Caudate Data

Models were also fit to real-world data from an ongoing clinical longitudinal pediatric autism study [32]. Ten subjects each from the autistic and typical groups were chosen and their segmented MRI scans from age four used to test the correspondence optimization. Volumetric segmentations of voxel objects were transformed into surface mesh models and parametrized by SPHARMs [33], with boundary correspondence given by aligning their first-order ellipsoids. This could be replaced by any other correspondence established via analysis of surface geometry or by additional measurements reflecting anatomical or functional geometry. The SPHARM surface was then converted to a triangle mesh and ϕ_j was chosen to map to their average after Procrustes alignment. Ray-triangle intersections computed with the algorithm in [34] were used to project $m+rU$ onto the SPHARM surface, and OBB trees [35] were used to reduced the number of triangles that needed to be tested. To speed up these tests even further, the most recent triangle intersecting each ray was cached, and the OBB tree was searched only if the intersection test against the cached triangle failed. The same scales, iteration limits, and subdivision thresholds were used during optimization as for the ellipse data. The results in the bottom row of Fig. 3 are even more striking than for the ellipse data, especially in the tail region.

4 Conclusion

Sect. 2.1 developed medial integrals as a fundamental tool for taking advantage of the link between the medial axis and the boundary. This allows properties of the boundary to be expressed on the boundary but be evaluated in medial coordinates. This gives continuous medial models advantages of both representations. Although Damon introduced the concept, this work is the first application to demonstrate that they are easily computable and to apply them to computational problems. These medial integrals are applied for computing volume overlap to evaluate goodness-of-fit and for computing second-order moments to align models to a common position, orientation and scale, demonstrating the way medial integrals can be used to compute basic object properties. Most important is the demonstration that these properties can be computed without first converting to a boundary representation, avoiding the additional complexity and approximation error such a conversion would involve.

This paper describes a new correspondence optimization method that works in tandem with the model fitting process to produce a group of models with a common parameterization. Key is a fitting process of a continuous medial model to a population of objects. We show how specific knowledge of correspondence can be incorporated into the model fitting process. This eliminates excess variability in the parameterization of the objects which could mask real statistical effects of the shape change. The correspondence match optimization introduced does not sacrifice the quality of the fit. Instead, it operates transversely to the fitting process up to the tolerance of the model, requiring no tuning parameter to trade off between the two.

The procedure described here serves as a good example of the reasons to use a continuous medial representation over a discrete one and is a non-trivial example of how the link between the medial axis and the boundary can be exploited to give a medial model the advantages of the latter without sacrificing those of the former. The sliding process used to remove ambiguities in the parameterization of the axis would not be possible with a discrete representation. Although the amount of variability this process eliminates is visually remarkable, little has been done to evaluate the quantitative effect this has on the power of statistical tests, and more work needs to be done in this area.

Acknowledgments. This research is supported by the NIH NIBIB grant P01 EB002779. The MRI images of infants, caudate images and expert manual segmentations are funded by NIH RO1 MH61696 and NIMH MH64580.

References

1. Kotcheff, A.C.W., Taylor, C.J.: Automatic construction of eigenshape models by direct optimization. Medical Image Analysis (MEDIA) 2(4), 303–314 (1998)
2. Davies, R.H., Twining, C.J., Cootes, T.F., Waterton, J.C., Taylor, C.J.: A minimum description length approach to statistical shape modeling. IEEE Transactions on Medical Imaging 21(5), 525–537 (2002)
3. Heimann, T., Wolf, I., Williams, T., Meinzer, H.P.: 3D active shape models using gradient descent optimization of description length. In: Christensen, G.E., Sonka, M. (eds.) IPMI 2005. LNCS, vol. 3565, pp. 566–577. Springer, Heidelberg (2005)
4. Cates, J., Meyer, M., Fletcher, P.T., Whitaker, R.T.: Entropy-based particle systems for shape correspondence. In: Proc. of the International Workshop on Mathematical Foundations of Computational Anatomy (MFCA'06), Copenhagen, Denmark, (October 2006) pp. 90–99 (2006)
5. Pizer, S.M., Siddiqi, K., Székely, G., Damon, J.N., Zucker, S.W.: Multiscale medial loci and their properties. International Journal of Computer Vision 55(2–3), 155–179 (2003)
6. Näf, M., Kübler, O., Kikinis, R., Shenton, M.E., Székely, G.: Shape characterization and recognition of 3D organ shape in medical image analysis using skeletonization. In: Proc. of the IEEE/SIAM Workshop on Mathematical Methods in Biomedical Image Analysis (MMBIA'96), San Francisco, California, (June 1996) pp. 139–150 (1996)
7. Zhang, J., Siddiqi, K., Macrini, D., Shokoufandeh, A., Dickinson, S.: Retrieving articulated 3-D models using medial surfaces and their graph spectra. In: Proc. of the 5th International Workshop on Energy Minimization Methods in Computer Vision and Pattern Recognition, St. Augustine, Florida, November 2005 (2005)
8. Malandain, G., Ayache, N., Bertrand, G.: Topological segmentation of discrete surfaces. In: Proc. of IEEE CVPR'91, Maui, Hawaii, (June 1991), pp. 444–449 (1991)
9. Golland, P., Grimson, W.E.L., Kikinis, R.: Statistical shape analysis using fixed topology skeletons: Corpus callosum study. In: Kuba, A., Sámal, M., Todd-Pokropek, A. (eds.) IPMI 1999. LNCS, vol. 1613, pp. 382–387. Springer, Heidelberg (1999)
10. Golland, P., Grimson, W.E.L.: Fixed topology skeletons. In: Proc. of IEEE CVPR'00. vol. 1., Head Island, South Carolina, (June 2000), pp. 10–17 (2000)
11. Pizer, S.M., Fritsch, D.S., Yushkevich, P.A., Johnson, V.E., Chaney, E.L.: Segmentation, registration, and measurement of shape variation via image object shape. IEEE Transactions on Medical Imaging 18, 851–865 (1999)

12. Joshi, S.C., Pizer, S.M., Fletcher, P.T., Thall, A., Tracton, G.S.: Multi-scale 3-D deformable model segmentation based on medial description. In: Insana, M.F., Leahy, R.M. (eds.) IPMI 2001. LNCS, vol. 2082, pp. 64–77. Springer, Heidelberg (2001)
13. Bouix, S., Pruessner, J.C., Collins, D.L., Siddiqi, K.: Hippocampal shape analysis using medial surfaces. NeuroImage 25(4), 1077–1089 (2005)
14. Styner, M.A., Gerig, G., Joshi, S.C., Pizer, S.M.: Automatic and robust computation of 3D medial models incorporating object variability. International Journal of Computer Vision 55(2–3), 107–122 (2003)
15. Giblin, P.J., Kimia, B.B.: A formal classification of 3D medial axis points and their local geometry. IEEE PAMI 26(2), 238–251 (2004)
16. Damon, J.N.: Smoothness and geometry of boundaries associated to skeletal structures I: Sufficient conditions for smoothness. Annales de l'Institut Fourier 53(6), 1941–1985 (2003)
17. Damon, J.N.: Smoothness and geometry of boundaries associated to skeletal structures II: Geometry in the Blum case. Compositio Mathematica 140(6), 1657–1674 (2004)
18. Thall, A.: Deformable Solid Modeling via Medial Sampling and Displacement Subdivision. PhD thesis, University of North Carolina at Chapel Hill (2004)
19. Han, Q., Pizer, S.M., Damon, J.N.: Interpolation in discrete single figure medial objects. In: Proc. of the IEEE Workshop on Mathematical Methods in Biomedical Image Analysis (MMBIA'06), New York City, New York June 2006 (2006)
20. Yushkevich, P.A.: Statistical shape characterization using the medial representation. PhD thesis, University of North Carolina at Chapel Hill Department of Computer Science (2003)
21. Yushkevich, P.A., Zhang, H., Gee, J.C.: Parametric medial shape representation in 3-D via the Poisson partial differential equation with non-linear boundary conditions. In: Christensen, G.E., Sonka, M. (eds.) IPMI 2005. LNCS, vol. 3565, pp. 162–173. Springer, Heidelberg (July 2005)
22. Yushkevich, P.A., Zhang, H., Gee, J.C.: Continuous medial representation for anatomical structures. IEEE TMI 25(12), 1–18 (2006)
23. Terriberry, T.B., Gerig, G.: A continuous 3-D medial shape model with branching. In: Proc. of the International Workshop on Mathematical Foundations of Computational Anatomy (MFCA'06), Copenhagen, Denmark, (October 2006), pp. 80–89 (2006)
24. Terriberry, T.B.: Continuous Medial Models in Two-Sample Statistics of Shape. PhD thesis, University of North Carolina at Chapel Hill (2006)
25. Stam, J.: Exact evaluation of Catmull-Clark subdivision surfaces at arbitrary parameter values. In: Zorin, D., Schröder, P.(eds.): Lecture Notes for the SIGGRAPH'99 Course on Subdivision for Modeling and Animation, pp. 89–110 (1999)
26. Damon, J.N.: Global geometry of regions and boundaries via skeletal and medial integrals (2005) Preprint: `http://www.math.unc.edu/Faculty/jndamon/Skel.Str.IV.r.pdf`
27. Joshi, S.C., Davis, B., Jomier, M., Gerig, G.: Unbiased diffeomorphic atlas construction for computational anatomy. NeuroImage; Supplemental issue on Mathematics in Brain Imaging 23(Supp. 1), S151–S160 (2004)
28. Škrinjar, O., Tagare, H.: Symmetric, transitive, geometric deformation and intensity variation invariant nonrigid image registration. In: Proc. of IEEE ISBI'04, Arlington, Virginia, April 2004, pp. 920–923 (2004)

29. Loop, C.: Second order smoothness over extraordinary vertices. In: Proc. of the 2004 Eurographics/ ACM SIGGRAPH Symposium on Geometry Processing, Nice, France, July 2004, pp. 165–174 (2004)
30. Halstead, M., Kass, M., DeRose, T.: Efficient, fair interpolation using Catmull-Clark surfaces. In: Proc. of the 20th Annual SIGGRAPH Conference on Computer Graphics and Interactive Techniques, Anaheim, California, August 1993, pp. 35–44 (1993)
31. Han, Q.: Personal communication (2006)
32. Styner, M.A., Gorczowski, K., Fletcher, P.T., Jeong, J.Y., Pizer, S.M., Gerig, G.: Statistics of pose and shape in multi-object complexes using prinipal geodesic analysis. In: Yang, G.-Z., Jiang, T., Shen, D., Gu, L., Yang, J. (eds.) Medical Imaging and Augmented Reality. LNCS, vol. 4091, pp. 1–8. Springer, Heidelberg (August 2006)
33. Brechbühler, C., Gerig, G., Kübler, O.: Parameterization of closed surfaces for 3-D shape description. Computer Vision, Graphics, and Image Processing: Image Understanding 61(2), 195–170 (1995)
34. Möller, T., Trumbore, B.: Fast, minimum storage ray/triangle intersection. Journal of Graphics Tools 2(1), 21–28 (1997)
35. Gottschalk, S., Lin, M.C., Manocha, D.: OBB-tree: A hierarchical structure for rapid interference detection. In: Proc. of the 23rd Annual SIGGRAPH Conference on Computer Graphics and Interactive Techniques, August 1996, pp. 171–180 (1996)

Robust Parametric Modeling Approach Based on Domain Knowledge for Computer Aided Detection of Vertebrae Column Metastases in MRI

A.K. Jerebko[1], G.P. Schmidt[2], X. Zhou[1], J. Bi[1], V. Anand[1], J. Liu[1], S. Schoenberg[2], I. Schmuecking[1], B. Kiefer[3], and A. Krishnan[1]

[1] Siemens Medical Solutions, Inc., Malvern, PA, United States
[2] Department of Clinical Radiology, University of Munich, Munich, Germany
[3] Siemens AG Medical Solutions, Erlangen, Germany

Abstract. This study evaluates a robust parametric modeling approach for computer-aided detection (CAD) of vertebrae column metastases in whole-body MRI. Our method involves constructing a model based on geometric primitives from purely anatomical knowledge of organ shapes and rough variability limits. The basic intensity range of primary 'simple' objects in our models is derived from expert knowledge of image formation and appearance for certain tissue types. We formulated the classification problem as a multiple instance learning problem for which a novel algorithm is designed based on Fisher's linear discriminant analysis. Evaluation of metastases detection algorithm is done on a separate test set as well as on the training set via leave-one-patient-out approach.

Keywords: vertebrae metastases, computer aided diagnosis.

1 Introduction

Whole-body MRI has high sensitivity and specificity for detection of bone-marrow metastases [1],[2]. Spine metastases detection is one of the most important and time-consuming tasks. In recent years, computer aided detection (CAD) has proven to be efficient help for radiologists if used as a second reader in various applications of computed tomography (CT) and X-rays, such as colonic polyp, lung nodule, breast mass calcification detection, etc. Although lately MRI is becoming a popular screening modality, development of MRI CAD applications is more complicated than that of CT because of intensity in-homogeneity problem and higher noise level. This study evaluates a robust parametric modeling approach based on image formation and anatomical knowledge for computer-aided detection (CAD) of vertebrae column metastases in whole-body MRI.

Radiologists usually use T2 STIR pulse sequence for primary vertebrae metastases detection [1],[2]. Although a standard non-contrast protocol of the bone marrow usually implies T1-weighted SE-sequences to discriminate between benign (hemangiomas, osteochondrosis, etc.) and malignant lesions, it is not always acquired in all hospitals. Therefore our CAD scheme was developed for T2 STIR as primary pulse

N. Karssemeijer and B. Lelieveldt (Eds.): IPMI 2007, LNCS 4584, pp. 713 – 724, 2007.
© Springer-Verlag Berlin Heidelberg 2007

sequence, while resulting CAD marks are shown on T2 STIR and, if available, on T1 images for radiologist review and final diagnosis.

Our goal was to develop an algorithm suited to work with alterations in scanning protocols and pulse sequences, such as changes in the level of fat suppression, image resolution, acquisition plane (sagittal or coronal) and tolerant to severe pathological changes in organ appearance. The few methods for vertebrae column segmentation in MR images available in recent literature, such as normalized cuts approach in [3], are not suitable in the case of severe metastases where dissimilarity between healthy and affected vertebrae could be much greater than between vertebrae and other tissue. Our approach involves constructing a model based on geometric primitives from purely anatomical knowledge of organ shape and rough variability limits. The basic intensity range of primary 'simple' objects is derived from expert knowledge of image formation for certain tissue types. Our assumptions include the following: 1) spinal cord, tumors and blood vessels are among the brightest structures in the image for number of MRI pulse sequences (par ex. T2, T2 STIR, HASTE) and, 2) bones are surrounded by cortical bone that does not generate signal in MR images, and therefore it is appears black (it looks like black contour around each bone). The spinal cord detection algorithm presented in section 2 relies only on these basic assumptions. The vertebrae segmentation algorithm described in section 3 also takes into account natural periodicity within vertebral column and requires minimal amount of training data to construct vertebrae column active shape model. The candidate lesion detection and feature extraction scheme are fairly simple and therefore only briefly outlined in section 4, while the main focus is made on a novel classification scheme. The reason for development of specialized classification algorithm is the following: bone metastases detection problem is characterized by multiple manifestation of *multifocal* or *diffuse* metastatic disease, while only one CAD detection per vertebrae column segment (cervical, thoracic and lumbar) is enough to bring the structure with *multifocal* or *diffuse* pathology into radiologist attention. In case of the *focal* metastatic disease, each *focal* lesion should be indicated to the radiologist by a separate mark. We designed a novel classification algorithm for detecting at least one hit from multiple hits associating with a lesion based on Fisher's linear discriminant (FLD) analysis. Aggregation of multiple classifiers was conducted to reduce the variability of the detection system. Evaluation of metastases detection algorithm on a separate unseen test set is described in section 5. The conclusion is given in Section 6.

2 Robust Algorithm for Spinal Cord Detection

Spinal cord is one of the most reliable reference objects in the MR images and it appears consistently bright in common MRI pulse sequences (scanning protocols), for example, HASTE, T2, and T2 STIR. Other tissue intensities however vary significantly with minor changes in the scanning protocols and levels of fat suppression. The number and shape of hyperintense objects in the image other than spinal cord is not known a priory, it varies from patient to patient depending on the primary tumor location, severity of the metastatic process, amount of body fat, condition of intervertebrae disks, pathological changes in the organ appearance, etc. The method presented below allows robust fitting and segmentation of spinal cord without extraction of full collection of other objects present in the image. The preprocessing steps include image intensity in-homogeneity correction, scaling and intensity thresholding.

Naturally, the spinal cord follows three curves presented in human spine: cervical curve - convex forward, thoracic – concave forward and lumbar - convex forward. It is convinient to model it with a curve having 3 extrema points. We modeled the spinal cord as a global 4 th-order 3D-polynomial:

$$\begin{cases} x(t) = \sum_{i=0}^{n} a_{xi} t^i \\ z(t) = \sum_{i=0}^{n} a_{zi} t^i \\ y(t) \approx t \end{cases} \qquad (1)$$
$$n = 4$$

where $x(t)$ represents the variation in the spinal curve from patient side to side (coronal orientation), $z(t)$ represents the variation in the spinal curve from patient's back to front (saggittal orientation).

In this parametric representation, polynomial could be easily constrained to have sacrum (end of the vertebrae column) always pointing back:

$$if \begin{cases} a_{zn} < 0 \\ n = 4 \ (is\ even) \end{cases} \qquad (2)$$
$$then\ z(t) \to -\infty$$

Polynomial extrema points in saggittal orientation correspond to cervical, thoracic and lumbar curves. If the patient's spine also has a lateral curvature (pathology called scoliosis), it will be reflected in $x(t)$ variations. Polynomial extrema points are computed from:

$$\begin{aligned} x'(t) &= \sum_{i=1}^{n} a_{xi} i t^{i-1} = 0 \Rightarrow (x_{cj}, y_{cj}) \\ z'(t) &= \sum_{i=1}^{n} a_{zi} i t^{i-1} = 0 \Rightarrow (z_{sj}, y_{sj}) \end{aligned} \qquad (3)$$

where (x_{cj}, y_{cj}) are extrema points in coronal orientation, (z_{sj}, y_{sj}) saggittal orientation, $j=1,2,3$.

Next, we constrain the distances between polynomial extrema points in saggittal orientaion to be within natural limits of longitudinal $[D_{j,j+1\ min}, D_{j,j+1\ max}]$ and the poterior-anterior (lordotic and kyphotic) $LK_{j,j+1}$ distances between cervical, thoracic and lumbar curves:

$$\begin{aligned} &|z_{sj} - z_{sj+1}| < LK_{j,j+1} \\ &D_{j,j+1\ min} < |y_{sj} - y_{sj+1}| < D_{j,j+1\ max} \end{aligned} \qquad (4)$$

The $[D_{j,j+1\ min}, D_{j,j+1\ max}]$ and $LK_{j,j+1}$ limits were set by expert radiologist.

We also constrain the lateral distances between coronal extrema points to be within the scoliosis pathology limit *Sc*, observed from our training set.

$$|x_{sj} - x_{sj+1}| < Sc; \tag{5}$$

Scanned patient section does not necessarily contain all three curves described above, but this modeling approach allows to extrapolate and guess their approximate location. The 4th short curve, pelvic, extends from sacrovertebral articulation to coccyx and, most often, is not visible in thoracic section of the whole body scan. It could be segmented together with pelvic bones using the spinal cord points as reference points. Pelvic bone segmentation is a subject of our future work and it is not addressed in this paper.

The model parameters are estimated using random sample consensus (RANSAC) algorithm [4] with subsequent least squares based fitting refinement. The RANSAC method was adapted for parametric shape fitting with a priori knowledge of the approximate object scale in the presence of highly correlated outliers that often constitute more than 50% of the image.

n+1 sample points are needed to define n^{th} order polynomial. To speed up fitting of a polynomial of an approximately known scale (defined by the limits on the distances between the extrema points, see eq. (4)), we split the image into *M*(n+1)* sampling bins. Bins are longitudinally evenly spaced throughout the image; each bin *b* contains all axial (horizontal) slices in the region $[y_b,\ y_b + \max(y)/(M(n+1))]$. Factor *M* constraints scaling/warping degree of freedom for polynomial. The model fitting is an iterative process:

1. For each iteration *(n+1)* bins are randomly selected.
2. Then one sample point is randomly selected from each bin.
3. $\overline{a_z}$ and $\overline{a_x}$ coefficient vectors are computer by solving equations 1.
4. If condition in equations 2 is satisfied, the polynomial extrema points are computed from equations 3.
5. If all extrema constraints are satisfied, then the fitting function is evaluated within the local vicinity of the parametric model as volume *V* of bright voxels within curved cylinder built around the polynomial. The size of the vicinity is the average human spinal cord radius *R + delta*.
6. If *V>minimal_cord_volume* the least-squares method is used to refine the fitting, taking into account only the voxels within *R + delta* vicinity of the spinal cord model (this shifts model more towards the actual spinal cord center-line).
7. The fitness function is estimated again and compared to the current best model fitness.
8. The iterations 1-7 are repeated until *V/V_total_bright_voxels>Threshold* or *number_of_iterations>k*.

The convergence speed of the algorithm depends on the percentage of outliers in the image: hyperintense points in the image not belonging to the spinal cord (which, in turn, depends on the exact pulse sequence, quality of fat suppression and degree of metastatic process). Maximum number of iterations *k* is estimated as:

$$k = \frac{\log(P_o)}{\log(1 - w^m)} + \frac{\sqrt{1 - w^m}}{w^m}; \quad (6)$$

where $m=n+1$, P_o is the probability of seeing only bad samples (in our experiments it was up to 80% for some data sets), w – probability of good (inlier) samples.

The detection results were visually evaluated in 77 T2 STIR and 5 HASTE images from different hospitals. Results appeared satisfactory in all images. Segmentation accuracy was numerically evaluated using manually segmented ground truth (GT) in 35 T2 STIR images with average voxel size of 1.25x1.25x6mm. The average segmentation accuracy, estimated as ratio of overlapping of automatically detected (AD) and GT spinal cord volumes to the GT volume, was 91% with standard deviation (STD) of 14%. The accuracy of centerline position evaluated as average distance from all GT spinal cord voxels to the AD centerline was 4.4mm with STD of 1.9mm. The presence of collapsed vertebrae and edema in 1 patient (see Fig. 1) and multiple vertebrae metastasis in 12 patients did not affect the segmentation accuracy in all cases but one, where all vertebrae had severe metastatic changes of similar image intensity as spinal cord with no visible boundary. As a result spinal cord centerline was shifted toward the center of the vertebral body.

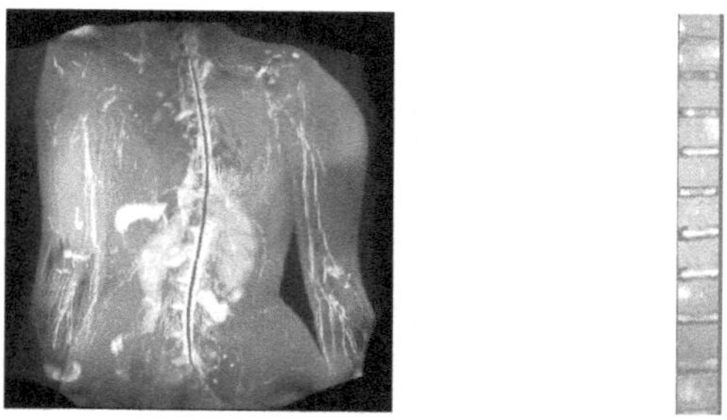

a) b)

Fig. 1. a). Spinal cord detection result shown in a maximum intensity projection image of a patient with collapsed vertebrae and edema. b) Curved MPR view of vertebrae column of another patient with several metastatic lesions. Curved MPR view was computed based on detected spinal cord.

3 Parametric Model Based Vertebrae Segmentation

Our vertebrae model is aimed to fit only the vertebrae body, excluding the processes and pedicles. It can be represented by a section of a curved cylinder adjacent to the spinal cord. The main motivations for this model are as follows. First, metastases that are present only in the pedicles but not vertebrae body are very rare and, second, processes and pedicles are not distinctly visible at the resolutions with slice thickness of ~6mm that are common for metastases screening protocols. On the other hand, when higher resolution screening images are available, vertebrae segmentation algorithm described in this paper can be used for rough vertebrae location at reduced resolution (sub-sampled images) and then other methods can be applied for refined vertebrae segmentation.

We assume that imaginary planes that separate vertebrae from each other and from inter-vertebrae disks are orthogonal to the spinal cord (see Fig. 2).

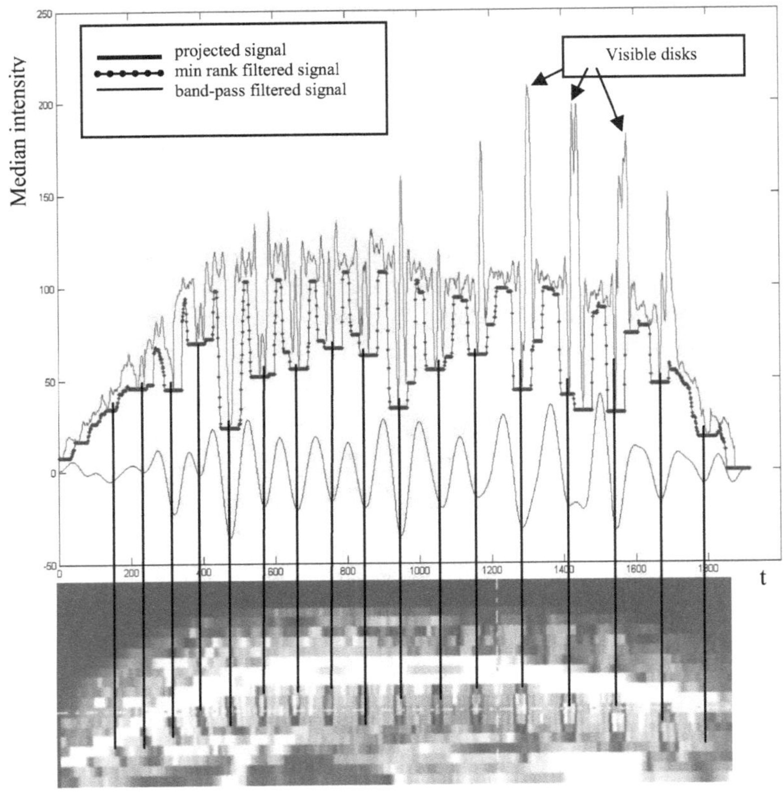

Fig. 2. Plot of projected median intensity along spinal cord and filtered signal

Vertebrae separating planes are detected by analyzing the one-dimensional signal representing the spinal column. The signal is extracted by projecting the median intensity values along the spinal cord inside the small sample circles adjacent to the front edge of the spinal cord within the planes orthogonal to it.

Normal vertebra is composed of spongy bone, containing bone marrow, which is surrounded by compact (cortical) bone. The most interesting property of cortical bone from MRI point of view is that it does not generate signal in MRI and therefore appears consistently hypointense in any pulse sequence, while vertebra and disks may change their appearance depending on the presences of metastases or other diseases (sometimes inter-vertebrae disks are not visible in the whole vertebral column).

To extract reliable information from the projected signal and skip inconsistent high intensity peaks like disks and lesions, we apply minimum rank filter with the width between the largest inter-vertebra space and shortest vertebrae that we want to detect. Next, band-pass filtering with frequency band derived from the height range of normal vertebrae body is applied to determine vertical vertebrae boundaries.

While different band of frequencies (or height thresholds) could be used in cervical, thoracic and lumbar areas for higher precision, in the current implementation we used the same band for the whole vertebrae column. Discrete Fourier transform (DFT) of the input signal is computed with a fast Fourier transform algorithm. Next, we set all the elements of the resulting vector Y to zero, which correspond to the frequencies outside of desired range. Finally, inverse Fourier transform $f(y)$ is obtained from the vector Y. The advantage of the filtered signal is that it is smooth, therefore differentiable. It is easy to find local minimums and maximums in this signal; minimums correspond to inter-vertebrae spaces and maximums to vertebrae body. Local maximums $f(m_i)$ and minimums $f(n_i)$of filtered signal are computed from:

$$\frac{\partial f}{\partial y}=0;\frac{\partial^2 f}{\partial y^2}<0;f(y)>0;\Rightarrow f(m_i); \qquad \frac{\partial f}{\partial y}=0;\frac{\partial^2 f}{\partial y^2}>0;f(y)<0;\Rightarrow f(n_i); \tag{7}$$

where y is the distance along spinal cord.

Then the precise locations of lower and upper boundary of each vertebra are found from the original signal, as two local minima $f(u_i)$ and $f(d_i)$ around the middle of each vertebra m_i, which represent the upper and lower boundary of each vertebra. The local minima that are caused by noise are removed by setting the adaptive amplitude threshold t_i for each vertebra: $f(u_i)<t_i;\quad f(d_i)<t_i$;

where $t_i = mean(f(n_{1-1}),..., f(n_{i+1})) - std(f(n_{1-1}),..., f(n_{i+1}))$.

Constraints are applied to maintain minimum height of the vertebrae T_v and inter-vertebrae space T_s: $u_i - d_i > T_v;\quad d_{i+1} - u_i > T_s$.

The next step is aimed at creating a parametric model [5] for estimating the horizontal extent of the vertebrae through fitting ellipse to the middle section of each vertebra (see Fig. 3). First, we align all training samples x based on the second extrema (thoracic curve) of the polynomial models of each spinal cord, that approximately corresponds to 8th thorasic vertebrae. We manually acquire measurements of minor b and major axis a for each vertebra though out the training set. Then, PCA is applied for all aligned and completed samples x_j. $x_j = [a_{j1},..., a_{jn}, b_{j1},..., b_{jn}]^T$;

where a_i – major axes (mm), b_i – minor axes (mm), $i=1,...,n$, n is number of vertebrae, j is the sample number.

Next, mean shape $\bar{x}$ is computed:

$$\bar{x} = \frac{1}{m}\sum_{j=1}^{m} x_j; \qquad S=\frac{1}{m}\sum_{j=1}^{m}(x_j-\bar{x})(x_j-\bar{x})^T; \qquad Sp_k = \lambda_k p_k \tag{8}$$

where m is the number of training samples, λ_k is k_{th} eigenvalue, p_k is k_{th} eigenvector, $k=1,..,2n$ and t is the number of modes.

$$\sum_{j=1}^{t} \lambda_j \geq \frac{confidence\_level}{100\%} \sum_{j}^{2n} \lambda_j ; \tag{9}$$

where *confidence_level* was set to 95%.

$x = \bar{x} + Pd$. $P=(p_1,\ldots,p_t)$ is a matrix of t eigenvectors, $d = (d_1,\ldots, d_t)^T$ is the model parameter vector. $-w\sqrt{\lambda_j} \leq d_j \leq w\sqrt{\lambda_j}$, where $j=1,\ldots,t$. w was set to 1. Generate new $x = \bar{x} + Pd$.

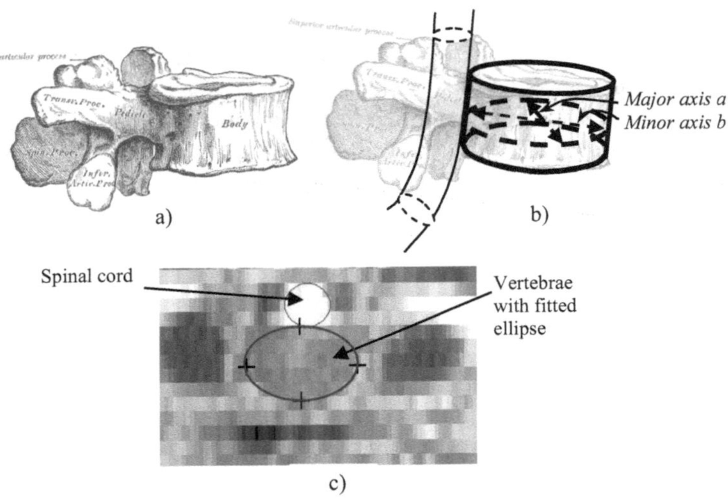

Fig. 3. a). The picture of thoracic vertebra from Henry Gray's Anatomy of the Human Body (1918). b). Schematic representation of vertebra and spinal cord. c) Axial slice through a vertebra with fitted ellipse. Locations of manually acquired reference points at the ends of major and minor axis are shown as +.

The vertebra body extent in axial planes is estimated through an ellipse-fitting algorithm [6]. Resulting vector: $x' = [a'_1 ,\ldots, a'_n , b'_1 ,\ldots, b'_n]^T$.
Project x' to model space: $d' = (x' - \bar{x}) / P$. If x' is reasonable, d' will satisfy the model constraints $-w\sqrt{\lambda_i} \leq d_i' \leq w\sqrt{\lambda_i}$.($i=1,\ldots,t$). Otherwise bring d' to the range $-w\sqrt{\lambda_i} \leq d_i' \leq w\sqrt{\lambda_i}$. Next, compute $x = \bar{x} + Pd'$.

$$b = (x_{new} - \bar{x}) / P ; \quad -\sqrt{\lambda_k} \leq b_k \leq \sqrt{\lambda_k} ; \tag{10}$$

The vertebrae segmentation algorithm was visually evaluated on 77 T2 STIR images with different levels of fat suppression and on 5 HASTE images (HASTE pulse sequence is mainly used for abdominal organs like liver). In all cases segmentation results appeared satisfactory (see Fig. 4). Although intensity distributions for majority of organs are very different for T2 STIR and HASTE images, it had no effect on the segmentation results. No changes were made to the algorithm developed originally for T2 STIR images to adapt it for the HASTE pulse sequence.

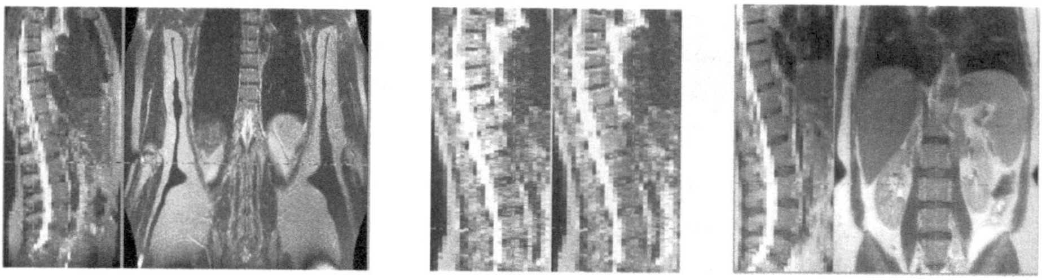

a) b) c)

Fig. 4. Vertebrae segmentation results for: a) Coronal T2 STIR image b). Original (left) and segmented (right) T2 STIR image with metastases. c) HASTE image.

4 Computer-Aided Detection of Vertebrae Metastases

The fully automatic metastases detection algorithm (research prototype) involved primary lesion detection and false positive reduction steps. Osteoblastic metastases, unlike osteolytic, appear hypointense in STIR images, and require similar detection approach, but with inverse thresholds. Our data set does not contain enough samples of osteoblastic metastases (4 patients only) for reliable training and testing, therefore all the results and conclusions below are targeted towards osteolytic metastatic lesions.

Primary lesion candidate detection inside segmented vertebrae was performed using adaptive intensity thresholds to search for any suspicious regions. Multiple features characterizing intensity, texture (moments of intensity), volume, shape (euler number, eccentricity, orientation, solidity, diameter of a circle with the same area as the region in coronal slice, orientation - the angle between the x-axis and the major axis of the ellipse that has the same second-moments as the region), and location of candidate lesions were extracted from 3D image data. Finally, a classifier constructed using the training set was applied to the candidate detections to reduce the number of false positives (FP). The classifier was constructed by taking into account the fact that a lesion may associate with several detections and if any of them is correctly classified, the lesion is considered being identified.

Let m be the number of total candidates that are identified in the lesion candidate detection step, d be the number of features that are evaluated for each of the candidates. With a little abuse of notation, we use x_i to denote a feature vector representation of the ith candidate. We then label the detected candidates (hits) by consulting the markers provided by expert radiologists. A candidate receives +1 label if it overlays with a lesion, or otherwise, it receives -1 label. We use C^+, C^- to denote the index sets that contain all candidates that are labeled +1, and -1, respectively.

In the classification task, a classifier needs to be constructed based on the training sample to predict the label for any candidate detected from unseen patient data. Standard machine learning algorithms such as *support vector machines* (SVM), and *Fisher's linear discriminant (FLD)*, are often used for CAD, but our detection task has specific characteristics that cannot be employed in the standard algorithm. In particular, there can be many hits or candidate regions that refer to unique underlying malignant structure, and even if one of the hits is correctly highlighted to the radiologist, the entire structure can be easily traced out by the radiologist. Hence correct classification of every candidate instance is not as important as the ability to detect *at least one* candidate that points to a malignant region. We thus formulate our problem as a problem of learning with multiple hits.

We design a novel classification algorithm based on Fisher's linear discriminant (FLD) analysis that aims to detect at least one hit for each lesion. FLD [7] has been successfully applied to many medical applications, and it fits the separation boundary between true hits and negative detections with a linear function $w^T x + b$. Recently, FLD has been recast into an equivalent optimization problem [8] as follows: minimize $\sum_{i=1}^{m} \xi_i + \gamma\|w\|_2^2$, subject to the constraints: $w^T x_i + b = y_i + \xi_i,\ i = 1, \cdots, m$, $\sum_{i \in C^+} \xi_i = 0,\ \sum_{i \in C^-} \xi_i = 0$, where y_i denotes the label, ξ_i is a residual error of the model fitting, $\|w\|_2^2$ is the so-called regularization term that controls the classifier complexity, and γ plays the trade-off between the residual error and the complexity regularization.

Assume in total n_i hits, each represented as a feature vector x_{ij}, are segmented for the ith lesion. Let S_i be the index set of all candidates pointing to the ith lesion. For each lesion, we form a convex hull using these vectors x_{ij} in the feature space. Any point in the convex hull can be represented as a convex combination of x_{ij}, that is, $\sum_{j \in S_i} \lambda_{ij} x_{ij}$, where $\lambda_{ij} \geq 0,\ \sum \lambda_{ij} = 1$. The goal of our learning algorithm is to determine a decision boundary that can separate, with high accuracy, any possible part of each of the convex hulls on one side and as many as possible negative detections on the other side. It implies that we do not require the entire convex hull to correctly classified, but only any possible part of it. In other words, our algorithm solves the following optimization problem based on the FLD formulation:

$$\begin{aligned} &\text{minimize} \quad \sum_{i=1}^{m} \xi_i + \gamma\|w\|_2^2, \text{ subject to:} \\ &w^T\left(\sum_{j \in S_i} \lambda_{ij} x_{ij}\right) + b = y_i + \xi_i,\ \lambda_{ij} \geq 0,\ \sum \lambda_{ij} = 1,\ \forall i \in C^+, \\ &w^T x_i + b = y_i + \xi_i, \quad \forall i \in C^-, \\ &\sum_{i \in C^+} \xi_i = 0, \quad \sum_{i \in C^-} \xi_i = 0. \end{aligned} \tag{11}$$

The classifier obtained by solving the formulation (11) can dramatically reduce false detections in comparison with standard classification algorithms, such as FLD.

Aggregation of multiple classifiers is used to get an average aggregated prediction for an unseen sample. It has been shown that the aggregation is effective on ``unstable" learning algorithms where small changes in the training set result in large changes in predictions [9]. Particularly, in our case, even though FLD itself may not be so unstable, reasonably small changes on the training sample set often cause undesirable changes on the classifier constructed due to an extremely limited size of patient data available. Hence, aggregation is necessary in order to reduce the variance of the learned classifier over various sample patient sets, thus enhancing accuracy.

We carry out T trials, and in each trial, 70% of the training cases are randomly sampled, and used in the training. A linear function $f_t(x) = w_t^T x + b_t$ is then constructed in the trial t. The final classifier is based on the averaged model $f(x) = \frac{1}{T}\sum_{t=1}^{T} f_t(x) = \frac{1}{T}(\sum_{t=1}^{T} w_t)^T x + \frac{1}{T}\sum_{t=1}^{T} b_t$. Thresholding on the value of $f(x)$ with an appropriate cut-off value a provides the final findings where a is tuned according to the desired false positive rate. If a candidate x gets $f(x) \geq a$, then it is classified as a true hit, or otherwise it is removed from the final findings.

5 Evaluation of Metastases Detection Algorithm

The patient population included 42 patients with different histologically clarified primary tumors examined with MRI of the spine for staging and follow-up of known skeletal metastases. The gold standard was constituted by histology and/or clinical radiological follow up within at least 6 months.

MRI was performed at 1.5 Tesla on a 32-channel scanner (Magnetom Avanto, Siemens). All patients underwent STIR-imaging of the complete spine in sagittal orientation. The data was split into training and test sets.

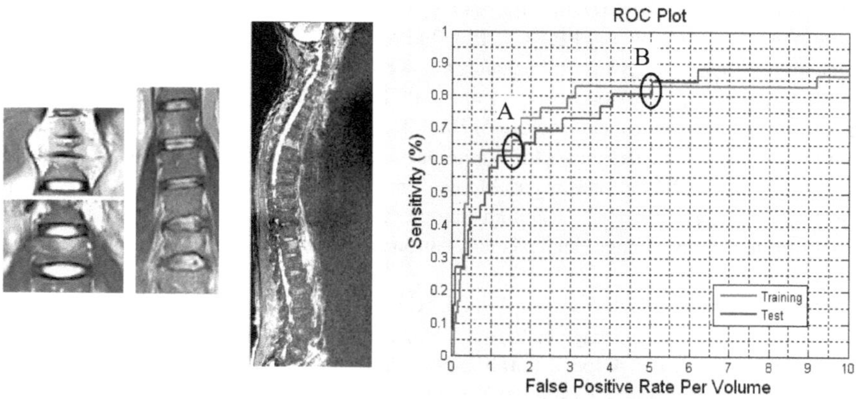

a) b) c) d)

Fig. 5. a) and b). Examples of metastases detection results on the images from the development set (coronal STIR images with less fat suppression). The left image is from the same patient with collapsed vertebrae and edema as in figure 1a. c). Test set image example: sagittal STIR image of the spine. Focal lesions detected by CAD are highlighted in red. d) ROC curves for training and test sets. A. Sensitivity at 1.5 FPs per patient: training – 66.32%, test - 61.61%. B. Sensitivity at 5.0 FPs per patient: training – 82.89%, test - 84.61%.

Training set included 21 patients, in which 12 had osteolytic spine metastases (13 focal, 6 diffuse and 10 multifocal lesions). The test set included 21 patients, of which 9 had osteolytic spine metastases (12 focal, 6 diffuse and 8 multifocal lesions). Each spine section (cervical, thoracic and lumbar) with diffuse or multifocal infiltration was counted as one lesion. Training and test set sensitivity was 82.76% and 84.61%, respectively, with 5 false positive detections per patient. The CAD algorithm missed 3 focal lesions in the training set and 3 focal lesions in the test set. One diffuse lesion (spine section) was missed in one patient from the test set and one multifocal and one diffuse lesion were missed in two patients from the training set. However, other lesions or infiltrated spine sections were successfully detected in the same patients, so that 'per patient' sensitivity was 100%.

6 Conclusion

Spine metastases CAD showed high standalone sensitivity at a relatively low FP rate. The run time was ~2 min on average in MATLAB implementation. While this study confirmed CAD feasibility, the next step is to incorporate additional features from T1-weighted SE-sequences to further reduce the number of false positives. Furthermore, the additive benefits of CAD as a second reader should be investigated.

References

1. Schmidt, G.P., Schoenberg, S.O., Schmid, R., Stahl, R., Tiling, R., Becker, C.R., Reiser, M.F., Baur-Melnyk, A.:Screening for bone metastases: whole-body MRI using a 32-channel system versus dual-modality PET-CT. Eur Radiol. Sep 2; [Epub] (2006)
2. Ghanem, N., Uhl, M., Brink, I., Schäfer, O., Kelly, T., Moser, E., Langer, M.: Diagnostic value of MRI in comparison to scintigraphy, PET, MS-CT and PET/CT for the detection of metastases of bone. European Journal of Radiology 55(1), 41–55 (2005)
3. Carballido-Gamio, J., Belongie, S., Majumdar, S.: Normalized Cuts in 3D for Spinal MRI Segmentation. IEEE Transactions on Medical Imaging 23(1), 36–44 (2004)
4. Fischler, M.A., Bolles, R.C.: Random Sample Consensus: A Paradigm for Model Fitting with Applications to Image Analysis and Automated Cartography. Comm. of the ACM 24, 381–395 (1981)
5. Cootes, T., Hill, A., Taylor, C., Haslam, J.: Use of active shape models for locating structures in medical images. Image & Vision Computing 12(6), 355–366 (1994)
6. Saha, P.: Tensor scale: A local morphometric parameter with applications to computer vision and image processing. Computer Vision and Image Understanding, 99(3), 384–413
7. Johnson, R.A., Wichern, D.W.: Applied Multivariate Statistical Analysis. Prentice-Hall, New Jersey (1998)
8. Mika, S., Ratsch, G., Muller, K.: A mathematical programming approach to the kernel Fisher algorithm. Advances in Neural Information Processing Systems 13, 591–597 (2001)
9. Breiman, L.: Bagging predictors. Machine Learning 24(2), 123–140 (1996)

Nonrigid Image Registration Using Conditional Mutual Information

Dirk Loeckx[1], Pieter Slagmolen[1,2], Frederik Maes[1],
Dirk Vandermeulen[1], and Paul Suetens[1]

[1] Medical Image Computing, Faculties of Medicine and Engineering,
[2] Department of Radiation Oncoloy, Faculty of Medicine,
Katholieke Universiteit Leuven, University Hospital Gasthuisberg,
Herestraat 49 - bus 7003, B-3000 Leuven, Belgium
Dirk.Loeckx@uz.kuleuven.ac.be

Abstract. We propose conditional mutual information (cMI) as a new similarity measure for nonrigid image registration. We start from a 3D joint histogram incorporating, besides the reference and floating intensity dimensions, also a spatial dimension expressing the location of the joint intensity pair in the reference image. cMI is calculated as the expectation value of the conditional mutual information between the reference and floating intensities given the spatial distribution.

Validation experiments were performed comparing cMI and global MI on artificial CT/MR registrations and registrations complicated with a strong bias field; both a Parzen window and generalised partial volume kernel were used for histogram construction. In both experiments, cMI significantly outperforms global MI. Moreover, cMI is compared to global MI for the registration of three patient CT/MR datasets, using overlap and centroid distance as validation measure. The best results are obtained using cMI.

1 Introduction

Since its introduction for medical image registration in 1995 [1,2], mutual information (MI) has gained wide interest in the field [3]. MI is a basic concept from information theory that measures the amount of information one image contains about the other. Starting from a reference image R and floating image F with intensities respectively r and f, the mutual information $I(R,F)$ is calculated from the joint and marginal probabilities $p(r,f)$, $p(r)=\sum_f p(r,f)$ and $p(f)=\sum_r p(r,f)$:

$$I(R,F) = H(R) + H(F) - H(R,F) = \sum_{r\in R}\sum_{f\in F} p(r,f)\ln\left(\frac{p(r,f)}{p(r)p(f)}\right), \qquad (1)$$

with $H(A) = -\sum_a p(a)\log(p(a))$ the entropy of a random variable A.

The maximisation of mutual information (MMI) registration criterion assumes that the images are correctly aligned when the MI between corresponding voxels

N. Karssemeijer and B. Lelieveldt (Eds.): IPMI 2007, LNCS 4584, pp. 725–737, 2007.
© Springer-Verlag Berlin Heidelberg 2007

is maximal. Because it assumes only a statistical relationship between both images, image registration using MMI is widely applicable, also when it cannot be assumed that corresponding intensities are one-to-one related. MMI has been applied to a wide range of registration problems [4], covering as well monomodal as multimodal applications and its accuracy and robustness has been demonstrated for rigid body image registration of CT, MR and PET brain images [5].

Extending MMI to nonrigid image registration is an active field of research both for mono and for multimodal applications. This extension is not trivial. Calculation of MI is based upon a global joint histogram, expressing the joint intensity probabilities over the whole image. During optimisation, the registration algorithm tends to minimise minor peaks in the histogram in favour of major peaks. While this does not cause a problem in affine image registration, a nonrigid transformation model, with a higher number of degrees of freedom, might be tempted to reduce smaller image details. This can happen e.g. when the intensity correspondence is inhomogeneous over the images, as in CT/MR registration. Another example is the registration of images complicated by a strong bias field. Registration guided by maximisation of global MI might be tempted to align the bias field rather than the image features.

Both problems can be reduced using a local estimation of the joint histogram. This can be obtained by progressively subdividing the image and performing a set of local registrations [6,7,8]. However, when the image parts are too small, the small number of samples limits the statistical power of the local joint histogram. Several adaptations have been proposed to overcome this problem. Likar and Pernuš [7] combine the local and global intensity distribution. Andronache *et al.* [8] present a local intensity re-mapping to allow for the use of cross correlation as similarity measure in the smaller sub-images.

An alternative approach has been proposed by Studholme *et al.* [9]. They present a nonrigid viscous fluid registration scheme, using a similarity measure that is calculated over a set of overlapping subregions of the image. This is achieved by extending the intensity joint histogram with a third channel representing a spatial label. Several extensions of calculation of mutual information to multiple dimensions exist; Studholme *et al.* choose the total correlation

$$C(R, F, X) = H(R) + H(F) + H(X) - H(R, F, X) \tag{2}$$

$$= \sum_{r \in R} \sum_{f \in F} \sum_{\mathbf{x} \in X} p(r, f, \mathbf{x}) \ln \left(\frac{p(r, f, \mathbf{x})}{p(r)p(f)p(\mathbf{x})} \right) \tag{3}$$

as similarity measure (see figure 1), with X expressing the spatial position in the reference image. The image is subdivided in cubic regions of 10-50 voxels, overlapping 50% in each dimension (i.e. every voxel belongs to 8 regions). The joint intensity histogram within each region is constructed using B-spline Parzen windows [10].

Within this article, we propose to use the conditional mutual information (cMI) [11] as similarity measure. The cMI $I(R, F|X)$ is calculated between the reference and floating intensities distributions R and F, given a certain spatial distribution X. While the two-variate MI $I(R, F)$ expresses the reduction in the

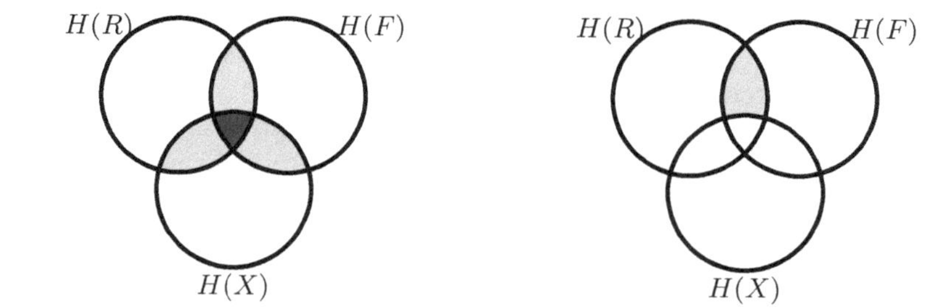

$H(R) + H(F) + H(X) - H(R, F, X)$ $\quad$ $H(R|X) + H(F|X) - H(R, F|X)$

(a) total correlation $\quad$ (b) conditional MI

Fig. 1. Comparison of entropies included in the total correlation (a) and conditional mutual information (b). The dark colour in (a) signifies that the area is counted twice.

uncertainty of R due to the knowledge of F (and vice-versa), cMI expresses the reduction in the uncertainty of R due to knowledge of F (and vice-versa) when the spatial location X is known:

$$I(R, F|X) = H(R|X) + H(F|X) - H(R, F|X) \tag{4}$$

$$= \sum_{\mathbf{x} \in X} p(\mathbf{x}) \sum_{r \in R} \sum_{f \in F} p(r, f|\mathbf{x}) \ln \left(\frac{p(r, f|\mathbf{x})}{p(r|x)p(f|\mathbf{x})} \right), \tag{5}$$

We think cMI corresponds to the actual situation in medical image registration, where the spatial location of each voxel is indeed known a priori.

Similar to [9], we calculate cMI by extending the joint histogram with a third dimension representing the spatial distribution of the joint intensities. For the construction of the joint histogram, we treat the intensity and spatial dimensions equivalently, considering the spatial regions as spatial bins. We incorporate cMI in a tensor-product B-spline registration algorithm [12], using the same kernel to interpolate between the B-spline deformation coefficients and to construct the joint histogram. In the next section, we provide a detailed explanation of our method.

In section 3, we present a validation of our method on two artifical datasets, representing multimodal CT/MR registration and registration in the presence of a strong bias field. We also provide initial results of our method on the multimodal registration of CT/MR datasets, as required for radiotherapy planning.

2 Methods

2.1 Similarity Measure

Mutual information. To calculate the global MI between a reference image I with intensity $\mathcal{I}_R(\mathbf{x}_R)$ and a floating image F with intensity $\mathcal{I}_F(\mathbf{x}_F)$ using a transformation $\mathbf{g}(\mathbf{x}_R; \boldsymbol{\mu})$ that maps every reference position $\mathbf{x}_R$ to the corresponding floating position $\mathbf{x}_F = \mathbf{g}(\mathbf{x}_R; \boldsymbol{\mu})$ given a set of parameters $\boldsymbol{\mu}$, we start from the joint histogram $\mathcal{H}(r, f; \boldsymbol{\mu})$ using a set of reference bin centres r and floating bin centres f. Two popular methods exist to obtain a derivable histogram (see also section 2.4), namely Parzen window (PW) interpolation [10] and generalised partial volume (PV) estimation [13,14]. In the following, we present the formulation for Parzen window interpolation only, although we have implemented both approaches. The formulas for global PV are described in [15].

The Parzen window joint histogram is given by

$$\mathcal{H}(r, f; \boldsymbol{\mu}) = \sum_{\mathbf{x}_R \in R} w_r(\mathcal{I}_R(\mathbf{x}_R) - r) w_f(\mathcal{I}_F(\mathbf{g}(\mathbf{x}_R; \boldsymbol{\mu})) - f), \tag{6}$$

where w_r and w_f are the Parzen window kernels used to distribute an intensity over the neighbouring bins. Because of their attractive mathematical properties, we have chosen to use second-degree B-splines for the Parzen window kernels $w_r(x) = w_f(x) = \beta_\epsilon^2(x)$ with ϵ the (constant) spacing between neighbouring bins and $\beta_\epsilon^n(x) = \beta^n(\frac{x}{\epsilon})/\epsilon$ the expanded B-spline of degree n. Thus, each joint intensity pair contributes to a 3×3 region in the joint histogram. When the floating intensity $\mathcal{I}_F(\mathbf{x}_F)$ is sought at a non-integer position $\mathbf{x}_F = \mathbf{g}(\mathbf{x}_R; \boldsymbol{\mu})$, it is obtained using second degree B-spline intensity interpolation.

The joint probability distribution can now be calculated as

$$p(r, f; \boldsymbol{\mu}) = \frac{\mathcal{H}(r, f; \boldsymbol{\mu})}{\sum_{r,f} \mathcal{H}(r, f; \boldsymbol{\mu})}, \tag{7}$$

which immediately leads to the mutual information as described in (1).

Conditional mutual information. To extend the joint histogram with spatial information, we overlay a regular lattice with knots $\mathbf{x}_{ijk} = (x_i^x, x_j^y, x_k^z)$ over the reference image. The joint histogram (6) is extended by a spatial kernel $w_\mathbf{x}$:

$$\mathcal{H}_s(r, f, \mathbf{x}; \boldsymbol{\mu}) = \sum_{\mathbf{x}_R \in R} w_r(\mathcal{I}_R(\mathbf{x}_R) - r) w_f(\mathcal{I}_F(\mathbf{g}(\mathbf{x}_R; \boldsymbol{\mu})) - f) w_\mathbf{x}(\mathbf{x}_R - \mathbf{x}), \tag{8}$$

with $\mathbf{x} \in \{\mathbf{x}_{ijk}\}$. Using second degree B-spline kernels for the spatial kernel in each dimension, and mesh spacing Δ_x, Δ_y and Δ_z, $w_\mathbf{x}$ is given by

$$w_\mathbf{x}(\mathbf{x}_R - \mathbf{x}) = \beta_{\Delta_x}^2(x_{R,x} - x_x)\beta_{\Delta_y}^2(x_{R,y} - x_y)\beta_{\Delta_z}^2(x_{R,z} - x_z) \tag{9}$$

with $\mathbf{x}_R = (x_{R,x}, x_{R,y}, x_{R,z})$ and $\mathbf{x} = (x_x, x_y, x_z)$.

Note that for the construction of the joint histogram, we put all spatial bins on a single axis. This is similar to [9], considering the spatial bins as a set of labels associated with each intensity pair. As the mutual information is independent of the bin order (in the spatial as well as in the intensity dimensions), the ordering of the spatial bins can be chosen arbitrarily. The correspondence between neighbouring spatial labels is encoded by the spatial kernel (9). This also holds for the intensity domain, where the intensity bins can be ordered at random to calculate the mutual information, while the correspondence is encoded in the PW or PV kernel.

Due to the limited span properties of B-splines, the extent of the image region contributing to the joint histogram for a given spatial bin $\mathbf{x}$ is a cube of $3\Delta_x$ by $3\Delta_y$ by $3\Delta_z$, centred around $\mathbf{x}$, with a higher contribution for the voxels closer to $\mathbf{x}$. The mesh spacing Δ regulates the locality of the cMI. To represent a more global histogram, a large Δ is chosen, yielding a limited number of spatial bins containing contributions from the whole image area. A fine mesh with small Δ and many spatial bins is used to calculate a more local histogram.

Starting from (8), the conditional probability can be obtained similar to (7), replacing $p(r, f; \boldsymbol{\mu})$ with

$$p(r, f|\mathbf{x}; \boldsymbol{\mu}) = \frac{\mathcal{H}_s(r, f, \mathbf{x}; \boldsymbol{\mu})}{p(\mathbf{x}; \boldsymbol{\mu})}, \text{ using } p(\mathbf{x}; \boldsymbol{\mu}) = \frac{\sum_{r,f} \mathcal{H}_s(r, f, \mathbf{x})}{\sum_{r,f,\chi} \mathcal{H}_s(r, f, \chi)}. \tag{10}$$

Finally, the above equations can be substituted in (5) to obtain the cMI.

2.2 Transformation Model

Several transformation models have been proposed for nonrigid image registration. We adopt a tensor-product B-spline model, as proposed by Rueckert *et al.* [12]. The B-spline model is situated between a global rigid registration model and a local nonrigid model at voxel-scale. Its locality or nonrigidity can be adopted to a specific registration problem by varying the mesh spacing and thus the number of degrees of freedom.

Using second degree B-splines, the 3D transformation field is given by

$$\mathbf{g}(\mathbf{x}_R; \boldsymbol{\mu}) = \sum_{ijk} \boldsymbol{\mu}_{ijk} \beta^2_{\Delta_x}(x - k_i^x) \beta^2_{\Delta_y}(y - k_j^y) \beta^2_{\Delta_z}(z - k_k^z), \tag{11}$$

with Δ_x, Δ_y, Δ_z the mesh spacing. The transformation is governed by the displacement vectors $\boldsymbol{\mu}_{ijk}$ located at the tensor-product knots $\mathbf{k}_{ijk} = (k_i^x, k_j^y, k_k^z)$. Note that the transformation parameters $\boldsymbol{\mu}$ are 3D vectors, and thus (11) models a different function for each dimension: $g_x(\mathbf{r}; \boldsymbol{\mu}^x)$, $g_y(\mathbf{r}; \boldsymbol{\mu}^y)$ and $g_z(\mathbf{r}; \boldsymbol{\mu}^z)$.

2.3 Spatial Resolution

Equation (9) and (11) both stipulate the spatial resolution of the algorithm. The latter governs the region of influence of a registration parameter and the former the scale at which the cMI is calculated. Therefore, we choose to use the same settings for the mesh knots and spacing in both formulas. Thus, the local transformation around a certain displacement vector is guided by the local joint histogram, both using the same concept and scale of locality.

2.4 Derivatives and Optimisation

A limited memory quasi Newton method [16] is adopted for the optimisation, using analytical derivatives to avoid discretisation errors. Using

$$\frac{\partial w_f(\mathcal{I}_F(\mathbf{g}(\mathbf{x}_R;\boldsymbol{\mu}))-f)}{\partial \mu^{\xi}_{ijk}} = \left.\frac{\partial w_f(i-f)}{\partial i}\right|_{i=\mathcal{I}_F(\mathbf{g}(\mathbf{x}_R;\boldsymbol{\mu}))} \left.\frac{\partial \mathcal{I}_F(\mathbf{r})}{\partial \mathbf{r}}\right|^T_{\mathbf{r}=\mathbf{g}(\mathbf{x}_R;\boldsymbol{\mu})} \frac{\partial \mathbf{g}(\mathbf{x}_R;\boldsymbol{\mu})}{\partial \mu^{\xi}_{ijk}} \tag{12}$$

$$\text{and } \frac{\partial \mathbf{g}(\mathbf{x};\boldsymbol{\mu})}{\partial \mu_{ijk}^{\xi}} = [\delta_{\xi x}, \delta_{\xi y}, \delta_{\xi z}]^T \cdot \beta_{\Delta_x}^2(x - k_i^x) \cdot \beta_{\Delta_y}^2(y - k_j^y) \cdot \beta_{\Delta_z}^2(z - k_k^z), \quad (13)$$

the derivative of (8) with respect to a transformation parameter μ_{ijk}^{ξ} is given by

$$\frac{\partial \mathcal{H}(r,f,\mathbf{x};\boldsymbol{\mu})}{\partial \mu_{ijk}^{\xi}} = \sum_{\mathbf{x}_R \in R} w_r(\mathcal{I}_r(\mathbf{x}_R) - r) \frac{\partial w_f(\mathcal{I}_F(\mathbf{g}(\mathbf{x}_R;\boldsymbol{\mu})) - f)}{\partial \mu_{ijk}^{\xi}} w_x(\mathbf{x}_R - \mathbf{x}). \quad (14)$$

3 Experiments and Results

3.1 Multimodal Registration

For the first experiment, we created 200 artificial 2D image pairs simulating a slice through a lower limb in CT and MR (see figure 2). Each image, measuring 256×256 pixels, consists of a dark background ($I = 0$) and two concentric polygons. The larger polygon is a hexagon with a medium intensity ($I = 200$), representing soft tissue. The smaller polygon is a pentagon, high intense ($I = 400$) in the CT image and dark ($I = 0$) in the MR image. We have added uniform Gaussian noise ($\sigma = 50$) to the images. A mesh spacing of $\Delta_x = \Delta_y = 32$ voxels was used for the B-spline transformation and the conditional joint histogram estimation; 32 bins were used in the joint histogram for the floating and the reference intensity.

For each image pair, the transformation field was initialised choosing $\boldsymbol{\mu}$ from a uniform distribution with a maximum amplitude of 30 pixels. Starting from this transformation, the MR images were registered to the original CT image. The registration quality was measured as the average intensity difference between the original (noise-free) CT image and the final transformation applied to this image. We also calculated the warping index, which is the root mean square of the local registration error in each voxel. However, even for a perfect registration (according to MI or cMI), the final transformation might contain nonzero components within homogeneous regions that have no influence on the final image, leading to an increased warping index. Both validation measures were calculated over a region of interest 10% larger than the outer polygon.

Figure 2 represents an example of the CT image, transformed MR image, and the registration results obtained using the different methods to calculate the similarity. The global methods typically reduce the size of the inner circle. The validation measures evaluated over the 200 registrations are summarised in figure 3, showing a clear improvement using conditional MI over global MI. Moreover, conditional PV seems to outperform conditional PW.

3.2 Bias Field Registration

For the second experiment, we started from the Lena image (8 bit, 256 × 256 voxels). It was used unmodified for the reference image, for the floating images it was distorted with a second-degree multiplicative bias field $ax^2 + bxy + cx +$

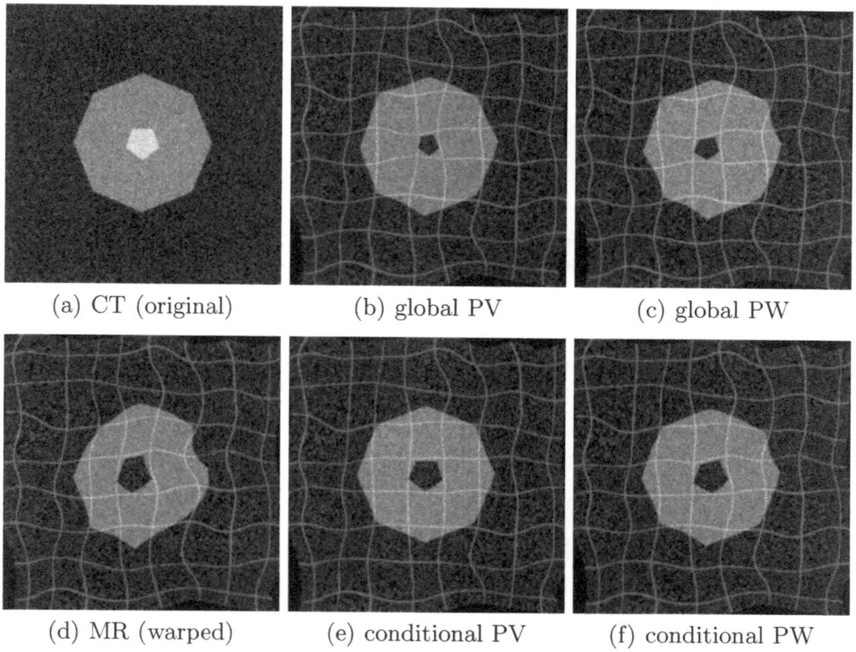

Fig. 2. Example of the registration results obtained for CT/MR registration

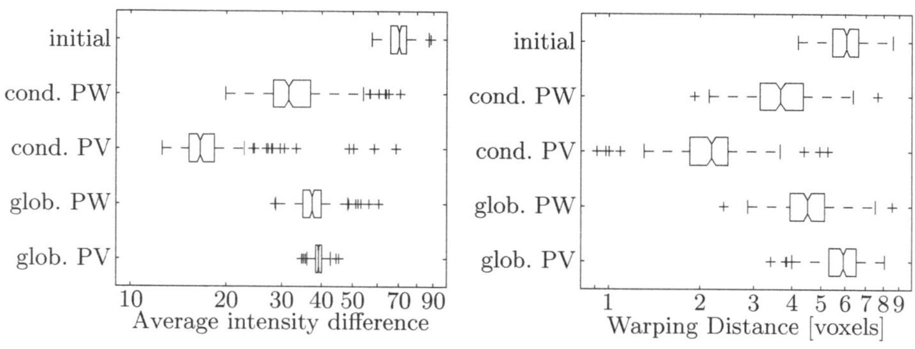

Fig. 3. Boxplot of the registration results obtained for 200 artificial CT/MR pairs

$dy^2 + e$, with a to e uniformly sampled from $\{[-0.75, -0.25], [0.25, 0.75]\}$. Next, the floating image was deformed and registered and the results were validated similar to the previous section. An example of a pair of reference and floating images and the obtained registration results is presented in figure 4. Quantitative results obtained over 200 image pairs are summarised in figure 5. Again, cMI clearly outperforms global MI.

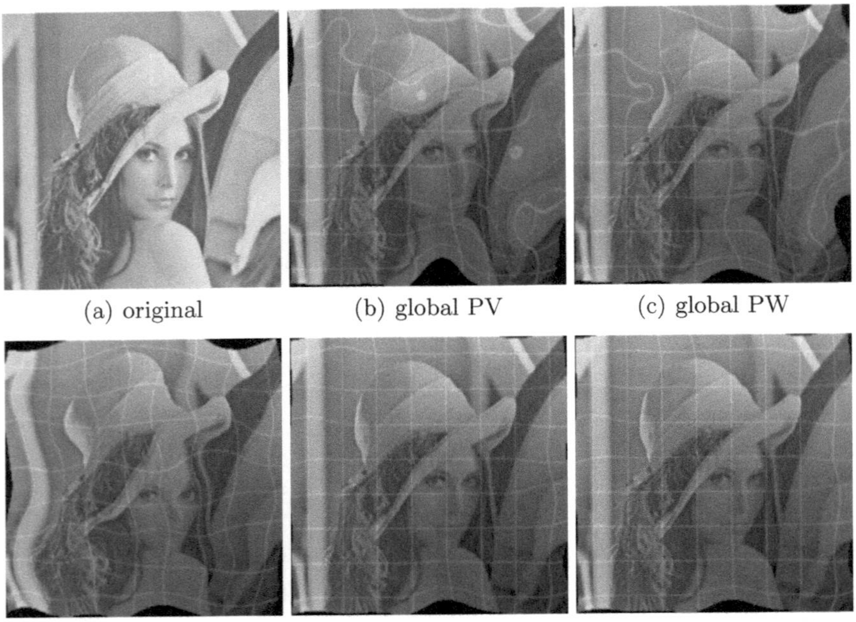

(a) original (b) global PV (c) global PW

(d) warped + bias field (e) conditional PV (f) conditional PW

Fig. 4. Example of the registration results obtained after bias field contortion

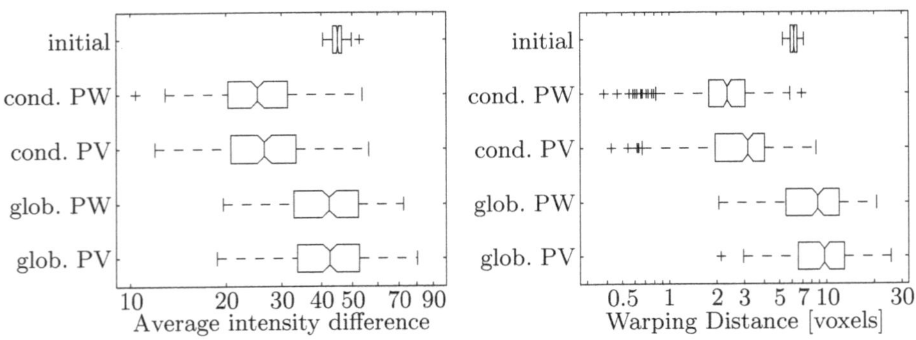

Fig. 5. Boxplot of the registration results obtained for 200 bias field distortion pairs

3.3 Clinical CT/MR

In our last experiment, we have applied global and conditional MI to MR/CT registration for colorectal cancer treatment [17]. The clinical goal of the registration is to transfer expert delineations of structures of interest from the MR scan to the CT scan. Both structures (and the tumour) are better visible in the MR scan, yet the CT scan is required to perform the actual planning and dose distribution calculation.

Table 1. Validation results for global and conditional MI registration of clinical MR and CT datasets for the manual delineation of the rectum and mesorectum, showing the Dice similarity overlap criterium (DSC) and centroid distance (cD, in mm) for image pairs P1-P3. Better results have a higher DSC and lower cD.

(a) rectum

	affine		global MI		cond. MI	
	DSC	cD	DSC	cD	DSC	cD
P1	0.52	5.5	0.65	4.4	0.67	2.4
P2	0.69	3.1	0.75	2.8	0.77	2.3
P3	0.58	8.0	0.65	6.4	0.77	2.8

(b) mesorectum

	affine		global MI		cond. MI	
	DSC	cD	DSC	cD	DSC	cD
P1	0.78	4.0	0.83	2.9	0.83	3.7
P2	0.82	3.5	0.82	4.6	0.83	5.4
P3	0.70	7.5	0.73	7.4	0.84	3.8

For the experiment, we start from three pairs of patient MR and CT scans and manual delineations of the rectum and mesorectum in both scans. A multiresolution registration scheme is adopted, using the CT image as reference image. The mesh spacing, as well for the cMI calculation as for the tensor product B-spline field, is gradually decreased, starting from $512 \times 512 \times 128$ voxels ($500 \times 500 \times 384$ mm) in the first stage to $32 \times 32 \times 32$ voxels ($62.5 \times 62.5 \times 48$ mm) in the fifth and last stage. Best results were obtained using 64 bins for the floating and reference intensities in the joint histogram and conditional PW interpolation.

Those results were compared to the results using the same registration settings but global PW interpolation. As validation measure, the Dice similarity criterium (DSC) and centroid distance (cD) between corresponding segmentations were evaluated. The results are provided in table 1. An example comparing segmentations obtained by global and conditional MI is shown in figure 6. Both cMI and global MI improve the results obtained using affine registrations. For the rectum segmentation, which is the most difficult part to register, cMI clearly outperforms global MI. For the mesorectum, global and conditional MI show similar results. Registration validation based on manual segmentations may suffer from significant inaccuracies in the manual delineations. This can explain the apparent inconsistencies, as e.g. the increase in both DSC and cD for the mesorectum of P2.

4 Discussion

In the context of nonrigid registration, registration by maximisation of mutual information may lead to undesired results. We have shown that global MI, an established similarity measure for rigid registration, can be outperformed by conditional MI for nonrigid applications.

In experiment 1, we have seen that global MI has a tendency to reduce the size of the inner circle in the MR image. This can be explained by manually constructing the joint and marginal entropies. We start from a square image picturing two concentric circles, as shown in figure 7(a). The surface areas A_1 (light gray), A_2 (medium gray) and A_3 (dark gray) are chosen such that

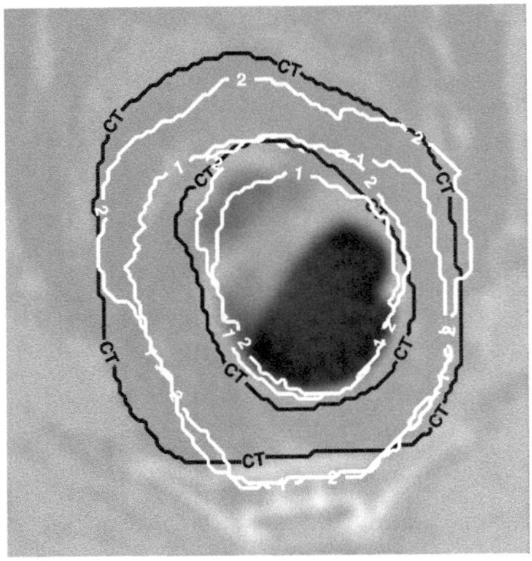

Fig. 6. Overview of the contours obtained using global and conditional MI registration. The inner and outer set of contours represent respectively the rectum and mesorectum segmentation. The black contour is the original (ground truth) contour as delineated by the clinical expert in the CT image. The white contours are obtained by nonrigid registration of the MR image using (1) global and (2) conditional MI.

$A_1 + A_2 + A_3 = 1$. Using I_R^1, I_R^2 and I_R^3 (I_F^1, I_F^2 and $I_F^3 = I_F^1$) for the reference (floating) intensities corresponding with the three regions, the joint histogram and marginal histograms are given by

$$\mathcal{H}_1(r, f) = \begin{bmatrix} 0 & A_2 & 0 \\ A_1 & 0 & A_3 \end{bmatrix}, \ \mathcal{H}_1(r) = [A_1, A_2, A_3], \ \text{and} \ \mathcal{H}_1(f) = [A_1 + A_3, A_2]. \quad (15)$$

When the conditional mutual information is calculated, a smaller region will contribute to the joint histogram. For simplicity, we assume a zeroth degree B-spline mesh overlaid over the reference image, as indicated by the dashed line in figure 7(a). A perturbation of A_3 will influence the central region only. Thus, the conditional joint and marginal histograms are obtained by

$$\mathcal{H}_2(r, f) = \begin{bmatrix} 0 & A_2' & 0 \\ 0 & 0 & A_3' \end{bmatrix}, \ \mathcal{H}_2(r) = [0, A_2', A_3'], \ \text{and} \ \mathcal{H}_2(f) = [A_3', A_2']. \quad (16)$$

Again, we assume $A_2' + A_3' = 1$. The influence of a perturbation ϵ on the floating surface A_3 on the global and conditional mutual information is shown in figure 7(c). Both $I(\mathcal{H}_1)$ and $I(\mathcal{H}_2)$ have a maximum for $\epsilon = 0$. However, the maximum of $I(\mathcal{H}_1)$ is only a local maximum. Global MI reaches a local minimum for $\epsilon = -A_3A_2/(A_1 + A_2)$, after which it rises again to reach its global maximum at $\epsilon = -A_3$, thus when the central region has completely disappeared.

The effect of the bias field on the global and conditional MI can be explained as follows. Global MI estimates the joint probability by combining contributions

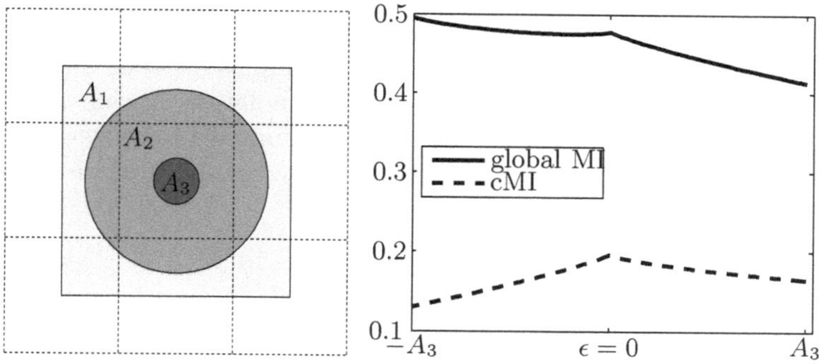

(a) (b)

Fig. 7. (a) Schematic representation of the figures used for experiment 1. (b) Evolution of the global and conditional MI for a perturbation on A_3 in the floating image.

from different spatial locations in the images, thus implicitly assuming the joint intensity distribution is spatially homogeneous. However, a non-uniform bias field will provoke an artificial widening of the histogram causing an increased number of spurious local optima. Therefore, nonrigid registration using global MI might look for a transformation that narrows this histogram without aligning corresponding structures. Using cMI, the extend of the assumed spatial homogeneity of the joint intensity distribution is limited to a single spatial bin.

In a real-life case, when the course of the similarity measure is influenced by a combination of noise, bias fields and intensity disagreements between the reference and floating image, conditional MI might not only increase the capture range of the registration, but also provide better registration results, as shown in the CT/MR registration experiments.

When the number of spatial bins increases, the number of joint intensity pairs contributing to a single bin in the joint histogram diminishes, thus imposing a lower limit on the resolution of the mesh spacing. This reduction is curbed as the spatially overlapping B-spline windows increase the number of joint intensity pairs (partially) contributing to each spatial bin. These windows also impose a certain relationship between neighbouring histograms.

Also, as the number of features present in a small spatial window decreases with decreasing mesh spacing, the number of nonzero bins will decrease as well. The available information is distributed over a smaller number of bins, increasing the statistical power of the joint histogram. On the other hand, image artefacts such as noise or a bias field, will widen the intensity range corresponding to a single feature, thus increasing the number of bins and minimum number of voxels required for a representative joint histogram.

The 2D registration experiments were performed using a 32×32 voxel mesh, thus actually including only $32 \times 32 \times 3 \times 3 = 9216$ voxels in each spatial bin. The same number of voxels is obtained in 3D using a mesh spacing as low as 10 voxels. Further research will show wether this extension can be made.

In our current implementation, cMI is calculated independently for each spatial bin, leading to an increase in registration time by a factor 10 for the 2D images. However, we are currently working on an implementation sharing calculation of the transformation mesh and image interpolation in each voxel. Thus, the extra steps required to calculate the cMI are limited to the weighing of the hits according to the spatial bins and the increased number of histograms for which the MI has to be calculated.

5 Conclusion

We have proposed conditional mutual information (cMI) as a new similarity measure for nonrigid image registration. We have shown that cMI can overcome several problems inherent to the use of global MI, using artificial and clinical images, and provided a theoretical foundation to explain the results.

References

1. Collignon, A., Maes, F., Delaere, D., Vandermeulen, D., Suetens, P., Marchal, G.: Automated multi-modality image registration based on information theory. In: Computational Imaging and Vision. Proceedings XIVth international conference on information processing in medical imaging - IPMI'95, June 26-30, vol. 3, pp. 263–274. Kluwer Academic Publishers, Boston, MA (1995)
2. Viola, P., Wells, W.M.: Alignment by maximization of mutual information. In: ICCV '95. Proceedings of the Fifth International Conference on Computer Vision, pp. 16–23. IEEE Computer Society, Los Alamitos (1995)
3. Maes, F., Vandermeulen, D., Suetens, P.: Medical image registration using mutual information. Proceedings of the IEEE, vol. 91(10), pp. 1699–1722 (October 2003)
4. Pluim, J., Maintz, J., Viergever, M.: Mutual-information-based registration of medical images: A survey. IEEE Trans. Med. Imag. 22(8), 986–1004 (2003)
5. West, J., et al.: Comparison and evaluation of retrospective intermodality brain image registration techniques. J Comput Assist Tomogr 21(4), 554–566 (1997)
6. Gaens, T., Maes, F., Vandermeulen, D., Suetens, P.: Non-rigid multimodal image registration using mutual information. In: Wells, W.M., Colchester, A.C.F., Delp, S.L. (eds.) MICCAI 1998. LNCS, vol. 1496, pp. 1099–1106. Springer, Heidelberg (1998)
7. Likar, B., Pernuš, F.: A hierarchical approach to elastic registration based on mutual information. Image and Vision Computing 19(1-2), 33–44 (2001)
8. Andronache, A., Cattin, P., Székely, G.: Local intensity mapping for hierarchical non-rigid registration of multi-modal images using the cross-correlation coefficient. In: Pluim, J.P.W., Likar, B., Gerritsen, F.A. (eds.) WBIR 2006. LNCS, vol. 4057, pp. 26–33. Springer, Heidelberg (2006)
9. Studholme, C., Drapaca, C., Iordanova, B., Cardenas, V.: Deformation-based mapping of volume change from serial brain MRI in the presence of local tissue contrast change. IEEE Trans. Med. Imag. 25(5), 626–639 (2006)
10. Thévenaz, P., Unser, M.: Optimization of mutual information for multiresolution image registration. IEEE Trans. Signal Processing 9(12), 2083–2099 (2000)
11. Cover, T.M., Thomas, J.A.: Elements of information theory. John Wiley & Sons, Chichester (1991)

12. Rueckert, D., Sonoda, L.I., Hayes, C., Hill, D.L., Leach, M.O., Hawkes, D.J.: Nonrigid registration using free-form deformations: application to breast MR images. IEEE Trans. Med. Imag. 18(8), 712–721 (1999)
13. Maes, F., Collignon, A., Vandermeulen, D., Marchal, G., Suetens, P.: Multimodality image registration by maximization of mutual information. IEEE Trans. Med. Imag. 16(2), 187–198 (1997)
14. Chen, H.M., Varshney, P.K.: Mutual information-based CT-MR brain image registration using generalized partial volume joint histogram estimation. IEEE Trans. Med. Imag. 22(9), 1111–1119 (2003)
15. Loeckx, D.: Automated Non-Rigid Intra-Patient Image Registration Using B-Splines. PhD thesis, Katholieke Universiteit Leuven (2006)
16. Byrd, R., Lu, P., Nocedal, J., Zhu, C.: A limited memory algorithm for bound constrained optimization. SIAM J. Sci. Comput. 16(5), 1190–1208 (1995)
17. Slagmolen, P., Loeckx, D., Roels, S., Geets, X., Maes, F., Haustermans, K., Suetens, P.: Nonrigid registration of multitemporal CT and MR images for radiotherapy treatment planning. In: Pluim, J.P.W., Likar, B., Gerritsen, F.A. (eds.) WBIR 2006. LNCS, vol. 4057, pp. 26–33. Springer, Heidelberg (2006)

Non-parametric Surface-Based Regularisation for Building Statistical Shape Models

Carole Twining, Rhodri Davies, and Chris Taylor

Imaging Sciences, University of Manchester, Manchester, UK

Abstract. Determining groupwise correspondence across a set of unlabelled examples of either shapes or images, by the use of an optimisation procedure, is a well-established technique that has been shown to produce quantitatively better models than other approaches. However, the computational cost of the optimisation is high, leading to long convergence times. In this paper, we show how topologically non-trivial shapes can be mapped to regular grids (called shape images). This leads to an initial reduction in computational complexity. By also considering the question of regularisation, we show that a non-parametric fluid regulariser can be applied in a principled manner, the fluid flowing on the shape surface itself, whilst not loosing the computational gain made by the use of shape images. We show that this non-parametric regularisation leads to a further considerable gain, when compared to previous parametric regularisation methods. Quantitative evaluation is performed on biological datasets, and shown to yield a substantial decrease in convergence time, with no loss of model quality.

1 Introduction

Statistical models of shape and appearance have proven to be powerful tools for image interpretation and morphological analysis. A key step in the construction of such a model is establishing a dense correspondence across a training set of examples of the object to be modelled. It is important that the correct correspondence is chosen, otherwise the model built from this correspondence will not truly represent the actual variation seen in the training set, for example, by not being specific enough, or by having poor generalisation ability.

It has been shown previously that for either shapes or images, this fundamental problem of groupwise correspondence can be solved by treating it as an integral part of the learning process (e.g, [3,4]). The key idea is that the quality of the correspondence can be evaluated by measuring the quality of the model build using that correspondence. This then casts model-building into the form of an optimisation problem. The required framework consists of: an *objective function* (which provides a quantitative measure of model quality), a method of *manipulating* the groupwise correspondence (which enables movement in the search space of our optimisation problem), and finally an *optimisation algorithm*.

It has been shown that an objective function based on the information theoretic concept of Minimum Description Length (MDL, [12]) produces models

N. Karssemeijer and B. Lelieveldt (Eds.): IPMI 2007, LNCS 4584, pp. 738–750, 2007.
© Springer-Verlag Berlin Heidelberg 2007

which are quantitatively better than those produced using other methods, including manual annotation [3,4]. Such an MDL approach can be applied to the groupwise correspondence problem for either shapes or images, but in this paper we will focus on the case of MDL groupwise correspondence for shapes.

In previous approaches, each shape in the training set was first parameterised by mapping it to a topological primitive (e.g., the unit sphere). The groupwise correspondence was then manipulated by re-parameterising each shape in turn, by means of re-parameterisations of the sphere. Although this allowed the topology of the shape to be maintained, it entailed the computationally-costly step of interpolating triangulated shape meshes on the surface of a sphere. In this paper, we adapt ideas from the computer graphics literature, which show how triangulated shape surfaces can be mapped onto regular grids, which we call *shape images*. Interpolation and numerical differentiation are much simpler and faster on regular grids, which leads to an order of magnitude decrease in convergence times.

The final issue is the optimisation algorithm used. The groupwise correspondence problem is in general ill-posed, and insoluble without some form of regularisation. Previous approaches to shape correspondence used parametric regularisation, confining the allowed re-parameterisation transformations to some set of parametric transformations (e.g., Cauchy functions [3], B-splines [10], or polynomials [9]). But the limited nature of the allowed transformations can also make the optimum correspondence difficult to find and represent. By analogy with techniques in image registration [2], we show that it is possible to use a non-parametric, fluid regularisation method. We also show that it is possible to introduce this regulariser in a principled way, so that the fluid regulariser acts on the shape surface itself, whilst retaining all the computational advantages of the shape image representation[1]. We perform a quantitative evaluation on biological datasets, and show that it converges several orders of magnitude faster than previous approaches.

2 Building Statistical Shape Models

We start with a training set of shapes $\{S_i : i = 1, \dots n_S\}$, where S_i represents the entire surface of the ith shape in $\mathbb{R}^3$. An initial chart/parameterisation $\mathfrak{X}$ is constructed for each shape, so that $\boldsymbol{S}_i(\boldsymbol{x}) \in \mathbb{R}^3$ is a single point on the ith shape, with parameter value $\boldsymbol{x} \in \mathfrak{X}$, and shape function $\boldsymbol{S}_i(\cdot)$. The dense pointwise correspondence between any two shapes is then: $\boldsymbol{S}_i(\boldsymbol{x}) \sim \boldsymbol{S}_j(\boldsymbol{x})$ for all $\boldsymbol{x} \in \mathfrak{X}$. The statistical properties of the distribution of shapes are then captured by the mean shape $\overline{\boldsymbol{S}}$, and by the shape covariance matrix $\boldsymbol{D}$ (with elements D_{ij}):

$$\overline{\boldsymbol{S}}(\boldsymbol{x}) \doteq \frac{1}{n_S} \sum_{i=1}^{n_S} \boldsymbol{S}_i(\boldsymbol{x}),\ D_{ij} \doteq \int dA(\boldsymbol{x})(\boldsymbol{S}_i(\boldsymbol{x}) - \overline{\boldsymbol{S}}(\boldsymbol{x})) \bullet (\boldsymbol{S}_j(\boldsymbol{x}) - \overline{\boldsymbol{S}}(\boldsymbol{x})), \quad (1)$$

[1] A preliminary version of this work was presented in [6], but did not include this important step, of fluid regularisation on the shape itself.

where $\bullet$ is the usual vector dot product in $\mathbb{R}^3$, and $dA(\boldsymbol{x})$ is the area measure defined on the mean shape (see [4] for further details). For a linear model, PCA is performed on the covariance matrix, which yields the eigenvectors (representing the modes of shape variation), and the corresponding eigenvalues $\{\lambda_\alpha\}$.

2.1 Manipulating Correspondence

The groupwise correspondence across the set of shapes is then manipulated by re-parameterising each shape. For the ith shape, we have the re-parameterisation function $\phi_i(\boldsymbol{x})$, where:

$$\boldsymbol{x} \overset{\phi_i}{\longmapsto} \boldsymbol{x}' \doteq \phi_i(\boldsymbol{x}) \ \& \ \boldsymbol{S}_i \overset{\phi_i}{\longmapsto} \boldsymbol{S}'_i, \text{ where } \boldsymbol{S}'_i(\boldsymbol{x}') \doteq \boldsymbol{S}_i(\boldsymbol{x}). \tag{2}$$

Hence both the shape-functions $\{\boldsymbol{S}_i(\cdot)\}$ and the groupwise correspondence change under re-parameterisation. For re-parameterising just the ith shape:

$$\boldsymbol{S}_j(\boldsymbol{x}) \sim \boldsymbol{S}_i(\boldsymbol{x}) \overset{\phi_i}{\longmapsto} \boldsymbol{S}_j(\boldsymbol{x}) \sim \boldsymbol{S}'_i(\boldsymbol{x}) \doteq \boldsymbol{S}_i\left(\phi_i^{-1}(\boldsymbol{x})\right). \tag{3}$$

The re-parameterisation is hence valid provided that ϕ_i is a homeomorphic mapping. Manipulating the groupwise correspondence changes the mean shape and the shape covariance matrix (1), hence leads to a different model.

Note that the re-parameterisation function ϕ_i acts on the space of the original chart $\mathfrak{X}$, *not* on the shape surface itself. Hence the problem of constructing valid re-parameterisation functions depends on the initial chart construction (See §3).

2.2 The Objective Function

A general objective function for model-building will be denoted by $\mathcal{L}_S(\{\boldsymbol{S}_i(\cdot)\})$, where the notation indicates that it depends *explicitly* on the set of shape functions $\{\boldsymbol{S}_i(\cdot)\}$, hence only *implicitly* on the set of re-parameterisation functions $\{\phi_i(\cdot)\}$, as described above. In this paper, we will focus on objective functions based on the MDL principle (e.g., [3,4]), where the explicit dependance is on the set of eigenvalues $\{\lambda_\alpha\}$ of $\boldsymbol{D}$ (1), which we will denote by $\mathcal{L}_S = \mathcal{L}_{\text{MDL}}(\{\lambda_\alpha\})$.

3 Coordinate Charts for Surfaces: Shape Images

The training set of shapes is typically represented as a set of triangulated meshes. In previous work [3], the initial chart $\mathfrak{X}$ was constructed by mapping each mesh to the surface of a unit sphere. Re-parameterising the shapes then involved manipulating points on the surface of the sphere, and then interpolating between the points of the triangulated mesh as mapped to the sphere to recover the shape positions of these manipulated points. The problem with this approach is that although it is relatively easy to maintain the topology of the shape, it entails a computationally-intensive interpolation step, which forms a major bottleneck in the optimisation algorithm.

The computational cost of the interpolation could be considerably decreased if our chart was a region of the plane, with a regular grid of sample points, which

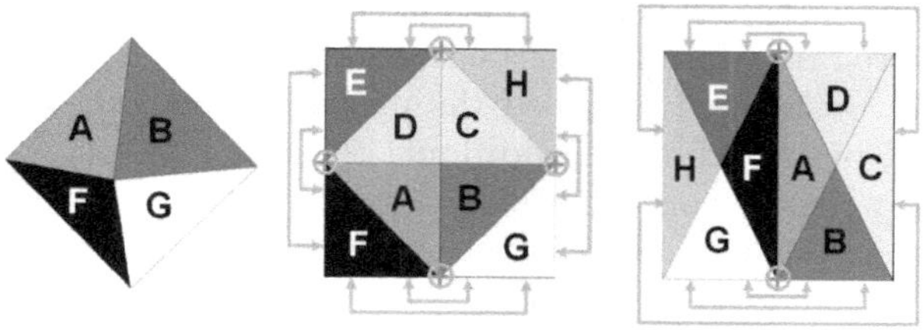

Fig. 1. Left: The octahedron, **Centre & Right:** Two unfoldings. The labels show the faces, the gray lines the boundary conditions, and the gray circles the singular points.

then allows much more straightforward methods of interpolation. It is a well-known result that a sphere cannot be covered by a single chart, so that any such single chart will have at least one point where derivatives cannot be defined. The naive approach would be to take as our chart a square, with cartesian coordinates on the chart being the usual polar angles on the sphere. However, this has the problem that two edges of this chart are identified with single points on the sphere.

A better chart can be constructed by using the work of Praun and Hoppe [11]. The sphere is not mapped directly to the plane, but first onto the inscribed regular octahedron, using a gnomic projection. The octahedron is then cut open and flattened to construct the final chart (see Figure 1). There are points where derivatives cannot be defined (the points where an edge of the chart folds back on itself, marked by plus symbols in the Figure), but these are just a few points[2]. A regular pixel grid is then constructed on this chart. Praun and Hoppe stored information about texture, colour and geometry at each pixel, and hence christened them *geometry images*. We instead store the coordinates of the corresponding point on the physical shape for each pixel, hence call these *shape images*.

4 Non-parametric Regularisation

As mentioned previously, the correspondence problem is ill-posed, and cannot be solved unless some regularisation is introduced. There are two basic approaches to regularisation, the parametric and the non-parametric.

The parametric approach reduces the dimensionality of the search space by considering only a finite-dimensional subspace of parameterised transformations. For shape correspondence, examples include transformations of the sphere based on Cauchy kernels [3], B-splines [10], and polynomials [9]. This parametric approach can be thought of as *hard* regularisation, since the subspace of allowed transformations is held fixed at a given level of resolution. Various optimisation algorithms can then be used to solve the optimisation problem (e.g., genetic algorithms [4], a generic local optimisation algorithm [3] or gradient descent [7]).

[2] Some such points will always remain, since an everywhere differentiable atlas for the sphere requires at least two coordinate charts.

The alternative approach can be thought of as *soft* regularisation, where the subspace of allowed transformations is not held fixed, but instead, more extreme transformations are allowed provided the evidence from the data warrants it. This is achieved by including an additional term $\mathcal{L}_\phi(\{\phi_i(\cdot)\})$ in the objective function, which weights transformations.

There are many possible choices for this weighting function $\mathcal{L}_\phi$, typically involving the curvature or bending energy of the transformation, which keep the transformation smooth. However, such forms have the disadvantage that they tend to penalize large-amplitude transformations.

A mathematically equivalent formulation is to express the problem not in terms of the objective function, but in terms of forces derived from it. We define the displacement field $\boldsymbol{u}(\boldsymbol{y})$ where $\phi(\boldsymbol{y}) \doteq \boldsymbol{y} + \boldsymbol{u}(\phi(\boldsymbol{y}))$ (for clarity, we drop the index i denoting the shape example). Note that $\phi(\boldsymbol{y})$ is defined so that the point $\boldsymbol{y}$ maps to $\phi(\boldsymbol{y})$, whereas the displacement field represents the inverse mapping, so that $\boldsymbol{x} = \phi(\boldsymbol{y}) = \boldsymbol{y} + \boldsymbol{u}(\boldsymbol{x}) \Rightarrow \boldsymbol{y} = \boldsymbol{x} - \boldsymbol{u}(\boldsymbol{x})$.

The driving force from the shape part of the objective function is then:

$$\boldsymbol{F}^S(\boldsymbol{u}) \propto \frac{\delta \mathcal{L}_S(\{\boldsymbol{S}_i\})}{\delta \boldsymbol{u}(\boldsymbol{x})}, \tag{4}$$

where the optimum value of the displacement field for just this part of the objective function corresponds to a zero driving force. The sign of the driving force is determined so that it tends to resist departures from this optimum.

The addition of the regulariser also provides a force. For a regulariser based on the displacement field $\boldsymbol{u}(\boldsymbol{x})$:

$$F_\phi = \frac{\delta \mathcal{L}_\phi(\{\boldsymbol{u}_i(\cdot)\})}{\delta \boldsymbol{u}(\boldsymbol{x})}. \tag{5}$$

But again, this form tends to penalise large displacements. Also, the regularising force is not zero for non-zero displacements, so that the position of the optimum (zero *net* force) is now shifted with respect to that defined by the shape term alone.

An alternative approach is to introduce an additional time coordinate t, so that we now have a time-dependant displacement field $\boldsymbol{u}(\boldsymbol{x}, t)$. And rather than penalizing $\boldsymbol{u}$ directly, we instead consider the derivatives of $\boldsymbol{u}$. This approach now does not explicitly penalise large displacements, whilst retaining all the advantages of a soft regulariser, and is the fluid-registration approach as introduced by Christensen et al. [2].

4.1 The Fluid Equations

Let us consider a fluid, where a particle of the fluid starts at $\boldsymbol{y}$ at $t = 0$, and is at a point $\phi(\boldsymbol{y}, t)$ after a time t. Rather than follow the dynamics of a tracked particle (the Lagrangian approach), we instead consider a fixed position with respect to some external coordinate frame, and consider the forces at this point as fluid moves past it (the Eulerian approach).

Consider a point $\boldsymbol{x}$ at time t. The fluid passing $\boldsymbol{x}$ originated at $\boldsymbol{y}$ at $t=0$, where:

$$\boldsymbol{y} = \phi(\boldsymbol{y},0),\ \ \boldsymbol{x} = \phi(\boldsymbol{y},t),\ \ \boldsymbol{y} = \boldsymbol{x} - \boldsymbol{u}(\boldsymbol{x},t) = \phi(\boldsymbol{y},t) - \boldsymbol{u}(\phi(\boldsymbol{y},t),t). \quad (6)$$

Hence the Eulerian velocity at point $\boldsymbol{x}$ at time t (the velocity of the fluid particles passing that point at that time) is:

$$\boldsymbol{v}(\boldsymbol{x},t) \doteq \left.\frac{\partial}{\partial t}\right|_{\boldsymbol{y}} \phi(\boldsymbol{y},t) = \left.\frac{\partial}{\partial t}\right|_{\boldsymbol{y}} \boldsymbol{u}(\phi(\boldsymbol{y},t),t) = \frac{\partial \boldsymbol{u}(\boldsymbol{x},t)}{\partial t} + (\boldsymbol{v}(\boldsymbol{x},t)\bullet\boldsymbol{\nabla})\boldsymbol{u}(\boldsymbol{x},t). \quad (7)$$

The regulariser is based on the physical model of a compressible viscous fluid, with viscous forces:

$$\boldsymbol{F}^{visc}(\boldsymbol{x},t) = \mu\boldsymbol{\nabla}^2\boldsymbol{v}(\boldsymbol{x},t) + (\lambda+\mu)\boldsymbol{\nabla}(\boldsymbol{\nabla}\bullet\boldsymbol{v}(\boldsymbol{x},t)), \quad (8)$$

where μ is the shear viscosity, and λ is the second viscosity coefficient, which is related to the bulk viscosity. Shear viscosity acts to resist non-uniform velocity gradients, whereas the bulk viscosity term acts to resist non-uniform compression/rarefaction. For a physical fluid, we would also have pressure terms and inertial terms, but for the purposes of regularisation, these terms are neglected. The only forces acting are then the viscous forces and the driving force:

$$\boldsymbol{F}^{visc} + \boldsymbol{F}^{S} = 0. \quad (9)$$

The required solution is found in the limit $\boldsymbol{v}(\boldsymbol{x},t) \to 0$ as $t \to \infty$, hence the point where the displacement field becomes static, and $\boldsymbol{F}^S = 0$, which is the same optimum as in the unregularised case. See Christensen et al. [2] for a full derivation and discussion.

The remaining question is the frame in which the viscous forces are calculated (8). If the shape image frame was used, it could be argued that the regulariser was not applied evenly across the surface of the shape, but depends on the particulars of the initial parameterisation $\mathfrak{X}$. The principled approach is hence to calculate the viscous effects on the shape surface itself, and the mathematical tools necessary for this are the subject of the next section.

4.2 The Shape Manifold

The mathematics of calculating derivatives on a shape, where we have a parameterisation of the shape (the shape image), is just the usual mathematics of changing coordinate frames in Riemannian differential geometry. What is slightly more complicated is deriving the form of the metric. We therefore present this derivation in some detail, for the benefit of readers who may not be familiar with such techniques.

Let $\mathcal{S}$ be a 2D shape manifold, with a definite fixed topology (e.g., a sphere, a torus). A physical shape $\boldsymbol{S} \subset \mathbb{R}^3$ is then an embedding of the shape manifold $\mathcal{S}$ into 3D Euclidean space. This induces a metric on the shape manifold, where distances on the shape surface are defined using the Euclidean metric of $\mathbb{R}^3$.

We construct a chart $\mathfrak{X}$ on the shape manifold, with associated cartesian coordinates (i,j). This is the basis for the shape image, where the value of the shape image function $\boldsymbol{S}(i,j)$ at point (i,j) in the chart is just the inverse of the chart mapping:

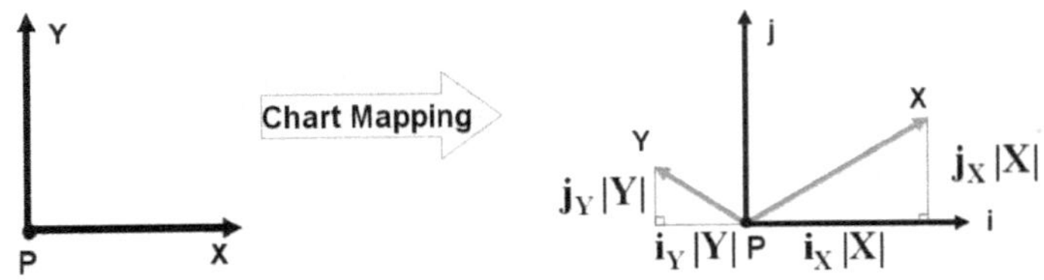

Fig. 2. The mapping of the tangent plane axes (left) into the shape image axes, showing the elements of the matrix J_P

$$\boldsymbol{S}(i,j) \underset{\mathfrak{X}}{\longmapsto} (i,j) \in \mathfrak{X}(\boldsymbol{S}).$$

Consider a general point P on the shape $\boldsymbol{S}$, with position $\boldsymbol{S}_P$. We denote the tangent space/plane at P by T_P, with tangent plane cartesian coordinates (X,Y). In the local neighbourhood of P, the shape is described by a shape function $\boldsymbol{S}(X,Y)$, with $\boldsymbol{S}(0,0) \doteq \boldsymbol{S}_P$. The induced metric means that within some neighbourhood of P, we have the distance relation:

$$\begin{aligned} X^2+Y^2 &\approx (\boldsymbol{S}(X,Y)-\boldsymbol{S}(0,0)) \bullet (\boldsymbol{S}(X,Y)-\boldsymbol{S}(0,0)) \\ &= (\boldsymbol{S}(X,Y)-\boldsymbol{S}_P) \bullet (\boldsymbol{S}(X,Y)-\boldsymbol{S}_P) \doteq \widetilde{\boldsymbol{S}}(X,Y) \bullet \widetilde{\boldsymbol{S}}(X,Y), \end{aligned} \tag{10}$$

where $\bullet$ is the usual vector dot product in $\mathbb{R}^3$, and $\widetilde{\boldsymbol{S}}(X,Y)$ is the shape difference function at P. This relation rests on the fact that the shape is locally euclidean, and flat. We then also have the approximate linear relation between the tangent plane coordinates (X,Y), and the shape image coordinates (i,j):

$$\begin{aligned} i(X,Y) &= i_P + X\left.\frac{\partial i}{\partial X}\right|_Y + Y\left.\frac{\partial i}{\partial Y}\right|_X \doteq i_P + X i_X + Y i_Y, \\ j(X,Y) &= j_P + X\left.\frac{\partial j}{\partial X}\right|_Y + Y\left.\frac{\partial j}{\partial Y}\right|_X \doteq j_P + X j_X + Y j_Y, \end{aligned} \tag{11}$$

which can be rewritten in the form:

$$\begin{pmatrix} i(X,Y)-i_P \\ j(X,Y)-j_P \end{pmatrix} = \begin{pmatrix} i_X & i_Y \\ j_X & j_Y \end{pmatrix}\begin{pmatrix} X \\ Y \end{pmatrix} \doteq \mathrm{J}_P\begin{pmatrix} X \\ Y \end{pmatrix}. \tag{12}$$

where J_P is the Jacobian of the transformation $(X,Y) \longmapsto (i(X,Y), j(X,Y))$ evaluated at P (see Figure 2). Hence a vector $\widetilde{\boldsymbol{W}} \in \mathrm{T}_P$ in the shape manifold[3], with tangent-plane components $(\widetilde{W}_X, \widetilde{W}_Y)$, maps to the corresponding vector in the shape image with components (W_i, W_j), where:

$$\begin{pmatrix} W_i \\ W_j \end{pmatrix} = \mathrm{J}_P\begin{pmatrix} \widetilde{W}_X \\ \widetilde{W}_Y. \end{pmatrix}, \;\Rightarrow \boxed{\boldsymbol{W} = \mathrm{J}_P\widetilde{\boldsymbol{W}}.} \tag{13}$$

[3] In what follows, we will use $\tilde{\cdot}$ to denote vectors or operators in the tangent plane, when the distinction is important.

There is a corresponding transformation law for derivatives. Using the chain-rule:

$$\widetilde{\nabla}_X \doteq \left.\frac{\partial}{\partial X}\right|_Y = \left.\frac{\partial i}{\partial X}\right|_Y \left.\frac{\partial}{\partial i}\right|_j + \left.\frac{\partial j}{\partial X}\right|_Y \left.\frac{\partial}{\partial j}\right|_i \doteq i_X \nabla_i + j_X \nabla_j,$$

$$\widetilde{\nabla}_Y \doteq \left.\frac{\partial}{\partial Y}\right|_X = \left.\frac{\partial i}{\partial Y}\right|_X \left.\frac{\partial}{\partial i}\right|_j + \left.\frac{\partial j}{\partial Y}\right|_X \left.\frac{\partial}{\partial j}\right|_i \doteq i_Y \nabla_i + j_Y \nabla_j,$$

$$\therefore\ \widetilde{\boldsymbol{\nabla}} \doteq \begin{pmatrix} \widetilde{\nabla}_X \\ \widetilde{\nabla}_Y \end{pmatrix} = \begin{pmatrix} i_X & j_X \\ i_Y & j_Y \end{pmatrix} \begin{pmatrix} \nabla_i \\ \nabla_j \end{pmatrix} \Rightarrow \boxed{\widetilde{\boldsymbol{\nabla}} = \mathrm{J}_P^T \boldsymbol{\nabla}.} \tag{14}$$

All that remains is to calculate J_P. Note however that the chart mapping $\mathfrak{X}$ does not totally determine J_P; there is a local gauge degree of freedom corresponding to rotating the (X, Y) coordinate axes in the tangent plane, $\mathrm{J}_P \mapsto \mathrm{J}_P g$ where g is a rotation matrix in 2D. We could fix the gauge, by setting, for example, the direction of X to be that of i when mapped, and the (X, Y) axes to have the same orientation as (i, j). However, this is not necessary, as we will see.

Consider the distance relation (10):

$$X^2 + Y^2 = \widetilde{\boldsymbol{S}}(X, Y) \bullet \widetilde{\boldsymbol{S}}(X, Y). \tag{15}$$

and the second-order differential operators $\widetilde{\nabla}_X^2$, $\widetilde{\nabla}_Y^2$ & $\widetilde{\nabla}_X \widetilde{\nabla}_Y$. Applying these in turn to the above expression, and using the transformation law for derivatives given above, we find:

$$1 = i_X^2 (\nabla_i \widetilde{\boldsymbol{S}})^2 + 2 i_X j_X (\nabla_i \widetilde{\boldsymbol{S}}) \bullet (\nabla_j \widetilde{\boldsymbol{S}}) + j_X^2 (\nabla_j \widetilde{\boldsymbol{S}})^2 + 2^{\text{nd}} \text{ derivatives}$$

$$1 = i_Y^2 (\nabla_i \widetilde{\boldsymbol{S}})^2 + 2 i_Y j_Y (\nabla_i \widetilde{\boldsymbol{S}}) \bullet (\nabla_j \widetilde{\boldsymbol{S}}) + j_Y^2 (\nabla_j \widetilde{\boldsymbol{S}})^2 + 2^{\text{nd}} \text{ derivatives}$$

$$0 = i_X i_Y (\nabla_i \widetilde{\boldsymbol{S}})^2 + (i_X j_Y + i_Y j_X)(\nabla_i \widetilde{\boldsymbol{S}}) \bullet (\nabla_j \widetilde{\boldsymbol{S}}) + j_X j_Y (\nabla_j \widetilde{\boldsymbol{S}})^2 + 2^{\text{nd}} \text{ derivatives},$$

where we can neglect the terms which contain second derivatives of the shape (e.g., $\nabla_i \nabla_j \widetilde{\boldsymbol{S}}$), since the distance relation (10) is only true to leading order. These equations can be written in matrix form thus:

$$\begin{pmatrix} 1 & 0 \\ 0 & 1 \end{pmatrix} = \begin{pmatrix} i_X & j_X \\ i_Y & j_Y \end{pmatrix} \begin{pmatrix} (\nabla_i \widetilde{\boldsymbol{S}})^2 & (\nabla_i \widetilde{\boldsymbol{S}}) \bullet (\nabla_j \widetilde{\boldsymbol{S}}) \\ (\nabla_i \widetilde{\boldsymbol{S}}) \bullet (\nabla_j \widetilde{\boldsymbol{S}}) & (\nabla_j \widetilde{\boldsymbol{S}})^2 \end{pmatrix} \begin{pmatrix} i_X & i_Y \\ j_X & j_Y \end{pmatrix} \tag{16}$$

$$M_P \doteq \begin{pmatrix} (\nabla_i \widetilde{\boldsymbol{S}})^2 & (\nabla_i \widetilde{\boldsymbol{S}}) \bullet (\nabla_j \widetilde{\boldsymbol{S}}) \\ (\nabla_i \widetilde{\boldsymbol{S}}) \bullet (\nabla_j \widetilde{\boldsymbol{S}}) & (\nabla_j \widetilde{\boldsymbol{S}})^2 \end{pmatrix}, \quad \boxed{\therefore\ \mathrm{J}_P \mathrm{J}_P^T = M_P^{-1}.} \tag{17}$$

M_P is just the Riemannian metric at the point P. Note that this result is gauge-invariant, since for a 2×2 real matrix representation of 2D rotations:

$$g^T \equiv g^{-1} \;\Rightarrow (\mathrm{J}_P g)(g^T \mathrm{J}_P^T) \equiv \mathrm{J}_P \mathrm{J}_P^T.$$

The important point to note about this result is that M_P (and hence M_P^{-1}) is obtained by calculating derivatives of the shape image with respect to the shape image coordinates, hence working purely within the shape image itself.

Consider the viscous forces calculated on the shape:

$$\widetilde{\boldsymbol{F}}^{visc} = \mu \widetilde{\boldsymbol{\nabla}}^2 \widetilde{\boldsymbol{v}}(\boldsymbol{x},t) + (\lambda+\mu)\widetilde{\boldsymbol{\nabla}}(\widetilde{\boldsymbol{\nabla}} \bullet \widetilde{\boldsymbol{v}}(\boldsymbol{x},t)). \tag{18}$$

Applying the above transformation rules[4], we find that for components in the shape image (denoted by $\boldsymbol{v}_a$ for vector components, and ∇_a for the components of derivatives):

$$\begin{aligned}\left(\boldsymbol{F}^{visc}\right)_c &= \mu \left[(\mathrm{J}_P \mathrm{J}_P^T)_{ab} \nabla_a \nabla_b\right] \boldsymbol{v}_c + (\lambda+\mu)\left[\mathrm{J}_P \mathrm{J}_P^T\right]_{ca} \nabla_a \nabla_b \boldsymbol{v}_b \\ &= \mu \left[(M_P^{-1})_{ab} \nabla_a \nabla_b\right] \boldsymbol{v}_c + (\lambda+\mu)\left[(M_P^{-1})_{ca} \nabla_a \nabla_b\right] \boldsymbol{v}_b. \end{aligned} \tag{19}$$

We hence see that the effect of calculating the viscous forces on the shape itself is that the effective viscous forces on the shape image become a bit more complicated, where we have a position-dependant mixture of spatial derivatives. Although this mixture depends on position, M_P^{-1} has only to be calculated once for each sample point in the shape image, since the shape image (and hence M_P^{-1}), remains fixed as the displacement field evolves.

4.3 Implementation Details

The Objective Function: To calculate the driving force $\boldsymbol{F}^S$ for the kth shape, we need to differentiate the objective function wrt the displacement field for this shape. As in approximate-MDL gradient descent methods [7,8,9], this can be done by applying the chain-rule:

$$\frac{\delta \mathcal{L}_S(\{\boldsymbol{S}_i\})}{\delta \boldsymbol{u}_k} = \frac{\partial \mathcal{L}_{\mathrm{MDL}}(\{\lambda^m\})}{\partial \lambda^m} \cdot \frac{\partial \lambda^m}{\partial D_{ij}} \cdot \frac{\delta D_{ij}}{\delta \boldsymbol{S}_k} \cdot \frac{\delta \boldsymbol{S}_k}{\delta \boldsymbol{u}_k}. \tag{20}$$

The first term just means differentiating the objective function written in terms of the eigenvalues of the model. The second term was calculated for the form of the covariance matrix given in (1) by Hladůvka and Bühlerit, and is a simple function of the eigenvectors [9]. The third term is obtained by differentiating the covariance matrix (1). The last term is the motion of points on the kth shape with respect to movement in the kth shape image, and hence can be calculated numerically using a simple finite-difference scheme on the shape image.

The Chart: We consider shapes which are topologically equivalent to spheres. Each shape is then mapped to the unit sphere using the method of Brechbühler et al. [1]. Points on the unit sphere are then mapped to the inscribed regular octahedron by using a gnomonic projection [11]. The octahedron is then unfolded,

[4] Note that we are making a further approximation here, that the shape is piecewise linear, so that we can pass the matrices through the derivatives. If we had not made this simplifying assumption, we would also have additional terms containing derivatives of the matrices. These are in effect the Christoffel symbols that would be obtained using standard differential geometry, where our expression $\boldsymbol{F}^{visc}$ would be calculated by just replacing the ordinary derivatives in eqn. (18) by covariant derivatives.

using either of the methods shown in Figure 1. A regular grid of sample points is then constructed on this chart, the total pixel grid being denoted by $\mathbf{X} = \{\boldsymbol{x}\}$. For each shape in the training set, the set of shape values is sampled on this grid, and the collected values denoted by $\mathbf{S}_i$, the entire pixellated shape image, with value $\boldsymbol{S}_i(\boldsymbol{x})$ at pixel $\boldsymbol{x} \in \mathbf{X}$.

Fluid Equations: For each shape example, the set of values of the fluid velocity field, the displacement field, and the viscous forces acting are collected into variables $\mathbf{V}(t) \doteq \{\boldsymbol{v}(\boldsymbol{x},t) : \boldsymbol{x} \in \mathbf{X}\}$, $\mathbf{U}(t) \doteq \{\boldsymbol{u}(\boldsymbol{x},t)\}$, and $\mathbf{F}^{visc}(t) \doteq \{\boldsymbol{F}^{visc}(\boldsymbol{x},t)\}$. Similarly, $\boldsymbol{\nabla}$ will be taken to represent either the derivative at a point, or the derivative operator acting across the entire grid. Approximating derivatives by a finite-differencing scheme, the equation for the viscous force (19) can now be written as a simple matrix operation:

$$\mathbf{F}^{visc}(t) = \mathbf{A}\mathbf{V}(t). \tag{21}$$

It is important to note that $\mathbf{A}$ is a *sparse* matrix that depends only on the initial chart $\mathfrak{X}$, remains fixed as the fluid evolves, hence can be pre-computed. The fluid algorithm can then be written symbolically as follows:

Initialize with $\mathbf{U} = 0, \mathbf{V} = 0$.
Repeat
- ► Given $\mathbf{U}$, find $\mathbf{F}_S(\mathbf{U})$ — % **Eqns (4) &(20)**
- ► Compute $\mathbf{V}$ using: $\mathbf{F}^{visc}(\mathbf{V}) \doteq -\mathbf{F}^S(\mathbf{U})$ & $\mathbf{F}^{visc} = \mathbf{A}\mathbf{V}$ — % **Eqns (9) & (21)**
- ► Update $\mathbf{U}$: $\mathbf{U} \Leftarrow \mathbf{U} + dt(\mathbf{V} - (\mathbf{V}\cdot\boldsymbol{\nabla})\mathbf{U})$ — % **Eqn (7)**
- ► Check if re-gridding is required

Until convergence

In [2], equation (21) was solved for $\mathbf{V}$ using an iterative method. However, since our shape images are only 2-dimensional we instead use the (pre-computed) LU decomposition with permutation, which gives a quicker solution within the loop:

$\mathbf{A} = \mathbf{PLUQ}$, Permutation matrices: $\mathbf{P}, \mathbf{Q}$, Triangular matrices: $\mathbf{L}, \mathbf{U}$
To solve: $\mathbf{F}^{visc} = \mathbf{AV} \Longrightarrow$ Solve: $\mathbf{F}^{visc} = \mathbf{PLW}$ for $\mathbf{W}$, then: $\mathbf{W} = \mathbf{UQV}$ for $\mathbf{V}$.

The time-step dt is scaled at each iteration so that the maximum additional displacement (as measured in shape image pixel units) is equal to a pre-defined value. From equation (8), we see that scaling the viscosities μ & λ for fixed driving force just gives a universal scaling of the velocity field. However, this scaling is then removed in our implementation, by the scaling of the timestep above. Hence the only free parameters are the ratio of the viscosities $\frac{\mu}{\lambda}$ (which was set to 1 in all our experiments), and the maximum permissible displacement. Note that the maximum permissible displacement should not be set too large, since we are using just a first-order finite difference approximation to the temporal derivative of the displacement field. Also, if this is set too large, the displacement field can cause the mapped grid to fold, entailing frequent re-gridding. Note that this implementation also means that fluid registration on the shape can depend on

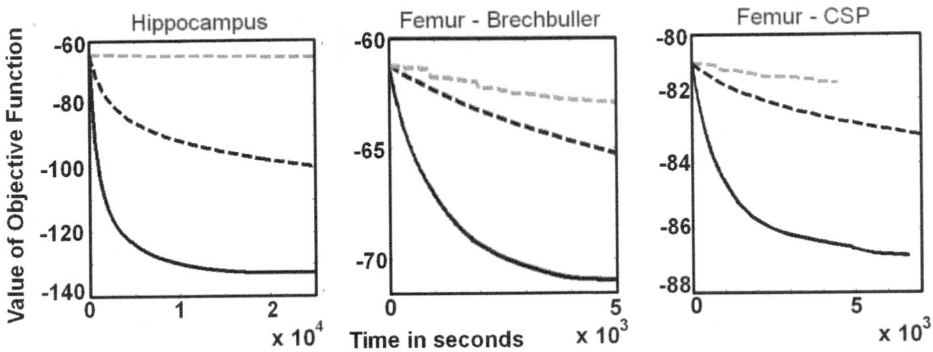

Fig. 3. Values of the objective function plotted as a function of time.**Left:** Hippocampus dataset, **Centre & Right:** Femur dataset with varying initial mappings to the sphere.
Gray dashed line: Parametric regularisation on the sphere.
Black dashed line: Parametric regularisation on the shape image.
Black solid line: Fluid regularisation on the shape.

Table 1. A table showing the convergence rate of the methods for the various datasets, compared to the parametric case on the sphere. Higher values indicate faster convergence.

	Hippocampus	Femur	
		Brechbuller	CSP
Parametric on sphere	1	1	1
Parametric on shape image	24	4	9
Fluid on the shape	**384**	**56**	**153**

the initial chart. Imagine a section of the shape, with the same body forces, but with two different mappings, one where the mapped pixels are smaller on the shape itself, and the other where they are larger. The criteria we have chosen depends on the suggested displacement in pixel units, hence the mapping with smaller pixels will lead to a smaller rate of physical shape displacement in this area wrt computational time.

5 Experiments

The aim of these experiments was to perform a direct comparison of the charting method of shape images as compared to other techniques, and to compare parametric with fluid regularisation, using the same MDL objective function. The datasets used were a set of 82 surfaces of the left hippocampus, and a set of 15 examples of the distal third of the human femur. Both were segmented from 3D MR images.

We used several methods to map shapes to the unit sphere, the method of Brechbühler et al. [1], as well as the Consistent Spherical Parameterisation (CSP) method of Davies et al. [5]. For parametric regulariser, we used a set of parametric transformations based on clamped-plate splines, applied either on the surface of the sphere (which is very similar to the method used by Heimann et al. [8]) or on the shape image, with gradient descent optimisation. The final comparison is then with the non-parametric fluid regularisation on the shape.

In Figure 3, we show the values of the objective function plotted as a function of time in seconds. Note that the algorithm was implemented in MATLAB and run on a Pentium-3 PC, and a implementation in C++ on a modern PC would be considerably faster!

In Table 1, we show the results for a quantitative comparison of the convergence rates for the graphs shown in Figure 3, with higher values indicating faster convergence.

Starting with the hippocampus dataset (Figure 3, **Left**), we can see that for parametric regularisation (dashed lines), the chart mapping to the shape image improves the convergence rate considerably when compared to using the sphere. This result is repeated for the femur data, for both methods of mapping to the sphere.

When we compare fluid with parametric regularisation (solid line compared to dashed lines), we see that fluid regularisation gives an appreciable advantage. If we compare the two methods for mapping the shape to the sphere (**centre & right** Figure 3 & Table 1), it can be seen that for this particular dataset, the exact result for fluid regularisation and rate of convergence does depend on the choice of chart. Note that for fluids, we would expect a possible difference in convergence rates for different parameterisations, since the scaling criterion depends on pixel size. Hence a region of the shape where the mapped pixels are small in terms of shape units will give a slower flow that a mapping where the pixels are larger. But we also might expect an additional effect, given that different initial sphere mappings lead to a different initial correspondence, hence we have to follow a different path in the space of groupwise correspondence. We also have to allow for the probability that the algorithm may get stuck in a local minimum. Note however that the degradation in performance for the Brechbühler et al. mapping as opposed to CSP is seen for both parametric regularisation on the shape image, and non-parametric regularisation.

We cannot however make a direct comparison between the two methods of mapping to the sphere, since the values of the objective function cannot be directly compared, as the differing scales on the y-axes show.

6 Discussion and Conclusions

The results clearly show that for parametric regularisation, the use of shape images improves the convergence rate by about an order of magnitude. It is clear that using fluid regularisation can give a further improvement, leading to an overall improvement by up to two orders of magnitude.

What is not clear from this data is the exact effect of choice of initial sphere mapping. It should also be noted that the femur dataset contains only 15 examples, whereas the hippocampus set contained 82. It could be that some of the results we are seeing on the femur dataset are the result of this small sample size, and not indicative of the behaviour for larger datasets.

The possibility of getting stuck in a local minimum should also be considered, and we intend to investigate techniques for introducing a stochastic element, so that the fluid can be moved out of such a minimum.

Finally, it would also be desirable to perform a full quantitative evaluation of the final models obtained, and analyse the differences (if any) in groupwise correspondence that these methods give, for a range of biological datasets.

Investigating the detailed behaviour of the fluid regularisation approach, and further refinement of the algorithm forms the basis of our future research.

Acknowledgements. Our thanks to Tomos Williams and Chris Wolstenholme for processing the femur dataset. Also, thanks to Anna Mills for suggesting the use of the LU decomposition.

References

1. Brechbühler, C., Gerig, G., Kübler, O.: Parameterisation of closed surfaces for 3D shape description. Computer Vision, Graphics and Image Processing 61, 154–170 (1995)
2. Christensen, G.E., Rabbitt, R.D., Miller, M.I.: Deformable templates using large deformation kinematics. IEEE Transactions on Image Processing 5, 1435–1447 (1996)
3. Davies, R.H., Twining, C.J., Cootes, T.F., Waterton, J.C., Taylor, C.J.: 3D statistical shape models using direct optimisation of description length. In: Heyden, A., Sparr, G., Nielsen, M., Johansen, P. (eds.) ECCV 2002. LNCS, vol. 2352, pp. 3–20. Springer, Heidelberg (2002)
4. Davies, R.H., Twining, C.J., Cootes, T.F., Waterton, J.C., Taylor, C.J.: A minimum description length approach to statistical shape modelling. IEEE Transactions on Medical Imaging 21, 525–537 (2002)
5. Davies, R.H., Twining, C.J., Taylor, C.J.: Consistent spherical parameterisation for statistical shape modelling. In: Proceedings of ISBI 2006, pp. 1388–1391(2006)
6. Davies, R.H., Twining, C.J., Williams, T.G., Taylor, C.J.: Building MDL statistical shape models using shape images and non-parametric regularisation. In: Proceedings of ISBI 2007 (2007)
7. Ericsson, A., Åström, K.: Minimizing the description length using steepest descent. In: Proceedings of BMVC 2003, pp. 93–102 (2003)
8. Heimann, T., Wolf, I., Williams, T.G., Meinzer, H.P.: 3D active shape models using gradient descent optimization of description length. In: Proceedings of IPMI 2005, pp. 566–577 (2005)
9. Hladůvka, J., Bühler, K.: MDL spline models: gradient and polynomial reparameterisations. In: Proceedings of BMVC 2005, pp. 869–878 (2005)
10. Horkaew, P., Yang, G.: Optimal deformable surface models for 3D medical image analysis. In: Proceedings of IPMI 2003, pp. 12–24 (2003)
11. Praun, E., Hoppe, H.: Spherical reparameterization and remeshing. In: Proceedings of SIGGRAPH 2003, pp. 340–349 (2003)
12. Rissanen, J.: Stochastic Complexity in Statistical Inquiry. World Scientific Press, Singapore (1989)

Geometrically Proper Models in Statistical Training

Qiong Han, Derek Merck, Josh Levy, Christina Villarruel,
James N. Damon, Edward L. Chaney, and Stephen M. Pizer

Medical Image Display & Analysis Group,
University of North Carolina, Chapel Hill, North Carolina 27599, USA
http://midag.cs.unc.edu

Abstract. In deformable model segmentation, the geometric training process plays a crucial role in providing shape statistical priors and appearance statistics that are used as likelihoods. Also, the geometric training process plays a crucial role in providing shape probability distributions in methods finding significant differences between classes. The quality of the training seriously affects the final results of segmentation or of significant difference finding between classes. However, the lack of shape priors in the training stage itself makes it difficult to enforce shape legality, i.e., making the model free of local self-intersection or creases. Shape legality not only yields proper shape statistics but also increases the consistency of parameterization of the object volume and thus proper appearance statistics. In this paper we propose a method incorporating explicit legality constraints in training process. The method is mathematically sound and has proved in practice to lead to shape probability distributions over only proper objects and most importantly to better segmentation results.

1 Introduction

Image segmentation, the main target problem of this paper, is an important task upon which many other medical image processing applications are based. The goal is to delineate image regions corresponding to certain anatomical structures from the background. Deformable model based methods tackle the segmentation problem by representing anatomical objects with geometric models and deform them into images via object shape and object-relative image intensity information. Shape and intensity statistics have been used respectively as priors and likelihoods in segmentations and have become a standard component in deformable model methods. In order to get trained statistics, we need to extract deformable models from a set of training images and calculate shape statistics and related appearance statistics from the trained models. This process of extracting models and calculating prior and likelihood statistics is called training.

Given a set of segmented images, a typical training step includes converting those segmentations into deformable models in a specific representation. The conversion is often realized by fitting a deformable template into a batch of binary characteristic images typically produced manually from the training greyscale images. Therefore the training step is also a fitting process but without any shape prior statistics. The lack of priors in training can cause illegal shapes, with local self-intersection or creases, which will yield unrealistic shape statistics and then defected appearance statistics relative

N. Karssemeijer and B. Lelieveldt (Eds.): IPMI 2007, LNCS 4584, pp. 751–762, 2007.
© Springer-Verlag Berlin Heidelberg 2007

to objects coordinates. Even in an iterative bootstrapping process [4] the results from the first pass training affects the final ones after multiple passes. Existing solutions to this challenge require humans to directly enforce smoothness on extracted deformable models [3]. This approach is time consuming and defeats the purpose of having an automatic training step given the binary images. Furthermore, human interferences might bring undesirable biases in the trained shapes and thus in the trained statistics.

In our framework, the deformable model is medial based. It has been argued that medial based models have strong descriptive power because they capture not only local positional information but also local orientational and size information [11]. Medial methods represent and parameterize both object surfaces and interior volumes. A particular strength of this representation is that powerful mathematics exists on the relation of the medial geometry and the geometry of the implied boundary and interior of objects [5]. In this paper we use this mathematics to provide a set of geometric constraints that can be explicitly applied to our deformable models in order to maintain the legality of the surfaces and interiors of the trained shapes.

The proposition this paper is designed to establish is that attention to model legality in fitting the models used in forming proper statistics on object geometry and on object-relative image intensity patterns is decisive for the quality of applications of the probability densities derived from the training process. Recall that achieving such legality by automatic means in Point Distribution Models (PDMs) of object boundaries required mathematics and serious computation [1]. The mathematics now available on medial representations lowers the computation necessary to assure legality from that required for PDMs.

The rest of the paper is organized as the follows. Sec. 2 covers background on the deformable method using a medial representation and medial mathematics. Sec. 3 details the proposed method for achieving medial legality and proper statistics in training. Sec. 4 shows how we generate synthetic test data and the results from application of our method to both synthetic and real world data. Sec. 5 concludes the paper.

2 Background

We begin with a brief review on deformable model based methods and medial representations. We then address some mathematical background necessary for the detailed description of the proposed method.

2.1 Medially Represented Deformable Model

Deformable models are probabilistic shape descriptions. Under the Gaussian model, the distribution of the training data is modeled by several modes of deformation about a point in the shape space. This distribution describes all shapes in the training data and moreover, for a sufficiently large training set, estimates the full ambient shape space from which the training data are drawn. This statistical framework has been shown [12] to provide a powerful basis for studies finding shape differences between classes of shape or, together with probabilistic models on image appearance via object-relative intensity patterns, to provide a powerful means of segmentation by posterior optimization.

The classical model representation is landmarks or its extension to surfaces, the point distribution model (PDM) with shape variance described by principal component analysis (PCA) of the feature space [3]. PDMs assume feature correspondence by fixed sampling, or attempt to induce correspondence post hoc by minimizing variability in the parameterization [7]. While it is possible to provide local legality constraints with such boundary representations, the literature shows little attention to this issue, perhaps because legality checks require extracting information about surface normals. Another surface representation uses spherical harmonic (SPHARM) basis functions, which guarantees local shape legality at serious computational expense but handles surface locality with difficulty. Legal PDMs can, however, be derived from the SPHARM fits to training images [13].

Our segmentation and shape analysis methodology uses the multi-scale discrete m-rep representation proposed in [11]. Medial representations provide a model-centric volumetric coordinate system for the object interior and hence, a framework for volumetric correspondence. As described in Sec. 2.2, the mathematics of m-reps based on [5] provides the means for legality guarantees over the whole object interior.

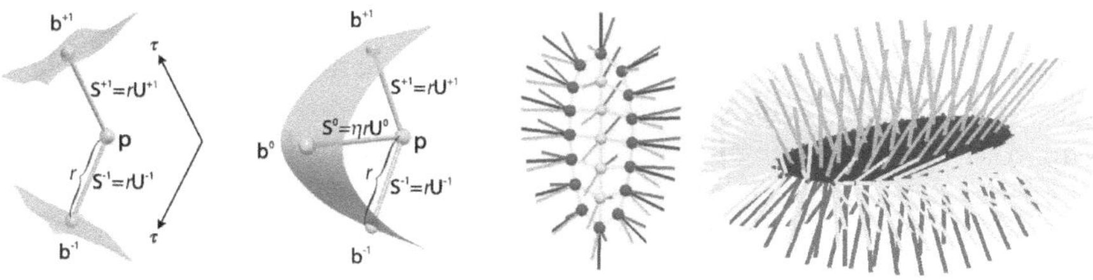

Fig. 1. From left to right: an internal atom of two spokes $\mathbf{S}^{+1}$ and $\mathbf{S}^{-1}$, with τ to parameterize the object interior along the spokes; an end atom with an extra bisector spoke $\mathbf{S}^0$; a discrete m-rep as a mesh of internal atoms (with white hubs) and end atoms (with red hubs); an interpolated spoke field on a smooth medial sheet (in dark blue).

An m-rep figure is a mesh of samples of an object's medial axis, as shown in Fig. 1. Each internal medial sample, or medial atom $\mathbf{m} = (\mathbf{p}, r, \mathbf{U}^{+1}, \mathbf{U}^{-1}) \in \mathbf{M} = \mathbb{R}^3 \times \mathbb{R}^+ \times \mathcal{S}^2 \times \mathcal{S}^2$ has eight parameters: 3 in hub position $\mathbf{p}$, 4 in two medial spoke directions $\mathbf{U}^{+1/-1}$, and 1 in scale r.

In order to have more stability in the representation, each end atom can be considered as the compound of an internal atom $\{\mathbf{p}, r, \mathbf{U}^{+1}, \mathbf{U}^{-1}\}$ plus the bisector spoke corresponding to the crest line on the object boundary. The hub position and two regular spokes $\mathbf{S}^{+1/-1}$ of each end atom are treated as one internal atom. An interpolation method can be applied to an m-rep to generate a continuous medial representation as a smooth double-sided spoke field [10], and the interpolated hub positions forms its own smooth surface called *medial sheet*, shown in dark blue in Fig. 1-rightmost.

Given that each atom lies on a Riemannian manifold [9], the distance between two atoms, $d(\mathbf{m}, \mathbf{o})$, is derived by a local flattening *Log*-map defined to map points on the manifold to the local tangent plane. This leads to a Riemannian distance $d(\mathbf{m}, \mathbf{o})$. The squared distance between two m-rep models $\mathbf{M}$ and $\mathbf{O}$ with samples $\mathbf{m}_i$ and $\mathbf{o}_i$ respectively is defined as the sum of the squared distances between corresponding samples $d^2(\mathbf{M}, \mathbf{O}) = \sum_i d^2(\mathbf{m}_i, \mathbf{o}_i)$. These metrics allow for the extension of PCA into non-Euclidean domains such as m-reps [9].

The medial atom is the basic building block in m-rep representation, and the derivatives of the medial sheet and the two spoke directions in each medial atom contain sufficient information to tell whether any illegal shape exists or is about to appear [5]. The next subsection reviews the mathematics that enable us to put legality constraints on m-reps, detailed in Sec. 3.4.

2.2 Radial Shape Operator $\mathbf{S}_{rad}$ and $r\mathbf{S}_{rad}$

Differential geometry reveals how a surface normal curves in its local surface tangent plane. The derivatives of surface normals can be summarized by a 2×2 symmetric matrix called the *shape operator*. Analogously, the *radial shape operator* [5] tells how a medial spoke changes while walking on the medial sheet. Since each m-rep atom has a spoke on both sides of the medial sheet, the spoke field on the medial sheet should be considered as double valued. Thus there are two radial shape operators defined for each atom: one for each side of the medial sheet.

Let us only consider one side of the medial sheet since the same method applies to the other. Assume that there is a continuous spoke field $\mathbf{S}(\mathbf{u})$ with unit length spoke direction $\mathbf{U}(\mathbf{u})$ and spoke length $r(\mathbf{u})$ on the continuous medial sheet $\mathbf{p}(\mathbf{u})$, where $\mathbf{u} = (v_1, v_2)$ parameterizes the 2D medial sheet and the spoke field. $\mathbf{S}(\mathbf{u}) = r(\mathbf{u}) \cdot \mathbf{U}(\mathbf{u})$. The derivatives of the unit length spoke direction $\mathbf{U}(\mathbf{u})$ wrt (v_1, v_2) are calculated as follows, with $\mathbf{U}$ and $\mathbf{p}_{v_1/v_2}$ being 1×3 row vectors.

$$\frac{\partial \mathbf{U}}{\partial v_i} = a_{0,i}\mathbf{U} - a_{i,1}\mathbf{p}_{v_1} - a_{i,2}\mathbf{p}_{v_2}, \text{ where } i = 1, 2, \tag{1}$$

or rewriting in matrix form,

$$\frac{\partial \mathbf{U}}{\partial \mathbf{u}} = \begin{pmatrix} a_{0,1} \\ a_{0,2} \end{pmatrix} \mathbf{U} - \begin{pmatrix} a_{1,1} & a_{1,2} \\ a_{2,1} & a_{2,2} \end{pmatrix} \begin{pmatrix} \mathbf{p}_{v_1} \\ \mathbf{p}_{v_2} \end{pmatrix} \tag{2}$$

where $\frac{\partial \mathbf{U}}{\partial \mathbf{u}}$ is a 2×3 matrix with row i as the vector $\frac{\partial \mathbf{U}}{\partial v_i}$ and $\mathbf{p}_{v_1}$ and $\mathbf{p}_{v_2}$ are the derivatives of the medial sheet $\mathbf{p}$ wrt parameters v_1 and v_2. In these equations, the derivative of $\mathbf{U}$ is decomposed by a generally non-orthogonal projection along the spoke direction $\mathbf{U}$ to the tangent plane of the medial sheet spanned by $\mathbf{p}_{v_1}$ and $\mathbf{p}_{v_2}$.

Let $\mathbf{A}_\mathbf{u} = \begin{pmatrix} a_{0,1} \\ a_{0,2} \end{pmatrix}$ and $\mathbf{S}_{rad} = \begin{pmatrix} a_{1,1} & a_{2,1} \\ a_{1,2} & a_{2,2} \end{pmatrix}$. $\mathbf{S}_{rad}$ is called the radial shape operator. The radial shape operator is a 2×2 matrix and in general not self-adjoint.

Then (2)$\Rightarrow$

$$\frac{\partial \mathbf{U}}{\partial \mathbf{u}} = \mathbf{A}_\mathbf{u}\mathbf{U} - \mathbf{S}_{rad}^T \begin{pmatrix} \mathbf{p}_{v_1} \\ \mathbf{p}_{v_2} \end{pmatrix} \tag{3}$$

$\mathbf{U}(\mathbf{u})$ is of unit length, $\frac{\partial \mathbf{U}}{\partial \mathbf{u}} \cdot \mathbf{U}^T = \begin{pmatrix} 0 \\ 0 \end{pmatrix}$ and $\mathbf{U} \cdot \mathbf{U}^T = 1$, so by [5]-Sec.2

$$\mathbf{A_u} = \mathbf{S}_{rad}^T \begin{pmatrix} \mathbf{p}_{v1} \\ \mathbf{p}_{v2} \end{pmatrix} \mathbf{U}^T \tag{4}$$

Substituting (4) into (3) yields the means of computing $\mathbf{S}_{rad}$ given $\frac{\partial \mathbf{U}}{\partial \mathbf{u}}$, $\mathbf{U}$ and $\begin{pmatrix} \mathbf{p}_{v1} \\ \mathbf{p}_{v2} \end{pmatrix}$. That is, $\mathbf{S}_{rad}$ depends on the spoke direction $\mathbf{U}$, and the derivatives of $\mathbf{U}$ and $\mathbf{p}$.

Furthermore, the derivative of $\mathbf{S} = r\mathbf{U}$ can be expressed using $r\mathbf{S}_{rad}$ and elementary linear algebra [12]-Ch.3. An explicit matrix expression for $r\mathbf{S}_{rad}$ is obtained as follows.

$$\frac{\partial \mathbf{S}}{\partial \mathbf{u}} = \frac{\partial (r\mathbf{U})}{\partial \mathbf{u}} = r\frac{\partial \mathbf{U}}{\partial \mathbf{u}} + \begin{pmatrix} r_{v1} \\ r_{v2} \end{pmatrix} \mathbf{U} \tag{5}$$

Substituting (3) and (4) into (5) yields

$$\frac{\partial \mathbf{S}}{\partial \mathbf{u}} = r\mathbf{S}_{rad}^T \begin{pmatrix} \mathbf{p}_{v1} \\ \mathbf{p}_{v2} \end{pmatrix} (\mathbf{U}^T\mathbf{U} - \mathbf{I}) + \begin{pmatrix} r_{v1} \\ r_{v2} \end{pmatrix} \mathbf{U} \tag{6}$$

The spokes being orthogonal to the boundary formed by their envelope requires [5] that $r_{v1/v2} = -\mathbf{p}_{v1/v2}\mathbf{U}^T$. Let $Q = \begin{pmatrix} \mathbf{p}_{v1} \\ \mathbf{p}_{v2} \end{pmatrix} (\mathbf{U}^T\mathbf{U} - \mathbf{I})$ be a 2×3 matrix. Then

$$r\mathbf{S}_{rad} = \left(\left(\frac{\partial \mathbf{S}}{\partial \mathbf{u}} + \begin{pmatrix} \mathbf{p}_{v1}\mathbf{U}^T \\ \mathbf{p}_{v2}\mathbf{U}^T \end{pmatrix} \mathbf{U} \right) \mathbf{Q}^T(\mathbf{Q}\mathbf{Q}^T)^{-1} \right)^T \tag{7}$$

(7) shows how to compute $r\mathbf{S}_{rad}$ given the derivatives of $\mathbf{p}$, $\mathbf{U}$ and $\mathbf{S}$ wrt (v_1, v_2).

Analogously with calling the eigenvalues and eigenvectors of the shape operator at a surface point the *principal curvatures* and *principal directions*, Damon named the eigenvalues of the radial shape operator $\mathbf{S}_{rad}$ the *principal radial curvatures* $\kappa_{ri}, i = 1, 2$, and he named the eigenvectors the *principal radial directions* [5].

Considering a local radial flow from the medial sheet $\mathbf{p}$ along one of the two spokes $\mathbf{S}$ to the implied boundary as $\varphi(\mathbf{p}, t) = \mathbf{p} + t\mathbf{S}, t \in [0, 1]$. φ can be generalized to a global radial flow via the doubled-sided spoke field on the medial sheet. The spoke field is legal if and only if the Jacobian matrix of the global radial flow φ is never singular. This implies that for a legal spoke field, i.e., one free of any intersections among the spokes, it has to fulfill a legality condition [5]:

$$\lambda_{ri} < 1, \text{ where } \lambda_{ri} = r\kappa_{ri}, \text{ for all positive real eigenvalues } \lambda_{ri,i=1,2} \text{ of } r\mathbf{S}_{rad}. \tag{8}$$

This relatively simple legality condition can be converted into a geometric constraint in our training process, which allows direct control on the legality of the model interior and implied boundary. We will talk about our training process in general and then come back to how to use this legality condition explicitly in the training.

3 Method

3.1 Binary Training

As described in the introduction, the binary training starts with a fitting process. The task for binary fitting is to find the best member of the shape space for each binary training image. Members of the shape space are parametric models, $\mathbf{M}$, with implied surfaces Ω. Training images, $\mathbf{I}$, are expert binary segmentations of 3D patient data, each with boundary voxels $\mathbf{B}$. We want to find the best $\mathbf{M}$ for a given $\mathbf{I}$: $\arg\min_{\mathbf{M}} F_{obj}(\mathbf{M}|\mathbf{I})$. The objective function $F_{obj}(\mathbf{M}|\mathbf{I})$ is the sum of two parts: the data match measures the fit of $\mathbf{M}$ to data including the image $\mathbf{I}$ and image landmarks, and the geometric penalty measures the geometric appropriateness of $\mathbf{M}$. The data match has two terms, the image match term F_{img} and the landmark match term F_{ilm}.

3.2 Data Match

Image Match. F_{img} enforces that the surface implied by model $\mathbf{M}$ is in accordance with the boundary voxels $\mathbf{B}$, in the binary image. We define the image match as an integral over $\mathbf{B}$ of the minimum distance to the implied model surface Ω as the follows.

$$F_{img}(\mathbf{M}, \mathbf{I}) \propto \sum_{b_i \in \mathbf{B}(\mathbf{I})} \min_{\Omega}(d^2(b_i, \Omega(M))) \tag{9}$$

In our current implementation, Ω is generated via a modified Catmull-Clark algorithm with additional normal constraints [14]. Ideally, we want to measure the distance of the label boundary surface from the model, $d^2(\mathbf{B}, \Omega)$. However, this is computationally expensive given finely sampled subdivision surfaces required for accurate matches and the large number of candidate surfaces generated during optimization.

Furthermore, we note that when $\mathbf{B}$ and Ω are very close, the distance function is nearly symmetric, $|d(\mathbf{B}, \Omega) - d(\Omega, \mathbf{B})| < \epsilon$ except when in a neighborhood the normals of $\mathbf{B}$ and Ω strongly differ. So we simplify by approximating our ideal function with the more tractable $d(\Omega, \mathbf{B})$.

In implementation, we generate a single space filling lookup table for distance from the label boundary by Danielsson's algorithm [6]. Trilinear interpolation gives a very fast measure of the distance at any point in space to the closest boundary point on $\mathbf{B}$. Then we let $d(\omega_i, \mathbf{B})$ be the lookup of the position of ω_i in the distance map and $d(\Omega, \mathbf{B}) = \sum_{\omega_i \in \Omega} d(\omega_i, \mathbf{B})$.

At a boundary location where the surface normal differs from the distance gradient, i.e. the normal to Ω, by more than a certain threshold, $d(\omega_i, \mathbf{B})$ is replaced by the distance along the surface normal to the nearest binary boundary location on $\mathbf{B}$.

Thin object regions also pose a challenge for the image match term. An advantage of the m-rep parameterization is that the medial skeleton can be thought of as the limiting case of a morphological erosion. This allows us to segment very thin object, the image of which is less than a voxel in thickness. We fit an initially dilated model to a dilation of the initial binary labels in the training image, and then we contract the model surface by the same amount via an inverse scaling of the spoke length (radius) parameter.

Landmark Match. F_{ilm} allows for identified explicit feature correspondences. An expert may identify a few anatomically important and easily identifiable landmarks in the training image population, and we penalize the distance from a medially specified point on the model to these landmarks images. Each image landmark $\mathbf{LI}_i$ identified in $\mathbf{I}$ has a real tolerance value ϕ_i that reciprocally weights the associated distance to the specified model point.

In detail, landmarks **LM** in an m-rep model **M** are identified as spoke ends of medial atoms. Corresponding image landmarks in the image data **I** are identified as points in image volumetric space. In our implementation, the Euclidean squared distance from the corresponding spoke ends to the image points is computed and summed, weighted by individual confidence factors $1/\phi_i^2$:

$$F_{ilm}(\mathbf{M}, \mathbf{I}) \propto \sum_{\mathbf{LM}_i \in \mathbf{LM}} \frac{1}{\phi_i^2} d^2(\mathbf{LM}_i, \mathbf{LI}_i) \tag{10}$$

3.3 Geometry Penalty

Besides the measure of the dissimilarity between the model and the image data, we also put geometric constraint on the shapes to measure the appropriateness of **M**.

The geometric penalty typically penalizes parameterizations that lead to irregular coverage of the boundary implied by **M**, via the irregularity penalty F_{reg}. We argue that it should also include a term to penalize illegality of the interior and boundary implied by **M**, which will be detailed in Sec. 3.4.

Irregularity Penalty. The irregularity penalty F_{reg} of a discrete structure, such as a discrete m-rep may reasonably measure the deviation of every atom from the average of its symmetrically placed neighbors. This term penalizes non-uniform spacing and changes in spoke length and direction of medial atoms. It contributes to proper object geometry and to correspondence across the training cases. For each medial atom $\mathbf{m}_i$, the regularity is calculated as the squared Riemannian distance between $\mathbf{m}_i$ and the Fréchet mean of its neighboring atoms N($\mathbf{m}_i$), where the Fréchet mean is defined as $FMean(\{\mathbf{o}_i\}) = \arg\min_{\mathbf{m}} \sum_i d^2(\mathbf{m}, \mathbf{o}_i)$ [9]. The penalties are then accumulated for all the medial atoms of the object:

$$F_{reg}(\mathbf{M}) \propto \sum_{i=1}^{n} d^2(\mathbf{m}_i, FMean(N(\mathbf{m}_i))) \tag{11}$$

3.4 Incorporation of $r\mathbf{S}_{rad}$ into F_{obj} as a Geometric Penalty

As described in Sec. 2.2, a fulfilled legality condition guarantees there is no local self-intersection or creases in a medial spoke field. In order to use the condition as a geometric penalty on a discrete m-rep, we need to calculate the $r\mathbf{S}_{rad}$ matrix and its eigenvalues $\lambda_{ri}, i = 1, 2$ first, and design a function $F_{leg}(\lambda_{ri})$ as the illegality penalty.

Calculating $r\mathbf{S}_{rad}$. According to (7), $r\mathbf{S}_{rad}$ can be calculated from the derivatives of the medial sheet **p** and spoke **S**.

We calculate the derivatives of the medial sheet and spoke by the finite differences between neighboring atoms. $r\mathbf{S}_{rad}$ is then calculated by (7). Eigen-decomposition is applied to the $r\mathbf{S}_{rad}$ to get both the eigenvalues λ_{ri}. Recall that the spoke field is double-sided on the medial sheet, and thus there are two $r\mathbf{S}_{rad}$ matrices and corresponding four eigenvalues for each medial atom.

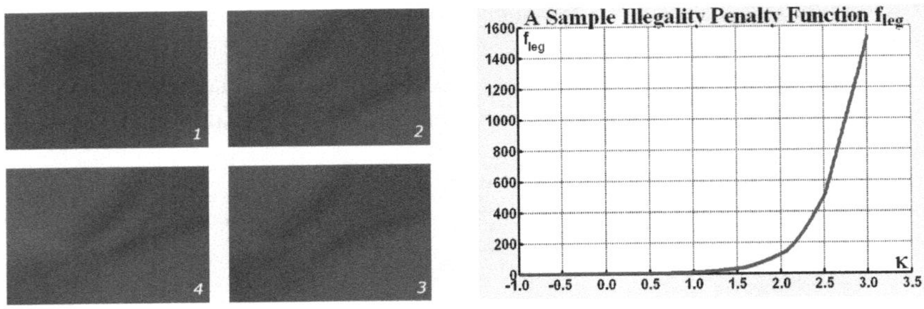

Fig. 2. Left: gradual formation of a self-intersection on a surface portion, rendered by the maximal λ_r of corresponding spokes to surface points. Blue/red means legal($\lambda_r \leq 0$)/illegal($\lambda_r \geq 1$) and any intermediate color shows the tendency for corresponding surface points to become illegal; **Right**: a sample illegality function f_{leg} as a cubic Hermite curve.

Fig. 2-Left shows a visualization of λ_r on the implied boundary of an m-rep. λ_r serves as a distinct indicator of local shape illegalities. Next we show the design of a penalty function on λ_r that will be used in the illegality penalty.

Illegality Penalty. Recall that in (8), legality holds iff $\lambda_{ri} < 1$ for all real eigenvalues of $r\mathbf{S}_{rad}$. Theoretically it is a binary condition that the sign of $\lambda_{ri} - 1$ determines the legality of the implied boundary. However, in practice smaller λ_{ri} desirably leads to smoother surface and binary fit. In order to incorporate this into the objective function $F_{obj}(\mathbf{M}|\mathbf{I})$ as a penalty term, we define a smooth function $f_{leg}(\lambda_{ri})$ that has the following properties.

1. Strictly monotonically increasing;
2. Does not penalize negative λ_{ri};
3. Increasingly penalizes when $\lambda_{ri} > 0$ approaches or passes 1.

Ideally f_{leg} should approach ∞ when λ_{ri} approaches 1. In practice we choose f_{leg} to be smooth at $\lambda_{ri} \in [1, \infty]$ in order to simplify the gradient-based optimizations on the objective function. We use a cubic Hermite curve to define f_{leg} with the luxury of freely picking the function slopes at desired control points, which in our case are $\lambda_{ri} = 0, 1$. A cubic Hermite curve is C^2 continuous.

A sample f_{leg} is shown in Fig. 2-Right. The penalties of all n atoms' λ_{ri} in an m-rep M are then summed up and combined into the objective function $F_{obj}(\mathbf{M}|\mathbf{I})$ as an explicit illegality penalty F_{leg} for training.

$$F_{leg}(\mathbf{M}) \propto \sum_{i \in [1,4]; j \in [1,n]} f_{leg}(\lambda(\mathbf{m}_j)_{ri}) \tag{12}$$

The objective function for binary training is then defined as

$$F_{obj}(\mathbf{M}|\mathbf{I}) = \alpha F_{img}(\mathbf{M}, \mathbf{I}) + \beta F_{ilm}(\mathbf{M}, \mathbf{I}) + \gamma F_{reg}(\mathbf{M}) + \delta F_{leg}(\mathbf{M}) \tag{13}$$

where $\alpha, \beta, \gamma, \delta$ are the parameters controlling the relative weights of the penalty terms.

As a normalization, the binary image **I** is uniformly scaled into a unit cube before the fitting process, and thus the calculated values of the four penalty terms are unitless. The binary fitting starts with a gross alignment step typically via a similarity transformation implied by the moments of the model and binary volumetric image, followed by an optimization on the objective function over m-rep parameters.

After fitting the deformable template into all binary images, the shape statistics are calculated by the Principal Geodesic Analysis (PGA) [9] on the fit models. The fit models are mapped back to their corresponding grayscale images, which are divided into regions using model coordinates provided by m-reps. Intensity histograms are then collected and converted into Regional Intensity Quantile Functions (RIQFs) [2]. PCA is applied to the RIQFs to form the appearance statistics. The PGA shape statistics and the RIQFs appearance statistics form the trained statistics that are used in applications such as segmentation or shape discrimination.

This paper focuses on image segmentation. We show some training and segmentation results based on the methods we proposed, using both synthetic and real world data. The synthetic binary images are generated by warping a standard ellipsoid by diffeomorphic deformations, and the real world data are male pelvic CT images. The next section starts by describing the generation of the synthetic data and ends with results of training on both synthetic and real world data and segmentations on male pelvis CT images of prostates and bladders.

4 Results

Adding an illegality penalty has led to better model fits hence to better statistics on geometry and intensity patterns. Our experience is that this led to considerably better segmentation results, indeed ones so good that on bladder and prostate segmentation from CT images the computer results compared to the manual segmentations by the human who did the training were closer than another human's manual segmentations were to the trainer's.

4.1 Synthetic Data

We applied a diffeomorphic deformation to the ambient space $\mathbb{R}^3$ in order to generate the synthetic ellipsoid models. Given the implicit form for the original ellipsoid $\frac{x^2}{a^2} + \frac{y^2}{b^2} + \frac{z^2}{c^2} \leq 1$, the ambient diffeomorphic deformation is defined as: $x\prime = x$; $y\prime = (y\cos(\rho_{twist}x) - z\sin(\rho_{twist}x))e^{\rho_{taper}x}$; $z\prime = (y\sin(\rho_{twist}x) + z\cos(\rho_{twist}x))$ $e^{\rho_{taper}x} + \rho_{bend}x^2$, where $\rho_{bend}, \rho_{twist}, \rho_{taper}$ are three independent normally-distributed variables that control the three types of deformations: bending, twisting and tapering, as shown in Fig. 3-Left. The standard ellipsoid gives an initial binary volumetric image to start with. By sampling three normal distributions we get a set of the three values. We then apply the deformation based on each set of $\{\rho_{bend}, \rho_{twist}, \rho_{taper}\}$ to the initial binary image and get a warped binary image. By this means we get a set of 150 sample binary images of warped ellipsoids.

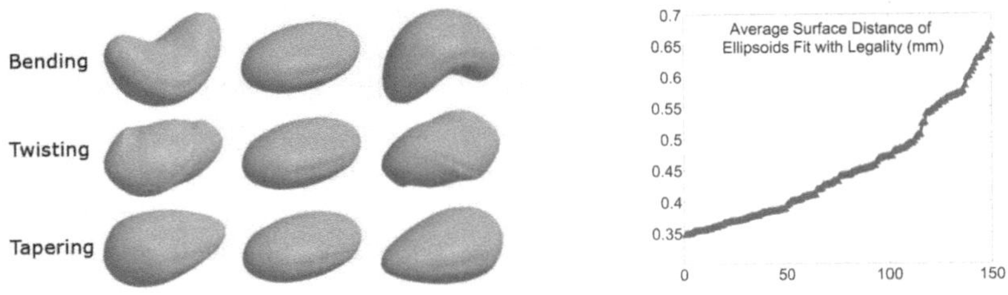

Fig. 3. Left: warped ellipsoids by three deformations of bending, twisting and tapering. Each deformation is shown as -2λ/0/+2λ away from the mean; **Right**: fitting results of 150 sample images shown as the average surface distances from model to binary boundary.

For each sampled binary image, landmarks are also picked automatically as the four extreme points on the middle section of the ellipsoid boundary, plus two vertices at the two warped tips. A template model was generated by sampling the medial axis of the standard ellipsoid. The template was then fit into all the sample binary images using our binary fitting with the geometric illegality penalty. In this study we only measure the quality of the binary fit in term of the average surface distance between model and binary boundaries. Since the synthetic binary images are generated independently from our medial representation, this study serves as a consistency test on our fitting method. The fit results in Fig. 3-Right show that the m-rep surface is on the average, over the boundary, closer than one voxel from the binary boundaries as the truth, while the three axes (a, b, c) of the original ellipsoid are approximately $(50, 30, 23)$ voxels in the binary image. Furthermore in some test cases, our proper training shows more robustness by providing good fit shapes that we failed to get without the illegality penalty. Next on real world data, we will show both training and segmentation results.

4.2 Real World Data

We used CT images $(1 \times 1 \times 3mm)$ of prostates and bladders from 5 patients (80 images) as the real world test data. Each patient has from 13-18 images from multiple days. For each patient, we successively left each day out, trained on all remaining days using both our proper training method and the training without legality constraints, and segmented the left-out day image using the trained shape and appearance statistics from both training methods from all other days. The results show that the trained shapes not only have smoother surfaces (Fig. 4-Left) but also fit better (Fig. 4-Right) into the binary images. The robustness that our proper training process provides allows us to get good fits even from the images that we failed to fit without the legality constraint.

Sorted statistics over all 80 images are given in Fig. 4-Right. For comparison, m-rep fits to humans average 93%, and the average agreement between two humans' segmentations of 16 prostates is 81% volume overlap and $1.9mm$ average closest point surface separation. For the majority of cases, the segmented results for both the bladder and prostate were judged qualitatively good.

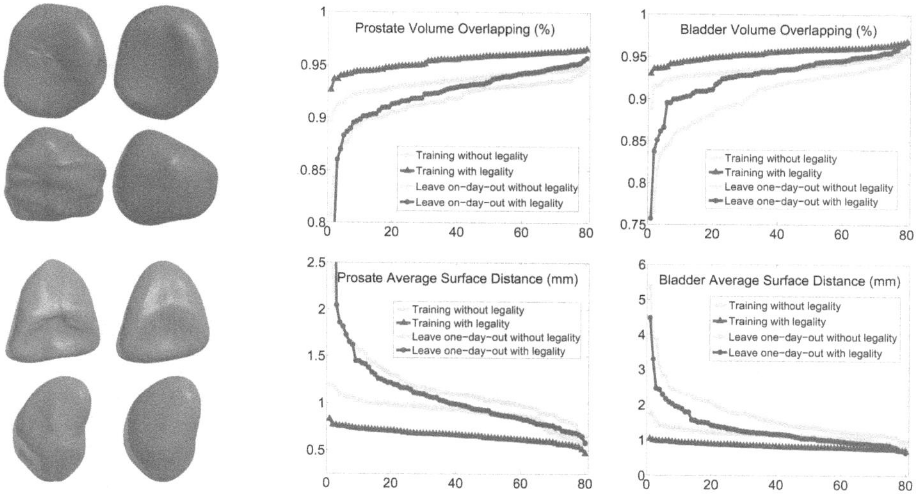

Fig. 4. Left: sample trained shapes from training without/with legality constraints, shown in the left/right column; **Right**: sorted measures (volume overlapping as *Dice similarity coefficients* [8] and average surface distance in mm) comparing m-rep segmentations (circle) and trained m-reps (triangle) to human segmentations, using training methods without (light color) and with (dark color) illegality penalty.

5 Conclusion and Future Work

The results in Fig. 4 suggest that the segmentations results based on our proper training process are improved from the results based on training without illegality penalty. Our training process incorporated with the legality constraint helps us to get proper shape and appearance statistics and lead to segmentation results that are as good as human segmentations. This shows that our method is not only mathematically sound but also proves in practice to improve segmentation results.

In the current implementation, we use adapted Catmull-Clark subdivision to generate the implied boundary used in the training, and legality constraints are applied to sample medial atom spokes. A medial spoke interpolation method [10] is also being adopted to generate both a smooth spoke field and implied boundary, which can further improve the legality of the interior and boundary of trained shapes. We are also working on extending the same framework to train models for anatomical objects with multiple parts, such as livers and hearts. Application of the properly trained shape statistics in methods finding significant differences between classes is in progress.

Acknowledgement

The authors are grateful to all members in MIDAG group, especially Joshua Stough for the latest segmentation results and the help in creating some of the figures, and Graham Gash, Gregg Tracton, Eli Broadhurst, Ja-Yeon Jeong, Xiaoxiao Liu and Rohit Saboo for conceptual, algorithmic, code, and operations contributions. The work was done under the support of NIH grant P01 EB02779.

References

1. Brechbuhler, C., Gerig, G., Kubler, O.: Parametrization of closed surfaces for 3-d shape description. Computer Vision and Image Understanding 61(2), 154–170 (1995)
2. Broadhurst, R., Stough, J., Pizer, S., Chaney, E.: A statistical appearance model based on intensity quantiles. In: International Symposium on Biomedical Imaging (ISBI), pp. 422–425 (2006)
3. Cootes, T., Cooper, D., Taylor, C., Graham, J.: Active shape models - their training and application. Computer Vision and Image Understanding 61(1), 18–59 (1995)
4. Dam, E., Fletcher, P.T., Pizer, S.M., Tracton, G., Rosenman, J.: Prostate shape modeling based on principal geodesic analysis bootstrapping. In: Barillot, C., Haynor, D.R., Hellier, P. (eds.) MICCAI 2004. LNCS, vol. 3217, pp. 1008–1016. Springer, Heidelberg (2004)
5. Damon, J.N.: Smoothness and geometry of boundaries associated to skeletal structures I: Sufficient conditions for smoothness. Annales de Institut Fourier 53(6), 1941–1985 (2003)
6. Danielsson, P.: Euclidean distance mapping. Computer Graphics and Image Processing, pp. 227–248 (1980)
7. Davies, R., Twining, C., Cootes, T., Taylor, C.: A minimum description length approach to statistical shape modelling. IEEE Transactions on Medical Imaging 21(5), 525–537 (2002)
8. Dice, L.R.: Measures of the amount of ecologic association between species. Ecology 26, 297–302 (1945)
9. Fletcher, P.T., Lu, C., Pizer, S.M., Joshi, S.: Principal geodesic analysis for the nonlinear study of shape. Transactions on Medical Imaging 23(8), 995–1005 (2004)
10. Han, Q., Pizer, S.M., Damon, J.N.: Interpolation in discrete single figure medial objects. In: IEEE CVPR Workshop on Mathematical Methods in Biomedical Image Analysis (MMBIA 2006), p. 85 (2006)
11. Pizer, S.M., Fletcher, T., Fridman, Y., Fritsch, D.S., Gash, A.G., Glotzer, J.M., Joshi, S., Thall, A., Tracton, G., Yushkevich, P., Chaney, E.L.: Deformable m-reps for 3d medical image segmentation. International Journal of Computer Vision Special UNC-MIDAG issue 55(2), 85–106 (2003)
12. Siddiqi, K., Pizer, S.M. (eds.): Medial Representations: Mathematics, Algorithms and Applications. Springer, Heidelberg (in press, 2007)
13. Styner, M., Oguz, I., Xu, S., Brechbuhler, C., Pantazis, D., Levitt, J., Shenton, M., Gerig, G.: Framework for the statistical shape analysis of brain structures using spharm-pdm. In: Open Science Workshop at MICCAI (2006), `http://hdl.handle.net/1926/215`
14. Thall, A.: Deformable solid modeling via medial sampling and displacement subdivision. PdD thesis, Dept. of Comp. Sci., UNC @ Chapel Hill (2004)

Registration-Derived Estimates of Local Lung Expansion as Surrogates for Regional Ventilation

Joseph M. Reinhardt[1], Gary E. Christensen[2], Eric A. Hoffman[3,1], Kai Ding[1], and Kunlin Cao[2]

[1] Department of Biomedical Engineering
[2] Department of Electrical and Computer Engineering
[3] Department of Radiology
The University of Iowa, Iowa City, IA 52242
{joe-reinhardt, gary-christensen, eric-hoffman, kai-ding, kunlin-cao}@uiowa.edu

Abstract. The main function of the respiratory system is gas exchange. Since many disease or injury conditions can cause biomechanical or material property changes that can alter lung function, there is a great interest in measuring regional lung ventilation. We describe a registration-based technique for estimating local lung expansion from multiple respiratory-gated CT images of the thorax. The degree of regional lung expansion is measured using the Jacobian of the registration displacement field. We compare lung expansion estimated across five pressure changes to a xenon CT based measure of specific ventilation, and have shown good agreement (linear regression, $r^2 = 0.89$ during gas wash-in) in one animal.

1 Introduction

The main function of the respiratory system is gas exchange. Regional ventilation depends on the mechanical relationships between the lungs, rib cage, diaphragm, and abdomen, which work together to generate expansile forces. Since many disease or injury conditions can change lung material properties, lung mechanics, and lung function, it is useful to understand the both the global and local functional behavior of lungs.

Attempts have been made to measure regional ventilation directly and indirectly with a variety of invasive techniques and with radioisotope imaging [1,2,3,4,5], but these methods have been greatly limited by invasiveness, poor spatial and temporal resolution, qualitative nature, and/or complexity.

Xenon-enhanced CT (Xe-CT) is a non-invasive method for the measurement regional pulmonary ventilation. With Xe-CT, radiodense, non-radioactive gas xenon gas is inhaled and exhaled during imaging, and local ventilation time constants are calculated by observing the gas wash-in and wash-out rates on serial CT images [6,7]. Xenon gas provides enhancement on the CT proportional to the concentration of xenon in the region being imaged; enhancements as much as 150 to 200 Hounsfield units (HU) are possible with high concentrations of xenon [7]. Xe-CT is not without shortcomings, however. Xe-CT requires the use

N. Karssemeijer and B. Lelieveldt (Eds.): IPMI 2007, LNCS 4584, pp. 763–774, 2007.
© Springer-Verlag Berlin Heidelberg 2007

of expensive xenon gas and the associated hardware to control delivery of the gas and harvest the gas from expired air for recycling. In addition, it is known that xenon gas has a strong anesthetic effect that must be carefully monitored [6]. Finally, Xe-CT imaging protocols require high temporal resolution imaging, so typically axial coverage is limited to just a few slices at a time. Nonetheless, recent work with the Xe-CT technique has re-established the interest in these methods for measuring regional ventilation. When combined with the unique capability of CT to describe lung anatomic detail, Xe-CT can provide detailed information on lung structure and respiratory function [6,7].

Imaging has long been used study lung mechanics, and some investigators have studied the linkage between estimates of regional lung expansion and local lung ventilation [8,9,10,11,12]. Gee et al. have applied serial magnetic resonance imaging to the problem of studying lung mechanics. Using static breath-hold imaging they acquired a single sagittal cross-section of the lung at different inflations [10]. Using non-linear image registration, they estimated a dense displacement field from one image to the other; from the displacement field they computed regional lung strain. Guerrero et al. use two CT images, acquired at different lung inflations, and optical flow image registration to estimate regional ventilation to identify functioning vs. non-functioning lung tissue for radiotherapy treatment planning [11,12]. While they were able to show a close correlation with global measurements of lung ventilation, their experimental methods did not allow them to compare local estimates of lung expansion with regional lung ventilation.

We describe a technique that uses multiple respiratory-gated CT images of the lung acquired at different levels of inflation, along with 3D image registration, to make local estimates of lung tissue expansion. We compare these lung expansion estimates to Xe-CT derived measures of regional ventilation to validate our measurements and establish their physiological significance. The ability to estimate regional ventilation maps for the entire lung from quickly and easily obtained respiratory-gated images is a significant contribution to functional lung imaging because of the potential increase in resolution, and large reductions in imaging time, radiation, and contrast agent exposure.

2 Methods

Figure 1 shows a block diagram of the entire process. Two or more respiratory-gated data sets are gathered at different points in the respiratory cycle, reflecting the state of the lung at two different pressures (and therefore, volumes). 3D image registration is used to create a voxel-by-voxel displacement map that shows the motion of the lung tissue as a function of respiratory state. The Jacobian of the displacement field is calculated for each voxel in the lung and is used to represent local tissue expansion. This index of tissue expansion is compared to Xe-CT based measures of lung ventilation.

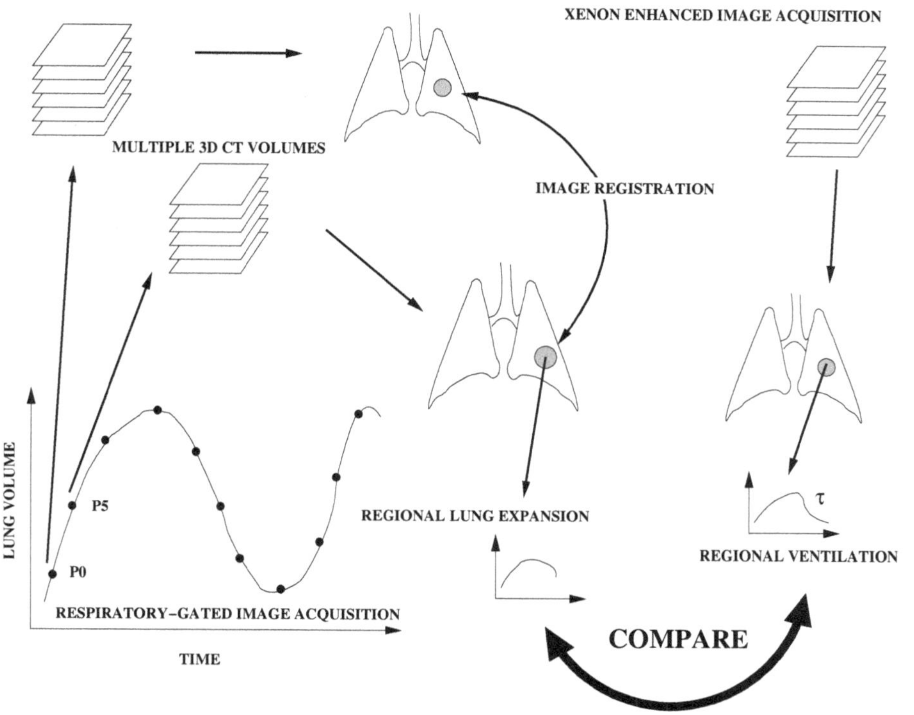

Fig. 1. Multiple volumetric CT images (in this case images $P0$ and $P5$) are acquired at two different points in the respiratory cycle and analyzed to compute a voxel-by-voxel transformation from one image to another. The Jacobian of the transformation is used to estimate regional lung expansion. Xenon-enhanced CT imaging is used to estimate local time constants associated with ventilation. We compare the registration-derived measure of lung expansion with the xenon-based estimate of regional ventilation.

2.1 Data Sets and Image Acquisition

Appropriate animal ethics approval was obtained for these protocols and the study adhered to NIH guidelines for animal experimentation. One adult male 42 kg sheep was used for these experiments. All images were acquired with the animal in the supine orientation on a Siemens Sensation 64 multi-detector CT scanner (MDCT) (Siemens Medical Solutions; Malverne, PA). The animal was anesthetized and mechanically ventilated during the experiments.

Respiratory-Gated Volumetric CT: Volumetric CT scans covering the thorax were acquired at 0, 5, 10, 15, 20, and 25 cm H_2O (herein denoted as the $P0$, $P5$, $P10$, $P15$, $P20$, and $P25$ images) airway pressures with the animal held apneic. The scanning protocol used a tube current of 100 mAs, a tube voltage

120 kV, slice collimation of 1 mm, an effective slice thickness of 0.65 mm, a slice separation of 0.5 mm, a pitch of 1, a 512 by 512 reconstruction matrix, and a field of view selected to fit the lung field of interest. All of the images are acquired without moving the animal between scans, so after acquisition the data sets are almost in rigid alignment.

Xenon CT: Six axial locations for Xe-CT studies are selected from the whole lung volumetric scan performed near end-expiration. Images are acquired with the scanner set in ventilation triggering mode, typically using 80 keV energy (for higher Xe signal enhancement), 120 mAs tube current, a 360° rotation, a 0.33 sec scan time, a 512 by 512 reconstruction matrix, and a field of view adjusted to fit the lung field of interest. The Xe-CT slice collimation is approximately 3 mm thick, or about six times as thick as the volumetric CT data. The six xenon slices give approximately 1.8 cm of coverage along the axial direction. Respiratory gating during image acquisition is achieved by replacing the standard ECG gating signal with a trigger signal from a LabView program. The program was set to trigger the scanner at end inspiratory and/or end expiratory points during the respiratory cycle. A respiratory tidal volume of 8 cc/kg (336 ml for 42 kg) was used for the Xe-CT acquisition.

The image acquisition sequence is as follows. Acquisition starts and images are gathered as the animal breathes six to eight breaths of room air. Next, the xenon delivery system is turned on and approximately 40 breaths of pure Xe are delivered while imaging, and then the air source is switched back to room air for another 40 breaths. Thus, axial images are acquired for approximately 90 breaths as the xenon gas washes in and out of the lungs.

2.2 Image Registration

The volumetric images are registered pairwise according to airway pressure, so that we register $P0$ to $P5$, $P5$ to $P10$, etc., up to $P20$ to $P25$, resulting in 5 pairs of registered images. In this section we shall refer to the images under consideration as I_0 and I_1, where I_0 is the image from the image pair acquired at the lower pressure (i.e., $P0$ from the pair $P0$–$P5$) and I_1 refers to the image acquired at the higher pressure (i.e., $P5$).

The I_0 and I_1 volumetric images are registered using an intensity-based inverse consistent image registration algorithm [13]. In this approach, the forward and reverse transformations between the two images are jointly estimated subject to the constraints that minimize the inverse consistency error, the intensity mismatch error, and the smoothness of the image transformation function. No explicit lung region segmentation is required prior to registration, however, we do perform a rigid image alignment based on the location of the branch point of the trachea (the carina) and the locations of the endpoints of the left and right mainstem bronchi.

The inverse consistent intensity registration is accomplished by minimizing this cost function:

$$C = C_{SIM}(I_0 \circ h, I_1) + C_{SIM}(I_1 \circ g, I_0) + C_{ICC}(u, \tilde{w}) + C_{ICC}(w, \tilde{u}) + C_{REG}(u) + C_{REG}(w), \tag{1}$$

where C_{SIM}, C_{ICC}, and C_{REG} are cost functions defined below. The functions $u, w, \tilde{u}, \tilde{w}$ are voxel displacement fields and are related to the forward and reverse transformations by the equations: $h(x) = x + u(x)$, $g(x) = x + w(x)$, $h^{-1}(x) = x + \tilde{u}(x)$, $g^{-1}(x) = x + \tilde{w}(x)$.

The forward transformation h is used to deform the image I_0 into the shape of the image I_1, and the reverse transformation g is used to deform the shape of I_1 into that of I_0. The deformed template and target images are denoted by $(I_0 \circ h)$ and $(I_1 \circ g)$, respectively.

The C_{SIM} term of the cost function in equation 1 defines the symmetric intensity similarity. This term is designed to minimize the squared error intensity differences between the images. The C_{ICC} term is the inverse consistency constraint or inverse consistency error cost and is minimized when the forward and reverse transformations are inverses of each other. The C_{REG} term is used to regularize the forward and reverse displacement fields. This term is used to force the displacement fields to be smooth and continuous.

When the registration process is complete, the displacement fields u and w (and $\tilde{u}$ and $\tilde{w}$) are voxel-by-voxel displacements between images I_0 and image I_1 that can be used to track arbitrary regions of interest across the portion of the respiratory cycle represented by the transition from I_0 to I_1.

2.3 Xenon CT Ventilation Analysis

Prior to Xe-CT data analysis, the lung region was semi-automatically defined in the Xe-CT data by tracing the strong gradient around the lung boundary (see Figure 3a for an example). After lung segmentation, 8×8 pixel regions of interest (ROIs) were defined in the lung region on each 2D slice.

The Xe-CT times series data shows an exponential rise and fall in lung density during the wash-in and wash-out phases of image acquisition. To quantify regional ventilation, a single-compartment exponential model is fit to the rise and decay portions of the data using a least-squares fit. For each ROI to be analyzed, the mean region density, $D(t)$, is calculated versus time (or equivalently, image number). For the wash-in phase, the compartment model gives [6]:

$$D(t) = \begin{cases} D_0 & 0 \leq t < t_0 \\ D_0 + (D_f - D_0)(1 - e^{-\frac{t-t_0}{\tau}}) & t \geq t_0, \end{cases} \tag{2}$$

where D_0 is the baseline density in the ROI prior to switching to xenon gas, D_f is the density that would be observed if xenon was inspired until equilibrium, t_0 is the start time of the switchover from room air to xenon, and τ is the model time

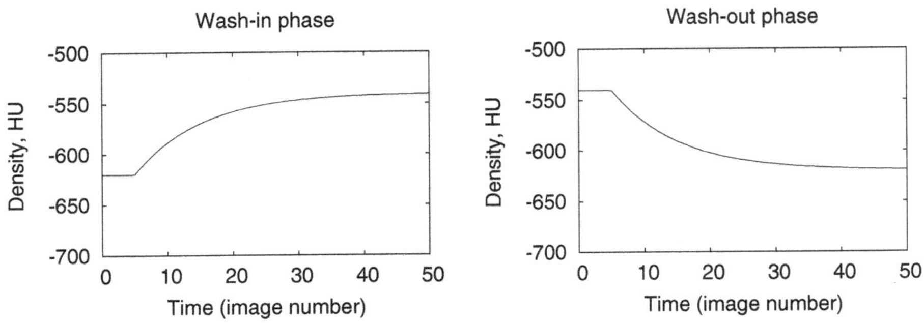

Fig. 2. Wash-in and wash-out behaviors predicted by compartment model for $t_0 = 5$ seconds, $\tau = 10$ seconds, $D_0 = -620$ HU, and $D_f = -540$ HU

constant. Thus, using this model, the $D_f - D_0$ term represents the enhancement due to the inspired xenon. The model gives a similar expression for the wash-out phase:

$$D(t) = \begin{cases} D_f & 0 \leq t < t_0 \\ D_0 + (D_f - D_0)e^{-\frac{t-t_0}{\tau}} & t \geq t_0, \end{cases} \quad (3)$$

where for the wash-out phase t_0 denotes that time that of switchover from xenon back to room air. Figure 2 shows the density–time variation predicted by the model. The time constants of the rising and falling phases curves may be fitted separately or may be forced to be equal. In our analysis, the wash-in and wash-out phases of the cycle were analyzed separately, resulting in two different estimates of τ. To reduce aberrations in the time series data due to the ROIs overlapping with large blood vessels or regions of atelectasis (see for example, the bottom left side of the lungs shown in Figure 3a), we eliminated from consideration any ROI that had more than 40% of its pixels above -300 HU. Time series data was measured and analyzed for the remaining ROIs. Specific ventilation (sV, ventilation per unit lung air volume in min^{-1}) for each ROI was calculated as the inverse of the time constant τ.

Figures 3a–b shows screen shots from the software tool used to analyze the Xe-CT data [14]. This tool facilitates lung segmentation, region of interest specification, and allows control over the curve fitting parameters during the exponential fits.

2.4 Assessment of Image Registration Accuracy

To assess the accuracy of the image registration, 13 manually-defined anatomic landmarks were manually selected and matched between the all five pairs of images for one animal. These landmarks were selected as recognizable branch-points of the vascular and airway branches. None of the registration landmarks were used for this accuracy assessment. Care was taken to obtain a sampling of landmarks that covered the apex, base, ventral, and dorsal regions of the lung.

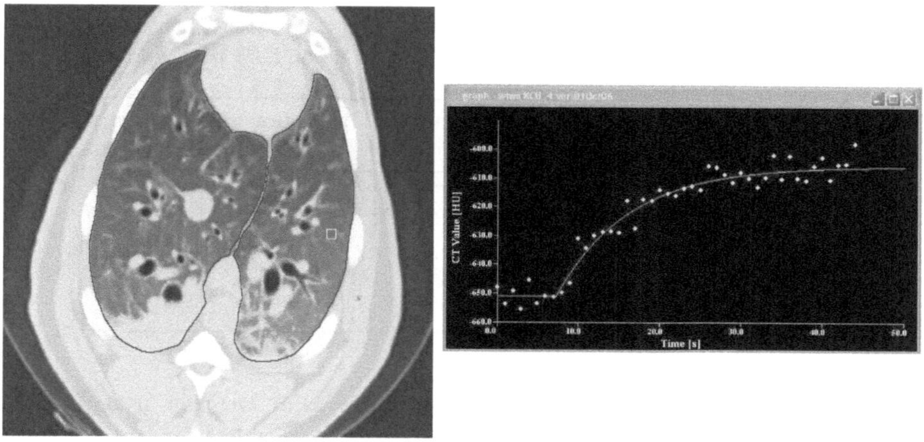

(a) (b)

Fig. 3. Time series data from Xe-CT study. (a) shows the Xe-CT image of the lungs, with the lung boundaries marked in blue and a rectangular region of interest in yellow. (b) shows the raw time series data for this region of interest (wash-in phase) and the associated exponential model fit.

For each image pair, the manually-defined landmarks in the higher pressure image were mapped to the lower pressure image using the transformation determined during the image registration step. The actual landmark position was compared to the registration-predicted landmark position and the landmark positioning error was calculated.

2.5 Comparing Lung Expansion to Xe-CT Estimates of sV

Local lung volume change is calculated using the Jacobian of the transformation that maps image I_0 to image I_1. Consider the vector displacement function $\boldsymbol{u}(x, y, z)$ (with x, y, and z components) that transforms a voxel from image I_0 into its corresponding location in image I_1, so that the voxel at location (x, y, z) in image I_0 is displaced by a vector function $\boldsymbol{u}(x, y, z)$ to map it to its corresponding location in image I_1. The Jacobian $J(x, y, z)$ of the transformation $\boldsymbol{u}(x, y, z)$ is

$$J(x,y,z) = \begin{vmatrix} \frac{\partial u_x(x,y,z)}{\partial x} & \frac{\partial u_x(x,y,z)}{\partial y} & \frac{\partial u_x(x,y,z)}{\partial z} \\ \frac{\partial u_y(x,y,z)}{\partial x} & \frac{\partial u_y(x,y,z)}{\partial y} & \frac{\partial u_y(x,y,z)}{\partial z} \\ \frac{\partial u_z(x,y,z)}{\partial x} & \frac{\partial u_z(x,y,z)}{\partial y} & \frac{\partial u_z(x,y,z)}{\partial z} \end{vmatrix},$$

where $u_x(x, y, z)$ is the x component of $\boldsymbol{u}(x, y, z)$, $u_y(x, y, z)$ is the y component of $\boldsymbol{u}(x, y, z)$, and $u_z(x, y, z)$ is the z component of $\boldsymbol{u}(x, y, z)$. The displacement field is analyzed in the Eulerian framework. The Jacobian measures the differential expansion at position (x, y, z) in the image. If the Jacobian is unity, there is

Table 1. Registration accuracy as assessed by using the image registration to predict the motion of manually-defined landmarks across lung inflation. Registration pair 0–5 indicates that the registration was performed on the $P0$ and $P5$ pair of images.

Registration Pair (cm H_2O)	Mean landmark error (mm)	Maximum landmark error (mm)
0−5	0.98 ± 0.41	1.87
5−10	0.55 ± 0.23	1.15
10−15	0.42 ± 0.20	0.93
15−20	0.30 ± 0.19	0.85
20−25	0.40 ± 0.17	0.70

no expansion or contraction in the function $\boldsymbol{u}(x, y, z)$ at location (x, y, z) in I_0. If the Jacobian is greater than one, there is local tissue contraction; if the Jacobian is less than one, there is local tissue expansion. Note that regional specific volume change can be estimated from the Jacobian as $J(x, y, z) - 1$.

To compare the Xe-CT ventilation measurements to the Jacobian from the image registration transformation, we compute the mean and standard deviation of each parameter as a function of lung height (y coordinate) by averaging over all x and z in the lung regions. The most dependent lung region (region closest to the direction of gravity) is defined $y = 0$ cm. A scatter plot showing mean sV and mean Jacobian is created and a linear regression line is fit to this data.

3 Results

3.1 Registration Accuracy

Table 1 shows the registration accuracy as assessed by predicting the motion of the 13 manually-defined landmarks across the five pressure pairs. Overall the registration accuracy is on the order of 0.5 to 1 mm, or about 1 to 2 voxels.

3.2 Lung Expansion and Xe-CT Estimates of sV

Figures 4a–b show color-coded maps of the sV and Jacobian of the registration transformation at approximately the same anatomic axial location. Figure 6a shows the average Jacobian vs. lung height for all pressure change pairs. Figure 6b shows the average sV vs. lung height calculated from the xenon study. Figure 5 shows sV vs. average Jacobian the $P10$ to $P15$ and $P5$ to $P10$ pressure transitions. The figure gives the slope of the regression line equations and r^2 values for the linear fits between average sV and the average Jacobian.

4 Discussion

Table 1 shows the registration algorithm accuracy is on the order of 1 or 2 voxels at the manually-selected validation landmarks. We expect that similar accuracy would be obtained in between landmarks, but this has not been examined.

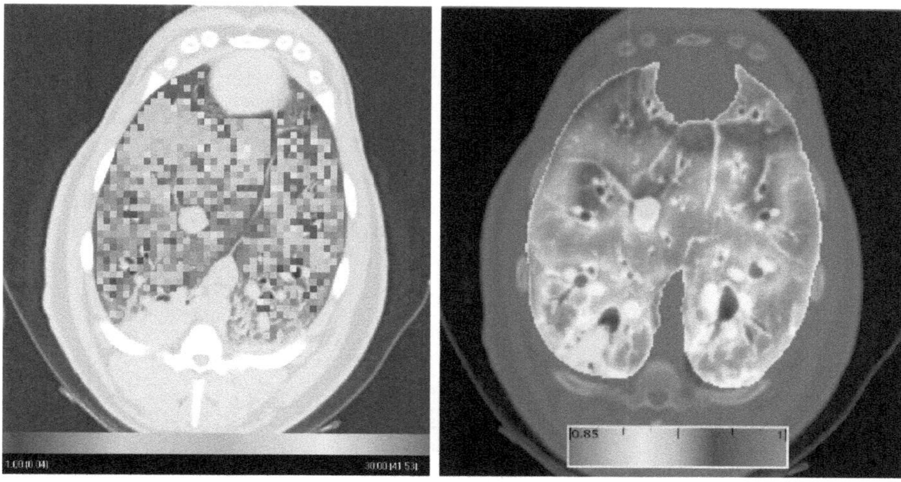

(a) (b)

Fig. 4. Color-coded maps showing (a) wash-in time constant (seconds) and (b) the Jacobian of the image registration transformation (unitless) for approximately the same anatomic slice. Note that the color scales are different for (a) and (b). Dark blue regions on the time constant image (a) are regions that have high ventilation while green and yellow regions have lower ventilation; Bright red and orange regions on the Jacobian image (b) have large lung deformation. while blue and purple regions are deforming less.

The results show good agreement between the Xe-CT derived specific ventilation and the registration-based estimates of local lung expansion. Figure 5a shows the sV-Jacobian scatter plot for the pressure change pair $P10$ to $P15$. For this case, the r^2 value for the linear regression is 0.89 for the wash-in phase and 0.82 for the wash-out phase. This pressure change pair gave highest correlation; the $P5$ to $P10$ pressure change pair is shown in Figure 5b for comparison. r^2 values as low as 0.5 were obtained for the highest pressure change pairs. Overall, the regression analysis shows a relationship between the average sV and average Jacobian exists at the lowest pressure change pairs, but that relationship is diminished as the lung volume increases.

Figure 6 shows that the sV measurements are have a large coefficient of variation (almost 50%) during the wash-in phase. The reasons for this are unclear; it could be that the curve-fitting and ROI processing is noisy, or it could be an indication that the underlying physiology is not homogeneous. In comparison, the coefficient of variation for the Jacobian measurements is on the order of 5% to 10%, but this smoothness might be artificially induced by the model constraints used during the registration process.

While the correlations are not perfect, these data are confirmatory of known physiology in that we expect a greater degree of ventilation in the dependent

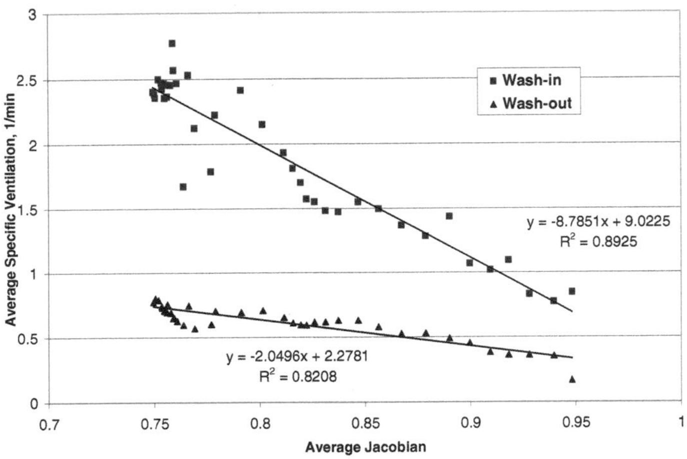

(a)

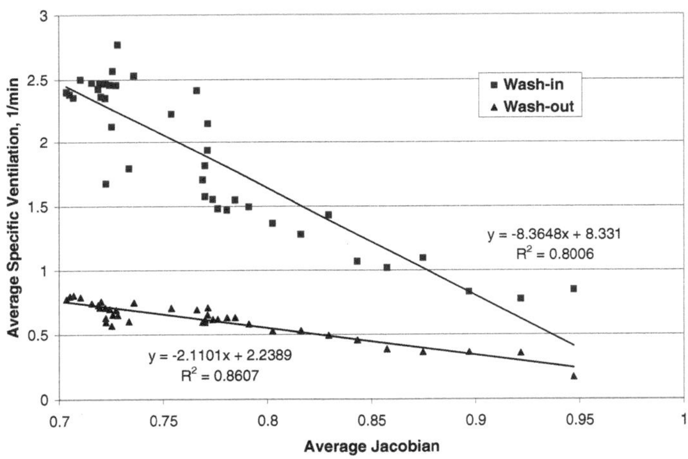

(b)

Fig. 5. Scatter plot of average sV and average Jacobian for (a) $P10$ to $P15$ pressure change pair and (b) $P5$ to $P10$ pressure change pair

region of the lung (i.e., the region that is closest to the direction of gravity). Figures 4 and 6 demonstrate ventral-dorsal gradients in both the ventilation time constants (inverse of sV) and in the Jacobian. Regions with high ventilation are regions that are receiving more gas during respiration than regions with low ventilation, and should have a correspondingly higher rate of expansion. This increased deformation shows up as smaller value of the Jacobian (indicating a bigger deformation to transition from a higher lung volume to a lower lung volume). As expected, Figure 6a shows that the largest lung deformation happens at the smallest lung volumes; i.e., the lung expands the most at low lung volumes (pressure), so the $P0$ to $P5$ transformation shows the most expansion (smallest

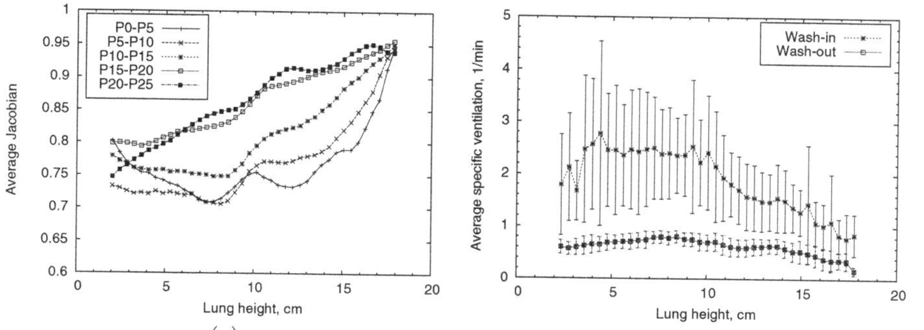

(a) (b)

Fig. 6. (a) Average Jacobian values for all pressure pairs and (b) average sV vs. lung height.

Jacobian values), while the $P20$ to $P25$ transformation shows the least expansion (Jacobian values closest to unity).

It is not possible to generalize from these results using a single subject to a population of subjects, but if this proof of concept were to be experimentally confirmed in a larger population, it would be a very important result. Xe-CT is a fairly expensive technique that requires special equipment, has fairly low resolution, and has very limited axial coverage of the lung so that multiple scans with increased radiation dose are required to cover the entire lung. A complete Xe-CT of the human lung is probably impractical due to time, cost, and radiation dose considerations. However, if a registration-based analysis using just two easy-to-acquire volumetric images of the lung acquired at different lung volumes could be registered, a high-resolution map of lung expansion may serve as a surrogate for local specific ventilation.

5 Summary and Conclusions

We have described a registration-based technique for estimating local lung expansion from multiple respiratory-gated CT images of the thorax. The degree of lung expansion is measured using the Jacobian of the registration displacement field. We have compared lung expansion estimated across five pressure changes to a xenon CT based measure of specific ventilation, and have shown good agreement in one animal. Additional studies are needed to characterize the level of agreement between the sV and Jacobian across a population, to estimate the confidence intervals for the lung expansion index, and to determine the optimal respiratory-gated scanning protocol for image acquisition.

Acknowledgments

This work was supported in part by grant HL079406 from the National Institutes of Health.

References

1. Bunow, B., Line, B., Horton, M., Weiss, G.: Regional ventilatory clearance by xenon scintigraphy: A critical evaluation of two estimation procedures. J. Nucl. Med. 20(7), 703–710 (1979)
2. Hubmayr, R., Walters, B., Chevalier, P., Rodarte, J., Olson, L.: Topographical distribution of regional lung volume in anesthetized dogs. J. Applied Physiology 54(4), 1048–1056 (1983)
3. van der Mark, T.W., Rookmaker, A.E., Kiers, A., Peset, R., Vaalburg, W., Paans, A.M., Woldring, M.G.: Nitrogen-13 and xenon-133 ventilation studies. J. Nucl. Med. 25(11), 1175–1182 (1984)
4. Robertson, H.T., Glenny, R.W., Stanford, D., McInnes, L.M., Luchtel, D.L., Covert, D.: High-resolution maps of regional ventilation utilizing inhaled fluorescent microspheres. J. Applied Physiology 82(3), 943–953 (1997)
5. Tajik, J.K., Chon, D., Won, C.H., Tran, B.Q., Hoffman, E.A.: Subsecond multisection CT of regional pulmonary ventilation. Acad. Radiol. 9, 130–146 (2002)
6. Simon, B.A., Marcucci, C.: Parameter estimation and confidence intervals for Xe-CT ventilation studies: A Monte Carlo approach. J. Applied Physiology 84(2), 709–716 (1998)
7. Marcucci, C., Nyhan, D., Simon, B.A.: Distribution of pulmonary ventilation using Xe-enhanced computed tomography in prone and supine dogs. J. Applied Physiology 90(2), 421–430 (2001)
8. Rodarte, J.R., Hubmayr, R.D., Stamenovic, D., Walters, B.J.: Regional lung strain in dogs during deflation from total lung capacity. J. Applied Physiology 58(1), 164–172 (1985)
9. Hubmayr, R.D., Rodarte, J.R., Walters, B.J., Tonelli, F.M.: Regional ventilation during spontaneous breathing and mechanical ventilation in dogs. J. Applied Physiology 63(6), 2467–2475 (1987)
10. Gee, J., Sundaram, T., Hasegawa, I., Uematsu, H., Hatabu, H.: Characterization of regional pulmonary mechanics from serial magnetic resonance imaging data. Acad. Radiol. 10, 1147–1152 (2003)
11. Guerrero, T., Sanders, K., Noyola-Martinez, J., Castillo, E., Zhang, Y., Tapia, R., Guerra, R., Borghero, Y., Komaki, R.: Quantification of regional ventilation from treatment planning CT. Int. J. Radiation Oncology Biol. Phys. 62(3), 630–634 (2005)
12. Guerrero, T., Sanders, K., Castillo, E., Zhang, Y., Bidaut, L., Komaki, T.P.R.: Dynamic ventilation imaging from four-dimensional computed tomography. Phys Med Biol. 51(4), 777–791 (2006)
13. Johnson, H., Christensen, G.: Consistent landmark and intensity-based image registration. IEEE Transactions on Medical Imaging 21(5), 450–461 (2002)
14. Chon, D., Simon, B.A., Beck, K.C., Shikata, H., Saba, O.I., Won, C., Hoffman, E.A.: Differences in regional wash-in and wash-out time constants for xenon-CT ventilation studies. Respiratory Physiology & Neurobiology 148, 65–83 (2005)

Author Index

Lecture Notes in Computer Science

For information about Vols. 1–4474

please contact your bookseller or Springer

Vol. 4600: H. Comon-Lundh, C. Kirchner, H. Kirchner (Eds.), Rewriting, Computation and Proof. XVI, 273 pages. 2007.

Vol. 4591: J. Davies, J. Gibbons (Eds.), Integrated Formal Methods. IX, 660 pages. 2007.

Vol. 4590: W. Damm, H. Hermanns (Eds.), Computer Aided Verification. XV, 562 pages. 2007.

Vol. 4588: T. Harju, J. Karhumäki, A. Lepistö (Eds.), Developments in Language Theory. XI, 423 pages. 2007.

Vol. 4584: N. Karssemeijer, B. Lelieveldt (Eds.), Information Processing in Medical Imaging. XX, 777 pages. 2007.

Vol. 4583: S.R. Della Rocca (Ed.), Typed Lambda Calculi and Applications. XI, 395 pages. 2007.

Vol. 4581: A. Petrenko, M. Veanes, J. Tretmans, W. Grieskamp (Eds.), Testing of Software and Communicating Systems. XII, 379 pages. 2007.

Vol. 4574: J. Derrick, J. Vain (Eds.), Formal Techniques for Networked and Distributed Systems – FORTE 2007. XI, 375 pages. 2007.

Vol. 4573: M. Kauers, M. Kerber, R. Miner, W. Windsteiger (Eds.), Towards Mechanized Mathematical Assistants. XIII, 407 pages. 2007. (Sublibrary LNAI).

Vol. 4572: F. Stajano, C. Meadows, S. Capkun, T. Moore (Eds.), Security and Privacy in Ad-hoc and Sensor Networks. X, 247 pages. 2007.

Vol. 4569: A. Butz, B. Fisher, A. Krüger, P. Olivier, S. Owada (Eds.), Smart Graphics. IX, 237 pages. 2007.

Vol. 4549: J. Aspnes, C. Scheideler, A. Arora, S. Madden (Eds.), Distributed Computing in Sensor Systems. XIII, 417 pages. 2007.

Vol. 4548: N. Olivetti (Ed.), Automated Reasoning with Analytic Tableaux and Related Methods. X, 245 pages. 2007. (Sublibrary LNAI).

Vol. 4547: C. Carlet, B. Sunar (Eds.), Arithmetic of Finite Fields. XI, 355 pages. 2007.

Vol. 4546: J. Kleijn, A. Yakovlev (Eds.), Petri Nets and Other Models of Concurrency – ICATPN 2007. XI, 515 pages. 2007.

Vol. 4543: A.K. Bandara, M. Burgess (Eds.), Inter-Domain Management. XII, 237 pages. 2007.

Vol. 4542: P. Sawyer, B. Paech, P. Heymans (Eds.), Requirements Engineering: Foundation for Software Quality. IX, 384 pages. 2007.

Vol. 4541: T. Okadome, T. Yamazaki, M. Makhtari (Eds.), Pervasive Computing for Quality of Life Enhancement. IX, 248 pages. 2007.

Vol. 4539: N.H. Bshouty, C. Gentile (Eds.), Learning Theory. XII, 634 pages. 2007. (Sublibrary LNAI).

Vol. 4538: F. Escolano, M. Vento (Eds.), Graph-Based Representations in Pattern Recognition. XII, 416 pages. 2007.

Vol. 4537: K.C.-C. Chang, W. Wang, L. Chen, C.A. Ellis, C.-H. Hsu, A.C. Tsoi, H. Wang (Eds.), Advances in Web and Network Technologies, and Information Management. XXIII, 707 pages. 2007.

Vol. 4536: G. Concas, E. Damiani, M. Scotto, G. Succi (Eds.), Agile Processes in Software Engineering and Extreme Programming. XV, 276 pages. 2007.

Vol. 4534: I. Tomkos, F. Neri, J. Solé Pareta, X. Masip Bruin, S. Sánchez Lopez (Eds.), Optical Network Design and Modeling. XI, 460 pages. 2007.

Vol. 4531: J. Indulska, K. Raymond (Eds.), Distributed Applications and Interoperable Systems. XI, 337 pages. 2007.

Vol. 4530: D.H. Akehurst, R. Vogel, R.F. Paige (Eds.), Model Driven Architecture- Foundations and Applications. X, 219 pages. 2007.

Vol. 4529: P. Melin, O. Castillo, L.T. Aguilar, J. Kacprzyk, W. Pedrycz (Eds.), Foundations of Fuzzy Logic and Soft Computing. XIX, 830 pages. 2007. (Sublibrary LNAI).

Vol. 4528: J. Mira, J.R. Álvarez (Eds.), Nature Inspired Problem-Solving Methods in Knowledge Engineering, Part II. XXII, 650 pages. 2007.

Vol. 4527: J. Mira, J.R. Álvarez (Eds.), Bio-inspired Modeling of Cognitive Tasks, Part I. XXII, 630 pages. 2007.

Vol. 4526: M. Malek, M. Reitenspieß, A. van Moorsel (Eds.), Service Availability. X, 155 pages. 2007.

Vol. 4525: C. Demetrescu (Ed.), Experimental Algorithms. XIII, 448 pages. 2007.

Vol. 4524: M. Marchiori, J.Z. Pan, C.d.S. Marie (Eds.), Web Reasoning and Rule Systems. XI, 382 pages. 2007.

Vol. 4523: Y.-H. Lee, H.-N. Kim, J. Kim, Y. Park, L.T. Yang, S.W. Kim (Eds.), Embedded Software and Systems. XIX, 829 pages. 2007.

Vol. 4522: B.K. Ersbøll, K.S. Pedersen (Eds.), Image Analysis. XVIII, 989 pages. 2007.

Vol. 4521: J. Katz, M. Yung (Eds.), Applied Cryptography and Network Security. XIII, 498 pages. 2007.

Vol. 4519: E. Franconi, M. Kifer, W. May (Eds.), The Semantic Web: Research and Applications. XVIII, 830 pages. 2007.

Vol. 4517: F. Boavida, E. Monteiro, S. Mascolo, Y. Koucheryavy (Eds.), Wired/Wireless Internet Communications. XIV, 382 pages. 2007.

Vol. 4516: L. Mason, T. Drwiega, J. Yan (Eds.), Managing Traffic Performance in Converged Networks. XXIII, 1191 pages. 2007.

Vol. 4515: M. Naor (Ed.), Advances in Cryptology - EUROCRYPT 2007. XIII, 591 pages. 2007.

Vol. 4514: S.N. Artemov, A. Nerode (Eds.), Logical Foundations of Computer Science. XI, 513 pages. 2007.

Vol. 4513: M. Fischetti, D.P. Williamson (Eds.), Integer Programming and Combinatorial Optimization. IX, 500 pages. 2007.

Vol. 4511: C. Conati, K. McCoy, G. Paliouras (Eds.), User Modeling 2007. XVI, 487 pages. 2007. (Sublibrary LNAI).

Vol. 4510: P. Van Hentenryck, L. Wolsey (Eds.), Integration of AI and OR Techniques in Constraint Programming for Combinatorial Optimization Problems. X, 391 pages. 2007.

Vol. 4509: Z. Kobti, D. Wu (Eds.), Advances in Artificial Intelligence. XII, 552 pages. 2007. (Sublibrary LNAI).

Vol. 4508: M.-Y. Kao, X.-Y. Li (Eds.), Algorithmic Aspects in Information and Management. VIII, 428 pages. 2007.

Vol. 4507: F. Sandoval, A. Prieto, J. Cabestany, M. Graña (Eds.), Computational and Ambient Intelligence. XXVI, 1167 pages. 2007.

Vol. 4506: D. Zeng, I. Gotham, K. Komatsu, C. Lynch, M. Thurmond, D. Madigan, B. Lober, J. Kvach, H. Chen (Eds.), Intelligence and Security Informatics: Biosurveillance. XI, 234 pages. 2007.

Vol. 4505: G. Dong, X. Lin, W. Wang, Y. Yang, J.X. Yu (Eds.), Advances in Data and Web Management. XXII, 896 pages. 2007.

Vol. 4504: J. Huang, R. Kowalczyk, Z. Maamar, D. Martin, I. Müller, S. Stoutenburg, K.P. Sycara (Eds.), Service-Oriented Computing: Agents, Semantics, and Engineering. X, 175 pages. 2007.

Vol. 4501: J. Marques-Silva, K.A. Sakallah (Eds.), Theory and Applications of Satisfiability Testing – SAT 2007. XI, 384 pages. 2007.

Vol. 4500: N. Streitz, A. Kameas, I. Mavrommati (Eds.), The Disappearing Computer. XVIII, 304 pages. 2007.

Vol. 4499: Y.Q. Shi (Ed.), Transactions on Data Hiding and Multimedia Security II. IX, 117 pages. 2007.

Vol. 4498: N. Abdennahder, F. Kordon (Eds.), Reliable Software Technologies – Ada Europe 2007. XII, 247 pages. 2007.

Vol. 4497: S.B. Cooper, B. Löwe, A. Sorbi (Eds.), Computation and Logic in the Real World. XVIII, 826 pages. 2007.

Vol. 4496: N.T. Nguyen, A. Grzech, R.J. Howlett, L.C. Jain (Eds.), Agent and Multi-Agent Systems: Technologies and Applications. XXI, 1046 pages. 2007. (Sublibrary LNAI).

Vol. 4495: J. Krogstie, A. Opdahl, G. Sindre (Eds.), Advanced Information Systems Engineering. XVI, 606 pages. 2007.

Vol. 4494: H. Jin, O.F. Rana, Y. Pan, V.K. Prasanna (Eds.), Algorithms and Architectures for Parallel Processing. XIV, 508 pages. 2007.

Vol. 4493: D. Liu, S. Fei, Z. Hou, H. Zhang, C. Sun (Eds.), Advances in Neural Networks – ISNN 2007, Part III. XXVI, 1215 pages. 2007.

Vol. 4492: D. Liu, S. Fei, Z. Hou, H. Zhang, C. Sun (Eds.), Advances in Neural Networks – ISNN 2007, Part II. XXVII, 1321 pages. 2007.

Vol. 4491: D. Liu, S. Fei, Z.-G. Hou, H. Zhang, C. Sun (Eds.), Advances in Neural Networks – ISNN 2007, Part I. LIV, 1365 pages. 2007.

Vol. 4490: Y. Shi, G.D. van Albada, J. Dongarra, P.M.A. Sloot (Eds.), Computational Science – ICCS 2007, Part IV. XXXVII, 1211 pages. 2007.

Vol. 4489: Y. Shi, G.D. van Albada, J. Dongarra, P.M.A. Sloot (Eds.), Computational Science – ICCS 2007, Part III. XXXVII, 1257 pages. 2007.

Vol. 4488: Y. Shi, G.D. van Albada, J. Dongarra, P.M.A. Sloot (Eds.), Computational Science – ICCS 2007, Part II. XXXV, 1251 pages. 2007.

Vol. 4487: Y. Shi, G.D. van Albada, J. Dongarra, P.M.A. Sloot (Eds.), Computational Science – ICCS 2007, Part I. LXXXI, 1275 pages. 2007.

Vol. 4486: M. Bernardo, J. Hillston (Eds.), Formal Methods for Performance Evaluation. VII, 469 pages. 2007.

Vol. 4485: F. Sgallari, A. Murli, N. Paragios (Eds.), Scale Space and Variational Methods in Computer Vision. XV, 931 pages. 2007.

Vol. 4484: J.-Y. Cai, S.B. Cooper, H. Zhu (Eds.), Theory and Applications of Models of Computation. XIII, 772 pages. 2007.

Vol. 4483: C. Baral, G. Brewka, J. Schlipf (Eds.), Logic Programming and Nonmonotonic Reasoning. IX, 327 pages. 2007. (Sublibrary LNAI).

Vol. 4482: A. An, J. Stefanowski, S. Ramanna, C.J. Butz, W. Pedrycz, G. Wang (Eds.), Rough Sets, Fuzzy Sets, Data Mining and Granular Computing. XIV, 585 pages. 2007. (Sublibrary LNAI).

Vol. 4481: J. Yao, P. Lingras, W.-Z. Wu, M. Szczuka, N.J. Cercone, D. Ślęzak (Eds.), Rough Sets and Knowledge Technology. XIV, 576 pages. 2007. (Sublibrary LNAI).

Vol. 4480: A. LaMarca, M. Langheinrich, K.N. Truong (Eds.), Pervasive Computing. XIII, 369 pages. 2007.

Vol. 4479: I.F. Akyildiz, R. Sivakumar, E. Ekici, J.C.d. Oliveira, J. McNair (Eds.), NETWORKING 2007. Ad Hoc and Sensor Networks, Wireless Networks, Next Generation Internet. XXVII, 1252 pages. 2007.

Vol. 4478: J. Martí, J.M. Benedí, A.M. Mendonça, J. Serrat (Eds.), Pattern Recognition and Image Analysis, Part II. XXVII, 657 pages. 2007.

Vol. 4477: J. Martí, J.M. Benedí, A.M. Mendonça, J. Serrat (Eds.), Pattern Recognition and Image Analysis, Part I. XXVII, 625 pages. 2007.

Vol. 4476: V. Gorodetsky, C. Zhang, V.A. Skormin, L. Cao (Eds.), Autonomous Intelligent Systems: Multi-Agents and Data Mining. XIII, 323 pages. 2007. (Sublibrary LNAI).

Vol. 4475: P. Crescenzi, G. Prencipe, G. Pucci (Eds.), Fun with Algorithms. X, 273 pages. 2007.

SPRINGER NATURE

GPSR Compliance

The European Union's (EU) General Product Safety Regulation (GPSR) is a set of rules that requires consumer products to be safe and our obligations to ensure this.

If you have any concerns about our products, you can contact us on ProductSafety@springernature.com

In case Publisher is established outside the EU, the EU authorized representative is:

Springer Nature Customer Service Center GmbH
Europaplatz 3
69115 Heidelberg, Germany

FSC
www.fsc.org
MIX
Papier | Fördert gute Waldnutzung
FSC® C083411

Kolibri 360 GmbH
Ferdinand-Jühlke-Straße 7
99095 Erfurt, Deutschland
produktsicherheit@kolibri360.de